W9-BTL-597

339.15/set

Fraser and Paré's

Diagnosis of
Diseases
of the
CHEST

Fraser and Paré's

Diagnosis of
Diseases
of the
CHEST

Fourth Edition

Volume II

R. S. Fraser, M.D.
Professor of Pathology
McGill University Health Centre
Royal Victoria Hospital
Montreal, Quebec

Neil Colman, M.D.
Associate Professor of Medicine
McGill University Health Centre
Montreal General Hospital
Montreal, Quebec

Nestor L. Müller, M.D., Ph.D.
Professor of Radiology
University of British Columbia
Vancouver Hospital and Health
  Sciences Centre
Vancouver, British Columbia

P. D. Paré, M.D.
Professor of Medicine
University of British Columbia
St. Paul's Hospital
Vancouver, British Columbia

W.B. SAUNDERS COMPANY
A *Harcourt Health Sciences Company*
Philadelphia London New York St. Louis Sydney Toronto

W.B. SAUNDERS COMPANY
A Harcourt Health Sciences Company

The Curtis Center
Independence Square West
Philadelphia, Pennsylvania 19106

Library of Congress Cataloging-in-Publication Data

Fraser and Paré's Diagnosis of diseases of the chest / Richard S. Fraser . . . [et al.].—4th ed.

p.   cm.

ISBN 0–7216–6194–7

1. Chest—Diseases—Diagnosis.   I. Fraser, Richard S.
   [DNLM: 1. Thoracic Diseases—diagnosis.   2. Diagnostic Imaging.
   WF 975D536 1999]

RC941.D52   1999   617.5′4075—dc21

DNLM/DLC   98–36145

ISBN 0–7216–6194–7 (set)
ISBN 0–7216–6195–5 (vol. I)
ISBN 0–7216–6196–3 (vol. II)
ISBN 0–7216–6197–1 (vol. III)
ISBN 0–7216–6198–X (vol. IV)

FRASER AND PARÉ'S DIAGNOSIS OF DISEASES OF THE CHEST

Printed in the United States of America.

Last digit is the print number: 9   8   7   6   5   4   3   2

This book is dedicated to

ROBERT G. FRASER AND J. A. PETER PARÉ
who had the inspiration to recognize the importance of radiologic findings in
the diagnosis of chest disease, the dedication and perseverance to document
these and other findings in the initial editions of this book, and the grace to
teach us the value of both

and to

OUR WIVES AND CHILDREN
without whose encouragement and patience during our many hours of
reading, writing, and editing this edition would not have been completed.

Preface to the Fourth Edition

Previous editions of this book were based on the principle that the radiograph is the "focal point" or "first step" in the diagnosis of chest disease. We agree with the fundamental importance of the radiograph in this respect; however, we feel that it is best considered as one of two "pillars" of diagnosis, the other being the clinical history. Although it is of course possible to render an opinion about the nature of a patient's illness on the basis of only one of these pillars, this is fraught with potential error and should be avoided in most cases. Instead, it is our belief that the combination of a good clinical history and high-quality posteroanterior and lateral chest radiographs provides the respiratory physician or radiologist with sufficient information to significantly limit the differential diagnosis in the vast majority of patients who have chest disease and to enable a specific (and often correct) diagnosis in many. Additional information derived from ancillary radiologic procedures, laboratory tests, pulmonary function tests, and pathologic examination enables further refinement of differential diagnosis and a confident diagnosis in almost all patients. Of these additional tests, one that has undergone significant advance in the recent past is computed tomography (CT), particularly with the advent of high-resolution (HRCT) and spiral CT. The former has enabled much clearer delineation of the location and extent of disease in the lungs, pleura, and mediastinum, and the latter has greatly improved the ability to image the airways and vessels. The current edition of this book has changed to reflect the increased availability and diagnostic accuracy of these procedures; in addition, numerous figures have been added to illustrate the various abnormalities that they can identify.

Some might argue that a knowledge of the etiology, pathogenesis, and pathologic characteristics of disease is unnecessary for the clinician or radiologist to diagnose chest disease. It is our belief, however, that a thorough understanding of the overall nature of such disease will result in improved diagnostic skill. This potential refinement may be apparent in several areas, including better appreciation of the nature of radiologic abnormalities (*e.g.*, via a knowledge of gross pathologic findings), improved knowledge of the potential value of new diagnostic tests (*e.g.*, via an understanding of the molecular and genetic abnormalities associated with certain diseases and with the techniques by which these are identified), and a more thorough understanding of the associations between certain diseases or disease processes (*e.g.*, viral infection and neoplasia). For these reasons, we have included a significant amount of material that is not directly relevant to diagnosis. We recognize the limitations of this approach, particularly with respect to a consideration of disease pathogenesis—the remarkable amount of research in chest disease, especially that related to cellular and molecular mechanisms, is difficult to summarize accurately, particularly since three of us have limited involvement in fundamental research. Moreover, it is inevitable that the progress that is currently being made in this research is such that some of the material in the text will be outdated at the time it is published. Despite these limitations, we consider an understanding of the etiology and pathogenesis of chest disease to be of sufficient importance to describe them to the best of our ability.

The organization of this book is based on a fairly consistent consideration of specific diseases under the headings of epidemiology, etiology and pathogenesis, pathologic characteristics, radiologic manifestations, clinical manifestations, laboratory findings (including pulmonary function tests), and prognosis and natural history. As with previous editions, a discussion of treatment has been omitted because of the rapidity with which therapeutic strategies may change and the implications that this may have. The scope of the book is such that it is meant primarily for specialists in chest disease, including pneumologists, thoracic surgeons, chest radiologists, and pathologists whose interest lies in this field. However, we believe that residents in training for these specialties will also find the text useful.

What will our readers find that is different from previous editions? Allusion has already been made to the extensive expansion of the discussion of HRCT and the addition of numerous new illustrations. Many new pathologic illustrations, both gross and microscopic, have also been included in an attempt to better explain the anatomic basis of disease. In addition to extensive updating of the material in previous editions, new sections have been written on CT of the normal lung, pulmonary transplantation, the effects on the chest of human immunodeficiency virus (HIV) infection, and pulmonary hemorrhage syndromes. The discussion of pulmonary neoplasia has been reorganized to conform more closely to the latest World Health Organization Classification of Lung Tumors. The Tables of Differential Diagnosis have been simplified to include primarily those diseases that are likely to be encountered by most pulmonary physicians; along with an increase in the number of illustrative examples, it is hoped that this version will provide a more simple and practical guide to differential diagnosis of the commonly enountered radiographic patterns of chest disease.

To make the text more accessible to the reader, the 21 chapters of the previous three editions have been expanded to 79. The subdivision is somewhat arbitrary and has necessitated repetition of material in some areas; for example, the inclusion of a chapter on chest disease in HIV infection necessarily involves a discussion of pulmonary infections and neoplasms that are also included in other, more comprehensive chapters on these subjects. As much as possible, we have tried to limit discussion of a particular topic to one place in the text; nevertheless, we have sometimes repeated material in order to minimize the necessity for the reader to refer to other sections of the book. We have also grouped chapters into larger categories based on anatomic location or presumed etiology and pathogenesis of disease; such grouping is again somewhat arbitrary, but hopefully will provide the reader easier access to appropriate information.

The reference list of the previous editions has been culled in an attempt to include those articles that are most relevant to the points we have chosen to emphasize; however, numerous reports published before 1990 have been retained. As might be expected, many references to articles published in the 1990s have also been added in an attempt to bring the text as up to date as possible. The resulting reference list contains a somewhat daunting total of approximately 31,000 citations! The inclusion of a list such as this might be questioned in light of the relatively easy availability of personal computers and electronic reference archives. However, we feel it is useful to have such references accessible to those who wish quick access to literature sources in book form. In addition, and perhaps more important in a book compiled by only four authors, we wish to provide a "factual" basis for our assertions as much as possible. As will be appreciated by those who publish in medical journals, it is inevitable that there are errors in our reference list, sometimes with respect to omission of an author or the spelling of his or her name and sometimes with respect to inappropriate attribution of statements or to omission of a key article. We apologize for these errors in advance and ask for our readers' understanding and the feedback to correct them. (Correspondence may be sent to [DDC@pathology.lan.mcgill.ca].)

The last edition of this book included a quotation from Ecclesiastes concerning the passage of time. We would also like to offer a quote of general philosophic interest, although one that is perhaps more directly related to the subject matter of this book. It derives from Maimonides, the great twelfth century scholar and physician:

Do not consider a thing as proof because you find it written in books: . . . there are fools who accept a thing as (such), because it is in writing.

What we offer in the following pages are a concept of disease of the chest and an approach to its diagnosis based on the combined experience and knowledge of reported observations of four individuals. As in our everyday practice, we have attempted to be as open-minded to new ideas and as unbiased in our selection of material as possible. Despite this, such bias is to some extent inevitable and errors of commission or omission must be present. We do not, of course, advocate the unequivocal acceptance of Maimonides' aphorism; however, we trust that our readers will take his words to heart and consider the following pages and indeed the entire subject of chest disease with a questioning and open mind.

RSF
NLM
NC
PDP

Acknowledgments

The production of a book such as *Fraser and Paré's Diagnosis of Diseases of the Chest* is a huge task, and we have been fortunate in having the support and encouragement of many colleagues and friends in our endeavor. The availability and efficiency of modern computers have meant that much writing and editing have been performed directly by us; nevertheless, we could not have accomplished our task without secretarial help from Laura Fiorita, Stella Totilo, and Andrea Sanders at the McGill University Health Centre (MUHC); Catherine Goyette and Tamara Eigendorf at St. Paul's Hospital and the University of British Columbia; and Jenny Silver at the Vancouver Hospital and Health Sciences Centre. The diligence with which these individuals carried out their tasks shows in the final product and is deeply appreciated.

The majority of the case histories and radiologic illustrations reproduced in the text are derived from patients of staff members of the MUHC (particularly the Royal Victoria Hospital, the Montreal General Hospital, and the Montreal Chest Hospital Institute) and the Vancouver Hospital and Health Sciences Centre. Almost all illustrations of pathology are related to patients from the MUHC. We are indebted to our colleagues who cared for these patients, not only for their generosity in permitting us to publish the illustrations of various diseases but also for the benefit of their experience and guidance over the years. A number of these colleagues deserve particular mention for their comments and help on selected topics; these include Drs. Richard Menzies and John Kosiuk at the MUHC; Drs. Pearce Wilcox, John Fleetham, Brad Munt, and Hugh Chaun and Ms. Elisabeth Baile at the University of British Columbia; and Drs. A. Jean Buckley, John Aldrich, John Mayo, and Daniel Worsley at the Vancouver Hospital and Health Sciences Centre.

The photographic work throughout these volumes was the accomplishment of many individuals. Illustrations from former editions were provided by members of the Department of Visual Aids of the Royal Victoria Hospital; Susie Gray at the Department of Radiology, University of Alabama; Joseph Donohue, Anthony Graham, and Michael Paré of Montreal; and Sally Osborne at St. Paul's Hospital, Vancouver. Those involved in the production of new illustrations for this edition include Marcus Arts and Helmut Bernhard at the Montreal Neurological Institute Photography Department; Diane Minshall and Stuart Greene at St. Paul's Hospital, University of British Columbia; and Janis Franklin and Michael Robertson at the Vancouver Hospital Sciences Centre.

Throughout our writing and editing, we received support and cooperation from several individuals at W.B. Saunders, notably our Chief Editor, Lisette Bralow, our developmental editors Janice Gaillard and Melissa Messersmith, and our copy editors Sue Reilly and Lee Ann Draud, all of whom helped us overcome a number of the obstacles we encountered at various times. Finally, we acknowledge and thank our wives and children, without whose patience and encouragement this book would not have been completed.

RSF
NLM
NC
PDP

Contents

VOLUME ONE

VOLUME TWO

VOLUME THREE

VOLUME FOUR

PART V
PULMONARY
INFECTION

General Features of Pulmonary Infection

Infection of the lower respiratory tract is one of the most common and important causes of human disease from the points of view of morbidity, mortality, and economic cost to society. In the United States, pneumonia is the sixth leading cause of death and the number one cause of death from infection;[1, 2] in developed countries as a whole, it has been estimated that it is associated with an annual death rate of approximately 50 to 60 per 100,000.[3] It has also been estimated that the total cost for hospitalization for pneumonia approaches $4 billion per year in the United States,[4] whereas direct costs for the management of outpatient pneumonia exceed $1 billion per year.[5]

The clinical and radiologic manifestations associated with infection of the lower respiratory tract can mimic those of virtually all other lung diseases; as a result, infection enters into the differential diagnosis of many pulmonary afflictions. The pathologic basis of these manifestations includes tracheitis, bronchitis, bronchiolitis, and pneumonitis (pneumonia), the last of which is by far the most important. The general features of these processes are discussed in this chapter under patterns of pulmonary infection; in addition, there is also a discussion of the general principles of microbiologic diagnosis and of certain epidemiologic features of pneumonia. The causative organisms responsible for infection of the lower respiratory tract are almost too numerous to list, and for ease of discussion and reference, they have been grouped into several chapters largely according to standard microbiologic classification schemes.

GENERAL EPIDEMIOLOGIC FEATURES OF PNEUMONIA

Because pneumonia is not a reportable disease, data regarding its incidence are suboptimal. It has been estimated that there are approximately 4 million cases of community-acquired pneumonia annually in the United States,[4, 6] resulting in 600,000 hospitalizations.[4] The elderly ambulatory patient who comes to the emergency department with fever is likely to have a serious pneumonia and in most instances requires hospitalization.[7] Even in young, healthy naval personnel, pneumonia has been found to be a major medical cause of lost workdays.[8]

Despite its frequency, pneumonia is the cause of acute lower respiratory tract symptoms in only a small minority of patients from the community. In one prospective study of lower respiratory infections requiring antibiotics in adults seeking attention from a physician, an incidence of 44 per 1,000 was found; however, only 12% had pneumonia.[9] The overall attack rate for pneumonia is about 10 to 12 cases per 1,000 persons per year; however, the incidence varies considerably with age, sex, race, and socioeconomic condition.[1, 10, 11] For example, in a review of all episodes of pneumonia requiring hospitalization in two counties in Ohio in 1991, the overall incidence was 266.8 per 100,000 population.[12] The incidence was higher among African Americans (337.7 per 100,000 versus 253.9 per 100,000 in whites), men (291.4 versus 244.8 in women) and older individuals (92 per 100,000 in those less than 45 years old and 1,012 per 100,000 for persons over the age of 65). The incidence is also greater in individuals residing in a nursing home. For example, in a study from Halifax, Nova Scotia, the rate of hospitalization for pneumonia in the general population was found to be 1 per 1,000, whereas it was 33 per 1,000 for nursing home residents.[13]

The authors of an extensive meta-analysis of the prognosis and outcome of 33,148 patients who had community-acquired pneumonia found an overall mortality rate of 13.7%.[14] As with incidence figures, however, those related to mortality also vary considerably in specific groups of patients. As might be expected, the mortality rate in patients not requiring hospitalization is generally low, in the range of 0.1%.[4] Among patients who have pneumonia of sufficient severity to require admission to the hospital, reported mortality rates range from 4% to as high as 37%[11, 12, 14, 15] and increase with increasing age.[1] In fact, pneumonia accounts for nearly half of all deaths resulting from infectious disease in the geriatric population, and 90% of all deaths from respiratory tract infection occur in persons older than 64 years of age.[5]

Hospital-acquired pneumonia occurs in about 5 to 10 per 1,000 hospitalized patients[17, 18] and has been found to complicate the course of as many as 18% of patients undergoing surgery.[19] The incidence is also significantly greater in patients undergoing mechanical ventilation, occurring in 10% to 25% of such patients.[17, 18, 20] Crude rates for ventilator-acquired pneumonia range from 1% to 3% per day of intubation and mechanical ventilation.[18] Among nosocomial infections, pneumonia has the highest mortality and morbidity,[18] and its presence increases length of stay in survivors by an average of 7 to 9 days per patient,[17] with its attendant increase in cost.[21, 22] Mortality in such patients is high, being estimated at 30% to 70% in different series.[23] It is believed that only one third to one half of deaths in this setting are due to the infection itself, however, the remainder being the result of comorbid disease.[17] By contrast, in the setting of ventilator-associated pneumonia, attributable mortality is, on average, less; for example, in two matched cohort studies, it was believed to be only 27% to 33%.[24, 25] In fact, some authors have estimated that the development of pneumonia may not increase mortality at all, after correction is made for confounding factors that independently influence mortality.[26]

There is evidence that the death rate from pneumonia is increasing. For example, in the 15-year period from 1979 to 1994, the overall crude death rate from pneumonia and influenza in the United States increased from 20.0 to 31.8 per 100,000 (59%);[16] the age-adjusted rate increased from 20.4 to 24.8 (22%). The increased mortality was particularly marked in individuals older than 65 years, in whom the death rate increased from 145 to 209 per 100,000.

PATHOGENESIS AND PATTERNS OF PULMONARY INFECTION

Organisms can enter the lung and cause infection by three routes: the tracheobronchial tree, the pulmonary vasculature, and directly from the mediastinum or neck or across the diaphragm or chest wall. Although there is overlap, infection acquired by each of these routes results in fairly characteristic pulmonary abnormalities that may be recognized both pathologically and radiologically.

Infection Via the Tracheobronchial Tree

Infection acquired via the tracheobronchial tree occurs most commonly by aspiration or inhalation of microorganisms; occasionally, it follows direct physical implantation from an infected source, such as a bronchoscope,[28] or extension of disease into the airway from a peribronchial lymph node (e.g., in tuberculosis). With respect to pulmonary infection, we use the terms *inhalation* to refer to the breathing of air that contains potentially infectious material, such as droplet nuclei contaminated by microorganisms, and *aspiration* to refer to the introduction of solid or liquid material into the lungs. When the latter material consists of a foreign body or is copious (as is often the case with aspirated gastric contents), it usually causes pulmonary damage directly by chemical or physical mechanisms (*see* page 2491); we use the term *aspiration pneumonia* to refer to such damage. Aspiration of smaller amounts of nasal or oral secretions that contain microorganisms is also a common cause of pneumonia, in this case as a result of the organisms themselves. Although such a process has also been termed *aspiration pneumonia*, we prefer to refer to this form of disease by the specific type of causative organism (e.g, anaerobic pneumonia, actinomycosis). (It should be remembered that the aspirated material in aspiration pneumonia as defined here may contain microorganisms or become secondarily infected, so that it is sometimes not possible to know what the original pathogenetic mechanism was in a specific case.)

Coughing or sneezing by an individual whose respiratory tract is either colonized or infected produces a myriad of minute droplets that are laden with microorganisms. On exposure to air, the droplets lose water and become droplet nuclei, which, because of their extremely small size, can remain suspended in air for an extended period of time; exposure to such contaminated air by another individual can then result in spread of organisms.[29, 30] In general, inhaled droplet nuclei larger than 5 μm are deposited on the upper airways, whereas those smaller than 0.5 μm are exhaled; nuclei between these extremes, especially those measuring 1 to 2 μm, are likely to affect peripheral airway epithelium, where they may proliferate and cause disease. Depending on their virulence, a substantial number of organisms may be necessary for this to occur because small numbers may be effectively cleared by host defenses;[31] however, some organisms (e.g., *Mycobacterium tuberculosis*) are capable of producing disease with only a small inoculum. In addition to the inhalational transmission of organisms from person to person, some forms of microorganisms of appropriate size, such as the microconidia of *Histoplasma capsulatum* or the arthroconidia of *Coccidioides immitis*, are inhaled as airborne particles originating in contaminated soil.

As indicated, aspiration of oropharyngeal secretions is also a common mechanism by which pathogenic organisms gain access to the lungs. The normal adult oropharyngeal flora consists of a variety of aerobic and anaerobic microorganisms.[32] Most are commensals of low virulence that never cause pulmonary infection; however, some (e.g., *Actinomyces israelii* and a variety of anaerobic bacteria) can cause pulmonary disease if aspirated in sufficient quantity in the susceptible host. In addition, it is not uncommon for the upper airways to be colonized by pathogenic organisms, such as *Streptococcus pneumoniae* or *Staphylococcus aureus* (in otherwise healthy individuals), or by potentially virulent gram-negative bacteria (in hospitalized or chronically ill patients). In either situation, aspiration of contaminated saliva or nasal secretions may deliver a bacterial inoculum sufficient to cause infection. It is likely that asymptomatic aspiration occurs occasionally in a high proportion of normal individuals and with even greater frequency in patients who are comatose, who have ingested excessive alcohol, or whose nasopharyngeal secretions are increased as a result of upper respiratory tract viral infection. For example, in one study, approximately 45% of normal subjects and 70% of patients who had impaired consciousness were found to aspirate during sleep.[33]

Deposition of microorganisms on the airway or alveolar epithelial surface by inhalation or aspiration may be followed by one of three events: (1) destruction and clearance of organisms with restoration of the original sterile lung; (2) limited but prolonged proliferation of organisms unassociated with significant transepithelial invasion (colonization); and (3) marked proliferation of organisms associated with an acute inflammatory reaction and, often, tissue necrosis. Which of these events ensues depends on a number of factors, including the size of the organism inoculum, the virulence of the organism, the status of the host inflammatory and immune reactions, and the presence or absence of underlying lung disease.[33a] Many substances are produced by the microorganisms to enhance the likelihood of colonization or invasion, including proteases and other chemicals that directly damage epithelial cells or connective tissue,[33b, 33c] substances such as pyocyanin that cause a reduction in mucociliary clearance,[33d] adhesion molecules that promote attachment to the epithelial surface, proteases that damage IgA,[33e] and substances that inhibit the host inflammatory reaction.[33f]

Infection of the lower respiratory tract acquired via the airways may be confined predominantly to the airways themselves (tracheitis, bronchitis, or bronchiolitis) or to the lung parenchyma (pneumonia). The latter can, in turn, be subdivided into three types, each with fairly typical pathologic and radiologic characteristics: nonsegmental air-space (lobar*) pneumonia, bronchopneumonia (lobular pneumonia*), and interstitial pneumonia. These patterns can be recognized with sufficient frequency and are associated with different etiologic organisms in enough cases that their recognition is diagnostically useful in the appropriate clinical context. For example, nonsegmental air-space pneumonia is usually of bacterial origin, most commonly *S. pneumoniae* or *Klebsiella pneumoniae*, whereas diffuse interstitial pneumonia commonly results from *Pneumocystis carinii*.[34, 34a–c]

Despite these observations, there is variation in the radiologic manifestations of pneumonia caused by specific organisms, and it is not always possible to fit an individual case into one of the three types; for example, the pattern of mycoplasmal pneumonia has been found by some investigators to be similar to that of bacterial air-space pneumonia in as many as 50% of cases.[34, 35] Moreover, in one study, a panel of six radiologists who had no prior knowledge of clinical data were only 67% accurate in the identification of 16 bacterial pneumonias and 65% correct in 9 viral pneumonias.[35]

There is also considerable interobserver variability in the assessment of radiographic findings in pneumonia. For example, in one study in which two independent radiologists interpreted the initial chest radiographs in 282 patients who had community-acquired pneumonia, there was agreement on the presence of parenchymal abnormalities in 79% of cases and on the absence of abnormalities in 6%;[35a] the two disagreed in the remaining 15% of cases. When an abnormality was detected, the two observers agreed that it was unilobar in 41% of cases and multilobar in 34%, disagreeing in the remaining 25%. Although they also agreed that the pattern of abnormality consisted of air-space consolidation in 96% of cases, there was no agreement between the observers in the diagnosis of interstitial pneumonia. There was also considerable disagreement in the recognition of air bronchograms, the two radiologists agreeing on their absence in 53% of cases and on their presence in 8% but disagreeing in the remaining 39%.

Thus, although many pulmonary infections can be recognized as nonsegmental air-space pneumonia, bronchopneumonia, or interstitial pneumonia, in some cases the superimposition of shadows makes it difficult to assess the pattern of abnormality on the plain radiograph. A better correlation between the radiologic and pathologic findings in pneumonia in both the immunocompetent and the immunocompromised patient is obtained with HRCT.[35b–e] For example, in one study of 32 patients who had community-acquired pneumonia, including 18 who had bacterial pneumonia and 14 who had nonbacterial pneumonia (12 *Mycoplasma pneumoniae*, 1 *Chlamydia pneumoniae*, and 1 influenza virus), the main feature differentiating the two was the presence of small centrilobular nodular opacities (seen in 64% of patients who had nonbacterial pneumonia and only 11% who had bacterial disease).[35b] A lobular distribution (corresponding to bronchopneumonia) was present in 33% of patients who had bacterial pneumonia and 86% of patients

---

*Although nonsegmental air-space pneumonia is sometimes referred to as *lobar pneumonia*, because the abnormality seldom involves a whole lobe we prefer to use the former term. Because the consolidation affects some secondary lobules and spares adjacent ones, bronchopneumonia has also been referred to as *lobular pneumonia*.

who had nonbacterial pneumonia. (The authors did not use interstitial or nonsegmental air-space consolidation as radiologic patterns.) All of the aforementioned studies have to be interpreted with caution; the power of the radiologic findings for predicting a causative agent is strongly influenced by the prevalence of the different organisms in the study population. Because most studies of community-acquired pneumonia include only patients who require hospitalization or in whom a definitive diagnosis was established by culture of blood or pleural fluid, there is an inevitable bias toward patients who have bacterial infection. This selection bias tends to increase the apparent diagnostic value of the radiographic pattern.

A number of factors can modify the radiologic and clinical manifestations of pulmonary infections,[36] including age, immunologic status, and the state of the underlying lung. Of greatest importance with regard to the last of these is emphysema, a condition that can result in a sponge-like appearance of consolidated lung parenchyma (Fig. 25–1). In fact, this abnormality accounts for at least some of the varied appearance of pneumonia described in the literature. For example, in one review of 40 patients who had pneumococcal pneumonia, nonsegmental air-space consolidation was present in 12, patchy consolidation in 12, an interstitial pattern in 9, and a mixed pattern in 7;[37] three of the cases chosen to illustrate atypical patterns of acute air-space pneumonia showed clear-cut evidence of emphysema. The severity and cause of pneumonia are also clearly influenced by the immunologic status, immunosuppressed patients being prone to develop widespread pneumonia, often by opportunistic organisms. In addition, there is evidence that the typical pattern of parenchymal consolidation may not develop in the presence of agranulocytosis.[38]

Clinical considerations that are helpful in the etiologic differential diagnosis of pneumonia include age of the patient, presence and severity of comorbid disease, rapidity of progression, and whether the infection is nosocomial or community acquired. For example, a community-acquired pneumonia that is abrupt in onset and is associated with rigor and a white blood count greater than 20,000/mm³ may well be pneumococcal in origin; however, these features are not specific enough to distinguish this infection reliably from pneumonia caused by *Legionella* species or other organisms in any given patient.[39] Only hyponatremia and the finding of a high creatine phosphokinase owing to rhabdomyolysis are helpful in individual cases in suggesting the diagnosis of *Legionella* pneumonia;[41] in the absence of these findings, there are no reliable clinical features that distinguish this infection from infection caused by other community-acquired or nosocomial organisms.[41, 42] In younger patients, pneumonia is more likely to be caused by viruses, *Chlamydia pneumoniae*, or *Mycoplasma pneumoniae*.[40] The presentation of bacterial pneumonia in the elderly may be subtle. "Classic" features of disease may be absent, and pneumonia may be confused with or confounded by other common medical problems, such as congestive heart failure, pulmonary thromboembolism, or malignancy.[43]

Although it is occasionally possible to detect pneumonia on the basis of physical examination of the chest when the chest radiograph is normal, more often there is complete absence of physical signs of lung disease in cases showing major areas of parenchymal consolidation. For example, in one study of 200 patients who had pneumonia, correlation of radiographic evidence of parenchymal consolidation with physical signs was evident in only 83 patients (42%).[44] In addition, in some cases, there is radiographic evidence of pneumonia without accompanying physical signs in one area and vice versa in other areas. Similarly, no single feature of

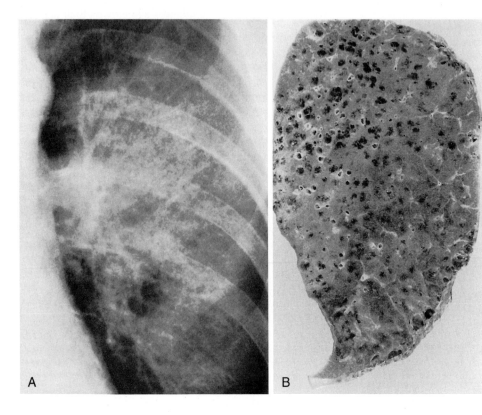

A **B**

Figure 25–1. Acute Air-Space Pneumonia Superimposed on Emphysema. A view of the left midlung zone from a posteroanterior radiograph *(A)* reveals a poorly defined opacity in the superior segment of the left lower lobe. Instead of the homogeneous opacity characteristic of acute air-space pneumonia, this consolidation contains a large number of small radiolucencies. A slice of an upper lobe *(B)* from another patient shows essentially homogeneous consolidation of the apical and posterior lung parenchyma. Within this region, there are numerous well-defined emphysematous spaces unaffected by the pneumonia. Such incomplete consolidation is responsible for the appearance in *A*.

the clinical history accurately predicts the presence or absence of radiographically detectable pneumonia.[48g]

Tracheitis, Bronchitis, and Bronchiolitis

Infection involving predominantly the airways may be limited to the trachea, bronchi, or bronchioles or affect two or three of these sites simultaneously. Viral and mycoplasmal organisms are the most frequent pathogenic agents. In fact, some degree of tracheitis is probably not uncommon in many upper respiratory tract infections caused by viruses, including those responsible for "common colds"; although such infection is usually relatively harmless, causing no more than cough, it may be followed by more ominous bacterial superinfection (*see* farther on). Of greater importance in terms of morbidity is bronchiolitis, particularly in children.[45, 46] Respiratory syncytial virus and parainfluenza viruses are the most common agents to cause serious disease,[47] which is characterized clinically by wheezing and dyspnea and, in the most severely affected, cyanosis, prostration, and death. Viral bronchiolitis in children is also well recognized as a precursor of adult bronchiectasis and unilateral hyperlucent lung (Swyer-James syndrome) and has been hypothesized to be a contributing factor in the development of asthma. Persistent adenoviral infection has been found in some patients after an acute bronchiolitis, and it has been hypothesized that this might be related to subsequent chronic airway obstruction in childhood[47a] and the development of chronic obstructive pulmonary disease (COPD) in adults.[48]

Although relatively uncommon, localized bacterial tracheitis is potentially a serious infection, particularly in children and occasionally in adults.[48a–c] *S. aureus* and *Haemophilus influenzae* appear to be the most common causative agents;[48d] however, anaerobes and other aerobic organisms are seen occasionally. Rarely, *Corynebacterium diphtheriae* has been the cause in the apparent absence of disease of the upper respiratory tract.[48e] The condition is often seen after viral upper airway infection, possibly as a result of viral mediated alteration of tracheal mucosal defense. The infection can lead to life-threatening airway obstruction as a result of granulation tissue and inflammatory exudate in the tracheal lumen; additional complications include toxic shock syndrome, septic shock, and adult respiratory distress syndrome (ARDS).[48c, f]

As in viral respiratory tract infection, bacterial bronchitis can be an isolated abnormality or can be seen with tracheitis, bronchiolitis, or both. In children, concomitant involvement of both proximal and distal airways is a relatively common manifestation of pertussis. In adults, bronchial infection occurs most often in patients who have underlying airway disease, usually COPD, bronchiectasis, or cystic fibrosis. In the first two of these, it is typically episodic and relatively mild in severity; in patients who have cystic fibrosis, however, chronic infection by *Pseudomonas aeruginosa* or *Burkholderia cepacia* is likely to be important in the pathogenesis of the progressive bronchiectasis seen in many individuals.

Pathologic manifestations of tracheobronchial infection include ulceration and the formation of pseudomembranes (Fig. 25–2) or occlusive masses of inflammatory exudate within the airway lumen. If large enough and located in the trachea, the last-named can cause severe respiratory distress

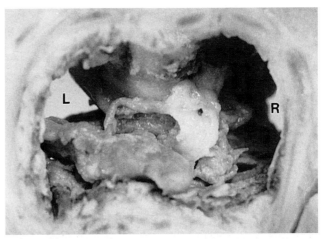

Figure 25–2. Acute Tracheitis with Pseudomembrane Formation—*Aspergillus*. A cross section through the lower trachea just proximal to the carina (the left and right main bronchi are indicated by L and R, respectively) shows a shaggy inflammatory exudate covering most of the airway surface and partly occluding its lumen. *Aspergillus* was identified in the exudate and the adjacent mucosa; extension outside the tracheal wall and pulmonary parenchymal aspergillosis were not evident.

and death. Viral or mycoplasmal associated bronchiolitis is associated with a variably severe inflammatory infiltrate, usually characterized by a predominance of lymphocytes, in the airway wall and adjacent parenchymal interstitium (Fig. 25–3); epithelial ulceration may ensue, in which case a neutrophilic exudate may partially occlude the lumen.

Acute bronchitis usually is associated with a normal radiograph or nonspecific radiographic findings; occasionally, it leads to bronchial wall thickening, bronchial dilation, and peribronchial inflammation apparent on the chest radiograph and HRCT.[48h, i] Bronchiolitis also may be associated with a normal radiograph[49] or may result in accentuation of lung markings or a reticulonodular pattern.[50a] On HRCT, inflammation of the bronchiolar wall and filling of the bronchiolar lumen by exudate results in a pattern of small centrilobular nodules and branching lines (Fig. 25–4).[35b, 48i, 50b] The pattern of centrilobular nodular and branching linear opacities has been aptly referred to as resembling a "tree in bud" and is seen most commonly in infectious bronchiolitis and endobronchial spread of tuberculosis.[50c–g] These abnormalities may be evident on HRCT even in patients who have normal radiographs.[48i] The distribution may be focal[48h, i] or diffuse.[50b]

Air-Space Pneumonia

Nonsegmental air-space pneumonia is most commonly caused by *S. pneumoniae* but can also occur with other organisms, such as *K. pneumoniae*. The most important pathogenetic feature of this form of pneumonia appears to be the rapid production of edema fluid with relatively minimal cellular reaction; the cellular and molecular mechanisms behind this reaction are not entirely clear but may be related to properties of the organism's cell wall or capsule (*see* page 736). The pneumonic consolidation tends to occur initially in the periphery of the lung beneath the visceral pleura.[51] As it increases in amount, edema fluid flows directly from acinus to acinus; because it usually contains abundant organ-

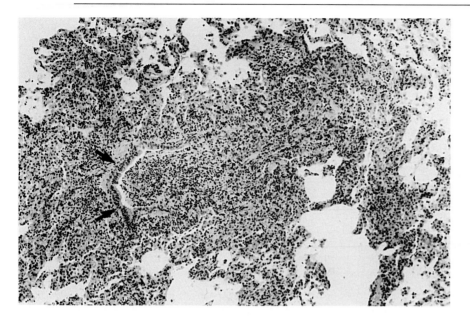

Figure 25–3. Acute Bronchiolitis—*Mycoplasma pneumoniae.* The section shows a small membranous bronchiole whose lumen is filled with an inflammatory exudate and whose wall is partly destroyed (residual epithelium is indicated by *arrows*). An inflammatory infiltrate is present in the bronchiolar wall; although this also extends into the adjacent lung parenchyma, the airway is the major focus of disease.

isms, infection spreads concomitantly. Thus, the infection does not localize in discrete foci (as in bronchopneumonia) but instead comes to occupy a confluent portion of the lung parenchyma (Fig. 25–5) limited only by pleural boundaries and, eventually, by the host's cellular inflammatory reaction.

Radiographically, nonsegmental air-space pneumonia appears as homogeneous consolidation that is relatively sharply demarcated from adjacent uninvolved parenchyma (Fig. 25–6). As the term implies, the consolidation characteristically crosses segmental boundaries, a finding of major importance in differentiating the process from bronchopneumonia.[52] It usually abuts an interlobar fissure but seldom involves the entire lobe (hence the preference for the term *acute air-space* rather than *lobar* pneumonia). The larger bronchi often remain patent and air containing, thus creating an air bronchogram. The amount of inflammatory exudate may be such that it results in expansion of a lobe and a *bulging fissure* sign (Fig. 25–7).[52a]

The clinical diagnosis of acute air-space pneumonia related to *S. pneumoniae* often is suggested by cough, expectoration, chills and fever, and (particularly) pleural pain. In many cases, physical signs indicate the location of the disease, although the classic signs of parenchymal consolidation—inspiratory lag, impaired percussion, bronchial breathing, fine crackles, and whispering pectoriloquy—are heard much less often than formerly, presumably because of the prompt institution of antibiotic therapy. In fact, physical examination of the chest usually reveals only fine crackles and decreased breath sounds.

Bronchopneumonia

Bronchopneumonia is exemplified by infection by *S. aureus*, most gram-negative bacteria, and some fungi. It differs pathogenetically from nonsegmental air-space pneumonia by the production of a relatively small amount of fluid

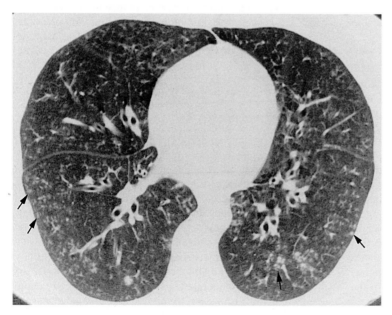

Figure 25–4. Acute Bronchiolitis—*Mycoplasma pneumoniae.* HRCT demonstrates small nodular opacities *(arrows)* in a centrilobular distribution involving mainly the lower lobes. The patient was a 40-year-old woman.

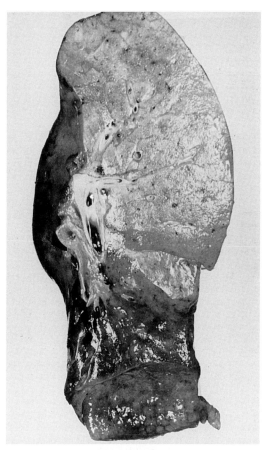

Figure 25–5. Acute Air-Space Pneumonia. A slice of an unfixed left lung near the hilum shows homogeneous consolidation of the upper lobe; histologic examination showed extensive air-space filling by neutrophils (gray hepatization). The pneumonia in this case is unusual in that involves an entire lobe (true lobar pneumonia). Premortem blood specimens grew *Streptococcus pneumoniae.*

and by the rapid exudation of numerous polymorphonuclear leukocytes, typically in relation to small membranous and respiratory bronchioles. The neutrophils appear to limit the spread of organisms, at least initially, resulting in a patchy appearance of the disease (Fig. 25–8). The initial reaction probably occurs in the airway mucosa and is associated with epithelial ulceration and the formation of an intraluminal fibrinopurulent exudate. A transmural inflammatory reaction follows and spreads into peribronchiolar alveoli, which become filled with hemorrhagic edema fluid and neutrophils (*see* Fig. 25–8). With progression of disease, the inflammatory reaction may spread to involve entire lobules, giving rise to confluent bronchopneumonia; usually, however, the patchy nature of the process can still be distinguished pathologically by the variable intensity of inflammation, the most severe foci being centered on the airways (*see* Fig. 25–8).

The pattern of healing of bronchopneumonia differs from that of acute air-space pneumonia (at least that caused by *S. pneumoniae*). Since air-space pneumonia caused by the latter organism usually is not associated with tissue destruction, restoration of normal lung architecture is the rule once host defenses are in control. By contrast, bronchopneumonia is typically associated with virulent organisms and some degree of tissue destruction. Thus, if the patient survives the infection, organization of the inflammatory fo-

cus is inevitable, manifested in the early stage as plugs of fibroblastic tissue in airway and alveolar air spaces (organizing pneumonia [Fig. 25–9]) and later on as mature fibrous tissue associated with a variable degree of loss of normal lung architecture.

The radiologic manifestations of bronchopneumonia can range from focal, peribronchial, and peribronchiolar areas of consolidation involving one or more segments of a single lobe (Fig. 25–10) to multilobar, bilateral consolidation.[52b, c] Consolidation involving the terminal and respiratory bronchioles and adjacent alveoli results in poorly defined centrilobular nodular opacities measuring 4 to 10 mm in diameter (air-space nodules)[50a, 53] or may extend to involve the entire secondary lobule (lobular consolidation).[35b] Because it involves the airways, bronchopneumonia frequently results in loss of volume of the affected segments or lobes.[52c] Confluence of pneumonia in adjacent lobules may be extensive and may result in a pattern simulating nonsegmental air-space pneumonia; distinction from the latter can be made in most cases by the presence of segmental or lobular distribution of the abnormalities in other areas.

Bronchopneumonia is typically caused by highly pathogenic organisms and is associated with the exudation of abundant neutrophils; the combined action of microbial toxins and leukocyte enzymes leads to tissue destruction,[54] which may result in several morphologic and radiologic manifestations, including abscess formation, pneumatocele, and pulmonary gangrene.

Pulmonary Abscess

Pulmonary abscesses vary in size from those that can be seen only with the microscope to those that occupy a large area of a pulmonary lobe. Grossly, they contain semisolid or liquid pus (Fig. 25–11); depending on their duration, they may be surrounded by a rim of granulation or fibrous tissue. Larger abscesses typically erode into bronchi, resulting in drainage of their necrotic material and the formation of a cavity. These may be solitary or multiple and, in cases of relatively long-standing disease, may be associated with considerable pulmonary destruction.

The radiologic manifestations of lung abscesses consist of single or multiple masses that are often cavitated (Fig. 25–12). They may be isolated or occur within areas of consolidation. In one review of the radiographic findings in 50 patients, the internal margins of the abscesses were smooth in 88% of cases and shaggy in 12%.[55] Air-fluid levels were present in 72% of cases and adjacent parenchymal consolidation in 48%. Maximal wall thickness was equal or less than 4 mm in 4% of cases, between 5 and 15 mm in 82%, and greater than 15 mm in 14%. The presence of shaggy internal margins and a maximal wall thickness greater than 15 mm results in a resemblance to cavitated pulmonary carcinoma.[55, 56]

Clinically, a pulmonary abscess may develop in the course of known pneumonia or may be the initial manifestation of disease. Many cases are caused by anaerobic bacteria,[57, 58] in which situation the patient is often elderly and has poor oral hygiene and an underlying condition predisposing to aspiration (*see* page 778); signs and symptoms of the disease may be remarkably mild, although fever is common. Other relatively common agents are *S. aureus* and *P. aerugi-*

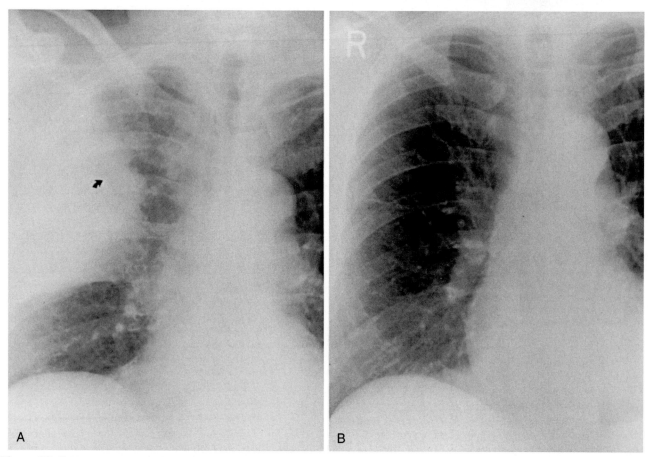

Figure 25–6. Nonsegmental Acute Air-Space Pneumonia—*Streptococcus pneumoniae.* A detail view of the right lung from a posteroanterior chest radiograph *(A)* discloses dense consolidation in the axillary portion of the right upper lobe. The irregular margin of the lesion superomedially and a faint air bronchogram *(curved arrow)* define the more typical signs of an air-space lesion. Follow-up radiograph 2 months after appropriate antibiotic therapy *(B)* shows resolution of the pneumonia. The patient was a middle-aged alcoholic man.

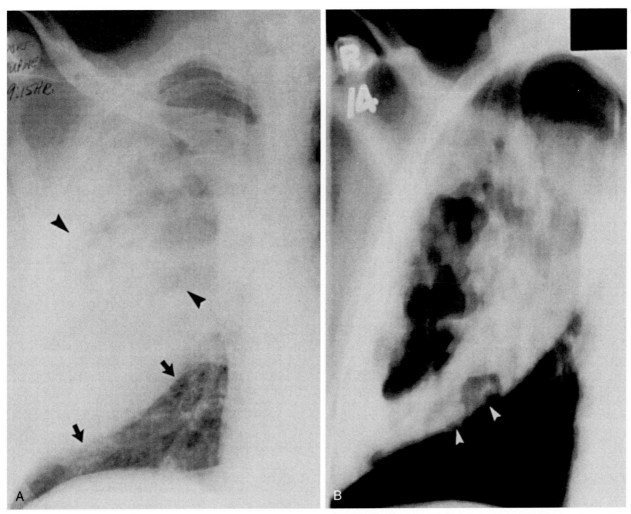

Figure 25–7. Acute Necrotizing *Klebsiella* Pneumonia with Bulging Fissure. A view of the right lung from a posteroanterior chest radiograph *(A)* reveals massive air-space consolidation involving most of the upper lobe. Note the downward-displaced, bulging minor fissure *(arrows)* indicating lobar expansion; numerous central radiolucencies *(between arrowheads)* suggest parenchymal necrosis. Five days later, an anteroposterior tomogram *(B)* taken with the patient in the supine position reveals a large abscess cavity with a thick, shaggy wall. One focus of necrosis *(arrowheads)* abuts the visceral pleura, a prelude to the development of a bronchopleural fistula. Subsequent films taken 2 days later (not illustrated) confirmed the development of pyopneumothorax.

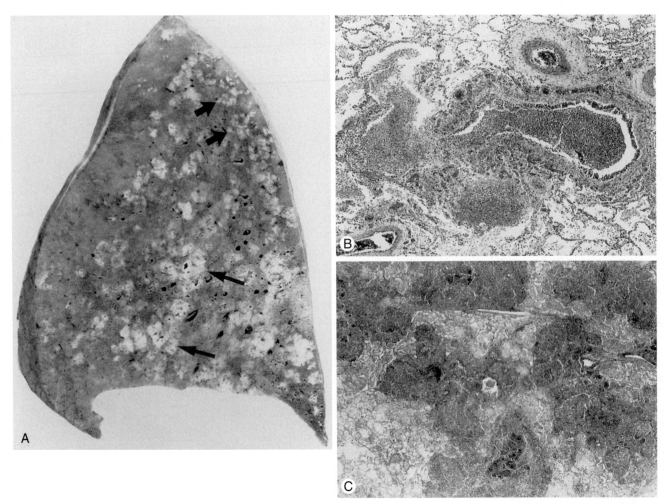

Figure 25–8. Acute Bronchopneumonia—*Pseudomonas aeruginosa.* A slice of left lower lobe *(A)* shows patchy consolidation throughout the lung parenchyma. In some areas *(short arrows),* there is a discrete, finely branching pattern, indicating early infection confined to a peribronchiolar location. In other sites *(long arrows),* there is confluent pneumonia; despite the more solid appearance, an underlying nodularity is easily appreciated. *B,* Histologic appearance of early disease (corresponding to short arrows in *A*), showing an acute inflammatory exudate within the lumen of a terminal bronchiole and immediately adjacent lung parenchyma. Surrounding air spaces are as yet unaffected. *C,* More advanced disease from the area indicated by *long arrows* in *A* showing extensive parenchymal consolidation, representing confluence of infection originating about several bronchioles. The patchy nature of the process is still identifiable. Postmortem lung culture demonstrated *Pseudomonas aeruginosa.* (*B,* ×40; *C,* ×12.)

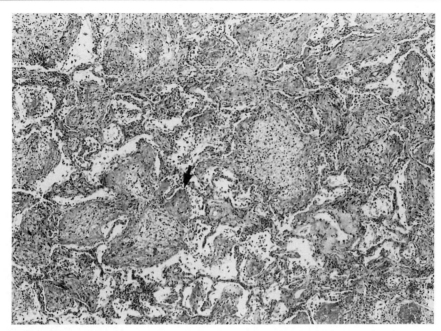

Figure 25–9. Organizing Bronchopneumonia. Air spaces are filled with fibroblastic connective tissue, lymphocytes, macrophages, and occasional polymorphonuclear leukocytes. The interstitium is only mildly thickened. Small foci of more homogeneous proteinaceous material *(arrow)* represent fibrinous exudate undergoing organization. Causative organism was undetermined. (×48.)

nosa. Hemoptysis is seen in some cases and may be the initial and sometimes fatal manifestation.[59] As with tuberculosis, spread of infection may occur by drainage of necrotic abscess contents into other lobes.[60]

Pulmonary Gangrene

A relatively uncommon complication of pneumonia is the development of fragments of necrotic lung within an abscess cavity (pulmonary sequestrum or gangrene) (Fig. 25–13). The pathogenesis of the pulmonary necrosis in these cases may be related to a direct action of bacterial toxins, to ischemia secondary to thrombosis of pulmonary arteries adjacent to the focus of pneumonia, or to a combination of the two.[61] Whatever the process leading to necrosis, it is likely that separation of necrotic from adjacent viable lung tissue is mediated at least partly by leukocyte enzymes.

The radiologic manifestations of pulmonary gangrene initially consist of small lucencies within an area of consolidated lung, usually developing within lobar consolidation associated with enlargement of the lobe and outward bulging of the fissure.[61a] The small lucencies rapidly coalesce into a large cavity containing fluid and sloughed lung.[61a, b] Lateral decubitus views demonstrate the necrotic lung fragment to be freely mobile within the cavity. The majority of cases are secondary to *K. pneumoniae*; other causative organisms include *S. pneumoniae*, *H. influenzae*, *S. aureus*, and anaerobic bacteria.[61a]

Pneumatocele

As discussed previously (*see* page 508), pneumatoceles are thin-walled, gas-filled spaces that usually develop in association with infection; characteristically, they increase in size over a period of days to weeks and almost invariably resolve. Of the several mechanisms proposed for their forma-

tion, the most likely is drainage of a focus of necrotic lung parenchyma followed by check-valve obstruction of the airway subtending it; the "valve," which may be inflammatory exudate or necrotic airway wall (or both), enables air to enter the parenchymal space during inspiration but prevents its egress during expiration (Fig. 25–14).[61c] The complication is usually caused by *S. aureus* in infants and children or *P. carinii* in patients with acquired immunodeficiency syndrome (AIDS);[62] however, other organisms are occasionally responsible.

Interstitial Pneumonia

Interstitial pneumonia is caused typically by viruses and *P. carinii* and is characterized by edema and an inflammatory cellular infiltrate situated predominantly within interstitial tissue. The pathologic reaction may take two forms, depending to some extent on the virulence of the organism and the rapidity with which the infection develops: (1) relatively long-standing or insidious infection is manifested predominantly by lymphocytic infiltration of alveolar septa without significant air-space abnormality (Fig. 25–15); (2) more rapidly progressive or virulent disease is often characterized by diffuse alveolar damage in which involvement of both interstitial and air-space components is prominent (Fig. 25–16). The underlying pathogenetic mechanism in the latter form of disease is related to damage to the alveolar-capillary membrane. Interstitial thickening by edema, capillary congestion, and an inflammatory cellular infiltrate; Type II cell hyperplasia; and a proteinaceous exudate within air spaces are characteristic histologic findings. In alveolar ducts and respiratory bronchioles, the exudate typically becomes concentrated and flattened, resulting in hyaline membranes.

The radiographic manifestations of interstitial pneumonia resulting from viral or mycoplasmal infection consist of a reticular or reticulonodular pattern (Fig. 25–17).[63–65] Septal

Text continued on page 713

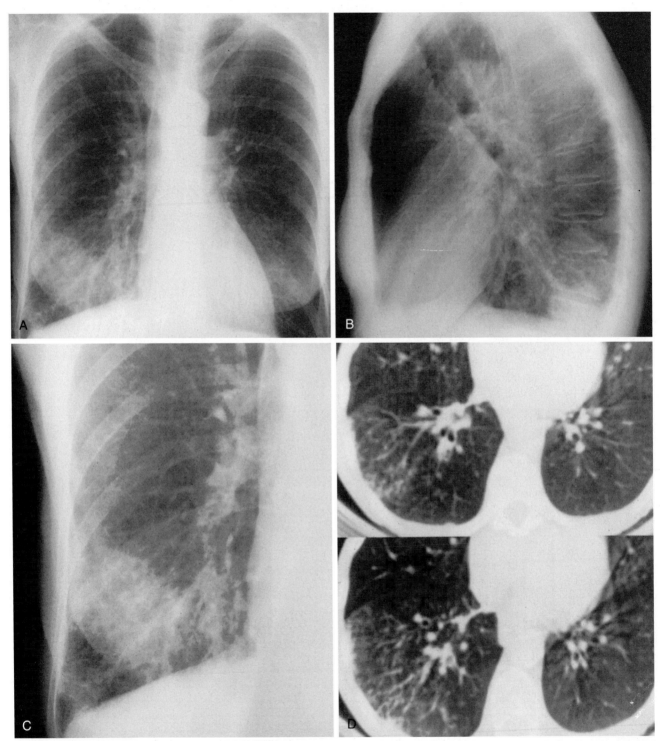

Figure 25–10. Acute Bronchopneumonia—*Staphylococcus aureus.* Posteroanterior *(A)* and lateral *(B)* chest radiographs disclose a triangular area of inhomogeneous consolidation in the right lower lobe. A detail view of the affected region *(C)* shows thickening and loss of definition of the bronchovascular bundles, areas of more confluent consolidation, and septal lines in the costophrenic angle. (The last feature is caused by distention of lymphatics and interstitial tissue of interlobular septa by inflammatory edema.) Contiguous CT scans through the lower lobes *(D)* reveal a fan-shaped area of increased attenuation and nodulation along the course of the three basal segments; note the patency of the anterior, lateral, and posterior segmental bronchi.

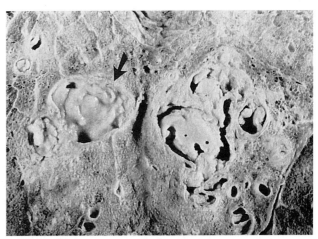

Figure 25–11. Pulmonary Abscesses—*Staphylococcus aureus.*
A magnified view of an upper lobe shows several irregularly shaped foci of necrotic lung, one of which is semisolid pus *(arrow)*. Early cavitation is present in the abscess on the right. (Interlobular septa are thickened as a result of lymphangitic spread of breast carcinoma.)

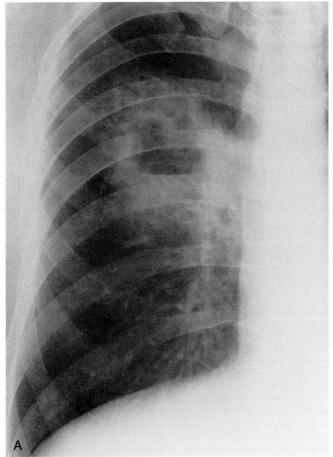

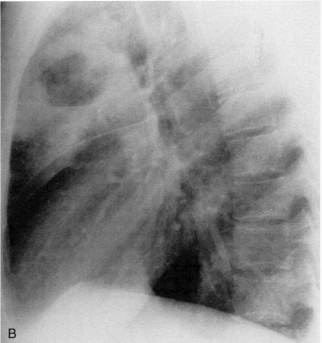

Figure 25–12. Lung Abscess. Views of the right lung from postero-anterior *(A)* and lateral *(B)* chest radiographs demonstrate a large abscess with an air-fluid level in the anterior segment of the right upper lobe. The internal margin of the abscess is irregular. There is minimal surrounding consolidation. The patient was a 38-year-old alcoholic man who customarily slept on his stomach. Gram stain of the sputum revealed gram-positive and gram-negative bacteria; no cultures were taken. The abscess resolved following treatment with antibiotics.

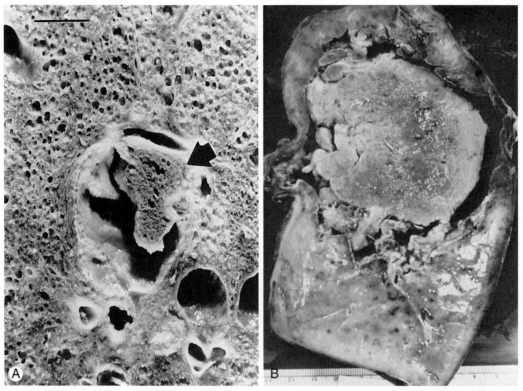

Figure 25–13. Pulmonary Sequestra—Early and Advanced. A highly magnified view of lung *(A)* shows a small cavity lined by a pyogenic exudate. Attached to one corner *(arrow)* is a small fragment of necrotic lung; the lower portion of the fragment has partially separated from the abscess wall; extension of this process to involve the entire fragment would result in a sequestrum. This process is dramatically illustrated in a slice of left lung from another patient *(B),* in which a large fragment of the necrotic upper lobe can be seen to lie within a cavity. The cause of the abscess in *A* is unknown but is presumed to be bacterial; *Klebsiella pneumoniae* was isolated from the sputum of the patient in *B.* (*A,* Bar = 0.75 cm.)

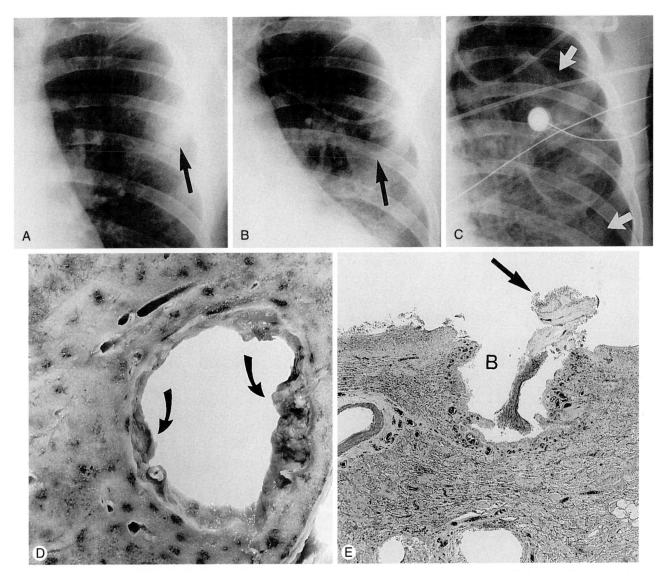

Figure 25–14. Pulmonary Pneumatocele. A chest radiograph *(A)* from a 28-year-old man with acute myelocytic leukemia and leukopenia shows an ill-defined opacity in the peripheral parenchyma of the left upper lobe. Twelve days later *(B)*, the opacity has been replaced by a smooth, thin-walled cavity approximately 4 cm in diameter. The following day *(C)*, the lesion measured 5.5 cm, even in the presence of partial collapse of the left lung as a result of pneumothorax *(arrows)*. At autopsy *(D)*, the cavity was seen to have a shaggy inner lining related to the presence of necrotic tissue *(arrows)*. A section through an airway (B) entering the cavity *(E)* showed a partially obstructing "flap" of mucus and inflammatory exudate; this was mobile in the gross specimen and was hypothesized to permit entry of air into the cavity during inspiration and prevent its egress on expiration. The cause of the cavity was believed to be most likely anaerobic organisms related to aspiration. *(A* to *E* from Quigley MJ, Fraser RS: Pulmonary pneumatocele: Pathology and pathogenesis. Am J Roentgenol 150:1275, 1988.)

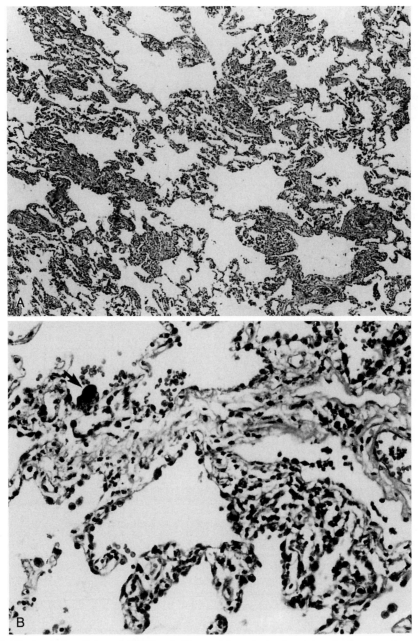

Figure 25–15. Interstitial Pneumonia—Cytomegalovirus. A 68-year-old man had a thymoma and subsequent development of red cell aplasia for which he was treated with transfusions and prednisone. He subsequently developed cough and increasing dyspnea. A posteroanterior chest radiograph showed a fine reticular pattern. Open lung biopsy *(A)* shows more or less diffuse interstitial pneumonitis; the air spaces are unaffected. Higher magnification *(B)* shows a lymphocytic infiltrate and a single large cell *(arrow)*, representing a cytomegalovirus-infected type II pneumocyte. *(A,* ×48; *B,* ×250.)

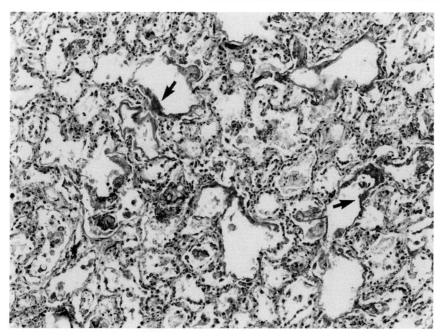

Figure 25–16. Diffuse Alveolar Damage—Herpes Zoster. Section shows mild interstitial thickening, extensive Type II cell hyperplasia, and proteinaceous material within air spaces. Well-defined hyaline membranes are present *(arrows).* (×100.)

(Kerley B) lines may be seen.[66] Associated bronchiolitis may result in centrilobular linear and nodular opacities, best seen on HRCT;[67] bronchitis may be manifested by peribronchial thickening and accentuation of lung markings.[50] Pneumonia caused by *P. carinii* typically presents radiographically as a bilateral, symmetric, fine granular or poorly defined reticulonodular pattern (Fig. 25–18).[68–70] With more severe infection, the findings progress to more homogeneous parenchymal opacification ranging from ground-glass opacities to consolidation; a heterogeneous reticulonodular pattern is often apparent at the periphery of the homogeneous opacity.[71] On HRCT, the predominant abnormality consists of extensive bilateral areas of ground-glass attenuation (Fig. 25–19); small nodules, reticular opacities, and interlobular septal thickening are seen in 20% to 40% of patients (Fig. 25–20).[72–74] Similar radiographic and HRCT findings may be seen in patients who have cytomegalovirus pneumonia.[75, 76, 76a] The findings in the more virulent form of viral or *P. carinii* pneumonia (corresponding to diffuse alveolar damage pathologically) are those of ARDS.

Several investigators have assessed the value of the chest radiograph and HRCT in distinguishing *P. carinii* pneumonia from other pneumonias as well as other complications seen in patients who have AIDS.[74, 77–79] In one study, the radiographic findings in 34 episodes of pyogenic pulmonary infection were compared with those in 30 episodes of *P. carinii* pneumonia in 30 HIV-positive patients.[78] Nonsegmental consolidation was present in 17 of the former infections (50%) and in only one episode of *P. carinii* pneumonia. Bilateral diffuse opacities were present in 28 episodes (93%) of *P. carinii* infection and only 6 (18%) of bacterial pneumonia. In another review of the HRCT scans of 102 patients who had AIDS and a variety of intrathoracic complications, including 35 cases of *P. carinii* pneumonia, two independent observers made a correct first-choice diagnosis of *P. carinii* pneumonia based on the presence of extensive bilateral areas of ground-glass attenuation in 29 of the 35 (83%) cases.[74]

Many viral infections that involve the lungs begin insidiously with fever, headache, and malaise, although other features (e.g., rash, pharyngitis, arthralgias) are not infrequently seen in association with specific organisms. The major symptom of lower respiratory tract involvement is cough; although initially nonproductive, it may become associated with mucoid or frankly purulent sputum if infection is prolonged. The latter feature should raise the possibility of bacterial superinfection. More severe disease may be manifested by dyspnea and, rarely, respiratory failure. Distinction of infection by viruses from that caused by bacteria or other organisms is usually not possible on a clinical basis.

Infection Via the Pulmonary Vasculature

Infection via the pulmonary vasculature usually occurs in association with an extrapulmonary focus of infection. In many cases, the source of such infection is evident from the clinical findings. Sometimes, however, as in endocarditis or minute foci of infection in the skin or an internal organ,[80] it is not immediately apparent. The organisms responsible for the pulmonary infection may be found free in the blood (sepsis) or may be associated with thrombus (septic emboli). Rarely, microbial spread follows extension of an intrapulmonary focus of infection into a pulmonary artery (e.g., tuberculosis), leading to disease in the specific portion of lung parenchyma supplied by that vessel.

Because of the vascular origin of the infecting organisms, the pattern of parenchymal involvement tends to be patchy and random in distribution (although there is sometimes a lower lobe predominance as a result of the greater blood flow to these regions). A nodular appearance of the individual foci of disease is typical. When the infection is associated with sepsis, it typically takes the form of innumerable nodules 1 to 5 mm in diameter (miliary infection) (Fig.

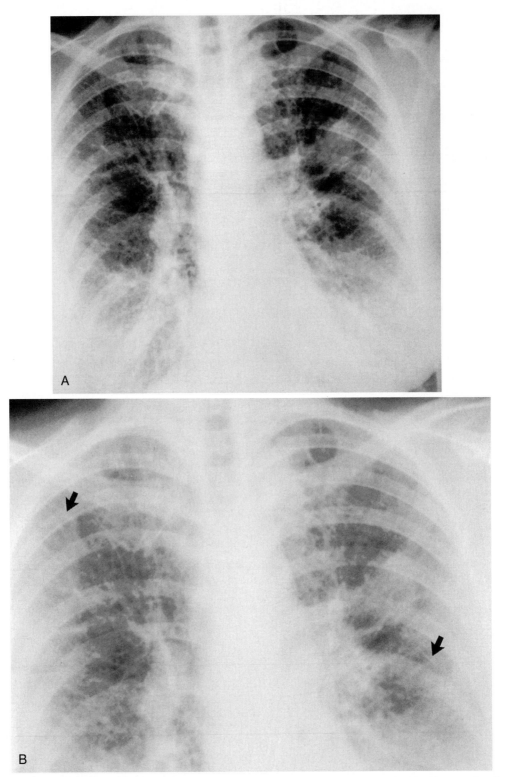

Figure 25–17. Acute Interstitial Pneumonia—*Mycoplasma pneumoniae*. A posteroanterior chest radiograph *(A)* and a closeup of the upper lobes *(B)* reveal thickening of the bronchovascular bundles and a ground-glass opacity throughout both lungs. Kerley A lines *(arrows)* and bilateral hilar lymph node enlargement are present. Also noted is a focal area of consolidation in the left upper lobe. The patient was a previously healthy 17-year-old girl.

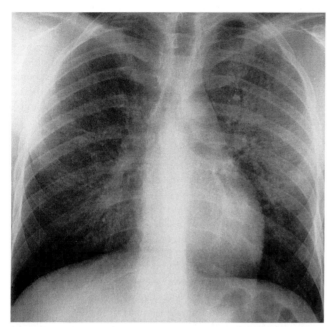

Figure 25–18. *Pneumocystis carinii* **Pneumonia.** A posteroanterior chest radiograph demonstrates bilateral ground-glass opacities and a poorly defined reticulonodular pattern. The patient was a 24-year-old man who had acquired immunodeficiency syndrome and *P. carinii* pneumonia.

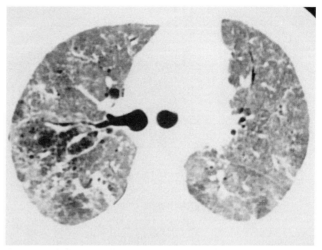

Figure 25–20. *Pneumocystis carinii* **Pneumonia.** HRCT shows extensive bilateral areas of ground-glass attenuation, localized areas of low attenuation, irregular linear, and small nodular opacities. The patient was a 37-year-old man who developed *P. carinii* pneumonia after bone-marrow transplantation.

25–21); when associated with septic emboli, multiple but substantially less numerous abscesses are characteristic.

The radiologic appearance of miliary disease is usually caused by tuberculosis. The pattern is distinctive and consists of discrete, pinpoint opacities usually evenly distributed throughout both lungs;[81, 82] sometimes, there is a slight basal predominance reflecting the gravity-induced increased blood flow (Fig. 25–22). When first visible, the nodules measure 1 to 2 mm in diameter (hence the term *miliary*, which refers to the similarly sized millet seed); in the absence of adequate therapy, they may increase to 3 to 5 mm in diameter, a finding seen in approximately 10% of cases.[82]

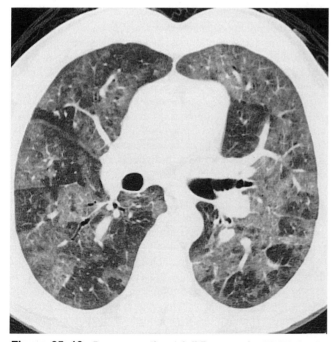

Figure 25–19. *Pneumocystis carinii* **Pneumonia.** HRCT demonstrates a characteristic appearance consisting of bilateral areas of ground-glass attenuation and areas of normal-appearing lung causing a mosaic pattern. The patient was a 46-year-old man who had acquired immunodeficiency syndrome and *P. carinii* pneumonia.

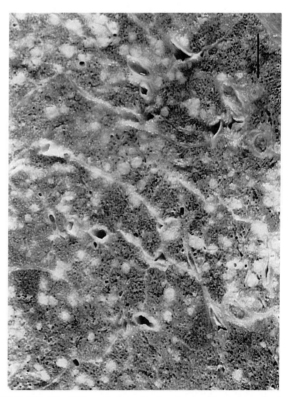

Figure 25–21. Miliary Tuberculosis. A magnified view of a lower lobe shows numerous randomly distributed nodules approximately 1 to 3 mm in diameter, representing hematogenous spread of tubercle bacilli. (Bar = 1 cm.)

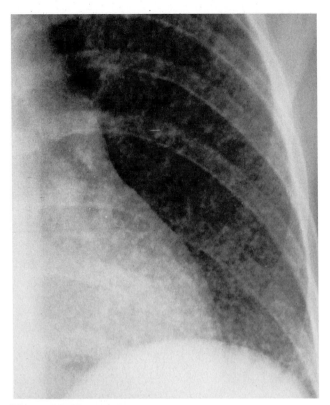

Figure 25–22. Miliary Tuberculosis. A view of the left lung from an anteroposterior chest radiograph in a 22-year-old woman demonstrates numerous sharply defined nodules measuring 1 to 3 mm in diameter. The nodules are most abundant in the lung base. The diagnosis of miliary tuberculosis was proven by bone marrow biopsy.

Septic emboli are characterized radiologically by the presence of nodules usually measuring 1 to 3 cm in diameter (Fig. 25–23), which are frequently cavitated. CT also frequently shows subpleural wedge-shaped areas of consolidation, often with central areas of necrosis or frank cavitation (Fig. 25–24).[83, 84] In approximately two thirds of patients who have multiple septic emboli, at least some of the nodules can be seen on CT to have vessels leading into the nodule, the so-called feeding vessel sign.

Infection by Direct Spread from an Extrapulmonary Site

Direct spread across the chest wall or diaphragm or from the mediastinum may occur in contaminated thoracic wounds[85] or by extension of infection from an extrapulmonary source, such as intra-abdominal abscess or a focus of mediastinitis secondary to esophageal rupture (Fig. 25–25). In these cases, the pulmonary disease is usually localized to an area contiguous with the extrapulmonary source of infection and often takes the form of an abscess. The source of such infections sometimes is not immediately apparent, such as an adrenal abscess or pyelonephritis with retroperitoneal or nephrobronchial fistula.[86, 87]

MICROBIOLOGIC AND GENERAL DIAGNOSTIC CONSIDERATIONS

Drawing accurate conclusions concerning the cause of pneumonia and predicting its outcome is problematical. One

major impediment is the lack of an acceptable gold standard for the diagnosis of pneumonia in many studies;[10] as a result, conclusions based on their results are suspect. Although there is little doubt that most previously healthy individuals who have the new onset of fever, systemic symptoms, cough, purulent sputum production, neutrophilia, and air-space consolidation on the chest radiograph likely have pneumonia,[88] differentiating infarction and edema from pneumonia in patients who have underlying chronic cardiopulmonary disease can be difficult.[10] In the setting of the mechanically ventilated patient who has ARDS, confirmation of the diagnosis of pneumonia on purely clinical and radiographic grounds may be impossible.[19, 27]

In one study, 39 patients who died after a mean of 14 days of mechanical ventilation were studied within 1 hour of death to evaluate the histologic, microbiologic, and clinical criteria of ventilator-associated pneumonia.[89] Temperature greater than 38.5° C during the 48 hours before death, WBC count greater than 15,000/mm[3] in the 48 hours before death, the presence of a bacterial or fungal pathogen on the last sputum culture, radiographic worsening in the week before death, and worsening gas exchange in the 72 hours before death were compared to histologic and microbiologic findings in specific areas of lung parenchyma. No single clinical criterion or combination of criteria correlated with the presence or absence of pneumonia documented histologically. In another study in which the reliability of clinical judgment in identifying ventilator-acquired pneumonia was evaluated by a number of physicians, only 27 of 84 patients suspected of having pneumonia on clinical grounds had the diagnosis confirmed by strict microbiologic or histologic criteria.[90] Those in whom the diagnosis was rejected were found to have other causes for their symptoms. The absence of clinical findings of pneumonia did not preclude its presence; 50 (38%) of 131 predictions of the absence of pneumonia based on clinical findings were wrong.

In fact, many other infectious and noninfectious causes of fever and radiographic opacities have been recognized in mechanically ventilated patients.[91] For example, in those managed with mechanical ventilation for ARDS, clinical assessment may fail to recognize the proliferative (organizing) phase of ARDS, empyema, nosocomial sinusitis, or catheter-related infection as sources of fever, wrongly attributing it to the presence of pneumonia.[91] Other nonpulmonary causes of fever that have been identified in mechanically ventilated patients who have pulmonary radiographic opacities include urinary tract infection, intra-abdominal abscess, and acalculous cholecystitis.[91] Similarly, purulent tracheal secretions are seldom caused by pneumonia in patients receiving prolonged mechanical ventilation;[92] such secretions can originate from both the upper and the lower respiratory tract in the absence of pneumonia.[93]

Even the use of histopathology as a gold standard for the diagnosis of pneumonia presents some difficulties. A review of the pathologic findings in 39 patients who died after a mean of 14 days of mechanical ventilation revealed important variability in the diagnosis of pneumonia by four pathologists.[94] A histologic diagnosis of pneumonia was given in 18% to 38% of the patients by individual pathologists; a consensus diagnosis of pneumonia (three of the four pathologists) was achieved in only 9 cases (23%) initially and 14 (36%) when predefined histologic criteria were rigor-

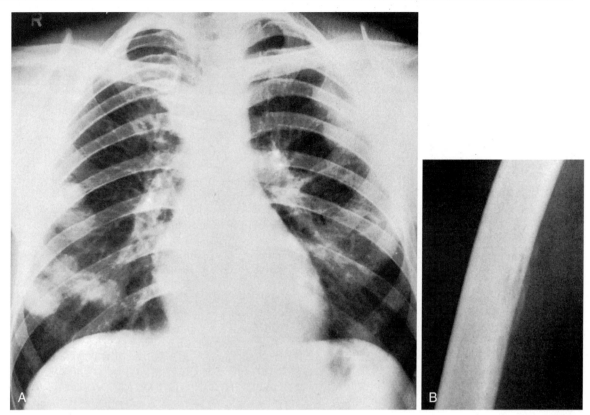

Figure 25–23. Septic Embolism. A posteroanteriorchest radiograph *(A)* reveals several sharply defined nodules ranging from 2 to 3 cm in diameter and situated predominantly in the right lower lobe and the left upper lobe. The masses are homogeneous in density and show no evidence of cavitation (although cavitation eventually occurred in the majority). A lateral view of the midshaft of the right femur *(B)* shows an irregular area of rarefaction in the cortex, associated with the subperiosteal new bone formation along the posterior aspect. *Staphylococcus aureus* was cultured from the sputum and from pus obtained from the thigh at incision and drainage.

ously applied. Other difficulties also arise in the interpretation of postmortem culture specimens (*see* page 351).

The radiographic diagnosis of ventilator-associated pneumonia also lacks sensitivity and specificity.[95] In one

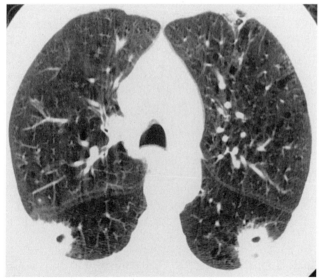

Figure 25–24. Septic Embolism. HRCT scan in a 65-year-old man demonstrates subpleural cavitated nodules in the superior segments of the lower lobes and a wedge-shaped area of consolidation in the left upper lobe. Blood cultures grew *Staphylococcus aureus*.

investigation of 69 ventilated patients, three reviewers interpreted the last radiograph before autopsy. Radiographic findings of air bronchograms, air-space opacities, silhouette sign, cavities, abutment of a fissure, atelectasis, and asymmetric opacities superimposed on diffuse bilateral opacities were evaluated for their accuracy in predicting pneumonia, individually, in combination with other radiographic signs, or in combination with clinical parameters. By stepwise logistic regression, the presence of an air bronchogram was the only radiographic sign that correlated with pneumonia, correctly predicting 64% of cases; however, the validity of the finding was confined to patients who did not have underlying ARDS. Only 7 of 22 of worsening parenchymal opacities were related to pneumonia. At autopsy, it was appreciated that pulmonary infarction or lung hemorrhage had been confused with pneumonia radiographically before death.

Apart from the difficulties in diagnosis based on clinical and radiographic features of disease, the precise identification of a specific microorganism responsible for a pneumonia is hampered by the lack of sensitivity and specificity of commonly used laboratory tests. There is little evidence that microbial investigation influences choice of treatment in most patients who have community-acquired pneumonia; moreover, mortality in this setting does not seem to be related to the determination of a specific cause for the pneumonia.[96, 97]

Several examples serve to illustrate these conclusions. In a survey of 116 nonimmunocompromised adults who had

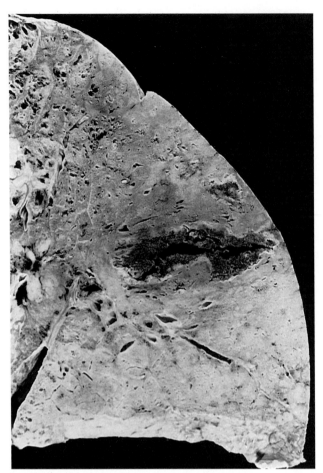

Figure 25–25. Pneumonia with Abscess Formation Secondary to Esophageal Perforation. A slice of the left lung shows extensive consolidation of the lower lobe associated with two irregularly shaped abscesses in the superior segment. The larger of these was in direct continuity with necrotic tissue in the mediastinum and a perforated esophageal carcinoma (esophagopulmonary fistula).

pneumonia, quantitative sputum culture and blood culture were able to establish a bacteriologic cause in 44% of cases;[97] the prognosis was identical whether a bacteriologic diagnosis was made or not. In another prospective study of 453 adults admitted to the hospital for community-acquired pneumonia, a specific cause was identified in two thirds of the patients;[98] again, mortality was not linked to ascertainment of cause in the 26 patients who died. In a third study of similar design, a microbiologic diagnosis was achieved in 281 of 510 patients (55%), 462 of whom were admitted to the hospital and 31 of whom died;[99] the failure to identify cause again did not appear to place a patient at increased risk for death. These results must be interpreted with caution because a small but real difference in mortality may not have been detected because of insufficient statistical power. It is also likely that patients in whom a specific bacteriologic diagnosis was made may have differed in important respects from those in whom no organism was isolated. Despite these caveats, it is likely that the conclusions derived from these studies are valid. In all probability, most of the patients in whom an organism was not identified had pneumonia caused by *S. pneumoniae* or *M. pneumoniae*, viruses, and other "atypical" organisms such as *Chlamydia* species. Most such

patients likely received antibiotics suitable for therapy or did not require antibiotics because the infection was of viral origin. In view of the previous discussion, the value of routine sputum culture and Gram stain, as recommended by practice guidelines,[2, 45] should be considered critically (*see* farther on).

In contrast to the mildly ill patient who has community-acquired pneumonia, the early and correct identification of the organism responsible for infection more likely improves the prognosis of severely ill patients, especially those who have nosocomial ventilator-associated pneumonia. In a study of 113 consecutive adults who had ventilator-associated pneumonia, those patients who had an inadequate initial selection of antibiotics, as determined by invasive culture methods, had a mortality of 37%;[100] this compared to a mortality of 15% in patients in whom the initially chosen antibiotics were effective against the organisms identified. In another study of approximately 17,000 patients admitted to the intensive care unit (ICU) in 30 Spanish hospitals, 530 patients developed 565 episodes of pneumonia;[101] the attributable mortality was approximately 16% in patients whose initial antibiotic selection was appropriate for the organism responsible for the infection, in contrast to 25% when the antibiotic selection was inappropriate. (These two studies may have been subject to selection bias because patients who were initially inappropriately treated could have had more virulent organisms, a marker of more severe underlying illness.) Using a more rigorous multiple logistic regression analysis for studying risk factors for death in ventilator-associated pneumonia, a third group of investigators found an odds ratio for fatality of 3.5 in those patients treated inappropriately.[102]

The effects of unnecessary empiric treatment of patients who do not have pneumonia are not without risk. In a study of 277 consecutive patients requiring mechanical ventilation, prior administration of antibiotics was an independent risk factor for developing pneumonia during the course of mechanical ventilation;[105] these patients had a higher mortality (37%) compared with those who did not have pneumonia (8.5%). Patients treated with antibiotics, whether necessary or not, may later develop infection resulting from resistant organisms, which has a higher mortality than that developing in patients who have not received previous antibiotic therapy.[104] Recognizing this phenomenon, one group of investigators applied decision analysis to a hypothetical group of immunocompetent individuals who had suspected bacterial pneumonia that developed during mechanical ventilation.[105] They concluded, in an admittedly counterintuitive fashion, that empiric therapy of purported infection, in the absence of invasive testing to establish an accurate diagnosis of pneumonia and its cause, would be associated with a poorer survival than if no therapy were given at all!

Several groups of investigators have attempted to determine the relative contributions of pneumonia and associated illness to mortality. For example, in some studies of patients who developed pneumonia and who were carefully matched to control patients for the severity of underlying illness, age, indication for ventilatory support, and duration of mechanical ventilation, analysis indicated that the mortality attributable to ventilator-associated pneumonia exceeded 25%.[24, 106] However, in another cohort study in which two groups of patients in a medical-surgical ICU were matched for diagnosis, indication for mechanical ventilation, age, sex, duration of mechanical ventilation, Apache II score on admission, and date of admission to the ICU, the mortality in patients who had pneumonia (34 of 85 patients [40%]) was the same as that of those in the control group (33 of 85 patients [39%]).[26] Similar results have been found by other workers.[107] It is possible that attributable death occurring in patients who have ventilator-associated pneumonia is confined to those whose infection is due to certain "high-risk" pathogens, such as *P. aeruginosa*, *Acinetobacter* species, and *Xanthomonas maltophilia*.[108]

This inconsistency in data likely accounts for the diverse approaches that have been proposed for the management of patients who have ventilator-acquired pneumonia.[109, 110] We favor attempting to establish diagnosis as firmly as possible and to define the cause of the infection so that therapy can be optimized. A variety of techniques have been described to do so; their use must depend on the expertise and inclination of consultants in any given institution.

Sputum Culture and Gram Stain

There is no doubt that sputum culture and Gram stain are not ideal diagnostic tests. Patient cooperation is required to obtain an adequate specimen, and less than half of patients who have pneumonia are able to produce sputum.[110a] Many specimens that are obtained are unsatisfactory because of contamination by upper airway flora or because of failure to produce purulent secretions from the lower airways. A number of pathogens are also eradicated from sputum by prior utilization of antibiotics. As a result of all these features, unless special precautions are taken, sputum culture is neither a sensitive nor a specific test for the identification of the causative organism of pneumonia. For example, in a study of 172 patients who had bacteremic nosocomial pneumonia, only 49% of the sputum samples contained the organism recovered from blood.[111] In a more comprehensive meta-analysis of sputum Gram stain in community-acquired pneumococcal pneumonia, a sensitivity of 15% to 100% and specificity of 11% to 100% were found in the various studies.[112]

The diagnostic yield of Gram stain and culture improves in an impressive manner when high-quality sputum—purulent sputum uncontaminated by upper airway secretions—can be obtained before the institution of antibiotics. For example, in one study in which a positive blood culture was used as the gold standard, the sensitivity of Gram stain for the diagnosis of pneumococcal pneumonia was 85%.[113] Similarly, insistence on the evaluation of only high-quality samples increases the specificity of the finding of gram-positive diplococci in the identification of *S. pneumoniae* in sputum.[10] The usefulness of this information increases with increasing prevalence of penicillin-resistant organisms in the community (*see* page 736). Gram staining of sputum has a high negative predictive value with respect to culture; for example, in one study of 800 sputum isolates, the sensitivity of the Gram stain was 78%.[114] Although information derived from these sputum studies is not likely to influence management in most patients who have community-acquired pneumonia, nevertheless, we favor performing a Gram stain and culture of sputum when a purulent sample

uncontaminated by upper airway secretions can be obtained before initiating antibiotic therapy. As has been pointed out, the use of this and other simple tests may allow modification of antibiotics, have prognostic importance, influence the duration of therapy, and provide information concerning the local epidemiology of infection.[115] This recommendation is especially strong for those patients whose illness is severe enough to warrant admission to the hospital.

Endotracheal Aspiration

In an intubated patient, lower airway secretions are easily obtained by endotracheal aspiration. Nonquantitative analysis of specimens obtained by this procedure is a sensitive, albeit nonspecific, means of determining the cause of pneumonia.[89, 93, 116, 117] In a baboon model of ventilator-acquired pneumonia, tracheal aspirates contained 78% of the organisms identified by culture of lung homogenates, although 14 (40%) of 35 species identified were not present in lung tissue.[116] In another study on humans, endotracheal aspiration identified 87% of bacterial species present in lung tissue simultaneously cultured immediately postmortem;[89] however, the specificity was only 31%.

Quantitative bacterial culture of endotracheal aspirates may improve specificity. Using a 10^6 cfu/ml cutoff point, the operating characteristics of the endotracheal aspirate compared favorably with those of the protected specimen brush in one study.[118] Although there was agreement between the two tests in approximately 85% of samples from 52 ventilated patients, the sensitivity of the aspirates was higher than that of the protected specimen brush (82% vs. 64%); however, the specificity was somewhat lower (83% vs. 96%). Among 26 patients already receiving empirically chosen antibiotics for what was subsequently proven to be pneumonia (positive pleural fluid or blood culture; compatible histopathologic or autopsy findings; isolation of a definite respiratory pathogen such as *Legionella, M. tuberculosis*, or *M. pneumoniae*) and using 10^5 cfu/ml as a cutoff point, endotracheal aspiration had a sensitivity of 70%, a specificity of 72%, and a negative predictive value of 72%. The specificity was only modestly lower than that obtained by invasive methods, and the negative predictive value was substantially higher. Similar results were reported by another group of investigators in a study of ventilated patients receiving antibiotics, although the threshold used to define a significant result was 10^6 cfu/ml.[119] Endotracheal aspiration has been shown to be the best technique to identify the causative organism of ventilator-acquired pneumonia in an animal model.[119a] Manipulation of the threshold for determination of a positive test can alter the test's performance; improvement in sensitivity sacrifices its specificity. Whether invasive methods can perform in a more precise fashion warrants examination.

Bronchoscopy with Protected Brush Specimens

In an attempt to improve the sensitivity and specificity of culture or Gram stain for the diagnosis of pneumonia, material has been obtained bronchoscopically by bronchoalveolar lavage or protected specimen brush in some centers.[17]

Quantification of the growth of the bacteria recovered has been used to help define the presence or absence of pneumonia and to aid in the identification of the causative pathogen.[119b] The wide application and utility of such testing, however, have been limited by lack of standardization and by the paucity of studies demonstrating improvement in mortality, morbidity, or other outcome variables compared to less invasive methods of diagnosis.[17]

The accuracy of the protected specimen brush technique has been assessed in a number of studies by comparing quantitative cultures of material obtained by the protected specimen brush to quantitative cultures and histopathologic findings of simultaneously sampled lung tissue from the same area.[89, 116, 120–122] The sensitivity of the protected specimen brush has varied from less than 50%[89, 116, 122] to as high as 82%.[121] The specificity of the test has been better—generally in excess of 80%.[89, 120, 121, 123] Despite these apparent limitations, some workers have found the protected specimen brush extraordinarily useful.[92, 119b, 121] Using a threshold of 10^3 cfu/ml for the diagnosis of pneumonia, only 45 of 147 ventilated patients suspected of nosocomial pneumonia had confirmation of the diagnosis.[92] In only four of these patients was the culture a false-positive one; no patient with less than this colony count was shown to have pneumonia, the absence of pneumonia at autopsy or resolution of signs and symptoms without antibiotics being demonstrated in most. As indicated earlier, however, others have not attained this success.

Culture using protected specimen brush may fail to yield an organism in patients who have pneumonia for a number of reasons, including culture early in the evolution of the infection, sampling the wrong area of the lung, processing the specimen incorrectly, or obtaining the sample after initiation of antibiotics.[124, 124a] In patients in whom the clinical suspicion of pneumonia remains high, repeating the protected specimen brush may reveal higher titers of the pathogen at a later time.[125] Although this may reflect progression of infection, it may also be related to inherent variability in test findings, as has been demonstrated by repeated sampling at the same time in the same patient.[126, 127]

It may be inappropriate and futile to attempt to fix threshold values of quantitative cultures for the diagnosis of pneumonia by protected specimen brush. Even if a test is reproducible, the significance of a positive result should be interpreted in the light of the pretest probability of disease, and consideration should be given both to the potential harm that could be done by not treating the pneumonia and to the risk of unnecessary therapy.[128] Although quantitative data concerning the risks and benefits of giving or withholding treatment are largely unavailable in the setting of the critically ill patient, given a fixed risk-to-benefit ratio for antibiotic therapy, it is evident that as the pretest probability for pneumonia increases, the threshold used to define an abnormal test result should decrease (i.e., fewer organisms would be necessary before one would embark on a course of therapy).[128]

Bronchoalveolar Lavage

Bronchoalveolar lavage, including protected bronchoalveolar lavage,[129] with quantitative culture of distal lung se-cretions has been found to yield similar results for the diagnosis of pneumonia as those derived from protected specimen brush.[129a] The sensitivity of the procedure has been found to be 47% to 70% and the specificity between 48% and 87% when cultures of bronchoalveolar lavage samples obtained either shortly before[120] or immediately after[89, 122] the death of mechanically ventilated patients were compared to histologic evidence of pneumonia as the gold standard. Using a *simplified bacterial index* (the sum of the whole numbers of each bacterial concentration expressed as a logarithm), quantitative bronchoalveolar lavage has yielded excellent results in some studies, with a sensitivity of 89% to 93% and specificity of 83% to 100% (despite the fact that many patients in some of the studies were receiving antibiotics at the time of the test).[130, 131] Some workers have found that the diagnostic yield of bronchoalveolar lavage in mechanically ventilated patients is not diminished by the prior administration of antibiotics,[121, 132] whereas others have found that it decreases the yield.[122, 124]

Some of the information obtained by analysis of bronchoalveolar lavage fluid is highly specific for the diagnosis of pneumonia, whereas the absence of some other findings is associated with a high negative predictive value for the diagnosis. Identification of intracellular organisms in phagocytic cells has a specificity for pneumonia of greater than 95% in most studies; the reported sensitivity has generally varied from 60% to greater than 75%,[121, 131, 133–137] although some investigators have reported a markedly lower yield.[120, 138] The morphology and Gram staining of organisms identified by bronchoalveolar lavage have correlated closely with the results of culture, allowing early and appropriate antibiotic selection.[27, 134, 137] The percentage of cells that contain intracellular organisms necessary to be considered diagnostic for pneumonia has varied widely in different reports, from a minimum of 2% to more than 25%; moreover, some investigators have been unable to establish any diagnostic threshold[130] and the quantitative reproducibility of a positive test has been found to be poor.[130a] Nevertheless, in one study, the absence of bronchoalveolar lavage neutrophilia predicted the absence of pneumonia within 2 days of specimen collection in 97% of patients,[139] while the finding of less than 50% neutrophils in bronchoalveolar lavage fluid had a negative predictive value of 100% in another.[89]

Miscellaneous Techniques for Sampling Airway Secretions

Because of the expense and potential morbidity of fiberoptic bronchoscopy,[93] a variety of other techniques for sampling distal secretions for culture have been developed. These include nonbronchoscopic lavage using a tracheal suction catheter,[139] blind nonbronchoscopic bronchoalveolar lavage sampling using a wedged catheter,[131, 140] blind distal bronchial sampling without lavage,[138] blind protected specimen brush sampling,[89, 141, 142] and blind sampling using a telescoping plugged catheter.[142, 143] Concordance between "invasive" and noninvasive sampling is good but imperfect; in particular, sampling of the upper lobes or left lung can be deficient.[144] Bronchoscopy itself may also provide a clue to the presence of infection: visualization of pus in the airway and the persistence of distal secretions emanating from distal bronchi during exhalation have been strongly associated with pneumonia.[145]

Transthoracic Needle Aspiration

Percutaneous fine needle aspiration of the lung using an ultrathin needle has been used for the identification of pathogens in nonventilated[146–148] and (occasionally) ventilated[146] patients who have pneumonia. As might be expected, the specificity and positive predictive value of a positive culture have been reported to be as high as 100%,[147] whereas the sensitivity and negative predictive values are poor (approximately 61% and 34%[147]). Results are better when the radiographic opacity is more extensive and when the patient has not yet received antibiotics.[148] In one study, antibiotics were modified after a positive culture in 29 of 97 patients (30%);[147] in 12 of these, the empirically chosen antibiotics were ineffective for the organism identified. Many of the patients had been chosen for the procedure because of their failure to improve in response to the initially selected antibiotics. Unfortunately, confirmation of these results is not yet available and whether outcome is favorably altered has not been determined.

There is controversy whether the methods described here should be the standard of care for patients who are severely ill due to pneumonia, especially ventilator-acquired pneumonia; in addition, if used at all, it is uncertain which of the tests is best.[109, 110, 149, 150] Most previously healthy individuals who are mildly ill are managed in an empiric fashion. Critiques of the widespread application of invasive diagnostic techniques have underscored the uncertainties in the literature.[109] It is not clear which of the many procedures provides the most reproducible and accurate results, what the bacteriologic threshold for diagnosis should be, how common false-negative results are, and whether overall antibiotic use can be reduced. Most importantly, it is not known whether application of any of these techniques results in a reduction in mortality and morbidity in a cost-effective fashion, compared to a less invasive and simplified approach (e.g., clinical assessment and culture and Gram stain of endotracheal aspirates).[150a]

Other diagnostic methods have been described for patients who have pneumonia. Some, such as the identification of endotoxin in bronchoalveolar lavage fluid for the rapid diagnosis of gram-negative pneumonia,[151] are applicable to specific forms of infection. Others, such as the identification of bacterial genome by the polymerase chain reaction,[152–155] the detection of antigen in secretions by latex agglutination,[156–158] or the determination of immune response by serologic testing,[159] are highly focused. Each of these is discussed in the sections of the text concerned with individual microorganisms.

PNEUMONIA IN SPECIFIC PATIENT GROUPS

A useful approach to the diagnosis of pneumonia is to consider infections as community acquired or as developing in patients who are hospitalized (nosocomial pneumonia). Because the type of organism and clinical manifestations of disease often differ in patients who have deficient immune or inflammatory reactions, it is also useful to consider pulmonary infections in this group separately (pneumonia in the compromised host).

Community-Acquired Pneumonia

The conclusions of studies investigating the microbiologic causes of community-acquired pneumonia have been subject to considerable bias.[160] Most reports are from academic centers and have been restricted to the minority of patients requiring hospitalization. Many studies have been restricted to immunocompetent hosts, and only the more recent ones reflect the impact of HIV infection on the epidemiology of the disease. Some investigators have excluded residents of nursing homes or patients who were recently hospitalized, whereas others have included such patients; some have had age limitations, and others have included patients of all ages.[10]

Absolute confirmation that pneumonia is caused by a particular pathogen requires culture from a normally sterile site, such as blood, pleural fluid, lung (by direct aspiration), or a metastatic site of infection.[160] (Blood culture, however, seldom reveals the cause of a pneumonia. In a review of its efficacy in establishing diagnosis, only 330 of 2,935 patients [11%] hospitalized for community-acquired pneumonia had a positive culture;[160] of these, S. pneumoniae accounted for two thirds.) Detection of a pathogen that does not normally colonize the airway, such as Legionella species, M. tuberculosis, or many fungal species, in sputum also constitutes reliable proof of infection. Serologic tests may also identify the causative organism, but their availability varies from center to center. Culture of sputum for some of the more common causes of community-acquired pneumonia, such as M. pneumoniae and Chlamydia species is not routinely performed, and the quality of testing for Legionella species is uneven.[160] Lastly, prior administration of antibiotics precludes successful identification of many organisms.[10, 160–163] These and other factors account for the failure to establish the causative organism in 50% or more of patients who have community-acquired pneumonia, even when special efforts are made to do so.[2, 6, 162, 164–167]

The frequency with which different organisms responsible for community-acquired pneumonia has been reported varies widely in different series.[10] As indicated, this variation is the result of several factors, including the techniques used for diagnosis, the age of the patients, the presence or absence of additional significant disease, and the severity of the pneumonia.[2] Despite this limitation, some important general observations may be made.

S. pneumoniae is the most commonly identified pathogen in most investigations;[9, 10, 98, 99, 168, 169] although the proportion varies widely as a function of which diagnostic tests are used, the median is about 35%. In patients admitted to the hospital for pneumonia, anaerobic bacteria have been isolated in approximately 20% to 35%,[170–172] the organisms being second only to S. pneumoniae as a cause of community-acquired pneumonia. Between 2% and 8% of patients have H. influenzae infection;[10] most of these have underlying chronic air-flow obstruction or are elderly, although younger, healthy adults can also be affected.[8, 10, 73] Community-acquired S. aureus pneumonia is uncommon; when it occurs in this setting, it frequently follows influenza virus infection. The infection is often associated with bacteremia and high mortality[10, 174] and should be considered in severely ill patients admitted to the ICU for the management of pneumonia.[175] Methicillin-resistant *S. aureus* can be a particularly serious cause of pneumonia in residents of nursing homes.[2, 176] *Moraxella catarrhalis* is a not uncommon cause of pneumonia in the elderly and in patients who have chronic air-flow obstruction.[177] The importance of *Legionella* species as a cause of community-acquired pneumonia shows marked regional variation. Although *Legionella* species account for only 2% or less of community-acquired pneumonia overall,[10] they are an important cause of pneumonia among patients sick enough to require hospitalization and care in an ICU.[2, 46, 174, 178–180] Gram-negative enteric organisms are an uncommon cause of pneumonia in the general population, but should also be considered in severely ill patients, especially in those who are older, who have aspirated[180a] or who have significant underlying disease.[10, 179–183]

Although often not considered among the causes of community-acquired pneumonia in epidemiologic surveys, it is clear that tuberculosis must be considered in outpatients who have pneumonia; its prevalence is greater in certain populations, such as residents of nursing homes, alcoholics, the homeless, drug addicts, HIV-infected individuals, as well as individuals from populations in which tuberculosis has a high prevalence.[2, 184]

When analysis is confined to ambulatory patients who do not require hospitalization, the proportion of bacterial species identified as the cause of community-acquired pneumonia decreases dramatically; for example, in one study of 149 patients, only 3 (2%) were found to have bacterial pneumonia.[6] Many of these patients have "atypical pneumonia," of which one of the most common causes is *M. pneumoniae*. In fact, this organism has been identified as the cause of pneumonia in up to 29% of patients in different series,[6, 10, 185] although it has been quite uncommon in some others.[9] The variability in the relative importance of *M. pneumoniae* might be partly explained by the epidemic behavior of the organism. *Chlamydia pneumoniae* is also an important cause of "atypical" community-acquired pneumonia, having been identified in up to 21% of patients.[1, 6, 10, 186] Other chlamydia-like organisms have also been recognized as a cause of community-acquired pneumonia.[98, 99] Q-fever pneumonia (caused by *Coxiella burnetti*) demonstrates important geographic variations in incidence, its discovery generally being confined to rural settings.[6] In adults, influenza virus is the most important cause of community-acquired viral pneumonia;[98, 99] in infants and children, respiratory syncytial virus and parainfluenza virus are the most common agents.

As might be expected, when patients infected with HIV have been included in studies of community-acquired pneumonia, the spectrum of causative organisms in those requiring hospitalization is significantly altered.[162] For example, in one investigation of 180 such patients, *P. carinii* was identified in 48 (27%), whereas *S. pneumoniae* was found in only 38 (21%). Other bacterial organisms frequently identified in HIV-infected patients include *Haemophilus* species, *S. aureus*, and gram-negative enteric bacteria.[188]

The severity of pneumonia influences the necessity for admission (whether to a ward or to the ICU), the use of diagnostic techniques, and the choice of antibiotics. Severe pneumonia has been defined as that requiring admission to an ICU.[2] Features that warrant consideration of such admission include the presence of a respiratory rate greater than 30 breaths/min at admission, severe respiratory failure (defined by a PaO_2-to-FIO_2 ratio < 250 mm Hg), necessity of mechanical ventilation, radiographic evidence of disease in more than one lobe or on both sides, rapid progression of disease radiographically within 48 hours of admission, shock, requirement for vasopressors for more than 4 hours, and urine output less than 20 ml/hr or less than 80 ml in 4 hours (unless another explanation is apparent) or acute renal failure requiring dialysis.[2]

In addition to these findings, a number of other clinical features have been associated with an increased risk of mortality or a complicated course.[2, 189] Their presence warrants serious consideration for admission to the hospital, at least until a favorable response to therapy can be established. These features include any history of significant underlying disease, age greater than 65 years, altered mental status, previous splenectomy, suspicion of aspiration, elevation of temperature greater than 38.3° C (101° F), and evidence of metastatic infection. A variety of laboratory findings have also been associated with increased morbidity and mortality, including a white blood cell count less than 4×10^9 or greater than 30×10^9, an absolute neutrophil count less than 1×10^9, a PaO_2 less than 60 or a $PaCO_2$ greater than 50 mm Hg while breathing room air, elevated blood urea nitrogen (BUN) and creatinine, serum hemoglobin less than 9 gm/dl, metabolic acidosis, and findings of disseminated intravascular coagulation. Additional radiographic findings that should encourage extra vigilance include cavitation and pleural effusion.

In the absence of the risk factors listed previously, a complicated clinical course is unlikely.[4, 190] Based on an analysis of clinical and laboratory data from 14,199 adult inpatients who had community-acquired pneumonia, a prediction rule that stratified patients into five classes with respect to risk for death within 30 days was developed and applied to an additional 40,236 patients.[4] The mortality rate among patients in the first three classes was found to be sufficiently low that outpatient treatment could reasonably be considered. This was especially true for class I patients (< 50 years of age, absence of comorbid disease, normal mental status, heart rate < 125 beats/min, respiratory rate < 30 breaths/min, systolic blood pressure > 90 mm Hg, and temperature between 35 and 40° C).

A variety of similar criteria have been used by other investigators for the same purpose. In a smaller study of 101 elderly patients who required admission to the hospital for community-acquired pneumonia, poor prognosis was associated with the patient being previously bedridden, having a history of a swallowing disorder, having a body temperature less than 37° C, having a respiratory rate greater than 30 breaths/min, and having three or more affected lobes present on the chest radiograph.[191] Of 255 patients admitted to the hospital in New Zealand for community-acquired pneumonia, the presence on admission of any two adverse criteria (respiratory rate ≥ 30 breaths/min, diastolic BP ≤ 60 mm Hg, blood urea nitrogen > 7 mmol/L, or confusion) identified 19 of 20 patients who died and 6 of 8 admitted to the ICU.[192] Similar conclusions were reported in an American series.[193] These findings imply that simple clinical and laboratory observations are of value in assessing risk of death in patients who have community-acquired pneumonia. No single criterion or group of criteria, however, can replace overall clinical judgment; social factors and clinical circumstances, such as persistent vomiting, should influence any decision regarding the need for hospitalization in the individual patient.[194]

Recurrent pneumonia is defined as two or more episodes of lower respiratory tract infection separated by an asymptomatic interval of at least 1 month or by radiographic clearing.[195] In the community setting, it usually denotes some underlying predisposing illness;[196] in one series that antedated the AIDS era in which 158 patients experienced 612 episodes of pneumonia, roughly one half of patients had chronic bronchitis, bronchiectasis, or congestive heart failure;[196] the remainder had a variety of extrathoracic illnesses, most commonly alcoholism, diabetes mellitus, chronic sinusitis, and malignancy. An organism considered pathogenic was isolated in 518 of the pneumonias.

Currently, by far the most important underlying abnormality associated with recurrent pneumonia is HIV infection. In fact, otherwise unexplained recurrent pneumonia is a reason to order a test for the presence of this virus.[195] Many other conditions associated with an abnormal immune or inflammatory reaction also have an increased risk of recurrent pneumonia; examples include chemotherapy in patients who have cancer and immunosuppression after organ transplantation. A number of systemic illnesses, such as diabetes mellitus and chronic renal failure, have recurrent pneumonia as one of their manifestations.

Hospital-Acquired Pneumonia

Hospital-acquired (nosocomial) pneumonia can be defined as pneumonia occurring 48 hours or more after admission, excluding infection that is incubating at the time of admission.[17] The true incidence of such pneumonia is difficult to ascertain and is probably greater than generally appreciated as a result of lack of recognition or misclassification of pulmonary disease. These diagnostic errors can occur for a variety of reasons, including manifestation of disease shortly after discharge from the hospital, atypical presentations of disease as a result of underlying immunosuppression or prior use of antibiotics, failure to perform postmortem examination, and failure to perform appropriate culture in some infections (such as in legionellosis or anaerobic infection).[197]

As discussed previously (*see* page 699), one of the most common mechanisms by which pathogens gain access to the lower respiratory tract is aspiration of upper airway secretions; as a result, the cause of hospital-acquired pneumonia depends largely on the type of organisms that colonize the oropharynx.[17] Many cases of nosocomial pneumonia are polymicrobial in origin.[19, 198] The specific cause depends, in part, on the presence of absence of certain risk factors, such as the duration of hospitalization, the use of mechanical ventilation, the severity of comorbidity, and the prior use of antibiotics. As might be expected, the reported frequency of causative organisms also depends on the diagnostic methods employed.[199]

Bacteria are the most frequently isolated pathogens in patients who have nosocomial pneumonia. Early in the hospital course (within the first 4 days), the more frequent organisms include *S. pneumoniae*, *Moraxella catarrhalis*, methicillin-sensitive *S. aureus*, and *H. influenzae*.[197, 200–202] Later on, enteric gram-negative organisms, such as *Enterobacter* species, *Escherichia coli*, *Klebsiella* species, *Proteus* species, and *S. aureus*, predominate.[17] In one study of 1,000 patients admitted to a medical-surgical ICU, of whom 264 required mechanical ventilation for more than 48 hours, 58 (22%) developed pneumonia.[107] A causative organism was identified by protected brush catheter, blood culture, or autopsy lung culture in 47 of these cases; gram-negative bacilli were isolated in 63% and *S. aureus* in 23%. Similar results have been reported in a study of 31 patients who developed pneumonia during the course of mechanical ventilation instituted in the management of ARDS.[202a]

The presence of specific risk factors increases the likelihood that certain organisms are responsible for the pneumonia.[17] For example, anaerobic bacteria are more likely to be the causative organisms in patients who develop pneumonia after witnessed aspiration or who have poor dentition or altered consciousness.[198] More severe illness is another factor associated with the presence of these organisms. *P. aeruginosa* infection should be considered in patients who have received corticosteroids or broad-spectrum antibiotics, who have had a prolonged stay in the ICU, or who have underlying lung disease such as bronchiectasis.[203, 203a] *S. aureus* is more common in patients who have coma,[203] head injury, recent influenza infection, renal failure, or a history of intravenous drug abuse. *Legionella* species are endemic in some hospitals;[204, 205] pneumonia caused by these organisms is favored by the prior administration of corticosteroids.[205] A prolonged hospitalization or prior use of antibiotics also favors the development of hospital-acquired pneumonia resulting from infection by antibiotic-resistant organisms, such as *S. aureus*, *Acinetobacter* species, *Serratia marcescens*, and *P. aeruginosa*.[206, 206a] Similar organisms should be suspected when pneumonia is severe (i.e., requiring mechanical ventilation or ICU admission).[207]

Viruses are much less common causes of hospital-acquired pneumonia than bacteria. Nevertheless, influenza pneumonia has occurred in acute outbreaks with attack rates of 25% to 80% among both patients and hospital personnel.[208] Both primary influenza pneumonia and secondary bacterial infection can cause significant morbidity and mortality, with chronically ill and elderly individuals being most at risk.[208, 209]

The risk factors for the development of nosocomial pneumonia have been examined by many groups of investigators[102, 103, 203, 205, 206, 210–217] and their features reviewed.[17, 20, 197, 199] They have been grouped into five general categories:[199] (1) host factors, such as age, underlying disease, and immunosuppression; (2) factors that favor microbial colonization of the upper airway or stomach (prior use of antibiotics being especially important in this regard); (3) factors that favor aspiration of upper airway or stomach secretions; (4) duration of mechanical ventilation (prolonged ventilation being associated with an increased risk of exposure to contaminated equipment or to the colonized hands of health care workers); and (5) factors that prevent adequate clearance of airway secretions, such as surgical procedures involving the head and neck, thorax, and upper abdomen as well as immobilization resulting from trauma or illness. Some examples of studies in which the importance of these risk factors have been analyzed suffice for illustrative purposes.

In one investigation, 20 patients who developed pneumonia in the surgical and medical/respiratory ICUs of a North Carolina teaching hospital were compared with a control group of 40 ICU patients who did not develop pneumonia for the presence or absence of 25 risk factors for hospital-acquired pneumonia.[212] The strongest predictor was the use of mechanical ventilation for more than 24 hours, for which there was a 12-fold increase in risk compared to nonventilated patients. Surgical ICU patients had a relative risk of 2.2 for developing nosocomial pneumonia compared to medical ICU patients; in the former group, the Apache III score was also correlated with the risk of developing hospital-acquired pneumonia. In another study of 78 episodes of hospital-acquired pneumonia in 322 consecutive mechanically ventilated patients, multivariate and univariate statistical techniques were applied to assess risk factors for pneumonia;[102] higher risk was associated with more than one intubation during mechanical ventilation ($P = 0.001$), a prior episode of gastric aspiration ($P < 0.001$), mechanical ventilation exceeding 3 days' duration ($P < 0.015$), and the presence of COPD ($P < 0.05$). In a third study, of elderly patients who either had or did not have hospital-acquired pneumonia, patients who developed pneumonia were more severely ill on admission to the hospital and had more preexisting (2.8 versus 1.3) and in-hospital risk factors (4.7 versus 1.6) than did controls.[213] Logistic regression analysis revealed low serum albumin, the presence of neuromuscular disease, and tracheal intubation to be strong independent predictors of risk for hospital-acquired pneumonia in this population.

Pneumonia in the Compromised Host

Abnormal immune or inflammatory function is an important manifestation of many diseases and is a complication of the therapy used in numerous others. For obvious reasons, both the incidence and severity of infection, including that of the lungs, is increased in patients who have these disorders. In addition, the organisms responsible for infection often differ from those associated with infection in the "normal" host. For example, invasive aspergillosis, *P. carinii* pneumonia, and cytomegalovirus pneumonia are relatively common diseases in patients who have acute myelogenous leukemia, AIDS, and organ transplants, respectively; however, each of these is seen rarely in patients whose immune and inflammatory systems are normal.

Disorders of immune or inflammatory function can be inherited or acquired, the latter being by far the most common. Discussion of the various clinical, radiologic, and pathologic features of pulmonary infection associated with most acquired abnormalities of host defense can be found in the appropriate chapters elsewhere in the text; particular attention is given to infections in patients who have had organ transplants (*see* Chapter 45, page 1713) or who have AIDS (*see* Chapter 44, page 1643).

Malakoplakia is a rare and unusual condition of uncertain etiology that is conveniently discussed at this point. The

abnormality is an inflammatory process associated with an impairment of bactericidal action of phagocytes, including both neutrophils and monocytes.[217a-c] Pathologically, it is characterized by single or, occasionally, multiple tumor-like aggregates of inflammatory cells. Most of the latter are histiocytes that contain cytoplasmic inclusions, often having a laminated internal structure and prominent calcification (Michaelis-Gutmann bodies).[271a, d] Ultrastructural studies have shown these bodies to be composed of bacteria in various stages of decomposition within histiocyte lysosomes.[217d]

The condition occurs most often in the colon and the urinary tract (particularly the bladder), where it is usually associated with the presence of gram-negative bacilli such as *E. coli*, *Klebsiella*, and *Enterobacter*;[217d] however, it has also been described in a number of other organs, including the lungs and mediastinum.[217a, b, e] The process is usually manifested by solitary or multiple parenchymal or endobronchial nodules, either confined to the thorax or in association with malakoplakia tumors elsewhere in the body; the latter combination may lead to an erroneous diagnosis of metastatic carcinoma to the lungs.[217e] The disorder can occur in otherwise apparently healthy individuals or in patients who have underlying immunosuppression, such as may be associated with malignancy or organ transplantation;[217b] it is a particularly common manifestation of *Rhodococcus equi* infection in patients with AIDS (*see* page 1645).

Inherited disorders are most often discovered in infancy and childhood; although many are fatal, some persist into or are identified in adulthood. They have been classified into six categories:[218] (1) combined immunodeficiencies; (2) predominant antibody deficiencies; (3) miscellaneous well-defined immunodeficiency syndromes, comprising Wiskott-Aldrich syndrome, ataxia-telangiectasia, and the third and fourth pouch/arch syndrome (DiGeorge's syndrome); (4) immunodeficiency associated with other diseases (e.g., hyper-IgE syndrome, hereditarily determined susceptibility to Epstein-Barr virus); (5) complement deficiencies; and (6) defects of phagocytic function.

Combined Immunodeficiencies

Combined immunodeficiencies include disorders such as severe combined immunodeficiency, adenosine deaminase deficiency, and purine nucleoside phosphorylase deficiency. In the absence of immune reconstitution by bone marrow transplantation or other interventions, patients who have these disorders do not survive past childhood.

Predominant Antibody Deficiencies

The four major disorders in predominant antibody deficiencies are X-linked agammaglobulinemia, IgA deficiency, IgG subclass deficiency, and common variable immunodeficiency.[218] Affected patients tend to have recurrent pyogenic infections of the upper and lower respiratory tract.

X-Linked Agammaglobulinemia

The most common form of congenital agammaglobulinemia (Bruton's agammaglobulinemia, infantile sex-linked agammaglobulinemia) is transmitted as an X-linked recessive trait and thus is seen exclusively in males. The disorder arises because of a block in early B-cell maturation, most likely in the pre–B cell stage.[218] Although levels of serum immunoglobulins are reduced, small amounts can usually be detected. Cell-mediated immunity is normal.

The onset of symptoms is usually late in the first year of life after passive immunity has worn off; some patients survive to adulthood.[219] Infants are particularly susceptible to infection by staphylococci, streptococci, and *H. influenzae*. Although capable of dealing with other bacteria, fungi, parasites, and many viruses, patients may develop recurrent measles, mumps, and varicella infections[219] and are prone to persistent enterovirus infection.[220] Lymph node germinal centers are absent or poorly developed, and there is a paucity of plasma cells; this lack of reaction in lymphatic tissue may be manifested radiographically by virtual absence of the shadow of adenoid tissue in the posterior nasopharynx (Neuhauser's sign).[221] As the child grows older, lymph nodes may become evident as a result of hyperplasia of dendritic or other non-B cells.[222] Associated conditions include a rheumatoid-like disorder (seen in about 30% of such patients), a dermatomyositis-like syndrome, and leukemia.[219, 220]

Selective IgA Deficiency

Selective IgA deficiency is not uncommon: population surveys have recorded it in 1 per 700 persons in Sweden,[223] 1 per 500 in England,[224] and 1 per 1,000 in North America.[225] There is a familial incidence,[226, 227] the mode of inheritance probably being autosomal dominant. For reasons that are unclear, some affected individuals appear to be healthy, whereas others have recurrent sinopulmonary infections, gastrointestinal disorders, atopy, and autoimmune disease.[228–230] It is possible that other immunoglobulins (mainly IgM but also IgG) play a role in protection in the former individuals. It has also been suggested that infection in some patients may be related to a concomitant IgG2 subclass deficiency.[231] No correlation has been found between susceptibility to infection and serum or skin IgE concentrations.[232, 233]

IgG Subclass Deficiency

Rare patients who have normal levels of gamma globulins and IgG have recurrent lower respiratory tract infections that result in bronchiectasis; these patients have a deficiency of one of the subclasses of IgG, typically IgG2, IgG3, or IgG4.[218, 234, 235] IgG2 deficiency with or without IgG4 deficiency is more common in children; in adults, IgG3 is the most frequent deficiency and the consequences are usually mild.[218] Recurrent upper respiratory tract infection, pneumonia, and asthma are the most common clinical problems, especially when IgA deficiency is also present.[218] Isolated IgG4 deficiency is also associated with serious sinopulmonary infections.[218]

Common Variable Immunodeficiency

Common variable immunodeficiency is the most prevalent specific immunodeficiency after IgA deficiency.[218] The term refers to a group of disorders that has in common a defect in the formation of a specific antibody.[218] The onset of symptoms varies from childhood to midadulthood.[218]

There is a high incidence of other immunologic abnormalities in the relatives of many patients, and multiple cases have been described in a single kindred, in keeping with the inherited nature of this disorder in most cases. Occasionally, such as after renal transplantation,[236] the condition is acquired.

Common variable immunodeficiency is a disorder of terminal differentiation of B cells; some cases may result from defective function of regulatory T cells or from an impairment of monocyte-macrophage surveillance.[237] B cells may be normal in number but defective in function; they are either incapable of developing into plasma cells and producing immunoglobulins or are unable to secrete immunoglobulins once they are produced.[238, 239] Low levels of IgG and IgA are seen, but IgM levels are usually normal.[218] There is often an associated abnormality of cellular immunity.

The great majority of affected patients have a particular susceptibility to infection of the lungs and paranasal sinuses.[240] Non-necrotizing granulomas can be seen in the lungs, spleen, liver, and skin, sometimes associated with hepatosplenomegaly and superficial lymph node enlargement. Such patients usually have deficient T-cell proliferation to mitogens, a clinical feature that is associated with an increased severity of disease.[241] Nodular lymphoid hyperplasia within the lamina propria of the small intestine may also result in a sprue-like disorder, and the pattern of lymphoid interstitial pneumonia may be seen in the lung.[218, 242] A single case of bronchiolitis obliterans organizing pneumonia has been described.[243] Autoimmune disease occurs commonly in this deficiency state, especially in patients who have T-cell dysfunction,[218] and approximately 10% of patients die of malignancy.[220] Bronchiectasis was once an inevitable feature;[240] however, early recognition of the disease and prompt institution of intravenous gamma globulin therapy has prevented both this complication and the recurrent lung infection that causes it.[244]

IgE Deficiency

IgE deficiency has been demonstrated to be an autosomal dominant trait with variable penetrance in one kindred.[245] Fourteen family members over three generations had a history of recurrent sinopulmonary infection; 12 of these had severe IgE deficiency.

Immunodeficiency Associated with Other Diseases

Hyperimmunoglobulin E Syndrome

This syndrome (Job's syndrome) is characterized by poor antibody and cell-mediated responses to neoantigens; defective neutrophil function; high serum IgE and IgD levels; blood and sputum eosinophilia; and normal concentrations of IgG, IgA, and IgM. The clinical presentation consists of severe staphylococcal abscesses of the lung and other sites, sometimes associated with eczema.[220, 246] One patient presented in adulthood with a cavitated fungal lung abscess.[247]

Chronic Mucocutaneous Candidiasis

Chronic mucocutaneous candidiasis is a relatively benign condition that is characterized by increased susceptibility to infection by *Candida* organisms; as the name suggests, skin and mucous membrane involvement is particularly common. Some patients develop endocrinopathies affecting the parathyroid, thyroid, adrenal, or pancreatic glands. Respiratory tract symptoms are generally absent.[218] Cell-mediated immunity is usually impaired, although seldom to the extent found in aplasia or hypoplasia of the thymus (in which extensive mucosal and cutaneous candidiasis may also occur).[229, 230]

Chromosomal Abnormalities

Bloom's syndrome and Fanconi's anemia may present with recurrent respiratory tract infections, depending on the degree of deficiency in immunoglobulin production and T-lymphocyte function. Patients who have Down's syndrome typically have recurrent sinopulmonary infections associated with mild defects in antibody response, T-lymphocyte function, and phagocytic cell function.[218]

Multiple Organ System Abnormalities

Partial albinism, short-limbed dwarfism, cartilage hypoplasia, and agenesis of the corpus callosum can be associated with varying degrees of immunoglobulin, T-lymphocyte, or combined immunodeficiency.[218]

Hereditary Metabolic Defects

Acrodermatitis enteropathica, biotin-dependent carboxylase deficiency, transcobalamin II deficiency, and Type 1 oroticaciduria are rare disorders that are typically manifested in infancy. Early recognition of immunodeficiency in association with these metabolic defects may allow for reversal by appropriate therapy.[218]

Hypercatabolism of Immunoglobulins

A kindred has been described in which there was hypercatabolism of immunoglobulins and recurrent sinopulmonary infections.[218] Individuals who have intestinal lymphangiectasia and lose immunoglobulins and lymphocytes in the gut may have also recurrent upper and lower respiratory tract disease.[218] Patients who have myotonic dystrophy have selective IgG hypermetabolism.[218]

Thymoma

Thymoma has been associated with defects in both humoral and T cell–mediated immune function. Recurrent sinopulmonary disease has been associated with the former and cytomegalovirus pneumonia or candidiasis with the latter.[218]

Hereditarily Determined Susceptibility to Epstein-Barr Virus

Most cases of hereditarily determined susceptibility to Epstein-Barr virus have occurred in males, and it appears to be an X-linked recessive trait. Agammaglobulinemia, aplastic anemia, and lymphoma may follow severe infectious mononucleosis-like illnesses in affected patients. Approximately 20% of individuals have the first of these complications; in these, symptoms of respiratory tract infection are common.[218]

Complement Deficiencies

Genetically determined deficiencies of all complement components, including C3, C5, C6, C7, C8, Factor I, Factor H, and properdin, have been associated with susceptibility to bacterial infection.[218] Patients who have deficiencies of the terminal complement components (C5, C6, C7, and C8) are especially prone to episodes of meningococcal and gonococcal infection and may also have a lupus-like syndrome.[218] C2, C3, Factor I, and Factor H deficiencies are characterized by recurrent infection and sepsis with encapsulated organisms, such as *S. pneumoniae*, *Neisseria meningitidis*, *Klebsiella* species, *E. coli*, and *Streptococcus pyogenes*.[218] Combinations of hypocomplementemia, susceptibility to infection, and other host defense defects, such as common variable immunodeficiency[248] and bronchial ciliary abnormalities, have occasionally been reported.[249] A normal level of total serum hemolytic complement virtually excludes the possibility that a complement deficiency led to infection.[230]

Defects of Phagocytic Function

Chronic Granulomatous Disease of Childhood

Chronic granulomatous disease of childhood is the most common phagocytic deficiency syndrome involving the microbicidal phase of macrophage function.[250, 251] The term encompasses a group of disorders with varying disturbances at the cellular level that result in chronic inflammation and recurrent infections with catalase-positive microorganisms.[218, 252–254] The phagocytic cells do not respond to particulate or soluble stimuli with a respiratory burst; as a result, they fail to reduce molecular oxygen to the free radical superoxide that is needed for the generation of other toxic cellular metabolites (e.g., hydrogen peroxide and hydroxyl radical) from the activation of the hexose monophosphate shunt.[254]

The organisms that infect patients with chronic granulomatous disease include *S. aureus*; *Staphylococcus epidermidis*; gram-negative bacteria such as *K. pneumoniae*, *E. coli*, *Serratia marcescens*, *Proteus*, and *Salmonella* species; and fungi such as *Aspergillus* and *Candida*. Less commonly implicated organisms include *Chromobacterium violaceum*,[255] *Burkholderia gladioli*,[256] and *Mycobacterium flavescens*.[257] Infection with hydrogen peroxide–producing organisms, such as streptococci and pneumococci, is rare, and there does not appear to be an increased susceptibility to virus infection.[258, 259] A single case of pulmonary botryomycosis has been described in a 19-year-old woman.[260] The importance of the phagocyte in host defense against fungi has been emphasized by the frequency with which patients with chronic granulomatous disease develop mycotic infections; these are usually fatal unless treated promptly.[261]

As the name of the disease implies, the pathologic reaction to infection is usually granulomatous, a reaction that is thought to be related to the persistence of intracellular bacteria in mononuclear cells. In many cases, the granulomas consist of a neutrophilic microabscess surrounded by a layer of palisaded epithelioid histiocytes.[263a] In addition to granulomas, the pulmonary interstitium may be thickened by fibrous tissue and an infiltrate of lymphocytes and plasma cells. Pigmented, lipid-laden histiocytes are often present, sometimes in large numbers.[262, 263]

The radiographic hallmark of chronic granulomatous disease is recurrent pneumonia that typically resolves incompletely or progresses to abscess formation; hilar lymph node enlargement is usually striking (Fig. 25–26). Multiple areas of parenchymal consolidation may coalesce into large, relatively discrete masses in which calcification may occur.[262, 263] Fibrosis and cellular infiltration of alveolar walls may produce a local or general reticulonodular pattern;[264] occasionally, the pattern is honeycomb in type, both radio-

logically and pathologically.[265] Two cases have been reported in which primary pulmonary aspergillosis was complicated by extension into the thoracic wall and destruction of ribs.[265a]

Although patients are usually identified in the first few years of life with severe recurrent bacterial and fungal infection, presentation in adolescence and early adulthood is well documented.[266] Recurrent pneumonia and infection of lymph nodes, bone, and sometimes the pericardium are frequent; hepatosplenomegaly and a seborrheic rash over the postauricular, periorbital, nasal, scalp, axillary, and inguinal areas are also common.[262] Occasional patients have minimal problems.[267] Suspicion should be aroused whenever a patient, particularly a young man, manifests repeated staphylococcal or gram-negative infections that slowly resolve with antibiotic therapy despite normal or raised immunoglobulin levels.

Chronic granulomatous disease is usually fatal, death generally resulting from extensive lung involvement and, in some cases, from liver disease.[262, 268] Some patients, however, enjoy long infection-free intervals and survive into adulthood.[269–271]

Chédiak-Higashi Syndrome

Chédiak-Higashi syndrome is a rare disorder with an autosomal recessive mode of inheritance in which neutrophils, monocytes, and lymphocytes contain basophilic staining cytoplasmic inclusion bodies.[272, 273] There is an associated defect in granule fusion, which results in abnormal intracellular microbicidal function. Recurrent skin abscesses and progressive pulmonary disease are the major clinical features.[218] Other clinical findings include photophobia, retinal albinism, horizontal nystagmus, fever, and, terminally, splenomegaly and (sometimes) hepatomegaly. Few patients survive beyond the age of 10 years, death in most cases being caused by pneumonia and septicemia.

Schwachman's Disease

Schwachman's disease is a rare disorder associated with exocrine pancreatic insufficiency, malabsorption, failure to thrive, metaphyseal chondrodysplasia, and frequent sinopulmonary infections.[218] The primary defects appear to be phagocytic locomotion and adhesion that affect a number of functions, including the release of neutrophils from bone marrow, endothelial adhesion, tissue migration, and chemotactic response; other functions remain normal.[218, 274]

Other Disorders of Adhesion and Mobility

The syndrome of leukocyte adhesion deficiency is usually related to defects in the CD-18 adhesion molecule subunit. Most patients present early in life with recurrent sinopulmonary infection, which frequently progresses to sepsis.[218]

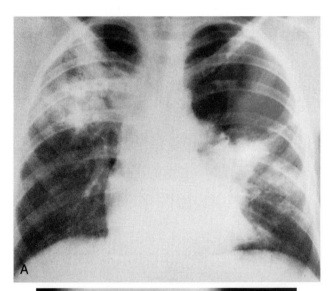
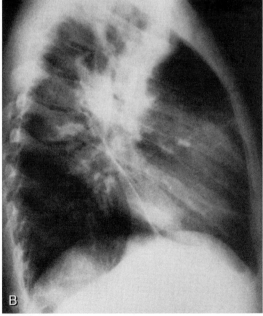

Figure 25–26. Chronic Granulomatous Disease of Childhood. Posteroanterior *(A)* and lateral *(B)* radiographs of this young man reveal extensive patchy consolidation of the right upper lobe and the superior segment of the left lower lobe. At least one cavity is visible in the right upper lobe. Right paratracheal and left hilar lymph node enlargement are present. Culture of the sputum produced a heavy growth of *Staphylococcus aureus*. The nitroblue tetrazolium test was positive.

Idiopathic Cd4+ T Lymphocytopenia

A number of cases have been reported of patients who presented with opportunistic infections characteristic of those seen in patients with AIDS but in whom there is no evidence of or risk for HIV infection.[275–281] CD4+ T lymphopenia is characteristic of the immunologic dysfunction described in these patients. The cause of the syndrome is unknown.

Miscellaneous Immunodeficiency Syndromes

Wiskott-Aldrich Syndrome

Wiskott-Aldrich syndrome is an X-linked, recessive disorder characterized by thrombocytopenic purpura, eczema, immunodeficiency, and recurrent infection. Cell-mediated immunity is abnormal. There is considerable variation in immunoglobulin levels because of increased synthesis and hypercatabolism of IgG, IgM, and IgA; however, IgM levels are usually low and IgA and IgE levels usually high. Patients die in the first few decades of life from overwhelming hemorrhage, lymphoreticular malignancy, or infection; the most common causes of infection are polymicrobial pneumonias, often associated with cytomegalovirus. With the use of antibiotic prophylaxis, *P. carinii* has become much less prevalent than previously.[218, 282] Bacterial infection caused by organisms such as *S. pneumoniae*, *H. influenzae*, or *P. aeruginosa* may be fulminant.[218]

Ataxia-Telangiectasia

Ataxia-telangiectasia is inherited in an autosomal recessive pattern and is characterized by cerebellar ataxia, oculocutaneous telangiectasia, recurrent sinopulmonary infection, and a high incidence of neoplasia. Affected patients have evidence of both T-cell and B-cell dysfunction. Endocrine, hepatic, and renal complications are seen in late childhood and early adulthood.[218] Progressive pulmonary insufficiency associated with bronchiectasis and chronic interstitial pneumonitis leads to death in the teens and twenties.[218] The thymus may be absent or underdeveloped; B cells and helper T cells are defective, particularly in the production of IgA, IgE, and IgG2 and IgG4 subclasses.[218–220, 283] The finding of an elevated level of serum α-fetoprotein and certain characteristic rearrangements of T-cell receptor and immunoglobulin genes on chromosomes 7 and 14 aid in diagnosis.[218]

DiGeorge's Syndrome

DiGeorge's syndrome includes aplasia or hypoplasia of the thymus; aplasia of the parathyroid glands; and malformations of the face, ears, nose, and heart. The abnormality is believed to occur as a result of embryonic maldevelopment of the third and fourth pharyngeal cleft pouches. Most affected individuals die within the first 3 months of life.[218]

REFERENCES

1. Mandell LA: Community-acquired pneumonia—etiology, epidemiology and treatment. Chest 108:35, 1995.
2. American Thoracic Society: Guidelines for the initial management of adults with community-acquired pneumonia: Diagnosis, assessment of severity, and initial antimicrobial therapy. Am Rev Respir Dis 148:1418, 1993.
3. Örtqvist A: Initial investigation and treatment of the patient with severe community-acquired pneumonia. Semin Respir Infect 9:166, 1994.
4. Fine MJ, Auble TE, Yealy DM, et al: A prediction rule to identify low-risk patients with community-acquired pneumonia. N Engl J Med 336:243, 1997.
5. Fein AM: Improving outcomes in pneumonia: Existing barriers and potential solutions. ATS Continuing Education Monograph Series, September 1997.
6. Marrie TJ, Peeling RW, Fine MJ, et al: Ambulator patients with community-acquired pneumonia: The frequency of atypical agents and clinical course. Am J Med 101:508, 1996.
7. Keating HG III, Klimex JJ, Levine DS, et al: Effect of aging on the clinical significance of fever in ambulatory adult patients. J Am Geriatr Soc 32:282, 1984.
8. Gray GC, Mitchell BS, Tueller JE, et al: Pneumonia hospitalizations in the US Navy and Marine Corps: Rates and risk factors for 6,522 admissions. Am J Epidemiol 15:139, 1994.
9. Macfarlane JT, Colville A, Guion A, et al: Prospective study of aetiology and outcome of adult lower-respiratory-tract infections in the community. Lancet 341:511, 1993.
10. Macfarlane J: An overview of community acquired pneumonia with lessons learned from the British Thoracic Society study. Semin Respir Infect 9:153, 1994.
11. Jokinen C, Heiskanen L, Juvonen H, et al: Evidence of community-acquired pneumonia in the population of four municipalities in Eastern Finland. Am J Epidemiol 137:977, 1993.
12. Marston BJ, Plouffe JF, File TM Jr, et al: Incidence of community-acquired pneumonia requiring hospitalization: Results of a population-based active surveillance study in Ohio. The Community-Based Pneumonia Incidence Study Group. Arch Intern Med 157:1709, 1997.
13. Marrie TJ: Epidemiology of community-acquired pneumonia in the elderly. Semin Respir Infect 5:260, 1990.
14. Fine MJ, Smith MA, Carson CA, et al: Prognosis and outcomes of patients with community-acquired pneumonia: A meta-analysis. JAMA 10:275, 1996.
15. Leeper KV Jr: Severe community-acquired pneumonia. Semin Respir Infect 11:96, 1996.
16. Anonymous. Pneumonia and influenza death rates—United States, 1979–1994. MMWR 44:535, 1995.
17. American Thoracic Society: Hospital-acquired pneumonia in adults: Diagnosis, assessment of severity, initial antimicrobial therapy and preventative strategies. Am J Respir Crit Care Med 153:1711, 1995.
18. Craven DE, Steger KA: Nosocomial pneumonia in mechanically ventilated adult patients: Epidemiology and prevention in 1996. Semin Respir Infect 11:32, 1996.
19. Baker AM, Meredith JW, Haponik EF: Pneumonia in intubated trauma patients—microbiology and outcomes. Am J Respir Crit Care Med 153:343, 1996.
20. Cassiere HA, Niederman MS: New etiopathogenic concepts of ventilator-associated pneumonia. Semin Respir Infect 11:13, 1996.
21. Anonymous: Public health focus: Surveillance, prevention, and control of nosocomial infections. MMWR 41:783, 1992.
22. Haley RW, Schaberg DR, Crossley KB, et al: Extra charges and prolongation of stay attributable to nosocomial infections: A prospective interhospital comparison. Am J Med 70:51, 1981.
23. Bassin AS, Niederman MS: New approaches to prevention and treatment of nosocomial pneumonia. Semin Thorac Cardiovasc Surg 7:70, 1995.
24. Fagon JY, Chastre J, Hance AJ, et al: Nosocomial pneumonia in ventilated patients: A cohort study evaluating attributable mortality and hospital stay. Am J Med 94:281, 1993.
25. Leu HS, Kaiser DL, Mori M, et al: Hospital-acquired pneumonia: Attributable mortality and morbidity. Am J Epidemiol 129:1258, 1989.
26. Papazian L, Bregeon F, Thirion X, et al: Effect of ventilator-associated pneumonia on mortality and morbidity. Am J Respir Crit Care Med 154:91, 1996.
27. Fagon JY, Chastre J, Hance AJ, et al: Evaluation of clinical judgement in the identification and treatment of nosocomial pneumonia in ventilated patients. Chest 103:547, 1993.
28. Transmission of tuberculosis by flexible fiberbronchoscopes. Am Rev Respir Dis 127:97, 1983.
29. Comstock GW: Epidemiology of tuberculosis. Am Rev Respir Dis 125:8, 1982.
30. Riley RL: Indoor spread of respiratory infection by recirculation of air. Bull Eur Physiopathol Resp 15:699, 1979.
31. Onofrio JM, Toews GB, Lipscomb MF, et al: Granulocyte-alveolar-macrophage interaction in the pulmonary clearance of S. aureus. Am Rev Respir Dis 127:335, 1983.
32. Johanson WG Jr, Harris GD: Aspiration pneumonia, anaerobic infections and lung abscess. Med Clin North Am 64:385, 1980.
33. Huxley EJ, Viroslav J, Gray WRT, et al: Pharyngeal aspiration in normal adults and patients with depressed consciousness. Am J Med 64:546, 1978.
33a. Stockley RA: Role of bacteria in the pathogenesis and progression of acute and chronic lung infection. Thorax 53:58, 1998.
33b. Pittet J-F, Kudoh I, Wiener-Kronish JP: Endothelial exposure to *Pseudomonas aeruginosa* proteases increases the vulnerability of the alveolar epithelium to a second injury. Am J Respir Cell Mol Biol 18:129, 1998.
33c. Wilson R, Sykes D, Rutman A: The effect of *Haemophilus influenzae* lipopolysaccharide on human respiratory epithelium *in vitro*. Thorax 41:728, 1986.
33d. Wilson R, Pitt T, Taylor G, et al: Pyocyanin and 1-hydroxyphenazine produced by *Pseudomonas aeruginosa* inhibit the beating of human respiratory cilia *in vitro*. J Clin Invest 79:221, 1987.
33e. Kilian M, Mestecky J, Kullhevy R, et al: IgA proteases from *Haemophilus influenzae, Streptococcus pneumoniae, Neisseria meningitidis,* and *Streptococcus sanguis*: Comparative immunochemical studies. J Immunol 124:2596, 1980.
33f. Cundell DR, Taylor GW, Kanthakumar K, et al: Inhibition of human neutrophil migration *in vitro* by low-molecular-mass products of nontypeable *Haemophilus influenzae*. Infect Immun 61:2419, 1993.
34. Macfarlane JT, Miller AC, Roderick-Smith WH, et al: Comparative radiographic features of community acquired Legionnaires disease, pneumococcal pneumonia, mycoplasma pneumonia, and psittacosis. Thorax 39:28, 1984.
34a. Wollschlager CM, Khan FA, Khan A: Utility of radiography and clinical features in the diagnosis of community-acquired pneumonia. Clin Chest Med 8:393, 1987.
34b. Lévy M, Dromer F, Brion N, et al: Community-acquired pneumonia: Importance of initial noninvasive bacteriologic and radiographic investigations. Chest 92:43, 1988.
34c. Moine P, Vercken JB, Chevret S, et al: Severe community-acquired pneumonia: Etiology, epidemiology, and prognosis factors. Chest 105:1487, 1994.
35. Tew J, Calenoff L, Berlin BS: Bacterial or nonbacterial pneumonia: Accuracy of radiographic diagnosis. Radiology 124:607, 1977.
35a. Albaum MN, Hill LC, Murphy M, et al: Interobserver reliability of the chest radiograph in community-acquired pneumonia. Chest 110:343, 1996.
35b. Tanaka N, Matsumoto T, Kuramitsu T, et al: High-resolution CT findings in community-acquired pneumonia. J Comput Assist Tomogr 20:600, 1996.
35c. Janzen DL, Padley SPG, Adler BD, et al: Acute pulmonary complications in immunocompromised non-AIDS patients: Comparison of diagnostic accuracy of CT and chest radiography. Clin Radiol 47:159, 1993.
35d. Brown MJ, Miller RR, Müller NL: Acute lung disease in the immunocompromised host: CT and pathologic examination findings. Radiology 190:247, 1994.
35e. Kang EY, Staples CA, McGuinness G, et al: Detection and differential diagnosis of pulmonary infections and tumors in patients with AIDS: Value of chest radiography versus CT. Am J Roentgenol 166:15, 1996.
36. Goodman LR, Goren RA, Teptick SK: The radiographic evaluation of pulmonary infection. Med Clin North Am 64:553, 1980.
37. Kantor HG: The many radiologic facies of pneumococcal pneumonia. Am J Roentgenol 137:1213, 1981.
38. Zornoza J, Goldman AM, Wallace S, et al: Radiologic features of gram-negative pneumonias in the neutropenic patient. Am J Roentgenol 127:989, 1976.
39. Granados A, Podzamczer D, Gudiol F, et al: Pneumonia due to Legionella pneumophila and pneumococcal pneumonia: Similarities and differences on presentation. Eur Respir J 2:130, 1989.
40. Editorial: Causes of primary pneumonia. Lancet 2:1212, 1981.
41. Roig J, Domiongo C, Morera J: Legionnaires' disease. Chest 105:1817, 1994.
42. Muder RR, Liu VL, Fang GD: Community-acquired Legionnaires' disease. Semin Respir Infect 4:32, 1989.
43. Musgrave T, Verghese A: Clinical features of pneumonia in the elderly. Semin Respir Infect 5:269, 1990.
44. Osmer JC, Cole BK: The stethoscope and roentgenogram in acute pneumonia. South Med J 59:75, 1966.
45. Penn CC, Liu C: Bronchiolitis following infection in adults and children. Clin Chest Med 14:645, 1993.
46. Panitch HB, Callahan CW Jr, Schidlow DV: Bronchiolitis in children. Clin Chest Med 14:715, 1993.
47. Taussig LM, Wright AL, Morgan WJ, et al: The Tucson Children's Respiratory Study: I. Design and implementation of a prospective study of acute and chronic respiratory illness in children. Am J Epidemiol 129:1219, 1989.
47a. Macek V, Sorli J, Kopriva S: Persistent adenoviral infection and chronic airway obstruction in children. Am J Respir Crit Care Med 150:7, 1994.
48. Matsuse T, Hayashi S, Kuwano K, et al: Latent adenoviral infection in the pathogenesis of chronic airways obstruction. Am Rev Respir Dis 148:177, 1992.
48a. Johnson JT, Liston SL: Bacterial tracheitis in adults. Arch Otolaryngol Head Neck Surg 113:204, 1987.
48b. Valor RR, Polnitsky CA, Tanis DJ, et al: Bacterial tracheitis with upper airway obstruction in a patient with the acquired immunodeficiency syndrome. Am Rev Respir Dis 146:1598, 1992.
48c. Dann EJ, Weinberger M, Gillis S: Bacterial laryngotracheitis associated with toxic shock syndrome in an adult. Clin Infect Dis 18:437, 1994.
48d. Brook I: Aerobic and anaerobic microbiology of bacterial tracheitis in children. Pediatr Emerg Care 13:16, 1997.
48e. Berner R, Leititis JU, Furste HO: Bacterial tracheitis caused by *Corynebacterium diphtheriae*. Eur J Pediat 156:207, 1997.
48f. Britto J, Habibi P, Walters S: Systemic complications associated with bacterial tracheitis. Arch Dis Child 74:249, 1996.
48g. Metlay JP, Kapoor WN, Fine MJ: Does this patient have community-acquired

pneumonia? Diagnosing pneumonia by history and physical examination. JAMA 278:1440, 1997.

48h. Logan PM, Primack SL, Miller RR, et al: Invasive aspergillosis of the airways: Radiographic, CT, and pathologic findings. Radiology 193:383, 1994.

48i. McGuinness G, Gruden JF, Bhalla M, et al: AIDS-related airway disease. Am J Roentgenol 168:67, 1997.

49. Louria DB, Blumenfeld HL, Ellis JT, et al: Studies on influenza in the pandemic of 1957–1958: II. Pulmonary complications of influenza. J Clin Invest 38:213, 1959.

50. Wenzel RP, McCormick DP, Beam WE Jr: Parainfluenza pneumonia in adults. JAMA 221:294, 1972.

50a. Itoh H, Tokunaga S, Asamoto H, et al: Radiologic-pathologic correlations of small lung nodules with special reference to peribronchiolar nodules. Am J Roentgenol 130:223, 1978.

50b. Müller NL, Miller RR: State-of-the-Art. Diseases of the bronchioles: CT and histopathologic findings. Radiology 196:3, 1995.

50c. Akira M, Kitatani F, Lee Y-S, et al: Diffuse panbronchiolitis: Evaluation with high-resolution CT. Radiology 168:433, 1988.

50d. Im J-G, Itoh H, Shim Y-S, et al: Pulmonary tuberculosis: CT findings—early active disease and sequential change with antituberculous therapy. Radiology 186:653, 1993.

50e. Aquino SL, Gamsu G, Webb WR, et al: Tree-in-bud pattern: Frequency and significance on thin-section CT. J Comput Assist Tomogr 20:594, 1996.

50f. Worthy SA, Müller NL: Small airway diseases. Radiol Clin North Am 36:163, 1998.

50g. Collins J, Blankenbaker D, Stern EJ: CT patterns of bronchiolar disease: What is "tree-in-bud"? Am J Roentgenol 171:365, 1998.

51. Genereux GP, Stillwell GA: The acute bacterial pneumonias. Semin Roentgenol 15:9, 1980.

52. Fraser RG, Wortzman G: Acute pneumococcal lobar pneumonia: The significance of nonsegmental distribution. J Can Assoc Radiol 10:37, 1959.

52a. Barnes DJ, Naraqi S, Igo JD: The diagnostic and prognostic significance of bulging fissures in acute lobar pneumonia. Aust NZ J Med 18:130, 1988.

52b. Kaye MG, Fox MJ, Bartlett JG, et al: The clinical spectrum of *Staphylococcus aureus* pulmonary infection. Chest 97:788, 1990.

52c. Macfarlane J, Rose D: Radiographic features of staphylococcal pneumonia in adults and children. Thorax 51:539, 1996.

53. Itoh H, Murata K, Konishi J, et al: Diffuse lung disease: Pathologic basis for the high-resolution computed tomography findings. J Thorac Imaging 8:176, 1993.

54. Melby K, Toews GB, Pierce AK: Pulmonary elastase activity in response to S. pneumoniae and P. aeruginosa. Am Rev Respir Dis 131:559, 1985.

55. Groskin SA, Panicek DM, Ewing DK, et al: Bacterial lung abscess: A review of the radiographic and clinical features of 50 cases. J Thorac Imaging 6:62, 1991.

56. Machiels P, Haxhe JP, Trigaux JP: Chronic lung abscess due to *Pasteurella multocida*. Thorax 50:1017, 1995.

56a. Woodring JH, Fried AM, Chuang VP: Solitary cavities of the lung: Diagnostic implications of cavity wall thickness. Am J Roentgenol 135:1269, 1980.

57. Hammond JM, Potgieter PD, Hanslo D: The etiology and antimicrobial susceptibility patterns of microorganisms in acute community-acquired lung abscess. Chest 108:937, 1995.

58. Mori T, Ebe T, Takahashi M: Lung abscess: Analysis of 66 cases from 1979 to 1991. Intern Med 32:278, 1993.

59. Philpott NJ, Woodhead MA, Wilson AG, et al: Lung abscess: A neglected cause of life threatening haemoptysis. Thorax 48:674, 1993.

60. Boon ES, Grupa N, Langenberg CJ, et al: Concealed lung abscesses in critically ill, mechanically ventilated patients. Nether J Med 48:100, 1996.

61. Reich JM: Pulmonary gangrene and the air crescent sign. Thorax 48:70, 1993.

61a. Penner C, Maycher B, Long R: Pulmonary gangrene: A complication of bacterial pneumonia. Chest 105:567, 1994.

61b. Padmanabhan K, Rajgopalan K, Yeo K, et al: Intracavitary mass in a patient with *Klebsiella* pneumonia. Chest 93:187, 1988.

61c. Quigley MJ, Fraser RS: Pulmonary pneumatocele: Pathology and pathogenesis. Am J Roentgenol 150:1275, 1988.

62. Feuerstein IM, Archer A, Pluda JM, et al: Thin-walled cavities, cysts, and pneumothorax in P. carinii pneumonia: Further observations with histopathologic correlation. Radiology 174:697, 1990.

63. Rosmus HH, Pare JAP, Masson AM, et al: Roentgenographic patterns of acute Mycoplasma and viral pneumonitis. J Can Assoc Radiol 19:74, 1968.

64. Borthwick RC, Cameron DC, Philp T: Radiographic patterns of pulmonary involvement in acute mycoplasmal infections. Scand J Respir Dis 59:190, 1978.

65. Cameron DC, Borthwick RN, Philp T: The radiographic patterns of acute mycoplasma pneumonitis. Clin Radiol 28:173, 1977.

66. Putman CE, Curtis AM, Simeone JF, et al: Mycoplasma pneumonia: Clinical and roentgenographic patterns. Am J Roentgenol 124:417, 1975.

67. Müller NL, Miller RR: State-of-the-art. Diseases of the bronchioles: CT and histopathologic findings. Radiology 196:3, 1995.

68. DeLorenzo LJ, Huang CT, Maguire GP, et al: Roentgenographic patterns of P. carinii pneumonia in 104 patients with AIDS. Chest 91:323, 1987.

69. Naidich DP, McGuinness G: Pulmonary manifestations of AIDS: CT and radiographic correlations. Radiol Clin North Am 29:999, 1991.

70. Kuhlman JE: Pneumocystic infections: The radiologist's perspective. Radiology 198:623, 1996.

71. Goodman PC: P. carinii pneumonia. J Thorac Imaging 6:16, 1991.

72. Bergin CJ, Wirth RL, Berry GJ, et al: P. carinii pneumonia: CT and HRCT observations. J Comput Assist Tomogr 14:756, 1990.

73. Kuhlman JE, Kavuru M, Fishman EK, et al: P. carinii pneumonia: Spectrum of parenchymal CT findings. Radiology 175:711, 1990.

74. Hartman TE, Primack SL, Müller NL: Diagnosis of thoracic complications in AIDS: Accuracy of CT. Am J Roentgenol 162:547, 1994.

75. Janzen DL, Padley SPG, Adler BD, et al: Acute pulmonary complications in immunocompromised non-AIDS patients: Comparison of diagnostic accuracy of CT and chest radiography. Clin Radiol 47:159, 1993.

76. McGuinness G, Scholes JV, Garay SM, et al: Cytomegalovirus pneumonitis: Spectrum of parenchymal CT findings with pathologic correlation in 21 AIDS patients. Radiology 192:451, 1994.

76a. Kang E-Y, Patz EF Jr, Müller NL: Cytomegalovirus pneumonia in transplant patients: CT findings. J Comput Assist Tomogr 20:295, 1996.

77. Kang EY, Staples CA, McGuinness G, et al: Detection and differential diagnosis of pulmonary infections and tumors in patients with AIDS: Value of chest radiography versus CT. Am J Roentgenol 166:15, 1996.

78. Amorosa JK, Nahass RG, Nosher JL, et al: Radiologic distinction of pyogenic pulmonary infection from P. carinii pneumonia in AIDS patients. Radiology 175:721, 1990.

79. Amin Z, Miller RF, Shaw PJ: Lobar or segmental consolidation on chest radiographs of patients with HIV infection. Clin Radiol 52:541, 1997.

80. Buwalda M, Speelberg B: Metastatic staphylococcal lung abscess due to a cutaneous furuncle. Nether J Med 47:291, 1995.

81. Gelb AF, Leffler C, Brewin A, et al: Miliary tuberculosis. Am Rev Respir Dis 108:1327, 1973.

82. Kwong JS, Carignan S, Kang EY, et al: Miliary tuberculosis: Diagnostic accuracy of chest radiography. Chest 110:339, 1996.

83. Huang RM, Naidich D, Lubat E, et al: Septic pulmonary emboli: CT radiographic correlation. Am J Roentgenol 153:41, 1989.

84. Kuhlman JE, Fishman EK, Teigen C: Pulmonary septic emboli: Diagnosis with CT. Radiology 174:211, 1990.

85. Biocina B, Sutlic Z, Husedzinovic I, et al: Penetrating cardiothoracic war wounds. Eur J Cardiothorac Surg 11:399, 1997.

86. Pointe HD, Osika E, Montagne JP, et al: Adrenobronchial fistula complicating a neonatal adrenal abscess: Treatment by percutaneous aspiration and antibiotics. Pediatr Radiol 27:184, 1997.

87. O'Brien JD, Ettinger NA: Nephrobronchial fistula and lung abscess resulting from nephrolithiasis and pyelonephritis. Chest 108:1166, 1995.

88. Heckerling PS, Tape TG, Wigton RS, et al: Clinical prediction rule for pulmonary infiltrates. Ann Intern Med 113:664, 1990.

89. Kirtland SH, Corley DE, Winterbauer RH, et al: The diagnosis of ventilator-associated pneumonia—a comparison of histologic, microbiologic, and clinical criteria. Chest 112:445, 1997.

90. Fagon JY, Chastre J, Hance AJ, et al: Evaluation of clinical judgment in the identification and treatment of nosocomial pneumonia in ventilated patients. Chest 103:547, 1993.

91. Louthan FB, Meduri U: Differential diagnosis of fever and pulmonary densities in mechanically ventilated patients. Semin Respir Infect 11:77, 1996.

92. Fagon JY, Chastre J, Hance AJ, et al: Detection of nosocomial lung infection in ventilated patients—use of a protected specimen brush and quantitative culture techniques in 147 patients. Am Rev Respir Dis 138:110, 1988.

93. Meduri GU: Diagnosis and differential diagnosis of ventilator-associated pneumonia. Clin Chest Med 16:61, 1995.

94. Corley DE, Kirtland SH, Winterbauer RH, et al: Reproducibility of the histologic diagnosis of pneumonia among a panel of four pathologists—analysis of a gold standard. Chest 112:458, 1997.

95. Wunderink RG, Woldenberg LS, Ziess J, et al: The radiologic diagnosis of autopsy-proven ventilator-associated pneumonia. Chest 101:458, 1992.

96. Chalasani NP, Valdecanas MAL, Gopal AK, et al: Clinical utility of blood cultures in adult patients with community-acquired pneumonia without defined underlying risks. Chest 108:932, 1995.

97. Lévy M, Dromer F, Brion N, et al: Community-acquired pneumonia—importance of initial noninvasive bacteriologic and radiographic investigations. Chest 92:43, 1988.

98. Anonymous: Community-acquired pneumonia in adults in British hospitals in 1982–1983: A survey of aetiology, mortality, prognostic factors and outcome. The British Thoracic Society and the Public Health Laboratory Service. QJM 62:195, 1987.

99. Blanquer J, Blanquer R, Borras R, et al: Aetiology of community acquired pneumonia in Valencia, Spain: A multicentre prospective study. Thorax 46:508, 1991.

100. Rello J, Gallego M, Mariscal D, et al: The value of routine microbial investigation in ventilator-associated pneumonia. Am J Respir Crit Care Med 156:196, 1997.

101. Alvarez-Lerma F: Modification of empiric antibiotic treatment in patients with pneumonia acquired in the intensive care unit. ICU-Acquired Pneumonia Study Group. Intensive Care Med 22:387, 1996.

102. Torres A, Aznar R, Gatell JM, et al: Incidence, risk, and prognosis factors of nosocomial pneumonia in mechanically ventilated patients. Am Rev Respir Dis 142:523, 1990.

103. Kollef MH: Ventilator-associated pneumonia: A multivariate analysis. JAMA 270:1965, 1993.

104. Rello J, Ausina V, Ricart M, et al: Impact of previous antimicrobial therapy on the etiology and outcome of ventilator-associated pneumonia. Chest 104:1230, 1993.

105. Sterling TR, Ho EJ, Brehm WT, et al: Diagnosis and treatment of ventilator-associated pneumonia—impact on survival. Chest 110:1025, 1996.

106. Fagon JY, Chastre J, Vuagnat A, et al: Nosocomial pneumonia and mortality among patients in intensive care units. JAMA 20:275, 1996.

107. Rello J, Quintana E, Ausina V, et al: Incidence, etiology, and outcome of nosocomial pneumonia in mechanically ventilated patients. Chest 100:439, 1991.

108. Kollef MH, Silver P, Murphy DM, et al: The effect of late-onset ventilator-associated pneumonia in determining patient mortality. Chest 108:1655, 1995.

109. Niederman MS, Torres A, Summer W: Invasive diagnostic testing is not needed routinely to manage suspected ventilator-associated pneumonia. Am J Respir Crit Care Med 150:565, 1994.

110. Chastre J, Fagon JY: Invasive diagnostic testing should be routinely used to manage ventilated patients with suspected pneumonia. Am J Respir Crit Care Med 150:570, 1994.

110a. MacDonald KS, Scriver SR, Skulnick M, et al: Community-acquired pneumonia: the future of microbiology focused diagnosis and syndromic management? Sem Respir Infect 9:180, 1994.

111. Bryan CS, Reynolds KL: Bacteremic nosocomial pneumonia: Analysis of 172 episodes from a single metropolitan area. Am Rev Respir Dis 129:668, 1984.

112. Reed WW, Byrd GS, Gates RH Jr, et al: Sputum gram's stain in community-acquired pneumococcal pneumonia: A meta-analysis. West J Med 165:197, 1996.

113. Gleckman R, DeVita J, Hibert D, et al: Sputum gram stain assessment in community-acquired bacteremic pneumonia. J Clin Microbiol 26:846, 1988.

114. Glaister D: Early detection of lower respiratory tract infection: The value of the gram-stained sputum smear. Med Lab Sci 48:175, 1991

115. Skerrett SJ: Diagnostic testing to establish a microbial cause is helpful in the management of community-acquired pneumonia. Semin Respir Infect 12:308, 1997.

116. Johanson WG Jr, Seidenfeld JJ, Gomez P, et al: Bacteriologic diagnosis of nosocomial pneumonia following prolonged mechanical ventilation. Am Rev Respir Dis 137:259, 1988.

117. Rumbak MJ, Bass RL: Tracheal aspirate correlates with protected specimen brushing long-term ventilated patients who have clinical pneumonia. Chest 106:531, 1994.

118. Marquette CH, Georges H, Wallet F, et al: Diagnostic efficiency of endotracheal aspirates with quantitative bacterial cultures in intubated patients with suspected pneumonia—comparison with the protected specimen brush. Am Rev Respir Dis 148:138, 1993.

119. Jourdain B, Novara A, Joly-Guillou ML, et al: Role of quantitative cultures of endotracheal aspirates in the diagnosis of nosocomial pneumonia. Am J Respir Crit Care Med 152:241, 1995.

119a. Wermet D, Marquette C-H, Copin M-C, et al: Influence of pulmonary bacteriology and histology on the yield of diagnostic procedures in ventilator-acquired pneumonia. Am J Respir Crit Care Med 158:139, 1998.

119b. Bonten MJ, Bergmans CJ, Stobberingh EE, et al: Implementation of bronchoscopic techniques in the diagnosis of ventilator-associated pneumonia to reduce antibiotic use. Am J Respir Crit Care Med 156:1820, 1997.

120. Marquette CH, Copin MC, Wallet F, et al: Diagnostic tests for pneumonia in ventilated patients: Prospective evaluation of diagnostic accuracy using histology as a diagnostic gold standard. Am J Respir Crit Care Med 151:1878, 1995.

121. Chastre J, Fagon JY, Bornet-Lesco M, et al: Evaluation of bronchoscopic techniques for the diagnosis of nosocomial pneumonia. Am J Respir Crit Care Med 152:231, 1995.

122. Torres A, El-Ebiary M, Padro L, et al: Validation of different techniques for the diagnosis of ventilator-associated pneumonia—comparison with immediate postmortem pulmonary biopsy. Am J Crit Care Med 149:324, 1994.

123. Torres A, Martos A, De La Bellacase JP, et al: Specificity of endotracheal aspiration, protected specimen brush, and bronchoalveolar lavage in mechanically ventilated patients. Am Rev Respir Dis 147:952, 1993.

124. Dotson RG, Pingleton SK: The effect of antibiotic therapy on recovery of intracellular bacteria from bronchoalveolar lavage in suspected ventilator-associated nosocomial pneumonia. Chest 103:541, 1993.

124a. Mertens AH, Nagler JM, Galdermans DI, et al: Quality assessment of protected specimen brush samples by microscopic cell count. Am J Respir Crit Care Med 157:1240, 1998.

125. Dreyfuss D, Mier L, Le Bourdelles G, et al: Clinical significance of borderline quantitative protected brush specimen culture results. Am Rev Respir Dis 147:946, 1993.

126. Timsit JF, Misset B, Francoual S, et al: Is protected specimen brush a reproducible method to diagnose ICU-acquired pneumonia? Chest 104:104, 1993.

127. Marquette CH, Herengt F, Mathieu D, et al: Diagnosis of pneumonia in mechanically ventilated patients. Am Rev Respir Dis 147:211, 1993.

128. Baker AM, Bowton DL, Haponik EF: Decision making in nosocomial pneumonia—an analytic approach to the interpretation of quantitative bronchoscopic cultures. Chest 107:85, 1995.

129. Meduri GU, Beals DH, Maijub AG, et al: Protected bronchoalveolar lavage—a new bronchoscopic technique to retrieve uncontaminated distal airway secretions. Am Rev Respir Dis 143:855, 1991.

129a. Jourdain B, Joly-Guillou M-L, Dombret M-C, et al: Usefulness of quantitative cultures of BAL fluid for diagnosing nosocomial pneumonia in ventilated patients. Chest 111:411, 1997.

130. Aubas S, Aubas P, Capdevila X, et al: Bronchoalveolar lavage for diagnosing bacterial pneumonia in mechanically ventilated patients. Am J Respir Crit Care Med 149:860, 1994.

130a. Gerveaux P, Ledoray V, Boussuges A, et al: Diagnosis of nosocomial pneumonia in mechanically ventilated patients. Am J Respir Crit Care Med 157:76, 1998.

131. Pugin J, Auckenthaler R, Mili N, et al: Diagnosis of ventilator-associated pneu-

monia by bacteriologic analysis of bronchoscopic and nonbronchoscopic "blind" bronchoalveolar lavage fluid. Am Rev Respir Dis 143:1121, 1991.

132. Timsit JF, Misset B, Renaud B, et al: Effect of previous antimicrobial therapy on the accuracy of the main procedures used to diagnose nosocomial pneumonia in patients who are using ventilation. Chest 108:1036, 1995.

133. Timsit JF, Misset B, Goldstein FW, et al: Reappraisal of distal diagnostic testing in the diagnosis of ICU-acquired pneumonia. Chest 108:1632, 1995.

134. Solé-Violan J, Rodriguez de Castro F, Rey A, et al: Usefulness of microscopic examination of intracellular organisms in lavage fluid in ventilator-associated pneumonia. Chest 106:889, 1994.

135. Chastre J, Fagon JY, Soler P, et al: Quantification of bronchoalveolar lavage cells containing intracellular bacteria rapidly identifies ventilated patients with nosocomial pneumonia. Chest 95:188, 1989.

136. Allaouchiche B, Jaumain H, Dumontet C, et al: Early diagnosis of ventilator-associated pneumonia—is it possible to define a cutoff value of infected cells in bronchoalveolar lavage fluid? Chest 110:1558, 1996.

137. Meduri GU, Wunderink RG, Leeper KV, et al: Management of bacterial pneumonia in ventilated patients—protected bronchoalveolar lavage as a diagnostic tool. Chest 101:500, 1992.

138. Papazian L, Martin C, Meric B, et al: A reappraisal of blind bronchial sampling in the microbiologic diagnosis of nosocomial bronchopneumonia—a comparative study in ventilated patients. Chest 103:236, 1993.

139. Garrard CS, A'Court CD: The diagnosis of pneumonia in the critically ill. Chest 108:17, 1995.

140. Kollef MH, Bock KR, Richards RD, et al: The safety and diagnostic accuracy of minibronchoalveolar lavage in patients with suspected ventilator-associated pneumonia. Ann Intern Med 122:743, 1995.

141. Marik PE, Brown WJ: A comparison of bronchoscopic versus blind protected specimen brush sampling in patients with suspected ventilator-associated pneumonia. Chest 108:203, 1995.

142. Pham LH, Brun-Biosson C, Legrand P, et al: Diagnosis of nosocomial pneumonia in mechanically ventilated patients—comparison of a plugged telescoping catheter with the protected specimen brush. Am Rev Respir Dis 143:1055, 1991.

143. Torres A, De La Bellacasa JP, Rodriguez-Roisin R, et al: Diagnostic value of telescoping plugged catheters in mechanically ventilated patients with bacterial pneumonia using the Metras catheter. Am Rev Respir Dis 138:117, 1988.

144. Chastre J, Trouillet JL, Fagon JL: Diagnosis of pulmonary infections in mechanically ventilated patients. Semin Respir Infect 11:65, 1996.

145. Timsit JF, Misset B, Azoulay E, et al: Usefulness of airway visualization in the diagnosis of nosocomial pneumonia in ventilated patients. Chest 110:172, 1996.

146. Torres A, Jiménez P, de la Bellacasa JP, et al: Diagnostic value of nonfluoroscopic percutaneous lung needle aspiration in patients with pneumonia. Chest 98:840, 1990.

147. Dorca J, Manresa F, Esteban L, et al: Efficacy, safety, and therapeutic relevance of transthoracic aspiration with ultrathin needle in nonventilated nosocomial pneumonia. Am J Respir Crit Care Med 151:1491, 1995.

148. Zalacain R, Lorente JL, Gaztelurrutia L, et al: Influence of three factors on the diagnostic effectiveness of transthoracic needle aspiration in pneumonia. Chest 107:96, 1995.

149. Timsit JF, Chevret S, Valcke J, et al: Mortality of nosocomial pneumonia in ventilated patients: Influence of diagnostic tools. Am J Respir Crit Care Med 154:116, 1996.

150. Luna CM, Vujacich P, Niederman MS, et al: Impact of bronchoalveolar lavage data on the therapy and outcome of ventilator-associated pneumonia. Chest 111:676, 1997.

150a. Sanchez-Nieto JM, Torres A, Garcia-Cordoba F, et al: Impact of invasive and noninvasive quantitative culture sampling on outcome of ventilator-associated pneumonia. Am J Respir Crit Care Med 157:371, 1998.

151. Kollef MH, Eisenberg PR, Ohlendorf MF, et al: The accuracy of elevated concentrations of endotoxin in bronchoalveolar lavage fluid for the rapid diagnosis of gram-negative pneumonia. Am J Respir Crit Care Med 154:1020, 1996.

152. Schluger NW, Rom WN: The polymerase chain reaction in the diagnosis and evaluation of pulmonary infections. Am J Respir Crit Care Med 152:11, 1995.

153. Naber SP: Molecular medicine—molecular pathology—diagnosis of infectious disease. N Engl J Med 331:1212, 1994.

154. Falguera M, Nogues A, Ruiz-Gonzales A, et al: Detection of Mycoplasma pneumoniae by polymerase chain reaction in lung aspirates from patient with community-acquired pneumonia. Chest 110:972, 1996.

155. Ma TS: Applications and limitations of polymerase chain reaction amplification. Chest 108:1393, 1995.

156. Boersma WG, Löwenberg A, Holloway Y, et al: Pneumococcal capsular antigen detection and pneumococcal serology in patients with community acquired pneumonia. Thorax 46:902, 1991.

157. Boersma WG, Löwenberg A, Holloway Y, et al: Pneumococcal antigen persistence in sputum from patients with community-acquired pneumonia. Chest 102:422, 1992.

158. Bella F, Tort J, Morera MA, et al: Value of bacterial antigen detection in the diagnostic yield of transthoracic needle aspiration in severe community acquired pneumonia. Thorax 48:1227, 1993.

159. Peeling RW: Laboratory diagnosis of chlamydia pneumoniae infections. Can J Infect Dis 6:198, 1995.

160. Bartlett JG, Mundy LM: Current concepts: Community-acquired pneumonia. N Engl J Med 333:1618, 1995.

161. Bohte R, van Furth R, van den Broek PJ: Aetiology of community acquired pneumonia: A prospective study among adults requiring admission to hospital. Thorax 50:543, 1995.

162. Mundy LM, Auwaerter PG, Oldach D, et al: Community-acquired pneumonia: Impact of immune status. Am J Respir Crit Care Med 152:1309, 1995.
163. Boerner DF, Zwady P: The value of the sputum Gram's stain in community-acquired pneumonia. JAMA 247:642, 1982.
164. File TM Jr, Tan JS: Incidence, etiologic pathogens, and diagnostic testing of community-acquired pneumonia. Curr Opin Pulm Med 3:89, 1997.
165. Davies BI: Critical review of microbiological data and methods in diagnosis of lower respiratory tract infections. Monaldi Arch Chest Dis 49:52, 1994.
166. Gomez J, Banos V, Ruiz Gomez J, et al: Prospective study of epidemiology and prognostic factors in community-acquired pneumonia. Eur J Clin Microbiol Infect Dis 15:556, 1996.
167. Ewig S, Bauer T, Hasper E, et al: Value of routine microbial investigation in community-acquired pneumonia treated in a tertiary care center. Respiration 63:164, 1996.
168. Pareja A, Bernal C, Leyva A, et al: Etiologic study of patients with community-acquired pneumonia. Chest 101:1207, 1992.
169. Örtqvist A, Hedlund J, Grillner L, et al: Aetiology, outcome and prognostic factors in community-acquired pneumonia requiring hospitalization. Eur Respir J 3:1105, 1990.
170. Ries K, Levison ME, Kaye D: Transtracheal aspiration in pulmonary infection. Arch Intern Med 133:453, 1974.
171. Pollock HM, Hawkins EL, Bonner JR, et al: Diagnosis of bacterial pulmonary infections with quantitative protected catheter cultures obtained during bronchoscopy. J Clin Microbiol 17:255, 1983.
172. Kato T, Ueemura H, Murakami N, et al: Incidence of anaerobic infections among patients with pulmonary diseases: Japanese experience with transtracheal aspiration and immediate bedside anaerobic inoculation. Clin Infect Dis 23:87, 1996.
173. Ostergaard L, Andersen PL: Etiology of community-acquired pneumonia—evaluation by transtracheal aspiration, blood culture or serology. Chest 104:1400, 1993.
174. Woodhead MA: The aetiology, management and outcome of severe community-acquired pneumonia on the intensive care unit. Respir Med 86:7, 1992.
175. Feldman C, Ross S, Mahomed AG, et al: The aetiology of severe community-acquired pneumonia and its impact on initial, empiric, antimicrobial chemotherapy. Respir Med 89:187, 1995.
176. Johnston BL: Methicillin-resistant S. aureus as a cause of community-acquired pneumonia—a critical review. Semin Respir Infect 9:199, 1994.
177. Carr B, Walsh JB, Coakley D, et al: Prospective hospital study of community acquired lower respiratory tract infection in the elderly. Respir Med 85:185, 1991.
178. Rello J, Quintana E, Ausina V, et al: A three-year study of severe community-acquired pneumonia with emphasis on outcome. Chest 103:232, 1993.
179. Woodhead MA: The aetiology, management and outcome of severe community-acquired pneumonia on the intensive care unit. Respir Med 86:7, 1992.
180. Pachon J, Prados MD, Capote F, et al: Severe community-acquired pneumonia—etiology, prognosis and treatment. Am Rev Respir Dis 142:369, 1990.
180a. Leroy O, Vandenbussche C, Coffinier C, et al: Community-acquired aspiration pneumonia in intensive care units. Am J Respir Crit Care Med 156:1922, 1997.
181. Potgieter PD, Hammond JMJ: Etiology and diagnosis of pneumonia requiring ICU admission. Chest 101:199, 1992.
182. Moine P, Vercken JB, Chevret S, et al: Severe community-acquired pneumonia—etiology, epidemiology and prognosis factors. Chest 105:1487, 1994.
183. Leroy O, Santre C, Beuscart C, et al: A five-year study of severe community-acquired pneumonia with emphasis on prognosis in patients admitted to an intensive care unit. Intensive Care Med 21:24, 1995.
184. Chan CHS, Cohen M, Pang J: A prospective study of community-acquired pneumonia in Hong Kong. Chest 101:442, 1992.
185. Porath A, Schlaeffer F, Lieberman D: The epidemiology of community-acquired pneumonia among hospitalized adults. J Infect 34:41, 1997.
186. Maartens G, Lewis SJ, de Goveia C, et al: 'Atypical' bacterial are a common cause of community-acquired pneumonia in hospitalized adults. S Afr Med J 84:678, 1994.
187. Lieberman D, Kahane S, Lieberman D, et al: Pneumonia with serological evidence of acute infection with the Chlamydia-like microorganism "Z." Am J Respir Crit Care Med 156:578, 1997.
188. Burack JH, Hahn JA, Saint-Maurice D, et al: Microbiology of community-acquired bacterial pneumonia in persons with and at risk for human immunodeficiency virus type 1 infection: Implications for rational empiric antibiotic therapy. Arch Intern Med 28:154, 1994.
189. Gilbert K, Fine MJ: Assessing prognosis and predicting patient outcomes in community-acquired pneumonia. Semin Respir Infect 9:140, 1994.
190. Fine MJ, Smith DN, Singer DE: Hospitalization decision in patients with community-acquired pneumonia: A prospective cohort study. Am J Med 89:713, 1990.
191. Riquelme R, Torres A, El-Ebiary M, et al: Community-acquired pneumonia in the elderly. Am J Respir Crit Care Med 154:1450, 1996.
192. Neill AM, Martin IR, Weir R, et al: Community acquired pneumonia: Aetiology and usefulness of severity criteria on admission. Thorax 51:1010, 1996.
193. Farr BM, Sloman AJ, Fisch MJ: Predicting death in patients hospitalized for community-acquired pneumonia. Ann Intern Med 115:428, 1991.
194. Fine MJ, Hough LJ, Medsger AR, et al: The hospital admission decision for patient with community-acquired pneumonia: Results from the pneumonia Patient Outcomes Research Team cohort study. Arch Intern Med 13:157, 1997.
195. Geppert EF: Chronic and recurrent pneumonia. Semin Respir Infect 7:282, 1992.

196. Winterbauer RH, Bedon GA, Ball WC Jr: Recurrent pneumonia: Predisposing illness and clinical patterns in 158 patients. Ann Intern Med 70:689, 1969.
197. Craven DE, Steger KA: Epidemiology of nosocomial pneumonia—new perspectives on an old disease. Chest 108:1, 1995.
198. Doré P, Robert R, Grollier G, et al: Incidence of anaerobes in ventilator-associated pneumonia with use of a protected specimen brush. Am J Respir Crit Care Med 153:1292, 1996.
199. Anonymous: Guidelines for prevention of nosocomial pneumonia. Centers for Disease Control and Prevention. MMWR 46:1, 1997.
200. Rello J, Torres A: Microbial causes of ventilator-associated pneumonia. Semin Respir Infect 11:24, 1996.
201. Cazzadori A, Di Perri G, Vento S, et al: Aetiology of pneumonia following isolated closed head injury. Respir Med 91:193, 1997.
202. Barreiro B, Dorca J, Esteban L, et al: Risk factors for the development of Haemophilus influenzae pneumonia in hospitalized adults. Eur Respir J 8:1543, 1995.
202a. Chastre J, Trouillet JL, Vuagnat A, et al: Nosocomial pneumonia in patients with acute respiratory distress syndrome. Am J Respir Crit Care Med 157:1165, 1998.
203. Rello J, Quintana E, Ausina V, et al: Risk factors for S. aureus nosocomial pneumonia in critically ill patients. Am Rev Respir Dis 142:1320, 1990.
203a. Talon D, Mulin B, Rouget C, et al: Risks and routes for ventilator-associated pneumonia with Pseudomonas aeruginosa. Am J Respir Crit Care Med 157:978, 1998.
204. Crossley KB, Thurn JR: Nursing home-acquired pneumonia. Semin Respir Infect 4:64, 1989.
205. Carratala J, Gudiol F, Pallares R, et al: Risk factors for nosocomial Legionella pneumophila pneumonia. Am J Respir Crit Care Med 149:625, 1994.
206. Rello J, Torres A, Ricart M, et al: Ventilator-associated pneumonia by S. aureus—comparison of methicillin-resistant and methicillin-sensitive episodes. Am J Respir Crit Care Med 150:1545, 1994.
206a. Trouillet J-L, Chastre J, Vuagnat A, et al: Ventilator-associated pneumonia caused by potentially drug-resistant bacteria. Am J Respir Crit Care Med 157:531, 1998.
207. Canadian Hospital Acquired Pneumonia Consensus Conference Group: Initial antimicrobial treatment of hospital acquired pneumonia in adults: A conference report. Can Respir J 1:110, 1994.
208. Graman PS, Hall CB: Nosocomial viral respiratory infections. Semin Respir Infect 4:253, 1989.
209. Avery RK, Longworth DL: Viral pulmonary infections in thoracic and cardiovascular surgery. Semin Thorac Cardiovasc Surg 7:88, 1995.
210. Celis R, Torres A, Gatell JM, et al: Nosocomial pneumonia—a multivariate analysis of risk and prognosis. Chest 93:318, 1988.
211. Torres A, Gatell JM, Aznar E, et al: Re-intubation increases the risk of nosocomial pneumonia in patients needing mechanical ventilation. Am J Respir Crit Care Med 152:137, 1995.
212. Cunnion KM, Weber DJ, Broadhead WE, et al: Risk factors for nosocomial pneumonia: Comparing adult critical-care populations. Am J Respir Crit Care Med 153:158, 1996.
213. Hanson LC, Weber DJ, Rutala WA: Risk factors for nosocomial pneumonia in the elderly. Am J Med 92:161, 1992.
214. Antonelli M, Moro ML, Capelli O, et al: Risk factors for early onset pneumonia in trauma patients. Chest 105:224, 1994.
215. Bonten MJM, Bergmans CJJ, Ambergen AW, et al: Risk factors for pneumonia, and colonization of respiratory tract and stomach in mechanically ventilated ICU patients. Am J Respir Crit Care Med 154:1339, 1996.
216. Joshi N, Localio AR, Hamroy BH: A predictive risk index for nosocomial pneumonia in the intensive care unit. Am J Med 93:135, 1992.
217. Kollef MH, Von Harz B, Prentice D, et al: Patient transport from intensive care increases the risk of developing ventilator-associated pneumonia. Chest 112:765, 1997.
217a. Colby TV, Hunt S, Pelzmann K, et al: Malakoplakia of the lung: A report of two cases. Respiration 30:295, 1980.
217b. Hodder RV, St. Georgy-Hyslop P, Chalvardjian A, et al: Pulmonary malakoplakia. Thorax 39:70, 1984.
217c. Abdou NI, NaPombejara C, Sagawa A, et al: Malakoplakia: Evidence for monocyte lysosomal abnormality correctable by cholinergic agonist in vitro and in vivo. N Engl J Med 297:1413, 1977.
217d. Lou TY, Teplitz C: Malakoplakia: Pathogenesis and ultrastructural morphogenesis. Hum Pathol 5:191, 1974.
217e. Crouch E, White V, Wright J, et al: Malakoplakia mimicking carcinoma metastatic to lung. Am J Surg Pathol 8:151, 1984.
218. Regelmann WE, Filipovich AH: Lung involvement in the primary immunodeficiency syndromes. Semin Respir Med 13:190, 1992.
219. Bardana EJ Jr: A conceptual approach to immunodeficiency. Med Clin North Am 65:959, 1981.
220. Cooper MD, Buckley RH: Developmental immunology and the immunodeficiency diseases. JAMA 248:2658, 1982.
221. Rosen S, Janeway CA: The gamma globulins: III. The antibody deficiency syndromes. N Engl J Med 275:709, 1966.
222. Margulis AR, Feinberg SB, Lester RG, et al: Roentgen manifestations of congenital agammaglobulinemia. Radiology 69:354, 1957.
223. Bachmann R: Studies on the serum gamma-A-globulin level: III. The frequency of A-gamma-A-globulinemia. Scand J Clin Lab Invest 17:316, 1965.
224. Hobbs JR: Immune imbalance in dysgammaglobulinaemia type IV. Lancet 1:110, 1968.

225. Gatti RA, Good RA: The immunological deficiency diseases. Med Clin North Am 54:281, 1970.

226. Tomkin GH, Mawhinney H, Nevin NC: Isolated absence of IgA with autosomal dominant inheritance. Lancet 2:124, 1971.

227. Vassallo CL, Zawadzki ZA, Simons JR: Recurrent respiratory infections in a family with immunoglobulin A deficiency. Am Rev Respir Dis 101:245, 1970.

228. Strober W: The regulation of mucosal immune system. J Allergy Clin Immunol 70:225, 1982.

229. Bardana EJ Jr: A conceptual approach to immunodeficiency. Med Clin North Am 65:959, 1981.

230. Cooper MD, Buckley RH: Developmental immunology and the immunodeficiency diseases. JAMA 248:2658, 1982.

231. Sandler SG, Trimble J, Mallory DM: Coexistent IgG2 and IgA deficiencies in blood donors. Transfusion 36:256, 1996.

232. Schwartz DP, Buckley RH: Serum IgE concentrations and skin reactivity to anti-IgE antibody in IgA-deficient patients. N Engl J Med 284:513, 1971.

233. Good RA, Choi YS: Relation of IgA and IgE to bodily defenses. N Engl J Med 284:552, 1971.

234. Heiner DC, Myers A, Beck CS: Deficiency of IgG4: A disorder associated with frequent infections and bronchiectasis may be familial. Clin Rev Allergy 1:259, 1983.

235. Beck CS, Heiner DC: Selective immunoglobulin G4 deficiency and recurrent infections of the respiratory tract. Am Rev Respir Dis 124:94, 1981.

236. Miller BW, Brennan DC, Korenblat PE, et al: Common variable immunodeficiency in a renal transplant patient with severe recurrent bacterial infection: A case report and review of the literature. Am J Kidney Dis 25:947, 1995.

237. Eibl MM, Mannhalter JW, Zlabinger G, et al: Defective macrophage function in a patient with common variable immunodeficiency. N Engl J Med 307:803, 1982.

238. Geha RS, Schneeberger E, Merler E, et al: Heterogeneity of "acquired" or common variable agammaglobulinemia. N Engl J Med 291:1, 1974.

239. Cooper MD, Lawton AR, Bockman DE: Agammaglobulinemia with B lymphocytes: Specific defect of plasma-cell differentiation. Lancet 2:791, 1971.

240. Dukes RJ, Rosenow EC III, Hermans PE: Pulmonary manifestations of hypogammaglobulinemia. Thorax 33:603, 1978.

241. Mechanic LJ, Dikman S, Cunningham-Rundles C, et al: Granulomatous disease in common variable immunodeficiency. Ann Intern Med 127:613, 1997.

242. Popa V: Lymphocytic interstitial pneumonia of common variable immunodeficiency. Ann Allergy 60:203, 1988.

243. Kaufman J, Komorowski R: Bronchiolitis obliterans organizing pneumonia in common variable immunodeficiency syndrome. Chest 100:552, 1991.

244. Sweinberg SK, Wodell RA, Grodofsky MP, et al: Retrospective analysis of the incidence of pulmonary disease in hypogammaglobulinemia. J Allergy Clin Immunol 88:96, 1991.

245. Schoettler JJ, Schleissner LA, Heiner DC: Familial IgE deficiency associated with sinopulmonary disease. Chest 96:516, 1989.

246. de la Torre FM, Garcia RJC, Bonnet MC, et al: Hyper-IgE syndrome: Presentation of three cases. Allergol Immunopathol (Madr) 25:30, 1997.

247. Hall RA, Salhany KE, Lebel E, et al: Fungal pulmonary abscess in an adult secondary to hyperimmunoglobulin E (Job's) syndrome. Ann Thorac Surg 59:759, 1995.

248. Seligmann M, Brouet J-C, Sasportes M: Hereditary C2 deficiency associated with common variable immunodeficiency. Ann Intern Med 91:216, 1979.

249. Starke ID, Corrin B, Selby PJ, et al: Recurrent chest infections, ciliary abnormalities and partial complement deficiency in a Jordanian family. Thorax 36:502, 1981.

250. Berendes H, Bridges RA, Good RA: A fatal granulomatosis of childhood: The clinical study of a new syndrome. Minn Med 40:309, 1957.

251. Landing BH, Shirkey HS: A syndrome of recurrent infection and infiltration of viscera by pigmented lipid histiocytes. Pediatrics 20:431, 1957.

252. Tauber AI: Current views of neutrophil dysfunction: An integrated clinical perspective. Am J Med 70:1237, 1981.

253. Tauber AI, Borregaard N, Simons E, et al: Chronic granulomatous disease: A syndrome of phagocyte oxidase deficiencies. Medicine 62:286, 1983.

254. Gallin JI, Buescher ES, Seligmann BE, et al: Recent advances in chronic granulomatous disease. Ann Intern Med 99:657, 1983.

255. Macher AM, Casale TB, Fauci AS: Chronic granulomatous disease of childhood and *Chromobacterium violaceum* infections in the southeastern United States. Ann Intern Med 97:51, 1982.

256. Ross JP, Holland SM, Gill VJ, et al: Severe Burkholderia (pseudomonas) gladioli infection in chronic granulomatous disease: Report of two successfully treated cases. Clin Infect Dis 21:1291, 1995.

257. Allen DM, Chng HH: Disseminated *Mycobacterium flavescens* in a probable case of chronic granulomatous disease. J Infect 26:83, 1993.

258. Miller ME: Enhanced susceptibility to infection. Med Clin North Am 54:713, 1970.

259. Dent PB, Larke RPB: Viral infection and immunity. Med Clin North Am 56:353, 1972.

260. Paz HL, Little BJ, Ball WC, et al: Primary pulmonary botryomycosis—a manifestation of chronic granulomatous disease. Chest 101:1160, 1992.

261. Cohen MS, Isturiz RE, Malech HL, et al: Fungal infection in chronic granulomatous disease: The importance of the phagocyte in defense against fungi. Am J Med 71:59, 1981.

262. Carson MJ, Chadwick DL, Brubaker CA, et al: Thirteen boys with progressive septic granulomatosis. Pediatrics 35:405, 1965.

263. Caldicott WJH, Baehner RL: Chronic granulomatous disease of childhood. Am J Roentgenol 103:133, 1968.

263a. Moskaluk CA, Pogrebniak HW, Pass HI, et al: Surgical pathology of the lung in chronic granulomatous disease. Am J Clin Pathol 102:684, 1994.

264. Wolfson JJ, Quie PG, Laxdal SD, et al: Roentgenologic manifestations in children with a genetic defect of polymorphonuclear leukocyte function: Chronic granulomatous disease of childhood. Radiology 91:37, 1968.

265. Fleming GM, Kleinerman J, Doershuk CF, et al: Chronic granulomatous disease of childhood, unusual cause of honeycombing lung. Chest 68:834, 1975.

265a. Altman AR: Thoracic wall invasion secondary to pulmonary aspergillosis: A complication of chronic granulomatous disease of childhood. Am J Roentgenol 129:140, 1977.

266. Liese JG, Jendrossek V, Jansson A, et al: Chronic granulomatous disease in adults. Lancet 347:220, 1996.

267. Cline MJ, Craddock CG, Gale RP, et al: Granulocytes in human disease. Ann Intern Med 81:801, 1974.

268. Good RA, Quie PG, Windhorst DB, et al: Fatal (chronic) granulomatous disease of childhood: A hereditary defect of leukocyte function. Semin Hematol 5:215, 1968.

269. Stossel TP: Phagocytosis. N Engl J Med 290:833, 1974.

270. Balfour HH Jr, Shehan JJ, Speicher CE, et al: Chronic granulomatous disease of childhood in a 23-year-old man. JAMA 217:960, 1971.

271. Frayha HH, Biggar WD: Chronic granulomatous disease of childhood: A changing pattern? J Clin Immunol 23:287, 1983.

272. Kritzler RA, Terner JY, Lindenbaum J, et al: Chediak-Higashi syndrome: Cytologic and serum lipid observations in a case and family. Am J Med 36:583, 1964.

273. Weary PE, Bender AS: Chediak-Higashi syndrome with severe cutaneous involvement: Occurrence in two brothers 14 and 15 years of age. Arch Intern Med 119:381, 1967.

274. Gabig TG: Leukocyte abnormalities. Med Clin North Am 64:647, 1980.

275. Duncan RA, von Reyn CF, Alliegro GM, et al: Idiopathic CD4+ T-lymphocytopenia—four patients with opportunistic infections and no evidence of HIV infection. N Engl J Med 328:393, 1993.

276. Lalonde RG, Rene P, Wainberg MA: Opportunistic infections and CD4+ T-lymphocytopenia without HIV infection: Report of two cases. Can Med Assoc J 149:179, 1993.

277. Kaczmarski RS, Webster AD, Moxham J, et al: CD4+ lymphocytopenia due to common variable immunodeficiency mimicking AIDS. J Clin Pathol 47:364, 1994.

278. Sinicco A, Maiello A, Raiteri R, et al: P. carinii in a patient with pulmonary sarcoidosis and idiopathic CD4+ T lymphocytopenia. Thorax 51:446, 1996.

279. Anzalone G, Cei M, Vizzaccaro A, et al: *M. kansasii* pulmonary disease in idiopathic CD4+ T-lymphocytopenia. Eur Respir J 9:1754, 1996.

280. Venzor J, Hua Q, Bressler RB, et al: Behcet's-like syndrome associated with idiopathic CD4+ T-lymphocytopenia, opportunistic infections, and a large population of TCR alpha beta+ CD4-CD8-T cells. Am J Med Sci 313:236, 1997.

281. Prekates A, Kyprianou T, Paniara O, et al: P. carinii pneumonia in a HIV-seronegative patient with untreated rheumatoid arthritis and CD4+ T-lymphocytopenia. Eur Respir J 10:1184, 1997.

282. Diaz-Buxo JA, Hermans PE, Ritts RE Jr: Wiskott-Aldrich syndrome in an adult. Mayo Clin Proc 49:455, 1974.

283. Waldman TA, Misiti J, Nelson DL, et al: Ataxia-telangiectasia: A multisystem hereditary disease with immunodeficiency, impaired organ maturation, x-ray hypersensitivity, and a high incidence of neoplasia. Ann Intern Med 99:367, 1983.

CHAPTER 26

Bacteria Other than Mycobacteria

Classification, nomenclature, and identification are three separate but interrelated areas of taxonomy. *Classification* is defined as the arrangement of organisms into taxonomic groups (taxa) on the basis of similarities or relationships. *Nomenclature* is the naming of an organism by international rules according to its characteristics. *Identification* refers to the practical use of a classification scheme, for example, to isolate and identify a specific pathogen.[1] Although many different schemes have been proposed and are in use, the one employed in this chapter is based on the most common, which organizes bacteria into various groups according to cultural, metabolic, morphologic, and staining characteristics (Table 26–1).

Information on the incidence of specific organisms that cause pneumonia and bacteremia has been obtained largely through retrospective analysis of "passive surveillance" data,[2] in which identification of pneumonia is limited to bacteremic patients. In fact, even vigorous attempts to diagnose the specific bacterial etiology of pneumonia lead to the identification of a specific organism in only 30% to 75% of

Table 26–1. NOMENCLATURE, TAXONOMY, AND CLASSIFICATION OF BACTERIA (OTHER THAN MYCOBACTERIA) CAUSING RESPIRATORY TRACT INFECTION

CURRENT NAME	SYNONYM	CURRENT NAME	SYNONYM
Aerobic and Facultative Bacteria		Non-enterobacteriaceae–nonfermentative bacilli	
Gram-positive cocci		*Acinetobacter* sp.	
Catalase positive		*Alcaligenes* sp.	*Pseudomonas cepacia*
Staphylococcus aureus		*Burkholderia cepacia*	*Pseudomonas mallei*
Staphylococcus cohnii		*Burkholderia mallei*	*Pseudomonas pseudomallei*
Staphylococcus epidermis	*Staphylococcus albus*	*Burkholderia pseudomallei*	
Stomatococcus mucilaginosus		*Pseudomonas aeruginosa*	
Catalase negative		*Pseudomonas fluorescens*	*Pseudomonas maltophila,*
Enterococcus faecalis	*Streptococcus faecalis* (group D enterococcus)	*Stenotrophomonas maltophila*	*Xanthomonas maltophila*
Streptococcus algalactiae	Group B streptococci (group D nonenterococcus)	*Chryseobacterium meningosepticum*	*Burkholderia pickettii,*
Streptococcus bovis		*Ralstonia pickettii*	*Pseudomonas pickettii*
Streptococcus milleri group	*Viridans* streptococci		
Streptococcus mitis	*Viridans* streptococci	Gram-negative coccobacilli	*Rochalimaea henselae*
Streptococcus pneumoniae	*Diplococcus pneumoniae*	*Bartonella henselae*	
Streptococcus pyogenes	Group A streptococci	*Brucella* sp.	
Gram-negative cocci		*Bordetella pertussis*	
Moraxella catarrhalis	*Branhamella catarrhalis*	*Campylobacter* sp.	
	Neisseria catarrhalis	*Chlamydia pneumoniae*	
Gram-positive bacilli		*Chlamydia psittaci*	
Bacillus anthracis		*Chlamydia trachomatis*	
Bacilus cereus		*Coxiella burnetii*	*Pasteurella tularensis*
Bacillus subtilis		*Francisella tularensis*	
Corynebacterium diphtheriae		*Haemophilus* sp.	
Corynebacterium pseudodiphtheriticum	*Corynebacterium hofmannii*	*Legionella* sp.	
Corynebacterium pseudotuberculosis		*Rickettsia* sp.	
Listeria monocytogenes		Mycoplasma	
Nocardia sp.		Treponemataceae (spiral organisms)	
Rhodococcus equi	*Corynebacterium equi*	*Borrelia burgdorferi*	
		Borrelia recurrentis	
Gram-negative bacilli		*Leptospira* sp.	
Enterobacteriaceae		*Treponema pallidum*	
Citrobacter sp.			
Enterobacter sp.		*Anaerobic Bacteria*	
Escherichia sp.			
Klebsiella sp.		Gram-negative bacilli	
Morganella morganii	*Proteus morganii*	Bacteroidaceae	
Proteus sp.		*Bacteroides fragilis*	
Providencia sp.		*Fusobacterium*	
Salmonella sp.		Non–spore-forming gram-positive bacilli	
Serratia marcescens		*Actinomyces israelii*	
Shigella sp.		*Propionibacterium*	
Yersinia pestis	*Pasteurella pestis*	Endospore-forming gram-positive bacilli	
Non-enterobacteriaceae–fermentative bacilli		*Clostridium* sp.	
Aeromonas sp.		Gram-positive cocci	
Pasteurella multocida	*Pasteurella septica*	*Peptostreptococcus* sp.	
Vibrio sp.			
Chromobacterium violaceum			

Adapted from Bruckner DA, Colonna P: Nomenclature for aerobic and facultative bacteria. Clin Infect Dis 21:263, 1995.

patients.[3–7] This limitation should be kept in mind as the clinical and radiologic findings of pneumonia caused by specific organisms are described in the following sections.

AEROBIC AND FACULTATIVE BACTERIA

Gram-Positive Cocci

Streptococcus pneumoniae

Streptococcus pneumoniae (Diplococcus pneumoniae) is a gram-positive, oval or lancet-shaped organism that is usually arranged in pairs and occasionally in short chains. It is surrounded by a well-defined polysaccharide capsule, which permits typing with specific antisera.[1] On the basis of chemical differences and polysaccharide composition, about 84 antigenic variants have been identified in the United States. In decreasing order of frequency, the majority of the pneumonias are caused by Types 3, 19F, 23F, 6B, 14, 4, and 6A;[8] Types 1, 6B, 8, 7F, and 18C have been implicated less commonly.[9] Similar findings have been reported from Canada,[10, 10a] England and Wales,[11, 12] Spain,[13] and Norway.[14]

The organism is a common human commensal that has been estimated to be present normally in up to 20% of the population.[15, 16] In certain groups, such as patients with asthma or chronic obstructive pulmonary disease (COPD)[17] or children in day-care centers,[18] colonization rates may be substantially higher.

The organism grows readily on blood agar and has the properties of a facultative anaerobe; its growth is enhanced by 5% to 10% CO_2. Serotypes can be identified by capsular swelling in the presence of specific antibody (the *quellung reaction*), by latex agglutination[19, 20] or coagglutination,[20] by enzyme-linked immunosorbent assay (ELISA) techniques,[21, 22] and by fluorescent antibody techniques.[23] Pulsed-field gel electrophoresis of genomic DNA[24] and other molecular biologic techniques[25, 25a] can be helpful in subdividing *Streptococcus pneumoniae* serotypes.

Epidemiology

S. pneumoniae is the most common pathogenic organism identified in patients admitted to the hospital, accounting for about 40% of all isolated species.[26, 26a] For several reasons, this is likely to be a significant underestimation of the importance of this organism as a cause of pneumonia.[26] It has been estimated, for example, that blood culture identifies only one patient in four with the infection; on the basis of this, it has been suggested that the attack rate for *S. pneumoniae* pneumonia is about 1 to 5 per 1000 persons per annum.[2] It is also important to remember that most of the information on etiology and prognosis of community acquired pneumonia is derived from patients with sufficiently severe illness to require hospitalization. Conclusions drawn from such patients may not apply to the relatively healthy outpatient, and diagnostic and treatment strategies must be modified accordingly.

There are several risk factors for the development of pulmonary infection by *S. pneumoniae*. One of the most important is age, elderly individuals having a much higher incidence of infection than younger ones.[27–30] Although esti-

mates of the increased risk for pneumonia with advancing age are confounded by the common presence of other risk factors (*see* farther on), one multivariate logistic regression analysis of 4,175 elderly Finnish patients confirmed the independent relationship between age and pneumonia risk.[30] This age-related risk appears to be substantial; for example, in one investigation from Ohio, the annual incidence of *S. pneumoniae* bacteremia in patients older than 65 years of age was 83.0 per 100,000, whereas it was only 9.6 per 100,000 in young adults.[28] Disease is also more common in African Americans[28] and Native Americans[31] than in whites. Extrapolation of this and similar data has led to estimates of approximately 40,000 to 45,000 cases of bacteremic pneumococcal pneumonia annually in the United States, of which 16,000 occur in the elderly.[32] The presence of chronic heart or lung disease, the use of immunosuppressive therapy, alcoholism,[30] and institutionalization[30, 33] confer increased risk for the development of pneumonia. The risk of infection is also greater in patients who have cirrhosis, renal failure,[34] lymphoma or leukemia,[35] multiple myeloma,[36] human immunodeficiency virus (HIV) infection,[28] a history of intravenous drug abuse,[37] sickle cell disease,[38–40] and prior splenectomy.[41] An outbreak of acute pneumonia in an American prison[36] illustrates the importance of overcrowding and inadequate ventilation in the propagation of infection.

Of particular concern in the epidemiology of *S. pneumoniae* infection is the emergence of drug-resistant strains.[42, 43, 43a] The frequency of such isolates varies in different areas of the world. For example, approximately 30% of cultured strains have been found to be penicillin resistant in Barcelona,[43] Atlanta,[30] Oklahoma,[33] and Japan;[44] by contrast, penicillin resistance has been documented in only 3% to 4% of isolates in England and Wales,[11, 45] in 1.4% of isolates causing invasive disease in New Zealand,[46] and in 3.8% of isolates in Alaska.[47] The prevalence of antibiotic-resistant organisms is particularly high in select groups of patients;[47a] for example, 25 (74%) of 34 HIV-infected patients[48] and 17 (53%) of 32 people in a Nebraska day-care facility[49] were colonized with a resistant strain. Thus, each physician must be aware of the pattern of resistance in his or her community when considering the choice of antibiotics in the treatment of pneumonia and other respiratory tract infections. Genetic analysis of antibiotic-resistant *S. pneumoniae* serotypes indicates that some isolates have a recent "common ancestor" and that certain serotypes (e.g., 6, 9, 14, 15, 19, and 23) are more likely to develop penicillin resistance.[12, 13, 44, 50–53]

Pathogenesis

Infection of the lower respiratory tract usually follows aspiration of organisms from a focus of colonization in the nasopharyngeal mucosa.[54] Virulence depends in part on their ability to adhere to lung cells by surface macromolecules (adhesins),[55] a property that is enhanced by a variety of cytokines induced by the organism's cell wall and (sometimes) antecedent viral infection.[54, 56] Exposure of respiratory epithelial cells to the organism also up-regulates their expression of platelet activating factor receptors, which are also important in bacterial adhesion.[54] Adherence of the organism to pulmonary epithelial cells has several consequences, including the production of cytokines capable of initiating an inflammatory reaction.[57, 57a] The cell wall of the bacterium also causes a decrease in endothelial barrier function, which leads to the development of intra-alveolar edema[54] and stimulates endothelial cells to initiate a procoagulant cascade. These processes are associated with the development of intra-alveolar fibrin-rich edema fluid and hemorrhage (corresponding to the histologic stages of congestion and red hepatization). Under the influence of cytokines,[58] leukocytes subsequently move into the lung via the leukocyte-adhesion molecules of the integrin family (CD18)[54, 58a] and by a PAF-dependent pathway initiated by the organism itself.[54]

The subsequent course of disease depends largely on the interaction between the organisms and neutrophils. *S. pneumonia* has the ability to counteract the killing effects of reactive oxygen species released by neutrophils[59] and to abrogate their production of oxidants.[60] The death of the bacteria leads to the release of cell wall and intracellular substances with a variety of proinflammatory functions. The inflammatory response is augmented by the activation of complement. The bacterium's death also releases pneumolysin, whose cytolytic and complement activating features facilitate both bacterial growth and invasion of the blood.[61] Other bacterial proteins, including pneumococcal surface protein A, neuraminidase, hyaluronidase, and IgA1 protease, increase the virulence of the organism by facilitating both colonization and invasion.[62]

In contrast with the strong inflammation-inducing properties of the cell wall, the polysaccharide capsule surrounding the organism has no proinflammatory function. However, by protecting the organism from phagocytosis, it is important in determining virulence.[54, 63] The capsule becomes the target for serotype-specific antibodies protective for the host. Despite the presence of a capsule, the cell wall remains accessible to some components of the acute inflammatory reaction; for example, it is able to fix complement and thereby further augment leukocyte recruitment.[54] Resolution of consolidation occurs with the appearance of anticapsular antibodies, which facilitate the phagocytosis of the organism by alveolar macrophages. The latter also rid the air spaces of fibrin and other debris, leading in most cases to a return to normal anatomic and functional characteristics of the lung parenchyma.[54]

Pathologic Characteristics

The pathology of pneumonia caused by *S. pneumoniae* has been well described in both humans[64, 65] and various experimental animals.[66, 67] The infection tends to begin in the lower lobes or the posterior segments of the upper lobes. Experimentally, the earliest findings occur in the terminal airways.[68] Instead of the host inflammatory reaction localizing the infection to this site, however, air-space edema fluid spreads rapidly to involve an increasing amount of pulmonary parenchyma. This centrifugal, contiguous spread accounts for the homogeneity of consolidation and nonsegmental distribution observed both morphologically and radiologically.

Classically, four pathologic stages can be recognized, representing the morphologic expression of the sequence of host inflammatory response to the organism: congestion, red hepatization, gray hepatization, and resolution. Different stages may be seen in the same lung, depending on the time in the course of the disease at which it is examined. The stage of *congestion* is usually seen in lung tissue at the advancing edge of the pneumonic zone and is manifested by alveolar capillary dilation and abundant intra-alveolar edema fluid containing numerous organisms and only occasional polymorphonuclear leukocytes (Fig. 26–1). In *red hepatization,* affected lung parenchyma is airless and possesses a striking brick red color; microscopically, the alveoli are filled with edema fluid containing numerous red blood cells, again with only scattered polymorphonuclear leukocytes. Airways are frequently patent, accounting for the air bronchogram seen radiographically; occasionally they are filled with edema or hemorrhagic fluid.[69] In the stage of *gray hepatization* (usually appearing 3 to 5 days after the onset of disease), the lung acquires a gray or grayish yellow color; microscopically, alveolar spaces are filled with numerous polymorphonuclear leukocytes and microorganisms are sparse. Fibrinous pleuritis is frequent at this time. During the stage of *resolution,* polymorphonuclear leukocytes decrease in number and are replaced by macrophages that phagocytose cellular and other debris. In patients who survive the acute infection, this is usually followed by reconstitution of normal lung; occasionally, the fibrinopurulent exudate organizes rather than resorbs, resulting in fibrosis of affected lung parenchyma.

The high incidence of complete resolution is probably related to the lack of toxins produced by the organism, a feature also reflected by the typical absence of tissue necrosis. Although experimental studies in dogs have shown that a considerable increase in proteolytic activity accompanies the accumulation of neutrophils, both in the circulation and in fluid obtained by bronchoalveolar lavage (BAL), a simultaneous and comparable rise in serum and lung fluid antiproteases seems to protect the lung parenchyma from damage.[70] As might be expected, therefore, abscess formation is rare in pneumococcal pneumonia and probably occurs only in association with particularly virulent strains[71] or with concomitant infection by anaerobic organisms.[70, 72]

Radiologic Manifestations

The characteristic radiographic pattern of acute pneumococcal pneumonia consists of homogeneous, nonsegmental consolidation involving one lobe (Fig. 26–2). Since the consolidation begins in the periphery of the lung, it almost invariably abuts against a visceral pleural surface, either interlobar or over the convexity. Occasionally, infection is manifested as a round (spherical) focus of consolidation that may simulate a pulmonary mass; although this pattern can be seen in adults (Fig. 26–3),[73] it is more common in children.[73, 74] Where consolidation is not related to a visceral pleural surface, its margin usually is fairly well defined. The lack of respect for segmental boundaries is of major importance in differentiating acute air-space pneumonia from bronchopneumonia. An air bronchogram is common, and its absence should cast doubt on the diagnosis unless the consolidation is confined to the periphery of the lung, where airways are too small to be clearly identifiable. Since the pathologic process is one of replacement of air by inflammatory exudate, loss of volume is either slight or absent during the acute stage of the disease; during resolution, however, some degree of atelectasis is common, presumably as a result of exudate within airways and resultant obstruction.

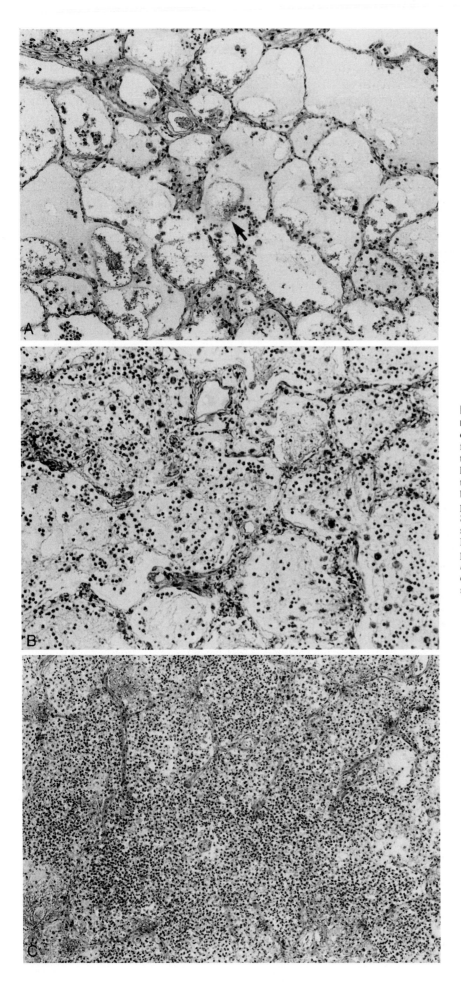

Figure 26–1. Acute Air-Space Pneumonia—*Streptococcus pneumoniae*. *A,* Stage of congestion showing air spaces filled with edema fluid and minimal cellular reaction. Numerous bacteria were evident within the fluid. *B,* Stage of red hepatization, showing alveolar walls expanded by tortuous capillaries and air spaces filled with red blood cells and finely filamentous fibrin. Polymorphonuclear leukocytes have begun to appear. *C,* Stage of gray hepatization, showing alveolar air spaces filled with polymorphonuclear leukocytes. Edema, fibrin, and capillary congestion are not prominent. Note that unlike the situation in *Staphylococcus aureus* infections and most pneumonias caused by gram-negative organisms, necrosis is absent. (*A,* ×100; *B,* ×130; *C,* ×100.)

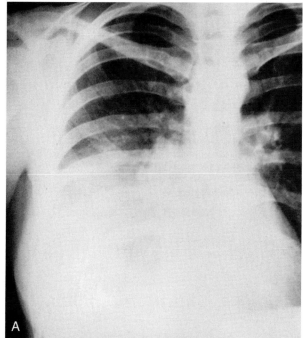

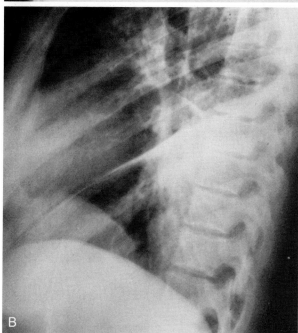

Figure 26–2. Acute Nonsegmental Air-Space Pneumonia—
Streptococcus pneumoniae. Posteroanterior *(A)* and lateral *(B)* radiographs reveal extensive consolidation of the right lower lobe, a portion of the anterior segment being the only portion of lung unaffected. An air bronchogram is visible in the lateral projection. There is little loss of volume. Sputum culture produced a heavy growth of *S. pneumoniae.*

As discussed previously (*see* page 701), contrary to the implication of the common term *lobar* pneumonia, because of early recognition and the availability of antibiotics, progression of the consolidation to involve an entire lobe is seen rarely.[75] Most frequently, the disease is confined to one lobe; however, it may develop simultaneously in two or more lobes, in which case it carries a poorer prognosis.

Although homogeneous, nonsegmental consolidation is

the most common radiographic manifestation of acute pneumococcal pneumonia, other patterns are not infrequent. For example, while 20 (67%) of 30 patients with pneumococcal pneumonia in one prospective survey had the typical pattern, 6 (20%) had patchy areas of consolidation and 4 (13%) had mixed air-space and interstitial opacities (Fig. 26–4).[76] In another review of 132 patients with severe community-acquired pneumonia treated in the intensive care unit (ICU), 28 (65%) of 43 patients with *S. pneumoniae* pneumonia had typical nonsegmental consolidation and 35% had bronchopneumonia; none had reticular or reticulonodular infiltrates.[77] Patients with *S. pneumoniae* bacteremia are more likely to have a radiographic pattern of bronchopneumonia; in one retrospective review of 26 patients, 15 (58%) had this pattern, as opposed to 7 (26%) with nonsegmental consolidation and one (4%) with a combined pattern (3 [12%] had normal chest radiographs).[78]

The radiographic pattern is also influenced by the presence of underlying lung disease, particularly emphysema. In patients with the latter abnormality, the homogeneity of consolidation is interrupted by a multitude of small air-containing "holes," representing large emphysematous spaces that have escaped consolidation.[79] In fact, the varied presentations of acute pneumococcal pneumonia described in some studies are probably attributable to the presence of COPD.[80]

Complications such as cavitation, pulmonary gangrene and pneumatocele formation are rare (Fig. 26–5). It is probable that many, if not all, of these are related to mixed

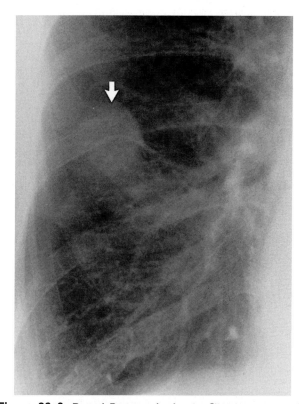

Figure 26–3. Round Pneumonia due to *Streptococcus pneumoniae.* A view of the right lung from a posteroanterior chest radiograph demonstrates a focal round area of consolidation *(arrow)* in the right lower lobe. Sputum cultures grew *S. pneumoniae.* The findings resolved following treatment with antibiotics.

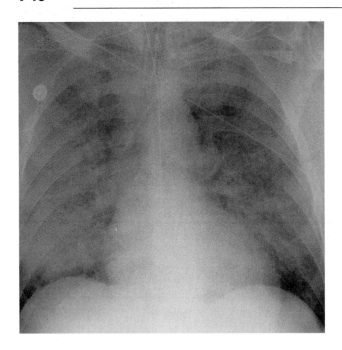

Figure 26–4. *Streptococcus pneumoniae* **Pneumonia.** A 50-year-old man presented with a 2-day history of high fever and progressive shortness of breath. An anteroposterior chest radiograph performed shortly after admission demonstrates extensive bilateral areas of consolidation. Sputum and blood cultures grew *S. pneumoniae.* The disease resolved within 2 weeks following treatment with antibiotics.

infections; anaerobic microorganisms in particular are likely to be undetected because of lack of appropriate culture methods.[72]

The reported incidence of pleural effusion varies with the radiographic technique used, the severity of infection, and the presence or absence of bacteremia. In one study, 14 (11%) of 123 patients considered to have pneumococcal pneumonia on the basis of smears and radiographic appear-

ance were found to have effusion or empyema detectable on conventional posteroanterior (PA) and lateral chest radiographs.[81] By contrast, in a prospective study of 35 patients judged to have pneumococcal pneumonia on the basis of sputum or blood culture results or both and on whom lateral decubitus as well as conventional PA and lateral radiographs were obtained, 20 (57%) were found to have parapneumonic effusions, 16 being evident on the PA and lateral projec-

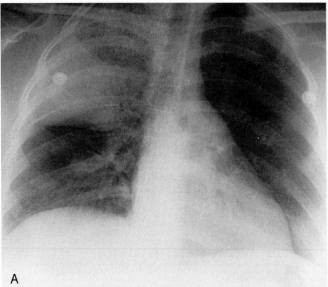

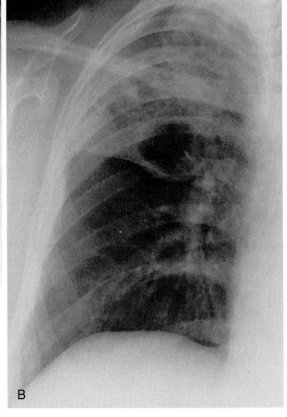

Figure 26–5. *Streptococcus pneumoniae* **Pneumonia.** A posteroanterior chest radiograph *(A)* in a 20-year-old woman shows extensive consolidation of the right upper lobe. Sputum cultures grew *S. pneumoniae.* A chest radiograph performed 1 week later, at a time when the patient had markedly improved clinically *(B),* shows focal lucency in the right upper lobe with bulging of the minor fissure. This subsequently resolved without complications. The appearance is consistent with a pneumatocele.

tions.[82] In the latter study, the presence of parapneumonic effusions correlated significantly with bacteremia, the duration of symptoms before admission, and prolonged fever after institution of therapy. In two additional investigations of 43 patients who had severe pneumonia requiring treatment in the ICU[77] and 26 who had bacteremia,[78] effusion was found in 13 (30%) and 10 (48%), respectively.

In our experience, resolution of pneumococcal pneumonia can be fairly rapid with appropriate therapy, complete clearing being apparent within 10 to 14 days in the majority of cases of community-acquired infections. In a prospective study of radiographic resolution in 81 patients who had community-acquired pneumonia due to a variety of organisms including S. pneumoniae, 51% of patients demonstrated complete clearing after 2 weeks, and 67% demonstrated clearing after 4 weeks.[83] Clearance was faster in patients who were treated as outpatients (mean 3.8 weeks) than in patients who required hospital admission (mean 9.1 weeks), and in nonsmokers compared with smokers (4.5 weeks vs. 8.4 weeks). The rate of clearance correlated inversely with age and with the number of lobes involved.

Clearance is slower in patients with bacteremia. For example, in one follow-up study of 72 patients with this complication, complete disappearance of radiographic consolidation took as long as 8 to 10 weeks.[84] Resolution occurred earlier in patients younger than 50 years of age and in those who were not alcoholics and had no underlying COPD regardless of age, whereas clearing was delayed when these complicating factors were present in patients older than 50 years of age. Other investigators have also recognized an association between the time of resolution and age.[85]

Clinical Manifestations

The usual clinical presentation of acute pneumococcal pneumonia is abrupt, with fever, shaking chills, cough, slight expectoration, and intense pleural pain. On close questioning, many patients give a history of an upper respiratory tract infection before the onset of the more dramatic symptoms. The temperature may be as high as 41° C. Cough may be nonproductive at first but soon produces bloody, "rusty," or greenish material. Debilitated or alcoholic patients may be deeply cyanosed, and shock may ensue rapidly. In the elderly, these classic features of disease may be absent and pneumonia may be confused with or confounded by other common medical problems, such as congestive heart failure, pulmonary thromboembolism, or malignancy.[86]

Typical findings on physical examination include decreased breath sounds, crackles, and impaired percussion over the site of the pneumonia; bronchial breathing, bronchophony, and whispering pectoriloquy are audible on auscultation in a small number of patients. During resolution, the crackles first increase and then slowly disappear as normal breath sounds return. In many cases, a friction rub is audible over the consolidated lung. There are no particular clinical features of this infection that distinguish it from pneumonia due to Legionella sp. or other organisms in any given patient.[87]

Meningitis and empyema are seen in fewer than 10% of cases;[82, 88, 89] pericarditis is uncommon and is usually detected only at autopsy.[90] Some complications, such as jaundice and disseminated intravascular coagulation,[91, 92]

have been correlated with high levels of pneumococcal capsular polysaccharide antigen in serum. In most patients, jaundice is caused by hepatocellular damage; occasionally, it is secondary to hemolysis, particularly in patients with glucose 6-phosphate dehydrogenase deficiency.[93] Metastatic foci of infection may occur in any tissue, but are usually clinically evident only in the heart, meninges, or joints. Rhabdomyolysis[94] and acute nephritis[95] have occasionally been described. Perhaps the most important complication of pneumococcal infection is superinfection, usually by gram-negative organisms in patients who have received broad-spectrum antibiotics.

Laboratory Findings and Diagnosis

Although the diagnosis of acute pneumococcal pneumonia may be suspected from the clinical picture and the radiographic pattern, isolation of the organism or the demonstration of a specific polysaccharide antigen is necessary for definitive diagnosis. The finding of cocci on smear of sputum and a positive quellung reaction are helpful;[96] however, the sensitivity of a good Gram stain for the diagnosis of pneumococcal pneumonia is only in the order of 15%, and sputum samples are often not obtained in a timely fashion.[26] Carriers of the organism can be distinguished from those truly infected by culture of the organism from normally sterile sources, such as lung (via transthoracic needle aspiration), blood, pleura, pericardium, joint space, or subarachnoid space.[2] It should be remembered, however, that prior administration of antibiotics seriously interferes with the ability to culture the organism.[26] Moreover, the reported incidence of negative sputum culture in patients with pneumococcal pneumonia proved by positive blood culture is as high as 45%.[97–100] The finding of capsular antigen in sputum also suggests the presence of infection; arguments in favor of this view have been reviewed.[26] Techniques used to demonstrate this antigen include counterimmunoelectrophoresis (CIE),[102] coagglutination,[103] latex agglutination,[102, 104, 105] and ELISA.[106] Polymerase chain reaction (PCR) has also been used to detect streptococcal DNA in blood[107, 108] and sputum.[109] Although not helpful in routine diagnosis, demonstration of a rise in antibodies to the organism suggests that recent infection has occurred.[110]

The white cell count usually is higher than 20,000/mm^3, in a range of 10,000 to 40,000/mm^3; polymorphonuclear leukocytosis, with many band forms, is common. Despite this, leukopenia develops in many extremely ill patients. Hyponatremia and hypobilirubinemia have been common in some studies.[110a] Analysis of arterial blood gas may show mild or even severe hypoxemia during the stage of red hepatization. In most cases, the PCO_2 is also reduced, and the minute ventilation indicates hyperventilation with small tidal volumes.

Prognosis and Natural History

In many series, S. pneumoniae is the most common cause of severe community-acquired pneumonia (defined as pneumonia causing death or requiring intensive care), occurring in about 15% to 45% of such cases.[40, 111] A number of risk factors have been identified that are associated with an increased risk of death due to pneumonia in general and

S. pneumoniae pneumonia in particular.[40, 111–118] These can be related to demographic factors (age, gender, and place of residence), clinical features (symptoms and signs, comorbid disease), and laboratory abnormalities.[117] In the absence of these risk factors, a good outcome can be anticipated. Some examples from the literature in which these criteria have been used are illustrative.

A prognostic index was applied to 14,199 patients admitted for pneumonia to three Pittsburgh hospitals; the index was derived from data obtained from 346 patients.[112] Patients were classified into five categories based on six predictors of mortality: age greater than 65 years, pleuritic chest pain (which, for unknown reasons, is protective), abnormalities in vital signs, altered mental status, the presence of underlying neoplastic disease, and a high-risk causative organism (which did not include *S. pneumoniae*). Mortality rates in the lowest- and highest-risk cohorts were 1% and 38%, respectively. In another review of 316 patients admitted to the hospital for pneumonia in New Zealand (many of whom had pneumococcal infection), patients with any two of the following abnormalities had a 36-fold increased risk of death:[115] respiratory rate higher than 30/min, diastolic blood pressure 60 mm Hg or lower, blood urea higher than 7 mmol/l, or confusion. Use of these criteria, derived from British Thoracic Society recommendations, enabled identification of 19 of the 20 patients who died, as well as 6 of the 8 admitted to the ICU who ultimately survived. In addition to findings of impaired renal function, other laboratory data that predict mortality in patients with pneumonia include a high white blood cell count, hypoalbuminemia, and multilobar involvement radiographically.[117]

Similar predictive strategies have been applied specifically to patients with *S. pneumoniae* infection. In one study of 102 patients with pneumococcal bacteremia, the risk for death and/or respiratory failure requiring mechanical ventilation was found to be increased in the presence of chronic lung disease, nosocomial infection, age older than 48 years, and temperature lower than 38° C at presentation.[113] In the absence of any of these risk factors, only 1 of 25 patients with bacteremia died; no other patient required intensive care. The adverse effect of older age was also shown in another series of 534 patients with bacteremia and *S. pneumoniae* pneumonia from Winnipeg;[114] although the overall case-fatality rate was 13%, it was 43% in patients older than 80 years of age.

The importance of comorbid disease to mortality risk has also been well documented. The "ALPS" mnemonic has been applied to a group of *a*lcoholic *l*euko*p*enic and *s*eptic patients with bacteremic infection; in one series of such patients, the mortality rate was 83%![119] Fulminant bacteremia can also occur in patients with splenectomy or functional asplenia or with reductions in serum IgG, such as occurs in multiple myeloma, hypogammaglobulinemia, and chronic lymphocytic leukemia.[40]

Many of the risk factors for development of pneumococcal infection are also associated with an adverse outcome. An exception is HIV infection; although the risk of developing pneumococcal pneumonia is much higher in patients with this abnormality than in the general population, the mortality rate in the absence of bacteremia is no different.[40] However, bacteremic patients with acquired immunodeficiency syndrome (AIDS) seem to have a very high mortality;

for example, in one report of such patients, 8 (57%) died.[120] Somewhat surprisingly, the increasing prevalence of antibiotic-resistant organisms has not been associated with an appreciable increase in mortality.[121, 122] The explanation is presumably related to the fact that most of these organisms show intermediate- rather than high-grade resistance, and high doses of antibiotics can still achieve tissue-killing levels.

Streptococcus pyogenes

Streptococcus pyogenes is a gram-positive organism (Lancefield group A β-hemolytic streptococcus) that appears on smear in chains. Culture on blood agar is very rapid, colonies being identifiable within 24 hours; typical β-hemolysis surrounds the colonies. The organism may be cultured from the sputum or from the pleural effusion that commonly accompanies the pneumonia.

Epidemiology

Until the advent of antibiotics, *S. pyogenes* was one of the most common causes of bronchopneumonia, predominantly of the young and the elderly. It often followed infection by measles virus or *Bordetella pertussis*; in the influenza pandemic following World War I, it was also a common and serious complication. Nowadays, streptococcal pneumonia is seldom seen, although cases are still reported following influenza[123] and childhood exanthems;[124, 125] outbreaks in relatively isolated populations such as in military barracks[126] or nursing homes[127] occur occasionally. A household cluster associated with toxic-shock syndrome has also been documented.[128] Pneumonia rarely follows streptococcal pharyngitis or tonsillitis. The infection is most common during the cold months.

Pathologic Characteristics

The morphologic characteristics of acute streptococcal pneumonia are almost identical to those of staphylococcal infection; as with the latter, the severity of the disease clinically correlates with the morphologic findings. In the preantibiotic era, many patients with fulminating disease died within 36 hours, autopsy revealing serosanguineous pleural effusion, hemorrhagic edema of the lung parenchyma (particularly in the lower lobes) and epithelial necrosis and neutrophil infiltration of bronchi and bronchioles.[129] Bacteria were easily identified in the hemorrhagic edema fluid. Edema and lymphatic dilatation within intralobular septa often were quite prominent. Cavities often developed in those who survived for 4 to 5 days. In patients with less severe disease—commonly associated with pertussis or measles—the pathologic picture is similar to that of acute purulent staphylococcal bronchopneumonia, often with peribronchial abscess formation, fibrinous pleuritis, and pleural effusion.

Radiologic Manifestations

In most respects the radiographic characteristics are indistinguishable from those of acute staphylococcal pneumonia: homogeneous or patchy consolidation in segmental

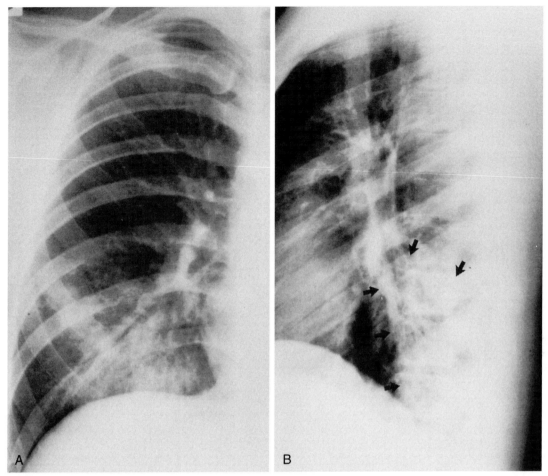

Figure 26–6. Acute Bronchopneumonia—*Streptococcus pyogenes*. Views of the right lung from posteroanterior *(A)* and lateral *(B)* radiographs show patchy consolidation of the posterior basal segment of the right lower lobe. The consolidation is inhomogeneous and possesses a roughly triangular configuration in lateral projection *(arrows* in *B),* indicating a segmental distribution. Sputum culture produced mixed flora but with a predominance of *S. pyogenes.*

distribution (Fig. 26–6) and some loss of volume that typically affects the lower lobes and sometimes is bilateral.[130] The tendency to form pneumatoceles or pyopneumothorax found in acute staphylococcal pneumonia is absent, although lung abscesses and cavities may develop and empyema is common (the latter was an invariable accompaniment before the advent of antibiotics).

Clinical Manifestations

The onset of acute streptococcal pneumonia is usually abrupt, with pleural pain, shaking chills, fever, and cough productive of purulent and often blood-tinged material. Patchy areas of decreased breath sounds may be appreciated at the lung bases, together with crackles and rhonchi; signs of pleural effusion are usually detectable. Rarely, pneumonia is associated with a desquamating skin rash characteristic of scarlet fever or toxic-shock syndrome.[128, 131]

Diagnosis depends on culture of the organism from sputum, pleural fluid, or (occasionally) blood. Antisera may be used to identify the type of organism. In the later stages of the disease, antibodies may be found in the serum, and an elevated titer of antistreptolysin O may suggest the diagnosis. There is commonly polymorphonuclear leukocytosis,

with a mixture of mature and immature cells. Complications include residual pleural thickening (in 15 of 20 patients in one series),[126] bronchiectasis (especially in children in whom the disease develops in conjunction with a viral exanthem), and (rarely) glomerulonephritis.[132]

Staphylococcus aureus

Staphylococcus aureus is a gram-positive, nonmotile, non–spore-forming coccus that characteristically appears on smear in pairs, short chains, tetrads, or clusters.[133] It grows readily on blood agar, usually as a golden-yellow colony surrounded by a zone of clear hemolysis. It is facultatively anaerobic; some strains produce a capsule or slime layer that contributes to the organism's virulence. It is distinguished from other *staphylococcal* species by its production of coagulase, a plasma-clotting enzyme.[133] In the chest, the organism most often causes bronchopneumonia in a variety of clinical settings. It is also responsible for localized tracheitis (particularly in children) as a complication of viral infection or (possibly) as a primary infection.[134, 135]

Epidemiology

The first and largest study of *S. aureus* pneumonia, reported in 1919, revealed the organism to be an important cause of death in soldiers following influenza virus infection.[136] The latter continues to be an important risk factor for the development of *S. aureus* pneumonia; for example, in one series of 61 patients with community-acquired staphylococcal infection, it preceded pneumonia in 32 (52%).[137] Despite this, *S. aureus* is an uncommon cause of community-acquired pneumonia, accounting for only about 3% of all cases[26] and about 3% to 12% of cases severe enough to require admission to hospital and care in an ICU.[40] Infection in the latter situation rarely occurs in healthy adults, most affected people being very young, elderly, or debilitated.[138]

S. aureus is a more important cause of nosocomial pneumonia, especially in the ICU. In this setting, it is one of the most common pathogenic organisms, being found in 15% or more of all cases.[133, 139] Methicillin-resistant *S. aureus* (MRSA) has been recognized as a nosocomial pathogen for more than 30 years[140] and now accounts for up to 38% of staphylococcal isolates in American hospitals.[140] However, although colonization with organisms of this strain is common in long-care treatment institutions, only a small percentage of affected people develop frank infection. For example, in one facility in which MRSA was endemic, the monthly colonization rate was about 23%;[141] most patients were already affected on admission to the unit, only 10% of newly admitted patients becoming colonized while in the institution. Most important, only 3% of patients developed clinically evident infection. Patients who do develop ventilator-associated pneumonia with MRSA are more likely than patients with methicillin-sensitive *S. aureus* infection to have been treated with steroids, to be older, to have underlying COPD, and (especially) to have received antibiotics.[142]

In addition to the intensive care setting, risk factors for the development of *S. aureus* pneumonia include alcoholism, chronic medical conditions such as COPD, influenza, age older than 60 years, AIDS, malnutrition, and bacteremia associated with soft-tissue infection or endocarditis.[133, 137, 143–149] The organism is also extremely common in the sputum of patients with cystic fibrosis.

Pathogenesis

The pathogenesis of pneumonia due to *S. aureus* is incompletely understood. The organism produces a variety of potent enzymes and toxins, including coagulase, hyaluronidase, α-toxin (α-hemolysin), β, γ-, and δ-toxins, and glucosiden.[150] Coagulase is related to pathogenicity, since coagulase-negative strains rarely cause disease in either humans or in murine models;[151] however, coagulase-negative, frequently antibiotic-resistant strains of *Staphylococcus epidermidis* can be pathogenic, usually in patients with severe granulocytopenia.[152, 153] As is true of other respiratory tract infections, binding and colonization with subsequent infection are more likely to occur in seriously ill, elderly patients than in those with less severe illness.[154] Local antibody response to the organism may be important in protection against disease; in immunosuppressed mice, inhalation and intravenous injection of gamma globulin protects against infection.[155]

Although *S. aureus* pneumonia is usually acquired via the tracheobronchial tree, a substantial proportion of cases are the result of hematogenous spread from an extrapulmonary site as, for example, in intravenous drug addicts with tricuspid endocarditis[149] and in malnourished children with skin infection in developing countries.[133]

Some patients with pneumonia caused by *S. aureus* develop one or more thin-walled cystic lesions adjacent to areas of parenchymal consolidation (*pneumatoceles*); for unknown reasons, the complication is much more common in children than in adults. Several theories have been proposed for their development:[156] (1) valvelike obstruction of small airways causing distal airtrapping and bronchiolar and parenchymal distention;[157] (2) the development of communications between alveolar air spaces and interlobular or peribronchial interstitial tissue, with formation of an interstitial or intrapleural air-containing space;[158] and (3) the development of a communication between an abscess and a bronchus or bronchiole as a result of necrosis of intervening tissue, with subsequent air trapping within the abscess due to check-valve obstruction by inflamed airway mucosa or intraluminal debris.[159] Support for the third hypothesis has been provided by experiments in rabbits with tuberculosis and by occasional case reports in humans.[156, 160]

Pathologic Characteristics

The pathologic findings in staphylococcal pneumonia depend on the rapidity of the disease process and can be conveniently grouped into three forms for descriptive purposes: acute hemorrhagic (fulminating) pneumonia, acute purulent pneumonia, and chronic organizing pneumonia.[161, 162] The first of these is commonly associated with influenza, although it also occurs sporadically without underlying disease in both children and adults.[162–164] Microscopically, the parenchyma resembles the stage of red hepatization in pneumococcal pneumonia, with extensive intraalveolar edema and hemorrhage, relatively sparse polymorphonuclear leukocytic infiltration, and little or no evidence of tissue necrosis. Organisms abound within the edema fluid and can easily be identified with Gram stain. Fibrin thrombi may be present within pulmonary vessels. It is possible that the fulminating course followed by these patients is associated with a massive production of bacterial toxins, since similar microscopic changes have been identified in rabbits injected intratracheally with filtrates of bacterial toxin.[165]

The acute purulent variety of *S. aureus* pneumonia is the most common form and is manifested as bronchopneumonia, frequently associated with abscess formation. Microscopically, the pulmonary parenchyma around terminal and respiratory bronchioles is most severely involved, and it is probably in this location that the abscesses first occur. As the disease progresses, individual microabscesses may enlarge and coalesce, producing a macroscopically visible abscess (Fig. 26–7); drainage of necrotic material may lead to cavitation. Rarely, infection is manifested by foci of coagulative necrosis surrounded by a neutrophil infiltrate.

The chronic organizing form of the disease is characterized by variably severe fibrosis in lung parenchyma and around abscess cavities (Fig. 26–8). The abscesses may or may not retain communication with airways, and there may be focal bronchiectasis. In most instances, hypertrophic bronchial arteries surround and supply the abscess wall.[166] Pneumonia associated with hematogenous spread of organisms is characterized by well- or ill-defined nodules, mostly

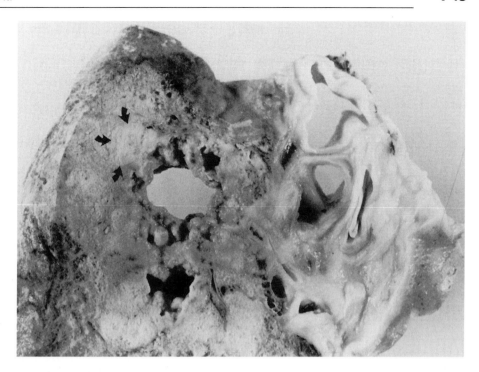

Figure 26–7. Confluent Broncho-pneumonia with Acute Abscess Formation—*Staphylococcus aureus.* A magnified view of the superior segment of a lower lobe shows extensive consolidation associated with multifocal areas of necrosis *(arrows).* Drainage of some of the latter via the airways has led to two irregularly shaped cavities.

0.5 to 3 cm in diameter. Focal parenchymal hemorrhage or infarction is seen in some cases.

Radiologic Manifestations

The parenchymal consolidation in acute staphylococcal bronchopneumonia is typically segmental in distribution. Depending on the severity of involvement, the process may be patchy or homogeneous, the latter representing confluent bronchopneumonia (Fig. 26–9). Since an inflammatory exu-

date fills the airways, segmental collapse may accompany the consolidation; for the same reason an air bronchogram is seldom observed, and its presence should cast some doubt on the diagnosis. The airway involvement is easier to appreciate on HRCT scan than on radiograph (Fig. 26–10). With this technique, bronchiolar involvement is manifested by centrilobular nodular and branching linear opacities ("tree-in-bud" pattern).[166a–c]

In a review of the radiographic abnormalities of 26 adults with staphylococcal pneumonia, 14 (54%) had homogeneous consolidation, 12 (46%) had patchy consolidation, and two (8%) had a mixed picture.[167] The consolidation involved a single lobe in 36% of cases, more than one lobe

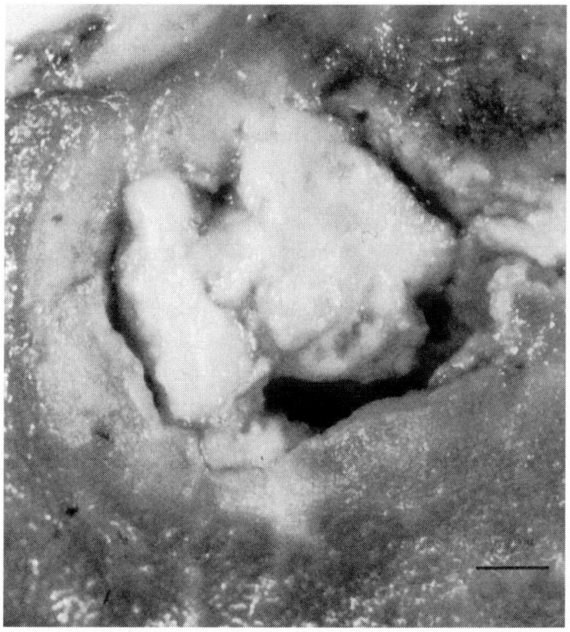

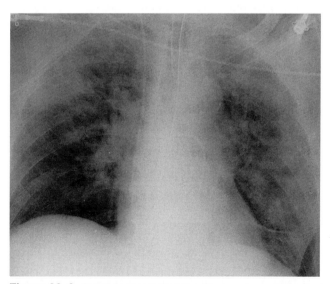

Figure 26–8. Chronic Abscess—*Staphylococcus aureus.* A mass of semisolid pus is surrounded by a wall of granulation tissue of variable thickness. (Bar = 5 mm.)

Figure 26–9. Staphylococcal Pneumonia. An anteroposterior chest radiograph in a 72-year-old man demonstrates poorly defined bilateral areas of consolidation. Sputum and blood cultures grew *Staphylococcus aureus.*

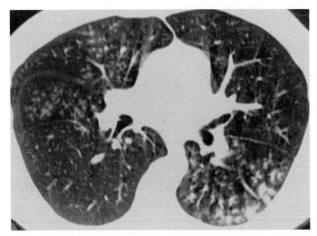

Figure 26–10. Staphylococcal Bronchopneumonia. An HRCT scan in a 32-year-old woman demonstrates centrilobular nodular and branching linear opacities in the right middle and upper lobes and in the left lower lobe. This pattern (which is often referred to as "tree in bud") and distribution are characteristic of bronchiolitis (early bronchopneumonia). In the left lower lobe, the process has progressed to parenchymal consolidation. Cultures from a bronchoscopic specimen grew *Staphylococcus aureus*.

in 54% of cases, and was bilateral in 35% of cases. In a second series of 31 adults, 15 (60%) had multilobar consolidation and 12 (39%) had bilateral pneumonia;[168] the consolidation involved predominantly or exclusively the lower lobes in 16 patients (64%).

As discussed previously, abscesses are not uncommon: they were seen in 7 (27%) of 26 patients in one series[167] and in 5 (16%) of 31 in a second.[168] Characteristically, they have an irregular, shaggy inner wall (Fig. 26–11). Although usually solitary, they may be multiple. Pneumatocele formation is also common, particularly in children in whom the incidence has been reported to be between 40% and 75%.[169–171] In one series of 26 adults, they were observed in 4 (15%).[167] Pneumatoceles present as thin-walled, gas-filled cystic spaces; many contain fluid levels. They usually appear during the first week of the pneumonia and disappear spontaneously within weeks[170] or months.[172, 173]

Other radiologic manifestations of staphylococcal pneumonia include lobar or segmental atelectasis (described in 5 [19%] of 26 adult patients in one series)[167] and, less commonly, lobar enlargement with bulging interlobar fissure.[167] Pleural effusions occur in 30% to 50% of patients, approximately half of which represent empyemas.[167, 168] Spontaneous pneumothorax occurs occasionally; since the complication is associated with pneumatoceles, it is less common in adults than in children.[167]

In pneumonia related to hematogenous spread of organisms, the radiologic appearance is one of multiple nodules or masses throughout the lungs. Sometimes they have poorly defined borders or are confluent (Fig. 26–12). Abscesses may erode into bronchi and produce air-containing cavities, frequently with fluid levels.[174] On CT, the majority of abnormalities can be seen to be in a subpleural location. In approximately two thirds of cases, some of the nodules have a vessel coursing into their substance ("feeding vessel" sign).[175, 176] The majority of nodules eventually cavitate. Septic infarcts result in subpleural, wedge-shaped areas of consolidation, which were reported in 11 (73%) of 15 patients in one series.[175]

Clinical Manifestations

The clinical picture of *S. aureus* pneumonia varies depending on the patient's age and degree of debilitation, and whether the pneumonia is superimposed on influenza infection. In children and adults who acquire the infection following influenza—up to 14 days after its onset[177]—and in the very occasional case in which the disease develops outside the hospital in an otherwise healthy person, the onset is abrupt, with pleural pain, cough, and expectoration of purulent yellow or brown sputum, sometimes streaked with blood. Rarely, primary pneumonia presents as a mild febrile illness with a remarkably benign, almost asymptomatic, clinical course; in two such cases, lung abscesses were present at the time of admission to the hospital (one patient had bronchiectasis and the other poorly controlled diabetes).[178] The clinical features of tracheitis resemble those of croup, with cough, stridor, and difficulty in swallowing.[179]

When the infection develops in the hospital, the clinical signs and symptoms are similar to those that occur with other virulent hospital-acquired bacterial infections. Fever, although not invariable, is frequently high grade. Cough may be dry but is commonly associated with the production of purulent, sometimes blood-streaked sputum.[133, 144] Physical signs include bronchial breathing, patchy areas of crackles, rhonchi, and decreased breath sounds; signs of pleural effusion are usually apparent. Large pneumatoceles may be associated with a hyperresonant percussion note.

Diagnosis

The diagnosis of staphylococcal pneumonia should be considered whenever pneumonia develops soon after influenza or in a hospitalized patient. Culture of expectorated sputum for *S. aureus* is a sensitive indicator of the presence of infection, being found in 92% of patients in one series;[144] however, since the organism may be a commensal, the test lacks specificity.[133] A purulent sputum specimen uncontaminated by saliva will show gram-positive cocci in clusters.[144] As discussed previously (*see* page 716), other techniques may help distinguish colonization from infection, especially in the ICU setting. The white blood cell count usually is elevated to between 16,000 and 25,000/ml and may be as high as 40,000/ml,[133] with polymorphonuclear leukocytosis; however, leukopenia may be present in severely ill patients. Positive results from blood cultures have been obtained in up to 50% of patients;[180] it is important to remember that this may represent either bacteremia secondary to the pneumonia or hematogenous spread of organisms from an extrapulmonary source.

Prognosis and Natural History

Complications of staphylococcal pneumonia include meningitis, metastatic abscesses (particularly to the brain and kidneys), and acute endocarditis, which may develop in patients without valvular disease. Rhabdomyolysis has been reported in one patient.[181] Pleural effusion is fairly common and may be complicated by empyema; for example, in one study of 31 patients with pneumonia, 15 (48%) had effusion, of whom 6 had frank empyema.[144] Given the common association of *S. aureus* pneumonia with underlying disease and

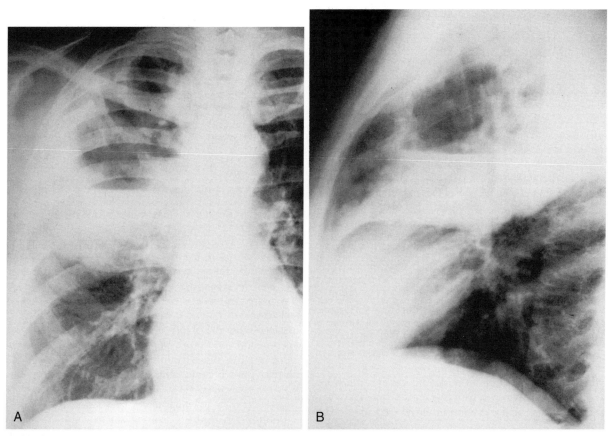

Figure 26–11. Acute Lung Abscess—*Staphylococcus aureus*. Posteroanterior *(A)* and lateral *(B)* radiographs reveal massive consolidation of the whole of the right upper lobe, a large ragged cavity being evident in its center. Volume of the lobe is increased, as indicated by the posterior bulging of the major fissure. Sputum culture produced a heavy growth of *S. aureus.*

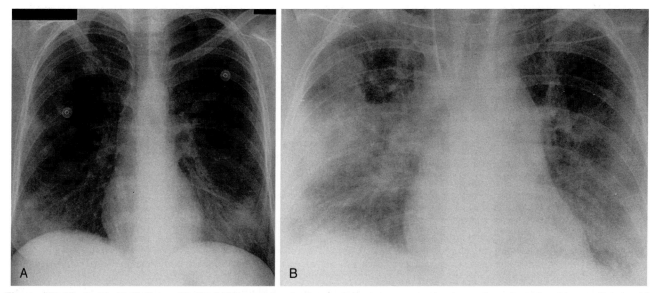

Figure 26–12. Septic Embolism with Rapid Progression to Pneumonia. An anteroposterior chest radiograph *(A)* in a 28-year-old drug addict demonstrates poorly defined bilateral nodular opacities. A radiograph performed 3 days later *(B)* shows progression to areas of consolidation, particularly in the right lung, as well as right pleural effusion. Blood cultures grew *Staphylococcus aureus.*

a hospital setting, it is not surprising that the mortality rate is very high, varying from about 20% to 85% in several series.[137, 140, 142, 144, 145]

Other Gram-Positive Cocci

A variety of streptococci other than *S. pneumoniae* and *S. pyogenes* occasionally cause pleuropulmonary disease. Lancefield group B organisms *(Streptococcus agalactiae)* in particular have been an increasing cause of serious infection, especially in infants; the birth canal appears to be the chief reservoir of this agent,[182] and nosocomial transmission to neonates can occur.[183] Delayed presentation of congenital diaphragmatic hernia, possibly caused by a "splinting effect" of consolidated lung on the diaphragmatic defect, has been noted in a number of neonates infected with this organism.[184] Adults, especially those with diabetes and those receiving antibiotic therapy, are also susceptible to infection with group B organisms.[185] The Lancefield group D bacterium *(Enterococcus, Streptococcus faecalis)* is an uncommon, but well-described respiratory pathogen, both in nosocomial and community settings.[186–191] The use of topical antimicrobial prophylaxis in the ICU setting may be a risk factor for the development of this infection.[192, 193] Reports have also appeared of pneumonia or empyema caused by group C,[194] group F,[195] and *Streptococcus viridans* group *(Streptococcus milleri)*[196, 197] streptococci.

Other rare pathogenic gram-positive cocci are *Staphylococcus cohnii,* a coagulase-negative organism that has been reported as a cause of pneumonia in an HIV-positive drug abuser,[198] and *Stomatococcus mucilaginosus,* a catalase-positive coccus that is a normal inhabitant of the oral cavity and upper respiratory tract and has caused fatal sepsis, meningitis, and pneumonia in neutropenic patients with malignancy.[191]

Gram-Negative Cocci

Gram-negative cocci occur singly or in pairs and clumps and are both catalase and oxidase positive.[1] The most important pulmonary pathogen is *Moraxella catarrhalis.*

Moraxella catarrhalis

M. catarrhalis (Branhamella catarrhalis, Neisseria catarrhalis) is an intracellular diplococcus that is similar if not identical in appearance to *Neisseria gonorrhoeae.*[199] Known for a long time as a commensal in the oral cavity, it has been increasingly recognized as an important pathogen in the upper and lower respiratory tract.[199–203] Although positive blood culture results have been reported in patients with pneumonia,[204] the diagnosis has generally been based on the presence of kidney-shaped, intraleukocytic, gram-negative diplococci on a good-quality Gram stain of sputum accompanied by a heavy growth of colonies on chocolate and sheep blood agars.[199, 200] Some affected patients develop an IgG antibody response during convalescence, which is directed against a variety of surface proteins.[205–207]

Infection usually occurs in patients with underlying pulmonary disease, particularly those with COPD who are receiving corticosteroid therapy.[26, 200, 208–210] Patients who are deficient in immunoglobulins also appear to be susceptible.[211, 212] Nosocomial outbreaks of infection have been described.[199, 213] Clinical disease takes the form of an acute febrile tracheobronchitis or bronchopneumonia.[203] In most patients, the infection is mild; however, it may be severe in immunocompromised patients.[199] Complications such as pleural effusion, empyema, or septicemia are uncommon.[203] Since the majority of organisms are β-lactamase producing, a good outcome has been associated with the use of appropriate antibiotics.[199]

Neisseria meningitidis

Neisseria meningitidis is a gram-negative diplococcus that in disease states is found largely intracellularly. It is exacting in its growth requirements and is sometimes difficult to culture. In fact, it has been suggested that the failure to recognize the organism as the causative agent of pneumonia can be accounted for both by its rapid eradication by antibiotics and by the difficulty in culturing the organism in expectorated sputum.[214, 215] Despite this, the organism can be isolated from the blood of patients with pneumonia without meningitis[216–218, 218a] or from transtracheal aspirates in patients with negative blood cultures.[214, 219] It has also been isolated in pure growth from patients with purulent exacerbations of chronic bronchitis.[220, 221]

Viral infection appears to be an important risk factor. During the 1918-to-1919 influenza pandemic, complicating meningococcal pneumonia occurred in the absence of meningococcemia and meningitis. More recently, most reported cases have occurred in adults with clinical, cultural, or serologic evidence of prior adenovirus[214, 219] or influenza virus infection.[222] Some patients have underlying hypogammaglobulinemia.[223] Young adults in military service appear to be particularly susceptible to meningococcal pneumonia, perhaps because of their close contact with carriers of *N. meningitidis* and the greater likelihood of their acquiring viral infection.

Published reproductions of chest radiographs show a pattern of acute air-space pneumonia, although some are described as segmental in distribution.[214] Cavitation has not been described, but bilateral pulmonary disease and pleural effusion may occur. In the majority of cases, pathologic features are those of typical bronchopneumonia. The typical history is of gradually increasing fever for 2 to 3 weeks, followed by pleural pain.[214, 224] The infection may be overwhelming, with leukopenia, systemic spread, and death within a few days,[225] despite presumably adequate therapy.

Other Neisseria Species

Some commensal species of *Neisseria,* such as *Neisseria sicca,*[226, 227] *Neisseria mucosa,*[228–230] and *Neisseria cinerea,*[231] have been considered to be potential pleuropulmonary pathogens in immunocompromised patients, including those with AIDS.[232] Rarely, gonococcemia has been associated with the development of acute respiratory distress syndrome (ARDS).[233]

Gram-Positive Bacilli

Bacillus anthracis

Bacillus anthracis is a large, gram-positive, spore-forming rod that appears in chains and is encapsulated.[1] Although preventative measures employed in the twentieth century have largely eradicated the disease in industrialized society, isolated outbreaks continue to occur in developing countries, where the organism is endemic.[234–237] The last reported patient in North America was a sheep shearer from Texas, who developed cutaneous anthrax in 1988.[238] The major clinical manifestation of anthrax is a cutaneous or gastrointestinal infection, either remaining limited to these sites or eventually disseminating.

Epidemiology

Spores are found in decaying soil and organic matter in which they germinate under proper conditions and are ingested by herbivorous livestock such as goats, sheep, and cattle. Thus, the disease tends to occur in farmers and others in contact with infected animals, such as butchers. In industrialized societies, anthrax is predominantly an occupational disease of persons involved with the handling of contaminated imported hides, such as in textile, tannery, and wool industries. Cases have also been reported occasionally in people living in the neighborhood of a tannery.[239] Uncommonly, veterinarians and laboratory workers come in contact with active disease and become infected. A case has also been reported in a bone charcoal worker, who contracted the disease from contaminated sacs used to transport the charcoal.[240] Although there is no seasonal predilection for industry-related anthrax, the incidence of agriculture-related disease is highest in summer and early fall.

Pathogenesis

After inhalation, the spores reach the alveoli where they are engulfed by macrophages that pass via the lymphatics to hilar lymph nodes.[241] Here, they germinate into the vegetative form of the organism, which is believed then to pass via efferent lymphatic channels into the systemic circulation.[241] The pathologic manifestations in the lungs and in other body organs are thus related to septicemia rather than to a direct action of the spore itself; as a consequence, septicemia originating from cutaneous or gastrointestinal infection can result in pulmonary effects indistinguishable from those of the inhalational form of disease. The organism produces a toxin complex that can cause edema and hemorrhage in certain laboratory animals, possibly by a direct effect on vascular endothelium, and that is believed to be of importance in the pathogenesis of anthrax-related death.[242]

Pathologic Characteristics

The most dramatic pathologic finding in the thorax is hemorrhagic edema of hilar and mediastinal lymph nodes and of surrounding mediastinal tissues;[243, 244] the lymph nodes are moderately to markedly enlarged. Sanguineous pleural effusion is also common. Grossly, the lungs are heavy and plum colored; airway lumens may be filled with mucus or hemorrhagic fluid. Microscopic examination shows intra-alveolar edema and hemorrhage, typically associated with only scattered neutrophils. Bacilli can easily be identified within lymph nodes and intra-alveolar fluid.

Radiologic Manifestations

The characteristic radiographic finding of anthrax is mediastinal widening resulting from lymph node enlargement.[245] Patchy, nonsegmental opacities may develop throughout the lungs, presumably caused by hemorrhagic edema. Pleural effusion is common.

Clinical Manifestations

The most common clinical manifestation of anthrax is a localized cutaneous papule, vesicle, or ulcer at the site of the initial infection. Adjacent soft-tissue hemorrhage and edema may be massive. Gastrointestinal infection is manifested by rapidly developing ascites and watery diarrhea. The initial symptoms following the inhalation of spores of *B. anthracis* are nonspecific, consisting of mild fever, myalgia, nonproductive cough, and (frequently) a sensation of precordial oppression. Acute dyspnea, cyanosis, tachycardia, fever, and sometimes shock characterize the second stage, which begins abruptly within a few days. Diffuse diaphoresis and subcutaneous edema of the chest and neck may develop, and stridor may result from compression of the airways by enlarged lymph nodes. Expectorated material is usually bloody and frothy. Physical examination may reveal widespread crackles and signs of pleural effusion; evidence of meningitis is present in some cases. Most patients die within 24 hours after onset of the second stage. Similar symptoms and course are occasionally seen in patients with primary cutaneous or gastrointestinal anthrax in whom the organisms become disseminated.

The organism can be cultured on peptone agar from the blood, cerebrospinal fluid, and sputum. However, if life-saving therapy is to be instituted promptly, the diagnosis cannot await positive culture results and must be made on the basis of a history of acute febrile illness in a person with potential occupational exposure whose radiographs show mediastinal widening.

Other Bacillus *Species*

Apart from *B. anthracis,* other members of the genus *Bacillus* are sometimes found in routine laboratory cultures and are usually dismissed as contaminants. Rarely, such organisms are pathogenic; species that have been implicated in human pneumonia include *Bacillus cereus,*[246–248] *Bacillus subtilis,*[246] and *Bacillus sphaericus.*[250] The organisms are ubiquitous and can be found in dust, soil, and water. All are rod shaped and spore forming but are otherwise somewhat variable in appearance, individual species being gram positive or gram variable, small or large, motile or nonmotile. Most cases appear to occur in compromised hosts.[251] Pathologically, the appearance is that of typical bronchopneumonia, often with multiple abscesses and sanguineous or serosanguineous pleural effusion.[251] One unusual case of *B. sphaericus* infection was associated with the presence of a large mucoid "tumor" that replaced part of the left upper lobe and extended into the mediastinum and subcutaneous tissues.[250]

Listeria monocytogenes

Listeria monocytogenes is a short, gram-positive, non–spore-forming, motile rod that grows well on most standard culture media.[1] It is a facultative intracellular organism that is widely distributed in nature and can be found in soil, water, sewage, many domestic animals, and (occasionally) the upper airways, genitalia, or lower gastrointestinal tract of asymptomatic human carriers. Most cases of adult human infection are sporadic and are not associated with an identifiable infectious source. Transmission is believed to occur by ingestion of or direct contact with contaminated food (especially pâté and unpasteurized cheese[252]) or animal products, or following contact with human carriers. Venereal transmission can also occur.[253] Neonatal disease can result from transplacental infection in the course of maternal bacteremia or during passage through an infected birth canal. Ingested organisms pass from the gastrointestinal tract to the reticuloendothelial system of the liver and spleen, from which they spread via the blood to the meninges and (occasionally) other organs.[254]

Listeriosis occurs predominantly in neonates, pregnant women, immunocompromised hosts, and older patients who have underlying chronic debilitating disease;[249, 255, 256] many patients have lymphoreticular malignancies.[253, 257, 258] Despite this, in one study of 64 juvenile and adult patients from Sweden, 22 had no obvious coexisting disorder.[258] In adults, disease usually takes the form of meningitis, frequently associated with septicemia. Pulmonary or pleural infection supervenes in a minority of cases;[253, 257, 259] for example, in one report of 80 patients who had *L. monocytogenes* infection, pneumonia was found in only 6.[260] ARDS has also been a complication in some patients.[261, 262]

Corynebacterium *Species*

Corynebacteria are gram-positive bacilli or coccobacilli that possess irregular swellings at one end, resulting in a club-shaped appearance.[1] They grow on blood agar as small, friable, nonhemolytic colonies with a sheen in reflected light.[263] *Corynebacterium diphtheriae* (the cause of diptheria) is the most important member of the genus to cause human disease. This is typically manifested by pharyngitis associated with a classic membrane that can extend to the larynx, resulting in upper airway obstruction;[264] the organism has not been reported to cause pneumonia. Sore throat is almost invariably present and any nonimmunized person who presents with this symptom and a membrane should have the latter cultured.[264]

Although members of the genus other than *C. diphtheriae* (termed *diphtheroides*) are usually judged to be commensals or contaminants when cultured, some have been documented to cause significant pulmonary disease. In 1976, a strain of *Corynebacterium* organisms normally abundant as a saprophyte on the skin and mucous membranes, was identified as a cause of infection in compromised hosts;[263] it was concluded that the bacterium entered through breaks in the skin–mucous membrane barrier. It was resistant to all antibiotics except vancomycin. In one study, opportunistic bacte-

remic infection with this organism occurred in 32 (11%) of 284 granulocytopenic recipients of bone marrow transplants;[265] the organism was also grown from the sputum of the seven patients who had pneumonia. More recently, *Corynebacterium pseudodiphtheriticum* has been reported to cause both bronchitis and pneumonia in two small case series.[266, 267] Most patients have significant chronic disease or are immunocompromised. Although the onset of infection is usually acute, fever may be absent.[267]

An unusual combination of pneumonia with tissue and blood eosinophilia occurred in a veterinary student that was ascribed to *Corynebacterium pseudotuberculosis,* a common pathogen that causes lymphadenitis in livestock.[268] Occasional cases have also been reported of pleuropulmonary disease caused by *Corynebacterium xerosis*[269] and *Corynebacterium striatum.*[270, 271]

Rhodococcus equi

Rhodococcus equi is a gram-positive, weakly acid-fast coccobacillus that has become increasingly recognized as an important human pathogen since the first case was noted in 1967 and the first series of patients reported in 1983.[272–275] Because the organism resembles commensal oropharyngeal diphtheroids, it is likely that many cases have been missed. It may also be confused with a mycobacterium because of its acid-fast staining properties.[274]

The organism causes disease most often in patients with AIDS; the features of this illness are discussed elsewhere (*see* page 1645). However, it has also been responsible for infection in other immunocompromised hosts[273, 276] and, rarely, in otherwise healthy individuals.[273, 274, 277] Pneumonia is usually insidious in onset and accompanied by fatigue, fever, and nonproductive cough. Cavitation is common.[272, 274, 278, 279] The underlying pathologic abnormality is often malakoplakia (*see* page 724), the features of which may be evident on cytologic specimens obtained by transthoracic needle aspiration (TTNA) or bronchial washing.[280, 281]

Tropheryma whippleii

Tropheryma whippleii is the cause of Whipple's disease, a rare, chronic systemic disorder characterized clinically by diarrhea, weight loss, fever, and arthritis; untreated disease is usually fatal. The organism is a gram-positive actinomycete not closely related to any known genus.[1] Biopsy specimens of proximal small bowel mucosa show characteristic blunted villi with numerous foamy macrophages and clumps of periodic acid–Schiff (PAS)-positive bacilli.

Pulmonary involvement in Whipple's disease has been documented rarely,[282–285] although chronic cough and autopsy-proven pleuritis, pleural effusion, and pleural adhesions have been noted in a high proportion of patients.[286] Abnormalities include interstitial pneumonitis[282] and rapidly enlarging pulmonary nodules.[285] The presence of numerous bacteria-laden macrophages within the media of pulmonary arteries without other significant pulmonary disease has also been reported.[284]

Other Gram-Positive Bacilli

A fatal case of community-acquired pneumonia with abscess formation due to *Lactobacillus casei* ss *rhamnosus* has been reported in an elderly patient with emphysema.[287]

Gram-Negative Bacilli

Gram-negative bacilli are important causes of nosocomial and, under certain conditions, community-acquired lung infection. (The diagnostic approach, epidemiologic features, and prognosis of patients with pneumonia developing in the community or in the hospital are discussed in detail elsewhere (*see* page 721). More than 50% of ventilator-associated pneumonias are caused by these organisms; moreover, when only lung superinfection is considered, they are also responsible for about two thirds of cases.[288–290] Nosocomial pneumonia occurs at a rate of between 5 to 10 cases per 1,000 hospital admissions, the incidence increasing to 30 to 200 cases in patients who receive mechanical ventilation.[290, 291] Although the mortality for such patients is an astounding 70%, it has been estimated that only about one third to one half of deaths are attributable to the pneumonia itself.[291]

Gram-negative bacilli are also the cause of community-acquired pneumonia in approximately 25% of patients requiring hospitalization for their infection.[40, 292, 293] Moreover, such infection is seen in patients who are less likely to recover.[291] The appreciation of the particular risk factors associated with the development of severe pneumonia is helpful in designing appropriate therapeutic strategies in these patients.

Gram-negative bacilli can be divided into three major groups: (1) the Enterobacteriaceae, including the *Klebsiella-Enterobacter-Serratia* group, *Escherichia coli, Yersinia pestis,* and the various species of *Morganella, Proteus, Shigella* and *Salmonella*; (2) the non-Enterobacteriaceae that ferment sugars, including species of *Aeromonas, Pasteurella,* and *Vibrio*; and (3) the non-Enterobacteriaceae that do not ferment sugars, including *Stenotrophomonas maltophilia* and species of *Acinetobacter, Alcaligenes, Burkholderia, Chryseobacterium,* and *Pseudomonas.*

The Enterobacteriaceae

The Enterobacteriaceae are a large group of gram-negative rods, often referred to as coliforms, whose natural habitat is the intestinal tract of humans and animals.[1] The family includes many genera, and their taxonomy is complex and rapidly changing;[1] some organisms are part of the normal flora and incidentally cause disease, whereas others are regularly pathogenic for humans. They are characterized biochemically by the ability to reduce nitrates to nitrites and to ferment glucose with the production of acid or acid and gas.[1] They are oxidase negative. On solid media *in vitro,* the organisms are chain-forming; however, their morphology is highly variable in biologic specimens. Most possess flagella over their entire surface and are motile; several forms produce capsules. Their antigenic structure is complex; however, all species have the capacity to produce endotoxin, whose polysaccharide component determines the O antigen. Other important antigenic determinants are labeled *K* (found in flagella) and *H* (present in the polysaccharide capsule). On the basis of O, K, and H antigens, numerous serotypes can be identified.

Although the Enterobacteriaceae are a well recognized cause of nosocomial pneumonias—accounting for approximately one third of all such cases[288]—their importance in community-acquired infection is a matter of some debate. On the one hand, British authors consider enteric gram-negative infection as a distinctly uncommon cause of community-acquired pneumonia and do not include consideration of these organisms in treatment guidelines.[26, 294, 295] On the other hand, both Canadian and American authors include coverage for Enterobacteriaceae in guidelines for the treatment of community-acquired pneumonia in patients who fit certain clinical profiles.[296, 297] As discussed in greater detail elsewhere (*see* page 722), the risk for enteric gram-negative pneumonia increases in the elderly, in the presence of significant comorbidity, and with clinical and radiographic markers of increased disease severity.[294]

Klebsiella, Enterobacter, *and* Serratia *Species*

Organisms of the genera *Klebsiella, Enterobacter* and *Serratia* are sometimes grouped together on the basis of colonial morphology and biochemical characteristics. The most important member of the group from a clinical point of view is *Klebsiella,* an encapsulated and nonmotile organism that is ubiquitous in the environment, particularly water; it is also found in the normal human gastrointestinal tract.[298] A number of species can be identified, including *Klebsiella pneumoniae, Klebsiella rhinoscleromatis, Klebsiella ozaenae, Klebsiella ornithinolytica, Klebsiella planticola, Klebsiella terrigena,* and *Klebsiella oxytoca.*[299] Although more than 80 serotypes have been delineated, primarily related to K antigen, they are not specified in most cases of pneumonia. The organism is a common cause of serious infection, being identified in more than 10% of patients with bacteremia; of these, up to 25% develop in hospital inpatients with pneumonia.[300, 301] Among outpatients presenting with bacteremia in one series, 7% were caused by *Klebsiella.*[300]

Pulmonary infection may follow colonization of the upper airway. In some cases, such colonization is secondary to ingestion of contaminated food. For example, in one study of 162 patients in a hospital in which *Klebsiella* infection was endemic, 31 became intestinal carriers while hospitalized;[302] infection developed in 15 of these, but in only 11 of 101 patients who were not colonized in this fashion. Moreover, in 14 of the 15 infected patients, the serotype causing the pneumonia was the same as the bowel organism.

K. pneumoniae is the most important *Klebsiella* species to cause human disease. Acute pneumonia caused by this organism occurs predominantly in men in the sixth decade of life, many of whom are chronic alcoholics.[303] In one series of 28 alcoholic patients admitted to the hospital with pneumonia, 11 (39%) had bacteremic *K. pneumoniae* pneumonia.[304] Among patients who developed pneumonia while residents in a nursing home, approximately 10% to 20% have infection caused by *K. pneumoniae.*[305] Chronic bronchopulmonary disease and, to a lesser extent, diabetes mellitus and debilitation also appear to predispose to infection.[40, 306]

K. rhinoscleromatis causes a chronic destructive infection that is usually confined to the nose; rare cases have been reported in which the process has extended into the upper respiratory tract and caused airway obstruction[307] or infection has been manifested as pneumonia and septicemia.[308] *K. oxytoca* has been isolated from patients with both community-acquired and nosocomial pneumonia; the latter cases are often fatal.[309] *K. ozaenae* has been found to be a long-term colonizer of patients with cystic fibrosis.[310]

The genus *Enterobacter* contains motile species but is otherwise similar to *Klebsiella* and can be grouped with the latter in routine laboratory testing. The organism most often responsible for infection is *Enterobacter aerogenes*. It causes bronchopneumonia that is usually nosocomial; the course of disease may be similar to that of less fulminant *K. pneumoniae* pneumonia, particularly in the elderly.[311, 312] A well-documented case of pneumonia caused by *Enterobacter agglomerans* has been reported in an immunocompromised host.[313]

Serratia marcescens is a common saprophyte of soil, water, and sewage.[314, 315] Most infections are acquired in the hospital by elderly, debilitated patients with malignancy, renal failure, or diabetes; the majority have been receiving antibiotic therapy.[314–316] In a few patients, the organism produces a red pigment in expectorated material that simulates blood (*pseudohemoptysis*).[314, 315] A single case of pneumonia due to *Serratia proteamaculans* ssp. *quinovora (Serratia liquefaciens)* has been described.[317]

Pathologic Characteristics

K. pneumoniae usually gains entry to the lung by aspiration of oral secretions, the areas most commonly affected being the posterior portion of an upper lobe and the superior portion of a lower lobe. Infection is usually unilateral and most frequently involves the right lung.

Grossly, the consolidated lung frequently has a mucoid appearance.[318] Homogeneous consolidation resembling that of acute air-space pneumonia caused by *S. pneumoniae* is seen in some cases (Fig. 26–13); a patchy distribution with abscess formation and cavitation may also be seen (Fig. 26–14). Experimentally, the earliest histologic changes resemble those of pneumococcal pneumonia: capillary congestion and abundant intra-alveolar edema that is teaming with organisms and that rapidly spreads centrifugally to involve multiple lobules.[319] In contrast with pneumococcal disease, however, parenchymal necrosis is a common event once an inflammatory cellular infiltrate supervenes; necrosis is microscopic at first, but eventually leads to the abscesses seen grossly. Vascular occlusion can result in the formation of large cavities containing fragments of necrotic lung (pulmonary gangrene).[311, 320] Extension of infection to the pleura with resultant empyema is common.

Pathologic features of *S. marcescens* pneumonia have been described in one report of 16 autopsied patients with pure, culture-proved disease.[321] The findings in neutropenic and nonneutropenic patients differed: the seven neutropenic patients showed extensive intra-alveolar hemorrhage and fibrinous exudate, occasionally associated with hyaline membrane formation; as might be expected, an inflammatory cellular reaction was minimal. In the nonneutropenic patients, the appearance was that of a necrotizing hemorrhagic bronchopneumonia, with microabscess and macroabscess formation.

Radiologic Manifestations

As an acute air-space pneumonia, *Klebsiella* pneumonia shows the same general radiographic features as acute pneu-

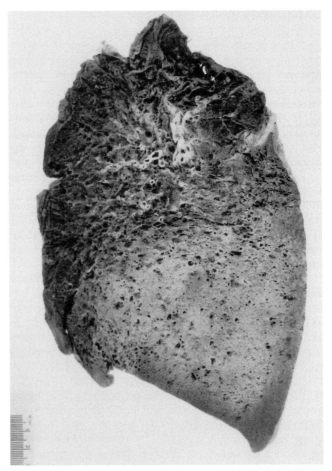

Figure 26–13. Acute Air-Space Pneumonia—*Klebsiella pneumoniae.* A sagittal slice through the mid-portion of the left lung shows severe apical emphysema and homogeneous consolidation of almost the entire lower lobe. Radiologically, the pneumonia appeared initially in the posterior basal segment and spread rapidly over the subsequent 48 hours; sepsis and death supervened. Postmortem lung and blood cultures demonstrated pure growth of *K. pneumoniae.*

mococcal pneumonia: homogeneous nonsegmental parenchymal consolidation containing an air bronchogram. Compared with pneumococcal pneumonia, however, acute *Klebsiella* pneumonia has a greater tendency for the formation of voluminous inflammatory exudate leading to lobar expansion with resultant bulging of interlobar fissures (Fig. 26–15),[101, 320, 322] a greater tendency to abscess and cavity formation (Fig. 26–16), and a greater frequency of pleural effusion and empyema.[322, 322a]

Bulging of interlobar fissures has been reported in approximately 30% of patients who have *Klebsiella* pneumonia,[101, 322a] compared with 10% or less of patients who have pneumococcal pneumonia.[101] However, because of the greater prevalence of pneumococcal pneumonia, lobar expansion in any given patient is more likely to be related to *S. pneumoniae* than to *Klebsiella*. In a study of 150 adult patients with pneumonia, 10 (7%) had bulging interlobar fissures; 8 of the cases were due to *S. pneumoniae,* 1 to *Klebsiella,* and 1 to *Acinetobacter calcoaceticus* var. *anitratus.*[101] Abscesses and unilocular or multilocular cavities usually develop rapidly if the patient survives the initial 48 hours. The complication develops in about 50% of patients

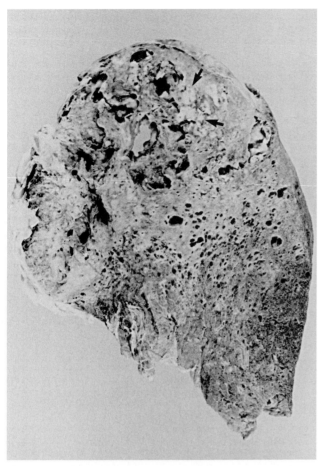

Figure 26–14. Confluent Bronchopneumonia with Abscess and Cavity Formation—*Klebsiella pneumoniae*. A parasagittal slice of the right lung shows extensive consolidation of the upper lobe associated with several irregularly shaped cavities. The white foci *(black arrows)* correspond to necrotic lung. The patient was a 55-year-old man with chronic alcoholism.

and in most can be recognized within 4 days of onset of the illness.[101, 306] Although pulmonary gangrene is infrequent,[323, 324] the organism is responsible for about 50% of reported cases of this complication.[325] Rupture of the abscess into the pleural space can result in the formation of empyema, bronchopleural fistula, and pneumothorax. Pleural effusion is seen in 60% to 70% of cases.[322a, b] Occasionally, acute *Klebsiella* pneumonia undergoes only partial resolution and passes into a chronic phase with cavitation and persistent positive cultures for *K. pneumoniae*; in this circumstance, the radiographic picture closely simulates tuberculosis.

The pattern of nonsegmental air-space consolidation is seen more commonly in patients with community-acquired than nosocomial pneumonia. In series consisting mainly of patients with community-acquired infection, the proportion of cases showing nonsegmental consolidation has been 70% or more[320, 322] (although associated bronchopneumonia may be observed in as many as 40% of cases).[322] In one study of 15 patients with *Klebsiella* infection, 13 of whom were considered to have hospital-acquired pneumonia, consolidation confined to one lobe was seen in 7 of 15 patients, patchy bilateral consolidation consistent with bronchopneumonia in 7, and patchy unilateral consolidation in 1;[322b] none of the 15 patients developed lobar expansion or cavitation.

The CT findings in *Klebsiella* pneumonia with abscess formation were assessed in a study of 11 patients.[322a] Nine patients had nonsegmental consolidation involving one or more lobes and 2 had segmental consolidation; abscess formation was suspected on the radiograph in all 11. Contrast-enhanced 10-mm-collimation CT demonstrated homogeneous peripheral enhancement of the areas of consolidation and central nonenhancing areas containing multiple abscesses 1 mm to 3 cm in diameter, often with air-fluid levels, in all cases. Follow-up CT scans showed coalescence of small-abscess cavities into a large cavity containing sloughed lung tissue (pulmonary gangrene) in 2 patients. Other CT findings included pleural effusion (in 8 of 11 patients) and hilar and mediastinal lymphadenopathy (in 3).

In a radiologic-pathologic correlative study of 18 patients who died of *S. marcescens* infection, the predominant radiologic findings consisted of focal bronchopneumonia in 13, lobar consolidation in 2, and diffuse inhomogeneous opacities in 10.[326] Small radiolucent areas were identified within the opacities in 5 patients; a large pulmonary abscess developed in 1 and pleural effusion occurred in 7. The predominant pathologic findings were necrotizing bronchopneumonia (in 14 patients) and diffuse hemorrhage (in 3).

Clinical Manifestations

The onset of acute *Klebsiella* pneumonia is usually abrupt, with prostration, pain on breathing, cyanosis, moderate fever, and severe dyspnea. Expectoration is often greenish, purulent, and blood streaked, and occasionally brick red and gelatinous ("currant jelly sputum").[40, 306, 327] Malaise, chills, and shortness of breath may be present for some time,[320] but on admission to the hospital many patients are in shock. Physical signs usually are those of parenchymal consolidation, including bronchial breathing, impaired percussion, whispering pectoriloquy, and crackles; breath sounds are decreased when pus in the airways results in bronchial obstruction. Extrapulmonary manifestations such as empyema, pericarditis, meningitis, gastroenteritis, erythematous rashes, and nonsuppurative polyarthritis occur occasionally.[306] The superior vena cava syndrome has been in a young alcoholic man.[327a] Acute renal failure and disseminated intravascular coagulation (DIC) may accompany septic shock.[304]

The white blood cell count usually is moderately elevated; when it is normal or reduced, the prognosis is unfavorable.[320] The total leukocyte count is within the normal range in approximately 25% of patients.[306] Bacteremia has been reported to occur in about 25% of cases.[306, 320, 328]

Pneumonia caused by *S. marcescens* in debilitated hosts is often fatal, particularly in bacteremic patients; however, the prognosis does not seem to be worse compared with other nosocomial infections in the same patient population.[316] The course of *K. pneumoniae* pneumonia may be also be fatal; in one series of 28 alcoholic patients, of whom 11 had bacteremic *K. pneumoniae* pneumonia, all 11 died in the hospital.[304]

Escherichia coli

E. coli is an important commensal of the small and large bowel; antigenic subtyping has identified more than

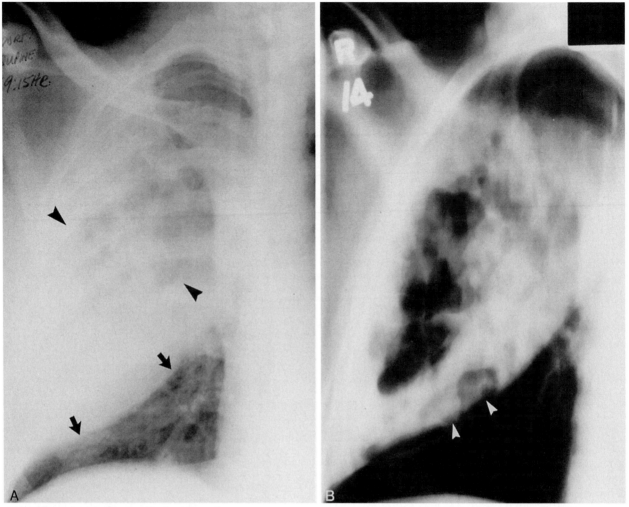

Figure 26–15. Acute Necrotizing *Klebsiella* Pneumonia. *A,* A view of the right lung from a posteroanterior chest radiograph reveals massive airspace consolidation involving most of the upper lobe. Note the downward displaced bulging minor fissure *(arrows)* indicating lobar expansion; numerous central radiolucencies (between *arrowheads*) suggest parenchymal necrosis. *B,* Five days later, an anteroposterior tomogram taken with the patient in the supine position reveals a large abscess cavity with a thick, shaggy wall. One focus of necrosis *(arrowheads)* abuts the visceral pleura, a prelude to the development of a bronchopleural fistula. Subsequent films taken 2 days later (not illustrated) confirmed the development of pyopneumothorax.

160 varieties. Pneumonia occurs chiefly in debilitated patients and (occasionally) neonates, in the latter presumably via aspirated amniotic fluid.[329] The organism is also responsible for a small but significant proportion of cases of pneumonia: among patients in whom this is acquired in a hospital or in a nursing home, it accounts for about 5% to 20% of cases;[305, 330] among patients with pneumonia of sufficient severity to require admission to the hospital, it is the cause of about 1% to 5%.[293, 331]

E. coli often becomes the predominant bacterium in the flora of the nose and throat during antibiotic therapy.[332] It is rare in this location otherwise; for example, in one study of 374 medical and surgical patients untreated with antibiotics, it was isolated from only 4.[332] Most cases of pneumonia are probably acquired by aspiration of contaminated secretions from such colonized airways. A single case has also been described in which acute pneumonia and pleuritis caused by E. coli was thought to be caused by direct extension from an abscess in the lesser peritoneal sac.[333]

Pathologically, the lungs of patients who have died of pulmonary disease generally show severe confluent broncho-pneumonia. Tissue necrosis and abscess formation may be evident, and empyema is not uncommon. As in staphylococcal pneumonia, fulminant cases may show only alveolar edema and hemorrhage, in which are situated numerous organisms but only a scanty inflammatory infiltrate (Fig. 26–17).[334]

The radiographic manifestations usually are those of bronchopneumonia (Fig. 26–18); rarely, a pattern of acute air-space pneumonia has been described.[335] Involvement is usually multilobar, with a strong lower lobe anatomic bias. Cavitation is uncommon, occurring in only one of the seven patients in one series. Pleural effusion is frequent.[336-338] Two cases have been described of massive lung gangrene.[101]

Clinically, the usual history is one of abrupt onset of fever, chills, dyspnea, pleuritic pain, cough, and expectoration of yellow, rarely blood-tinged, sputum in a patient with pre-existing chronic disease. Gastrointestinal symptoms, including nausea, abdominal pain, dysphagia, diarrhea, and vomiting, may be present. The onset may be fulminating, with shock leading rapidly to death.[334] The classic signs of consolidation may be lacking, the sole finding on physical examination being basal crackles; pleural effusion or empy-

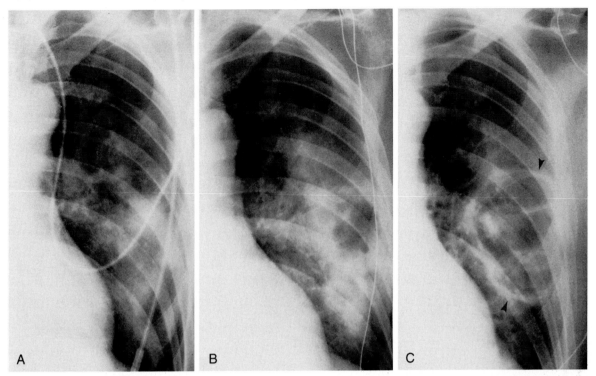

Figure 26–16. Acute Lung Abscess—*Klebsiella pneumoniae.* *A,* A view of the left lung from a posteroanterior chest radiograph discloses a poorly defined area of air-space consolidation in the lower lobe. *B,* Three days later, the consolidation is more extensive and several radiolucencies have appeared, indicating necrosis and bronchial communication. *C,* Five days later, the cavities have coalesced to form a smoothly contoured, multiloculated abscess *(arrowheads).* The patient was a 45-year-old alcoholic man.

ema may lead to decreased breath sounds and dullness on percussion. The white blood cell count may be decreased or may be increased to more than 20,000/mm³. Metabolic acidosis is common.[339]

A presumptive diagnosis requires a predominant or pure growth of *E. coli* on sputum culture; occasional colonies are of no significance, particularly in patients receiving antibiotic therapy. A positive culture from the blood or pleural fluid confirms that the organism is the cause of the concomitant pneumonia.

Salmonella *Species*

Pleuropulmonary infection caused by *Salmonella* species is uncommon. For example, in one review of 7,779 cases of salmonellosis caused by organisms other than *Salmonella typhi,* only 85 (1.1%) were found to affect the lungs or pleura;[340] many serotypes were implicated, most frequently *Salmonella paratyphi, Salmonella choleraesuis,* and *Salmonella typhimurium.*[340] Since this report, only occasional patients have been described.[341–343] However, *Salmonella* has also been described as an important cause of pneumonia in selected populations, such as children in rural Gambia during the rainy season.[344] Infections usually develop during the warm months, although sporadic cases may occur at any time. The disease was much more common in former years because of inadequate hygiene.[345] Patients with disseminated malignant disease apparently are predisposed to the infection.[346] Pleuropulmonary disease caused by nontyphoid strains of *Salmonella* generally occur in immunosuppressed hosts[341] or in HIV-infected individuals.[347–349, 349a]

Pneumonia can occur secondary to aspiration of infected gastrointestinal contents or by seeding during bacteremia. Empyema is most often secondary to pulmonary disease, but may also develop by transdiaphragmatic spread from an abdominal focus.[350]

Pulmonary manifestations include pneumonia, abscess formation, and ARDS.[344, 351, 352] Pathologic characteristics depend largely on the mode of infection, aspiration of organisms causing bronchopneumonia and bacteremic seeding resulting in more diffuse, often bilateral disease possessing a nodular appearance. Suppuration and necrosis may be followed by cavity formation and empyema.[354–357]

Radiographically, the typical pattern is one of segmental bronchopneumonia if the organism gains entry by aspiration;[345] cavitation and pleural effusion (empyema) are common.[355, 356] Occasionally, infection is manifested as an isolated lung abscess (Fig. 26–19). A miliary pattern has been described in cases of *Salmonella* bacteremia.[354]

Clinically, the course of the disease usually is prolonged, with chills, fever, and pleural pain; cough is often nonproductive, but purulent sputum may be expectorated eventually. The peripheral blood may show leukopenia or moderate leukocytosis. A chronic, low-grade infection with intermittent fever and bacteremia has been described in patients who had combined schistosomal and *Salmonella* infections.[358] The species type can be identified by biochemical and agglutination tests.

Proteus *and* Morganella *Species*

Organisms of the *Proteus* and *Morganella* genera are widely distributed in nature and may be isolated from the

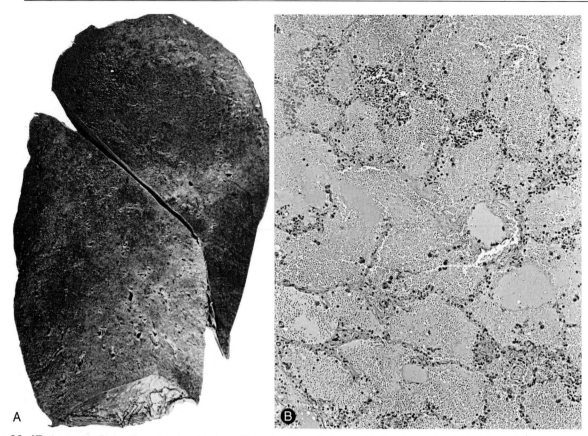

Figure 26–17. Acute Air-Space Pneumonia—*Escherichia coli.* A slice of left lung *(A)* shows extensive, fairly uniform hemorrhagic consolidation of the upper lobe and superior segment of the lower lobe. A representative histologic section *(B)* shows air-space hemorrhage and edema; occasional clusters of inflammatory cells are present adjacent to alveolar septa. Numerous bacilli were present in the hemorrhagic fluid; premortem blood and postmortem lung cultures showed a pure growth of *E. coli.* The patient was a 55-year-old man without underlying disease.

feces of healthy humans. The most common form associated with human infection is *Proteus mirabilis.* Other less common species that have been reported to cause pneumonia include *Proteus vulgaris* and *Morganella morganii* ssp. *morganii (Proteus morganii).*[40, 291] Like *E. coli, Proteus* is more often a cause of urinary tract and wound infections and is only occasionally the etiologic agent of pulmonary disease. A comprehensive report on acute *Proteus* pneumonia was published in 1968.[359]

Both morphologically and radiographically, the picture is one of acute air-space pneumonia similar in most respects to that caused by *S. pneumoniae.* Nonsegmental homogeneous consolidation occurs predominantly in the posterior portion of the upper lobes or the superior portion of the lower lobes; abscess formation is frequent, being observed in five of the six cases in one series,[359] and in five of the eight cases in a second.[337] Infection usually occurs in the setting of chronic suppurative respiratory disease, such as bronchiectasis, or in patients with tracheostomies.[360] One instance of pneumatocele formation has been reported.[361] Loss of volume of the affected lobe manifested by tracheal deviation toward the side of the lesion was seen in four of six cases in one review.[359]

Clinically, the onset and course of acute *Proteus* or *Morganella* pneumonia are more insidious than in other gram-negative pneumonias. For several weeks before admission to the hospital, patients may complain of a general lack of well-being and worsening of the symptoms of any underlying chronic pulmonary disease; as these symptoms become more severe, pleural pain develops, with cough productive of purulent yellow sputum, which is sometimes blood streaked. There is moderate fever but usually no evidence of shock. Physical signs of pulmonary consolidation were present in every case reviewed in one series;[359] moderate leukocytosis with a shift to the left was common.

Yersinia pestis

Y. pestis is a small, somewhat pleomorphic nonmotile rod that takes up stains more avidly at its two ends, giving it a bipolar appearance.[1] Capsules are usually present in organisms seen in living tissue but less often in culture. The organism grows well but slowly on blood agar.

Epidemiology

Y. pestis is the cause of plague, a disease that occurs both sporadically and in worldwide epidemics that have caused tremendous misery and loss of life. Largely as a result of public health measures, these disasters have essentially been controlled, although epidemics are still reported occasionally where public health measures have broken down;[362] in fact, some consider that the illness may be a "re-emerging" disease.[362a] The disease is endemic in many parts of the world, including South and East Africa, parts of

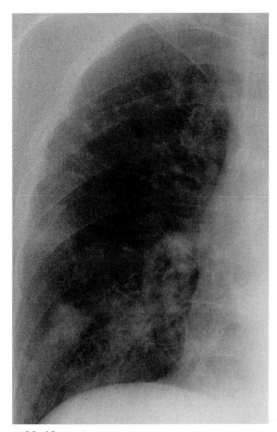

Figure 26–18. *Escherichia coli* **Pneumonia.** A view of the right lung from a posteroanterior chest radiograph in a 36-year-old alcoholic man demonstrates a poorly defined nodular area of consolidation in the right lung. Sputum cultures grew *E. coli*.

South America, China, and Russia, and the western United States. In the United States, 296 cases were reported from 1970 to 1991, mainly from New Mexico, Arizona, and Colorado;[363] of these, 295 were indigenous. The vast majority (almost 95%) of these cases had their onset between April and November; males were more frequently affected than females. Almost 19,000 cases were reported to the World Health Organization by 24 countries in Africa, the Americas, and Asia from 1980 to 1994.[363a]

The bacillus is primarily a parasite of wild rodents, of which more than 200 susceptible species have been identified; however, domestic animals such as dogs and (especially) cats are also at risk. In contrast with cats, dogs do not usually become clinically ill.[364, 365] In the United States, ground squirrels are the most important reservoir. Transmission of the disease occurs from animal to animal and from animal to humans by fleas or ticks (frequently the rat flea, *Xenopsylla cheopis,* or the common squirrel flea, *Diamanus montanus*), that abandon their host on its death. In endemic areas, sporadic disease (sylvatic plague) occurs in people such as small animal veterinarians and farmers or trappers who come in contact with rural animals.[366, 367] Workers at the Centers for Disease Control and Prevention (CDC) have stressed the frequency with which the late diagnosis of the disease in interstate travelers results in fatalities, a reflection of a lack of familiarity with the disease by medical practitioners who do not reside in an endemic area.[368]

Occasionally, and far more ominously, the disease spreads to urban rats (usually the common black rat, *Rattus rattus*) from which epidemics of human infection can result. Although usually acquired from a tick or flea bite, disease can also be transmitted to carnivores by ingestion of infected rodents and (rarely) to humans by inhalation from patients with pneumonic plague (*see* further on) or from laboratory exposure.[369] The history and additional aspects of the epidemiology of plague have been described in detail.[370]

Pathogenesis

Yersinia bacilli circulating in the blood of infected rodents are ingested by feeding fleas. They multiply within the flea's midgut and, with the help of a coagulase, block the entire gut; when the flea bites another animal, organisms become mixed with ingested blood and are regurgitated into the wound. In humans, the initial site of infection gives rise within 1 to 5 days to a local skin lesion, usually on the legs, although this is not always appreciated. Regional lymph nodes become enlarged and extremely tender, and the overlying skin becomes firm and purplish, forming the characteristic buboes of *bubonic plague.* The disease may then enter a septicemic phase with involvement of the lungs (*secondary pneumonic plague*), from which air-borne person-to-person transmission of organisms can lead directly to pneumonia (*primary pneumonic plague*). Rarely, the disease enters a primary septicemic phase without buboes.

Pathogenicity is related to capsule production associated with a considerable resistance to phagocytosis, and to the presence of V and W surface antigens that appear to enable monocyte-phagocytosed organisms to survive and multiply intracellularly.[371] The organism can also multiply extracellularly.[1]

Pathologic Characteristics

Pathologically, primary plague pneumonia is characterized initially by severe bronchitis and bronchiolitis, followed by bronchopneumonia that rapidly becomes confluent to form large areas of homogeneous consolidation.[372, 373] Microscopically, alveolar air spaces show hemorrhagic edema and, in patients who survive long enough, an infiltrate of polymorphonuclear leukocytes and macrophages. Alveolar necrosis is usually prominent and organisms are abundant. Regional lymph nodes are enlarged and edematous. Secondary plague pneumonia lacks the lobular distribution of the primary disease, affecting the lung parenchyma more or less diffusely; however, histologic changes are identical to the primary form.

Radiologic Manifestations

The radiographic pattern is one of nonsegmental, homogeneous consolidation, which may be extensive and occasionally simulates diffuse bilateral pulmonary edema; cavitation does not occur. In a review of 42 cases from New Mexico, the radiographic manifestations in the more severely involved patients simulated ARDS;[374] it was emphasized that in an endemic area and in the proper clinical setting, patients with this type of radiographic abnormality should be considered to have pneumonic plague until proved otherwise. Pleural effusion may be present. Occasionally, radiographic man-

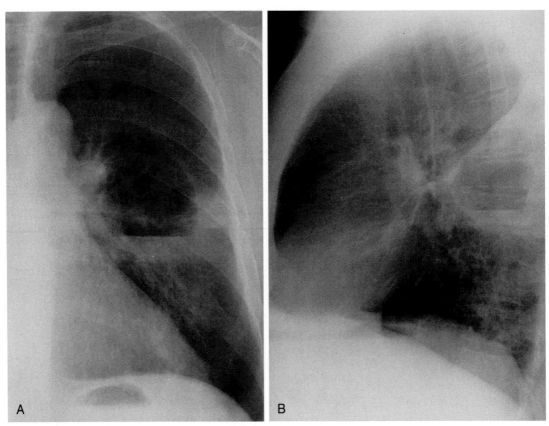

Figure 26–19. *Salmonella* **Abscess.** Views of the left lung from posteroanterior *(A)* and lateral *(B)* chest radiographs demonstrate a large cavity with an air-fluid level in the superior segment of the lower lobe. Cultures from bronchial washings and a needle biopsy specimen revealed pure growth of *Salmonella.* The patient was an alcoholic man who presented with a history of productive cough and low-grade fever.

ifestations within the thorax are restricted to hilar and paratracheal lymph node enlargement.[375]

Clinical Manifestations

Primary pneumonic plague is fulminating, with high fever, dyspnea, cyanosis, and a rapid downhill course. Cough and the expectoration of bloody, frothy material may occur. Pleural pain is common. Most patients have mild to moderate leukocytosis. Terminally, DIC often develops, manifested by cutaneous petechiae and eventually by massive ecchymoses (the Black Death).

The diagnosis should be suspected from the combination of confluent pneumonia; enlarged mediastinal lymph nodes; tender, enlarged peripheral lymph nodes; and a history of contact with rats, other rodents, or cats in an endemic area. It can be confirmed by culture of sputum, blood, or material aspirated from an enlarged lymph node. Antibodies are present during the second week of the illness and may be demonstrated by agglutination or complement fixation tests. If treatment is to be successful, however, antibiotic therapy must be initiated on the basis of an appropriate clinical presentation in a patient residing in an endemic area; it is hazardous to await the results of culture.[376]

Until the advent of antibiotics, plague pneumonia was invariably fatal within 2 to 4 days. Antibiotic therapy results in complete resolution in the majority of cases.[377] In cases reported in the United States between 1970 and 1991, the overall mortality was approximately 15%;[363] for unknown

reasons, the rate in males (17%) exceeded that in females (11%). The death rate of cases reported to the WHO between 1980 and 1994 was approximately 10%.[363a] Public health authorities should be promptly notified of any diagnosis.

Other Enterobacteriaceae

Pneumonia caused by *Yersinia enterocolitica* is uncommon but has been diagnosed in a number of immunocompromised patients, usually by positive blood culture.[378–380] The organism can also be found in feces, sometimes associated with diarrhea and abdominal pain; erythema nodosum and arthritis occur in a minority of patients.[378, 380] Rare cases of pneumonia have been caused by *Citrobacter* species[381, 382] and *Hafnia alvei* (in immunocompromised patients).[383]

Non-Enterobacteriaceae–Fermentative Bacilli

Aeromonas *Species*

Aeromonas species are free-living, gram-negative rods found in fresh water and (occasionally) in reptiles, amphibians, or fish and in soil or food.[1] The three most important species to affect humans are *Aeromonas hydrophilia, Aeromones sobria,* and *Aeromonas caviae.* They are an uncommon cause of human disease, usually in the form of gastroenteritis or wound infection as a result of ingestion of or contamination by infected water. About 10 cases of severe pneumonia have been described following near-drowning.[385, 386] In each case, a brief period of stability postimmersion was followed by the rapid development of severe bilateral pneumonia; there was a high rate of bacteremia and mortality. Acute necrotizing pneumonia due to *A. hydrophilia* has also been reported in an alcoholic patient with chronic hepatitis, diabetes, and diarrhea.[384] Rarely, pneumonia or lung abscess has developed in previously healthy individuals.[387, 388]

Chromobacterium violaceum

Chromobacterium violaceum is a gram-negative, motile, catalase-positive rod that has been isolated from soil and water and cultured from infected animals in a number of tropical and subtropical countries, including the southeastern United States.[389, 390] In 1970, a report was published of fatal pneumonia in two American servicemen in Vietnam.[391] Since then, the organism has been recognized as being responsible for serious infections in several young children in Florida and Louisiana;[389] in three of these, a diagnosis of chronic granulomatous disease had been made and there was circumstantial evidence to suggest that some of the others were similarly compromised. Of 12 children reported with this infection, cutaneous lesions were present in 10 and pneumonia in 6.[389] The chest radiographs were interpreted as showing "unilateral or bilateral patchy infiltrates, cavitary infiltrates, miliary nodules, and pleural effusion."[389]

Pasteurella multocida

Pasteurellae are nonmotile gram-negative bacilli with a biopolar appearance on stained smears. They are primarily animal pathogens, but can produce a number of forms of human disease.[1] *Pasteurella multocida* principally infects animals and is an important cause of disease in domestic cattle and fowl; most cats and approximately 25% of dogs harbor the organism.[392] Infected patients usually give a history of animal contact, and disease is especially common in farmers.[393] Among 1,234 isolates reported to the United Kingdom Communicable Disease Surveillance Centre between 1975 and 1979, 1,004 occurred after animal bites or scratches,[394] in which case the disease usually remained localized. When no history of bite or scratch is obtained, it is assumed that the organism enters the lungs by inhalation.[395] Very occasionally, the bacillus has been isolated from the throats of apparently healthy people,[396] and it has also been suggested that person-to-person transmission may occur.[393]

The organism is an uncommon respiratory pathogen, and its isolation from sputum usually occurs in the presence of chronic lung disease such as bronchiectasis, chronic bronchitis, and/or emphysema.[393, 397] Sometimes, such isolation is simply a reflection of colonization of the abnormal lung; however, occasional cases have been associated with exacerbation of these conditions, presumably by causing acute bronchitis.[398-400] The organism can also cause acute bronchopneumonia[394, 401] (often associated with empyema),[395, 402] lung abscesses[403, 404] and (in one case) Pancoast's syndrome.[404a] Positive blood culture results have also been documented.[392, 394, 401] Two cases of *Pasteurella* pneumonia have been reported in patients with AIDS; exposure to cats

is a risk for such infection.[405, 406] Pathologic, radiologic, and clinical features of any of these forms of infection are nonspecific.

Vibrio *Species*

Vibrios are curved, aerobic, motile rods that possess a polar flagellum. Although they are among the most common bacteria in surface waters,[1] they are an extremely rare cause of respiratory disease. *Vibrio fetus* has been reported to have caused a lung abscess in a patient with malabsorption syndrome and acquired agammaglobulinemia.[407]

Non-Enterobacteriacea–Nonfermentative Bacilli

Burkholderia pseudomallei

The genus *Burkholderia* comprises a group of small aerobic, gram-negative rods that contains several organisms responsible for human pulmonary disease, including *Burkholderia pseudomallei*, *Burkholderia mallei*, and *Burkholderia cepacia*. The first of these causes melioidosis, an endemic glanders-like disease of animals and humans. It is a natural saprophyte that has been cultured from soil, fresh water, rice paddies, and vegetable produce. Human infection originates from these sources by contamination of skin abrasions and (possibly) by inhalation or ingestion.[1]

Epidemiology

Melioidosis occurs principally in rodents, cats, and dogs and is endemic throughout Southeast Asia and northern Australia.[408-411] Sporadic cases have been reported in humans from Papua New Guinea, Korea, the Philippines, Central and South America, the West Indies, the Indian subcontinent, Africa, and Madagascar.[411-414] In some of these regions, such as Thailand, melioidosis is also a common cause of community-acquired sepsis and community-acquired pneumonia.[411] In fact, serologic tests have shown infection to be widespread in this region, most affected people being asymptomatic.[411] In North America, occasional cases have been discovered in veterans from Vietnam,[415] in refugees from Southeast Asia[416] and in tourists returning from Thailand.[417] Although the organism has been isolated from the soil in the United States, cases of infection in people without a history of travel to the usual endemic areas are extremely rare.[411, 418, 419]

In humans residing in endemic areas, infection occurs predominantly in adult men during the wet season, presumably via contact of damaged skin with infected soil or ground water.[408, 409, 420] Other routes of infection include inhalation and ingestion of food contaminated by animal excreta.[408, 409, 421] Although person-to-person transmission generally does not occur, a case in which the disease was apparently acquired venereally has been reported.[422] Laboratory transmission has also been described.[423, 424] The potential for epidemics to occur in nonendemic areas is illustrated by an outbreak in France in the 1970s, in which a link to importation of infected zoo animals was hypothesized.[417] Underlying disease, particularly diabetes mellitus and alcoholism, increases susceptibility to the infection.[409, 420, 425, 426] The incubation period of acute infection may be as short as 3 days; however, the disease is more typically latent, reactivation occurring months to years later, often concomitant with other illnesses or surgical procedures.[411, 427, 428]

The disease exists in two clinical-pathologic forms: an acute septicemic illness with multiorgan involvement and high mortality, and a chronic illness with a relatively indolent course; the lungs are commonly affected in both forms.[411] Although the authors of a review of more than 300 cases in 1957 found that the great majority of patients presented with acute fulminating disease, most cases documented since then have been chronic or subacute.[429]

Pathologic Characteristics

Acute melioidosis is characterized by abscesses ranging in size from microscopic to 2 to 3 cm in diameter. Although they can involve virtually any organ, they most frequently affect the lungs, liver, and spleen.[430, 431] In the lungs, the abscesses are randomly distributed throughout the parenchyma and appear grossly as yellow to tan-colored, rubbery nodules with hemorrhagic rims.[431] Microscopically, there is necrosis associated with a mixed mononuclear and polymorphonuclear inflammatory infiltrate. Organisms are abundant within the lesions and can best be demonstrated with Giemsa's and Brown-Hopps tissue Gram stain.[430]

The chronic lesion consists of stellate or serpiginous foci of granulomatous inflammation similar to those found in lymphogranuloma venereum. Within the granulomas, there is central necrosis that may be amorphous (resembling that seen in tuberculosis) or (more frequently) purulent.[430] Surrounding the necrotic areas is a zone of epithelioid histiocytes, multinucleated giant cells, and fibrous tissue. Organisms typically are difficult to identify.

Radiologic Manifestations

Acute melioidosis is characterized radiographically by irregular nodular opacities, 3 to 15 mm in diameter, widely disseminated throughout both lungs[432, 433] or by segmental or lobar areas of consolidation.[433, 434] Areas of consolidation may be multilobar or be limited to a single lobe and can be patchy or confluent.[433–435] The nodules tend to enlarge, coalesce, and cavitate as they progress;[432] although seldom seen at presentation, cavitation eventually develops in 40% to 60% of patients.[433, 434] CT and ultrasound frequently demonstrate abscesses in the liver and spleen.[434, 435] Pleural effusion or empyema is seen at the time of admission or within the first week thereafter in approximately 15% of patients.[433]

The chronic form of disease is characterized by nodular opacities, irregular linear opacities, areas of consolidation, and cavitation.[433] It usually involves predominantly or exclusively the upper lobes; in contrast with tuberculosis, however, it tends to spare the lung apex, is seldom associated with superior retraction of the hila, and rarely calcifies.[433]

Clinical Manifestations

The clinical spectrum of melioidosis is broad and includes acute fulminant septicemia, and subacute and chronic disease; subclinical infection also occurs in many people.[410, 411] The condition has been labeled a "medical time bomb" because of its propensity to recrudesce with a decrease in host defense following a prolonged and asymptomatic carrier state.[411] Disease may be localized or disseminated. Depending on its acute or chronic presentation, it can imitate other acute or chronic infections, including typhoid, malaria, tuberculosis, and fungal infections.[411]

The onset of acute melioidosis is usually abrupt, but may be preceded by a brief period of malaise, anorexia, and diarrhea. Symptoms can include high fever, chills, cough, expectoration of purulent blood-streaked material, dyspnea, and pleuritic pain. They are followed rapidly by evidence of bacteremic dissemination, including miliary visceral and osseous abscesses. However, the presentation is one of acute pneumonia in only a minority of patients; in most cases, features of septicemia dominate and lung infection is secondary to hematogenous spread of infection.[411] Prostration and death due to shock, respiratory failure, and multiorgan failure follow within a few days.[408, 411, 421, 436, 437]

The clinical picture of chronic melioidosis mimics pulmonary tuberculosis, patients usually presenting with fever, cough that is often productive, and weight loss.[438] Pleuritic chest pain and hemoptysis are frequent. A history of residence in or travel to an endemic area can usually be obtained. In most cases, the lungs appear to be the organ predominantly involved, although many patients also have foci of granulomatous inflammation in other sites, including viscera, bones, joints, genitourinary tract, orbit, central nervous system, and skin.[421, 436, 439–442] Occasionally, patients present with fever of unknown origin without any obvious localizing signs.[411, 443]

Laboratory Features and Diagnosis

The white blood cell count in melioidosis may be normal or may show moderate leukocytosis with neutrophilia. Cultures should be made of sputum, urine, blood, and if symptoms indicate meningeal spread, cerebrospinal fluid. A Gram stain of an appropriate specimen will show small gram-negative bacilli; bipolar staining is seen with Wright's or methylene blue stains.[1] Diagnosis by immunohistochemical techniques has also been described.[444] A positive culture is diagnostic; throat carriage of the organism in children indicates active infection.[445] Special media, such as Ashdown's agar and selective broth, are required for respiratory tract specimens to ensure isolation of the organism from normal flora.[446] A positive serologic test constitutes evidence for either current or past infection;[1] although the specificity of the finding for active disease declines with age, very high titers are diagnostically useful.[445] Use of ELISA on blood[447] or urine[448] samples enhances the sensitivity and specificity of serologic tests and provides a means for rapid diagnosis of infection. Latex agglutination testing of concentrated urine may also be useful in areas with limited laboratory capability.[449] PCR has been used to provide rapid identification of the organism in buffy coat specimens and pus.[450] There is no specific skin test. Most patients respond initially to appropriate antibiotic therapy;[438] however, relapse of infection is common despite prolonged treatment.[411]

Burkholderia mallei

B. mallei is the cause of glanders, a disease primarily of horses and rarely of humans. It has been reported from many areas throughout the world but appears to be controlled in developed countries. The disease can be communicated from horses to horses, from horses to people, and from person to person.

The usual manifestation of glanders is cellulitis of the face, commonly with extension to regional lymph nodes. Involvement of the lungs is characterized most often by acute pneumonia, frequently with abscess formation, empyema, and hilar lymph node enlargement. However, like melioidosis, the clinical picture includes chronic granulomatous disease simulating tuberculosis; it is also possible that the majority of those infected remain asymptomatic.

The disease should be suspected in persons residing in an endemic area who are exposed to horses and who develop oral and nasal ulcers associated with nodules along the lymphatics and acute or chronic pneumonia. The white blood cell count may be normal or low. The organism grows readily on ordinary culture media. Agglutination and complement fixation tests are available, and a skin test using a sterile culture filtrate known as *mallein* is highly specific.

Burkholderia cepacia

The major importance of *B. cepacia* and other multi–antibiotic-resistant organisms is as a cause of opportunistic infection in patients with cystic fibrosis (a complication discussed in Chapter 57 [*see* page 2301]).[451–454] The organism has become an important cause of infection in this group of patients, in whom its prevalence ranges from about 2.5% to 18% in different centers;[422, 455, 456] it has also been identified at autopsy in as many as 55% of cases.[452, 422] Colonization tends to occur in patients with more severe underlying disease.[452] A "cepacia" syndrome consisting of fulminant pneumonia and frequent septicemia occurs in about 20% of colonized patients, including some with initially mild disease.[457] There is good evidence that the organism is transmitted between patients with cystic fibrosis and that its presence worsens the prognosis of those who are infected.[453, 457–461]

The organism is also responsible for increased morbidity and mortality in patients undergoing lung transplantation[454, 462] and has been documented to cause nosocomial pneumonia in immunocompromised hosts as a result of contaminated nebulizing devices.[463, 464]

Burkholderia gladioli

Although this organism may do no more than colonize the airways of patients who have cystic fibrosis, its acquisition in the sputum of six such patients was associated with a fatal outcome in all but one.[465] Patient-to-patient transmission was documented, and there was support for nosocomial infection in the hospital and/or outpatient clinic. The organism has been responsible for rare cases of pneumonia in immunocompromised patients.[465a]

Pseudomonas aeruginosa

P. aeruginosa is a motile, gram-negative rod that may occur as a single bacterium, in pairs, and (occasionally) in short chains. It is an obligate aerobe and sometimes produces a sweet, or grapelike, odor on culture. The organism grows readily on many standard laboratory media, in which it may form smooth round colonies with a fluorescent greenish color; in addition, it often produces pyocyanin, a nonfluorescent pigment that diffuses into the agar. Cultures from patients with cystic fibrosis characteristically yield organisms that form very mucoid colonies as a result of overproduction of the exopolysaccharide alginate.[1] As with other pseudomonads, the organism occurs widely in soil, water, plants, and animals; *P. aeruginosa* is also frequently present in small numbers in the normal human intestinal flora and on the skin.[1]

Epidemiology

Pneumonia due to *P. aeruginosa* is the most common and most lethal form of nosocomial pulmonary infection:[466] data from the National Nosocomial Infections Surveillance System from 1986 to 1993 revealed that it caused approximately 18% of nosocomial pneumonia in adult patients in the ICU.[290] The organism thrives in moist environments such as sinks, water baths, nebulizers, and showers, and many infections are believed to be derived from such sources;[1] outbreaks of infection have also been traced to contaminated respiratory therapy equipment.[467, 468]

A number of risk factors have been observed that increase the likelihood of developing *P. aeruginosa* pneumonia in the ICU, including COPD (relative risk, 29.9), mechanical ventilation longer than 8 days (relative risk, 8.1), and prior use of antibiotics (relative risk, 5.5).[469] Risk factors noted in other studies include the use of corticosteroids, malnutrition, and prolonged hospitalization.[291] Tracheostomy also predisposes to infection, especially in the early postoperative period.[470] Patients with long-term tracheostomies may be colonized with *Pseudomonas* at the tracheostomy site in the absence of positive culture results from the oropharynx; some subsequently develop pneumonia.[471]

Although *P. aeruginosa* pneumonia is generally a nosocomial infection, it is sometimes community acquired,[472, 473] particularly in patients with advanced AIDS. The clinical spectrum of infection is broad in these patients and includes pneumonia that is acute and fulminating or (sometimes) indolent and relapsing (*see* Chapter 44, page 1645).[474–476]

Pathogenesis

As with many other nosocomial pneumonias, that caused by *P. aeruginosa* usually results from aspiration of the organism from a previously colonized upper airway. Leakage of subglottic secretions into the lower airways has also been strongly linked to the risk for developing pneumonia in intubated patients.[477] Colonization of the oropharynx is preceded by increased adherence of the airway epithelium for the organism or by its denudation; in a rat trachea model, the latter situation results in exposure of the organism to a distinct subepithelial receptor.[478] Adherence is also promoted by the organism's pili (fimbriae) that extend from its surface[1] and by the increased affinity for the organism by epithelial cells undergoing repair.[479]

P. aeruginosa produces a number of potent enzymes and toxic substances, including elastases, proteases, hemolysins, cytotoxins, alginate, lipids, and exotoxin A, which promote both local invasion and systemic disease by their inhibition of mucociliary, phagocytic, and inflammatory defense in the lung.[1, 477, 480–483, 483a, b] Lipopolysaccharide derived from the organism's capsule (endotoxin) plays a key role in causing fever, shock, oliguria, leukocytosis, DIC, and ARDS.[1] The role of cytokine expression by alveolar epithelial cells and macrophages in promoting lung injury in patients with cystic fibrosis[484, 485] and the means by which impairment of local defense permits colonization of the airways by *P. aeruginosa*[486] are discussed in Chapter 57 (*see* page 2301).

Pathologic Characteristics

The lungs of patients and of experimental animals that become infected in the course of *P. aeruginosa* bacteremia show a characteristic morphologic appearance.[487, 488] The lesions tend to be situated predominantly in the lower lobes or lower portions of the upper lobes and consist of poorly defined hemorrhagic nodules, frequently subpleural in location, or firm, yellowish brown, umbilicated nodules with lobulated borders; the latter are present throughout the parenchyma but are typically located around small- to medium-sized pulmonary arteries. Microscopically, many of these nodules show central coagulative necrosis of lung parenchyma in which numerous bacteria and only a few inflammatory cells can be identified (Fig. 26–20). In these regions, prominent bacterial invasion of the adventitia and media of small- to medium-sized pulmonary arteries and veins is frequently observed. Although it has been suggested that the parenchymal necrosis is the result of ischemia secondary to such vascular involvement,[489] vasculitis and thrombosis of the bacteria infiltrated vessels are rarely identified, and it is more likely that the necrosis is the result of bacterial toxins.[487] Whatever the pathogenesis, the prominent vascular involvement and coagulative necrosis are characteristic of bacteremia-related *Pseudomonas* pneumonia and, in the absence of a positive culture, provide evidence for its etiology.[490]

The morphologic appearance of pneumonia caused by inhalation of *Pseudomonas* organisms is one of typical bronchopneumonia—patchy, peribronchial foci of hemorrhage and microabscess formation associated with a mixed inflammatory cellular infiltrate.[491] Vascular infiltration by bacteria is usually absent.

Radiologic Manifestations

The radiologic manifestations of *P. aeruginosa* pneumonia are usually those of bronchopneumonia, consisting of multifocal bilateral areas of consolidation.[337, 492, 493] These may be lobular, subsegmental or segmental in distribution, and patchy or confluent (Fig. 26–21).[492, 493] The consolidation frequently involves all lobes,[492, 493] although it tends to predominate in the lower lobes.[337] Less common radiographic manifestations include multiple nodular opacities[494, 495] and (occasionally) a reticular pattern.[337, 493] The nodules usually are secondary to bacteremia[494] but occasionally follow aspiration.[495]

The reported incidence of abscess formation in acute *Pseudomonas* pneumonia is quite variable.[336, 337, 491, 496, 497, 499] In the largest and most recent study, based on a review of 56 patients with ventilator-associated *Pseudomonas* pneumonia documented at bronchoscopy,[493] 13 patients (23%) developed cavitation (in two, evident at CT scan but not at chest radiography). The cavities may be small or large,[492, 493] single or multiple, and have thin or thick walls (Fig. 26–22).[493] Pneumatocele formation was reported in 4 of 56 patients in one series.[493]

Unilateral or bilateral pleural effusions, usually small, were identified on chest radiographs in 16 (84%) of 19 patients in one early study[337] and 13 (23%) of 56 in a more recent series.[493] Empyema is seen in a small percentage of cases;[493] rarely, enlargement of the cardiopericardial silhouette is the result of purulent pericarditis.[502]

The radiographic manifestations of *P. aeruginosa* pneumonia are nonspecific and often difficult to distinguish from those of underlying lung disease, particularly in patients with ARDS.[493] In one study, 18 (33%) of 56 patients undergoing mechanical ventilation and diagnosed as having *Pseudomonas* pneumonia by fiberoptic bronchoscopy did not have any increase in the parenchymal opacities on radiographs obtained prior to bronchoscopy.[493]

A unique case has been reported of an asymptomatic 46-year-old man in whom a solitary pulmonary nodule was observed radiographically to grow slightly over a 20-year period of observation; the mass was finally resected and on sectioning was found to possess a necrotic, purulent center from which a pure growth of *P. aeruginosa* was obtained on culture.[503] Histologically, the wall of the abscess showed only chronic inflammation.

Clinical Manifestations

An upper respiratory tract infection may precede the pneumonia, whose onset is typically abrupt, with chills, fever, severe dyspnea, and cough productive of copious yellow or green, occasionally blood-streaked sputum. Although empyema is common, pleural pain is infrequent. Bradycardia is the rule. There are no special features that distinguish this pneumonia from that due to other bacteria;[466] however, the temperature curve is unusual in that it peaks in the mornings rather than in the evenings.[491] The white blood cell count usually is normal in the early stages but commonly rises to an average of about 20,000/mm³. Eosinophilia has been reported,[491] and leukopenia with neutropenia is not uncommon.[495]

In the bacteremic form of the disease, diagnosis may be extremely difficult during the early stages, and only the appearance of circulatory collapse or the typical skin lesions of ecthyma gangrenosum—lesions that begin as vesicles and rapidly progress to pustules and gangrenous ulcers with undermined purpuric edges—may suggest the etiology. When the disease is secondary to inhalation, the diagnosis usually is made by culture of heavy—sometimes pure—growth of *P. aeruginosa* in sputum. Blood cultures should be made whenever the diagnosis is suspected: in patients in whom the organism has gained entry via the bloodstream, positive culture may antedate by several days discovery of the organism in the sputum.

The mortality rate in ventilated patients who develop *Pseudomonas* pneumonia in the ICU is very high; for example, in one series of 38 patients, 26 (69%) died.[504] Mortality occurring in ventilated patients with *P. aeruginosa* pneumonia is in excess of that predicted by physiologic scores, up to 44% of such mortality being attributable to the pneumonia

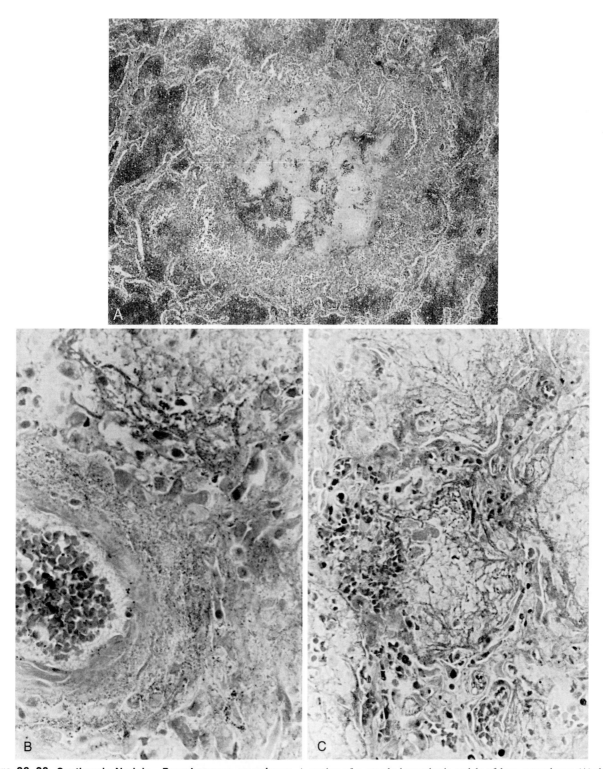

Figure 26–20. Septicemic Nodule—*Pseudomonas aeruginosa*. A section of a grossly hemorrhagic nodule of lung parenchyma *(A)* shows a central focus of coagulative necrosis surrounded by zones of acute inflammatory exudate and hemorrhage. A magnified view of the central area *(B)* show a small pulmonary artery with an indistinct wall and innumerable bacteria barely recognizable at this magnification as minute dots. Note the complete absence of vasculitis and thrombosis. A view of lung parenchyma distant from the vessel *(C)* shows necrotic alveolar septa and few identifiable bacteria. *(A, ×40; B* and *C, ×450).*

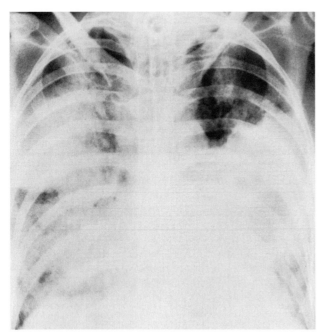

Figure 26–21. Acute Bronchopneumonia—*Pseudomonas aeruginosa.* This 38-year-old woman was admitted to the hospital in a deep coma as a result of an overdose of barbiturates. Several days after admission, an anteroposterior radiograph demonstrated massive air-space consolidation of all lobes of both lungs, the superior portion of the left upper lobe being least involved. An air bronchogram was present in all areas. The patient died 3 days after the radiograph was taken. *Pseudomonas aeruginosa* was recovered in pure culture from the sputum and directly from the lung at autopsy.

and the remainder to underlying disease.[466, 504, 505] Recurrent *Pseudomonas* pneumonia in this setting may be related to a failure to completely eradicate the strain responsible for the initial infection.[505a]

Stenotrophomonas maltophilia

Stenotrophomonas maltophilia (*Xanthomonas maltophilia, Pseudomonas maltophilia*) is a gram-negative rod that is widely distributed in the environment.[1] It has emerged as an important nosocomial pathogen in immunocompromised patients with cancer and organ transplants;[453, 506] it also colonizes the airways of patients who have severe cystic fibrosis.[507] As with *B. cepacia*, colonization by the organism may worsen the course of the latter disease; it is also resistant to many of the antibiotics commonly used in the treatment of cystic fibrosis.[507]

Acinetobacter *Species*

Acinetobacter species are encapsulated, nonmotile, aerobic gram-negative coccobacilli that are widely distributed in soil and water.[1] The most common species is *Acinetobacter baumannii*; others include *Acinetobacter johnsonii, Acinetobacter calcoaceticus, Acinetobacter haemolyticus, Acinetobacter junii,* and *Acinetobacter lwoffi.*[1] Colonization by the organism can be acquired by several means. In one retrospective study, one third of hospital personnel had transient hand colonization with multiple strains of *A. calcoaceticus*;[508] transmission in the ICU was considered to be from

person to person. There is also a significant association of colonization and infection with endotracheal tubes, tracheostomies, chest tubes, and vascular and urinary catheters, particularly in patients in the ICU who are receiving antibiotics.[508, 509, 509a] Although most affected patients are immunocompromised,[510] some are otherwise healthy;[510, 510a] for example, an unusual cluster was reported in three foundry workers, two of whom died.[511]

Although usually considered a contaminant or commensal when cultured in clinical specimens, *Acinetobacter* can cause an acute bacteremic pneumonia that is often fatal.[510–512, 512a] Pathologic findings in patients who die of pneumonia consist of confluent bronchopneumonia that may progress to abscess formation;[511, 513] organisms are usually easily identified. The chest radiograph may show air-space pneumonia or bronchopneumonia; associated pleural effusion or empyema is present in 50% of cases.[510, 512] Appropriate antibiotic therapy can result in complete recovery,[510] although the organism may be resistant to all antibiotics.[514]

Miscellaneous Non-Enterobacteriaceae–Nonfermentative Bacilli

The *Alcaligenes* group includes four species of oxidase-positive, motile, gram-negative rods with peritrichous flagella (present over the entire surface).[1] They may be part of the normal human bacterial flora and have also been isolated from ventilators, nebulizers, and renal dialysis systems.[1] The organisms have occasionally been reported to cause pneumonia[515, 516] and may colonize the airways of patients who have cystic fibrosis.[517]

Chryseobacterium meningosepticum is a ubiquitous gram-negative bacillus that has been associated with menin-

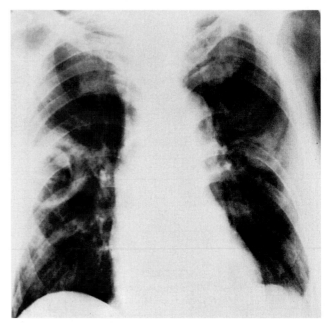

Figure 26–22. Lung Abscess—*Pseudomonas aeruginosa.* This 78-year-old man had an esophageal resection with esophagogastric anastomosis for esophageal ulcer and stricture 10 days prior to this anteroposterior radiograph. Abscesses are present in both lungs, situated in the superior segment of the lower lobes. Repeated sputum cultures revealed heavy growth of *P. aeruginosa.*

gitis in premature infants; it has also been reported to cause pneumonia in immunocompromised hosts.[518] *Chryseobacterium indologenes* has been reported as a cause of nosocomial pneumonia in Taiwan.[518a] Cases of pneumonia with positive blood[519] or pleural fluid[516] culture have been described with *Pseudomonas pseudoalcaligenes. Ralstonia pickettii, (Burkholderia pickettii, Pseudomonas pickettii)* has caused a nosocomial outbreak of infection in a pediatric ICU,[520] which was traced to contamination of vials of tracheal irrigant solution.[521]

Gram-Negative Coccobacilli

Bartonella henselae

Bartonella henselae is the agent responsible for cat-scratch disease, a common cause of lymph node infection in children. Organisms can be identified in infected tissue by the Warthin-Starry stain as very small rods located mainly in the walls of capillaries near foci of follicular hyperplasia or within microabscesses in the lymph nodes.[1] They are found in abundance in developing lesions, but become scarce as disease resolves. The disease develops about 2 weeks after contact with a cat and is usually a mild, self-limited illness characterized by fever and lymphadenopathy. A skin pustule or papule develops at the site of a bite, scratch, or even fleabite 3 to 10 days after the contact. More than 20,000 cases a year are believed to occur yearly in the United States.[1]

Several unusual manifestations of cat-scratch disease have been reported, including pneumonia.[522] Single cases of pleural effusion accompanied by anicteric hepatitis,[523] of life-threatening disease in an immunocompromised host who developed ARDS,[524] and of multiple pulmonary nodules in a renal transplant patient[525] have also been documented. In patients with AIDS, *B. henselae* also causes bacillary angiomatosis, a condition characterized by localized areas of vascular proliferation that may involve the skin, mucous membranes, and visceral organs, including the lungs (see Chapter 44, page 1647).[526, 527]

The diagnosis has traditionally been made on the basis of four criteria: (1) a history of animal contact (usually a cat), coupled with the presence of a primary skin or eye lesion; (2) positive results of a cat-scratch disease skin test (although development of a diagnostic titer may be delayed); (3) negative results of laboratory studies for other causes of lymph node enlargement; and (4) compatible histopathology on lymph node biopsy.[1, 524] Recent identification of the causative organism has led to new diagnostic tests, including serum assays for *B. henselae* antibodies.[528]

Brucella Species

Brucella organisms are small, nonmotile, nonencapsulated gram-negative coccobacilli that are obligate parasites of animals and humans (characteristically located intracellularly).[1] Four species—*Brucella melitensis* (goat), *Brucella abortus* (cow), *Brucella canis* (dog), and *Brucella suis* (pig)—are important causes of disease in domestic animals; each of these can also infect humans. The organism gains entry into the body by one of three mechanisms: penetration of abraded skin, absorption after ingestion, or inhalation.[1] Disease is usually acquired by ingestion of unpasteurized contaminated milk or milk products or by direct contact by occupationally exposed individuals (such as farmers, veterinarians, or workers in slaughterhouses).

Brucellosis is usually classified into three clinical types: acute (malignant) brucellosis, recurrent (or undulant) fever, and chronic brucellosis. Involvement of the lungs is rare in all three types. For example, in one review of 228 cases of bacteriologically proved infection, respiratory symptoms (cough, sputum, or chest pain) were noted in only a very small percentage of patients;[529] minor abnormalities were detected on physical examination of the chest in 34 patients (15%), but none showed radiographic evidence of pulmonary disease. Similarly, in a study of 160 patients with brucellosis who worked in an Iowa abattoir, none showed radiographic abnormality of the lungs or pleura, although 23% complained of cough.[530] Despite these observations, occasional cases of air-space pneumonia and bronchopneumonia, lung abscess, pleural effusion, and empyema have been reported.[531–537]

Pathologic features of bacteriologically proven cases of pulmonary involvement are those of necrotizing granulomatous inflammation similar to that seen in chronic tuberculosis.[538, 539]

Symptoms of brucellosis include musculoskeletal pain, sweats, chills, and malaise. Splenomegaly and peripheral lymph node enlargement are found in about 50% of patients. Hepatitis may be accompanied by jaundice. The white blood cell count is normal or low. Titers of agglutination antibodies are usually elevated,[540] although false-negative results may be seen as a result of blocking antibodies.[1] Skin tests are unreliable and rarely used; they may stimulate an increase in the agglutination titer.[1]

Bordetella Species

The genus *Bordetella* contains five species: *Bordetella pertussis, Bordetella parapertussis, Bordetella bronchiseptica, Bordetella hinzii,* and *Bordetella holmesii.*[299] The first two cause whooping cough (pertussis); *B. parapertussis* causes a relatively mild form of disease that is often subclinical.[1] *B. bronchiseptica* is primarily an animal pathogen (kennel cough) but has been reported as a cause of pneumonia in at least one normal host[541] and in several patients with AIDS.[542–544] The other species have been rarely isolated from humans.[545] All organisms are very small, gram-negative coccobacilli; *B. pertussis* is the only encapsulated one.

In nonimmunized populations, pertussis typically occurs in epidemics affecting infants and children younger than 2 years of age. Although it was generally assumed that the disease has been largely eradicated through immunization, it is now appreciated that immunity may not be very long lasting and that the disease may be occurring more frequently in adults.[546–548] Reported cases to the CDC have been increasing, almost 5,500 cases having been documented in the first 11 months of 1993;[549] since the reporting of pertussis is not mandatory, it is likely that the true number of cases is significantly larger. In 1991 to 1992, a reference laboratory was established in Germany as part of a study to assess vaccine efficacy.[550] Physicians submitted samples from coughing children and their household contacts. *B.*

pertussis was isolated in 601 of 3,629 samples (17%), an astounding result that suggests that the illness is much more common than was imagined. Although the probability of isolating the organism increased with duration of illness and with the observation of the characteristic whoop, approximately 25% of isolates were associated with an illness of less than 3 weeks' duration. There is also evidence that the proportion of older patients with pertussis has increased. For example, in two prospective studies in which the etiology of acute cough in adults was investigated, pertussis was identified as the cause in one fourth of cases![548]

Although the pathogenesis of pertussis is incompletely understood, the organism produces a number of virulence factors that explain some of the mechanisms. These include pertussis toxin A and B, filamentous hemagglutinin, agglutinogens, pertactin, tracheal cytotoxin, dermonecrotic toxin, and adenylate cyclase toxin.[548] Together, these factors promote adhesion of the bacillus to the respiratory epithelium, help the organism evade host defenses, cause damage to ciliated cells, and produce a variety of systemic effects.[548]

Pathologically, the disease is characterized grossly by abundant intraluminal mucus that results in partial or complete airway obstruction and patchy areas of hyperinflation and atelectasis. Microscopically, there is bronchitis and bronchiolitis associated with a mononuclear inflammatory infiltrate. Patchy and, sometimes, extensive epithelial necrosis may ensue, in which case neutrophils may be apparent. Organisms can be identified by Gram stain adjacent to epithelial cilia. Bronchopneumonia caused by superimposed bacterial infection may alter the typical pathologic appearance. Bronchiectasis develops in some patients if airway damage is severe.[551]

In a review of the chest radiographs of 556 children with pertussis, the findings consisted of various combinations of atelectasis (48%), segmental consolidation (26%, usually in the lower lobes or middle lobe), and hilar lymph node enlargement (30%).[552] However, because no autopsies were performed, there is no proof that the abnormalities were caused by *B. pertussis* alone and not by superinfecting organisms. A fairly common but not distinctive feature of the pulmonary disease is its tendency to conglomerate contiguous with the heart, obscuring the cardiac borders.

Acute pertussis is most common in children younger than 2 years of age, in whom the disease frequently is prolonged and debilitating. The characteristic clinical picture consists of a paroxysmal cough ending in a "whoop." The diagnosis may be more difficult to make in adults, since they are less likely to have the full-blown whoop and vomiting and often manifest little more than a short-lived, mild paroxysmal cough. The severity of the disease itself and of its complications appears to have been modified by vaccination and the use of antibiotics. When disease develops in vaccinated individuals, the coughing spasms are less severe and the course less prolonged.[553] Acute pertussis causes moderate to severe lymphocytosis.

Since it is probable that some cases of "whooping cough" are caused by Types 1, 2, 3, or 5 adenovirus,[554, 555] definitive diagnosis depends on positive culture from nasopharyngeal swabbing on Bordet-Gengou medium; this is most readily achieved during the initial catarrhal phase of the illness.[548] A direct fluorescent antibody test is a useful aid to diagnosis in questionable cases; however, culture or serology (especially ELISA) is required for confirmation.[548]

Worldwide, the disease is responsible for a small but significant number of respiratory deaths: although only 23 deaths were reported in the United States from 1992 to 1993,[556] the World Health Organization has estimated that more than 500,000 deaths occur yearly, mainly in children in developing countries.[548] Saccular bronchiectasis was a relatively common complication in patients prior to the availability of antibiotics; however, follow-up studies of patients treated with these agents have found this to be relatively infrequent.[557, 558] In some (albeit not all[557]) investigations, such patients have been found to show a deterioration in lung function.[558]

Francisella tularensis

Francisella tularensis is responsible for tularemia, a disease that is most common in rodents and small mammals; insects act as both reservoirs and vectors. The organism is a gram-negative, nonmotile, non–spore-forming, pleomorphic bacillus that grows best on blood-glucose-cysteine agar. Culture should be undertaken with special isolation techniques to avoid laboratory infection.[1]

Epidemiology

Humans can be infected by several mechanisms, including (1) penetration of the organism into an open sore on the hands while skinning infected animals such as rabbits or muskrats;[559] (2) transmission of the organism from animal to human through the bite of certain insects such as ticks, deer flies, and mosquitoes or directly from cat scratches or bites;[560, 561] (3) ingestion of contaminated water or meat from infected animals; and (4) inhalation of organisms derived from culture material in the laboratory.

The type of infectious mechanism is associated with a seasonal variation in the incidence of disease; for example, cases that develop after direct contact with rabbits and hares tend to occur during the late winter hunting season,[562] whereas those associated with ticks, mosquitoes, deer flies, and other biting insects occur predominantly in mid and late summer.[563] The majority of cases in the United States have been reported from four states (Missouri, Oklahoma, Arkansas, and Utah), in which ticks and deer flies appear to be the predominant vectors.[564, 565] In Canada[566, 567] and bordering states of the United States, particularly in the Quebec-Vermont area,[568, 569] the chief source of infection has been the muskrat, apparently by direct skin contact with moist carcasses. Because of the mechanism of transmission, most cases undoubtedly occur in rural endemic areas; however, a surprising number are detected in cities by astute observers who question the possibility of recent animal contact in parks, zoos, and adjacent wooded suburbs.[569–572]

Pathogenesis

Six forms of the disease have been described, depending in part on the site of entry: (1) an ulceroglandular form, consisting of ulcerated cutaneous lesions and regional lymph node enlargement; (2) a glandular form, identical to ulceroglandular disease but without skin lesions; (3) an oropharyngeal form, characterized by pharyngitis, tonsillitis, and cervical adenitis, that occurs most often in children and probably is caused by ingestion of contaminated water or food; (4) an oculoglandular form, in which the organism causes conjunctivitis and cervical and preauricular node enlargement; (5) a typhoidal form, which is associated with bacteremia and occurs chiefly following the ingestion of contaminated meat; and (6) a pulmonary form, which usually develops as a result of hematogenous dissemination of organisms in the ulceroglandular and typhoidal forms, but may be caused by the inhalation of organisms, chiefly by laboratory workers.[573] Although rare, the pneumonic form has been reported from all areas of the United States, Canada, and Scandinavia. It may be complicated by the development of pleural effusion.[574]

In one review of a 30-year experience with 88 cases of tularemia, it was concluded that the two major syndromes—ulceroglandular (associated only occasionally with pneumonia) and typhoidal (with a higher incidence of pneumonia)—reflected differences in host response.[575] Cellular immunity appears to play the predominant role in host defense; a vigorous T-lymphocyte proliferation occurs within 1 to 2 weeks of exposure, accompanied by the development of a positive intradermal skin test. This cell-mediated immunity is long lasting and is responsible for local containment of the lesion on repeated exposures to the antigen. Humoral immunity appears 2 to 3 weeks into the illness.

Pathologic Characteristics

Pathologically, the lungs show multiple gray-white nodules that may be necrotic and, depending on the stage of the disease, confluent. Microscopically, the nodules show coagulative necrosis associated with a largely mononuclear inflammatory infiltrate.[576] Organisms are typically difficult to identify. True granuloma formation is uncommon in the pulmonary parenchyma but is found occasionally in regional lymph nodes;[576] in one case it was identified in the pleura and was confused with tuberculosis.[577]

Radiologic Manifestations

The radiographic findings are variable and nonspecific.[578] The most common manifestation consists of airspace consolidation.[579, 580] In a review of the findings in 50 patients with pleuropulmonary disease, patchy air-space consolidation was present in 37 (74%) and nonsegmental or segmental consolidation in 9 (18%).[580] Oval areas of consolidation described as characteristic in the early literature[579, 581] are rarely seen today.[578, 580] Hilar lymph node enlargement occurs in 25% to 50% of cases (Fig. 26–23) and pleural effusions with about the same frequency.[579, 580, 582] The former is usually ipsilateral to the areas of consolidation. Cavitation occurs in approximately 15% to 20% of patients with consolidation.[579, 580] Less common manifestations include a miliary pattern, hilar lymphadenopathy without pulmonary consolidation, mediastinal lymphadenopathy, pneumothorax, and ARDS.[565, 578, 580, 583]

Clinical Manifestations

Exposure to the organism is followed by the development of peripheral cutaneous ulcers, enlarged draining lymph nodes, acute pulmonary infection, and/or typhoid-like symptoms. When transmission of the disease is by an insect vector the cutaneous lesion is almost invariably single,[564] whereas with direct contact with animals the ulcers are frequently multiple.[584] Ulcers may be up to 4 cm and regional lymph nodes 2 to 3 cm in diameter.[564] The location of the ulcers and enlarged lymph nodes can suggest the likely vector, lesions on the upper extremities being more commonly associated with mammalian contact and those of the head and neck and lower extremities with arthropod contact.[575] Erythema nodosum is seen occasionally. Hepatitis, usually of a mild degree and recognized by the results of liver function testing, has been reported in some cases.[571, 575]

Pneumonia develops in about one third of patients with the ulceroglandular form of the disease and three fourths of those with the typhoidal form. Rhabdomyolysis occurs occasionally.[585] Two variant strains of *F. tularensis* have caused bacteremic pneumonia in immunocompromised hosts.[586]

Symptoms related to pleuropulmonary infection appear within 1 to 14 days of exposure and consist of high septic fever (temperature usually is > 40° C), chills, malaise, weakness, and headaches. The throat frequently is affected, ranging from simple pharyngitis to ulcerative tonsillitis.[587] Physical findings in the chest are minimal in most patients. The white blood cell count usually is normal or low; however, mild leukocytosis may occur.[565]

Laboratory Findings and Diagnosis

Smears and culture of the organism are generally not contributory, and the diagnosis depends on serologic studies. A rise in agglutination titers taken 2 weeks apart confirms recent infection; a single titer of 1:160 is highly suggestive of the diagnosis when the history is compatible.[1] Serologic cross-reactivity with *Brucella* may occur, and antibodies to both organisms should be measured, the higher titer usually indicating the offending organism.[1] A highly specific tuberculin-like delayed reaction skin test has also been reported;[1] it becomes positive during the first week of the disease even prior to the development of agglutinins. However, the availability of the antigen is limited.

Haemophilus influenzae

The genus *Haemophilus* contains several species, of which by far the most important from a respiratory point of view is *Haemophilus influenzae*. For example, in one retrospective study of 473 instances of invasive infections caused by *Haemophilus* over a 13-year period, 460 were due to *H. influenzae*, 10 to *Haemophilus parainfluenzae*, and only 3 to *Haemophilus aphrophilus*.[588] The organism is a small, pleomorphic, nonmotile, non–spore-forming, gram-negative coccobacillus that sometimes occurs in pairs or short chains.[1] Culture requires the use of chocolate agar, brain-heart infusion agar, or staphylococcal streaking on blood agar, which enhances growth.[1]

Strains of the bacterium are classified on the basis of serotyping that requires a capsular swelling test with specific antisera or immunofluorescence.[1] Encapsulated strains are divided into Types a to f on the basis of antigenic differences in capsular polysaccharide composition. Type b[589] and

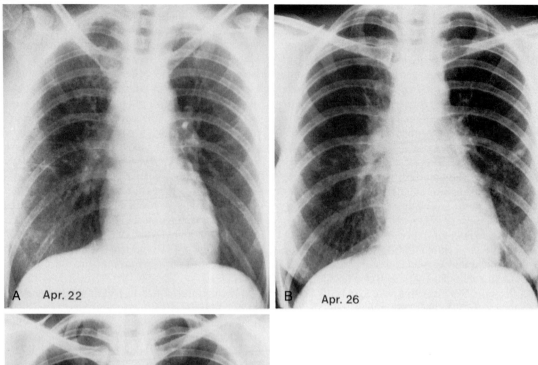

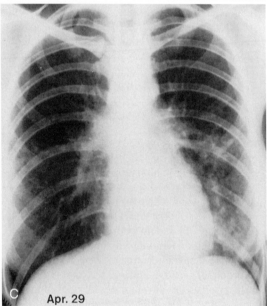

Figure 26–23. Acute Tularemia. Shortly before the radiograph illustrated in *(A)* was made, this 25-year-old microbiology laboratory worker noted the onset of dry cough, right pleuritic chest pain, and low-grade fever. The radiograph reveals evidence of right hilar and paratracheal lymph node enlargement and a poorly defined opacity in lung parenchyma contiguous to the right hilum. Four days later *(B),* the right paratracheal node enlargement had subsided but the right hilum was larger and a few patchy opacities had appeared in the right midlung zone and left lower lobe. Three days later *(C),* the consolidation of the left lower lobe had increased considerably. *Francisella tularensis* was recovered on sputum culture. Recovery was uneventful.

(rarely) Types e and f[590, 591] have been recognized as pathogens in human disease; there is little doubt that they are of greater virulence and are more frequently associated with bacteremia than are nonencapsulated strains. In one survey of *H. influenzae* serotypes associated with invasive disease, Type f was found to increase in importance, accounting for 17% of isolates in 1994 and only 1% in 1991;[592] this may have reflected the utilization of *H. influenzae* b vaccination in the community. Nontypeable strains of *H. influenzae* species have long been considered a cause of acute purulent exacerbations of chronic bronchitis;[593] more recently, they have also been identified as etiologic agents of pneumonia in both immunocompromised[594–596] and normal[597] hosts. In contrast with typeable strains—that can be found in the throats of about 0.5% to 6% of adults[512, 598]—one group of investigators found that throat cultures grew nonencapsulated organisms in 42% of adults.[599]

Claims of a pathogenic relationship in individual cases

have usually been based on the finding of heavy or pure culture from material obtained by transtracheal aspiration[595] or from the Gram stain of such specimens.[600] Additional circumstantial evidence for pathogenicity includes the following experience of some,[345, 594] albeit not all,[601] investigators: (1) antibiotics clear purulent expectoration; (2) antibodies to nonencapsulated strains are found in the sera of patients with tracheobronchitis and pneumonia;[594, 602] (3) an antigen related to *H. influenzae* can be detected by immunofluorescence in bronchial biopsy specimens from patients with chronic bronchitis;[603] and (4) the identification of the organism on blood culture in patients with pneumonia.[594]

Epidemiology

Infection of the respiratory tract by *H. influenzae* is seen in a wide variety of circumstances. Children—especially those between the ages of 2 months and 3 years—are especially at risk. In adults, the organism is usually isolated from patients who have COPD;[604, 605] for example, in one study of 68 patients requiring hospitalization for lower respiratory tract infection in whom *H. influenzae* was isolated from the sputum, 48 had this abnormality.[604] Other chronic underlying diseases, such as alcoholism, diabetes mellitus, anatomic or functional asplenia, and immunoglobulin defect,[596, 606–609] are also important risk factors.

The organism is also a common cause of bacterial pneumonia in drug addicts who are HIV negative,[610] in patients who are HIV positive or who have AIDS,[610–613] in children requiring hospitalization for pneumonia, in adult patients without apparent comorbidity,[26, 296, 589, 614–617] and in the elderly (as a community-acquired infection);[618] in fact, it is responsible for about 5% to 20% of community-acquired pneumonias in patients in whom an organism can be successfully identified.[331, 619–624] In one investigation of patients with pneumonia severe enough to require admission to the ICU, *H. influenzae* was the culpable organism in 15% of those in whom an etiology could be established.[293]

H. influenzae is an important cause of nosocomial pneumonia of mild to moderate severity in patients free of particular risk factors for pneumonia.[331] It is also a significant cause of severe nosocomial pneumonia in patients whose duration of hospitalization has been short prior to the development of pneumonia and in whom no antibiotics have been administered.[331] A review of reports of outbreaks of *H. influenzae* pneumonia in nursing homes underscore the potential for nosocomial transmission of this organism.[355]

Although chronic infectious pneumonia is usually caused by mycobacterial or fungal organisms,[625] commonly cultured bacteria, including *H. influenzae,* may be a more common cause than is generally appreciated. For example, in one series of 115 patients with symptoms of at least 1 month's duration and radiographic abnormalities, *H. influenzae* was identified by quantitative culture of protected specimen brush samples in 53 (46%);[626] two thirds of these patients had significant comorbidity, but one third were normal hosts.

In infants and children, *H. influenzae* can cause meningitis, epiglottitis, tracheitis, bronchitis, bronchiolitis, and pneumonia.[134, 627–632] In adults, the organism has been incriminated as the cause of pneumonia, bronchitis, meningitis, epiglottitis, septic arthritis, pericarditis, and endocarditis.[598, 633] As a pathogen in the lower respiratory tract, *H. influenzae* usually causes acute bronchitis only; however, when it follows respiratory viral disease, particularly by influenza virus, it can cause a typical bronchopneumonia.[372] A pathologic pattern of air-space pneumonia similar to that caused by *S. pneumoniae* can also occur.

In both children and adults, epiglottitis is a serious disease; in adults, there is a high incidence of complete airway obstruction and a mortality rate as high as 17%.[634] Many episodes of epiglottitis are undoubtedly unreported and are likely to be of viral origin, although the virus is seldom identified.[635–637] However, some are of bacterial origin, and it is this variety of infection that can result in rapid, life-threatening upper airway obstruction. In one review of this subject,[634] the authors found 29 cases in a total of 158 in which the cause of infection was identified: *H. influenzae* in 20, *S. pneumoniae* in 6, *H. parainfluenzae* in 2, and *S. pyogenes* in one. Symptoms include sore throat, dysphagia, and dyspnea;[634, 635, 638] stridor and cellulitis or tenderness of the neck may be present on physical examination.[634, 639] The diagnosis can be established by mirror or flexible fiberoptic laryngoscopy and by lateral radiography of the neck.[635, 638]

Radiologic Manifestations

The radiologic manifestations of *H. influenzae* are variable. In 50% to 60% of patients the pattern is that of bronchopneumonia (Fig. 26–24).[77, 640, 641] The consolidation may be unilateral or bilateral[77, 641] and tends to involve mainly the lower lobes.[640] In 30% to 50% of patients, the pattern is that of acute nonsegmental air-space consolidation similar to that of *S. pneumoniae*; this pattern may be seen alone or in combination with a pattern of bronchopneumonia.[77, 589, 640, 641] A reticular or reticulonodular interstitial pat-

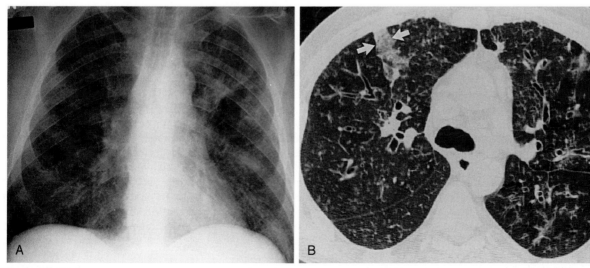

Figure 26–24. *Haemophilus influenzae* **Pneumonia.** An anteroposterior chest radiograph *(A)* in a 50-year-old man demonstrates poorly defined nodular opacities and patchy areas of consolidation. HRCT *(B)* shows that the small nodules have a centrilobular distribution consistent with bronchiolitis. An area of lobular consolidation *(arrows)* characteristic of early bronchopneumonia is also present. Sputum and blood cultures grew *H. influenzae.*

tern, by itself or in combination with air-space consolidation, occurs in 15% to 30% of cases.[77, 641] Cavitation has been reported in 15% or less of cases[77, 595, 641] and pleural effusion in approximately 50%;[590, 641, 642] empyema is uncommon. Rare manifestations include lobar expansion with a bulging fissure[643] and pneumatocele formation.[644]

Clinical Manifestations

Clinical features depend on the anatomic site of infection. In adults with pneumonia, symptoms of underlying chronic pulmonary disease are frequently predominant.[594–596] Pneumonia caused by typeable organisms tends to have a fulminant course, the duration of illness at presentation being only 1.5 days compared with about 5 days for patients whose organisms are nontypeable.[594]

The mortality rate from bacteremic *H. influenzae* pneumonia has been estimated to be as high as 57%, a reflection of the common severity of underlying comorbid disease.[645] Another important factor affecting the prognosis is antibiotic sensitivity: the degree of resistance to amoxicillin has increased dramatically over the years and is now estimated to be present in up to 36% of infected adults.[605]

Haemophilus parainfluenzae

Infection by *Haemophilus parainfluenzae* is rare and appears to have no predilection for any age group.[588] Epiglottitis,[646] lung abscess,[647] and empyema[648] have been described in immunocompromised adults.

Legionella *Species*

Legionella is a family of fastidious, weakly staining, gram-negative coccobacilli consisting of several species that can be distinguished by microbiologic, tinctorial, ultrastructural, gas-liquid chromatography, DNA homology, and serologic criteria. Cross-reactive antigenicity occurs between different species and (occasionally) with other organisms.[1] The use of monoclonal antibodies, latex slide agglutination reagents, DNA probe fingerprinting, plasmid analysis, and restriction endonuclease analysis by enzyme electrophoresis allows for the distinction of subtypes of particular species and serogroups.[649]

The identification of *Legionella* as the etiologic agent of the July 1976 epidemic of acute respiratory disease that occurred in Philadelphia at the National Convention of the American Legion[650] represented the first of many isolations of related pneumonia-causing pathogens over the subsequent two decades. The species of *Legionella* responsible for the original outbreak of legionnaires' disease has been designated as *Legionella pneumophila* serogroup 1. In retrospective studies using specimens of stored frozen serum, the Centers for Disease Control and Prevention (CDC) in Atlanta have ascertained that this microorganism was responsible for several minor "epidemics" in the past,[651–653] including a 1957 outbreak associated with a meat packing plant.[654] Following the recognition of legionnaires' disease in Philadelphia, many common source outbreaks[654–661] and sporadic cases[662–664] have been identified throughout the world.

L. pneumophila serogroup 1 accounts for the great majority of cases of legionellosis; for example, 84% of the

1,005 sporadic cases reported to the CDC in the United States by 1979 were of this type.[663] More than 10 other serotypes of this species have been isolated, either from the environment or from patients (often both).[665–672] The clinical presentation of patients infected with these various serogroups is similar to that seen with *L. pneumophila* serogroup 1: most patients develop pneumonia, which is usually severe and may be associated with evidence of liver, renal, or central nervous system disturbance;[673, 674] occasionally, the pneumonia is mild.[673] When associated with *Legionella* infection, this combination of clinical findings has been referred to as *legionnaires' disease*. A flulike syndrome is sometimes seen, unaccompanied by lower respiratory tract involvement;[673, 675–677] this manifestation is commonly referred to as *Pontiac fever,* since it was first recognized in an epidemic in Pontiac, Michigan.[654]

In addition to *L. pneumophila,* at least 42 distinct species of *Legionella* and 64 serogroups[299, 649, 678, 679, 679a] are now recognized, including *Legionella feelei,*[680] *Legionella gormanii,*[681, 682] *Legionella jordanis,*[683–685] *Legionella micdadei,*[686] *Legionella oakridgensis,*[687, 688] *Legionella wadsworthii,*[689] *Legionella cincinnatiensis,*[690] *Legionella bozemanii,*[691–694] *Legionella dumoffii,*[679] and *Legionella longbeachae.*[685, 695] The last three of these have each been shown to have two serotypes. *L. feelei* has been associated with the Pontiac fever syndrome and only rarely with community-acquired pneumonia.[696] The remaining species have been found to cause pneumonia that closely resembles that of *L. pneumophila.* Although most infections occur in immunosuppressed patients, disease may also develop in otherwise healthy individuals.[697, 698]

Originally isolated from injections into yolk sac or guinea pig, *Legionella* species are now best cultured on buffered charcoal yeast extract (BCYE) agar.[649] They have been isolated from material obtained by transtracheal aspiration,[699, 700] transthoracic needle aspiration,[700, 701] and bronchoalveolar lavage[702, 703] and from pleural fluid,[704, 705] blood,[706–708] and lung tissue.[705, 709] Tissue dilution has been advocated as a means of increasing the yield, presumably by decreasing the concentration of antimicrobial agents and antibacterial properties associated with lung host defense mechanisms.[710] Cultural isolation directly from sputum is not feasible because of overgrowth of oropharyngeal commensals on the media.[711]

Epidemiology

The precise incidence of *L. pneumophila* pneumonia in the United States is uncertain, estimates having ranged from 13,000[711a] to 50,000[712] to 250,000 cases per year.[652, 713] Prospective studies on consecutive patients hospitalized with pneumonia show an incidence ranging from 2% to 25%,[26, 292, 293, 620–622, 657, 659, 714–716] making the organism one of the more common in this setting; as a consequence, therapy for this organism is mandatory in patients with severe pneumonia in whom the responsible organism is not apparent after initial evaluation.[649] Among patients with nosocomial pneumonia, the reported incidence of *Legionella* species has varied from 1% to 40%.[649] This variation depends partly on the techniques used to diagnose the infection and partly on the presence or absence of an environmental source of infection.[291] Whenever *Legionella* is identified as the cause of nosocomial pneumonia, surveillance for other cases should be undertaken.[291] Despite its high frequency as a cause of nosocomial infection in some studies, the organism appears to be a distinctly uncommon cause of pneumonia in patients receiving mechanical ventilation.[717]

Data from seroreactivity studies suggest that infection by *Legionella* organisms is fairly common in the general population, although with significant geographic variation.[652] (Many variables must be taken into account in assessing the significance of the available epidemiologic data. Maximal detection of cases requires culture and the use of direct and indirect immunofluorescent antibody [IFA] techniques. A variety of culture methods are available, some having a greater yield than others [see farther on]. A search for antigen-antibody reaction using immunofluorescence requires appropriate matching and, despite the fact that the great majority of infections are caused by *L. pneumophila* serogroup 1 and that some degree of cross-reactivity exists, antigenic material that includes additional serotypes and species is desirable.)

A seroepidemiologic study in Iowa based on paired sera stored from 1972 to 1977 from 586 patients with community-acquired pneumonia revealed a fourfold rise in titer of IFA to *L. pneumophila* in 4%;[718] moreover, a presumptive diagnosis of legionnaires' disease could be made in about 11% of patients, if an IFA titer of 1:256 in one sample was accepted as being significant. By contrast, in a retrospective study of 500 patients in a prepaid medical group in Seattle, a fourfold rise in antibody titer was found in only 5 patients (1%).[712] The results of serosurveys of the apparently noninfected population vary considerably, probably because some were carried out around the sites of outbreaks of legionnaires' disease and others were not.[652] In an analysis of serum specimens from 4,320 healthy residents of New York City, in which *L. pneumophila* serogroup 1 was used as antigen and 1:64 was accepted as a titer reflecting infection, approximately 24% of subjects were found to be IFA positive.[719] A similar survey of outpatients at the Minneapolis Veterans Affairs Medical Center revealed antibody titers of 1/128 or higher to serogroups 1 through 6 in 143 (36%) of 396 patients.[720]

Legionnaires' disease shows a propensity for older men, the male-to-female ratio being in the order of 2 or 3 to 1.[651, 721] Most cases occur in patients with pre-existing disease. Malignancy (particularly hairy cell leukemia[722]) renal failure, and transplantation are the most common underlying conditions associated with nosocomial infection; COPD and malignancy are often present in patients who become infected in the community.[721] Corticosteroid use is also a risk factor, and many patients are immunosuppressed, often as a result of therapy for prevention of rejection of a transplanted kidney,[662, 724–727] heart,[728] heart-lung,[729] or bone marrow.[730, 731] Virulent organisms can also cause infection in previously healthy individuals; for example, the risk of infection during nosocomial epidemics of infection among hospital personnel has been about 2%.[649] Some investigations have shown a peak incidence in the summer and early fall, a finding that might be explained by the organism's preference for warm water.[732]

Legionella species are unique among the common causes of bacterial pneumonia in that they do not form part of normal human flora, infection occurring in the majority

of cases by spread from the organism's natural habitat, water.[732] *Legionella* species are ubiquitous in fresh water; for example, in an investigation of almost 800 20-liter samples of water obtained from 67 lakes and rivers in seven states in the United States and concentrated 500-fold, virtually all were found to contain the bacilli.[733, 734] When disease occurs in outbreaks, bacteria are frequently recovered from air-conditioning cooling towers and evaporative condensers.[654, 677, 735] The risk of infection appears to be directly related to the extent of exposure to the moisture-laden atmospheric drift;[736] tracer-smoke studies have demonstrated airborne transmission from cooling towers to the area in buildings where clinical cases have occurred.[735, 737] Contaminated cooling towers serving hospitals have been responsible not only for nosocomial cases but also for community-acquired disease in individuals living downwind from them.[737–739] Hotels,[654, 735] office buildings,[677] and even a shopping center[740] have also been the sites of "cooling tower miniepidemics." A temporal relationship has been noted between the turning on of air-conditioning systems and the appearance of the disease.[655, 737] Individuals have also developed legionnaires' disease following the cleaning of contaminated water tanks[675, 676] and exposure to a contaminated decorative fountain.[658]

Domestic water supplies are also recognized as a source of infection from *Legionella* species,[671, 741–746] although the risk from such sources seems to be low.[649] Organisms have been isolated from hot water storage tanks, showerheads, mixing valves, and taps.[741] In fact, *L. pneumophila* appears to have a particular predisposition to flourish in hot water distribution systems.[741] There is evidence that hyperchlorination and superheating of the hot water will eradicate this source of infection.[742–744, 747] Control of bacterial growth requires the temperature of the water to be lower than 20° C or higher than 60° C.

The mechanism by which *Legionella* bacilli reach the lungs from potable water is poorly understood. It is likely that aerosolization of tap water by showerheads,[656, 667, 748, 749] nebulizers,[746, 750] and even water heaters in private homes[751] can produce droplets small enough to be deposited in the lung parenchyma. However, the association of nosocomial *Legionella* infection with potable water rather than sources of aerosolization suggests that aspiration following upper airway colonization is the dominant mode of establishment of infection, at least in this setting.[660, 661, 727, 729, 752, 753]

Reports of the identification of identical strains of organisms from patients and from cooling towers or potable water clearly incriminate such foci as sources of infection;[691, 739, 743] however, such contamination has been seen in the absence of disease.[754–756] Equally puzzling is the ability of such a fastidious microorganism to survive in such environments. A partial explanation for the latter phenomenon may lie in the discovery that *Legionella* species can infect and multiply in amoebae present in water.[757, 758] In addition, the sediment at the bottom of stagnant water distribution tanks favors the growth of commensal microflora that appear to show a symbiotic relationship with *L. pneumophila*.[649]

Epidemiologic and clinical evidence, supported by animal research,[759] clearly points to the lungs as the portal of entry of the bacterium into the human body. To the best of our knowledge there have been no clinical episodes that suggest person-to-person spread of the disease; however, in one study the level of antibodies to *L. pneumophila* in hospital employees exposed to patients with the disease was higher than in a control group of employees that was not so exposed.[760]

Pathogenesis

As indicated previously, the natural habitat of *Legionella* appears to be biofilms or various protozoa within water, and it has been suggested that human infection is in essence a "mistake in the survival strategy" of the organism similar to that of some parasitic infestations.[761] Once organisms gain access to the lungs, they enter the cytoplasm of various cells, predominantly alveolar macrophages, via phagosomes. Such entry may be partly mediated by complement or immunoglobulin receptors on the macrophage surface;[762, 763] however, the observations that alveolar epithelial cells are also invaded and that virulent strains of the organism are 100 to 1000 times more invasive than avirulent strains suggest that bacterial-directed cell invasion is also important.[761] There is evidence that this effect may be mediated by a bacterial heat shock protein, Hsp60.[761]

Once inside the cell, it appears that the organism has the ability to prevent fusion of phagosomes with lysosomes, thus preventing effective macrophage killing; this effect may also be mediated by Hsp60.[764, 765] The phagosomes subsequently become intimately associated with cell endoplasmic reticulum, following which bacteria begin replicating. Once the phagosomes are full of bacteria (after about 10 to 12 hours of replication), the organisms undergo a variety of morphologic and, probably, functional alterations.[761] Such "mature" forms are 10 to 100 times more infectious than agar-grown bacteria,[761] and following cell death, it is presumably this property that enhances invasion of other cells and perpetuates the infection. Once invasion of new cells has occurred, the bacteria resume a "vegetative" form and undergo further intracellular replication.

Despite the protean clinical manifestations that characterize legionnaires' disease[674] and the occasional positive blood culture result,[706–708] bacterial invasion is usually confined to the lungs at autopsy;[766–768] only rarely is the infection widely disseminated and then usually (albeit not invariably[751]) in immunosuppressed patients.[768, 769] The rarity with which muscles, kidneys, gastrointestinal tract, liver, and brain are directly invaded by bacilli has led to the conclusion that impaired function of these organs is caused by an endotoxin. However, in applying accepted methods of assessing endotoxicity of gram-negative organisms,[770] it has been observed that *Legionella* is only mildly endotoxic, possibly as a result of a bacterial lipopolysaccharide with a unique chemical structure.[771] There is also experimental evidence that pulmonary damage is caused by a protease secreted by the organism.[772]

In addition to being a target cell of the bacterium, the alveolar macrophage is also an important effector cell in host resistance. Resistance to infection in experimental animals is related to macrophage activation and the resulting increased ability to inhibit replication of the organism.[772a] Lymphocytes from patients with legionnaires' disease that are challenged with Hsp60 antigen show a proliferative response[761] and produce IL-1β, IL-12,[773] 11 TNF-α[774] and interferon,[775] substances that are important in defense against the organism.[649]

Th-1 helper cells are particularly important in this cellular immune response.[772a] Although antibodies enhance opsonization of the microbe,[776] disease has occurred in patients with pre-existing antibodies, an effect that is not surprising considering the apparent invasive properties of the bacterium. The role of neutrophils in containing the infection is unclear; however, neutropenia does not appear to be associated with an increased risk of pneumonia.[649]

Pathologic Characteristics

Pathologic features of pneumonia due to *Legionella species* have been described in several reports.[777–784] Grossly, the typical appearance is that of a bronchopneumonia, which, when seen in autopsy specimens, is usually extensive and confluent. Occasionally, the pattern resembles acute air-space pneumonia. Macroscopic abscess formation has been noted in almost 25% of cases in some series.[780]

Microscopically, alveolar air spaces are more or less uniformly filled with a mixture of polymorphonuclear leukocytes, red blood cells, macrophages, fibrin, and necrotic debris; leukocytoclasis is typically prominent (Fig. 26–25). Alveolar septa can often be identified surrounding the exudate, but in some foci are themselves necrotic. Vasculitis and thrombosis of small vessels can occur. Some cases also show features of diffuse alveolar damage; however, in many of these there are complicating factors such as shock or oxygen therapy, which may explain this histologic reaction. Organizing pneumonia and interstitial fibrosis are seen in patients who have protracted or clinically resolved infection.[782, 783, 785]

Although the identification of gram-negative coccobacilli in respiratory secretions or tissue may be an important clue to the diagnosis,[706, 786] the organisms are seen to better advantage in lung specimens stained by the Gimenez or Dieterle silver impregnation techniques.[787] *L. micdadei* can be mildly acid-fast when stained by the Ziehl-Neelsen method.[686] and may also be identified with the Wolbach modification of the Giemsa stain.[788] Despite these reactions, the most reliable method of identifying *Legionella* is by direct immunofluorescent or immunohistochemical staining of respiratory tract secretions, TTNA, or tissue.[711, 789, 790]

Radiologic Manifestations

Acute *Legionella* pneumonia is usually accompanied by an abnormal chest radiograph, whether the illness develops in association with an outbreak[791] or sporadically.[662] For example, in the original Philadelphia outbreak, chest radiographs were abnormal in 90% of 182 patients with the disease.[791] Moreover, of the 1,005 cases of sporadic legionellosis reported in the United States by 1981, 984 had radiographically documented pneumonia;[662] of the remainder, three patients were reported to have had normal chest radiographs and the rest had not had radiographs taken.

The characteristic radiographic pattern is one of nonsegmental air-space consolidation that is initially peripheral and sublobar, similar to that seen in acute *S. pneumoniae* pneumonia (Fig. 26–26). In many cases, the area of consolidation subsequently enlarges to occupy all or a large portion of a lobe, or to involve contiguous lobes on the ipsilateral side.[724, 792–796] Progression of the pneumonia is usually

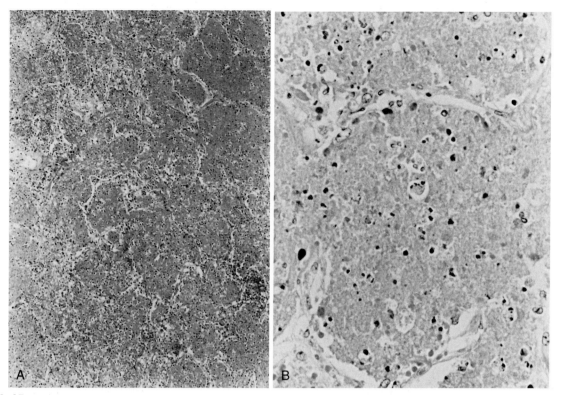

Figure 26–25. Acute Legionnaires' Disease. Alveolar septa are identifiable but poorly defined and focally necrotic. Air spaces are completely filled by amorphous proteinaceous debris containing macrophages and polymorphonuclear leukocytes. (*A* ×80; *B* ×250.)

rapid,[792] most of a lobe becoming involved within 3 or 4 days, often despite the institution of appropriate antibiotic therapy (*see* Fig. 26–26),[793] a behavior that is seldom seen in acute air-space pneumonia caused by *S. pneumoniae.*[724, 794, 797]

There is a tendency to bilateral involvement as the disease progresses; thus, of the 24 patients reported in one series,[792] the pneumonia was unilateral in 68% at the onset but was bilateral in 65% at the peak of the disease (ten days after the first occurrence of symptoms). In two other series, one with 61 patients,[724] and the other with 34,[795] 50% were found to have bilateral involvement at some time in their illness. A distinct lower lobe predilection has been reported in several[724, 798–800] (albeit not in all[801, 802]) series. No difference has been found in the radiographic findings between community-acquired and nosocomial infection.[796, 803]

In immunocompetent patients, abscess formation with subsequent cavitation is surprisingly infrequent.[804–809] For example, cavitation was identified in only 3 (4%) of 70 cases in one series[810] and 9 (6%) of 154 in a second.[796] In the latter study, there was no difference in the prevalence of abscess formation between nosocomial (7 of 122 cases) and community-acquired (2 of 32 cases) pneumonia.[796] On the other hand, cavitation is seen fairly frequently in immuno-compromised patients;[811–817] for example, in one series of the 10 patients who had received renal transplants, it was identified in 7, the interval between the first evidence of infection and cavitation ranging from 4 to 14 days (Fig. 26–27).[816] Pleural effusion may occur at the peak of the illness, as in 35% to 63% of cases in two series.[724, 795] Hilar lymph node enlargement,[800, 818] lobar expansion, and hydropneumotho-rax[819] are rare manifestations.

Occasionally, the focus of pneumonia is round, simulat-ing a pulmonary mass (Fig. 26–28).[820] Single or multiple nodules, which sometimes undergo rapid growth, may also be seen in addition to consolidation involving part or all of one or more lobes.[821] Most investigators have found the radiographic pattern associated with infection by various *Legionella* species to be similar to that of *L. pneumophila* (Fig. 26–29).[686, 691, 789, 822, 823]

Although radiographic resolution may be fairly rapid with appropriate therapy,[724, 793] it is often prolonged; for example, in one group of 10 patients reported from Great Britain, it took up to 8 weeks, with a mean of 5 weeks.[824] Radiographic resolution tends to lag far behind clinical im-provement.[825]

Clinical Manifestations

Infection by *Legionella* species usually causes pneu-monia; rarely, the clinical picture simulates an influenza-like illness (Pontiac fever) and is unassociated with radiographic evidence of pleuropulmonary involvement. In cases of pneu-monia, the incubation period has been estimated to range from 2 to 10 days;[651, 652] occasionally, an interval of 2 weeks has been documented between exposure and diagnosis.[724] Many patients with community-acquired disease are asymp-tomatic, the infection being documented by elevated anti-body titers in individuals with no history of pneumonia.[720, 826, 827] When symptoms are present, the typical patient is a middle-aged man with underlying COPD who presents dur-ing the period of June to October.[651, 652, 662, 721]

The severity of disease varies from a mild respiratory illness to fulminating infection.[649] Although some symptoms and signs are typical of legionellosis, none reliably distin-

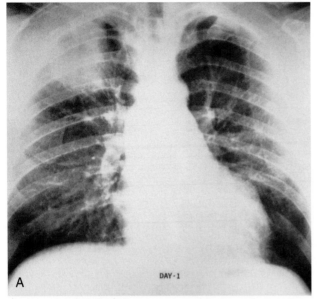

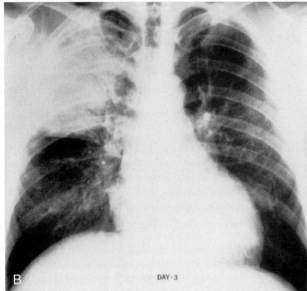

Figure 26–26. Acute Legionnaires' Pneumonia. On the day of admission of this 69-year-old man, a posteroanterior radiograph *(A)* revealed homogeneous consolidation of the axillary portion of the right upper lobe; an air bronchogram was clearly apparent. Radiographs 2 days later *(B)* showed marked worsening. *Legionella pneumophila* was recovered from the sputum.

guishes pneumonia by this agent from that caused by other community-acquired or nosocomial organisms.[649, 732] The usual presenting symptoms are fever (sometimes high and unremitting[663, 724]), malaise, myalgia, rigors, confusion, headaches, and diarrhea. The most common respiratory complaints are a nonproductive cough without prior upper respiratory tract symptoms and, as the pneumonia progresses, dyspnea.[673, 724, 828] In time, cough may become productive and can be associated with hemoptysis. Pleural pain develops in about one third of patients;[724] however, primary empyema is uncommon.[829] The combination of acute pleural pain and hemoptysis may suggest a diagnosis of pulmonary thromboembolism.[789] ARDS occurs as a complication of the infection in some cases.[830]

In patients who survive, fever has been shown to break by lysis, even when there is an adequate response to antibiotics.[791] Fever may persist for more than 2 weeks, and the chest radiograph usually does not begin to clear until the end of the second week.[651] *Legionella* pneumonia shows a greater tendency to organize than do other bacterial pneumonias,[831, 832] and patients may be left with some diminution in respiratory reserve and a reduction in diffusing capacity.[834, 835]

Symptoms reflecting involvement of other sites, notably the gastrointestinal tract, kidney, and central nervous systems, are more common in legionnaires' disease than in pneumonia caused by other microorganisms. Hyponatremia, a high creatine phosphokinase (as a result of rhabdomyolysis), the failure to respond to a β-lactam antibiotic, and the presence of diarrhea and headache are features that should suggest the diagnosis.[649, 833] Although hyponatremia is common,[715, 836] being identified in 50% of patients in one large series,[724] rhabdomyolysis, myoglobinuria, and consequent acute renal failure (unassociated with evidence of bacterial invasion of muscle) are rare.[766, 837, 838]

Patients may complain of watery diarrhea and (occasionally) abdominal pain. Hematuria and proteinuria may be present;[521, 674, 839] renal failure is usually (but not always[840, 841]) associated with shock.[673] Bilirubin levels may be elevated and liver function may be disturbed.[673, 674, 724, 839] Many patients become confused and even obtunded;[673, 674, 724, 828] in addition to this encephalopathy, other neurologic disturbances include cerebellar dysfunction,[834, 842, 843] peripheral neuropathy,[844] and neurogenic bladder.[843] In such patients, autopsy rarely reveals organisms within the central nervous

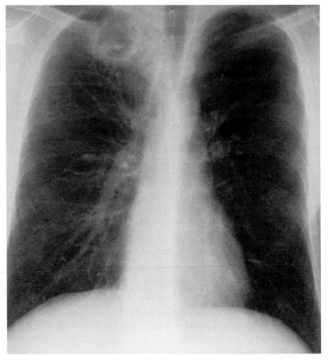

Figure 26–27. *Legionella pneumophila*—**Abscess Formation.** A posteroanterior chest radiograph in a 25-year-old renal transplant patient demonstrates a 3-cm-diameter cavity in the right lung apex. Cultures of a fine-needle aspiration specimen revealed *L. pneumophila*. The abnormality resolved following treatment with antibiotics.

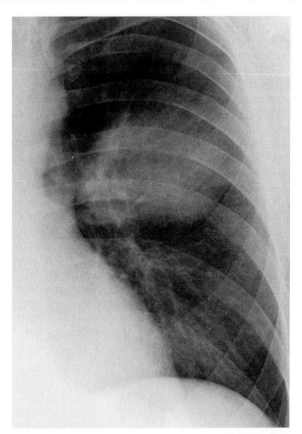

Figure 26–28. Round Pneumonia due to *Legionella pneumophila.* A view of the left lung from a posteroanterior chest radiograph in a 34-year-old man demonstrates a round area of consolidation. The patient presented with a 3-day history of fever and pleuritic chest pain. Sputum cultures grew *L. pneumophila.* The findings resolved within 2 weeks following treatment with erythromycin.

system and, in most cases, cerebrospinal fluid pressure is not elevated. Pericarditis,[845–848] myocarditis,[849] skin rash,[850, 851] pancreatitis, and retinitis[847] are additional occasional complications.

Laboratory Findings and Diagnosis

The white blood cell count is usually below 15,000/mm[3] with a shift to the left; in one review of 61 patients, it was higher than 14,000/mm[3] in 50% of patients.[724] Lymphopenia is frequent, the count often being 1,000/mm[3] or less.[791] As indicated previously, muscle and liver enzyme levels may be elevated. Cold agglutinins have been found rarely.[852] Autoimmune hemolytic anemia,[853] thrombocytopenic purpura,[854] and DIC[855] are also seen in some patients.

Confirmation of the diagnosis requires positive culture, positive direct (DFA) or indirect (IFA) immunofluorescent testing, a positive hemagglutination test for antibody, or the detection of antigen by DNA probe or radioimmunoassay. Confidence in the diagnosis will obviously increase when more than one test yields a positive result. Since the organism is not part of the normal human flora, a positive culture, with few exceptions, confirms infection.[1] However, careful handling of the specimen is required, and the sensitivity of culture for diagnosis has ranged from about 10% to 60%.[607, 649, 711a] Sensitivity is higher in specimens obtained from the

lower respiratory tract; for example, culture of BAL fluid has confirmed the diagnosis in up to 78% of cases.[649] DFA can be used for testing respiratory tract secretions, pleural fluid, or lung tissue; however, although fairly specific, it lacks sensitivity.[711, 856, 857] In addition, there has been one report of a "pseudoepidemic" secondary to contamination of DFA reagents.[858] Occasional false-positive results have also been reported even with newer monoclonal antibody reagents.[649]

IFA is the serologic technique that has been employed to identify most cases of legionellosis. However, although useful in epidemiologic studies, the inherent delay in achieving diagnosis makes it of little value in direct clinical care. The overall ability to detect *Legionella* infection varies with the particular type and number of antibodies used, the inclusion of those directed to a number of serogroups of *L. pneumophila* as well as other *Legionella* species obviously augmenting the yield of positive diagnosis. Demonstration of a fourfold rise in antibody to a titer of at least 1:128 between acute and convalescent phase sera (seroconversion) is generally considered necessary for confirmation of infection.[651] A titer of 1:256 on a single specimen has also been accepted by some as presumptive evidence of infection in the presence of an appropriate clinical illness, at least in epidemic situations.

Seroconversion occurs within 3 weeks of infection in 60% to 90% of culture-proven cases; for example, a follow-up study in 1978 of the surviving patients from the 1976 Philadelphia epidemic revealed 94% of patients to have significant antibody levels.[826] The sensitivity of IFA is approximately 90%;[651] however, as a result of cross-reactivity with other organisms, the specificity is somewhat less.[652, 711, 859–861] A microagglutination test, which employs heat-killed antigen, is simple, sensitive, and apparently specific.[651, 862, 863] Good results have also been obtained using ELISA methods, which are mainly used to detect antigen in urine specimens. The sensitivity of both ELISA and microagglutination tests is about 80%, and there is high specificity for the diagnosis of *L. pneumophila* serogroup 1.[864–868] DNA probes have also been developed but, to date, are associated with sensitivities and specificities similar to those with DFA.[649, 869–871] Unfortunately, a negative result cannot exclude infection in the individual patient with any of these tests.

Prognosis and Natural History

Pneumonia caused by *Legionella* species is a serious disease: approximately one third of patients require assisted ventilation, and many die. In four autopsy studies of consecutive patients with pneumonia in which DFA staining was used for diagnosis, *Legionella* species was found to be the etiologic agent in 1% to 6.6% of cases.[779, 872–874] Since most of these patients were compromised hosts, any extension of the findings to arrive at a national incidence of mortality of *L. pneumophila* pneumonia is probably unwarranted. Despite this, the mortality rate in patients is certainly significant, having been reported to range from 10% to 25%,[652, 662, 713, 875] with an overall rate of about 20%.[296] However, when erythromycin therapy is administered, the case fatality rate is closer to 5%.[296, 651, 721, 875, 876]

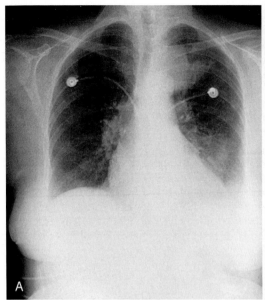

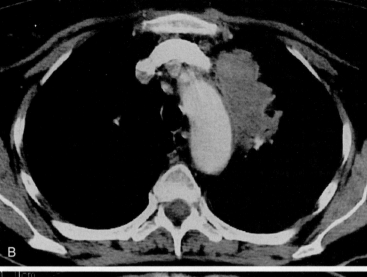

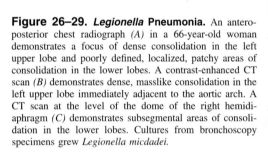

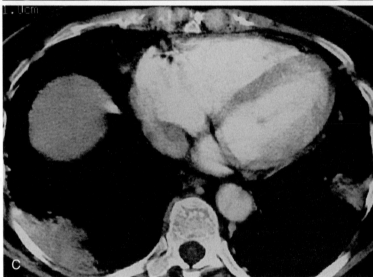

Figure 26–29. *Legionella* **Pneumonia.** An antero-posterior chest radiograph *(A)* in a 66-year-old woman demonstrates a focus of dense consolidation in the left upper lobe and poorly defined, localized, patchy areas of consolidation in the lower lobes. A contrast-enhanced CT scan *(B)* demonstrates dense, masslike consolidation in the left upper lobe immediately adjacent to the aortic arch. A CT scan at the level of the dome of the right hemidiaphragm *(C)* demonstrates subsegmental areas of consolidation in the lower lobes. Cultures from bronchoscopy specimens grew *Legionella micdadei.*

Miscellaneous Gram-Negative Coccobacilli

Actinobacillus actinomycetemcomitans is a small, gram-negative coccobacillus that is a normal commensal of the oral cavity. As a pathogen, it usually causes endocarditis; rare cases of pneumonia, mediastinal abscess, and empyema with chest wall abscess have also been described.[877–879]

Capnocytophaga is a genus of capnophilic gram-negative bacilli that includes *Capnocytophaga ochracea,* an organism that is generally associated with periodontitis; it has also been shown to cause pleuropulmonary disease in both immunocompromised and immunocompetent patients,[880, 881] especially younger ones.[882] In one study of 31 infections caused by *Capnocytophaga* species, three patients were found to have empyema, three bacteremia, and one a lung abscess;[881] the organism was frequently isolated as part of a polymicrobial infection along with other oral flora. *Capnocytophaga canimorsus* is a commensal in the saliva of cats and dogs that has caused pleural disease in humans during the course of septicemia following animal exposure.[883]

Eikenella corrodens is a facultatively anaerobic gram-negative rod that is part of the normal oral flora. In both immunocompromised and immunocompetent patients, it has been associated with lung abscess and empyema and presumably causes pulmonary infection following aspiration;[884, 885] the organism has been recovered in pure culture from blood and empyema fluid and by transtracheal aspiration.[886, 887]

Treponemataceae

The Treponemataceae are motile, spiral-shaped organisms that are usually quite thin and are seen to best advantage by dark-field microscopy, fluorescent antibody techniques, or silver staining of tissue sections. Two genera—*Leptospira* and *Treponema*—are associated with pulmonary disease in humans.

Leptospira interrogans

Leptospira interrogans is an aerobic, very slender (0.1 μm) spirochete that can be divided antigenetically into about 170 serotypes. For practical purposes, these are usually considered in larger serogroups, of which 18 are known to be pathogenic for humans or animals; four of these (*Leptospira icterohaemorrhagica, Leptospira canicola, Leptospira pomona,* and *Leptospira autumnalis*) are responsible for most cases of human disease. The organism is widely distributed in nature, primarily as a saprophyte or parasite of rodents and of many domestic animals including dogs, pigs, horses, sheep, goats, and cattle. In natural hosts, infection is usually mild and nonfatal, the organisms residing in renal convoluted tubules from which they are constantly shed into the urine. Human infection most often results from contact with contaminated water or damp soil and is most prevalent in the tropics; in southern Asia, about 15% to 25% of persons tested have serologic evidence of prior infection.[888] In developed countries, the incidence of clinically evident infection is very low; for example, in southwest France only 30 cases were described between 1980 and 1992.[889]

In industrialized countries, leptospirosis has been regarded largely as an occupational disease; for example, in Aberdeen, Scotland, fish workers appear to be at risk as a consequence of rats urinating on the fish food.[890] In the United States and Canada, the disease was formerly seen chiefly in workers in jobs such as sewer work, rice and sugar cane cultivation, farming, and slaughtering. However, in a study reported in 1973, approximately 60% of cases were found in children, students, and housewives, and only 17% in patients with a clearcut occupational exposure history.[891] This apparent change in risk may reflect an increased frequency of acquisition of the disease from family pets.[891, 892] The infecting sources in the cases documented in this series, in order of frequency, were rats, dogs, cattle, and swine;[891] some patients acquired the infection through swimming in stagnant water.

The pathologic findings of leptospiral pneumonia are poorly documented. One group of investigators injected *Leptospira* isolated from a patient intraperitoneally into 20 guinea pigs.[893] Initially, all lungs from the guinea pigs showed petechial hemorrhages approximately 1 mm in diameter; these progressed over several days to larger nodules and areas of confluent hemorrhage.

The radiologic manifestations were reviewed in a study of 58 patients from South Korea.[893] Abnormalities were evident on chest radiographs in 37 (64%) and could be grouped into three patterns: (1) multiple nodular opacities (air-space nodules) ranging from 1 to 7 mm in diameter with or without associated focal areas of consolidation (21 patients [57%]); (2) large confluent areas of consolidation (6 patients [16%]); and (3) diffuse, ill-defined areas of ground-glass opacity (10 patients [27%]). In all patients, the abnormalities were bilateral and nonlobar in distribution; in approximately 50%, they involved mainly the peripheral lung regions. Other findings included small pleural effusions (seen in 7 patients [19%]) and cardiomegaly (10 patients [27%]). Abscess formation has also been reported.[894] Consolidation has been seen less commonly in other series; for example, it was reported in only 39 (11%) of 345 cases in the United States prior to 1961[895] and in 10 (23%) of 44 patients in one review from Jamaica.[896]

The clinical manifestations of *Leptospirosis* are usually associated with symptoms and signs of kidney and liver failure (Weil's disease);[895] occasionally, pulmonary disease due to ARDS or diffuse lung hemorrhage dominates the clinical picture.[889, 897, 898] Patients often present with conjunc-

tivitis and muscle tenderness, features considered by some to be valuable clues to the diagnosis.[899] Other manifestations include headaches, chills, nausea and vomiting, pyuria, hematuria, and hepatomegaly. Respiratory symptoms include cough and (occasionally) hemoptysis; the latter may be severe.[900, 901] In such cases, hemorrhage may also occur into the gastrointestinal tract or skin. Signs of meningitis, usually aseptic, may be evident.

The diagnosis should be suspected from the clinical picture in a patient who has had possible exposure to contaminated water or to potentially infected animals. Although dogs can be immunized against *Leptospira,* the results of one study suggest that healthy immunized animals may still shed spirochetes in the urine.[891] Diagnosis can be confirmed by the culture of organisms from blood and urine, by isolation of the organism by animal inoculation, and by serologic testing.[1, 891]

Treponema pallidum

Treponema pallidum is a slender (0.15-mm wide), microaerophilic-to-aerophilic spirochete that has never been cultured on artificial media. It is responsible for syphilis, a disease of protean clinical manifestations that is usually acquired through sexual contact with an infected person and classically progresses through primary, secondary, and tertiary stages. The first two are themselves contagious and are manifested primarily as mucocutaneous disease. The tertiary form can affect virtually any organ, although central nervous system and cardiovascular diseases cause the most frequent symptomatic manifestations. Congenital syphilis results from transplacental spread of the organism.

Pulmonary syphilis classically occurs in both the congenital and acquired forms of disease. The former *(pneumonia alba)* occurs as part of a spectrum of syphilitic involvement of multiple organs and is usually associated with stillbirth or early death. Acquired disease is rarely associated with pulmonary involvement and is most often seen in the tertiary stage. It has two major manifestations: fibrogummatous parenchymal disease and pulmonary arteritis. Pleural effusion[902] and subacute pneumonitis with a radiographic pattern of reticulonodular infiltration[903] have also been described in patients with HIV infection and AIDS, respectively.

Fibrogummatous disease is the most variable in appearance and probably the most difficult to diagnose with conviction. Pathologically, the fibrosis can occur in a relatively well-defined interstitial pattern, or as dense, broad, irregular scars radiating through the parenchyma.[904] Gummas can be solitary or multiple and appear as gray-white, rubbery nodules surrounded by a rim of fibrous tissue. Microscopically, the nodules show a zone of central coagulative necrosis surrounded by an inflammatory infiltrate of plasma cells and scattered, multinucleated giant cells.[904] Organisms are rarely identifiable. Occasionally, gummas encroach on the wall of the trachea or major bronchi, causing ulceration or compression with secondary bronchiectasis.[905]

Syphilitic involvement of the main pulmonary artery has been reported rarely[906, 907] and is similar in appearance and course to syphilitic aortitis, with which it is invariably associated.[907] Macroscopically, there is aneurysmal dilatation accompanied by irregular intimal scarring and luminal thrombus formation. Histologic examination reveals medial fibrosis, disruption of elastic tissue, adventitial endarteritis, and a perivascular plasma cell infiltrate. Organisms are rarely identified. Occasionally, the vessel wall is the site of necrotic gummas[907] that may cause arterial rupture.[906] Pleuritis and pleural effusion unassociated with pulmonary or vascular disease have also been described in acquired syphilis,[908] as has rupture of an aortic aneurysm into a pulmonary artery.[909]

Since organisms are rarely found within the gummas and the pattern of fibrosis is nonspecific, confident diagnosis of a syphilitic etiology of acquired parenchymal disease may be difficult, even in surgically excised or autopsy material; particular difficulty may be encountered in distinguishing the abnormality from fibrocaseous tuberculosis. The absence of acid-fast organisms in both sputum specimens and histologic material, negative results of PCR examination, the presence of a positive syphilitic serology, the identification of tertiary syphilitic lesions in other sites, and the presence of histologic features typical of a gumma all must be considered in establishing a definitive diagnosis.[904]

ANAEROBIC BACTERIA

The renewed interest in anaerobic pleuropulmonary infection, which occurred in the late 1960s, resulted from two factors: (1) the development of sampling techniques that allowed the separation of lung pathogens from the normal (and contaminated) flora of the upper airway; and (2) the growth of research laboratories with an interest in defining the clinical manifestations of infection with these organisms.[910] The variety of terms used to describe these types of infection has been a source of some confusion.[911] *Aspiration pneumonia* is commonly defined as infection occurring in dependent lung zones in a patient with associated disease that predisposes to aspiration.[910] The fact that most such patients have infection with anaerobic organisms has led to the terms *anaerobic pneumonia* and *aspiration pneumonia* being used in an interchangeable fashion.[912] However, all persons aspirate on occasion, and the process is a major mechanism of many bacterial lung infections caused by aerobic or facultative organisms. We prefer to use the term *aspiration pneumonia* to refer to disease that follows aspiration of relatively large quantities of material from the upper airway, such as vomitus and acid gastric contents; such pneumonia may be the result of chemical injury (due to gastric acid) or to toxin-mediated bacterial damage, or both. By contrast, infection caused by anaerobic organisms in a patient with poor dentition and impaired consciousness is referred to as *anaerobic pneumonia*. Unfortunately, this is not a perfect solution to this particular semantic problem, and overlap between these conditions clearly exists.

Anaerobic organisms tend to cause tissue necrosis, which is manifested in the lung as cavitating abscesses and empyema. Although it is true that when patients present with the clinical and radiographic tableau of lung abscess, anaerobic organisms are usually responsible, a host of other organisms, including *M. tuberculosis, S. aureus,* and enteric organisms, can produce similar disease.[913, 914] The use of the terms *primary lung abscess* to describe patients with lung abscess in whom no antecedent pneumonia has been docu-

mented, and *nonspecific lung abscess*[915] to describe patients in whom no organism can be isolated, should be abandoned.

More than 30 genera and 200 species of anaerobes have been identified in human infection and, in fact, such infection of the lung is usually polymicrobial.[1] Among the most important agents are the gram-negative bacilli *Bacteroides, Fusobacterium, Porphyromonas* and *Prevotella*; the gram-positive bacilli *Actinomyces, Eubacterium,* and *Clostridium*; the gram-positive cocci *Peptostreptococcus* and *Peptococcus*; and the gram-negative cocci *Veillonella*.[910, 916–919]

Epidemiology

Because of the requirements for special sampling and microbiologic techniques, the precise incidence of anaerobic lung infection is difficult to determine. However, when particular efforts have been made, the high prevalence of anaerobic and mixed aerobic-anaerobic infection has been surprising. For example, in the absence of special effort, anaerobic bacteria are seldom identified as playing any role at all in ventilator-associated pneumonia;[920] however, in one study of 130 patients with such infection, they were recovered in significant concentrations by protected specimen brush sampling of the lower airways in 30 (23%).[916] Granted, such infections seem to have little impact on outcome, since common antibiotic regimens used in this situation are effective against anaerobic organisms,[916] and protected brush sampling is an imperfect means of diagnosing the infection.[921] Even so, it is likely that these organisms are pathogenic in many patients with ventilator-associated pneumonia. Among all patients admitted to the hospital with pneumonia, anaerobic bacteria have been isolated in approximately 20% to 35%,[922–924] the organisms being second only to *S. pneumoniae* as a cause of community-acquired pneumonia. They are undoubtedly also important in nosocomial lung infection in general; for example, in one careful and extensive study of 159 patients with this complication, including those in intensive care units, wards, and chronic care units, anaerobic organisms were found to be the cause of the infection in 59 (35%).[925]

There is a significant male predominance in pleuropulmonary anaerobic infection, men outnumbering women by three or four to one.[926, 927] As indicated previously, many cases are believed to be related to aspiration of contaminated oral secretions. As a result, clinical situations that increase the number of organisms in such secretions and that result in an increased risk of aspiration are risk factors for the disease. It has been estimated that anaerobes outnumber aerobes by at least ten to one in the normal flora of expectorated material;[928, 929] in the presence of poor oral hygiene, the number of such anaerobic commensals is even greater. Thus, periodontitis and gingivitis are found in two thirds of patients with lung abscesses;[928, 930, 931] in others, the initial nidus of anaerobic infection is the paranasal sinuses[929] or tonsils.[932, 933] Patients with adequate oral hygiene and an anaerobic pleuropulmonary infection may have an endobronchial-obstructing lesion that interferes with clearance of aspirated organisms harbored in distal parenchyma; this is the probable explanation for the unexpected association of pulmonary carcinoma and edentulous patients in one series of 143 cases of anaerobic infection.[928]

When precautions are taken to avoid contamination

from the oropharynx or when the material comes from a closed space, positive cultures usually reveal mixed anaerobes, alone or with aerobes; only rarely is pure culture of a single anaerobe obtained. On average, three bacterial species are obtained per case; isolates are exclusively anaerobic in 30% to 50% of patients and are mixed with facultative and (occasionally) aerobic bacteria in the remainder.[359, 934] The incidence of concomitant aerobes in cultures of material obtained by transtracheal aspiration (TTA) is higher in hospital-acquired than in community-acquired nonbacteremic anaerobic disease; for example, in one prospective study of 54 patients seen or predisposed to aspirate in whom the diagnosis was made by culture of TTA specimens, empyema fluid or blood, 67% of those who acquired infection during hospitalization had a mixture of aerobes and anaerobes, whereas 19 (63%) of 30 who acquired their infection outside the hospital had exclusively anaerobic flora.[934]

An unusual type of anaerobic infection known as *Lemierre's syndrome* was recognized fairly frequently a half century ago and has reappeared more recently.[936] The causative agent is a member of either the *Fusobacterium* or *Bacteroides* genera, and young adults appear to be particularly susceptible. The primary focus occurs in the pharynx, from which septicemic spread occurs, often to bones and joints but also to the lungs and pleura.[937–940] *Bacteroides fragilis* bacteremia is more commonly associated with abdominal surgery or with gynecologic or obstetric conditions.[941–949] In one investigation of 250 isolates from blood specimens, the site of entry was considered to be the gastrointestinal tract in 116, the genitourinary tract in 41, the lung in 30, and the oropharynx in 21.[941] Early invasion of regional veins is a hallmark of such infections, with consequent thrombophlebitis and, in many cases, pulmonary thromboemboli.[941] In blood cultures, *B. fragilis* usually is isolated with other organisms such as anaerobic and β-hemolytic streptococci, *S. faecalis, S. aureus, E. coli* and, less often, *Proteus* species and *Pseudomonas aeruginosa*.[943]

Members of the *Clostridium* genus, usually *Clostridium perfringens,* and rarely *Clostridium sordelli*[950] and *Clostridium sporogenes,*[951] are sometimes causes of pleuropulmonary infection, either as primary disease or in association with bacteremia following attempted criminal abortion.[952, 953] Primary pneumonia usually occurs in patients with underlying pulmonary or cardiac disease[953] or as a secondary infection following pulmonary thromboembolism.[954, 955] Empyema is relatively common; although it often follows thoracentesis,[956] it can occur spontaneously in an otherwise healthy person. Gas formation can result in pyopneumothorax.[955, 957]

The presence of risk factors for aspiration has frequently directed investigators to search for anaerobic organisms on a selective basis. About 25% of patients give a history of compromised consciousness associated with such conditions as general anesthesia, acute cerebrovascular accident, epileptic seizures, and drug ingestion;[912, 926, 931, 958] alcoholism has been reported in 40% to 75% of patients.[926, 931, 958] Dysphagia is also a predisposing factor, commonly in association with multiple sclerosis, vascular or malignant central nervous system disease, or esophageal disease.[912] Immunosuppressed patients and those with COPD are not particularly at risk for anaerobic infection, provided there are no additional predisposing factors;[359] however, this is not true for *Bacteroides* bacteremia, which occurs most commonly in patients who are immunocompromised or have undergone recent surgery.[941, 942]

Anaerobic bacteria are a particularly common cause of empyema. For example, in one study at three hospitals equipped with anaerobic research laboratories, they were recovered from pleural fluid in 63 (76%) of 83 adult patients who had not received antimicrobial therapy or undergone thoracic surgery;[959] the organisms were the exclusive isolates in 29 cases (35%). Most of the flora was complex, averaging 2.6 species per specimen. In order of prevalence, isolated organisms were anaerobic or microaerophilic streptococci, *S. aureus, Peptococcus, F. nucleatum, B. melaninogenicus, B. fragilis, Clostridium* species, *E. coli,* and *P. aeruginosa.* Other studies of the bacteriology of empyema have revealed anaerobic organisms in about 20% to 50% of cases.[910]

In developing countries a protracted, relapsing, suppurative, and cavitating infection presumably caused by anaerobic organisms and known as *chronic destructive pneumonia* has been described;[960] it usually necessitates resectional surgery and almost certainly reflects a lack of hygiene and poor patient compliance with medication regimens.

Pathogenesis

As indicated previously, the initial event in most cases of anaerobic pulmonary infection is aspiration of infected material from the upper airways. Anaerobic bacteria proliferate in areas of poor perfusion and in the presence of tissue necrosis, situations causing a lowering of the oxidation-reduction potential. Some species produce superoxide dismutase, which provides them with oxygen tolerance.[921, 961, 962] Potential mechanisms that might account for the virulence of these organisms and their propensity to cause tissue necrosis include the production of exotoxins, the formation of capsules, the action of superoxide dismutase, and the elaboration of low-molecular-weight products that inhibit killing by phagocytes.[910, 916]

Pathologic Characteristics

The pathologic findings of anaerobic bacterial infection are those of a confluent bronchopneumonia, frequently associated with extensive hemorrhage and abscess formation (Fig. 26–30). Colonies of bacteria and fragments of aspirated foreign material can sometimes be identified in the necrotic foci. Elastin fibers have occasionally been seen in sputum specimens, providing evidence of the necrotizing nature of the process.[962a]

Radiologic Manifestations

The distribution of pneumonia following aspiration of material contaminated by anaerobic organisms reflects gravitational flow: the posterior segments of the upper lobes or superior segments of the lower lobes tend to be involved with aspiration in the recumbent position and the basal segments of the lower lobes when aspiration occurs in an erect patient. The anterior segments of the upper lobes are involved less often, and the middle lobe and lingula rarely. The right lung is affected approximately twice as often as the left.[912, 928, 958, 963]

The typical radiographic pattern is that of bronchopneu-

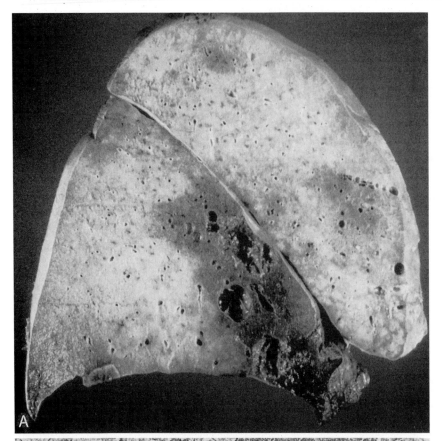

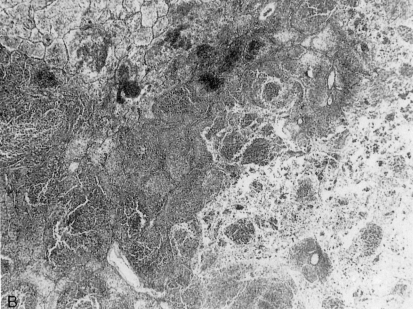

Figure 26–30. Anaerobic Bacterial Pneumonia. *A,* A sagittal slice of the left lung shows severe hemorrhage associated with multiple shaggy-walled cavities. Although the location is somewhat unusual, the appearance is otherwise typical of anaerobic bacterial lung infection. *B,* Histologic appearance, showing consolidation and necrosis of lung parenchyma; an early stage of cavity formation is seen in the lower right. (*B,* ×20.)

monia, ranging from localized segmental areas of consolidation to patchy bilateral consolidation to extensive, confluent, multilobar consolidation (Fig. 26–31). Cavitation has been reported in 20% to 60% of cases.[964, 965] In one study of 69 patients, approximately 50% had pulmonary parenchymal abnormalities, 30% had empyema without apparent parenchymal abnormalities, and 20% had combined parenchymal and pleural disease at presentation.[964] The parenchymal abnormalities consisted of consolidation without cavitation in

approximately 50% of cases and lung abscess (defined as a circumscribed cavity with relatively little surrounding consolidation) or necrotizing pneumonia (defined as areas of consolidation containing single or multiple cavities) in the remaining 50% of cases. The parenchymal abnormalities involved predominantly the posterior basal segments and the superior segments of the lower lobes. In all cases, the radiographic findings worsened in the first 3 days and in 30% of cases for at least 1 week. Of the 17 patients who

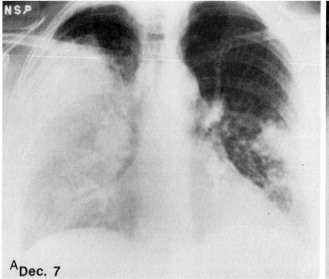

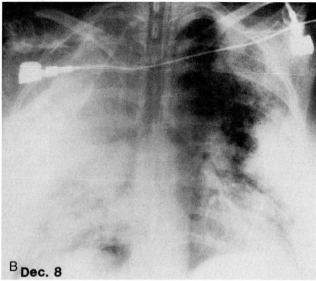

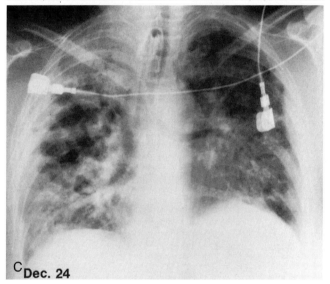

Figure 26–31. Anaerobic Pneumonia—Massive Air-Space Consolidation with Abscess Formation. The first examination *(A)* on this extremely ill 45-year-old woman alcoholic revealed massive, homogeneous consolidation of the right lower lobe and patchy consolidation of the left lung. Twenty-four hours later *(B)*, the pneumonia had extended throughout most of the right lung and much of the left. During the next 2 weeks on antibiotic therapy most of the pneumonia in the left lung resolved *(C)*. However, a large, ragged, thick-walled cavity had appeared in the right lung. A heavy growth of bacilli was present on anaerobic culture.

initially had solitary localized areas of consolidation, 2 developed a lung abscess and 3 other developed necrotizing pneumonias while on antibiotic therapy. In another series of 46 patients (which excluded those with radiographic evidence of abscess formation at the time of diagnosis as well as those with culture-positive pleural fluid), 9 (20%) developed lung abscess after initiation of antibiotic therapy.[965]

Like others,[966] we have occasionally seen hilar or mediastinal lymph node enlargement associated with an anaerobic abscess, a combination of findings that may resemble pulmonary carcinoma (Fig. 26–32). Rarely, an anaerobic abscess is associated with lung gangrene.[966a] Empyema caused by *B. fragilis* or *C. perfringens* may be associated with gas production and resultant pyopneumothorax.[955] In abdominal infections caused by *B. fragilis,* empyema may overlie a subphrenic abscess, suggesting transdiaphragmatic spread.[928]

When the infection is blood borne (most often from septic emboli in *Bacteroides* bacteremia), the disease usually is localized to the lower lobes and takes the form of patchy or confluent nonsegmental, homogeneous consolidation, generally with cavitation.[947] Abscess cavities can be small or

large.[926, 928] The cavitating mass that characterizes progressive massive fibrosis of various pneumoconioses is usually considered to be either aseptic or to contain tubercle bacilli but has also been shown to yield anaerobic organisms on culture of aspirated material.[967]

Clinical Manifestations

The clinical features of anaerobic pulmonary infection are variable. On the one hand, acute pneumonitis may be indistinguishable from that caused by infection with *S. pneumoniae*;[965] on the other, infection complicated by lung abscess or empyema may have a protracted, insidious course. For example, in one series of 87 presumed anaerobic lung abscesses, illness before admission to a hospital ranged from a few days to 10 months;[930] in another investigation of 54 patients with anaerobic pulmonary infection diagnosed by culture of TTA, empyema fluid, or blood, the duration of symptoms ranged from less than 1 day to 20 weeks.[912] Overall, the mean duration appears to be about 2 to 3 weeks.[928, 934, 963]

Patients with anaerobic pulmonary infection may be

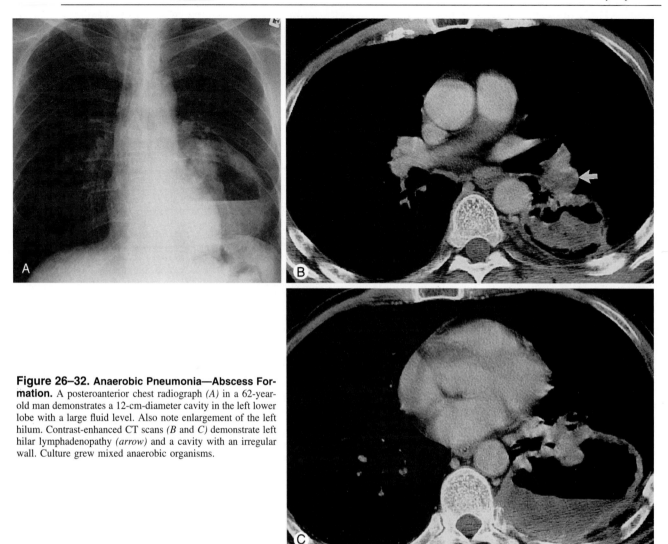

Figure 26–32. Anaerobic Pneumonia—Abscess Formation. A posteroanterior chest radiograph *(A)* in a 62-year-old man demonstrates a 12-cm-diameter cavity in the left lower lobe with a large fluid level. Also note enlargement of the left hilum. Contrast-enhanced CT scans *(B* and *C)* demonstrate left hilar lymphadenopathy *(arrow)* and a cavity with an irregular wall. Culture grew mixed anaerobic organisms.

virtually asymptomatic. In fact, the majority do not appear seriously ill when first seen, although occasionally the disease runs a fulminant course leading to death. Fever is present in 70% to 80% of cases,[926, 931] but is usually low grade. Chills are rare in disease acquired by aspiration,[931, 965] but are common in *Bacteroides* and *Fusobacterium* bacteremia, in which they are associated with high fever, diaphoresis, and malaise.[939, 941]

In the initial stages of infection, cough is frequently nonproductive and the expectorated material, if any, is seldom putrid. When cavitation occurs—usually 7 to 10 days or more after the onset of pneumonia[912]—expectoration increases and becomes putrid in 40% to 75% of cases.[926, 928, 931, 968] Foul-smelling sputum always indicates the presence of anaerobic organisms; however, in the absence of abscess formation, such putrid expectoration is present in only 5% of patients.[910] Pleural pain occurs in approximately 50% of patients and hemoptysis in 25%.[931] Physical findings are generally those of pneumonia of any cause; clubbing is common when the infection is chronic.[969]

Laboratory Findings and Diagnosis

In most cases of anaerobic pneumonia and lung abscess, the leukocyte count is mildly to moderately elevated, al-

though it may be within normal limits. One group of investigators reported white blood cell counts of 12,000/mm³ or higher in 40 (60%) of 66 patients;[931] in another study, values ranged from 7,800 to 32,000/mm³ (mean peak of 17,000/mm³).[970] Leukocytosis is even more common in *Bacteroides* bacteremia.[941, 947] In one review of 357 patients, it was documented in 235 (95%);[941] leukopenia was found in only 9. Anemia, commonly accompanied by weight loss, is additional evidence of the frequent chronicity of this infection.[928, 931, 934, 963]

A definitive diagnosis of anaerobic bacterial pulmonary infection can be made only with special effort. The pleomorphic character of organisms on Gram stain, particularly gram-positive and gram-negative bacilli, and a subsequent lack of aerobic growth may alert the physician to the possibility. However, culture of sputum may reveal potential aerobic pathogens, and there are many other causes for negative sputum cultures,[910] such that this combination of findings is clearly not diagnostic. In fact, cultures of expectorated material are of little value in diagnosis, since they are invariably contaminated by mouth flora. To be considered conclusively pathogenic, organisms must be isolated from a closed space such as the pleural or peritoneal cavity, a subcutaneous or intra-abdominal abscess, or blood. Providing aseptic precautions are taken, TTNA should also be accepted as a dependable source of pathogens, as should cultures of lung tissue obtained surgically.

One group of investigators carried out a study of other methods of eliminating contamination by oral flora by bypassing the oropharynx.[971] Using TTNA as a standard, they compared the bacterial yield from TTA and from wire brushing under direct vision through a fiberoptic bronchoscope in 10 patients with aerobic and anaerobic lung abscesses. The results underscored the relatively poor sensitivity and specificity of these techniques for determining the contribution of anaerobic bacteria to lung infection.[971] Caution is therefore warranted against unqualified acceptance of published data on anaerobic bacteriology in pulmonary infection, much of which is based on material obtained by TTA.

Specific fluorescent antibody staining techniques and selective differential culture media may be valuable in diagnosis.[921] In contrast with aerobic bacteria, most anaerobic organisms produce volatile fatty acids, so that gas-liquid chromatography of pleural fluid or respiratory secretions can prove useful.[972–976] The results are negative or only weakly positive in patients in whom the presence of anaerobes is clinically insignificant, probably as a result of contamination of sputum samples by saliva.[976] The identification of succinic acid is indicative of *Bacteroides* infection.[975]

Prognosis and Natural History

With early diagnosis and the prompt institution of therapy, the prognosis of anaerobic pulmonary infection is good.[930, 940] Antibiotic therapy markedly decreases the incidence of complicating abscess formation.[930, 969, 977] Currently, the mortality rate for lung abscess is 5% to 12%, with most of the deaths occurring in patients who have serious underlying disease.[978] A poor prognosis has been associated with inadequate drainage of subdiaphragmatic or pleural pockets of infection[928, 931, 979] and with multiple abscesses;[958] in such cases, the response to antibiotic therapy alone may be poor.

In patients who respond to therapy, cavity closure occurs steadily but may be prolonged. Long-term follow-up of patients with lung abscess has shown residual cystic and bronchiectatic abnormalities for as long as 7 years after an otherwise satisfactory response to therapy,[926] indicating irreversibility of lung damage. A lack of response and persistence of symptoms for more than 12 weeks have been correlated with large cavities.[926, 980]

REFERENCES

1. Brooks GF, Butel JS, Ornston LN et al (eds): Javetz, Melnick, & Adelberg's Medical Microbiology. Norwalk, CT, Appleton & Lange, 1995.
2. Austrian R: Pneumococcal pneumonia: Diagnostic, epidemiologic, therapeutic, and prophylactic considerations. Chest 90:736, 1986.
3. Gomez J, Banos V, Ruiz Gomez J, et al: Prospective study of epidemiology and prognostic factors in community-acquired pneumonia. Eur J Clin Microbiol Infect Dis 15:556, 1996.
4. Neill AM, Martin IR, Weir R, et al: Community-acquired pneumonia: Aetiology and usefulness of severity criteria on admission. Thorax 51:1010, 1996.
5. Pareja A, Bernal C, Leyva A, et al: Etiologic study of patients with community-acquired pneumonia. Chest 101:1207, 1992.
6. Hedlund J: Community-acquired pneumonia requiring hospitalisation: Factors of importance for the short- and long term prognosis. Scand J Infect Dis Suppl 97:1, 1995.
7. Bohte R, van Furth R, van den Broek PJ: Aetiology of community-acquired pneumonia: A prospective study among adults requiring admission to hospital. Thorax 50:543, 1995.
8. Jorgenson JH, Howell AW, Maher LA, et al: Serotypes of respiratory isolates of *Streptococcus pneumoniae* compared with the capsular types included in the current pneumococcal vaccine. J Infect Dis 163:644, 1991.
9. Marrie TJ: Bacteremic pneumococcal pneumonia mortality rate—is it really different in Sweden? Chest 103:658, 1993.
10. Jette LP, Lamothe F: Surveillance of invasive *Streptococcus pneumoniae* infection in Quebec, Canada, from 1984 to 1986: Serotype distribution, antimicrobial susceptibility, and clinical characteristics. J Clin Microbiol 27:1, 1989.
10a. Lovgren M, Spika JS, Talbot JA: Invasive *Streptococcus pneumoniae* infections: Serotype distribution and antimicrobial resistance in Canada, 1992–1995. Can Med Assoc J 158:327, 1998.
11. Johnson AP, Speller DC, George RC, et al: Prevalence of antibiotic resistance and serotypes in pneumococci in England and Wales: Results of observational surveys in 1990 and 1995. BMJ 312:1454, 1996.
12. Boswell TC, Frodsham D, Nye KJ, et al: Antibiotic resistance and serotypes of *Streptococcus pneumoniae* at Birmingham Public Health Laboratory, 1989–1994. J Infect 33:17, 1996.
13. Coffey TJ, Berron S, Daniels M, et al: Multiple antibiotic–resistant *Streptococcus pneumoniae* recovered from Spanish hospitals (1988–1994): Novel major clones of serotypes 14, 19F, and 15F. Microbiology 142:2747, 1996.
14. Magnus T, Andersen BM: Serotypes and resistance patterns of *Streptococcus pneumoniae* causing systemic disease in northern Norway. Eur J Clin Microbiol Infect Dis 14:229, 1995.
15. George WL, Finegold SM: Bacterial infections of the lung. Chest 81:502, 1982.
16. Mogdasy MC, Camou T, Fajardo C, et al: Colonizing and invasive strains of *Streptococcus pneumoniae* in Uruguayan children: Type distribution and patterns of antibiotic resistance. Pediatr Infect Dis J 11:648, 1992.
17. Boersma WG, Lowenberg A, Holloway Y, et al: The role of antigen detection in pneumococcal carriers: A comparison between cultures and capsular antigen detection in upper respiratory tract secretions. Scand J Infect Dis 25:51, 1993.
18. Boken DJ, Chartrand SA, Moland ES, et al: Colonization with penicillin-nonsusceptible *Streptococcus pneumoniae* in urban and rural child-care centers. Pediatr Infect Dis J 15:667, 1996.
19. Singhal A, Lalitha MK, John TJ, et al: Modified latex agglutination test for rapid detection of *Streptococcus pneumoniae* and *Haemophilus influenzae* in cerebrospinal fluid and direct serotyping of *Streptococcus pneumoniae*. Eur J Clin Microbiol Infect Dis 15:472, 1996.
20. Lalitha MK, Pai R, John TJ, et al: Serotyping of *Streptococcus pneumoniae* by agglutination assays: A cost-effective technique for developing countries. Bull World Health Organ 74:387, 1996.
21. Zielen S, Brokr M, Strnad N, et al: Simple determination of polysaccharide-specific antibodies by means of chemically modified ELISA plates. J Immunol Methods 193:1, 1996.
22. Konradsen HB, Sorensen UB, Henrichse J: A modified enzyme-linked immunosorbent assay for measuring type-specific anti-pneumococcal capsular polysaccharide antibodies. J Immunol Methods 164:13, 1993.
23. Wicher K, Kalinka C, Mlodozeniec P, et al: Fluorescent antibody technic used for identification and typing of *Streptococcus pneumoniae*. Am J Clin Pathol 77:72, 1982.
24. Lefevre JC, Faucon G, Sicard AM, et al: DNA fingerprinting of *Streptococcus pneumoniae* strains by pulsed-field gel electrophoresis. J Clin Microbiol 31:2724, 1993.
25. Hermans PW, Sluijter M, Hoogenboezem T, et al: Comparative study of five different DNA fingerprint techniques for molecular typing of *Streptococcus pneumoniae* strains. J Clin Microbiol 33:1606, 1995.
25a. Hall LMC: Application of molecular typing to the epidemiology of streptococcus pneumoniae. J Clin Pathol 51:270, 1998.
26. Macfarlane J: An overview of community-acquired pneumonia with lessons learned from the British Thoracic Society Study. Semin Respir Infect 9:153, 1994.
26a. Porath A, Schlaeffer F, Pick N, et al: Pneumococcal community-acquired pneumonia in 148 hospitalized adult patients. Eur J Clin Microbiol Infect Dis 16:863, 1997.
27. Sankilampi U, Herva E, Haikala R, et al: Epidemiology of invasive *Streptococcus pneumoniae* infections in adults in Finland. Epidemiol Infect 118:7, 1997.
28. Plouffe JF, Breiman RF, Facklam RR: Bacteremia with *Streptococcus pneumoniae*: Implication for therapy and prevention—Franklin County Pneumonia Study Group. JAMA 275:194, 1996.
29. Afessa B, Greaves WL, Frederick WR: Pneumococcal bacteremia in adults: A 14-year experience in an inner-city university hospital. Clin Infect Dis 21:345, 1995.
30. Koivula I, Sten M, Mäkelä PH: Risk factors for pneumonia in the elderly. Am J Med 96:313, 1994.
31. Davidson M, Parkinson AJ, Bulkow LR, et al: The epidemiology of invasive pneumococcal disease in Alaska, 1986–1990—ethnic differences and opportunities for prevention. J Infect Dis 170:368, 1994.
32. Fedson DS: Pneumococcal vaccination in the prevention of community-acquired pneumonia: An optimistic view of cost-effectiveness. Semin Respir Infect 8:285, 1993.
33. Haglund LA, Istre GR, Pickett DA, et al: Invasive pneumococcal disease in central Oklahoma: Emergence of high-level penicillin resistance and multiple antibiotic resistance—Pneumococcus Study Group. J Infect Dis 168:1532, 1993.
34. Mufson MA, Kruss DM, Wasil RE, et al: Capsular types and outcome of bacteremic pneumococcal disease in the antibiotic era. Arch Intern Med 134:505, 1974.
35. Armstrong D, Young LS, Meyer RD, et al: Infectious complications of neoplastic disease. Med Clin North Am 55:729, 1971.
36. Twomey JJ: Infections complicating multiple myeloma and chronic lymphocytic leukemia. Arch Intern Med 132:562, 1973.
37. Hoge CW, Reichler MR, Dominguez EA, et al: An epidemic of pneumococcal disease in an overcrowded, inadequately ventilated jail. N Engl J Med 331:643, 1994.
38. Kabins SA, Lerner C: Fulminant pneumococcemia and sickle cell anemia. JAMA 211:467, 1970.
39. Powers D, Overturf G, Weiss J, et al: Pneumococcal septicemia in children with sickle cell anemia: Changing trend of survival. JAMA 245:1839, 1981.
40. Leeper KV Jr: Severe community-acquired pneumonia. Semin Respir Infec 11:96, 1996.
41. Bisno AL, Freeman JC: The syndrome of asplenia, pneumococcal sepsis, and disseminated intravascular coagulation. Ann Intern Med 72:389, 1970.
42. Hofmann J, Cetron MS, Farley MM, et al: The prevalence of drug-resistant *Streptococcus pneumoniae* in Atlanta. N Engl J Med 333:481, 1995.
43. Pallares R, Liñares J, Vadillo M, et al: Resistance to penicillin and cephalosporin and mortality from severe pneumococcal pneumonia in Barcelona, Spain. N Engl J Med 333:474, 1995.
43a. Campbell GD Jr, Silberman R: Drug-resistant *Streptococcus pneumoniae*. Clin Infect Dis 26:1188, 1998.
44. Yoshida R, Kaku M, Kohno S, et al: Trends in antimicrobial resistance of *Streptococcus pneumoniae* in Japan. Antimicrob Agents Chemother 39:1196, 1995.
45. Ridgway EJ, Tremlett CH, Allen KD: Capsular serotypes and antibiotic sensitivity of *Streptococcus pneumoniae* isolated from primary-school children. J Infect 30:245, 1995.
46. Martin DR, Brett MS: Pneumococci causing invasive disease in New Zealand, 1987–1994: Serogroup coverage and antibiotic resistances. N Z Med J 109:288, 1996.
47. Parkinson AJ, Davidson M, Fitzgerald MA, et al: Serotype distribution and antimicrobial resistance patterns of invasive isolates of *Streptococcus pneumoniae*: Alaska 1986–1990. J Infect Dis 170:461, 1994.
47a. Nuorti JP, Butler JC, Crutcher JM, et al: An outbreak of multidrug-resistant pneumococcal pneumonia and bacteremia among unvaccinated nursing home residents. N Engl J Med 338:1861, 1998.
48. Rodriguez-Barradas MC, Tharapel RA, Groover JE, et al: Colonization by *Streptococcus pneumoniae* among human immunodeficiency virus–infected adults: Prevalence of antibiotic resistance, impact of immunization, and characterization by polymerase chain reaction with BOX primers of isolates from persistent *S. pneumoniae* carriers. J Infect Dis 175:590, 1997.
49. Boken DJ, Chartrand SA, Goering RV, et al: Colonization with penicillin-resistant *Streptococcus pneumoniae* in child-care center. Pediatr Infect Dis J 14:879, 1995.
50. Versalovic J, Kapur V, Mason EO Jr, et al: Penicillin-resistant *Streptococcus pneumoniae* strains recovered in Houston: Identification and molecular characterization of multiple clones. J Infect Dis 167:850, 1993.
51. Carvalho C, Geslin P, Vaz Pato MV: Pulsed-filed gel electrophoresis in *Streptococcus pneumoniae* isolated in France and Portugal. Pathol Biol 44:430, 1996.
52. Reichmann P, Varon E, Gunther E, et al: Penicillin-resistant *Streptococcus pneumoniae* in Germany: Genetic relationship to clones from other European countries. J Med Microbiol 43:377, 1995.
53. Coffey TJ, Daniels M, McDougal LK, et al: Genetic analysis of clinical isolates of *Streptococcus pneumoniae* with high-level resistance to expanded-spectrum cephalosporins. Antimicrob Agents Chemother 39:1306, 1995.
54. Tuomanen EI, Austrian R, Masure HR: Pathogenesis of pneumococcal infection. N Engl J Med 332:1280, 1995.
55. Wizman TM, Moskovitz J, Pearce BJ, et al: Peptide methionine sulfoxide reductase contributes to the maintenance of adhesions in three major pathogens. Proc Natl Acad Sci U S A 93:7985, 1996.

56. Hakansson A, Kidd A, Wadell G, et al: Adenovirus infection enhances in vitro adherence of *Streptococcus pneumoniae*. Infect Immun 62:2707, 1994.

57. Hakansson A, Carlstedt I, Davies J, et al: Aspects on the interaction of *Streptococcus pneumoniae* and *Haemophilus influenzae* with human respiratory tract mucosa. Am J Respir Crit Care Med 154:187, 1996.

57a. van der Poll T, Koegh CV, Buurman WA, et al: Passive immunization against tumor necrosis factor-α impairs host defense during pneumococcal pneumonia in mice. Am J Respir Crit Care Med 155:603, 1997.

58. Boutten A, Dehoux MS, Seta N, et al: Compartmentalized IL-8 and elastase released within the human lung in unilateral pneumonia. Am J Respir Crit Care Med 153:336, 1996.

58a. Smith JD, Cortes NJ, Evans GS, et al: Induction of beta$_2$ integrin–dependent neutrophil adhesion to human alveolar epithelial cells by type 1 *Streptococcus pneumoniae* and derived soluble factors. J Infect Dis 177:977, 1998.

59. Perry FE, Elson CJ, Mitchell TJ, et al: Characterisation of an oxidative response inhibitor produced by *Streptococcus pneumoniae*. Thorax 49:676, 1994.

60. Perry FE, Elson CJ, Greenham LW, et al: Interference with the oxidative response of neutrophils by *Streptococcus pneumoniae*. Thorax 48:364, 1993.

61. Rubins JB, Charboneau D, Fasching C, et al: Distinct roles for pneumolysin's cytotoxic and complement activities in the pathogenesis and pneumococcal pneumonia. Am J Respir Crit Care Med 153:1339, 1996.

62. Paton JC, Andrew PW, Boulnois GJ, et al: Molecular analysis of the pathogenicity of *Streptococcus pneumoniae*: The role of pneumococcal proteins. Annu Rev Microbiol 47:89, 1993.

63. Duguid JP, Marmion BP, Swain RHA: Medical Microbiology: A Guide to the Laboratory Diagnosis and Control of Infection. Edinburgh, Churchill Livingstone, 1978.

64. Robertson OH, Uhley CG: Changes occurring in the macrophage system of the lungs in *Pneumococcus* lobar pneumonia. J Clin Invest 15:115, 1936.

65. Loeschcke H: Untersuchungen über die krupposse Pneumonie. Beitr Pathol Anat Allgemeinen Pathol 86:201, 1931.

66. Wood WB Jr: Studies on the mechanism of recovery in pneumococcal pneumonia: I. The action of type-specific antibody upon the pulmonary lesion of experimental pneumonia. J Exp Med 73:201, 1941.

67. Robertson OH, Coggeshall LT, Terrell EE: Experimental *Pneumococcus* lobar pneumonia in the dog: II. Pathology. J Clin Invest 12:433, 1933.

68. Robertson OH, Coggeshall LT, Terrell EE: Experimental *Pneumococcus* lobar pneumonia in the dog: III. Pathogenesis. J Clin Invest 12:467, 1933.

69. Hamburger M, Robertson OH: Studies on pathogenesis of experimental *Pneumococcus* pneumonia in dogs: I. Secondary pulmonary lesions—relationship of bronchial obstruction and distribution of pneumococci to their inception. J Exp Med 72:261, 1940.

70. Lonky SA, Marsh J, Steele R, et al: Protease and antiprotease responses in lung and peripheral blood in experimental canine pneumococcal pneumonia. Am Rev Resp Dis 121:685, 1980.

71. Wood WB Jr, Smith MR: Host-parasite relationships in experimental pneumonia due to *Pneumococcus* type III. J Exp Med 92:85, 1950.

72. Leatherman JW, Iber C, Davies SF: Cavitation in bacteremic pneumococcal pneumonia: Causal role of mixed infection with anaerobic bacteria. Am Rev Resp Dis 129:317, 1984.

73. Hershey CO, Panaro V: Round pneumonia in adults. Arch Intern Med 148:1155, 1988.

74. Rose RW, Ward BH: Spherical pneumonias in children simulating pulmonary and mediastinal masses. Radiology 106:179, 1973.

75. Fraser RG, Wortzman G: Acute pneumococcal lobar pneumonia: The significance of non-segmental distribution. J Can Assoc Radiol 10:37, 1959.

76. Lévy M, Dromer F, Brion N, et al: Community-acquired pneumonia: Importance of initial noninvasive bacteriologic and radiographic investigations. Chest 92:43, 1988.

77. Moine P, Vercken JB, Chevret S, et al: Severe community-acquired pneumonia: Etiology, epidemiology, and prognosis factors. Chest 105:1487, 1994.

78. Lippmann ML, Goldberg SK, Walkenstein MD, et al: Bacteremic pneumococcal pneumonia: a community hospital experience. Chest 108:1608, 1995.

79. Ziskind MM, Schwarz MI, George RB, et al: Incomplete consolidation in pneumococcal lobar pneumonia complicating pulmonary emphysema. Ann Intern Med 721:835, 1970.

80. Kantor HG: The many radiologic facies of pneumococcal pneumonia. Am J Roentgenol 137:1213, 1981.

81. Brewin A, Arango L, Hadley WK, et al: High-dose penicillin therapy and pneumococcal pneumonia. JAMA 230:409, 1974.

82. Taryle DA, Potts DE, Sahn SA: The incidence and clinical correlates of parapneumonic effusions in pneumococcal pneumonia. Chest 74:170, 1978.

83. Mittl RL, Schwab RJ, Duchin JS, et al: Radiographic resolution of community-acquired pneumonia. Am J Respir Crit Care Med 149:630, 1994.

84. Goodman LR, Goren RA, Teplick SK: The radiographic evaluation of pulmonary infection. Med Clin North Am 64:553, 1980.

85. Tuazon CU: Gram-positive pneumonias. Med Clin North Am 64:343, 1980.

86. Musgrave T, Verghese A: Clinical features of pneumonia in the elderly. Semin Respir Infect 5:269, 1990.

87. Granados A, Podzamczer D, Gudiol F, et al: Pneumonia due to *Legionella pneumophila* and pneumococcal pneumonia: Similarities and differences on presentation. Eur Respir J 2:130, 1989.

88. Mufson MA, Oley G, Hughey D: Pneumococcal disease in a medium-sized community in the United States. JAMA 248:1486, 1982.

89. Camara DS, Beam TR, Perakos PG, et al: *Streptococcus pneumoniae* meningitis in two patients with peritoneovenous shunts. Am J Gastroenterol 79:287, 1984.

90. Berk SL, Rice PA, Reynolds CA, et al: Pneumococcal pericarditis: A persisting problem in contemporary diagnosis. Am J Med 70:247, 1981.

91. Rytel MW, Dee TH, Ferstenfeld JE, et al: Possible pathogenetic role of capsular antigens in fulminant pneumococcal disease with disseminated intravascular coagulation (DIC). Am J Med 57:889, 1974.

92. Tugwell P, Williams AO: Jaundice associated with lobar pneumonia: A clinical, laboratory, and histological study. Q J Med 46:97, 1977.

93. Tugwell P: Glucose-6-phosphate-dehydrogenase deficiency in Nigerians with jaundice associated with lobar pneumonia. Lancet 1:968, 1973.

94. Hroncich ME, Rudinger AN: Rhabdomyolysis with pneumococcal pneumonia: A report of two cases. Am J Med 86:467, 1989.

95. Kaehny WD, Ozawa T, Schwarz MI, et al: Acute nephritis and pulmonary alveolitis following pneumococcal pneumonia. Arch Intern Med 138:806, 1978.

96. Perlino CA: Laboratory diagnosis of pneumonia due to *Streptococcus pneumoniae*. J Infect Dis 150:139, 1984.

97. Kaiser AB, Schaffner W: Prospectus: The prevention of bacteremic pneumococcal pneumonia: A conservative appraisal of vaccine intervention. JAMA 230:404, 1974.

98. Barrett-Connor E: The nonvalue of sputum culture in the diagnosis of pneumococcal pneumonia. Am Rev Resp Dis 103:845, 1971.

99. Rathbun HK, Govani I: Mouse inoculation as a means of identifying pneumococci in the sputum. Johns Hopkins Med J 120:46, 1967.

100. Fiala M: A study of the combined role of viruses, mycoplasmas, and bacteria in adult pneumonia. Am J Med Sci 257:44, 1969.

101. Barnes DJ, Naraqi S, Igo JD: The diagnostic and prognostic significance of bulging fissures in acute lobar pneumonia. Aust NZ J Med 18:130, 1988.

102. Jimenez P, Meneses M, Saldias F, et al: Pneumococcal antigen detection in bronchoalveolar lavage fluid from patients with pneumonia. Thorax 49:872, 1994.

103. Menendez Villanueva R: The diagnostic evaluation of rapid sputum technics for *Pneumococcus* in community-acquired pneumonia: The usefulness of Bayes theorem for clinical application. Arch Broncopneumol 31:317, 1995.

104. Perkins MD, Mirrett S, Reller LB: Rapid bacterial antigen detection is not clinically useful. J Clin Microbiol 33:1486, 1995.

105. Boersma WG, Lowenberg A, Holloway Y, et al: Rapid detection of pneumococcal antigen in pleural fluid of patients with community-acquired pneumonia. Thorax 48:160, 1993.

106. Gillespie SH, Smith MD, Dickens A, et al: Diagnosis of *Streptococcus pneumoniae* pneumonia by quantitative enzyme-linked immunosorbent assay of C-polysaccharide antigen. J Clin Pathol 47:749, 1994.

107. Salo P, Ortqvist A, Leinonen M: Diagnosis of bacteremic pneumococcal pneumonia by amplification of pneumolysin gene fragment in serum. J Infect Dis 171:479, 1995.

108. Rudolph KM, Parkinson AJ, Black CM, et al: Evaluation of polymerase chain reaction for diagnosis of pneumococcal pneumonia. J Clin Microbiol 31:2661, 1993.

109. Gillespie SH, Ullman C, Smith MD, et al: Detection of *Streptococcus pneumoniae* in sputum samples by PCR. J Clin Microbiol 32:1308, 1994.

110. Leinonen M: Serological diagnosis of pneumococcal pneumonia—will it ever become a clinical reality? Semin Respir Infect 9:189, 1994.

110a. Torres JM, Cardenas O, Vasquez A, et al: *Streptococcus pneumoniae* bacteremia in a community hospital. Chest 113:387, 1998.

111. Moine P, Vercken JB, Chevret S, et al: Severe community-acquired pneumococcal pneumonia—The French Study Group of Community-Acquired Pneumonia in ICU. Scand J Infect Dis 27:201, 1995.

112. Fine MJ, Singer DE, Hanusa BH, et al: Validation of a pneumonia prognostic index using the MedisGroups comparative hospital database. Am J Med 94:153, 1993.

113. Marfin AA, Sporrer J, Moore PS, et al: Risk factors for adverse outcome in persons with pneumococcal pneumonia. Chest 107:457, 1995.

114. Mirzanejad Y, Roman S, Talbot J, et al: Pneumococcal bacteremia in two tertiary care hospitals in Winnipeg, Canada. Chest 109:173, 1996.

115. Neill AM, Martin IR, Weir R, et al: Community-acquired pneumonia: Aetiology and usefulness of severity criteria on admission. Thorax 51:1010, 1996.

116. Hedlund J: Community-acquired pneumonia requiring hospitalisation: Factors of importance for the short- and long-term prognosis. Scand J Infect Dis 97:1, 1995.

117. Watanakunakorn C, Greifenstein A, Stroh K, et al: Pneumococcal bacteremia in three community teaching hospitals from 1980 to 1989. Chest 103:1152, 1993.

118. Marrie TJ: Epidemiology of community-acquired pneumonia in the elderly. Semin Respir Infect 5:260, 1990.

119. Perlino CA, Rimland D: Alcoholism, leukopenia, and pneumococcal sepsis. Am Rev Respir Dis 132:757, 1985.

120. Pesola GR, Charles A: Pneumococcal bacteremia with pneumonia—mortality in acquired immunodeficiency syndrome. Chest 101:150, 1992.

121. Friedland IR: Comparison of the response to antimicrobial therapy of penicillin-resistant and penicillin-susceptible pneumococcal disease. Pediatr Infect Dis J 14:885, 1995.

122. Friedland IR, McCracken GH: Management of infections caused by antibiotic-resistant *Streptococcus pneumoniae*. N Engl J Med 331:377, 1994.

123. Gerber GJ, Farmer WC, Fulkerson LL: Beta-hemolytic streptococcal pneumonia following influenza. JAMA 240:242, 1978.

124. Kevy SV, Lowe BA: Streptococcal pneumonia and empyema in childhood. N Engl J Med 264:738, 1961.

125. Aebi C, Ahmed A, Ramilo O: Bacterial complications of primary varicella in children. Clin Infect Dis 23:698, 1996.

126. Welch CC, Tombridge TL, Baker WJ, et al: Beta-hemolytic streptococcal pneumonia: Report of an outbreak in a military population. Am J Med Sci 242:157, 1961.
127. Ruben FL, Norden CW, Heisler B, et al: An outbreak of *Streptococcus pyogenes* infections in a nursing home. Ann Intern Med 101:494, 1984.
128. Anonymous: A household cluster of fulminant group A *Streptococcus* pneumonia associated with toxic shock syndrome—Quebec. Can Commun Dis Rep 22:41, 1996.
129. MacCallum WG: Pathological anatomy of pneumonia associated with influenza. Johns Hopkins Hosp Rep 20:149, 1921.
130. Basiliere JL, Bistrong HW, Spence WF: Streptococcal pneumonia: Recent outbreaks in military recruit populations. Am J Med 44:580, 1968.
131. Hamour A, Bonnington A, Wilkins EG: Severe community-acquired pneumonia associated with a desquamating rash due to group A beta-haemolytic streptococcus. J Infect 29:77, 1994.
132. Burmeister RW, Overholt EL: Pneumonia caused by hemolytic streptococcus. Arch Intern Med 111:367, 1963.
133. al-Ujayli B, Nafziger DA, Saravolatz L: Pneumonia due to *Staphylococcus aureus* infection. Clin Chest Med 16:111, 1995.
134. Jones R, Santos JI, Overall JC Jr: Bacterial tracheitis. JAMA 242:721, 1979.
135. Kasian GF, Bingham WT, Steinberg J, et al: Bacterial tracheitis in children. Can Med Assoc J 140:46, 1989.
136. Chickering HT, Park JH: *Staphylococcus aureus* pneumonia. JAMA 72:617, 1919.
137. Woodhead MA, Radvan J, MacFarlane JT: Adult community-acquired staphylococcal pneumonia in the antibiotic era: A review of 61 cases. Q J Med 64:783, 1987.
138. Mostow SR: Pneumonias acquired outside the hospital—recognition and treatment. Med Clin North Am 58:555, 1974.
139. Spencer RC: Predominant pathogens found in the European Prevalence of Infection in Intensive Care Study. Eur J Clin Microbiol Infect Dis 15:281, 1996.
140. Johnston BL: Methicillin-resistant *Staphylococcus aureus* as a cause of community-acquired pneumonia—a critical review. Semin Respir Infect 9:199, 1994.
141. Bradley SF, Terpenning MS, Ramsey MA, et al: Methicillin-resistant *Staphylococcus aureus*: colonization and infection in a long-term care facility. Ann Intern Med 115:417, 1991.
142. Iwahara T, Ichiyama S, Nada T, et al: Clinical and epidemiologic investigations of nosocomial pulmonary infections caused by methicillin-resistant *Staphylococcus aureus*. Chest 105:826, 1994.
143. Rello J, Quintana E, Ausina V, et al: Risk factors for *Staphylococcus aureus* nosocomial pneumonia in critically ill patients. Am Rev Respir Dis 142:1320, 1990.
144. Kaye MG, Fox MJ, Bartlett JG, et al: The clinical spectrum of *Staphylococcus aureus* pulmonary infection. Chest 97:788, 1990.
145. Bergmans D, Bonten M, Gaillard C, et al: Clinical spectrum of ventilator-associated pneumonia caused by methicillin-sensitive *Staphylococcus aureus*. Eur J Clin Microbiol Infect Dis 15:437, 1996.
146. Moroni M, Franzetti F: Bacterial pneumonia in adult patients with HIV infection. J Chemother 7:292, 1995.
147. Miller RF, Foley NM, Kessel D, et al: Community-acquired lobar pneumonia in patients with HIV infection in AIDS. Thorax 49:367, 1994.
148. Fagbule DO: Bacterial pathogens in malnourished children with pneumonia. Trop Geogr Med 45:294, 1993.
149. Tsao TCY, Tsai YH, Lan RS, et al: Pulmonary manifestations of *Staphylococcus aureus* septicemia. Chest 101:574, 1992.
150. Kaplan MH, Tenenbaum MJ: *Staphylococcus aureus*: Cellular biology and clinical application. Am J Med 72:248, 1982.
151. Sawai T, Tomono K, Yanagihara K, et al: Role of coagulase in a murine model of hematogenous pulmonary infection induced by intravenous injection of *Staphylococcus aureus* enmeshed in agar beads. Infect Immun 65:466, 1997.
152. Wade JC, Schimpff SC, Newman KA, et al: *Staphylococcus epidermidis*: An increasing cause of infection in patients with granulocytopenia. Ann Intern Med 97:503, 1982.
153. Henrickson KJ, Shenep JL: Fulminating *Staphylococcus epidermis* bacteremia. South Med J 83:231, 1990.
154. Rikitomi N, Nagatake T, Sakamoto T, et al: The role of MRSA (methicillin-resistant *Staphylococcus aureus*) adherence and colonization in the upper respiratory tract of geriatric patients with nosocomial pulmonary infections. Microbiol Immunol 38:607, 1994.
155. Ramisse F, Szatanik M, Binder P, et al: Passive local immunotherapy of experimental staphylococcal pneumonia with human intravenous immunoglobulin. J Infect Dis 168:1030, 1993.
156. Quigley MJ, Fraser RS: Pulmonary pneumatocele: Pathology and pathogenesis. Am J Roentgenol 150:1275, 1988.
157. Conway DJ: The origin of lung cysts in childhood. Arch Dis Child 26:504, 1951.
158. Boisset GF: Subpleural emphysema complicating staphylococcal and other pneumonias. J Pediatr 81:259, 1972.
159. Dines DE: Diagnostic significance of pneumatocele of the lung. JAMA 204:79, 1968.
160. Yesner R, Bernstein S, D'Esopo ND: The evolution of bullous cavities in adequately treated experimental pulmonary tuberculosis. Am Rev Resp Dis 82:810, 1960.
161. Wollenman OJ Jr, Finland M: Pathology of staphylococcal pneumonia complicating clinical influenza. Am J Pathol 19:23, 1943.
162. Guthrie KJ, Montgomery GL: Staphylococcal pneumonia in childhood: Pathological considerations. Lancet 253:752, 1947.

163. Gresham GA, Gleeson-White MH: Staphylococcal bronchopneumonia in debilitated hospital patients: A report of fourteen fatal cases. Lancet 1:651, 1957.
164. Magner D, Kussner N: Staphylococcal pulmonary infection in infancy. Am J Clin Pathol 24:1391, 1954.
165. Jackson JR, Gibbons RJ, Magner D: The effects of staphylococcal toxin on the lungs of rabbits. Am J Pathol 34:1051, 1958.
166. Charan NB, Turk GM, Dhand R: The role of bronchial circulation in lung abscess. Am Rev Resp Dis 131:121, 1985.
166a. Akira M, Kitatani F, Lee Y-S, et al: Diffuse panbronchiolitis: Evaluation with high-resolution CT. Radiology 168:433, 1988.
166b. Aquino SL, Gamsu G, Webb WR, et al: Tree-in-bud pattern: Frequency and significance on thin-section CT. J Comput Assist Tomogr 20:594, 1996.
166c. Collins J, Blankenbaker D, Stern EJ: Patterns of bronchiolar disease: What is "tree-in-bud"? Am J Roentgenol 171:365, 1998.
167. MacFarlane J, Rose D: Radiographic features of staphylococcal pneumonia in adults and children. Thorax 51:539, 1996.
168. Kaye MG, Fox MJ, Bartlett JG, et al: The clinical spectrum of *Staphylococcus aureus* pulmonary infection. Chest 97:788, 1990.
169. Chartrand SA, McCracken GH: Staphylococcal pneumonia in infants and children. Pediatr Infect Dis 1:19, 1982.
170. Dines DE: Diagnostic significance of pneumatocele of the lung. JAMA 204:1169, 1968.
171. Huxtable KA, Tucker AS, Wedgwood RJ: Staphylococcal pneumonia in childhood: Long-term follow-up. Am J Dis Child 108:262, 1964.
172. Meyers HI, Jacobsen G: Staphylococcal pneumonia in children and adults. Radiology 72:665, 1959.
173. Flaherty RA, Keegan JM, Sturdevant HN: Post-pneumonic pulmonary pneumatoceles. Radiology 74:50, 1960.
174. Naraqi S, McDonnell G: Hematogenous staphylococcal pneumonia secondary to soft tissue infection. Chest 79:173, 1981.
175. Huang RM, Naidich DP, Lubat E, et al: Septic pulmonary emboli: CT-radiographic correlation. AJR 153:41, 1989.
176. Kuhlman JE, Fishman EK, Teigen C: Pulmonary septic emboli: Diagnosis with CT. Radiology 174:211, 1990.
177. Angeloni JM, Scott AW: Lung abscess and pneumonia complicating influenza. Lancet 1:1254, 1958.
178. Kuperman AS, Fernandez RB: Subacute staphylococcal pneumonia. Am Rev Resp Dis 101:95, 1970.
179. Kasian GF, Bingham WT, Steinberg J, et al: Bacterial tracheitis in children. Can Med Assoc J 140:46, 1989.
180. Fisher AM, Trever RW, Curtin JA, et al: Staphylococcal pneumonia: A review of 21 cases in adults. N Engl J Med 258:919, 1958.
181. Bando T, Fujimura M, Noda Y, et al: Rhabdomyolysis associated with bacteremic pneumonia due to *Staphylococcus aureus*. Intern Med 33:454, 1994.
182. Anthony BF: Carriage of group-B streptococci during pregnancy. J Infect Dis 145:789, 1982.
183. Easmon CSF, Hastings MJG, Clare AJ, et al: Nosocomial transmission of group-B streptococci. BMJ 283:459, 1981.
184. Banagale RC, Watters JH: Delayed right-sided diaphragmatic hernia following group B streptococcal infection: A discussion of its pathogenesis, with a review of the literature. Hum Pathol 14:67, 1983.
185. Bayer AS, Chow AW, Anthony BF, et al: Serious infections in adults due to group B streptococci. Am J Med 61:498, 1976.
186. Berk SL, Verghese A, Holtsclaw SA, et al: Enterococcal pneumonia: Occurrence in patients receiving broad-spectrum antibiotic regimens and enteral feeding. Am J Med 74:153, 1983.
187. Verghese A, Berk SL, Boelen LJ, et al: Group-B streptococcal pneumonia in the elderly. Arch Intern Med 142:1642, 1982.
188. Duma RJ, Weinberg AN, Medrek TF, et al: Streptococcal infections: A bacteriologic and clinical study of streptococcal bacteremia. Medicine 48:87, 1969.
189. Morris JE, Okies JE: Enterococcal lung abscess: Medical and surgical therapy. Chest 65:688, 1974.
190. Vassallo J, Galizia AC, Cuschieri P: Mixed pulmonary infection with *Nocardia, Candida,* methicillin-resistant *Staphylococcus aureus,* and group D *streptococcus* species. Postgrad Med J 72:680, 1996.
191. Henwick S, Koehler M, Patrick CC: Complications of bacteremia due to *Stomatococcus mucilaginosus* in neutropenic children. Clin Infect Dis 17:667, 1993.
192. Bonten MJ, van Tiel FH, van der Geest S, et al: Topical antimicrobial prophylaxis of nosocomial pneumonia in mechanically ventilated patients: Microbiological observations. Infection 21:137, 1993.
193. Bonten MJ, van Tiel FH, van der Geest S, et al: *Enterococcus faecalis* pneumonia complicating topical antimicrobial prophylaxis. N Engl J Med 328:209, 1993.
194. Mohr DN, Feist DJ, Washington JA II, et al: Infections due to group-C streptococci in man. Am J Med 66:450, 1979.
195. Shlaes DM, Lerner PI, Wolinsky E, et al: Infections due to Lancefield group-F and related streptococci (*S. milleri, S. anginosus*). Medicine 60:197, 1981.
196. Hocken DB, Dussek JE: *Streptococcus milleri* as a cause of pleural empyema. Thorax 40:626, 1985.
197. Shinzato T, Saito A: The *Streptococcus milleri* group as a cause of pulmonary infections. Clin Infect Dis 21:238, 1995.
198. Mastroianni A, Coronado O, Nanetti A, et al: Community-acquired pneumonia due to *Staphylococcus cohnii* in an HIV-infected patient: Case report and review. Eur J Clin Microbiol Infect Dis 14:904, 1995.
199. Wright PW, Wallace RJ Jr: Pneumonia due to *Moraxella (Branhamella) catarrhalis*. Semin Respir Infect 4:40, 1989.

200. Barreiro B, Esteban L, Prats E, et al: *Branhamella catarrhalis* respiratory infections. Eur Respir J 5:675, 1992.
201. Murphy TF: *Branhamella catarrhalis*: Epidemiology, surface antigenic structure, and immune response. Microbiol Rev 60:267, 1996.
202. Slevin NJ, Aitken J, Thornley PE: Clinical and microbiological features of *Branhamella catarrhalis* bronchopulmonary infections. Lancet 1:782, 1984.
203. Wallace RJ Jr, Musher DM: The realization of *Branhamella catarrhalis* as a respiratory pathogen. Chest 90:447, 1986.
204. Srinivasan G, Raff MJ, Templeton WC, et al: *Branhamella catarrhalis* pneumonia: Report of two cases and review of the literature. Am Rev Resp Dis 123:553, 1981.
205. Christensen JJ, Renneberg J, Bruun B, et al: Serum antibody response to proteins of *Moraxella (Branhamella) catarrhalis* in patients with lower respiratory tract infection. Clin Diagn Lab Immunol 2:14, 1995.
206. Helminen ME, Beach R, Maciver I, et al: Human immune response against outer membrane proteins of *Moraxella (Branhamella) catarrhalis* determined by immunoblotting and enzyme immunoassay. Clin Diagn Lab Immunol 2:35, 1995.
207. Chapman AJ Jr, Musher DM, Jonsson S, et al: Development of bactericidal antibody during *Branhamella catarrhalis* infection. J Infect Dis 151:878, 1985.
208. Thornley PE, Aitken J, Drennan CJ, et al: *Branhamella catarrhalis* infection of the lower respiratory tract: Reliable diagnosis by sputum examination. BMJ 285:1537, 1982.
209. McLeod DT, Ahmad F, Capewell S, et al: Increase in bronchopulmonary infection due to *Branhamella catarrhalis*. BMJ 292:1103, 1986.
210. Christensen JJ, Gadeberg O, Bruun B: *Branhamella catarrhalis*: Significance in pulmonary infections and bacteriological features. Acta Pathol Microbiol Immunol Scand 94:89, 1986.
211. Karnad A, Alvarez S, Berk SL: *Branhamella catarrhalis* pneumonia in patients with immunoglobulin abnormalities. South Med J 79:1360, 1986.
212. Diamond LA, Lorber B: *Branhamella catarrhalis* pneumonia and immunoglobulin abnormalities: A new association. Am Rev Resp Dis 129:876, 1984.
213. Richards SJ, Greening AP, Enright MC, et al: Outbreak of *Moraxella catarrhalis* in a respiratory unit. Thorax 48:91, 1993.
214. Irwin RS, Woelk WK, Coudon WL III: Primary meningococcal pneumonia. Ann Intern Med 82:493, 1975.
215. Barnes RV, Dopp AC, Gelberg HJ, et al: *Neisseria meningitidis*: A cause of nosocomial pneumonia. Am Rev Resp Dis 111:229, 1975.
216. Jacobs SA, Norden OW: Pneumonia caused by *Neisseria meningitidis*. JAMA 227:67, 1974.
217. Ball JH, Young DA: Primary meningococcal pneumonia. Am Rev Resp Dis 109:480, 1974.
218. Galaid EI, Cherubin CE, Marr JS, et al: Meningococcal disease in New York City, 1973 to 1978: Recognition of groups Y and W-135 as frequent pathogens. JAMA 244:2167, 1980.
218a. Jones EM, Brown NM, Harvey JE, et al: Three cases of meningococcal pneumonia. Thorax 52:927, 1997.
219. Ellenbogen C, Graybill JR, Silva J Jr, et al: Bacterial pneumonia complicating adenoviral pneumonia: A comparison of respiratory tract bacterial culture sources and effectiveness of chemoprophylaxis against bacterial pneumonia. Am J Med 56:169, 1974.
220. Davies BI, Spanjaard L, Dankert J: Meningococcal chest infections in a general hospital. Eur J Clin Microbiol Infect Dis 10:399, 1991.
221. Christensen JJ, Gadeberg O, Bruun B: *Neisseria meningitidis*: Occurrence in nonpneumonic pulmonary infections. APMIS 96:218, 1988.
222. Young LS, LaForce FM, Head JJ, et al: A simultaneous outbreak of meningococcal and influenza infections. N Engl J Med 287:5, 1972.
223. Salit IE: Meningococcemia caused by serogroup W-135: Association with hypogammaglobulinemia. Arch Intern Med 141:664, 1981.
224. Witt D, Olans RN: Bacteremic W-135 meningococcal pneumonia. Am Rev Resp Dis 125:255, 1982.
225. Ball JH, Young DA: Primary meningococcal pneumonia. Am Rev Resp Dis 109:480, 1974.
226. Gilrane T, Tracy JD, Greenlee RM, et al: *Neisseria sicca* pneumonia: Report of two cases and review of the literature. Am J Med 78:1038, 1985.
227. Gris P, Vincke G, Delmez JP, et al: *Neisseria sicca* pneumonia and bronchiectasis. Eur Respir J 2:685, 1989.
228. Thorsteinsson SB, Minuth JN, Musher DM: Postpneumonectomy empyema due to *Neisseria mucosus*. Am J Clin Pathol 64:534, 1975.
229. Hussain Z, Lannigan R, Austin TW: Pulmonary cavitation due to *Neisseria mucosa* in a child with chronic neutropenia. Eur J Clin Microbiol Infec Dis 7:175, 1988.
230. Claassen JL, Eppes SC, Buckley RH: Pulmonary coin lesion caused by *Neisseria mucosa* in a child with chronic granulomatous disease. Pediatr Infect Dis J 6:567, 1987.
231. Boyce JM, Taylor MR, Mitchell EB Jr, et al: Nosocomial pneumonia caused by a glucose-metabolizing strain of *Neisseria cinerea*. J Clin Microbiol 21:1, 1985.
232. Morla N, Guibourdenche M, Riou JY: *Neisseria* spp. and AIDS. J Clin Microbiol 30:2290, 1992.
233. Belding ME, Carbone J: Gonococcemia associated with adult respiratory distress syndrome. Rev Infec Dis 13:1105, 1991.
234. John TJ: Emerging and re-emerging bacterial pathogens in India. Indian J Med Res 103:4, 1996.
235. Meselson M, Guillemin J, Hugh-Jones M, et al: The Sverdlovsk anthrax outbreak of 1979. Science 266:1202, 1994.
236. George S, Mathai D, Balraj V, et al: An outbreak of anthrax meningoencephalitis. Trans R Soc Trop Med Hyg 88:206, 1994.
237. Anonymous: Anthrax control and research, with special reference to national programme development in Africa: Memorandum from a WHO meeting. Bull World Health Organ 72:13, 1994.
238. Taylor JP, Dimmitt DC, Ezzell JW, et al: Indigenous human cutaneous anthrax in Texas. South Med J 86:1, 1993.
239. Brachman PS, Pagano JS, Albrink WS: Two cases of fatal inhalation anthrax, one associated with sarcoidosis. N Engl J Med 265:203, 1961.
240. Enticknap JB, Galbraith NS, Tomlinson AJH, et al: Pulmonary anthrax caused by contaminated sacks. Br J Industr Med 25:72, 1968.
241. Ross JM: The pathogenesis of anthrax following the administration of spores by the respiratory route. J Pathol Bacteriol 73:485, 1957.
242. Dalldorf FG, Kaufmann AF, Brachman PS: Woolsorters' disease: An experimental model. Arch Pathol 92:418, 1971.
243. Cowdery JS: Primary pulmonary anthrax with septicemia: Case reports. Arch Pathol 43:396, 1947.
244. Albrink WS, Brooks SM, Biron RE, et al: Human inhalation anthrax: A report of three fatal cases. Am J Pathol 36:457, 1960.
245. Vessal K, Yeganehdoust J, Dutz W, et al: Radiological changes in inhalational anthrax: A report of radiological and pathological correlation in two cases. Clin Radiol 25:471, 1975.
246. Ihde DC, Armstrong D: Clinical spectrum of infection due to *Bacillus* species. Am J Med 55:839, 1973.
247. Jonsson S, Clarridge J, Young EJ: Necrotizing pneumonia and empyema caused by *Bacillus cereus* and *Clostridium bifermentans*. Am Rev Resp Dis 127:357, 1983.
248. Miller JM, Hair JG, Hebert M, et al: Fulminating bacteremia and pneumonia due to *Bacillus cereus*. J Clin Microbiol 35:514, 1997.
249. Garcia-Montero M, Rodriguez-Garcia JL, Calvo P, et al: Pneumonia caused by *Listeria monocytogenes*. Respiration 62:107, 1995.
250. Isaacson P, Jacobs PH, MacKenzie AMR, et al: Pseudotumour of the lung caused by infection with *Bacillus sphaericus*. J Clin Pathol 29:806, 1976.
251. Bekemeyer WB, Zimmerman GA: Life-threatening complications associated with *Bacillus cereus* pneumonia. Am Rev Resp Dis 131:466, 1985.
252. Farber JM, Ross WH, Harwig J: Health risk assessment of *Listeria monocytogenes* in Canada. Int J Food Microbiol 30:145, 1996.
253. Louria DB, Hensle T, Armstrong D, et al: Listeriosis complicating malignant disease: A new association. Ann Intern Med 67:261, 1967.
254. Schlech WF: Pathogenesis and immunology of *Listeria monocytogenes*. Pathol Biol 44:775, 1996.
255. Skidmore AG: Listeriosis at Vancouver General Hospital, 1965–1979. Can Med Assoc J 125:1217, 1981.
256. Paul ML, Dwyer DE, Chow C, et al: Listeriosis—a review of eighty-four cases. Med J Aust 160:489, 1994.
257. Ananthraman A, Israel RH, Magnussen CR: Pleural-pulmonary aspects of *Listeria monocytogenes* infection. Respiration 44:153, 1983.
258. Larsson S, Cronberg S, Winblad S: Clinical aspects on 64 cases of juvenile and adult listeriosis in Sweden. Acta Med Scand 204:503, 1978.
259. Buchner LH, Schneierson SS: Clinical and laboratory aspects of *Listeria monocytogenes* infections: With a report of ten cases. Am J Med 45:904, 1968.
260. Bowmer EJ, McKiel JA, Cockcroft WH, et al: *Listeria monocytogenes* infections in Canada. Can Med Assoc J 109:125, 1973.
261. Fulco OJ, Leggiadro RJ: *Listeria monocytogenes* sepsis complicated by the adult respiratory distress syndrome. NY State J Med 82:1857, 1982.
262. Boucher M, Yonekura ML, Wallace RJ, et al: Adult respiratory distress syndrome: A rare manifestation of *Listeria monocytogenes* infection in pregnancy. Am J Obstet Gynecol 149:686, 1984.
263. Young VM, Meyers WF, Moody MR, et al: The emergence of Coryneform bacteria as a cause of nosocomial infections in compromised hosts. Am J Med 70:646, 1981.
264. Dobie RA, Tobey DN: Clinical features of diphtheria in the respiratory tract. JAMA 242:2197, 1979.
265. Stamm WE, Tompkins LS, Wagner KF, et al: Infection due to *Corynebacterium* species in marrow transplant patients. Ann Intern Med 91:167, 1979.
266. Ahmed K, Kawakami K, Watanabe K, et al: *Corynebacterium pseudodiphtheriticum*: A respiratory tract pathogen. Clin Infect Dis 20:41, 1995.
267. Manzella JP, Kellogg JA, Parsey KS: *Corynebacterium pseudodiphtheriticum*: A respiratory tract pathogen in adults. Clin Infect Dis 20:37, 1995.
268. Keslin MH, McCoy EL, McCusker JJ, et al: *Corynebacterium pseudotuberculosis*: A new cause of infectious and eosinophilic pneumonia. Am J Med 67:228, 1979.
269. Wallet F, Marquette CH, Courcol RJ: Multiresistant *Corynebacterium xerosis* as a cause of pneumonia in a patient with acute leukemia. Clin Infect Dis 18:845, 1994.
270. Bowstead TT, Santiago SM: Pleuropulmonary infection due to *Corynebacterium striatum*. Br J Dis Chest 74:198, 1980.
271. Martinez-Martinez L, Suarez AI, Ortega MC, et al: Fatal pulmonary infection caused by *Corynebacterium striatum*. Clin Infect Dis 19:806, 1994.
272. Van Etta LL, Filice GA, Ferguson RM, et al: *Corynebacterium equi*: A review of 12 cases of human infection. Rev Infect Dis 5:1012, 1983.
273. Scott MA, Graham BS, Verrall R, et al: *Rhodococcus equi*—an increasingly recognized opportunistic pathogen: Report of 12 cases and review of 65 cases in the literature. Am J Clin Pathol 103:649, 1995.
274. Verville TD, Huycke MM, Greenfield RA, et al: *Rhodococcus equi* infections of humans: 12 cases and a review of the literature. Medicine 73:119, 1994.
275. Arlotti M, Zoboli G, Moscatelli GL, et al: *Rhodococcus equi* infection in HIV-

positive subjects: A retrospective analysis of 24 cases. Scand J Infect Dis 28:463, 1996.

276. Segovia J, Pulpon LA, Crespo MG, et al: *Rhodococcus equi*: First case in a heart transplant recipient. J Heart Lung Transplant 13:332, 1994.

277. Walsh RD, Cunha BA: *Rhodococcus equi*: Fatal pneumonia in a patient without AIDS. Heart Lung 23:519, 1994.

278. Berg R, Chmel H, Mayo J, et al: *Corynebacterium equi*: Infection complicating neoplastic disease. Am J Clin Pathol 68:73, 1977.

279. Savdie E, Pigott P, Jennis F: Lung abscess due to *Corynebacterium equi* in a renal transplant recipient. Med J Aust 1:817, 1977.

280. Sughayer M, Ali SZ, Erozan YS, et al: Pulmonary malacoplakia associated with *Rhodococcus equi* infection in an AIDS patient: Report of a case with diagnosis by fine-needle aspiration. Acta Cytol 41:507, 1997.

281. van Hoeven KH, Dookhan DB, Petersen RO: Cytologic features of pulmonary malakoplakia related to *Rhodococcus equi* in an immunocompromised host. Diag Cytopathol 15:325, 1996.

282. Winberg CD, Rose ME, Rappaport H: Whipple's disease of the lung. Am J Med 65:873, 1978.

283. Symmons DP, Shepherd AN, Boardman PL, et al: Pulmonary manifestations of Whipple's disease. J Med 56:497, 1985.

284. James TN, Bulkley BH: Whipple bacilli within the tunica media of pulmonary arteries. Chest 86:454, 1984.

285. Kelly CA, Egan M, Rawlinson J, et al: Whipple's disease presenting with lung involvement. Thorax 51:343, 1996.

286. Enzinger FM, Helwig EB: Whipple's disease: A review of the literature and report of fifteen patients. Virchows Arch Pathol Anat 336:238, 1963.

287. Namnyak SS, Blair AL, Hughes DF, et al: Fatal lung abscess due to *Lactobacillus casei* ss *rhamnosus*. Thorax 47:666, 1992.

288. George DL: Epidemiology of nosocomial pneumonia in intensive care unit patients. Clin Chest Med 16:29, 1995.

289. Rello J, Quintana E, Ausina V, et al: Incidence, etiology, and outcome of nosocomial pneumonia in mechanically ventilated patients. Chest 100:439, 1991.

290. Maloney SA, Jarvis WR: Epidemic nosocomial pneumonia in the intensive care unit. Clin Chest Med 16:209, 1995.

291. [This official statement of the American Thoracic Society was adopted by the ATS Board of Directors, November 1995.] Hospital-acquired pneumonia in adults: Diagnosis, assessment of severity, initial antimicrobial therapy, and preventative strategies. Am J Respir Crit Care Med 153:1711, 1995.

292. Pachon J, Prados MD, Capote F, et al: Severe community-acquired pneumonia—etiology, prognosis, and treatment. Am Rev Respir Dis 142:369, 1990.

293. Moine P, Vercken JB, Chevret S, et al: Severe community-acquired pneumonia—etiology, epidemiology, and prognosis factors. Chest 105:1487, 1994.

294. Anonymous: Guidelines for the management of community-acquired pneumonia in adults admitted to hospital: The British Thoracic Society. Br J Hosp Med 49:346, 1993.

295. Woodhead MA: Management of pneumonia. Respir Med 86:459, 1992.

296. Mandell LA: Community-acquired pneumonia—etiology, epidemiology, and treatment. Chest 108:358, 1995.

297. Niederman MS, Bass JB Jr, Campbell GD, et al: Guidelines for the initial management of adults with community-acquired pneumonia: Diagnosis, assessment of severity, and initial antimicrobial therapy: American Thoracic Society, Medical Section of the American Lung Association. Am Rev Respir Dis 148:1418, 1993.

298. Gorzynski EA: Enterobacteriaceae: II. *In* Milgrom F, Flanagan TD (eds): Medical Microbiology. New York, Churchill Livingstone, 1982, p 309.

299. Bruckner DA, Colonna P: Nomenclature for aerobic and facultative bacteria. Clin Infect Dis 21:263, 1995.

300. Yinnon AM, Butnaru A, Raveh D, et al: *Klebsiella* bacteraemia: Community versus nosocomial infection. QJM 89:933, 1996.

301. Lee KH, Hui KP, Tan WC, et al: *Klebsiella* bacteraemia: A report of 101 cases from National University Hospital, Singapore. J Hosp Infect 27:299, 1994.

302. Selden R, Lee S, Wang WLL, et al: Nosocomial *Klebsiella* infections: Intestinal colonization as a reservoir. Ann Intern Med 74:657, 1971.

303. Dorff GJ, Rytel MW, Farmer SG, et al: Etiologies and characteristic features of pneumonias in a municipal hospital. Am J Med Sci 266:349, 1973.

304. Jong GM, Hsiue TR, Chen CR, et al: Rapidly fatal outcome of bacteremic *Klebsiella* pneumoniae pneumonia in alcoholics. Chest 107:214, 1995.

305. Crossley KB, Thurn JR: Nursing home–acquired pneumonia. Semin Respir Infect 4:64, 1989.

306. Pierce AK, Sanford JP: Aerobic gram-negative bacillary pneumonias. Am Rev Resp Dis 110:647, 1974.

307. Williams I, Radcliffe G, Hetzel M, et al: Tracheal rhinoscleroma treated by argon laser. Thorax 37:638, 1982.

308. Porto R, Hevia O, Hensley GT, et al: Disseminated *Klebsiella rhinoscleromatis* infection. Arch Pathol Lab Med 113:1381, 1989.

309. Alvarez S, Stinnett JA, Shell CG, et al: *Klebsiella oxytoca* isolates in a general hospital. Infect Control 6:310, 1985.

310. McCarthy VP, Hubbard VS: *Klebsiella ozaenae* in a patient with cystic fibrosis. Arch Intern Med 144:408, 1984.

311. Reed WP: Indolent pulmonary abscess associated with *Klebsiella* and *Enterobacter*. Am Rev Respir Dis 107:1055, 1973.

312. Karnad A, Alvarez S, Berk SL: *Enterobacter* pneumonia. South Med J 80:601, 1987.

313. Al-Damluji S, Dickinson CM, Beck A: *Enterobacter agglomerans*: A new cause of primary pneumonia. Thorax 37:865, 1982.

314. Meltz DJ, Grieco MH: Characteristics of *Serratia marcescens* pneumonia. Arch Intern Med 132:359, 1973.

315. Wilkowske CJ, Washington JA II, Martin WJ, et al: *Serratia marcescens*: Biochemical characteristics, antibiotic susceptibility patterns, and clinical significance. JAMA 214:2157, 1970.

316. Haddy RI, Mann BL, Nadkarni DD, et al: Nosocomial infection in the community hospital: Severe infection due to *Serratia* species. J Fam Pract 42:273, 1996.

317. Bollet C, Grimont P, Gainnier M, et al: Fatal pneumonia due to *Serratia proteamaculans* subsp. *quinovora*. J Clin Microbiol 31:444, 1993.

318. Solomon S: Primary Friedländer pneumonia: Report of thirty-two cases. JAMA 108:937, 1937.

319. Sale L, Wood WB Jr: Studies on the mechanism of recovery in pneumonia due to Friedländer's bacillus: I. The pathogenesis of experimental Friedländer's bacillus pneumonia. J Exp Med 86:239, 1947.

320. Holmes RB: Friedlander's pneumonia. Am J Roentgenol 75:728, 1956.

321. Goldstein JD, Godleski JJ, Balikian JP, et al: Pathologic patterns of *Serratia marcescens* pneumonia. Hum Pathol 13:479, 1982.

322. Felson B, Rosenberg LS, Hamburger M Jr: Roentgen findings in acute Friedländer's pneumonia. Radiology 53:559, 1949.

322a. Moon WK, Im JG, Yeon KM, et al: Complications of *Klebsiella* pneumonia: CT evaluation. J Comput Assist Tomogr 19:176, 1995.

322b. Korvick AJ, Hackett AK, Yu VL, et al: *Klebsiella* pneumonia in the modern era: Clinicoradiographic correlations. South Med J 84:200, 1991.

323. Danner PK, McFarland DR, Felson B: Massive pulmonary gangrene. Am J Roentgenol 103:548, 1968.

324. Knight L, Fraser RG, Robson HG: Massive pulmonary gangrene: A severe complication of *Klebsiella* pneumonia. Can Med Assoc J 112:196, 1975.

325. Penner C, Maycher B, Long R: Pulmonary gangrene—a complication of bacterial pneumonia. Chest 105:567, 1994.

326. Balikian JP, Herman PG, Godleski JJ: *Serratia* pneumonia. Radiology 137:309, 1980.

327. Hammond JMJ, Potgieter PD, Linton DM, et al: Intensive care management of community-acquired *Klebsiella* pneumonia. Respir Med 84:11, 1990.

327a. Kim JY, Lim CM, Koh Y, et al: A case of superior vena cava syndrome caused by *Klebsiella pneumoniae*. Eur Respir J 10:2902, 1997.

328. Morse LJ, Williams HL, Grenn FP Jr, et al: Septicemia due to *Klebsiella pneumoniae* originating from a hand-cream dispenser. N Engl J Med 277:472, 1967.

329. Scotland Department of Health, Scientific Advisory Committee on Medical Administration and Investigation: Neonatal deaths due to infection: Report of a Subcommittee of the Scientific Advisory Committee, Edinburgh, HMSO, 1947.

330. Carson MJ, Chadwick DL, Brubaker CA, et al: Thirteen boys with progressive septic granulomatosis. Pediatrics 35:405, 1965.

331. Mundy LM, Auwaerter PG, Oldach D, et al: Community-acquired pneumonia: Impact of immune status. Am J Respir Crit Care Med 152:1309, 1995.

332. Philp JR, Spencer RC: Secondary respiratory infection in hospital patients: Effect of antimicrobial agents and environment. BMJ 2:359, 1974.

333. Faegenburg D, Saperstein, RL, Chiat H, et al: Colon bacillus pneumonia: A complication of lesser sac abscess. Am J Roentgenol 107:300, 1969.

334. Salomon PF, Tamlyn TT, Grieco MH: *Escherichia coli* pneumonia: Case report. Am Rev Resp Dis 102:248, 1970.

335. Jaffey PB, English PW II, Campbell GA, et al: *Escherichia coli* lobar pneumonia: Fatal infection in a patient with mental retardation. South Med J 89:628, 1996.

336. Tillotson JR, Lerner AM: Pneumonias caused by gram-negative bacilli. Medicine 45:65, 1966.

337. Unger JD, Rose HD, Unger GF: Gram-negative pneumonia. Radiology 107:283, 1973.

338. Tillotson JR, Lerner AM: Characteristics of pneumonias caused by *Escherichia coli*. N Engl J Med 277:115, 1967.

339. Jonas M, Cunha BA: Bacteremic *Escherichia coli* pneumonia. Arch Intern Med 142:2157, 1982.

340. Saphra I, Winter JW: Clinical manifestations of salmonellosis in man. N Engl J Med 256:1128, 1957.

341. Aguado JM, Obeso G, Cabanillas JJ, et al: Pleuropulmonary infections due to nontyphoid strains of *Salmonella*. Arch Intern Med 150:54, 1990.

342. Roberts FJ: Nontyphoidal, nonparatyphoidal salmonella septicemia in adults. Eur J Clin Microbiol Infect Dis 12:205, 1993.

343. Shahram F, Akbarian M, Davatchi F: *Salmonella* infection in systemic lupus erythematosus. Lupus 2:55, 1993.

344. O'Dempsey TJ, McArdle TF, Lloyd-Evans N, et al: Importance of enteric bacteria as a cause of pneumonia, meningitis, and septicemia among children in a rural community in the Gambia, West Africa. Pediatr Infect Dis J 13:122, 1994.

345. Balkin SS: Bronchopneumonia, empyema, pneumothorax, and bacteremia due to *Salmonella choleraesuis* (var. *kunzendorf*) treated with chloramphenicol. Am J Med 21:974, 1956.

346. Han T, Sokal JE, Neter E: Salmonellosis in disseminated malignant disease: A seven-year review (1959–1965). N Engl J Med 276:1045, 1967.

347. Ridha AG, Malbrain ML, Mareels H, et al: Lung abscess due to nontyphoid *Salmonella* in an immunocompromised host: Case report with review of the literature. Acta Clin Belg 51:175, 1996.

348. Riantawan P, Subhannachart P: *Salmonella* lung abscess and bacteraemia in an AIDS patient. J Med Assoc Thai 79:333, 1996.

349. Mussini C, Trenti F, Manicardi G, et al: Nontyphoid *Salmonella* subdural empyema in a patient with AIDS. Scand J Infect Dis 27:173, 1995.

349a. Casado JL, Navas E, Frutos B, et al: *Salmonella* lung involvement in patients with HIV infection. Chest 112:1197, 1997.

350. Burney DP, Fisher RD, Schaffner W: *Salmonella* empyema: A review. South Med J 70:375, 1977.

351. Sharma AM, Sharma OP: Pulmonary manifestations of typhoid fever—two case reports and a review of the literature. Chest 101:1144, 1992.

352. Chan JC, Raffin TA: *Salmonella* lung abscess complicating Wegener's granulomatosis. Respir Med 85:339, 1991.

353. O'Dempsey TJ, McArdle TF, Lloyd-Evans N, et al: Importance of enteric bacteria as a cause of pneumonia, meningitis, and septicemia among children in a rural community in The Gambia, West Africa. Pediatr Infect Dis J 13:122, 1994.

354. Greenspan RH, Feinberg SB: *Salmonella* bacteremia: A case with miliary lung lesions and spondylitis. Radiology 68:860, 1957.

355. Weiss W, Eisenberg GM, Flippin HF: *Salmonella* pleuropulmonary disease. Am J Med Sci 233:487, 1957.

356. Hahne OH: Lung abscess due to *Salmonella typhi*. Am Rev Resp Dis 89:566, 1964.

357. Kuncaitis J, Okutan AM: Empyema due to *Salmonella typhimurium*. Am Rev Resp Dis 83:741, 1961.

358. Rocha H, Kirk JW, Hearey CD Jr: Prolonged *Salmonella* bacteremia in patients with *Schistosoma mansoni* infection. Arch Intern Med 128:254, 1971.

359. Tillotson JR, Lerner AM: Characteristics of pneumonias caused by *Bacillus proteus*. Ann Intern Med 68:287, 1968.

360. Adler JL, Burke JP, Martin DF, et al: *Proteus* infections in a general hospital: II. Some clinical and epidemiological characteristics: With an analysis of 71 cases of *Proteus* bacteremia. Ann Intern Med 75:531, 1971.

361. Lysy J, Werczberger A, Globus M, et al: Pneumatocele formation in a patient with *Proteus mirabilis* pneumonia. Postgrad Med J 61:255, 1985.

362. John TJ: Emerging and re-emerging bacterial pathogens in India. Indian J Med Res 103:4, 1996.

362a. Galimand M, Guiyoule A, Berbaud G, et al: Multidrug resistance in *Yersinia pestis* mediated by a transferable plasmid. N Engl J Med 337:677, 1997.

363. Craven RB, Maupin GO, Beard ML, et al: Reported cases of human plague infections in the United States, 1970–1991. J Med Entomol 30:758, 1993.

363a. Dennis DT, Hughes JM: Multidrug resistance in plague. N Engl J Med 337:702, 1997.

364. Werner SB, Weidmer CE, Nelson BC, et al: Primary plague pneumonia contracted from a domestic cat at South Lake Tahoe, California. JAMA 251:929, 1984.

365. Weniger BG, Warren AJ, Forseth V, et al: Human bubonic plague transmitted by a domestic cat scratch. JAMA 251:927, 1984.

366. Plague pneumonia: California. MMWR 33:481, 1984.

367. Leads from the MMWR: Plague pneumonia: California. JAMA 252:1399, 1984.

368. Plague—South Carolina. MMWR 32:417, 1983.

369. Burmeister RW, Tigertt WD, Overholt EL: Laboratory-acquired pneumonic plague: Report of a case and review of previous cases. Ann Intern Med 56:789, 1962.

370. Gregg CT: Plague: An Ancient Disease in the Twentieth Century. Revised Edition, Albuquerque, University of New Mexico Press, 1985.

371. Cavanaugh DC, Randall R: The role of multiplication of *Pasteurella pestis* in mononuclear phagocytes in the pathogenesis of flea-borne plague. J Immunol 83:348, 1959.

372. Spencer H: Pathology of the Lung. 4th ed. Oxford, Pergamon, 1985.

373. Finegold MJ: Pneumonic plague in monkeys: An electron microscopic study. Am J Pathol 54:167, 1969.

374. Alsofrom DJ, Mettler FA, Mann JM: Radiographic manifestations of plague in New Mexico, 1975—1980: A review of 42 proved cases. Radiology 139:561, 1981.

375. Sites VR, Poland JD: Mediastinal lymphadenopathy in bubonic plague. Am J Roentgenol 116:567, 1972.

376. Barnes AM, Poland JD: Plague in the United States, 1983. MMWR CDC Surveill Summ 33:15SS, 21SS, 1984.

377. Conrad FG, LeCocq FR, Krain R: A recent epidemic of plague in Vietnam. Arch Intern Med 122:193, 1968.

378. Snyder JD, Christenson E, Feldman RA: Human *Yersinia enterocolitica* infections in Wisconsin: Clinical, laboratory and epidemiologic features. Am J Med 72:768, 1982.

379. Bigler RD, Atkins RR, Wing EJ: *Yersinia enterocolitica* lung infection. Arch Intern Med 141:1529, 1981.

380. Cropp AJ, Gaylord SF, Watanakunakorn C: Cavitary pneumonia due to *Yersinia enterocolitica* in a healthy man. Am J Med Sci 288:130, 1984.

381. Hodges GR, Degener CE, Barnes WG: Clinical significance of *Citrobacter* isolates. Am J Clin Pathol 70:37, 1978.

382. Shih CC, Chen YC, Chang SC, et al: Bacteremia due to *Citrobacter* species: Significance of primary intraabdominal infection. Clin Infect Dis 23:543, 1996.

383. Klapholz A, Lessnau KD, Huang B, et al: *Hafnia alvei*—respiratory tract isolates in a community hospital over a three-year period and a literature review. Chest 105:1098, 1994.

384. Takano Y, Asao Y, Kohri Y, et al: Fulminant pneumonia and sepsis due to *Aeromonas hydrophilia* in an alcohol abuser. Intern Med 35:410, 1996.

385. Reines HD, Cook FV: Pneumonia and bacteremia due to *Aeromonas hydrophila*. Chest 80:264, 1981.

386. Ender PT, Dolan MJ, Dolan D, et al: Near-drowning–associated *Aeromonas* pneumonia. J Emerg Med 14:737, 1996.

387. Hur T, Cheng KC, Hsieh JM: *Aeromonas hydrophila* lung abscess in a previously healthy man. Scand J Infect Dis 27:295, 1995.

388. Scott EG, Russell CM, Noell KT, et al: *Aeromonas hydrophila* sepsis in a previously healthy man. JAMA 239:1742, 1978.

389. Maki DG: Through a glass darkly: Nosocomial pseudoepidemics and pseudobacteremias. Arch Intern Med 140:26, 1980.

390. Richard C: *Chromobacterium violaceum*, opportunistic pathogenic bacteria in tropical and subtropical regions. Bull Soc Pathol Exot 86:169, 1993.

391. Ognibene AJ, Thomas E: Fatal infection due to *Chromobacterium violaceum* in Vietnam. Am J Clin Pathol 54:607, 1970.

392. Stein AA, Fialk MA, Blevins A, et al: *Pasteurella multocida* septicemia: Experience at a cancer hospital. JAMA 249:508, 1983.

393. Hubbert WT, Rosen MN: II. *Pasteurella multocida* infection in man unrelated to animal bite. Am J Public Health 60:1109, 1970.

394. Calverley PMA, Douglas NJ, Buchanan DR, et al: Ventilatory failure after *Pasteurella multocida* pneumonia. Thorax 36:954, 1981.

395. Schmidt ECH, Truitt LV, Koch ML: Pulmonary abscess with empyema caused by *Pasteurella multocida*: Report of a fatal case. Am J Clin Pathol 54:733, 1970.

396. Smith JE: Studies on *Pasteurella septica*: III. Strains from human beings. J Comp Pathol 69:231, 1959.

397. Holloway WJ, Scott EG, Adams YB: *Pasteurella multocida* infection in man: Report of 21 cases. Am J Clin Pathol 51:705, 1969.

398. Morris AJ, Heckler GB, Schaub IG, et al: *Pasteurella multocida* and bronchiectasis: Report of two cases. Bull Johns Hopkins Hosp 91:174, 1952.

399. Cawson RA, Talbot JM: The occurrence of *Pasteurella septica* (syn. *multocida*) in bronchiectasis. J Clin Pathol 8:49, 1955.

400. Inoue Y, Fujii T, Ohtsubo T, et al: [Three cases of *Pasteurella multocida* infection in the respiratory tract]. Kansenshogaku Zasshi 68:242, 1994.

401. Rose HD, Mathai G: Acute *Pasteurella multocida* pneumonia. Br J Dis Chest 71:123, 1977.

402. Nelson SC, Hammer GS: *Pasteurella multocida* empyema: Case report and review of the literature. Am J Med Sci 281:43, 1981.

403. Steyer BJ, Sobonya RE: *Pasteurella multocida* lung abscess: A case report and review of the literature. Arch Intern Med 144:1081, 1984.

404. Machiles P, Haxhe JP, Trigaux JP, et al: Chronic lung abscess due to *Pasteurella multocida*. Thorax 50:1017, 1995.

404a. Ribas J, Lores L, Ruiz J, et al: Pancoast's syndrome due to chronic pneumonia by *Pasteurella multocida*. Eur Respir J 10:2904, 1997.

405. Drabick JJ, Gasser RA Jr, Saunders NB, et al: *Pasteurella multocida* pneumonia in a man with AIDS and nontraumatic feline exposure. Chest 103:7, 1993.

406. Moritz F, Martin E, Lemeland JF, et al: Fatal *Pasteurella bettyae* pleuropneumonia in a patient infected with human immunodeficiency virus. Clin Infect Dis 22:591, 1996.

407. Buchanan TM, Hendricks SL, Patton CM, et al: Brucellosis in the United States, 1960–1972: An abattoir-associated disease: III. Epidemiology and evidence for acquired immunity. Medicine (Baltimore) 53:427, 1974.

408. Rode JW, Webling DDA: Melioidosis in the northern territory of Australia. Med J Aust 1:181, 1981.

409. Guard RW, Khafagi FA, Brigden MC, et al: Melioidosis in far North Queensland: A clinical and epidemiological review of 20 cases. Am J Trop Med Hyg 33:467, 1984.

410. Bovornkitti S, Nana A: The tropical lung. Semin Respir Med 9:425, 1988.

411. Lars MI, Osterberg LG, Chau PY, et al: Pulmonary melioidosis. Chest 108:1420, 1995.

412. Howe C, Sampath A, Spotnitz M: The *Pseudomallei* group: A review. J Infect Dis 124:598, 1971.

413. John TJ, Jesudason MV, Lalitha MK, et al: Melioidosis in India: The tip of the iceberg? Indian J Med Res 103:62, 1996.

414. Batchelor BI, Paul J, Trakulsomboon S, et al: Melioidosis survey in Kenya. Trans R Soc Trop Med Hyg 88:181, 1994.

415. Carruthers MM: Recrudescent melioidosis mimicking lung abscess. Am Rev Resp Dis 124:756, 1981.

416. Chan CK, Hyland RH, Leers WD, et al: Pleuropulmonary melioidosis in a Cambodian refugee. Can Med Assoc J 131:1365, 1984.

417. Wilks D, Jacobson SK, Lever AM, et al: Fatal melioidosis in a tourist returning from Thailand. J Infect 29:87, 1994.

418. Barnes PF, Appleman MD, Cosgrove MM: A case of melioidosis originating in North America. Am Rev Resp Dis 134:170, 1986.

419. Barnes PF, Appleman MD, Cosgrove MM: A case of melioidosis originating in North America. Am Rev Resp Dis 134:170, 1986.

420. Suputtamongkol Y, Hall AJ, Dance D, et al: The epidemiology of melioidosis in Ubon Ratchatani northeast Thailand. Int J Epidemiol 23:1082, 1994.

421. Sweet RS, Wilson ES Jr, Chandler BF: Melioidosis manifested by cavitary lung disease. Am J Roentgenol 103:543, 1968.

422. McCormick JB, Sexton DJ, McMurray JG, et al: Human-to-human transmission of *Pseudomonas pseudomallei*. Ann Intern Med 83:512, 1975.

423. Schlech WF III, Turchik JB, Westlake RE Jr, et al: Laboratory-acquired infection with *Pseudomonas pseudomallei* (melioidosis). N Engl J Med 305:1133, 1981.

424. Green RN, Tuffnell PG: Laboratory-acquired melioidosis. Am J Med 44:599, 1968.

425. Rimington RA: Meliodosis in North Queensland. Med J Aust 1:50, 1962.

426. Merianos A, Patel M, Lane JM, et al: The 1990–1991 outbreak of melioidosis in the Northern Territory of Australia: Epidemiology and environmental studies. Southeast Asian J Trop Med Public Health 24:425, 1993.

427. Sanford JP, Moore WL Jr: Recrudescent melioidosis: A Southeast Asian legacy. Am Rev Resp Dis 104:452, 1971.

428. Poe RH, Vassallo CL, Domm BM: Melioidosis: The remarkable imitator (case reports). Am Rev Resp Dis 104:427, 1971.

429. Prevatt AL, Hunt JS: Chronic systemic melioidosis: Review of literature and

report of a case with a note on visual disturbance due to chloramphenicol. Am J Med 23:810, 1957.

430. Piggott JA, Hochholzer L: Human melioidosis: A histopathologic study of acute and chronic melioidosis. Arch Pathol 90:101, 1970.

431. Greenwald KA, Nash G, Foley FD: Acute systemic melioidosis: Autopsy findings in four patients. Am J Clin Pathol 52:188, 1969.

432. James AE, Dixon GD, Johnson H: Melioidosis: A correlation of the radiologic and pathologic findings. Radiology 89:230, 1967.

433. Dhiensiri T, Puapairoj S, Susaengrat W: Pulmonary melioidosis: Clinical-radiologic correlation in 183 cases in Northeastern Thailand. Radiology 166:711, 1988.

434. Chong VFH, Fan YF: The radiology of melioidosis. Australas Radiol 40:244, 1996.

435. Tan APA, Pui MH, Tan LKA: Imaging patterns in melioidosis. Australas Radiol 39:260, 1995.

436. Sheehy TW, Deller JJ Jr, Weber DR: Melioidosis. Ann Intern Med 67:897, 1967.

437. Weber DR, Douglass LE, Brundage WG, et al: Acute varieties of melioidosis occurring in U.S. soldiers in Vietnam. Am J Med 46:234, 1969.

438. Everett ED, Nelson RA: Pulmonary melioidosis: Observations in thirty-nine cases. Am Rev Resp Dis 112:331, 1975.

439. Thin RNT, Brown M, Stewart JB, et al: Melioidosis: A report of ten cases. Q J Remia 39:115, 1970.

440. Koh KB. Melioidosis presenting as epididymo-orchitis. Singapore Med J 36:446, 1995.

441. Wong PK, Ng PH: Melioidosis presenting with orbital cellulitis. Singapore Med J 37:220, 1996.

442. Currie B, Howard D, Nguyen VT, et al: The 1990–1991 outbreak of melioidosis in the Northern Territory of Australia: Clinical aspects. Southeast Asian J Trop Med Public Health 24:436, 1993.

443. Handa R, Bhatia S, Wali JP: Melioidosis: A rare but not forgotten cause of fever of unknown origin. Br J Clin Pract 50:116, 1996.

444. Wong KT, Vadivelu J, Puthucheary SD, et al: An immunohistochemical method for the diagnosis of melioidosis. Pathology 28:188, 1996.

445. Kanaphun P, Thirawattanasuk N, Suputtamongkol Y, et al: Serology and carriage of *Pseudomonas pseudomallei*: A prospective study in 1000 hospitalized children in northeast Thailand. J Infect Dis 167:230, 1993.

446. Walsh AL, Wuthiekanun V: The laboratory diagnosis of melioidosis. Br J Biomed Sci 53:249, 1996.

447. Phung LV, Han Y, Oka S, et al: Enzyme-linked immunosorbent assay (ELISA) using a glycolipid antigen for the serodiagnosis of melioidosis. FEMS Immunol Med Microbiol 12:259, 1995.

448. Desakorn V, Smith MD, Wuthiekanun V, et al: Detection of *Pseudomonas pseudomallei* antigen in urine for the diagnosis of melioidosis. Am J Trop Med Hyg 51:627, 1994.

449. Smith MD, Wuthiekanun V, Walsh AL: Latex agglutination for rapid detection of *Pseudomonas pseudomallei* antigen in urine of patients with melioidosis. J Clin Pathol 48:174, 1995.

450. Dharakul T, Songsivilai S, Viriyachira S, et al: Melioidosis. Br J Biomed Sci 53:249, 1996.

451. Flume PA, Egan TM, Paradowski LJ, et al: Infectious complications of lung transplantation: Impact of cystic fibrosis. Am J Respir Crit Care Med 149:1601, 1994.

452. Taylor RFH, Hodson ME: *Pseudomonas cepacia*: Pulmonary infection in patients with cystic fibrosis. Respir Med 87:187, 1993.

453. Spencer RC: The emergence of epidemic, multiple-antibiotic–resistant *Stenotrophomas (Xanthomonas) maltophilia* and *Burkholderia (Pseudomonas) cepacia*. J Hosp Infect 30:453, 1995.

454. Snell GI, de Hoyos A, Krajden M, et al: *Pseudomonas cepacia* in lung transplant recipients with cystic fibrosis. Chest 103:466, 1993.

455. Revets H, Vandamme P, Van Zeebroeck A, et al: *Burkholderia (Pseudomonas) cepacia* and cystic fibrosis: The epidemiology. Acta Clin Belg 51:222, 1996.

456. Isles A, Maclusky I, Corey M, et al: *Pseudomonas cepacia* infection in cystic fibrosis: An emerging problem. J Pediatr 104:206, 1984.

457. Govan JR, Hughes JE, Vandamme P: *Burkholderia cepacia*: Medical, taxonomic, and ecological issues. J Med Microbiol 45:395, 1996.

458. Muhdi K, Edenborough FP, Gumery L, et al: Outcome for patients colonised with *Burkholderia cepacia* in a Birmingham adult cystic fibrosis clinic and the end of an epidemic. Thorax 51:374, 1996.

459. Sun L, Jiangh RZ, Steinbach S, et al: The emergence of a highly transmissible lineage of cbl+ *Pseudomonas (Burkholderia) cepacia* causing CF centre epidemics in North America and Britain. Nat Med 1:626, 1995.

460. Lipuma JJ, Marks-Austin KA, Holsclaw DS Jr, et al: Inapparent transmission of *Pseudomonas (Burkholderia) cepacia* among patients with cystic fibrosis. Pediatr Infect Dis J 13:716, 1994.

461. Govan Jr, Brown PH, Maddison J, et al: Evidence for transmission of *Pseudomonas cepacia* by social contact in cystic fibrosis. Lancet 342:15, 1993.

462. Herridge MS, de Hoyos AL, Chapparo C, et al: Pleural complications in lung transplant recipients. J Thorac Cardiovasc Surg 110:22, 1995.

463. Yamagishi Y, Fujita J, Takigawa K, et al: Clinical features of *Pseudomonas cepacia* pneumonia in an epidemic among immunocompromised patients. Chest 103:1706, 1993.

464. Conly JM, Klass L, Larson L, et al: *Pseudomonas cepacia* colonization and infection in intensive care units. Can Med Assoc J 134:363, 1986.

465. Wilsher ML, Kolbe J, Morris AJ, et al: Nosocomial acquisition of *Burkholderia gladioli* in patients with cystic fibrosis. Am J Respir Crit Care Med 155:1436, 1997.

465a. Graves M, Robin T, Chipman AM, et al: Four additional cases of *Burkholderia gladioli* infection with microbiological correlates and review. Clin Infect Dis 25:838, 1997.

466. Dunn M, Wunderlink RG: Ventilator-associated pneumonia caused by *Pseudomonas* infection. Clin Chest Med 16:95, 1995.

467. Pierce AK, Sanford JP, Thomas GD, et al: Long-term evaluation of decontamination of inhalation therapy equipment and the occurrence of necrotizing pneumonia. N Engl J Med 282:528, 1970.

468. Cobben NA, Drent M, Jonkers M, et al: Outbreak of severe *Pseudomonas aeruginosa* respiratory infections due to contaminated nebulizers. J Hosp Infect 33:63, 1996.

469. Rello J, Ausina V, Ricart M, et al: Risk factors for infection by *Pseudomonas* in patients with ventilator-associated pneumonia. Intensive Care Med 20:193, 1994.

470. Tinne JE, Gordon AM, Bain WH, et al: Cross-infection by *Pseudomonas aeruginosa* as a hazard of intensive surgery. Br Med J 4:313, 1967.

471. Niederman MS, Ferranti RD, Zeigler A, et al: Respiratory infection complicating long-term tracheostomy: The implication of persistent gram-negative tracheobronchial colonization. Chest 85:39, 1984.

472. Pennington JE, Reynolds HY, Carbone PP: *Pseudomonas* pneumonia: A retrospective study of 36 cases. Am J Med 55:155, 1973.

473. Govan J, Reiss-Levy E, Bader L, et al: *Pseudomonas* pneumonia with bacteremia. Med J Aust 1:627, 1977.

474. Schuster MG, Morris AH: Community-acquired *Pseudomonas aeruginosa* pneumonia in patients with HIV infection. AIDS 8:1437, 1994.

475. Miller RF, Foley NM, Kessel D, et al: Community-acquired lobar pneumonia in patients with HIV infection and AIDS. Thorax 49:367, 1994.

476. Baron AD, Hollander H: *Pseudomonas aeruginosa* bronchopulmonary infection in late human immunodeficiency virus disease. Am Rev Respir Dis 148:992, 1993.

477. Rello J, Soñora R, Jubert P, et al: Pneumonia in intubated patients: Role of respiratory airway care. Am J Respir Crit Care Med 154:111, 1996.

478. Yamaguchi T, Yamada H: Role of mechanical injury on airway surface in the pathogenesis of *Pseudomonas aeruginosa*. Am Rev Respir Dis 144:1147, 1991.

479. de Bentzmann S, Roger P, Puchelle E: *Pseudomonas aeruginosa* adherence to remodelling respiratory epithelium. Eur Respir J 9:2145, 1996.

480. Seybold ZV, Abraham WM, Gazeroglu H, et al: Impairment of airway mucociliary transport by *Pseudomonas aeruginosa* products. Am Rev Respir Dis 146:1173, 1992.

481. Ying QL, Kemme M, Simon SR: Alginate, the slime exopolysaccharide of *Pseudomonas aeruginosa*, binds human leukocyte elastase, retards inhibition by alpha$_1$-proteinase inhibitor, and accelerates inhibition by secretory leukoprotease inhibitor. Am J Respir Cell Mol Biol 15:283, 1996.

482. McClure CD, Schiller NL: Inhibition of macrophage phagocytosis by *Pseudomonas aeruginosa* rhamnolipids in vitro and in vivo. Curr Microbiol 33:109, 1996.

483. Azghani AO: *Pseudomonas aeruginosa* and epithelial permeability: Role of virulence factors elastase and exotoxin A. Am J Respir Cell Mol Biol 15:132, 1997.

483a. Pittet J-F, Kudoh I, Wiener-Kronish JP: Endothelial exposure to *Pseudomonas aeruginosa* proteases increases the vulnerability of the alveolar epithelium to a second injury. Am J Respir Cell Mol Biol 18:129, 1998.

483b. Hauser AR, Kang PJ, Engel JN: PepA, a secreted protein of *Pseudomonas aeruginosa*, is necessary for cytotoxicity and virulence. Mol Microbiol 27:807, 1998.

484. Schuster A, Haarmann A, Wahn V: Cytokines in neutrophil-dominated airway inflammation in patients with cystic fibrosis. Eur Arch Otorhinolaryngol Suppl 1:59, 1995.

485. Bonfield TL, Panuska JR, Konstan MW, et al: Inflammatory cytokines in cystic fibrosis lungs. Am J Respir Crit Care Med 152:2111, 1995.

486. Buret A, Cripps AW: The immunoevasive activities of *Pseudomonas aeruginosa*—relevance for cystic fibrosis. Am Rev Respir Dis 148:793, 1993.

487. Teplitz C: Pathogenesis of *Pseudomonas* vasculitis and septic lesions. Arch Pathol 80:297, 1965.

488. Fetzer AE, Werner AS, Hagstrom JWC: Pathologic features of pseudomonal pneumonia. Am Rev Resp Dis 96:1121, 1967.

489. Soave R, Murray HW, Litrenta MM: Bacterial invasion of pulmonary vessels: *Pseudomonas* bacteremia mimicking pulmonary thromboembolism with infarction. Am J Med 65:864, 1978.

490. McHenry MC, Baggenstoss AH, Martin WJ: Bacteremia due to gram-negative bacilli: Clinical and autopsy findings in 33 cases. Am J Clin Pathol 50:160, 1968.

491. Tillotson JR, Lerner AM: Characteristics of nonbacteremic *Pseudomonas* pneumonia. Ann Intern Med 68:295, 1968.

492. Renner RR, Coccaro AP, Heitzman ER, et al: *Pseudomonas* pneumonia: A prototype of hospital-based infection. Radiology 105:555, 1972.

493. Winer-Muram HT, Jennings SG, Wunderink RG, et al: Ventilator-associated *Pseudomonas aeruginosa* pneumonia: radiographic findings. Radiology 195:247, 1995.

494. Joffe N: Roentgenologic aspects of primary *Pseudomonas aeruginosa* pneumonia in mechanically ventilated patients. Am J Roentgenol 107:305, 1969.

495. Iannini PB, Claffey T, Quintiliani R: Bacteremic *Pseudomonas* pneumonia. JAMA 230:558, 1974.

496. Shooter RA, Faiers MC, Cooke EM, et al: Isolation of *Escherichia coli, Pseudomonas aeruginosa,* and *Klebsiella* from food in hospitals, canteens, and schools. Lancet 2:390, 1971.

497. McHenry MC, Hawk WA: Bacteremia caused by gram-negative bacilli. Med Clin North Am 58:623, 1974.

498. Sande MA: Antimicrobial therapy for two serious bacterial infections: Enterococcal endocarditis and nosocomial pneumonia. Arch Intern Med 142:2033, 1982.

499. McGowan JE Jr, Parrot PL, Duty VP: Nosocomial bacteremia: Potential for prevention of procedure-related cases. JAMA 237:2727, 1977.

500. Young VM, Meyers WF, Moody MR, et al: The emergence of *Coryneform* bacteria as a cause of nosocomial infections in compromised hosts. Am J Med 70:646, 1981.

501. Lowder JN, Lazarus HM, Herzig RH: Bacteremias and fungemias in oncologic patients with central venous catheters: Changing spectrum of infection. Arch Intern Med 142:1456, 1982.

502. Tirdel GB, Gibbons GH, Fishman RS: Pneumonia with an enlarged cardiac silhouette. Chest 109:1380, 1996.

503. Zwillich CW, Ellis JH: *Pseudomonas aeruginosa* abscess masquerading as a slowly growing solitary pulmonary nodule. Thorax 29:603, 1974.

504. Brewe SC, Wunderink RG, Jones CB, et al: Ventilator-associated pneumonia due to *Pseudomonas aeruginosa*. Chest 109:1019, 1996.

505. Rello J, Jubert P, Valles J, et al: Evaluation of outcome for intubated patients with pneumonia due to *Pseudomonas aeruginosa*. Clin Infect Dis 23:973, 1996.

505a. Rello J, Mariscal D, March F, et al: Recurrent *Pseudomonas aeruginosa* pneumonia in ventilated patients: Relapse or reinfection? Am J Respir Crit Care Med 157:912, 1998.

506. Fujita J, Yamadori I, Xu G, et al: Clinical features of *Stenotrophomonas maltophilia* pneumonia in immunocompromised patients. Respir Med 90:35, 1996.

507. Karpati F, Malmborg AS, Alfredsson H, et al: Bacterial colonisation with *Xanthomonas maltophilia*—a retrospective study in a cystic fibrosis patient population. Infection 22:258, 1994.

508. Buxton AE, Anderson RL, Werdegar D, et al: Nosocomial respiratory tract infection and colonization with *Acinetobacter calcoaceticus*: Epidemiologic characteristics. Am J Med 65:507, 1978.

509. Glew RH, Moellering RC Jr, Kunz LJ: Infections with *Acinetobacter calcoaceticus* (*Herellea vaginicola*): Clinical and laboratory studies. Medicine 56:79, 1977.

509a. Cox TR, Roland WE, Dolan ME: Ventilator-related *Acinetobacter* outbreak in an intensive care unit. Mil Med 163:389, 1998.

510. Rudin ML, Michael JR, Huxley EJ: Community-acquired *Acinetobacter* pneumonia. Am J Med 67:39, 1979.

510a. Yang CH, Chen KJ, Wang CK: Community-acquired *Acinetobacter* pneumonia: A case report. J Infect 35:316, 1997.

511. Cordes LG, Brink EW, Checko PJ, et al: A cluster of *Acinetobacter* pneumonia in foundry workers. Ann Intern Med 95:688, 1981.

512. Rudin ML, Michael JR, Huxley EJ: Community-acquired Acinetobacter pneumonia. Am J Med 67:39, 1979.

512a. Baraibar J, Correa H, Mariscal D, et al: Risk factors for infection by *Acinetobacter baumannii* in intubated patients with nosocomial pneumonia. Chest 112:1050, 1997.

513. Wands JR, Mann RB, Jackson D, et al: Fatal community-acquired *Herellea* pneumonia in chronic renal disease. Am Rev Resp Dis 108:964, 1973.

514. Fagon JY, Chastre J, Domart Y, et al: Mortality due to ventilator-associated pneumonia or colonization with *Pseudomonas* or *Acinetobacter* species: Assessment by quantitative culture of samples obtained by a protected specimen brush. Clin Infect Dis 23:538, 1996.

515. Cheron M, Abachin E, Guerot E, et al: Investigation of hospital-acquired infections due to *Alcaligenes denitrificans* subsp. *xylosoxydans* by DNA restriction fragment length polymorphism. J Clin Microbiol 32:1023, 1994.

516. Pedersen MM, Marso E, Pickett MJ: Nonfermentative bacilli associated with man: III. Pathogenicity and antibiotic susceptibility. Am J Clin Pathol 54:178, 1970.

517. Dunne WM Jr, Maisch S: Epidemiological investigation of infections due to *Alcaligenes* species in children and patients with cystic fibrosis: Use of repetitive-element-sequence polymerase chain reaction. Clin Infect Dis 20:836, 1995.

518. Bloch KC, Nadarajah R, Jacobs JR: *Chryseobacterium meningosepticum*: An emerging pathogen among immunocompromised adults. Medicine 76:30, 1997.

518a. Hsueh PR, Teng LJ, Yang PC, et al: Increasing incidence of nosocomial *Chryseobacterium indologenes* infections in Taiwan. Eur J Clin Microbiol Infect Dis 16:568, 1997.

519. Gilardi GL: Infrequently encountered *Pseudomonas* species causing infection in humans. Ann Intern Med 77:211, 1972.

520. Yabuuchi E, Kosako Y, Yano I, et al: Transfer of two *Burkholderia* and *Alcaligenes* species to *Ralstonia* gen. *Nov*: Proposal of *Ralstonia pickettii* (*Ralston, Palleroni*, and *Doudoroff* 1973) comb. *Nov, Ralstonia solanacearum* (Smith 1896) comb. *Nov*, and *Ralstonia eutropha* (Davis 1969) comb. *Nov*. Microbiol Immunol 39:897, 1995.

521. Gardner P, Schulman ST: A nosocomial common source outbreak caused by *Pseudomonas pickettii*. Pediatr Infect Dis 3:420, 1984.

522. Abbasi S, Chesney PJ: Pulmonary manifestations of cat-scratch disease: A case report and review of the literature. Pediatr Infect Dis J 14:547, 1995.

523. Katner HP, Treen B, Pankey GA, et al: Pleural effusion and anicteric hepatitis associated with cat-scratch disease: Documentation by cat-scratch bacillus. Chest 89:302, 1986.

524. Black JR, Harrington DA, Hadfield TL, et al: Life-threatening cat-scratch disease in an immunocompromised host. Arch Intern Med 146:394, 1986.

525. Caniza MA, Granger DL, Wilson KH, et al: *Bartonella henselae*: Etiology of pulmonary nodules in a patient with depressed cell-mediated immunity. Clin Infect Dis 20:1505, 1995.

526. Moore EH, Russell LA, Klein JS, et al: Bacillary angiomatosis in patients with AIDS: Multiorgan imaging findings. Radiology 197:67, 1995.

527. Coche E, Beigelman C, Lucidarme O, et al: Thoracic bacillary angiomatosis in a patient with AIDS. Am J Roentgenol 165:56, 1995.

528. Regnery RL, Olson JG, Perkins BA, et al: Serologic response to *"Rochalimaea henselae"* antigen in suspected cat-scratch disease. Lancet 339:1443, 1992.

529. Pfischner WCE Jr, Ishak KG, Neptune EM, et al: Brucellosis in Egypt: A review of experience with 228 patients. Am J Med 22:915, 1957.

530. Buchanan TM, Faber LC, Feldman RA: Brucellosis in the United States, 1960–1972: An abattoir-associated disease: I. Clinical features and therapy. Medicine (Baltimore) 53:403, 1974.

531. Greer AE: Pulmonary brucellosis. Dis Chest 29:508, 1956.

532. Harvey WA: Pulmonary brucellosis. Ann Intern Med 28:768, 1948.

533. Takahashi H, Tanaka S, Yoshida K, et al: An unusual case of brucellosis in Japan: Difficulties in the differential diagnosis from pulmonary tuberculosis. Intern Med 35:310, 1996.

534. Papiris SA, Maniati MA, Haritou A, et al: Brucella haemorrhagic pleural effusion. Eur Respir J 7:1369, 1994.

535. Kerem E, Diav O, Navon P, et al: Pleural fluid characteristics in pulmonary brucellosis. Thorax 49:89, 1994.

536. Mili N, Auckenthaler R, Nicod LP: Chronic *Brucella* emphysema. Chest 103:620, 1993.

537. Jubber AS, Gunawardana DRL, Lulu AR: Acute pulmonary edema in *Brucella* myocarditis and interstitial pneumonitis. Chest 97:1008, 1990.

538. Weed LA, Sloss PT, Clagett OT: Chronic localized pulmonary brucellosis. JAMA 161:1044, 1956.

539. Ramah SJ, Chomet B, McLean J, et al: Pulmonary granuloma due to brucellosis. JAMA 170:1665, 1959.

540. Buchanan TM, Sulzer CR, Frix MK, et al: Brucellosis in the United States, 1960–1972: An abattoir-associated disease: II. Diagnostic aspects. Medicine (Baltimore) 53:415, 1974.

541. Tamion F, Girault C, Chevron V, et al: *Bordetella bronchiseptica* pneumonia with shock in an immunocompetent patient. Scand J Infect Dis 28:197, 1996.

542. Libanore M, Rossi MR, Pantaleoni M, et al: *Bordetella bronchiseptica* in an AIDS patient: A new opportunistic infection. Infection 23:312, 1995.

543. Brisou P, De Jaureguiberry JP, Peyrade F, et al: Sinusitis and *Bordetella bronchiseptica* pneumonia in AIDS. Presse Med 23:1400, 1994.

544. de la Fuente J, Albo C, Rodriguez A, et al: *Bordetella bronchiseptica* pneumonia in a patient with AIDS. Thorax 49:719, 1994.

545. Funke G, Hess T, von Graevenitz A, et al: Characteristics of *Bordetella hinzii* strains isolated from a cystic fibrosis patient over a 3-year period. J Clin Microbiol 34:966, 1996.

546. Waggoner-Fountain L, Hayden GF: Pertussis in primary care practice: Recent advances in diagnosis, treatment, and prevention. Prim Care 23:793, 1996.

547. Cherry JD: Historical review of pertussis and the classical vaccine. J Infect Dis 174:259, 1996.

548. Keitel WA, Edwards KM: Pertussis in adolescents and adults: Time to reimmunize? Semin Respir Infect 10:51, 1995.

549. Anonymous: Resurgence of pertussis—United States, 1993. MMWR Morb Mortal Wkly Rep 42:952, 1993.

550. Heininger U, Cherry JD, Eckhardt T, et al: Clinical and laboratory diagnosis of pertussis in the regions of a large vaccine efficacy trial in Germany. Pediatr Infect Dis J 12:504, 1993.

551. Kissane JM: Pathology of Infancy and Childhood. St. Louis, CV Mosby, 1975.

552. Fawcitt J, Parry HE: Lung changes in pertussis and measles in childhood: A review of 1894 cases with a follow-up study of the pulmonary complications. Br J Radiol 30:76, 1957.

553. Grob PR, Crowder MJ, Robbins JF: Effect of vaccination on severity and dissemination of whooping cough. Br Med J 282:1925, 1981.

554. Connor JD: Evidence for an etiologic role of adenoviral infection in pertussis syndrome. N Engl J Med 283:390, 1970.

555. Connor JD: Communication in answer to a letter re: pertussis syndrome. N Engl J Med 283:1174, 1970.

556. Wortis N, Strebel PM, Wharton M, et al: Pertussis deaths: Report of 23 cases in the United States, 1992 and 1993. Pediatrics 97:607, 1996.

557. Johnston IDA, Anderson HR, Lambert HP, et al: Respiratory morbidity and lung function after whooping cough. Lancet 2:1104, 1983.

558. Respiratory sequelae of whooping cough: Swansea Research Unit of the Royal College of General Practitioners. Br Med J 290:1937, 1985.

559. Francis E: Sources of infection and seasonal incidence of tularemia in man. Public Health Rep 52:103, 1937.

560. Capellan J, Fong IW: Tularemia from a cat bite: Case report and review of feline-associated tularemia. Clin Infect Dis 16:472, 1993.

561. Liles WC, Burger RJ: Tularemia from domestic cats. West J Med 158:619, 1993.

562. Francis E: Sources of infection and seasonal incidence of tularemia in man. Public Health Rep 52:103, 1937.

563. Feldman RA, Koehler RE: Tularemia. JAMA 226:189, 1973.

564. Klock LE, Olsen PF, Fukushima T: Tularemia epidemic associated with the deerfly. JAMA 226:149, 1973.

565. Miller RP, Bates JH: Pleuropulmonary tularemia: A review of 29 patients. Am Rev Resp Dis 99:31, 1969.

566. Gattereau A, Gareau R, Diallo GS: Deux cas de tularémie dans la province de Québec. Can Med Assoc J 103:512, 1970.

567. Walker WJ, Moore CA: Tularemia: Experience in the Hamilton area. Can Med Assoc J 105:390, 1971.

568. Kozak AJ, Hall WH, Gerding DN: Cavitary pneumonia associated with tularemia. Chest 73:426, 1978.

569. Ford-Jones L, Delage G, Powell KR, et al: "Muskrat fever": Two outbreaks of tularemia near Montreal. Can Med Assoc J 127:298, 1982.
570. Martin T, Holmes IH, Wobeser GA, et al: Tularemia in Canada, with a focus on Saskatchewan. Can Med Assoc J 127:279, 1982.
571. Martone WJ, Marshall LW, Kaufmann AF, et al: Tularemia pneumonia in Washington, D.C.: A report of three cases with possible common-source exposures. JAMA 242:2315, 1979.
572. Preiksaitis JK, Crawshaw GJ, Nayar GSP, et al: Human tularemia at an urban zoo. Can Med Assoc J 121:1097, 1979.
573. Overholt EL, Tigertt WD: Roentgenographic manifestations of pulmonary tularemia. Radiology 74:758, 1960.
574. Pettersson T, Nyberg P, Norstrom D, et al: Similar pleural fluid findings in pleuropulmonary tularemia and tuberculous pleurisy. Chest 109:572, 1996.
575. Evans ME, Gregory DW, Schaffner W, et al: Tularemia: A 30-year experience with 88 cases. Medicine 64:251, 1985.
576. Terry LL, Reichle HS: Ulceroglandular tularemia: Report of three fatal cases with autopsies. Arch Pathol 29:473, 1940.
577. Leading article: Granulomatous pleuritis caused by *Francisella tularensis*: Possible confusion with tuberculous pleuritis. Am Rev Resp Dis 128:314, 1983.
578. Gill V, Cunha BA. Tularemia pneumonia. Semin Respir Infect 12:61, 1997.
579. Overholt EL, Tigertt WD: Roentgenographic manifestations of pulmonary tularemia. Radiology 74:758, 1960.
580. Rubin SA: Radiographic spectrum of pleuropulmonary tularemia. Am J Roentgenol 131:277, 1978.
581. Overholt EL, Tigertt WD, Kadull PJ, et al: An analysis of forty-two cases of laboratory-acquired tularemia: Treatment with broad-spectrum antibiotics. Am J Med 30:785, 1961.
582. Dennis JM, Boudreau RP: Pleuropulmonary tularemia: Its roentgen manifestations. Radiology 68:25, 1957.
583. Sunderrajan EV, Hutton J, Marienfeld RD: Adult respiratory distress syndrome secondary to tularemia pneumonia. Arch Intern Med 145:1435, 1985.
584. Young LS, Bicknell DS, Archer BG, et al: Tularemia epidemic—Vermont, 1968: Forty-seven cases linked to contact with muskrats. N Engl J Med 280:1253, 1969.
585. Kaiser AB, Rieves D, Price AH, et al: Tularemia and rhabdomyolysis. JAMA 253:241, 1985.
586. Clarridge JE III, Raich TJ, Sjosted A, et al: Characterization of two unusual clinically significant *Francisella* strains. J Clin Microbiol 34:1995, 1996.
587. Giddens WR, Wilson JW Jr, Dienst FT Jr, et al: Tularemia: An analysis of one hundred forty-seven cases. J Louisiana M Soc 109:93, 1957.
588. Trollfors B, Brorson JE, Claesson B, et al: Invasive infections caused by *Haemophilus* species other than *Haemophilus influenzae*. Infection 13:12, 1985.
589. Quintiliani R, Hymans PJ: The association of bacteremic *Haemophilus influenzae* pneumonia in adults with typable strains. Am J Med 50:781, 1971.
590. Wallace RJ Jr, Musher DM, Martin RR: *Haemophilus influenzae* pneumonia in adults. Am J Med 64:87, 1978.
591. Dworzack DL, Blessing LD, Hodges GR, et al: *Haemophilus influenzae* type F pneumonia in adults. Am J Med Sci 275:87, 1978.
592. Urwin G, Krohn JA, Deaver-Robinson K, et al: Invasive disease due to *Haemophilus influenzae* serotype f: Clinical and epidemiologic characteristics in the *H. influenzae* serotype b vaccine era. The *Haemophilus influenzae* Study Group. Clin Infect Dis 22:1069, 1996.
593. Bates JH: The role of infection during exacerbations of chronic bronchitis. Ann Intern Med 97:130, 1982.
594. Musher DM, Kubitschek KR, Crennan J, et al: Pneumonia and acute febrile tracheobronchitis due to *Haemophilus influenzae*. Ann Intern Med 99:444, 1983.
595. Berk SL, Holtsclaw SA, Wiener SL, et al: Nontypeable *Haemophilus influenzae* in the elderly. Arch Intern Med 134:537, 1982.
596. Trollfors B, Claesson B, Lagergard T, et al: Incidence, predisposing factors, and manifestations of invasive *Haemophilus influenzae* infections in adults. Eur J Clin Microbiol 3:180, 1984.
597. Klein JO: Role of nontypeable *Haemophilus influenzae* in pediatric respiratory tract infections. Pediatr Infect Dis J 16:5, 1997.
598. Norden CW: *Haemophilus influenzae* infections in adults. Med Clin North Am 62:1037, 1978.
599. Hirschmann JV, Everett ED: *Haemophilus influenzae* infections in adults: Report of nine cases and a review of the literature. Medicine 58:80, 1979.
600. Everett ED, Rham AE Jr, Adaniya R, et al: *Haemophilus influenzae* pneumonia in adults. JAMA 238:319, 1977.
601. Nicotra MB, Rivera M, Awe RJ: Antibiotic therapy of acute exacerbations of chronic bronchitis. Ann Intern Med 97:18, 1982.
602. Burns MW, May JR: *Haemophilus influenzae* precipitins in the serum of patients with chronic bronchial disorders. Lancet 1:354, 1967.
603. Clarke JR, Hannant CA, Scicchitano R, et al: Antigen of *Haemophilus influenzae* in bronchial tree. Thorax 36:665, 1981.
604. Johnson SR, Thompson RC, Humphreys H, et al: Clinical features of patients with beta-lactamase–producing *Haemophilus influenzae* isolated from sputum. J Antimicrob Chemother 38:881, 1996.
605. Farley MM, Stephens DS, Brachman PS, et al: Invasive *Haemophilus influenzae* disease in adults—a prospective, population-based surveillance. Ann Intern Med 116:806, 1992.
606. Eykyn SJ, Thomas RD, Philips I: *Haemophilus influenzae* meningitis in adults. Br Med J 2:462, 1974.
607. Alsever RN, Silver HG, Dinerman N, et al: *Haemophilus influenzae* pericarditis and empyema with thyroiditis in an adult. JAMA 230:1426, 1974.
608. Austrian R: Prevention of fatal bacterial infection in patients with anatomic or functional asplenia. Ann Intern Med 96:117, 1982.

609. Gillis S, Dann EJ, Berkman N, et al: Fatal *Haemophilus influenzae* septicemia following bronchoscopy in a splenectomized patient. Chest 104:1607, 1993.
610. Boschini A, Smacchia C, DiFine M, et al: Community-acquired pneumonia in a cohort of former injection drug users with and without human immunodeficiency virus infection: Incidence, etiologies, and clinical aspects. Clin Infect Dis 23:107, 1996.
611. Moroni M, Franzetti F: Bacterial pneumonia in adult patients with HIV infection. J Chemother 7:292, 1995.
612. Keller DW, Breiman RF: Preventing bacterial respiratory tract infections among persons infected with human immunodeficiency virus. Clin Infect Dis 21:77, 1995.
613. Falco V, Fernandez de Sevilla T, Alegre J, et al: Bacterial pneumonia in HIV-infected patients: A prospective study of 68 episodes. Eur Respir J 7:235, 1994.
614. Ashworth M, Ross G, Loehry C: Lobar pneumonia caused by *Haemophilus influenzae* type b. Br J Dis Chest 79:95, 1985.
615. Duncan GW, Randall WE Jr, Mulholland JH: *Haemophilus influenzae* type b, mediastinitis, cellulitis, bacteremia, and meningitis in an adult. Am Rev Resp Dis 123:333, 1981.
616. Woodhead MA, MacFarlane JT: *Haemophilus influenzae* pneumonia in previously fit adults. Eur J Resp Dis 70:218, 1987.
617. Patwari AK, Bisht S, Srinivasan A, et al: Aetiology of pneumonia in hospitalized children. J Trop Pediatr 42:15, 1996.
618. Rello J, Rodriguez R, Jubert P, et al: Severe community-acquired pneumonia in the elderly: Epidemiology and prognosis: Study Group for Severe Community-Acquired Pneumonia. Clin Infect Dis 23:723, 1996.
619. Gomez J, Banos V, Ruiz Gomez J, et al: Prospective study of epidemiology and prognostic factors in community-acquired pneumonia. Eur J Clin Microbiol Infect Dis 15:556, 1996.
620. Neill AM, Martin IR, Weir R, et al: Community-acquired pneumonia: Aetiology and usefulness of severity criterial on admission. Thorax 51:1010, 1996.
621. Lieberman D, Schlaeffer F, Boldur I, et al: Multiple pathogens in adult patients admitted with community-acquired pneumonia: A one-year prospective study of 346 consecutive patients. Thorax 51:179, 1996.
622. Bohte R, van Furth R, van den Broek PJ: Aetiology of community-acquired pneumonia: A prospective study among adults requiring admission to hospital. Thorax 50:543, 1995.
623. Burman LA, Leinonen M, Trollfors B: Use of serology to diagnose pneumonia caused by nonencapsulated *Haemophilus influenzae* and *Moraxella catarrhalis*. J Infect Dis 170:220, 1994.
624. Belliveau P, Hickingbotham N, Maderazo EG, et al: Institution-specific patterns of infection and Gram's stain as guides for empiric treatment of patients hospitalized with typical community-acquired pneumonia. Pharmacotherapy 13:396, 1993.
625. Geppert EF: Chronic and recurrent pneumonia. Sem Respir Infect 7:282, 1992.
626. Kirtland SH, Winterbauer RH, Dreis DF, et al: A clinical profile of chronic bacterial pneumonia—report of 115 cases. Chest 106:15, 1994.
627. Robbins JB, Schneerson R, Argaman M, et al: *Haemophilus influenzae* type b: Disease and immunity in humans. Ann Intern Med 78:259, 1973.
628. Holdaway MD, Turk DC: Capsulated *Haemophilus influenzae* and respiratory tract disease. Lancet 1:358, 1967.
629. Walker SH: The respiratory manifestations of systemic *Haemophilus influenzae* infection. J Pediatr 62:386, 1963.
630. Vinik M, Altman DH, Parks RE: Experience with *Haemophilus influenzae* pneumonia. Radiology 86:701, 1966.
631. Claesson B, Trollfors B, Ekstrom-Jodal B, et al: Incidence and prognosis of acute epiglottitis in children in a Swedish region. Pediatr Infect Dis 3:534, 1984.
632. Ward JI, Margolis HS, Lum MKW, et al: *Haemophilus influenzae* disease in Alaskan Eskimos: Characteristics of a population with an unusual incidence of invasive disease. Lancet 1:1281, 1981.
633. Crowe HM, Levitz RE: Invasive *Haemophilus influenzae* disease in adults. Arch Intern Med 147:241, 1987.
634. Khilanani U, Khatib R: Acute epiglottitis in adults. Am J Med Sci 287:65, 1984.
635. Ossoff RH, Wolff AP: Acute epiglottitis in adults. JAMA 244:2639, 1980.
636. Deeb ZE, Yenson AC, DeFries HO: Acute epiglottitis in the adult. Laryngoscope 95:289, 1985.
637. Mustoe T, Strome M: Adult epiglottitis. Am J Otolaryngol 4:393, 1983.
638. Cohen EL: Epiglottitis in the adult: Recognizing and treating the acute case. Postgrad Med 75:309, 1984.
639. Rose FB, Garman RF, Falkenberg KJ, et al: Adult epiglottitis, cellulitis, and *Streptococcus pneumoniae* bacteremia. Scand J Infect Dis 14:301, 1982.
640. Goldstein E, Daly AK, Seamans C: *Haemophilus influenzae* as a cause of adult pneumonia. Ann Intern Med 66:35, 1967.
641. Pearlberg J, Haggar AM, Saravolatz L, et al: *Haemophilus influenzae* pneumonia in the adult: Radiographic appearance with clinical correlation. Radiology 151:23, 1984.
642. Stratton CW, Hawley HB, Horsman TA, et al: *Haemophilus influenzae* pneumonia in adults: Report of five cases caused by ampicillin-resistant strains. Am Rev Resp Dis 121:595, 1980.
643. Francis JB, Francis PB: Bulging (sagging) fissure sign in *Haemophilus influenzae* lobar pneumonia. South Med J 71:1452, 1978.
644. Warner JO, Gordon I: Pneumatoceles following *Haemophilus influenzae* pneumonia. Clin Radiol 32:99, 1981.
645. Quinones CA, Memon MA, Sarosi GA: Bacteremic *Haemophilus influenzae* pneumonia in the adult. Semin Respir Med 4:12, 1989.
646. Schultes A, Agie GA: Acute *Haemophilus parainfluenzae* epiglottitis in an adult. Postgrad Med 75:207, 1984.

647. Israel RH, Magnussen CR, Greenblatt DW, et al: *Haemophilus parainfluenzae* lung abscess. Respiration 46:379, 1984.
648. Cooney TG, Harwood BR, Meisner DJ: *Haemophilus parainfluenzae* thoracic empyema. Arch Intern Med 141:940, 1981.
649. Roig J, Domiongo C, Morera J: Legionnaires' disease. Chest 105:1817, 1994.
650. McDade JE, Shepard CC, Fraser DW, et al: Legionnaires' disease: Isolation of a bacterium and demonstration of its role in other respiratory disease. N Engl J Med 297:1197, 1977.
651. Davis GS, Winn WC Jr, Beaty HN: Legionnaires' disease: Infections caused by *Legionella pneumophila* and *Legionella*-like organisms. Clin Chest Med 2:145, 1981.
652. Cordes LG, Fraser DW: Legionellosis: Legionnaires' disease—Pontiac fever. Med Clin North Am 64:395, 1980.
653. Osterholm MT, Chin TDY, Osborne DO, et al: A 1957 outbreak of Legionnaires' disease associated with a meat packing plant. Am J Epidemiol 117:60, 1983.
654. Fraser DW: Legionnaires' disease: Four summers' harvest. Am J Med 68:1, 1980.
655. Conwill DE, Werner SB, Dritz SK, et al: Legionellosis: The 1980 San Francisco outbreak. Am Rev Resp Dis 126:666, 1982.
656. Rosmini F, Castellani-Pastoris M, Mazzotti MF, et al: Febrile illness in successive cohorts of tourists at a hotel on the Italian Adriatic coast: Evidence for a persistent focus of *Legionella* infection. Am J Epidemiol 119:124, 1984.
657. Bozzoni M, Radice L, Frosi A, et al: Prevalence of pneumonia due to *Legionella pneumophila* and *Mycoplasma pneumoniae* in a population admitted to a department of internal medicine. Respiration 62:331, 1995.
658. Hlady WG, Mullen RC, Mintz CS, et al: Outbreak of Legionnaires' disease linked to a decorative fountain by molecular epidemiology. Am J Epidemiol 138:555, 1993.
659. Lieberman D, Porath A, Schlaeffer F, et al: *Legionella* species community-acquired pneumonia—a review of 56 hospitalized adult patients. Chest 109:1243, 1996.
660. Venezia RA, Agresta MD, Hanley EM, et al: Nosocomial legionellosis associated with aspiration of nasogastric feedings diluted in tap water. Infect Control Hosp Epidemiol 15:529, 1994.
661. Nechwatal R, Ehret W, Klatte OJ, et al: Nosocomial outbreak of legionellosis in a rehabilitation center: Demonstration of potable water as a source. Infection 21:235, 1993.
662. England AC III, Fraser DW, Plikaytis BD, et al: Sporadic legionellosis in the United States: The first thousand cases. Ann Intern Med 94:164, 1981.
663. Meenhorst PL, van der Meer JWM, Borst J: Sporadic cases of legionnaires' disease in the Netherlands. Ann Intern Med 90:529, 1979.
664. Bartlett CLR: Sporadic cases of legionnaires' disease in Great Britain. Ann Intern Med 90:592, 1979.
665. McKinney RM, Thacker L, Harris PP, et al: Four serogroups of legionnaires' disease bacteria defined by direct immunofluorescence. Ann Intern Med 90:621, 1979.
666. Nagington J, Wreghitt TG, Smith DJ: *Legionella pneumophila* serogroup 5 infections in the Cambridge area: A serological survey. J Infect 3:18, 1981.
667. Cordes LG, Wiesenthal AM, Gorman GW, et al: Isolation of *Legionella pneumophila* from hospital shower heads. Ann Intern Med 94:195, 1981.
668. Bibb WF, Arnow PM, Dellinger DL, et al: Isolation and characterization of a seventh serogroup of *Legionella pneumophila*. J Clin Microbiol 17:346, 1983.
669. Bissett ML, Lee JO, Lindquist DS: New serogroup of *Legionella pneumophila*, serogroup. Br J Clin Microbiol 17:887, 1983.
670. Edelstein PH, Bibb WF, Gorman GW, et al: *Legionella pneumophila* serogroup 9: A cause of human pneumonia. Ann Intern Med 101:196, 1984.
671. Meenhorst PL, Reingold AL, Groothuis AL, et al: Water-related nosocomial pneumonia caused by *Legionella pneumophila* serogroups 1 and 10. J Infect Dis 152:356, 1985.
672. Thacker WL, Benson RF, Wilkinson HW, et al: Eleventh serogroup of *Legionella pneumophila* isolated from a patient with fatal pneumonia. J Clin Microbiol 23:1146, 1986.
673. Tsai TF, Finn DR, Plikaytis BD, et al: Legionnaires' disease: Clinical features of the epidemic in Philadelphia. Ann Intern Med 90:509, 1979.
674. Van Arsdall JA II, Wunderlich HF, Melo JC, et al: The protean manifestations of legionnaires' disease. J Infect 7:51, 1983.
675. Fraser DW, Deubner DC, Hill DL, et al: Nonpneumonic, short-incubation-period legionellosis (Pontiac fever) in men who cleaned a steam turbine condenser. Science 205:690, 1979.
676. Girod JC, Reichman RC, Winn WC Jr, et al: Pneumonic and nonpneumonic forms of legionellosis: The result of a common-source exposure to *Legionella pneumophila*. Arch Intern Med 142:545, 1982.
677. Friedman S, Spitalny K, Barbaree J, et al: Pontiac fever outbreak associated with a cooling tower. Am J Public Health 77:568, 1987.
678. Editorial: Severe pneumonia: A continuing story. Lancet 1:1064, 1980.
679. Edelstein PH, Pryor EP: A new biotype of *Legionella dumoffii*. J Clin Microbiol 21:641, 1985.
679a. Benson RF, Fields BS: Classification of the genus *Legionella*. Semin Respir Infect 13:90, 1998.
680. Herwaldt LA, Gorman GW, McGrath T, et al: A new *Legionella* species, *Legionella feelei* species nova, causes Pontiac fever in an automobile plant. Ann Intern Med 100:333, 1984.
681. Morris GK, Steirgerwalt AG, Feeley JC, et al: *Legionella gormanii*, sp. nov. J Clin Microbiol 12:718, 1980.
682. Cordes LG, Wilkinson HW, Gorman GW, et al: Atypical *Legionella*-like organisms: Fastidious water-associated bacteria pathogenic for man. Lancet 2:927, 1979.
683. Cherry WB, Gorman GW, Orrison LH, et al: *Legionella jordanis*: A new species of *Legionella* isolated from water and sewage. J Clin Microbiol 15:290, 1982.
684. Thacker WL, Wilkinson HW, Benson RF, et al: *Legionella jordanis* isolated from a patient with fatal pneumonia. J Clin Microbiol 26:1400, 1988.
685. Svendsen JH, Jonsson V, Niebuhr U: Combined pericarditis and pneumonia caused by *Legionella* infection. Br Heart J 58:663, 1987.
686. Pasculle AW, Myerowitz RL, Rinaldo CR Jr: New bacterial agent of pneumonia isolated from renal-transplant recipients. Lancet 2:58, 1979.
687. Orrison LH, Cherry WB, Tyndall RL, et al: *Legionella oakridgensis*: Unusual new species isolated from cooling tower water. Appl Environ Microbiol 45:536, 1983.
688. Tang PW, Toma S, MacMillan LG: *Legionella oakridgensis*: Laboratory diagnosis of a human infection. J Clin Microbiol 21:462, 1985.
689. Edelstein PH, Brenner DJ, Moss CW, et al: *Legionella wadsworthii* species nova: A cause of human pneumonia. Ann Intern Med 97:809, 1982.
690. Jernigan DB, Sanders LI, Waites KB, et al: Pulmonary infection due to *Legionella cincinnatiensis* in renal transplant recipients: Two cases and implications for laboratory diagnosis. Clin Infect Dis 18:385, 1994.
691. Parry MF, Stampleman L, Hutchinson JH, et al: Waterborne *Legionella bozemanii* and nosocomial pneumonia in immunosuppressed patients. Ann Intern Med 103:205, 1985.
692. Tang PW, Toma S, Moss CW, et al: *Legionella bozemanii* serogroup 2: A new etiological agent. J Clin Microbiol 19:30, 1984.
693. Taylor TH, Albrecht MA: *Legionella bozemanii* cavitary pneumonia poorly responsive to erythromycin: Case report and review. Clin Infect Dis 20:329, 1995.
694. Schoousboe MI, Chereshsky A: Fatal pneumonia due to *Legionella bozemanii* serogroup 1 in a patient with occult malignant lymphoma. N Z Med J 108:127, 1995.
695. McKinney RM, Porschen RK, Edelstein PH, et al: *Legionella longbeachae* species nova, another etiologic agent of human pneumonia. Ann Intern Med 94:739, 1981.
696. Palutke WA, Crane LR, Wentworth BB, et al: *Legionella feeleii*–associated pneumonia in humans. Am J Clin Pathol 86:348, 1986.
697. Aronson MD, Komaroff AL, Pasculle AW, et al: *Legionella micdadei* (Pittsburgh pneumonia agent) infection in nonimmunosuppressed patients with pneumonia. Ann Intern Med 94:486, 1981.
698. Back E, Schvarcz R, Kallings I: Community-acquired *Legionella micdadei* (Pittsburgh pneumonia agent) infection in Sweden. Scand J Infect Dis 15:313, 1983.
699. Edelstein PM, Finegold SM: Isolation of *Legionella pneumophila* from a transtracheal aspirate. J Clin Microbiol 9:457, 1979.
700. Wing EJ, Schafer FJ, Pasculle AW: The use of tracheal and pulmonary aspiration to diagnose *Legionella micdadei* pneumonia. Chest 82:705, 1982.
701. Benson MK, Mitchell RG, Phillips PM: Postoperative *Legionella* pneumonia diagnosed by percutaneous lung aspiration. Br Med J 282:1585, 1981.
702. Chiodini PL, Williams AJ, Barker J, et al: Bronchial lavage and transbronchial lung biopsy in the diagnosis of legionnaires' disease. Thorax 40:154, 1985.
703. Kohorst WR, Schonfeld SA, Macklin JE, et al: Rapid diagnosis of legionnaires' disease by bronchoalveolar lavage. Chest 84:186, 1983.
704. Freedman AP, Coodley E, Johnston RF, et al: Loculated pleural effusion caused by *Legionella pneumophila*. Thorax 37:79, 1982.
705. Dumoff M: Direct *in vitro* isolation of the legionnaires' disease bacterium in two fatal cases: Cultural and staining characteristics. Ann Intern Med 90:694, 1979.
706. Ferrington M, French GL: *Legionella pneumophila* seen in Gram stains of respiratory secretions and recovered from conventional blood cultures. J Infect 6:123, 1983.
707. Martin RS, Marrie TJ, Best L, et al: Isolation of *Legionella pneumophila* from the blood of a patient with legionnaires' disease. Can Med Assoc J 131:1085, 1984.
708. Edelstein PH, Meyer RD, Finegold SM: Isolation of *Legionella pneumophila* from blood. Lancet 1:750, 1979.
709. Pasculle AW, Feeley JC, Gibson RJ, et al: Pittsburgh pneumonia agent: Direct isolation from human lung tissue. J Infect Dis 141:727, 1980.
710. Lattimer GL, Rhodes LV III, Salventi JF, et al: Isolation of *Legionella pneumophila* from clinical specimens: Salutary effects of lung tissue dilution. Am Rev Resp Dis 122:101, 1980.
711. Edelstein PH, Meyer RD, Finegold SM: Laboratory diagnosis of legionnaires' disease. Am Rev Resp Dis 121:317, 1980.
711a. Breiman RF, Butler JC: Legionnaires' disease: Clinical, epidemiological, and public health perspectives. Semin Respir Infect 13:84, 1998.
712. Foy HM, Broome CV, Hayes PS, et al: Legionnaires' disease in a prepaid medical-care group in Seattle 1963–1975. Lancet 1:767, 1979.
713. Bartlett JG: New developments in infectious diseases for the critical care physician. Crit Care Med 11:563, 1983.
714. MacFarlane JT, Finch RG, Laverick A, et al: Pittsburgh pneumonia agent and legionellosis in Nottingham. Br Med J 283:1222, 1981.
715. Yu VL, Kroboth FJ, Shonnard J, et al: Legionnaires' disease: New clinical perspective from a prospective pneumonia study. Am J Med 73:357, 1982.
716. Friis-Moller A, Rechnitzer C, Black FT, et al: Prevalence of legionnaires' disease in pneumonia patients admitted to a Danish department of infectious diseases. Scand J Infect Dis 18:321, 1986.
717. Craven DE, Steger KA: Nosocomial pneumonia in mechanically ventilated adult patients: Epidemiology and prevention in 1996. Semin Respir Infect 11:32, 1996.

718. Renner ED, Helms CM, Hierholzer WJ Jr, et al: Legionnaires' disease in pneumonia patients in Iowa: A retrospective seroepidemiologic study, 1972–1977. Ann Intern Med 90:603, 1979.

719. Poshni IA, Millian SJ: Seroepidemiology of *Legionella pneumophila* serogroup 1 in healthy residents of New York City. NY State J Med 85:10, 1985.

720. Nichol KL, Parenti CM, Johnson JE: High prevalence of positive antibodies to *Legionella pneumophila* among outpatients. Chest 100:663, 1991.

721. Helms CM, Viner JP, Weisenburger DD, et al: Sporadic legionnaires' disease: Clinical observations on 87 nosocomial and community-acquired cases. Am J Med Sci 288:2, 1984.

722. Cordonnier C, Farcet J-P, Desforges L, et al: Legionnaires' disease and hairy cell leukemia: An unfortuitous association? Arch Intern Med 144:2373, 1984.

723. Sarngadharan MG, Popovic M, Bruch L, et al: Antibodies reactive with human T-lymphotropic retroviruses (HTLV-III) in the serum of patients with AIDS. Science 224:506, 1984.

724. Kirby BD, Snyder KM, Meyer RD, et al: Legionnaires' disease: Report of sixty-five nosocomially acquired cases and review of the literature. Medicine 59:188, 1980.

725. Bauling PC, Weil R III, Schroter GP: *Legionella* lung abscess after renal transplantation. J Infect 11:51, 1985.

726. Moore EH, Webb WR, Gamsu G, et al: Legionnaires' disease in the renal transplant patient: Clinical presentation and radiographic progression. Radiology 153:589, 1984.

727. Prodinger WM, Bonatti H, Allerberger F, et al: *Legionella* pneumonia, in transplant recipients: A cluster of cases of eight years' duration. J Hosp Infect 26:191, 1994.

728. Fuller J, Levinson MM, Kline JR, et al: Legionnaires' disease after heart transplantation. Ann Thorac Surg 39:308, 1985.

729. Bangsborg JM, Uldum S, Jensen JS, et al: Nosocomial legionellosis in three heart-lung transplant patients: Case reports and environmental observations. Eur J Clin Microbiol Infect Dis 14:99, 1995.

730. Kugler JW, Armitage JO, Helms CM, et al: Nosocomial legionnaires' disease: Occurrence in recipients of bone marrow transplants. Am J Med 74:281, 1983.

731. Cordonnier C, Farcet J-P, Desforges L, et al: Legionnaires' disease and hairy cell leukemia: An unfortuitous association? Arch Intern Med 144:2373, 1984.

732. Muder RR, Liu VL, Fang GD: Community-acquired legionnaires' disease. Semin Respir Infect 4:32, 1989.

733. Fliermans CB, Cherry WB, Orrison LH, et al: Isolation of *Legionella pneumophila* from nonepidemic-related aquatic habitats. Environ Microbiol 37:1239, 1979.

734. Fliermans CB, Cherry WB, Orrison LH, et al: Ecological distribution of *Legionella pneumophila*. Appl Environ Microbiol 41:9, 1981.

735. Band JD, LaVenture M, Davis JP, et al: Epidemic legionnaires' disease: Airborne transmission down a chimney. JAMA 245:2404, 1981.

736. Editorial: *Legionella* by the legion. Lancet 2:716, 1983.

737. Dondero TJ Jr, Rendtorff RC, Mallison GF, et al: An outbreak of legionnaires' disease associated with a contaminated air-conditioning cooling tower. N Engl J Med 302:365, 1980.

738. Klaucke DN, Vogt RL, LaRue D, et al: Legionnaires' disease: The epidemiology of two outbreaks in Burlington, Vermont, 1980. Am J Epidemiol 119:382, 1984.

739. Garbe PL, Davis BJ, Weisfeld JS, et al: Nosocomial legionnaires' disease: Epidemiologic demonstration of cooling towers as a source. JAMA 254:521, 1985.

740. Nordstrom K, Kallings I, Dahnsjo H, et al: An outbreak of legionnaires' disease in Sweden: Report of sixty-eight cases. Scand J Infect Dis 15:43, 1983.

741. Stout J, Yu VL, Vickers RM, et al: Potable water supply as the hospital reservoir for Pittsburgh pneumonia agent. Lancet 1:471, 1982.

742. Shands KN, Ho JL, Meyer RD, et al: Potable water as a source of legionnaires' disease. JAMA 253:1412, 1985.

743. Neill MA, Gorman GW, Gibert C, et al: Nosocomial legionellosis, Paris, France: Evidence for transmission by potable water. Am J Med 78:581, 1985.

744. Fisher-Hoch SP, Bartlett CLR, Tobin J O'H, et al: Investigation and control of an outbreak of legionnaires' disease in a district general hospital. Lancet 1:932, 1981.

745. Stout J, Yu VL, Vickers RM, et al: Ubquitousness of *Legionella pneumophila* in the water supply of a hospital with legionnaires' disease. N Engl J Med 306:466, 1982.

746. Arnow PM, Chou T, Weil D, et al: Nosocomial legionnaires' disease caused by aerosolized tap water from respiratory devices. J Infec Dis 146:460, 1982.

747. Walter C: *Legionella pneumophila* in a hospital water supply. N Engl J Med 307:379, 1982.

748. Tobin J O'H, Beare J, Dunnill MS, et al: Legionnaires' disease in a transplant unit: Isolation of the causative agent from shower baths. Lancet 2:118, 1980.

749. Makela TM, Harders SJ, Cavanagh P, et al: Isolation of *Legionella pneumophila* (serogroup 1) from shower water in Ballarat. Med J Aust 1:293, 1981.

750. Gorman GW, Yu VL, Brown A, et al: Isolation of Pittsburgh pneumonia agent from nebulizers used in respiratory therapy. Ann Intern Med 93:572, 1980.

751. Joly J: *Legionella* and domestic water heaters in the Quebec City area. Can Med Assoc J 132:160, 1985.

752. Blatt SP, Parkinson MD, Pace E, et al: Nosocomial legionnaires' disease: Aspiration as a primary mode of disease acquisition. Am J Med 95:16, 1993.

753. Yu VL: Could aspiration be the major mode of transmission for *Legionella*? Am J Med 95:13, 1993.

754. Dennis PJ, Taylor JA, Fitzgeorge RB, et al: *Legionella pneumophila* in water plumbing systems. Lancet 1:949, 1982.

755. Muder RR, Yu VL, McClure JK, et al: Nosocomial legionnaires' disease uncovered in a prospective pneumonia study. JAMA 249:3184, 1983.

756. Tobin J O'H, Swann RA, Bartlett CLR: Isolation of *Legionella pneumophila* from water systems: Methods and preliminary results. Br Med J 282:515, 1981.

757. Editorial: *Legionella* and amoebae. Lancet 1:703, 1981.

758. Fields BS: *Legionella* and protozoa: Interaction of a pathogen and its natural host. *In* Barbaree JM, Breiman RF, Dufour AP, eds: *Legionella*: Current status and emerging perspectives. Washington: American Society for Microbiology, 1993, pp 129–136.

759. Baskerville A, Fitzgeorge RB, Broster M, et al: Experimental transmission of legionnaires' disease by exposure to aerosols of *Legionella pneumophila*. Lancet 2:1389, 1981.

760. Saravolatz L, Arking L, Wentworth B, et al: Prevalence of antibody to the legionnaires' disease bacterium in hospital employees. Ann Intern Med 90:601, 1979.

761. Hoffman PS: Invasion of eukaryotic cells by *Legionella pneumophila*: A common strategy for all hosts? Can J Infect Dis 8:139, 1997.

762. Payne NR, Horwitz MA: Phagocytosis of *Legionella pneumophila* is mediated by human monocyte complement receptors. J Exp Med 166:1377, 1987.

763. Bellinger-Kawahara CG, Horwitz MA: Complement component C3 fixes selectively to the major outer membrane protein (MOMP) of *Legionella pneumophila* and mediates phagocytosis of liposome-MOMP complexes by human monocytes. J Exp Med 172:1201, 1990.

764. Horwitz MA: Characterization of avirulent mutant *Legionella pneumophila* that survive but do not multiply within human monocytes. J Exp Med 166:1310, 1987.

765. Horwitz MA: The legionnaires' disease bacterium (*Legionella pneumophila*) inhibits phagosome-lysosome fusion in human monocytes. J Exp Med 158:2108, 1983.

766. Posner MR, Caudill MA, Brass R, et al: Legionnaires' disease associated with rhabdomyolysis and myoglobinuria. Arch Intern Med 140:848, 1980.

767. Pendlebury WW, Perl DP, Winn WC Jr, et al: Neuropathologic evaluation of 40 confirmed cases of *Legionella* pneumonia. Neurology 33:1340, 1983.

768. Johnson JD, Raff MJ, Van Arsdall JA: Neurologic manifestations of legionnaires' disease. Medicine 63:303, 1984.

769. Ampel NM, Ruben FL, Norden CW: Cutaneous abscess caused by *Legionella micdadei* in an immunosuppressed patient. Ann Intern Med 102:630, 1985.

770. Wong KH, Moss CW, Hochstein DH, et al: "Endotoxicity" of the legionnaires' disease bacterium. Ann Intern Med 90:624, 1979.

771. Zahringer U, Knirel YA, Lindner B et al: The lipopolysaccharide of *Legionella pneumophila* serogroup 1 (strain Philadelphia 1): Chemical structure and biological significance. Prog Clin Biol Res 392:113, 1995.

772. Williams A, Baskerville A, Dowsett AB, et al: Immunocytochemical demonstration of the association between *Legionella pneumophila*, its tissue-destructive protease, and pulmonary lesions in experimental legionnaires' disease. J Pathol 153:257, 1987.

772a. Friedman H, Yamamoto Y, Newton C, et al: Immunologic response and pathogenesis of *Legionella* infection. Semin Respir Infect 13:100, 1998.

773. Retzlaff C, Yamamoto Y, Hoffman PS, et al: Bacterial heat shock proteins directly induce cytokine mRNA and IL-1 secretion in macrophage cultures. Infect Immunol 62:5689, 1994.

774. Brieland JK, Remick DG, Freeman PT, et al: *In vivo* regulation of replicative *Legionella pneumophila* lung infection by endogenous tumor necrosis factor alpha and nitric oxide. Infect Immunol 63:3253, 1995.

775. Heath L, Chrisp C, Huffnagle G, et al: Effector mechanisms responsible for gamma interferon–mediated host resistance to *Legionella pneumophila* lung infection: The role of endogenous nitric oxide differs in susceptible and resistant murine hosts. Infect Immunol 64:5151, 1996.

776. Brieland JK, Heath LA, Huffnagle GB, et al: Humoral immunity and regulation of intrapulmonary growth of *Legionella pneumophila* in the immunocompetent host. J Immunol 157:5002, 1996.

777. Carrington CB: Pathology of legionnaires' disease. Ann Intern Med 90:496, 1979.

778. Winn WC Jr, Glavin FL, Perl DP, et al: Macroscopic pathology of the lungs in legionnaires' disease. Ann Intern Med 90:548, 1979.

779. Goldstein JD, Keller JL, Winn WC, et al: Sporadic Legionellaceae pneumonia in renal transplant recipients. Arch Pathol Lab Med 106:108, 1982.

780. Winn WC, Myerowitz RL: The pathology of the *Legionella* pneumonias. Hum Pathol 12:401, 1981.

781. Weisenburger DD, Helms CM, Renner ED: Sporadic legionnaires' disease. Arch Pathol Lab Med 105:130, 1981.

782. Hernandez FJ, Kirby BD, Stanley TM, et al: Legionnaires' disease: Postmortem pathologic findings of 20 cases. Am J Clin Pathol 73:488, 1980.

783. Blackmon JA, Harley RA, Hicklin MD, et al: Pulmonary sequelae of acute legionnaires' disease pneumonia. Ann Intern Med 90:552, 1979.

784. Winn WC, Glavin FL, Perl DP, et al: The pathology of legionnaires' disease: Fourteen fatal cases from the 1977 outbreak in Vermont. Arch Pathol Lab Med 102:344, 1978.

785. Sato P, Madtes DK, Thorning D, et al: Bronchiolitis obliterans caused by *Legionella pneumophila*. Chest 87:840, 1985.

786. Baptiste-Desruisseaux D, Duperval R, Marcoux JA: Legionnaires' disease in the immunocompromised host: Usefulness of Gram's stain. Can Med Assoc J 133:117, 1985.

787. Chandler FW, Hicklin MD, Blackmon JA: Demonstration of the agent of legionnaires' disease in tissue. N Engl J Med 297:1218, 1977.

788. Frenkel JK, Baker LH, Chonko AM: Autopsy diagnosis of legionnaires' disease in immunosuppressed patients: A paleodiagnosis using Giemsa stain (Wohlbach, modification). Ann Intern Med 90:559, 1979.

789. Rudin JE, Wing EJ: A comparative study of *Legionella micdadei* and other nosocomial-acquired pneumonia. Chest 86:675, 1984.

790. Theaker JM, Tobin JO, Jones SEC, et al: Immunohistological detection of *Legionella pneumophila* in lung sections. J Clin Pathol 40:143, 1987.

791. Fraser DW, Tsai TR, Orenstein W, et al: Legionnaires' disease: Description of an epidemic of pneumonia. N Engl J Med 297:1189, 1977.

792. Dietrich PA, Johnson RD, Fairbank JT, et al: The chest radiograph in legionnaires' disease. Radiology 127:577, 1978.

793. Storch GA, Sagel SS, Baine WB: The chest roentgenogram in sporadic cases of legionnaires' disease. JAMA 245:587, 1981.

794. Kroboth FJ, Yu VL, Reddy SC, et al: Clinicoradiographic correlation with the extent of legionnaires' disease. Am J Roentgenol 141:263, 1983.

795. Kroboth FJ, Yu VL, Reddy SC, et al: Clinicoradiographic correlation with the extent of legionnaires' disease. Am J Roentgenol 141:263, 1983.

796. Pedro-Botet ML, Sabria-Leal M, Haro M, et al: Nosocomial- and community-acquired *Legionella pneumonia*: Clinical comparative analysis. Eur Respir J 8:1929, 1995.

797. Meyer RD: Legionnaires' disease update: Be prepared for this summer. J Resp Dis 1:12, 1980.

798. Lo CD, MacKeen AD, Campbell DR, et al: Radiographic analysis of the course of *Legionella* pneumonia. J Can Assoc Radiol 34:116, 1983.

799. Helms CM, Viner JP, Weisenburger DD, et al. Sporadic legionnaires' disease: Clinical observations on 87 nosocomial- and community-acquired cases. Am J Med Sci 288:2, 1984.

800. Storch GA, Sagel SS, Baine WB: The chest roentgenogram in sporadic cases of legionnaires' disease. JAMA 245:587, 1981.

801. Fairbank JT, Patel MM, Dietrich PA: Legionnaires' disease. J Thorac Imaging 6:6, 1991.

802. Winn WC Jr, Glavin FL, Perl DP, et al: The pathology of legionnaires' disease. Arch Pathol Lab Med 102:344, 1978.

803. Lieberman D, Porath A, Schlaeffer F, et al: *Legionella* species community-acquired pneumonia: A review of 56 hospitalized adult patients. Chest 109:1243, 1996.

804. Venkatachalam KK, Saravolatz LD, Christopher KL: Legionnaires' disease: A cause of lung abscess. JAMA 241:597, 1979.

805. Lake KB, Van Dyke JJ, Gerberg E, et al: Legionnaires' disease and pulmonary cavitation. Arch Intern Med 139:485, 1979.

806. Gump DW, Frank RO, Winn WC Jr, et al: Legionnaires' disease in patients with associated serious disease. Ann Intern Med 90:538, 1979.

807. Lewin S, Brettman LR, Goldstein EJC, et al: Legionnaires' disease: A cause of severe abscess-forming pneumonia. Am J Med 67:339, 1979.

808. Fairbank JT, Mamourian AC, Dietrich PA, et al: The chest radiograph in legionnaires' disease: Further observations. Radiology 147:33, 1983.

809. Hughes JA, Anderson PB: Pulmonary cavitation, fibrosis, and legionnaires' disease. Eur J Resp Dis 66:59, 1985.

810. Fairbank JT, Mamourian AC, Dietrich PA, et al: The chest radiograph in legionnaires' disease. Radiology 147:30, 1983.

811. Copeland J, Wieden M, Feinberg W, et al: Legionnaires' disease following cardiac transplantation. Chest 79:669, 1981.

812. Edelstein PH, Meyer RD, Finegold SM: Long-term follow-up of two patients with pulmonary cavitation caused by *Legionella pneumophila*. Am Rev Resp Dis 124:90, 1981.

813. Gombert ME, Josephson A, Goldstein EJC, et al: Cavitary legionnaires' pneumonia: Nosocomial infection in renal transplant recipients. Am J Surg 147:402, 1984.

814. Meenhorst PL, Mulder JD: The chest x-ray in *Legionella* pneumonia (legionnaires' disease). Eur J Radiol 3:180, 1983.

815. Meenhorst PL, Mulder JD: The chest x-ray in *Legionella* pneumonia (legionnaires' disease). Eur J Radiol 3:180, 1983.

816. Moore EH, Webb RW, Gamsu G, et al: Legionnaires' disease in the renal transplant patient: Clinical presentation and radiographic progression. Radiology 163:589, 1984.

817. Mirich D, Gray R, Hyland R: *Legionella* lung cavitation. J Can Assoc Radiol 41:100, 1990.

818. MacFarlane JT, Miller AC, Roderick Smith WH, et al: Comparative radiographic features of community-acquired legionnaires' disease, pneumococcal pneumonia, mycoplasma pneumonia, and psittacosis. Thorax 39:28, 1984.

819. Bali A, Pierry AA, Bernstein A: Spontaneous pneumothorax complicating legionnaires' disease. Postgrad Med J 57:656, 1981.

820. Carter JB, Wolter RK, Angres G, et al: Nodular legionnaires' disease. Am J Roentgenol 137:612, 1981.

821. Pope TL Jr, Armstrong P, Thompson R, et al: Pittsburgh pneumonia agent: Chest film manifestations. Am J Roentgenol 138:237, 1982.

822. Muder RR, Reddy SC, Yu VL, et al: Pneumonia caused by Pittsburgh pneumonia agent: Radiologic manifestations. Radiology 150:633, 1984.

823. Mehta P, Patel JD, Milder JE: *Legionella micdadei* (Pittsburgh pneumonia agent): Two infections with unusual clinical features. JAMA 249:1620, 1983.

824. Evans AF, Oakley RH, Whitehouse GH: Analysis of the chest radiograph in legionnaires' disease. Clin Radiol 32:361, 1981.

825. Miller AC: Early clinical differentiation between legionnaires' disease and other sporadic pneumonias. Ann Intern Med 90:526, 1979.

826. Lattimer GL, Rhodes LV III, Salventi JS, et al: The Philadelphia epidemic of legionnaires' disease: Clinical, pulmonary, and serologic findings two years later. Ann Intern Med 90:522, 1979.

827. Buehler JW, Kuritsky JN, Gorman GW, et al: Prevalence of antibodies to *Legionella pneumophila* among workers exposed to a contaminated cooling tower. Arch Environ Health 40:207, 1985.

828. Helms CM, Viner JP, Sturm RH, et al: Comparative features of pneumococcal, mycoplasmal, and legionnaires' disease pneumonias. Ann Intern Med 90:543, 1979.

829. Randolph KA, Beekman JF: Legionnaires' disease presenting with empyema. Chest 75:404, 1979.

830. Shaw RA, Whitcomb ME, Schonfeld SA: Pulmonary function after adult respiratory distress syndrome associated with legionnaires' disease pneumonia. Arch Intern Med 141:741, 1981.

831. Kariman K, Shelburne JD, Gough W, et al: Pathologic findings and long-term sequelae in legionnaires' disease. Chest 75:736, 1979.

832. Blackmon JA, Harley RA, Hicklin MD, et al: Pulmonary sequelae of acute legionnaires' disease pneumonia. Ann Intern Med 90:552, 1979.

833. Sopena N, Sabria-Leal M, Pedro-Botet ML, et al: Comparative study of the clinical presentation of *Legionella* pneumonia and other community-acquired pneumonias. Chest 113:1195, 1998.

834. Maskill MR, Jordan EC: Pronounced cerebellar features in legionnaires' disease. Br Med J 283:276, 1981.

835. Lattimer GL, Rhodes LV III, Salventi JS, et al: The Philadelphia epidemic of legionnaires' disease: Clinical, pulmonary, and serologic findings two years later. Ann Intern Med 90:522, 1979.

836. Miller AC: Hyponatremia in legionnaires' disease. Br Med J 284:558, 1982.

837. Gross D, Willens H, Zeldis SM: Myocarditis in legionnaires' disease. Chest 79:232, 1981.

838. Hall SL, Wasserman M, Dall L, et al: Acute renal failure secondary to myoglobinuria associated with legionnaires' disease. Chest 84:633, 1983.

839. Helms CM, Viner JP, Renner ED, et al: Legionnaires' disease among pneumonias in Iowa (FY 1972–1978): II. Epidemiologic and clinical features of 30 sporadic cases of *L. pneumophila* infection. Am J Med Sci 282:2, 1981.

840. Fenves AZ: Legionnaires' disease associated with acute renal failure: A report of two cases and review of the literature. Clin Nephrol 23:96, 1985.

841. Allen FP, Fried JS, Wiegmann TB, et al: Legionnaires' disease associated with rash and renal failure. Arch Intern Med 145:729, 1985.

842. Bamford JM, Hakin RN: Chorea after legionnaires' disease. Br Med J 284:1232, 1982.

843. Bernardini DL, Lerrick KS, Hoffman K, et al: Neurogenic bladder: New clinical finding in legionnaires' disease. Am J Med 78:1045, 1985.

844. Morgan DJR, Gawler J: Severe peripheral neuropathy complicating legionnaires' disease. Br Med J 283:1577, 1981.

845. Landes BW, Pogson GW, Beauchamp GD, et al: Pericarditis in a patient with legionnaires' disease. Arch Intern Med 142:1234, 1982.

846. Mayock R, Skale B, Kohler RB: *Legionella pneumophila* pericarditis proved by culture of pericardial fluid. Am J Med 75:534, 1983.

847. Friedland L, Snydman DR, Weingarden AS, et al: Ocular and pericardial involvement in legionnaires' disease. Am J Med 77:1105, 1984.

848. Nelson DP, Rensimer ER, Raffin TA: *Legionella pneumophila* pericarditis without pneumonia. Arch Intern Med 145:926, 1985.

849. Gross D, Willens H, Zeldis SM: Myocarditis in legionnaires' disease. Chest 79:232, 1981.

850. Cheung M-T: Eight cases of legionnaires' disease. Can Med Assoc J 123:639, 1980.

851. Helms CM, Johnson W, Donaldson MF, et al: Pretibial rash in *Legionella pneumophila* pneumonia. JAMA 245:1758, 1981.

852. King JW, May JS: Cold agglutinin disease in a patient with legionnaires' disease. Arch Intern Med 140:1537, 1980.

853. Strikas R, Seifert MR, Lentino JR: Autoimmune hemolytic anemia and *Legionella pneumophila* pneumonia. Ann Intern Med 99:345, 1983.

854. Riggs SA, Wray NP, Waddell CC, et al: Thrombotic thrombocytopenic purpura complicating legionnaires' disease. Arch Intern Med 142:2275, 1982.

855. Oldenberger D, Carson JP, Gundlach WJ, et al: Legionnaires' disease: Association with mycoplasma pneumonia and disseminated intravascular coagulation. JAMA 241:1269, 1979.

856. Saravolatz LD, Russell G, Cvitkovich D: Direct immunofluorescence in the diagnosis of legionnaires' disease. Chest 79:566, 1981.

857. Giglia AR, Morgan PN, Bates JH: Rapid definitive diagnosis of legionnaires' disease. Chest 76:98, 1979.

858. Ristagno RL, Saravolatz LD: A pseudoepidemic of *Legionella* infections. Chest 88:466, 1985.

859. Collins MT, McDonald J, Hoiby N, et al: Agglutinating antibody titers to members of the family Legionellaceae in cystic fibrosis patients as a result of cross-reacting antibodies to *Pseudomonas aeruginosa*. J Clin Microbiol 19:757, 1984.

860. Grady GF, Gilfillan RF: Relation of *Mycoplasma pneumoniae* seroreactivity, immunosuppression, and chronic disease to legionnaires' disease: A twelve-month prospective study of sporadic cases in Massachusetts. Ann Intern Med 90:607, 1979.

861. Storch G, Hayes PS, Meyers JD, et al: Legionnaires' disease bacterium: Prevalence of antibody reacting with the organism in patients suspected of having infection with *Pneumocystis carinii*. Am Rev Resp Dis 121:483, 1980.

862. Edson DC, Stiefel HE, Wentworth BB, et al: Prevalence of antibodies to legionnaires' disease: A seroepidemiologic survey of Michigan residents using the hemagglutination test. Ann Intern Med 90:691, 1979.

863. Harrison TG, Dournon E, Taylor AG: Evaluation of sensitivity of two serological tests for diagnosing pneumonia caused by *Legionella pneumophila* serogroup 1. J Clin Pathol 40:77, 1987.

864. Kohler RB, Zimmerman SE, Wilson E, et al: Rapid radioimmunoassay diagnosis of legionnaires' disease: Detection and partial characterization of urinary antigen. Ann Intern Med 94:601, 1981.

865. Flesher AR, Jennings HJ, Lugowski C, et al: Isolation of a serogroup 1–specific antigen from *Legionella pneumophila*. J Infect Dis 145:224, 1982.

866. Naot Y, Brown A, Elder EM, et al: IgM and IgG antibody response in two immunosuppressed patients with legionnaires' disease: Evidence of reactivation of latent infection. Am J Med 73:791, 1982.

867. Kohler RB, Winn WC, Girod JC, et al: Rapid diagnosis of pneumonia due to *Legionella pneumophila* serogroup 1. J Infect Dis 146:444, 1982.

868. Sathapatayavongs B, Kohler RB, Wheat LJ, et al: Rapid diagnosis of legionnaires' disease by urinary antigen detection: Comparison of ELISA and radioimmunoassay. Am J Med 72:576, 1982.

869. Ramirez JA, Ahkee S, Tolentino A, et al: Diagnosis of *Legionella pneumophila*, *Mycoplasma pneumoniae*, or *Chlamydia pneumoniae* lower respiratory infection using the polymerase chain reaction on a single throat swab specimen. Diagn Microbiol Infec Dis 24:7, 1996.

870. Murdoch DR, Walford EJ, Jennings LC, et al: Use of the polymerase chain reaction to detect *Legionella* DNA in urine and serum samples from patients with pneumonia. Clin Infect Dis 23:475, 1996.

871. Koide M, Saito A: Diagnosis of *Legionella pneumophila* infection by polymerase chain reaction. Clin Infect Dis 21:199, 1995.

872. Sutherland GE, Tsai CC, Routburg M, et al: Prevalence of pneumonias caused by *Legionella* species among patients on whom autopsies were performed. Arch Pathol Lab Med 107:358, 1983.

873. Cohen ML, Broome CV, Paris AL, et al: Fatal nosocomial legionnaires' disease: Clinical and epidemiologic characteristics. Ann Intern Med 90:611, 1979.

874. Fay D, Baird IM, Aguirre A, et al: Unrecognized legionnaires' disease as a cause of fatal illness. JAMA 243:2311, 1980.

875. Falcó V, Fernández de Sevilla T, Alegre J, et al: *Legionella pneumophila*—a cause of severe community-acquired pneumonia. Chest 100:1007, 1991.

876. Broome CV, Goings SAJ, Thacker SB, et al: The Vermont epidemic of legionnaires' disease. Ann Intern Med 90:573, 1979.

877. Garland SM, Prichard MG: *Actinobacillus actinomycetemcomitans* causing a mediastinal abscess. Thorax 38:472, 1983.

878. Chen AC, Liu CC, Yao WJ, et al: *Actinobacillus actinomycetemcomitans* pneumonia with chest wall and subphrenic abscess. Scand J Infect Dis 27:289, 1995.

879. Morris JF, Sewell DL: Necrotizing pneumonia caused by mixed infection with *Actinobacillus actinomycetemcomitans* and *Actinomyces israelii*: Case report and review. Clin Infect Dis 18:450, 1994.

880. Shales DM, Dul MJ, Lerner PI: *Capnocytophaga* bacteremia in the compromised host. Am J Clin Pathol 77:359, 1982.

881. Parenta DM, Snydman DR: *Capnocytophaga* species: Infections in nonimmunocompromised and immunocompromised hosts. J Infect Dis 151:140, 1985.

882. Warren JS, Allen SD: Clinical, pathogenetic, and laboratory features of *Capnocytophaga* infections. Am J Clin Pathol 86:513, 1986.

883. Lion C, Escande F, Burdin JC: *Capnocytophaga canimorsus* infections in human: Review of the literature and cases report. Eur J Epidemiol 12:52, 1996.

884. Javaheri S, Smith RM, Wiltse D: Intrathoracic infections due to *Eikenella corrodens*. Thorax 42:700, 1987.

885. Kentos A, De Vuyst P, Stuelens MJ, et al: Lung abscess due to *Eikenella corrodens*: Three cases and review. Eur J Clin Microbiol Infect Dis 14:146, 1995.

886. Goldstein EJC, Kirby BD, Finegold SM: Isolation of *Eikenella corrodens* from pulmonary infections. Am Rev Resp Dis 119:55, 1979.

887. Suwanagool S, Rothkolf MM, Smith SM, et al: Pathogenicity of *Eikenella corrodens* in humans. Arch Intern Med 143:2265, 1983.

888. Sanford JP: Leptospirosis—time for a booster. N Engl J Med 310:524, 1984.

889. Ragnaud JM, Morlat P, Buisson M, et al: Epidemiological, clinical, biological, and developmental aspects of leptospirosis: Apropos of 30 cases in Aquitaine. Rev Med Interne 15:452, 1994.

890. Robertson MH, Clarke IR, Coghlan JD, et al: Leptospirosis in trout farmers. Lancet 2:626, 1981.

891. Felgin RD, Lobes LA Jr, Anderson D, et al: Human leptospirosis from immunized dogs. Ann Intern Med 79:777, 1973.

892. Fraser DW, Glosser JW, Francis DP, et al: Leptospirosis caused by serotype Fort Bragg: A suburban outbreak. Ann Intern Med 79:786, 1973.

893. Im JG, Yeon KM, Han MC, et al: Leptospirosis of the lung: Radiographic findings in 58 patients. Am J Roentgenol 152:955, 1989.

894. Winter RJD, Richardson A, Lehner MJ, et al: Lung abscess and reactive arthritis: Rare complications of leptospirosis. Br Med J 288:448, 1984.

895. Heath CW Jr, Alexander AD, Galton MM: Leptospirosis in the United States (concluded): Analysis of 483 cases in man, 1949–1961. N Engl J Med 273:915, 1965.

896. Lee REJ, Terry SI, Walker TM, et al: The chest radiograph in leptospirosis in Jamaica. Br J Radiol 54:939, 1981.

897. Teglia OF, Battagliotti C, Villavicencio RL, et al: Leptospiral pneumonia. Chest 108:872, 1995.

898. de Koning J, van der Hoeven JG, Meinders AE: Respiratory failure in leptospirosis (Weil's disease). Neth J Med 47:224, 1995.

899. Maze SS, Kirsch RE: Leptospirosis experience at Groote Schuur Hospital, 1969–1979. S Afr Med J 59:33, 1981.

900. Zaltzman M, Kallenbach JM, Goss GD, et al: Adult respiratory distress syndrome in *Leptospira canicola* infection. Br Med J 283:519, 1981.

901. Burke BJ, Searle JF, Mattingly D: Leptospirosis presenting with profuse haemoptysis. Br Med J 2:982, 1976.

902. Zaharopoulos P, Wong J: Cytologic diagnosis of syphilitic pleuritis: A case report. Diagn Cytopathol 16:35, 1997.

903. Dooley DP, Tomski S: Syphilitic pneumonitis in an HIV-infected patient. Chest 105:629, 1994.

904. Morgan AD, Lloyd WE, Price-Thomas C: Tertiary syphilis of the lung and its diagnosis. Thorax 7:125, 1952.

905. Pearson RSB, de Navasquez S: Syphilis of the lung. Guys Hosp Rep 88:1, 1938.

906. Segal AJ: Syphilitic (gummatous) pulmonary arteritis with rupture into the bronchial tree. Arch Pathol 30:911, 1940.

907. de Navasquez S: Aneurysm of the pulmonary artery and fibrosis of the lungs due to syphilis. J Pathol Bacteriol 54:315, 1942.

908. Impens N, Warson F, Roels P, et al: A rare cause of pleurisy. Eur J Respir Dis 68:388, 1986.

909. Pessotto R, Santini F, Bertolini P, et al: Surgical treatment of an aortopulmonary artery fistula complicating a syphilitic aortic aneurysm. Cardiovasc Surg 3:707, 1995.

910. Bartlett JG: Anaerobic bacterial pleuropulmonary infections. Semin Respir Med 13:158, 1992.

911. Martin WJ: Isolation and identification of anaerobic bacteria in the clinical laboratory: A two-year experience. Mayo Clin Proc 49:300, 1974.

912. Bartlett JG, Gorbach SL, Finegold SM: The bacteriology of aspiration pneumonia. Am J Med 56:202, 1974.

913. Bartlett JG: Antibiotics in lung abscess. Semin Respir Infect 6:103, 1991.

914. Hammond JMJ, Potgieter PD, Hanslo D, et al: The etiology and antimicrobial susceptibility patterns of microorganisms in acute community-acquired lung abscess. Chest 108:937, 1995.

915. Leading Article: Nonspecific lung abscess. Br Med J 3:120, 1970.

916. Doré P, Robert R, Grollier G, et al: Incidence of anaerobes in ventilator-associated pneumonia with use of a protected specimen brush. Am J Respir Crit Care Med 153:1292, 1996.

917. Marina M, Strong CA, Civen R, et al: Bacteriology of anaerobic pleuropulmonary infections. Clin Infect Dis 16:256, 1993.

918. Bartlett JG. Anaerobic bacterial infections of the lung and pleural space. Clin Infec Dis 16:248, 1993.

919. Brook I, Frazier EH: Aerobic and anaerobic microbiology of empyema: A retrospective review in two military hospitals. Chest 103:1502, 1993.

920. Rello J, Torres A: Microbial causes of ventilator-associated pneumonia. Semin Respir Infect 11:24, 1996.

921. Finegold SM: Pathogenic anaerobes. Arch Intern Med 142:1988, 1982.

922. Ries K, Levison ME, Kaye D: Transtracheal aspiration in pulmonary infection. Arch Intern Med 133:453, 1974.

923. Pollock HM, Hawkins EL, Bonner JR, et al: Diagnosis of bacterial pulmonary infections with quantitative protected-catheter cultures obtained during bronchoscopy. J Clin Microbiol 17:255, 1983.

924. Kato T, Ueemura H, Murakami N, et al: Incidence of anaerobic infections among patients with pulmonary diseases: Japanese experience with transtracheal aspiration and immediate bedside anaerobic inoculation. Clin Infect Dis 23:87, 1996.

925. Bartlett JG, O'Keefe P, Tally FP et al: Bacteriology of hospital-acquired pneumonia. Arch Intern Med 146:868, 1986.

926. Barnett TB, Herring CL: Lung abscess: Initial and late results of medical therapy. Arch Intern Med 127:217, 1971.

927. Hagan JL, Hardy JD: Lung abscess revisited: A survey of 184 cases. Ann Surg 197:755, 1983.

928. Bartlett JG, Finegold SM: State of the art: Anaerobic infections of the lung and pleural space. Am Rev Resp Dis 110:56, 1974.

929. Su W-Y, Liu C, Hung S-Y, et al: Bacteriological study in chronic maxillary sinusitis. Laryngoscope 93:931, 1983.

930. Abernathy RS, Antibiotic therapy of lung abscess: Effectiveness of penicillin. Dis Chest 53:592, 1968.

931. Gopalakrishna KV, Lerner PI: Primary lung abscess: Analysis of sixty-six cases. Cleve Clin Q 42:3, 1975.

932. Povolotskii YL, Fal NI, Smolnikova LI, et al: A bacteriological and/or immunological study of anaerobic streptococcal infection in chronic tonsillitis, paratonsillitis, and periodontitis patients. J Hyg Epidemiol Microbiol Immunol 26:308, 1982.

933. Brook I, Gober AE: *Bacteroides melaninogenicus*: Its recovery from tonsils of children with acute tonsillitis. Arch Otolaryngol 109:818, 1983.

934. Gorbach SL, Bartlett JG: Anaerobic infections. N Engl J Med 290:1237, 1974.

935. Malkamaki M, Honkanen E, Leinonen M, et al: *Branhamella catarrhalis* as a cause of bacteremic pneumonia. Scand J Infect Dis 15:125, 1983.

936. Lemierre A: On certain septicaemias due to anaerobic organisms. Lancet 1:701, 1936.

937. Henry S, DeMaria A Jr, McCabe WR: Bacteremia due to *Fusobacterium* species. Am J Med 75:225, 1983.

938. Kleinman PK, Flowers RA: Necrotizing pneumonia after pharyngitis due to *Fusobacterium necrophorum*. Pediatr Radiol 14:49, 1984.

939. Moore-Gillon J, Lee TH, Eykyn SJ, et al: Necrobacillosis: A forgotten disease. Br Med J 288:1526, 1984.

940. Seidenfeld SM, Sutker WL, Luby JP: *Fusobacterium necrophorum* septicemia following oropharyngeal infection. JAMA 248:1348, 1982.

941. Felner JM, Dowell VR Jr: "*Bacteroides*" bacteremia. Am J Med 50:787, 1971.

942. Bodner SJ, Koenig MG, Goodman JS: Bacteremic *Bacteroides* infections. Ann Intern Med 73:537, 1970.

943. Okubadejo OA, Green PJ, Payne DJH: *Bacteroides* infection among hospital patients. Br Med J 21:212, 1973.

944. Chow AW, Montgomerie JZ, Guze LB: Parenteral clindamycin therapy for severe anaerobic infections. Arch Intern Med 134:78, 1974.

945. Gorbach SL, Thadepalli H: Clindamycin in pure and mixed anaerobic infections. Arch Intern Med 134:87, 1974.

946. Volk TE: *Bacteroides.* Marquette Med Rev 22:78, 1959.

947. Tillotson JR, Lerner AM: *Bacteroides* pneumonias: Characteristics of cases with empyema. Ann Intern Med 68:308, 1968.

948. Dickinson PCT, Saphyakhajon P: Treatment of *Bacteroides* infection with clindamycin-2-phosphate. Can Med Assoc J 111:945, 1974.

949. Leigh DA: Clinical importance of infections due to *Bacteroides fragilis* and role of antibiotic therapy. Br Med J 3:225, 1974.

950. File TM, Fass RJ, Perkins RK: Pneumonia and empyema caused by *Clostridium sordelli.* Am J Med Sci 274:211, 1977.

951. Malmborg AS, Rylander M, Selanden M: Primary thoracic empyema caused by *Clostridium sporogenes.* Scand J Infect Dis 2:155, 1970.

952. Sweeting J, Rosenberg L: Primary clostridial pneumonia. Ann Intern Med 51:805, 1959.

953. Goldberg N, Rifkind D: Clostridial empyema. Arch Intern Med 115:421, 1965.

954. Spagnuolo PJ, Payne VD: Clostridial pleuropulmonary infection. Chest 78:622, 1980.

955. Raff MJ, Johnson JD, Nagar D, et al: Spontaneous clostridial empyema and pyopneumothorax. Rev Infect Dis 61:715, 1984.

956. Bayer AS, Nelson SC, Galpin JE, et al: Necrotizing pneumonia and empyema due to *Clostridium perfringens.* Am J Med 59:851, 1975.

957. Bentley DW, Lepper MH: Empyema caused by *Clostridium perfringens* (case reports). Ann Rev Resp Dis 100:706, 1969.

958. Shafron RD, Tate CF Jr: Lung abscesses: A five-year evaluation. Dis Chest 53:12, 1968.

959. Bartlett JG, Gorbach SL, Thadepalli H, et al: Bacteriology of empyema. Lancet 1:338, 1974.

960. Editorial: Chronic destructive pneumonia. Lancet 2:350, 1980.

961. McGowan K, Gorbach SL: Anaerobes in mixed infections. J Infect Dis 144:181, 1981.

962. Zaleznik DF, Kasper DL: The role of anaerobic bacteria in abscess formation. Annu Rev Med 33:217, 1982.

962a. Shlaes DM, Lederman M, Chmielewski R, et al: Elastin fibers in the sputum of patients with necrotizing pneumonia. Chest 83:885, 1993.

963. Gorbach SL, Bartlett JG: Anaerobic infections. N Engl J Med 290:1177, 1974.

964. Landay MJ, Christensen EE, Bynum LJ, et al: Anaerobic pleural and pulmonary infections. Am J Roentgenol 134:233, 1980.

965. Bartlett JG: Anaerobic bacterial pneumonitis. Am Rev Resp Dis 119:19, 1979.

966. Rohlfing BM, White EA, Webb WR, et al: Hilar and mediastinal adenopathy caused by bacterial abscess of the lung. Radiology 128:289, 1978.

966a. Penner C, Maycher B, Long R: Pulmonary gangrene: A complication of bacterial pneumonia. Chest 105:567, 1994.

967. Delcampo JM, Hitado J, Gea G, et al: Anaerobes: A new aetiology in cavitary pneumoconiosis. Br J Ind Med 39:392, 1982.

968. Bartlett JG, McGaughey MD, Kim WS: Lung abscess. Johns Hopkins Med J 150:141, 1982.

969. Schweppe HI, Knowles JN, Kane L: Lung abscess: An analysis of the Massachusetts General Hospital cases from 1943 through 1956. N Engl J Med 265:1039, 1961.

970. Friedenberg RM, Isaacs N, Elkin M: The changing roentgenologic picture in pulmonary tuberculosis under modern chemotherapy. Am J Roentgenol 81:196, 1959.

971. Irwin RS, Garrity FL, Erickson AD, et al: Sampling lower respiratory tract secretions in primary lung abscess: A comparison of the accuracy of four methods. Chest 79:559, 1981.

972. Gorbach SL, Mayhew JW, Bartlett JG, et al: Rapid diagnosis of anaerobic infections by direct gas-liquid chromatography of clinical specimens. J Clin Invest 57:478, 1976.

973. Phillips KD, Tearle PV, Willis AT: Rapid diagnosis of anaerobic infections by gas-liquid chromatography of clinical material. J Clin Pathol 29:428, 1976.

974. Abeysundere RL, Hodson ME: Pleuropulmonary lung infection by anaerobic bacteria. Br J Dis Chest 72:187, 1978.

975. Thadepalli H, Gangopadhyay PK: Rapid diagnosis of anaerobic empyema by direct gas-liquid chromatography of pleural fluid. Chest 77:507, 1980.

976. Hunter JV, Chadwick M, Hutchinson G, et al: Use of gas-liquid chromatography in the clinical diagnosis of anaerobic pleuropulmonary infection. Br J Dis Chest 79:1, 1985.

977. Wolcott MW, Coury ON, Baum GL: Changing concepts in the therapy of lung abscess: A twenty-year survey. Dis Chest 40:1, 1961.

978. Pohlson EC, McNamara JJ, Char C, et al: Lung abscess: a changing pattern of the disease. Am J Surg 150:97, 1985.

979. Lerner PI: Antimicrobial considerations in anaerobic infections. Med Clin North Am 58:533, 1974.

980. Vainrub B, Musher DM, Guinn GA, et al: Percutaneous drainage of lung abscess. Am Rev Resp Dis 117:153, 1978.

Mycobacteria

Mycobacteria are nonmotile, non–spore-forming rods that are strictly aerobic; a decrease in the ambient oxygen concentration results in a substantial decrease in the growth rate.[1] In comparison to other bacteria, they possess an exceptionally high lipid content ($> 25\%$ compared with 0.5% in gram-positive and 3.0% in gram-negative bacilli),[2] a feature that is important in explaining many of their properties, including resistance to drying, alcohol, alkali, some germicides, and acids.[2] The acid-fast quality is especially important in traditional laboratory identification because mycobacteria that have been stained bright red with carbol-fuchsin are able to resist decoloration by strong acid solutions (a property shared by only a few other organisms, including some *Nocardia* and *Corynebacterium* species and *Legionella micdadei*).[3] In smears and in tissue sections, the organisms typically stain irregularly, resulting in a beaded appearance. On routine nonfixed slides of sputum, *Mycobacterium tuberculosis* may be gram neutral or weakly gram positive;[4] in the former situation, organisms may be seen as "ghosts."[5]

Although mycobacteria are capable of growth on simple media, enrichment is usually necessary for adequate culture of clinical specimens and for identification of a specific organism. In the majority of species, such growth is slow, ranging from 3 to 8 weeks, and is related to an unusually long doubling time (12 to 18 hours for *M. tuberculosis* compared with 15 minutes for the Enterobacteriaceae).[2] On culture in solid media, the organism can be recognized by its characteristic colonial morphology, lack of pigmentation, slow or delayed catalase activity, positive niacin reaction, and ability to reduce nitrate.[6] The use of a liquid culture medium and a radiometric system that detects the metabolism of ^{14}C-labeled carbon dioxide (BACTEC) can significantly reduce the time necessary to document the presence of the organism.[7] *M. tuberculosis* is also highly pathogenic for guinea pigs, a feature that is still occasionally used in isolation and diagnosis, since drug-resistant bacilli grow poorly on standard media and fail to produce progressive disease in guinea pigs.[8] Organisms have also been identified by serology, chromatographic pattern analysis of cell wall mycolic acid, immunohistochemistry using monoclonal antibodies,[9, 10] and genetic probing for organism-specific DNA or RNA; phage typing and DNA fingerprinting have been used predominantly in epidemiologic investigations to detect various strains of *M. tuberculosis*.[11] The uses and limitations of these techniques are discussed in greater detail farther on (*see* page 845).

The genus *Mycobacterium* contains approximately 60 species, including saprophytic, parasitic, and pathogenic forms. Many birds, mammals, and cold-blooded animals are affected by one particular organism, although cross-species infection can occur. In humans, the organisms have been considered in two groups. The *tuberculosis complex* includes *M. tuberculosis*, *M. bovis*, *M. africanum*, and *M. microti*.[6] It is possible that *M. africanum* is, in fact, a strain of *M. tuberculosis* rather than a separate species; in any event, it is rarely identified as a cause of human disease, as the name implies, predominantly in Africa. Although *M. microti* is an established species, it is not pathogenic for humans.

Infection with *M. bovis* was formerly fairly common, particularly in children and often involving the lymph nodes, gastrointestinal tract, and bones; pulmonary involvement occurred chiefly by dissemination from these extrapulmonary foci. As a result of the control of the disease in cattle and the pasteurization of milk, the infection has all but disappeared from most areas of the world.[12] Sporadic cases, however, still occur;[13, 14] some of these are related to occupational exposure, as was the case in workers in an elk and deer slaughtering plant in Canada[15] and seal trainers in Australia.[16] The pathologic, radiologic, and clinical manifestations of pulmonary disease caused by *M. bovis* and *M. tuberculosis* are identical (including the presence of primary and postprimary disease[17]); however, it is important to distinguish the two on culture, partly because the former is insensitive to some drugs ordinarily employed in the treatment of tuberculosis and partly because its spread between humans is unlikely.

The *bacille Calmette-Guérin* (BCG) is an attenuated, relatively avirulent strain of *M. bovis* that has been widely used as a vaccine in the prophylaxis of tuberculosis and more recently as an immunostimulant in the treatment of various neoplasms. In both situations, it can cause pathologic and radiologic abnormalities, sometimes associated with significant clinical manifestations (*see* page 848).

In addition to *M. leprae*, nontuberculous (atypical) mycobacteria include three groups of slow-growing organisms (the photochromogens, the scotochromogens, and the non-photochromogens) and one of rapid growers. Although relatively uncommon causes of human disease in the past, these organisms (particularly those of the *M. avium* complex) have become increasingly important as a result of the acquired immunodeficiency syndrome (AIDS) epidemic (*see* page 1654).

MYCOBACTERIUM TUBERCULOSIS

Although any mycobacterial disease other than that caused by *M. leprae* can theoretically be designated *tuberculosis*, the term usually implies the presence of *M. tuberculosis*, and it is in that sense that it is used here. Such disease should be distinguished from simple infection by the organism in the absence of clinical or radiologic manifestations.

Epidemiology

Tuberculosis is and has been a disease of tremendous importance to the human race. It was evident in early civilizations and became epidemic in the crowded, impoverished cities of Europe in the 1600s and 1700s, in which as many as 25% of all deaths have been attributed to the disease (the "great white plague").[18] European settlers brought the disease to North America, and in large cities, such as New York, the mortality rate in 1800 was approximately 700 per 100,000.[18] Further settlement of North America in the 1800s was associated with rapid and devastating spread of disease to Native Americans; in some reservations, the mortality rate has been estimated to have been an astounding 9,000 per 100,000 around the year 1900.[18] Although these death rates have decreased steadily since that time in many populations, in some areas of the world they are still very high, and it has been estimated that about 3 million individuals succumb each year; with the increasing prevalence of HIV infection in many areas of the world, this figure is likely to increase.[19] Currently, approximately one third of the world's population is believed to be infected with the organism.[19, 20]

Although tuberculosis is a disease of worldwide distribution, it shows significant geographic differences in both incidence and prevalence, presumably as a result of differences in socioeconomic conditions and natural resistance of the host. The worldwide case rate was estimated to be about 60 to 70 per 100,000 in 1990;[21] however, rates vary from about 6 to 20 per 100,000 in Europe and North America[22, 23] to about 120 per 100,000 in Southeast Asia and as high as 200 to 300 per 100,000 in sub-Saharan Africa.[21] The case rate in "developed" countries has decreased significantly in the twentieth century.[23] For example, in the United States, the rate per 100,000 was approximately 55 in 1950, 30 in 1960, 18 in 1970, and 12 in 1980.[22] There was a decrease in this rate of decline in the 1980s, attributed to increased immigration of infected patients, the onset of the AIDS epidemic, and increased poverty and homelessness; thus, in 1990, the case rate was approximately 10 per 100,000. A further decrease has been noted since then, so that the rate in 1995 was 8.7 (approximately 22,860 cases).[22] Similar figures have been documented in other "developed" countries, such as Canada.[24]

A discussion of the epidemiologic features of tuberculous infection is best considered in two parts, that associated with the development of the infection and that with the development of clinically evident disease (tuberculosis). The particular features of tuberculosis associated with human immunodeficiency virus (HIV) infection are discussed in greater detail in Chapter 44 (*see* page 1648).

Development of Infection

In the majority of cases, infection is acquired by inhalation of droplet nuclei carrying the organisms.[23, 25] The risk of infection is related to the degree of contagiousness of the primarily infected individual, the adequacy of antimicrobial defense of the exposed individual, the frequency of contact between the two, and the environment in which the contact takes place.

The degree of source contagiousness is itself associated with several variables, including the extent and nature of the tuberculous disease, the frequency of coughing, and the virulence of the infecting organism. The presence of pulmonary cavities is an important factor determining contagiousness, a feature related to two mechanisms: (1) the creation of a more favorable local environment for bacterial growth and replication (possibly as a result of increased oxygen supply and loss of the relatively acid caseous necrotic material);[26] and (2) the formation of a relatively easy exit route out of the lung. Although the number of organisms that may be released to the atmosphere in cavitary disease may be quite low—for example, in one study, it was estimated that the ward of a tuberculosis sanitarium contained only one droplet nucleus per 13,000 cubic feet of air[25]—it is nevertheless sufficient to account for person-to-person spread of the organism. Although pulmonary cavities are an important source of tubercle bacilli, individuals may be smear positive without their formation. This may occur in association with a focus of parenchymal disease or with disease of the airway mucosa; for example, in laryngeal tuberculosis, the simple act of talking can cause shedding of organisms, thus greatly increasing contagiousness.[27] The extent of pulmonary involvement is also related to the risk of disease spread—the more extensive the disease, the larger the number of organisms, the greater the tendency to cavitation, and the more severe the cough.[28, 29] As might be expected, the last of these is particularly important as a means of creating bacteria-laden droplet nuclei.[30, 31]

The importance of these features in the transmission of the organism is illustrated by several clinical observations. For example, it is known that smear-positive patients are more contagious than those who are smear negative (presumably as a result of a greater number of organisms in sputum). There is also evidence that the greater the number of organisms in smear-positive specimens, the greater the degree of infectiousness.[32] The same principle applies to patients undergoing chemotherapy, many of whom rapidly become noncontagious.[33–35] Based on a review of the literature, one author concluded that respiratory secretions that are initially smear negative but culture positive should no longer have viable bacilli detectable by culture within 2 weeks of the onset of therapy;[36] however, it was also estimated that after 2 weeks of therapy almost all smear-positive patients would remain culture positive, and more than one half would re-

main smear positive. As might be expected, there is evidence that patients who have tuberculosis and are noncompliant with respect to therapy are an important source for the spread of disease in the community.[37]

Because the organism is transferred from person to person via droplets suspended in the air, contact between contagious and noninfected individuals is clearly a risk factor, particularly if it occurs in poorly ventilated locations. In fact, individuals who have had close contact with an infectious person have been shown to be twice as likely to be tuberculin positive as those who have only a casual acquaintance.[38] The increased incidence of infection in people who live in relatively crowded areas, such as prisons, hostels, slums of large metropolitan centers, and refugee camps, is at least partly explained by this observation. Workers in contact with individuals in these environments are also at increased risk.[39]

Transmission of the organism also occurs frequently in the home, and many cases of childhood infection can be traced to a parent or grandparent.[40] Infection, sometimes widespread, can develop from a single active case in school[41–43] or a day-care center.[44] Continued contact has also been clearly demonstrated to increase the risk of infection in relatively confined areas, such as ships, hospital wards, nursing homes, and chronic care units.[45–49] Contact with contagious individuals in less clearly confined settings, such as a neighborhood bar[50] or a church,[51, 51a] has also been shown to be associated with an increased risk. Guidelines for the prevention and control of tuberculosis in many of these settings have been published.[52]

Health care workers (including physicians, dentists, nurses, medical students, and support staff) constitute another group at increased risk; outbreaks of infection among these individuals are well documented,[53–57] and, in some settings, the incidence of purified protein derivative (PPD) conversion appears to be quite high.[58, 59] Despite this, it should be remembered that the acquisition of infection by hospital workers may also occur in the community at large, in which case other risk factors (e.g., socioeconomic) are important.[60] Biosafety guidelines for laboratory technicians working with *M. tuberculosis* have also been established.[61]

The effect of host factors on the acquisition of infection is poorly understood. Heredity appears to play an important role, as indicated by experimental animal studies in which strains have been bred that are either resistant or sensitive to the disease.[62–64] Certain ethnic groups, such as African Americans and native North Americans, have long been noted to have increased rates of infection and disease compared with white individuals.[22] Although it is likely that these observations are influenced to some extent by socioeconomic or other environmental factors, there is evidence that at least some of the difference is the result of heredity.[65] Similar statements may apply to individuals in some "developing" regions of the world. Despite this, the ethnic association has been questioned by some investigators; for example, in one study of a tuberculous outbreak in a racially mixed school, no difference in infection rate was identified between black and white children, although the former individuals more often had radiographic evidence of disease.[43] Whatever the pathogenetic basis, it is clear that immigrants to North America and Western Europe are much more likely to be infected than individuals among the general population in these regions and that they represent an important potential source of future illness.[22, 24]

Although the vast majority of tuberculous infections are acquired by transmission of bacteria-laden droplet nuclei from humans who have pulmonary disease, some have been transmitted via fiberoptic bronchoscopy,[66] organ transplantation,[67] and irrigation of a tuberculous abscess.[68] In addition, humans rarely transmit infection to or acquire infection from house pets,[69, 70] monkeys,[71] and farm animals.[72] Pathologists and laboratory technicians may also be infected after exposure to tissue in the course of autopsies or culture procedures. Although infection in these circumstances can result from direct inoculation,[73] the more common mechanism is probably inhalation of droplet nuclei; the latter is especially likely to occur in procedures such as the use of a cryostat to obtain frozen sections of surgical material in which compressed gas coolants are used.[74]

Development of Disease

Tuberculosis has been estimated to develop in only 5% to 15% of individuals who are infected with *M. tuberculosis*.[75, 76] Although the possibility for the development of disease exists for the lifetime of an infected individual, the risk is highest during the 2 years after initial infection, during which time the incidence has been estimated to be about 4% per year.[75] However, in an investigation of individuals who received placebo therapy in the Veterans Administration isoniazid prevention therapy trial, a reactivation rate of only 1% was found over a 7-year period and it is possible that this estimate is too high.[76a]

Disease may be associated either with progression of the primary focus of infection (*primary* or *progressive primary tuberculosis*) or with the development of new disease months or years after "healing" of the initial infection has occurred (*postprimary tuberculosis*). The latter is often the result of reactivation of an endogenous focus of infection acquired in earlier life;[77, 78] occasionally, an exogenous source is responsible (i.e., reinfection).[79–81] Although it has been difficult to prove whether a particular case of active tuberculosis is the result of endogenous reactivation or reinfection, the availability of techniques such as restriction fragment length analysis (DNA fingerprinting) is beginning to elucidate the relative importance of the two more precisely.[82]

Although the precise mechanisms by which infection develops into clinically evident disease are not well understood, a number of risk factors have been identified.[38, 83] Clearly, these are not all independent, and in many cases a combination of several factors is likely to be involved.[84]

Socioeconomic Factors

As with infection, some of the most important risk factors for the development of disease are socioeconomic, particularly overcrowded living conditions and malnutrition.[85, 85a] For example, the incidence of disease in North America is much higher in the inner-city areas of large metropolitan centers than in the continent as a whole;[86, 87] individuals in these areas are often homeless or can be found living in skid-row hostels, long-term care facilities, or prisons.[88–94] The prevalence of disease in such individuals

may be high: for example, in one investigation of homeless men in New York City, active disease (defined as a positive sputum or tissue culture) was diagnosed in 18%.[90] (However, 90% of individuals with a positive culture were also HIV positive, and it is likely that the prevalence of tuberculosis is lower in populations in which HIV is less common.) Although the association between homelessness and tuberculosis has been most thoroughly documented in the United States, it is likely that it applies in other countries.[95] The risk of both infection and clinically evident disease increases during conditions of war, in which a combination of factors—malnutrition, homelessness, overcrowding, and inadequate medical services—is probably implicated.[96]

An exception to the association with low socioeconomic status is the health care worker, in whom the incidence of tuberculosis is higher than in the general population, presumably because of increased risk of contact with the organism.[58, 97, 98] Similarly, exposure of individuals in relatively crowded environments, such as recreation centers,[99] schools,[41, 43] or army barracks,[100] can also lead to outbreaks of disease in the absence of other risk factors.

Drug and Alcohol Abuse

In many cases, drug or alcohol abuse is associated with one or more of the adverse socioeconomic conditions outlined previously, in which situation there may be a particularly high risk of disease; for example, in one investigation of indigent people in New York City who were alcoholics or drug abusers (or both), the case rate was almost 750 per 100,000.[84] Not all cases of alcohol-associated disease, however, can be explained by socioeconomic factors; for example, in one investigation of 97 individuals who came into contact with a contagious individual in a neighborhood bar, 27 developed infection and 14 developed disease.[50] It is possible that the pathogenesis of the increased risk in these individuals is related to an effect of alcohol on the immune system.[101]

Because drug abuse is a well-established risk factor for HIV infection, many cases of tuberculosis in addicts occur in patients who are also HIV positive.[102] Nevertheless, epidemiologic investigations performed before the era of AIDS also showed an increased risk of disease in addicts;[103] for example, in one review of the causes of death in drug addicts who were institutionalized in one center in the United States during the period 1935 to 1966, tuberculosis was identified in 18%.[104] Although the risk of tuberculosis in addicts is highest in those who inject drugs intravenously (probably because of the concomitant risk of HIV infection), the disease is also well associated with the use of other illicit drugs (e.g., crack cocaine[105]).

Sex and Age

Although pulmonary tuberculosis can develop at any age, case rates vary markedly in different groups. They are generally relatively high in the early years of life, decrease during adolescence, and increase markedly in middle and old age.[22, 106] Part of the reason for the increase in the 25- to 45-year-old group is the prevalence of AIDS in this population; however, in some areas of the world in which AIDS has been identified in relatively few individuals, the incidence of tuberculosis is still high in patients between 20 and 39 years of age.[107]

The reason for the relatively high proportion of cases in the elderly is complex and probably related to several factors, including the higher prevalence of infection and disease 50 to 70 years ago in some populations, decreased immunity, malnutrition, coexistent disease such as diabetes and malignancy and its therapy, and communal living in nursing homes.[108] Whatever the pathogenesis, the relatively large number of cases in this group is important: in the United States, the percentage of new cases of tuberculosis in patients aged 65 and over more than doubled from 1953 to 1979;[108] moreover, the overall case rate in 1995 was 16.0 per 100,000 (compared with 9.9 for those aged 25 to 45 and only 1.7 for those aged 5 to 14).[22] There is evidence that this situation may be particularly serious for individuals living in nursing homes; some investigators have found the case rate to be as high as 14 times that of the general population and 4 times that of noninstitutionalized patients of the same age.[88] Compounding the problem is the observation that the disease in the elderly tends to be advanced at the time of presentation, is more commonly associated with miliary disease, may be manifested by atypical clinical features, and is associated with a poor tolerance of therapy.[108–111]

Overall, the case rate of tuberculosis in men in the United States is about twice that in women.[22] This increase is largely seen in individuals 25 years of age and over; in younger patients, the rates are more or less equal.

Pregnancy

Data from several investigations suggest that pregnancy is not associated with an increased risk of developing tuberculosis or with its progression in cases of established disease.[112, 113] In some studies, this lack of risk has been found even in women infected with HIV.[114] There is also no evidence that tuberculosis alters the course of pregnancy, although the risk of acquiring the disease is clearly increased for the fetus and neonate.[112] Most investigators believe that the clinical manifestations of disease are no different in pregnant and nonpregnant women.[112, 115]

Ethnic Status

As with some of the other risk factors for tuberculosis, the reasons for the increased incidence of disease in certain ethnic groups is complex and probably multifactorial. Although socioeconomic factors undoubtedly have an important influence,[115a] it is likely that genetically related susceptibility is also important.[116]

In North America, case rates are highest in African Americans and Native Americans and recent immigrants from parts of the world with a high prevalence of the disease.[22, 24] For example, in the United States in 1995, case rates per 100,000 were as follows: white (non-Hispanic) individuals, 3.1; African Americans, 23.9; Hispanics, 18.0; and Native Americans, 16.5. Similarly, of 2,074 cases reported in Canada in 1994, 1,183 were in individuals born outside of the country;[24] of the 835 native-born patients, 398 were aboriginal and 437 nonaboriginal. The age distribution of affected patients also differs significantly between ethnic groups. For example, in the United States in 1995, approxi-

mately 24% of reported cases in white (non-Hispanic) individuals occurred between 25 and 44 years of age compared with 43% in those over age 65;[22] the corresponding figures for African Americans were 43% and 16%. African Americans also appear to be particularly susceptible to miliary tuberculosis.[117–119]

The emigration from "developing" countries to North America and Europe that has occurred in the recent past has had an important influence on the case rate in these regions;[120, 120a] for example, in the United States in 1995, approximately one third of all cases occurred in foreign-born patients.[22, 121] Although most such patients (approximately 60%) have been in their adopted country for 5 years or less when they develop disease, the potential for onset well after this time period cannot be overlooked;[122, 123] for example, of the 500,000 refugees who immigrated to the United States from Southeast Asia during the 1970s, 60% had a positive PPD reaction.[124] Compounding this problem is the fact that a significant number of immigrants who develop tuberculosis have been infected by drug-resistant organisms.[123, 125–127]

Genetic Factors

As indicated previously, genetic factors appear to play a major role in susceptibility and resistance to tuberculous infection in some animal models.[62, 64] Experimental observations in the mouse suggest that natural resistance is related to the presence of a gene that affects the ability of macrophages to kill intracellular organisms (including *Mycobacterium* species).[128] This gene (originally termed the *Bcg* gene) is associated with the production of natural resistance–associated macrophage protein (Nramp), which is in turn involved with transport of nitrite from the cytosol to phagolysozomes.[128a] Evidence that this process might be important in humans was provided in a study of macrophages derived from six African American and eight white individuals from Colorado, tubercle bacilli being found to grow significantly faster in cell cultures of the former group.[129]

A variety of epidemiologic observations also suggest that inherited susceptibility is an important risk factor in humans. For example, concordance for tuberculosis has been found to be significantly higher among monozygotic than dizygotic twin pairs.[130] Body build has also been shown to be associated with an increased risk of disease, individuals who are lean and underweight appearing to be more susceptible; although this might be partly the result of undernutrition, there is evidence that it is related to a familial trait.[131] A number of groups have shown a relationship between HLA phenotype (particularly HLA DR2) and the presence of tuberculosis in selected groups of patients.[132–136] An association between skin test responsiveness to tuberculin antigen and sibship has also been documented[137] and may be partly related to HLA type.[138]

Coexistent Disease

In addition to diseases characterized primarily by a derangement of immunocompetence (*see* farther on), a number of abnormalities have been associated with an increased risk for the development of tuberculosis. These include silicosis, diabetes mellitus, chronic renal failure, alveolar proteinosis, the postgastrectomy state, and iron overload.[139]

Several groups of investigators have found patients with *diabetes mellitus* to be more susceptible to tuberculosis, the overall increased risk being in the order of 2 to 3.5.[140, 141] Some have also documented an increased likelihood of lower lobe or multilobe disease, pleural effusion, and cavitation.[141] In one investigation of 106 patients who had both diabetes and tuberculosis, 48 were diagnosed as having tuberculosis before diabetes was recognized, and 40 were known to have diabetes at the time tuberculosis was discovered;[142] in the remaining 18 cases, the diagnoses were made simultaneously. The increased incidence of tuberculosis in patients with diabetes mellitus is paralleled by the incidence of diabetes in those with tuberculosis: in one investigation of 256 patients with the infection, blood glucose concentration 2 hours after eating was within the diabetic range in 41%.[143]

There is little question that *silicosis* predisposes to tuberculosis;[145–147] moreover, there is evidence that disease is apt to recur after treatment.[148] The prevalence of the complication in workers with silicosis depends to a large extent on the prevalence of tuberculosis in the population from which they come.[149] Although it is customary to associate the disease with the presence of progressive massive fibrosis (PMF), there is evidence that its risk increases with increasing profusion of simple nodular shadows;[150] in fact, the likelihood of developing tuberculosis is greater in workers with any degree of silicosis compared with similarly exposed workers without silicosis.[150] It may be extremely difficult to isolate tubercle bacilli during life in patients who have tuberculosis and silicosis, particularly those with PMF;[151] identification of organisms by polymerase chain reaction (PCR) might prove useful in this setting.[152]

A small increase in the risk of tuberculosis has been found by some investigators in patients who have had *partial gastrectomy* for peptic ulcer disease[153–155] or *jejunoileal bypass* for the treatment of obesity.[156, 157] In one study of the latter patients, the diagnosis was usually made 10 to 15 months after surgery, and the disease was often extrapulmonary, with a particular affinity for lymph nodes.[157] Hypothesized mechanisms for the postgastrectomy association include malnutrition and decreased immune function.[153] There is evidence that decreased gastric acidity and peptic ulcer disease itself are not involved.[153]

Another well-established risk factor for tuberculosis is *chronic renal failure*. Although patients who do not require dialysis are at increased risk,[158] the major association appears to be with those on hemodialysis, in whom the incidence has been estimated to be 6 to 16 times that expected.[159–162] The diagnosis is frequently not made during life because symptoms are often confused with those generally ascribed to uremia, and the PPD reaction is often negative. Persistent high fever is a valuable clue to the diagnosis in this setting.[159, 161, 163]

Coexistent tuberculosis and *pulmonary alveolar proteinosis* (PAP) was documented in 10 patients in a 1980 literature review.[164] (One group also found *Mycobacterium avium-intracellulare* in 8 of 19 consecutive patients who underwent therapeutic lung lavage for PAP.[165]) In most patients in whom *M. tuberculosis* was isolated, the infection was recognized before the appearance of the proteinosis; however, the infection has also been reported to develop after the diagnosis of PAP.[166] Experimental studies have shown that surfactant protein A from patients with PAP

appears to enhance the entry of mycobacteria into alveolar macrophages,[167] providing some rationale for the latter sequence. In some patients, both PAP and tuberculosis have resolved after antituberculous therapy.[166] Eleven patients have also been described in whom minute foci of histologically characteristic alveolar proteinosis were identified adjacent to surgically resected tuberculous lesions;[168] because none of these patients subsequently developed radiographic evidence of full-blown PAP, the significance of this observation is not clear.

Most specialists in pulmonary disease have encountered one or more patients who, despite a clinical and pathologic picture of *sarcoidosis*, subsequently have acid-fast organisms demonstrated in their sputum. In one remarkable investigation of 230 patients who had sarcoidosis reported in 1960, tuberculosis was believed to be present in 29 (13%).[169] There are at least three possible explanations for this association: (1) the tuberculosis is a complication of sarcoidosis (particularly in the setting of steroid therapy); (2) the diagnosis of sarcoidosis was incorrect; or (3) there is a pathogenetic relationship between a mycobacterial organism and sarcoidosis (*see* page 1534). Because of this uncertainty, it is recommended that the possibility of tuberculosis be considered in patients in whom a diagnosis of sarcoidosis has been made and who have atypical or progressive disease.

There is some evidence for an increased risk of tuberculosis in *systemic lupus erythematosus*;[170–172] to what extent this is related to therapy, the disease itself, or a combination of the two is not clear. Many of the reported cases have been from areas with a relatively high prevalence of tuberculosis in the general population. There is also evidence that *iron overload*, such as seen in some parts of Africa, may be associated with an increased risk.[173]

Immunosuppression

Immunocompromised patients are clearly at increased risk for mycobacterial disease.[174] By far the most important underlying immunosuppressive condition is HIV infection, which has become a major influence on the incidence and course of tuberculosis throughout the world.[175–177] The presence of the virus increases the likelihood that primary infection will progress to clinically evident disease and that latent disease will undergo reactivation.[175] Compounding these effects is the relatively high incidence of drug-resistant organisms (at least in some populations, such as those in U.S. urban areas) and an increased risk of disseminated and extrapulmonary disease. This subject is discussed in greater detail on page 804.

There is evidence that corticosteroid therapy is a risk factor for the development of tuberculosis,[178–180] and prophylactic use of isoniazid has been advocated for positive reactors to PPD who are to be given the medication. Paradoxically, there is also evidence that steroid therapy is beneficial in some forms of tuberculosis, such as meningitis and pericarditis.[180, 181] An association between the use of nonsteroidal anti-inflammatory drugs and the development of tuberculosis has also been suggested.[182]

Patients who have organ (including heart,[183, 184] liver,[185, 186] lung,[187, 188] and kidney[189–192]) or bone marrow[193] transplants are also at increased risk of developing tuberculosis. Most investigators have found the incidence to be about

1% to 2% of their transplant population; however, rates of 8% to 12% have been documented by some.[190, 191] Those with renal transplants appear to be particularly susceptible.[190, 191] As might be expected, the risk appears to be greater in regions in which the local prevalence of tuberculosis is higher.[190, 193] The majority of cases are discovered in the first year after transplantation; however, the complication has developed in some patients after 5 or 6 years.[185, 192] The performance of surveillance cultures has been advocated as a means to detect the disease in an early stage.[194]

Although the pathogenesis is probably complex, immunosuppression—either inherent or related to therapy—is also likely to be involved in the increased incidence of tuberculosis in patients who have malignant neoplasms.[195] In addition, patients with less well-characterized immune abnormalities, such as angioimmunoblastic lymphadenopathy,[196] also appear to be at increased risk.

Drug-Resistant Tuberculosis

One of the most important advances in the treatment of tuberculosis in the twentieth century has been the development of effective antimicrobial drugs, such as isoniazid, rifampin, streptomycin, ethambutol, and pyrazinamide. As with other bacteria, *M. tuberculosis* has the capacity to develop resistance to the effects of these drugs.[197] Such resistance may be primary (i.e., developing in individuals who have not received previous drug therapy) or secondary (acquired as a result of a patient not following appropriate therapy).[198] The problem may also be considered in terms of the number of drugs to which the organism is resistant, *multidrug resistance* being defined as resistance to two or more first-line medications (such as isoniazid and rifampin).[123]

Drug resistance has been known to occur for many years and has traditionally been a particular problem in developing countries, in which the cost and availability of medication and public health care programs have been such that secondary resistance was almost certain to develop in a significant number of patients.[123, 125, 126] Immigrants from these countries may bring resistant organisms with them, potentially contributing to the incidence of cases of primary resistance in the country to which they immigrate.[127]

Drug resistance was a relatively unimportant problem in the United States until the 1990s. National surveys by the Centers for Disease Control in the 1960s and 1970s showed primary drug resistance in approximately 3.5% and 7% of isolates for a single drug and approximately 1% and 2.5% for two or more drugs.[123] Investigations by workers from the same institution in the 1980s and early 1990s have shown resistance to one or more drugs in about 10% to 13% of patients.[123] In these and other studies, there has been a significant variation in likelihood of infection by resistant organisms between different age groups, ethnic populations, and hospital centers.[199] In fact, there are certain regions and population groups in which the incidence of drug resistance, particularly to multiple agents, is alarmingly high.[200, 200a] For example, in one review of patients in New York City in 1991, 33% of tuberculous isolates were found to be resistant to at least one drug (26% to isoniazid and 19% to rifampin).[201] The most important risk factor for the presence of

drug resistance in these individuals is previous treatment for tuberculosis;[200, 200a, 202] many patients also have a history of drug abuse and HIV infection.[203] In addition to these more general surveys, there have been a number of reports of isolated outbreaks of multidrug-resistant tuberculosis, most often in hospitalized patients with concomitant HIV infection.[204–206]

Primary Pulmonary Tuberculosis

Patients who become ill immediately following their first exposure to the tubercle bacillus have traditionally been thought to have pathologic, radiologic, and clinical features that differ from those associated with reactivation of previous disease or reinfection; consequently, it is customary to consider tuberculosis under the headings of *primary* and *postprimary* disease. It should be remembered, however, that the pathologic and radiologic abnormalities associated with postprimary disease are likely related, at least partly, to hypersensitivity and acquired immunity; because these features generally develop within 1 to 3 weeks of the onset of the initial infection, a "postprimary" form of disease can develop during the primary infection itself if the latter is not checked by the body's defense mechanisms. Moreover, there is evidence from some DNA fingerprinting studies that the radiologic features of active tuberculosis are similar in patients who have apparently acquired the infection recently and those who have evidence of remote infection (and, by inference, reactivation [postprimary] disease).[207] The descriptions that follow of the radiologic and pathologic features of primary and postprimary disease should be considered with these points in mind.

Primary pulmonary tuberculosis has traditionally been thought to occur predominantly in children and is particularly prevalent in regions in which the annual risk of infection is high. With the reduction in the incidence of the disease since the early part of the twentieth century in many regions, however, and the resulting increase in the number of nonsensitized individuals, the primary form of disease appears to have become more common in adults than it was previously.[208]

Pathogenesis and Pathologic Characteristics

M. tuberculosis produces no exotoxins or endotoxins and shows no effective resistance to phagocytosis. Although some strains of the organism are cytotoxic for alveolar type II cells,[208a] the significance of this effect to the development of disease is uncertain. Virulence has been related to growth in culture in the form of cords of bacilli arranged in parallel, which, in turn, correlates with the presence of trehalose-6, 6'-dimycolate, commonly known as *cord factor*. In its purified form, this substance possesses a variety of experimental effects, including lethality for mice, chemotaxis and stimulation of macrophages, activation of the alternative complement pathway, and induction of granulomas.[209] Despite these qualities, the mechanism by which cord factor relates to disease is not well understood, and it has been questioned whether any of these effects are of pathogenetic significance.[209] Sulfatides (trehalose glycolipids related chemically to cord factor) have been shown experimentally to inhibit fusion of lysosomes with phagosomes, and it has been suggested that this may be important in promoting intracellular survival of the organism.[209] A similar effect has been seen with ammonia produced by the bacillus.[209a] There is also evidence that virulent strains of *M. tuberculosis* are capable of lysing phagosomes even if they have been incorporated within these structures.[210] Production of catalase is also associated with virulence, as illustrated by the fact that isoniazid-resistant strains that typically lack this enzyme are not pathogenic for guinea pigs;[211, 212] again, however, the relationship of this substance to disease pathogenesis is not understood.

Whatever the precise cellular and molecular mechanisms, there appear to be two particularly important factors in the development of tuberculosis: (1) the ability of the organism to survive and multiply within macrophages and to persist for many years in unfavorable conditions in an inactive but viable state within necrotic tissue; and (2) the ability of the host to mount an effective cell-mediated immune response.[213, 214, 214a] The interplay between survival capacity of the organism and the efficiency with which T-cell–stimulated macrophages contain and kill the organism largely determines whether infection is established in an individual exposed to the organism and, once established, the extent of the ensuing disease. The development of such disease, as manifested pathologically by necrosis and eventually fibrosis, appears to be related principally to a delayed hypersensitivity reaction mediated by sensitized T lymphocytes;[214] as might be expected, the balance between specific T-cell subsets is likely to be important in determining the degree of macrophage activation and, ultimately, the course of the disease.[215, 216, 216a] There is also increasing evidence that cytotoxic T cells are directly involved in the immunologic response.[217, 218] Although the result of these reactions is clearly beneficial to the host in that they localize and destroy a substantial number of bacteria, they also possess the major disadvantage of causing tissue destruction.

As discussed previously, humans usually acquire primary pulmonary tuberculosis by inhaling droplet nuclei laden with bacilli. The nuclei measure less than 10 μm in diameter and are kept airborne by air currents normally present in any room;[25] many are small enough to avoid impaction in the upper airways and bronchi, and settle out instead in the lung parenchyma, usually close to the pleura, where the bacilli multiply. The organisms are initially phagocytozed by alveolar macrophages via a number of receptors (particularly those related to complement and mannose[218a]); interaction of organisms with surfactant protein A may also be important in this process.[218b] An exudative inflammatory reaction consisting of edema and an infiltrate of polymorphonuclear leukocytes soon follows.[219] Although the neutrophils are also capable of phagocytosis and have been shown to be able to kill the bacilli,[220] they are not able to contain the infection by themselves and are quickly replaced by macrophages derived from the adjacent interstitium. Under the influence of sensitized T cells recruited to the site of inflammation,[221] the macrophages undergo morphologic and functional alterations to become epithelioid cells and begin to aggregate into more or less discrete granulomas (Fig. 27–1).[222, 223] The molecular events underlying these reactions are complex and involve a number of chemokines and cytokines; among the most important are interleukin-8, tumor necrosis factor-alpha, interferon-gamma, and transforming growth factor-beta.[214a]

After several weeks (coinciding with the development of hypersensitivity), granulomas are well formed, and their central portions undergo necrosis.[224] At first, this is probably patchy, corresponding to multiple microscopic foci of granuloma formation. As the disease progresses, however, individual necrotic foci tend to enlarge and coalesce, resulting in relatively large areas of necrotic debris surrounded by a layer of epithelioid histiocytes and multinucleated giant cells (*see* Fig. 27–1). These cells are in turn surrounded by layers of mononuclear cells—both lymphocytes and blood-derived monocytes—and fibroblasts. These three zones—epithelioid cells, mononuclear cells, and fibroblasts—serve to isolate the tubercle bacilli within a relatively discrete region of the lung parenchyma, and in most cases, to prevent further spread of the disease. At this point, the inflammatory focus may be grossly visible, the central necrotic material being white and somewhat crumbly (similar to goat cheese); this appearance is known as *caseation necrosis* and is characteristic (albeit not diagnostic) of most forms of tuberculous necrosis.

The initial focus of parenchymal disease in primary tuberculosis is termed the *Ghon focus*. It either enlarges as the disease progresses or, much more commonly, undergoes healing. In the latter event, fibroblasts at the periphery of the necrotic foci proliferate and form collagen. Although this sometimes results in conversion of the entire area into a dense fibrous scar, more often the central necrotic material persists and becomes separated from the surrounding lung parenchyma by a well-developed fibrous capsule (Fig. 27–2). Dystrophic calcification is common in the necrotic material at this stage and is often of sufficient degree to be visible radiographically. Despite the fact that the disease is inactive, viable organisms may remain within the encapsulated necrotic areas and serve as a focus for reactivation in later life.

During the early phase of infection, spread of organisms to regional lymph nodes via lymphatic channels is common and results in granulomatous inflammation of both lymphatic vessels and the nodes themselves. The combination of the Ghon focus and affected lymph nodes is known as the *Ranke complex*. The course of the disease in lymph nodes is similar to that in the parenchyma, consisting initially of granulomatous inflammation and necrosis followed by fibrosis and calcification; however, the degree of inflammatory reaction typically is greater in lymph nodes than in the parenchyma, making this site of infection more obvious radiographically. Because of their anatomic location, such lymph nodes can be associated with a variety of complications.

1. Enlargement can be sufficient to compress adjacent airways and result in atelectasis. This can occur during active disease, the atelectasis resolving with the decrease in inflammation that accompanies healing. It can also be present with chronic (inactive) tuberculosis, in which case it is associated with either large foci of nodal necrosis or perinodal fibrosis resulting from local extension of disease (Fig. 27–3).

2. Extranodal extension of the inflammatory reaction can cause localized mucosal edema or actual granulomatous inflammation and ulceration of the airway wall; such tracheobronchial disease is not infrequent and may be visible at bronchoscopy.[225]

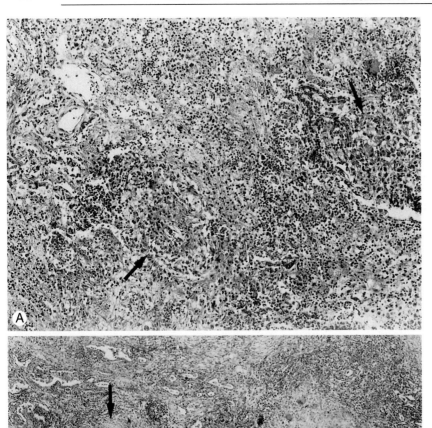

Figure 27–1. Tuberculosis—Development of Granulomatous Inflammation. Early stage *(A)*, showing lung parenchyma consolidated by mononuclear cells, many of which appear to be lymphocytes. Focally *(arrows)*, the cells are larger with more abundant cytoplasm and are beginning to form small aggregates, representing early granulomas. Note the absence of necrosis. Subsequent stage *(B)*, showing well-defined foci of granulomatous inflammation surrounded by a mononuclear inflammatory infiltrate. Necrosis is now apparent in the center of some granulomas *(arrow)*.

3. Rarely, the node ruptures into the adjacent bronchus or pulmonary artery, releasing liquefied necrotic material into the airway or vascular lumen.[226, 227] In the former instance, this may result in tuberculous bronchopneumonia; in the latter, there may be local or widespread miliary disease; if the bronchus and artery are affected simultaneously, there may be massive hemoptysis. Because the responsible lymph node reduces in size as a result of rupture, pre-existing segmental or lobar atelectasis may actually disappear.

In addition to lymphatic dissemination to regional lymph nodes, organisms also gain access to the bloodstream (and thus extrapulmonary tissues) via efferent nodal lymphatics or pulmonary veins in the vicinity of the Ghon focus. Although such hematogenous dissemination is probably common,[228] clinical manifestations of miliary or localized extrapulmonary tuberculosis in primary disease are usually absent, presumably as a result of the limited number of disseminated organisms and the adequacy of host defense. Nevertheless, this systemic dispersal of organisms is extremely important because the minute areas of infection it establishes remain as potential foci for subsequent disease reactivation.

In a small number of patients with primary tuberculosis, local parenchymal disease progresses, either at the site of the initial Ghon focus or elsewhere in the lung (usually the apical or posterior segments of the upper lobes). This is termed *progressive primary tuberculosis*[229] and is similar in both its morphology and course to postprimary disease (Fig. 27–4).

Radiologic Manifestations

Most individuals infected with *M. tuberculosis* do not have radiologic abnormalities. When primary infection leads

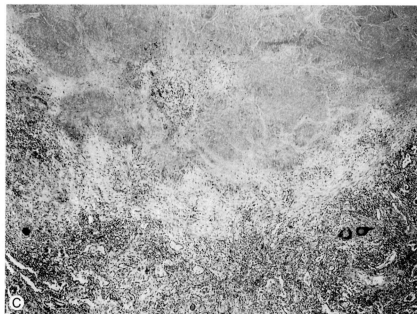

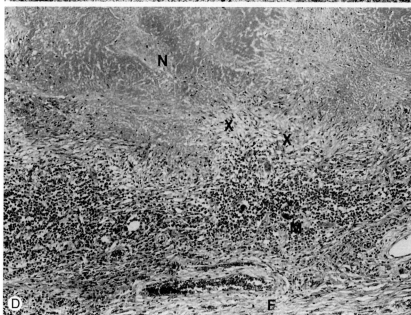

Figure 27–1 *Continued.* More advanced disease *(C)*, showing confluent foci of necrosis delineated by a zone of granulomatous inflammatory tissue. Magnified view of the latter region *(D)*, showing zones of necrosis (N), epithelioid histiocytes (X), mononuclear cells (M), and fibrosis (F). (*A*, ×100; *B*, ×40; *C*, ×40; *D*, ×100.)

to thoracic disease, it usually affects one or more of four structures: the pulmonary parenchyma, the mediastinal and hilar lymph nodes, the tracheobronchial tree, and the pleura.

Parenchymal Involvement

The largest recent study of the radiologic manifestations of primary tuberculosis in children is based on a review of 252 consecutive cases, for which chest radiographs were available in 191.[230] Air-space consolidation was identified in approximately 70% of these cases; it affected the right lung more often than the left, was bilateral in 15% of cases, and showed no significant predilection for any particular lung region. Previous studies of a smaller number of cases had shown a slight upper lobe predominance.[225, 231, 232]

In another review of chest radiographs of 103 adults with primary disease, evidence of air-space consolidation

was found in approximately 90%.[233] The consolidation involved the right upper lobe most commonly (30% of cases) and the right middle lobe least commonly (10% of cases); each of the remaining lobes and lingula were involved in approximately 20% of cases. The consolidation is usually homogeneous, dense, and anatomically confined to a segment (Fig. 27–5) or, more commonly, a lobe.[234] In approximately 25% of cases, it is multifocal, and in 10%, it is bilateral.[230, 233] Cavitation has been reported in approximately 2% of children and 6% of adults.[230, 233] Radiologic evidence of miliary disease has been reported in only about 3% of children and 6% of adults.[225, 233, 235]

Lymph Node Involvement

Evidence of lymphadenopathy is identified on the chest radiograph in about 90% to 95% of children with primary

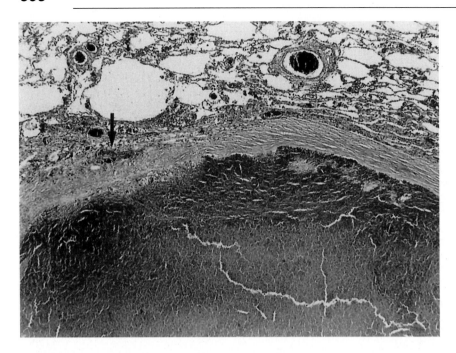

Figure 27–2. Inactive Tuberculous Granuloma. A well-developed fibrous capsule surrounds abundant granular necrotic material. Apart from occasional clusters of lymphocytes *(arrow)*, evidence of inflammation is absent. Although this nodule was caused by *M. tuberculosis*, an identical histologic apperance can be seen with fungi, such as *Coccidioides immitis* and *Histoplasma capsulatum.* (×25.)

disease.[225, 230] The majority have hilar involvement, most commonly on the right; approximately 50% have both hilar and mediastinal (usually the right paratracheal region) disease.[230]

Lymphadenopathy is seen less commonly in adults than in children; for example, in two studies of 103 and 19 adults with primary tuberculosis, it was evident radiographically in only 10 (10%)[233] and 6 (32%).[236] As with children, the lymphadenopathy is most commonly unilateral and hilar *(see* Fig. 27–5) or paratracheal (Fig. 27–6); however, it may be the only abnormality and, in both children and adults, unilateral lymphadenopathy should suggest the possibility of the

disease. The presence of bilateral lymphadenopathy or lymphadenopathy without parenchymal consolidation does not exclude tuberculosis, but is uncommon in adults with primary disease with the exception of patients who have AIDS.[233]

On CT, affected lymph nodes often shows relatively low attenuation of their central region and peripheral (rim) enhancement after intravenous administration of contrast material (Fig. 27–7).[234, 237, 237a, 238] In one study of 23 patients, such rim enhancement was usually seen in nodes larger than 2 cm in diameter;[237] smaller nodes usually showed inhomogeneous enhancement throughout. In a subsequent

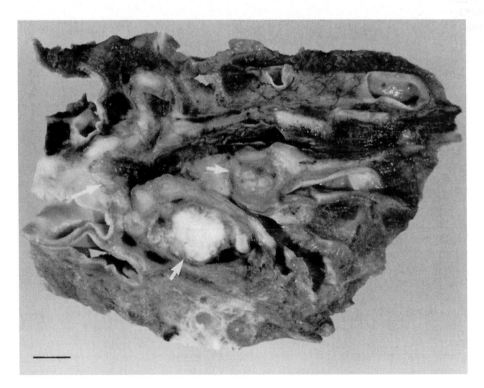

Figure 27–3. Bronchial Stenosis from Chronic Granulomatous Lymphadenitis. A magnified view of a portion of lung shows a lower lobe bronchus *(long arrow)* and its segmental divisions. One of these is compressed to a narrow slit by two well-demarcated foci of remote granulomatous inflammation within peribronchial lymph nodes *(short arrows)*. The lower one shows caseous necrosis; the upper is predominantly fibrotic. This complication can be seen in both tuberculosis and histoplasmosis; the cause in this case was not apparent. This was an incidental finding at autopsy in a 60-year-old woman. (Bar = 5 mm.)

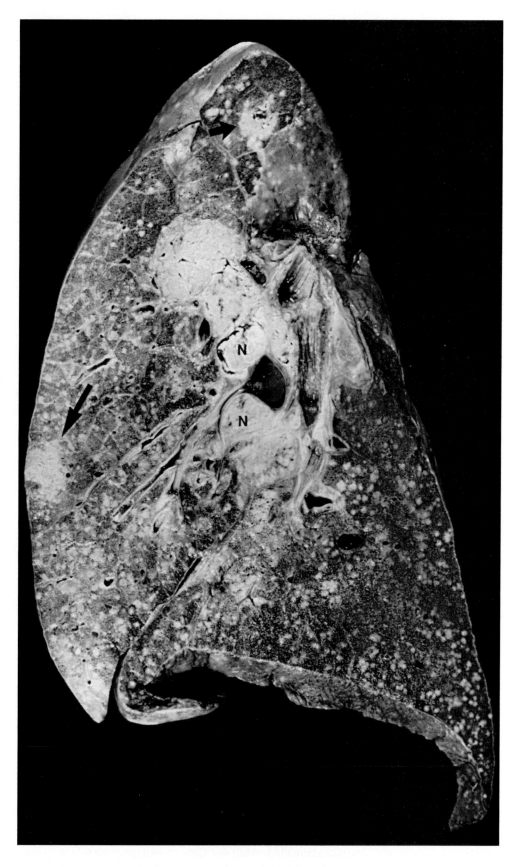

Figure 27–4. Progressive Primary Tuberculosis. A sagittal slice of the right lung near the hilum shows a 2-cm focus of consolidation in the subpleural region of the upper lobe *(long arrow)* (Ghon focus). Peribronchial lymph nodes (N) are enlarged and replaced by necrotic (caseous) tissue. The remaining lung parenchyma shows numerous randomly distributed nodules, 0.5 to 2 mm in diameter, representing miliary dissemination. A single ill-defined nodular focus of consolidation approximately 1.5 cm in diameter, possibly with early cavitation, is also evident in the apical portion of the upper lobe *(short arrow)*.

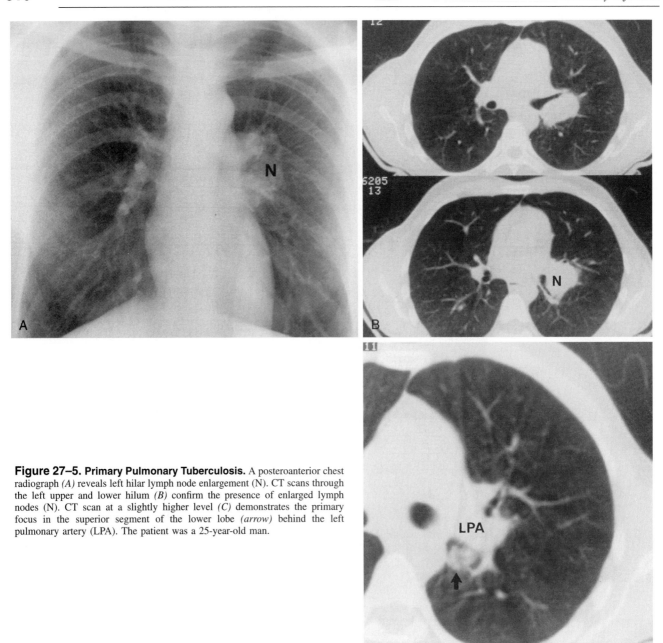

Figure 27–5. Primary Pulmonary Tuberculosis. A posteroanterior chest radiograph *(A)* reveals left hilar lymph node enlargement (N). CT scans through the left upper and lower hilum *(B)* confirm the presence of enlarged lymph nodes (N). CT scan at a slightly higher level *(C)* demonstrates the primary focus in the superior segment of the lower lobe *(arrow)* behind the left pulmonary artery (LPA). The patient was a 25-year-old man.

study, the attenuation values of enlarged lymph nodes before and after intravenous administration of contrast material were assessed in 38 patients.[237a] Approximately 50% of nodes had low attenuation (< 30 HU), and 50% had soft tissue attenuation (> 35 HU). Four patterns of contrast enhancement were identified: peripheral rim enhancement (57%), inhomogeneous enhancement (21%), homogeneous enhancement (16%), and homogeneous nonenhancing nodes (5%). The authors concluded that although neither the nodal attenuation values nor the patterns of enhancement were diagnostic of tuberculosis, the presence of peripheral rim enhancement with relative low attenuation centers should suggest the diagnosis in the appropriate clinical setting. Low attenuation nodes with peripheral enhancement, however, have also been described in infections caused by organisms

such as *M. avium* complex and *Histoplasma capsulatum* and, less commonly, in patients with lymph node enlargement secondary to pulmonary carcinoma or lymphoma.[238–240]

Airway Involvement

Atelectasis, usually lobar and right-sided, has been reported in 10% to 30% of children with primary tuberculosis.[225, 230, 241] It is usually the result of compression by enlarged lymph nodes; less commonly, endobronchial disease is responsible.[225, 242] Occasionally, enlarged lymph nodes result in obstructive overinflation of a lobe or lobes.[225, 230] Atelectasis is even more uncommon in adults than in children; when it occurs, it tends to involve the anterior segment

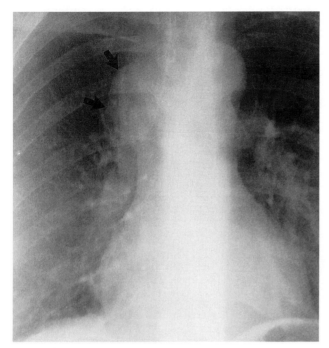

Figure 27–6. Primary Tuberculosis. A view of the mediastinum from a posteroanterior chest radiograph in a 46-year-old woman demonstrates right paratracheal lymphadenopathy *(arrows)*. Cultures from a lymph node biopsy specimen grew *Mycobacterium tuberculosis.*

of the upper lobes and may simulate pulmonary carcinoma.[243]

Pleural Involvement

Pleural effusions have been reported in 5% to 10% of children[225, 230] and 30% to 40% of adults[229, 233] with primary tuberculosis. Radiologic and other features are discussed in Chapter 69 (*see* page 2743).

Calcification

Follow-up chest radiographs in children with primary tuberculosis have demonstrated evidence of calcification in the pulmonary lesion in about 10% to 15% of cases and in the lymph nodes in about 5% to 35%.[225, 230] In one investigation, no calcification was identified before 6 months of follow-up.[230] Although a calcified Ranke complex constitutes reasonable evidence of primary tuberculosis (Fig. 27–8), the same radiographic finding may occur as a sequela to histoplasmosis or other fungal infection. The character of splenic calcifications can be useful in differentiating the cause: they tend to be multiple, small, punctate shadows in histoplasmosis and relatively few and larger in tuberculosis.[244]

Resolution of radiographic abnormalities in primary tuberculosis is a slow process. In one study, 33% of 125 children in whom follow-up radiographs were available demonstrated progression of disease with an increase in the extent of consolidation and enlargement or development of lymphadenopathy despite prompt and appropriate therapy.[230] Complete clearing within 6 months or less was seen in only two cases. Improvement of the air-space consolidation

preceded regression of enlarged lymph nodes, and complete resolution of consolidation was present in all cases within 2 years. In 14 cases (7%), residual lymphadenopathy was identified after 3 years; in 1 case, it persisted up to 9 years.

Clinical Manifestations

The decision to categorize a case of tuberculosis as primary has usually been based on young age, recent tuberculin conversion,[163, 245] radiographic evidence of bronchopulmonary or mediastinal lymph node enlargement,[163, 246] or pleural effusion.[245, 247] As discussed previously, however, the clinical and radiologic distinction between primary and postprimary disease is not always clear-cut.[207]

Few patients with primary infection are symptomatic. This fact was well illustrated in a study of 715 children whose tuberculin reaction became positive between birth and 5 years of age;[248] only 136 of the 611 children with adequate follow-up studies showed radiographic changes in the chest. Only 55 (9%) developed tuberculosis; the remaining patients were clinically well.

As many as 40% of children with primary tuberculosis in some series have symptoms, the most frequent being cough and fever.[249] By comparison, a review of the findings in 103 adults with primary disease demonstrated that 82% of patients were symptomatic.[233] The symptoms in adults consisted of fever in 40% of patients, cough in 37%, weight loss in 24%, and hemoptysis in 8%.[233] Other manifestations include sweating, chest pain, and lethargy.[225]

Additional manifestations may develop as a result of spread of disease to extrathoracic locations, such as the meninges. Involvement of extrathoracic structures by tuberculosis is not necessarily accompanied by radiographic abnormalities in the chest; for example, in two studies of 180 and 25 children with tuberculous meningitis,[250, 251] the chest radiograph was normal in 43% and 28%. Erythema nodosum is an occasional feature; in one investigation of 305 children, it was the initial manifestation of disease in 37 (12%).[235]

Postprimary Tuberculosis

As discussed previously, the term *postprimary (secondary, reactivation) tuberculosis* is used to describe a clinical, morphologic, and radiologic form of disease that is correlated pathogenetically with the presence of acquired hypersensitivity and immunity. Many cases occur in adults as a result of reactivation of a focus of infection acquired in earlier life. Although it used to be believed that this mechanism was responsible for the vast majority of cases of pulmonary tuberculosis, epidemiologic evidence based on DNA fingerprinting has shown that as many as 30% to 40% of cases of tuberculosis in selected populations are recently acquired.[252, 253] In addition, as discussed previously, the certainty of a distinction between the radiologic findings in patients who have primary and postprimary disease has been questioned.[207]

Pathogenesis and Pathologic Characteristics

Postprimary tuberculosis tends to be localized initially to the apical and posterior segments of the upper lobes

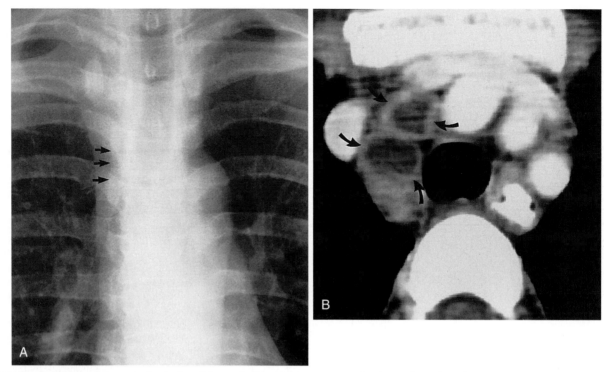

Figure 27–7. Primary Tuberculosis. A view of the mediastinum from a posteroanterior chest radiograph *(A)* in a 29-year-old woman shows widening of the right paratracheal stripe *(straight arrows)*. Contrast-enhanced CT scan 2 cm above the level of the aortic arch *(B)* demonstrates enlarged right paratracheal lymph nodes *(curved arrows)* with a low attenuation center and rim enhancement. Cultures from a lymph node biopsy specimen grew *Mycobacterium tuberculosis.*

and, to a lesser extent, the superior segment of the lower lobe.[254, 255] It has been postulated that this localization is related to the relatively high Po_2 in these zones as a result of a high ventilation-perfusion ratio[256, 257] or to impaired lymphatic drainage resulting from decreased pulmonary arterial blood flow.[1] Whatever the mechanism, it is believed that the vast majority of disease that arises in apical locations is

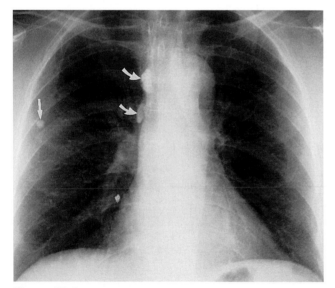

Figure 27–8. Calcified Ghon Focus and Lymph Nodes (Ranke Complex). A posteroanterior chest radiograph in a 35-year-old woman demonstrates a calcified right upper lobe nodule *(straight arrow)* and right paratracheal lymph nodes *(curved arrows).*

caused by organisms transmitted hematogenously to these sites during the primary infection. In most cases, the previously inactive site of reactivation is destroyed by the ensuing inflammatory reaction and cannot be definitely identified; occasionally, however, there is conclusive evidence of prior disease (Fig. 27–9). Although the apex of the lung is by far the most frequent location for postprimary tuberculosis, any focus of prior infection within the lung or lymph nodes can serve as a site of recrudescence, and an atypical anatomic distribution in no way excludes the diagnosis.

Histologically, the sequence of events in postprimary tuberculosis is similar to the primary infection except that necrosis probably occurs more rapidly as a result of the presence of hypersensitivity. The initial reaction consists of an exudate of edema fluid, fibrin, and polymorphonuclear leukocytes within alveolar air spaces. Shortly thereafter, the cellular infiltrate becomes largely mononuclear and is formed predominantly by necrotizing and non-necrotizing granulomas; as in primary disease, these frequently become confluent, resulting in the formation of a continuous layer of epithelioid and giant cells around one or more necrotic areas (*see* Fig. 27–1, page 807). Rarely, the macrophages assume a spindle shape without the formation of granulomas (*spindle cell pseudotumor*)[258] or contain numerous needle-like structures (*pseudo-Gaucher cells*).[259] Organisms can usually be identified within the necrotic tissue, but are often patchy in distribution so that examination of several sections may be required for their demonstration; they are usually scarce in well-formed granulomas.

The subsequent pathologic manifestations depend on a number of factors, including the degree of immunity and delayed hypersensitivity of the host, the presence or absence

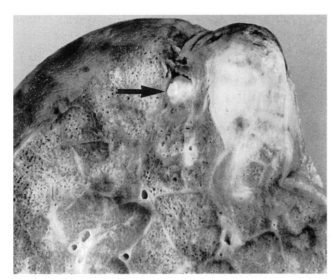

Figure 27–9. Early Postprimary Tuberculosis. A magnified view of the apex of the right upper lobe shows a 3-mm calcified nodule *(arrow)* associated with fibrosis and pleural retraction. This represents a focus of remote tuberculous disease acquired via hematogenous dissemination of organisms during the primary infection. The secondary lobule to the right shows uniform parenchymal consolidation related to the presence of necrotizing granulomatous inflammation and resulting from reactivation of disease in the adjacent calcified nodule. The abnormality was radiographically inapparent. This was an incidental finding in a 63-year-old man who died of metastatic colonic adenocarcinoma.

of therapy, and whether the disease remains localized to the initial site of reactivation or spreads to other parts of the lung or elsewhere in the body.

Local Parenchymal Disease

In contrast to primary tuberculosis, in which fibrosis and healing are the rule, the postprimary form of disease tends to progress, foci of inflammation and necrosis enlarging to occupy ever greater portions of lung parenchyma. During this process, communication with airways is frequent (Fig. 27–10), resulting in expulsion of necrotic material and cavity formation. Additional foci of necrotic lung are usually clearly evident grossly in such cases; occasionally, however, they are absent (Fig. 27–11), in which situation the cavity may be easily overlooked. In addition to erosion into an airway, the expanding infection may extend toward the periphery of the lung and rupture into the pleural space causing tuberculous empyema.

The formation of cavities depends on liquefaction of caseous material, a process that has been shown experimentally to occur only in the presence of hypersensitivity.[260] Hypersensitivity-related liquefaction may be mediated by enzymes derived from inflammatory cells in the vicinity of the necrotic tissue.[261, 262] In fact, there is evidence that *M. tuberculosis* itself may participate directly in the process of cavitation by stimulating the release of macrophage enzymes.[263]

The importance of cavity formation in tuberculosis lies in the communication it provides the organisms with the outside environment. This has two effects, neither of which is beneficial to the host: first, it leads to a continuous supply of well-oxygenated air to the interior of the cavity, theoreti-

cally resulting in increased extracellular bacterial multiplication; and second, it provides a means for spread of disease to other parts of the lung as well as to other individuals.

As in primary tuberculosis, the course of the disease from this point on depends largely on the interplay between host response and the virulence of the organism. When host factors prevail, there is gradual healing with the formation of parenchymal scars, often accompanied by adjacent irregular emphysema and bronchiectasis (Fig. 27–12). Although these abnormalities can occur alone, they are seen most frequently in association with foci of necrotic parenchyma (an appearance sometimes known as *chronic fibrocaseous tuberculosis*). The necrotic foci vary from less than 1 mm to several centimeters in diameter and may or may not communicate with the tracheobronchial tree (in the former situation forming a chronic cavity, and in the latter, a *tuberculoma*[264]) (Fig. 27–13). Depending on the stage of healing at which a tuberculoma is examined, it may have a wall lined by granulomatous inflammatory tissue or composed simply of fibrous tissue; the necrotic contents may be relatively uniform or may show prominent lamination similar to that of a histoplasmoma.[265] As in primary disease, even remote, apparently inactive tuberculomas can contain viable organisms within their necrotic contents.[266] The wall of a chronic cavity varies from 1 cm to less than 1 mm in thickness

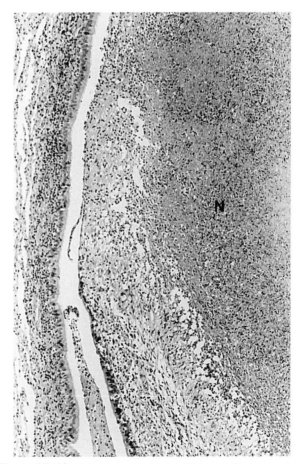

Figure 27–10. Tuberculosis—Airway Erosion. The section shows a small airway whose wall has been focally destroyed by an expanding focus of necrotizing granulomatous inflammation. Drainage of the necrotic material (N) via the airway leads to cavity formation and spread of organisms to other parts of the lung.

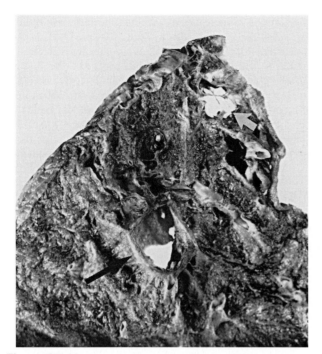

Figure 27–11. Early Tuberculosis with Cavitation. A magnified view of the apical portion of the right upper lobe shows emphysema and a well-circumscribed cavity approximately 1 cm in diameter *(long arrow)*. The cavity wall is only 0.5 to 1 mm in thickness, and there is no evidence of parenchymal consolidation elsewhere. On cursory examination, such an abnormality might be considered to represent no more than a bulla (an example of which is indicated by the *short arrow*). Histologic examination showed the cavity wall to be composed of granulomatous inflammatory tissue containing scattered acid-fast bacilli. (The white areas in the lung tissue represent a light artefact.)

and may be surprisingly smooth, sometimes simulating an emphysematous bulla (Fig. 27–14).[267]

Theoretically, cavities can heal in two ways:[268] (1) by apposition of granulation tissue at the opening of the draining bronchus and within the cavity itself, resulting in complete collapse of the cavity and its conversion to a scar (artificial pneumothorax and thoracoplasty were procedures formerly employed to collapse the draining airways and cavities to accelerate this apposition); and (2) by complete shedding of the lining of necrotic tissue and transformation of tuberculous granulation tissue into fibrous tissue. The development of saprophytic fungus balls (usually caused by *Aspergillus* species) within chronic cavities is relatively common. Sometimes, chronic cavities are incompletely healed and are lined, at least focally, by active granulomatous inflammatory tissue; such cavities may continue to disseminate organisms to other parts of the tracheobronchial tree and lung parenchyma (*see* farther on), to the gastrointestinal tract by expectoration and swallowing, and to other individuals by coughing and droplet nuclei dispersal.

When the organism overpowers host defenses, disease progresses, either locally by gradual expansion of the region of necrosis and inflammation or in other parts of the lung or body after spread of bacteria via the airways, lymphatics, or bloodstream. Local extension occurs when epithelioid histiocytes at the periphery of the necrotic material are unable to contain and kill the tubercle bacilli and are themselves destroyed. This process may continue until a consider-

able portion of a lobe or entire lung is involved;[269] in the latter situation, the left lung has been reported to be more frequently affected than the right.[270] Pathologically, the affected parenchyma shows irregularly sized foci of consolidation, fibrosis, and caseous necrosis interspersed by cavities of variable size and shape (Fig. 27–15).

Tuberculous Bronchopneumonia

Endobronchial spread of liquefied necrotic material from a cavity can result in tuberculous infection in the same lobe or in other lobes of either lung. Such infection occurs initially in the region of the transitional airways, giving the appearance of multiple, ill-defined parenchymal nodules (Figs. 27–16 and 27–17). Histologically, this usually takes the form of typical necrotizing granulomatous inflammation. In some individuals, however, the large amount of tuberculoprotein that suddenly fills the air spaces causes a prominent exudative reaction without a significant granulomatous component (Fig. 27–18); this can be associated with widespread necrosis, numerous organisms, and rapid destruction of whole lobules (*galloping consumption*). As in primary tuberculosis, endobronchial spread of disease in postprimary disease occasionally occurs by rupture of an affected lymph node into the adjacent airway lumen.[271, 272]

Miliary Tuberculosis

Dissemination of organisms by way of the lymphatics or pulmonary vasculature can result in innumerable small foci of infection (miliary tuberculosis). Although these are most commonly seen in the lungs, liver, spleen, and bone marrow, virtually any organ or tissue in the body may be affected; for example, cases have been reported of miliary disease involving a cardiac pacemaker pocket,[273] the placenta,[274] and tendon and fascia.[275]

In the lungs, the appearance is that of a multitude of spherical, gray-white nodules measuring from 1 mm to several millimeters and scattered more or less randomly throughout the parenchyma and on the pleura (Fig. 27–19). The appearance is characteristic, but can also be seen with miliary infection caused by other organisms (particularly fungi and occasionally bacteria[276]) and by malignancy. Histologically, the earliest finding is interstitial pneumonitis with or without an exudative inflammatory reaction in the adjacent air spaces.[277] With time, the appearance of the nodules can vary from well-formed necrotizing or non-necrotizing granulomas to poorly formed epithelioid cell aggregates with a prominent polymorphonuclear component (Fig. 27–19). Organisms may be difficult to identify, especially in the well-formed granulomas. Usually, the nodules are roughly the same size and have the same histologic appearance, implying a single episode of dissemination;[278] sometimes, however, both active and partly or completely healed foci can be observed at the same time, suggesting repeated episodes of hematogenous spread.[278] Occasionally, nodules become confluent, forming larger foci of inflammation.

The lungs can be the site of miliary tuberculosis without evidence of a pulmonary source of the infection, dissemination having occurred from an extrapulmonary location; according to some investigators, the frequency of such an

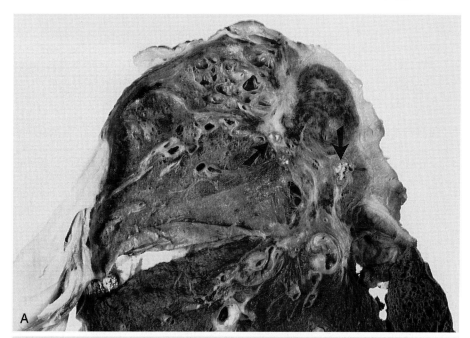

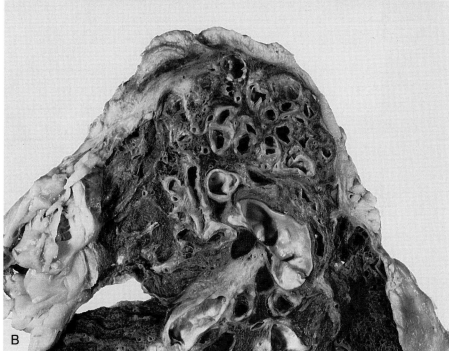

Figure 27–12. Healed Postprimary Tuberculosis. Two sides of a slice of the right upper lobe are shown. In *A*, there is patchy parenchymal fibrosis associated with a small focus of bronchiectasis in the most apical portion; several foci of calcified necrotic material are evident *(arrows)*. The bronchiectasis is more evident in *B*, where it is confined to the apical posterior region. Both slices show a moderate degree of pleural fibrosis.

occurrence has increased since the advent of antituberculous chemotherapy.[278] One remarkable case derived from the kidney was associated with shock wave lithotripsy.[279]

Rarely, miliary tuberculosis occurs in the virtual absence of cellular response *(nonreactive tuberculosis)*, often in association with underlying hematopoietic disease, HIV infection, or steroid therapy.[280, 281] Histologically, the abnormality consists of foci of necrotic parenchyma containing numerous bacteria; an acute inflammatory or granulomatous reaction in the surrounding lung parenchyma is minimal or absent. Miliary disease is also associated sometimes with histiocytosis in bone marrow, lymph nodes, liver, and spleen,

similar to that seen in virus-associated hemophagocytic syndrome.[282]

Tracheobronchial Tuberculosis

As in primary tuberculosis, involvement of the tracheobronchial tree in the postprimary form is frequent and may be seen either in chronic disease (with the development of bronchiectasis) or during the acute infection. The latter occurs especially when the disease is rapidly progressive or extensive; in autopsy series from the preantibiotic era in which the airways have been specifically examined, such

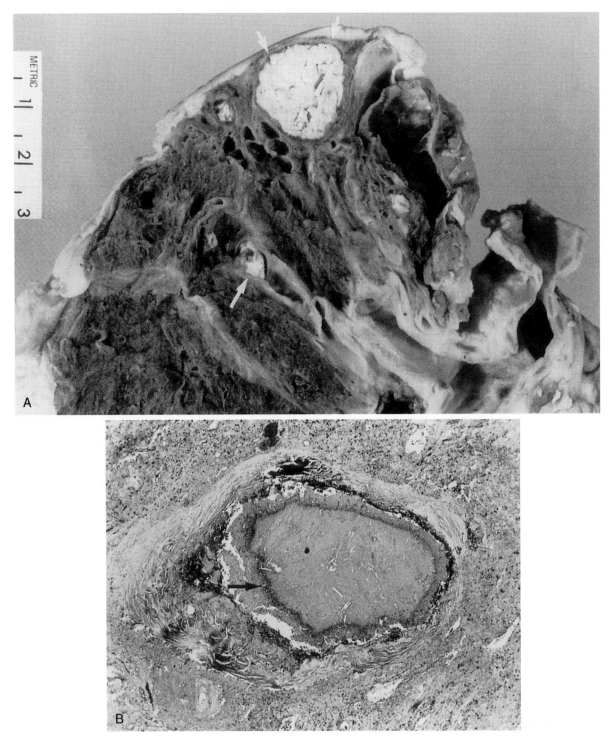

Figure 27–13. Healed Postprimary Tuberculosis. The apical portion of the left upper lobe *(A)* shows extensive parenchymal fibrosis and focal bronchiectasis. A 2-cm, well-circumscribed nodule of caseous necrotic material *(tuberculoma)* is present in the apex. Its inactive nature is indicated by the well-defined fibrous capsule *(short arrows)* completely surrounding the periphery. Smaller foci of necrosis representing remote granulomatous inflammation are also present, and a 5-mm broncholith is seen in a subsegmental airway *(long arrow)*. A section *(B)* from the area contiguous with the tuberculoma shows parenchymal fibrosis and a small focus of remote, inactive granulomatous inflammation. The dark rim adjacent to the fibrous capsule *(arrow)* represents dystrophic calcification. *(B, ×25.)*

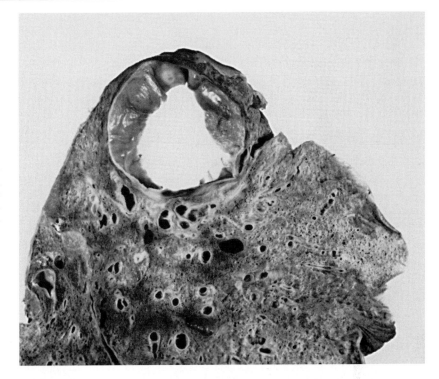

Figure 27–14. Tuberculosis—Residual Thin-Walled Cavity. A slice of left lung removed at autopsy shows a cavity with a smooth inner surface and a fibrous wall about 0.5 mm in thickness. Histologic sections showed no evidence of active granulomatous inflammation. Prior radiographs and smears had shown tuberculosis (*see* Fig. 27–31, page 829).

involvement has been identified in as many as 40% to 50% of cases.[283, 284] As might be expected, the abnormality is seen less commonly during life; in one study of 65 patients who had smear-negative disease, only 12 (8%) had bronchial disease demonstrated by fiberoptic bronchoscopy.[285]

In most cases, bronchial infection occurs by spread of organisms within the airway lumen or along peribronchial lymphatic channels from an area of cavitation or localized pneumonia. Occasionally, it is caused by direct extension of infection from a contiguous lymph node or from the parenchyma itself. Rarely, the airways are involved as part of hematogenous miliary tuberculosis (by way of the bronchial arteries).[283] Although airway involvement is usually associated with obvious parenchymal disease, active bronchial infection sometimes persists as peripheral disease heals, thus providing a potential source of bacteria-laden sputum in the absence of significant radiographic abnormality.[283] Occasionally, airway epithelium is destroyed, and the wall is replaced by granulomatous inflammatory tissue in the absence of significant parenchymal disease (bronchocentric granulomatosis) (Fig. 27–20).

Grossly, tracheobronchitis in active tuberculosis is variable in appearance and depends largely on the duration of the infection; there may be swelling or irregularity of the mucosa; ulceration; or, in the healed stage, fibrotic stenosis. The most common histologic changes occur in airways that drain an active cavity and consist of a mucosal lymphocytic infiltrate associated with variably severe edema and congestion; the epithelium may show squamous metaplasia in proximity to the cavity, but is usually unremarkable in more proximal regions.[226] Such histologic abnormalities most likely represent simply a reaction to intraluminal necrotic material rather than infection. Airways that are truly infected reveal typical necrotizing or non-necrotizing granulomatous inflammation. Healed lesions may show only fibrosis without histologic evidence of a tuberculous cause.

Although bronchiectasis in postprimary tuberculosis can be the result of cicatricial bronchostenosis after local infection, more commonly it occurs by destruction and fibrosis of lung parenchyma with secondary bronchial dilation (traction bronchiectasis) (Fig. 27–21). Because the majority of cases of postprimary tuberculosis affect the apical and posterior segments of an upper lobe, bronchiectasis is usually found in these sites; because of adequate bronchial drainage, symptoms are usually minimal (*bronchiectasis sicca*). As with residual tuberculous cavities, ectatic bronchi may become sites for the development of saprophytic fungus balls (Fig. 27–22).

Vascular Complications

Vascular abnormalities are also common in postprimary tuberculosis. Pulmonary arteries and veins in an area of active tuberculous infection may show vasculitis and thrombosis (Fig. 27–23); thus, an acid-fast stain should be performed in any case of necrotizing granulomatous pulmonary vasculitis to exclude a tuberculous cause. More frequently, pulmonary arteries in the vicinity of chronic tuberculous cavities or tuberculomas show endarteritis obliterans; a concomitant local increase in the number and size of bronchial artery branches is common.[286] Sometimes, occlusion of a pulmonary artery by thrombus results in the formation of an intracavitary mass of necrotic lung (*pulmonary gangrene*).[287, 288]

Occasionally, a small-to-medium-sized artery that is contiguous with a cavity wall undergoes localized dilation (Rasmussen's aneurysm).[289, 290] In one series of 1,114 autopsies of patients with chronic cavitary tuberculosis, this complication was identified in 45 (4%);[289] 38 of the 45 had died from rupture of the affected artery. Such patients may or may not have a history of prior hemoptysis; in fact, the hemorrhage is occasionally clinically occult, the patient un-

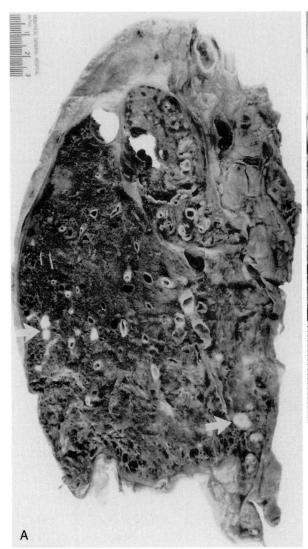

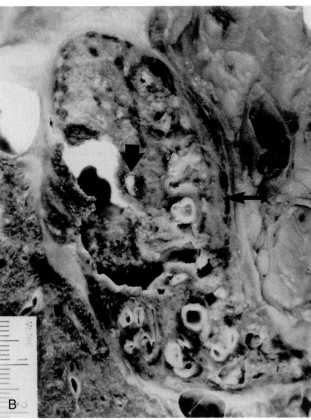

Figure 27–15. Chronic Fibrocaseous Tuberculosis. A sagittal section of the right lung *(A)* shows severe atelectasis and destruction of the upper lobe associated with a large cavity. The well-circumscribed foci of necrotic tissue in the lower and middle lobes *(arrows)* represent endobronchial spread. An enlarged view of upper lobe *(B)* shows an irregular shaggy-walled cavity, fibrosis *(long arrow)*, and foci of caseous necrosis *(short arrow)*.

expectedly being found dead as a result of massive pulmonary hemorrhage.[289] Chronic pulmonary artery stenosis is a rare complication that occurs as a result of vascular compression, thrombosis, or both.[291]

Treatment-Related Effects

Treatment can modify somewhat the typical pathologic features of postprimary pulmonary tuberculosis and occasionally results in additional complications many years later. Although rarely used nowadays, collapse therapy (by means of techniques such as thoracoplasty, induced pneumothorax, or extrapleural plombage) was extensively used in the first half of the twentieth century. Marked pleural fibrosis frequently accompanied these interventions *(see* Fig. 27–22) and should not necessarily be considered an indication of prior tuberculous empyema. Fluid can collect between the collapsed lung and the fibrotic pleura; although these effusions have sometimes been associated with bronchial fistula and superimposed infection, they are often sterile.[292] Lipid pneumonia secondary to seepage of lipid from the extrapleural tissue to the lung after oleothorax induction has also been reported.[293] Other complications of collapse therapy include

invasive aspergillus pleuritis,[294] primary pleural lymphoma (particularly in Japanese patients),[295–297] and (in one patient) squamous cell carcinoma.[298]

Chemotherapy tends to accelerate healing of pulmonary lesions; in fact, the radiographic clearing of acute exudative disease may be so rapid as to simulate resolution of nontuberculous pneumonia.[299, 300] Such therapy also alters the appearance and natural histopathologic progression of many of the lesions described previously.[268, 301] For example, in treated cavitary lesions, there tends to be a relative thinning of the capsular wall, decreased intensity of pericavitary disease, a decrease in inflammation of draining bronchi, and evidence of re-epithelialization; an appreciable increase in the incidence of open healed cavities also occurs. Although some investigators have found healing of encapsulated, partially necrotic nodules to be similar in both treated and untreated individuals,[301] others have noted a thinner capsule in treated cases.[268]

Radiologic Manifestations

Radiologists sometimes use the terms *active*, *inactive*, *quiescent*, and *healed* to describe pulmonary lesions in pa-

Figure 27–16. Postprimary Tuberculosis with Early Endobronchial Spread. A slice of the right upper lobe *(A)* shows an irregular focus of consolidation with small areas of cavitation. A focus of bronchopneumonia confined predominantly to a single lobule in the inferior aspect *(arrow)* is also evident. A section through the area of bronchopneumonia *(B)* shows a terminal bronchiole *(arrow)* largely destroyed and replaced by necrotizing granulomatous inflammation. (×40.)

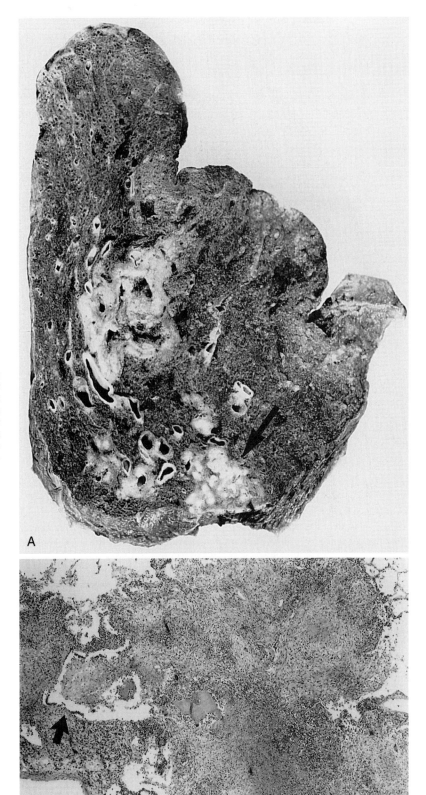

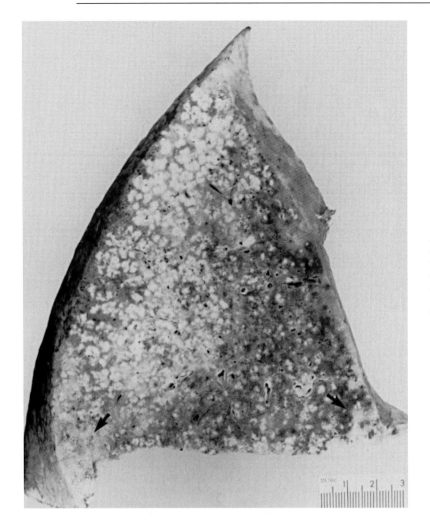

Figure 27–17. Tuberculous Bronchopneumonia.
A slice of lower lobe shows extensive, patchy consolidation centered about terminal airways. This differs from miliary tuberculosis by the irregular size and shape of the inflammatory foci (some of which resemble branching airways) and by the regions of confluence, seen best in the inferior aspect *(arrows)*. The patient was a 36-year-old woman with rapidly progressive pneumonia.

tients in whom the diagnosis of tuberculosis has been established or is strongly suspected. Although there is no question that the presence of consolidation can often be equated with activity and calcified nodules with inactivity, the radiologist must never be dogmatic about the activity of an assumed tuberculous lesion on the basis of a single radiograph. We have seen patients with focal consolidation in the apical and posterior segments of the upper lobes who have had repeated negative sputum cultures and whose lesions have remained unchanged, even with adequate chemotherapy. At the other end of the spectrum are calcified nodules that pathologically show active granulomatous inflammation and contain viable tubercle bacilli. Occasionally, even in cases of lesions showing little or no change for months or years, sputum culture is repeatedly positive. Therefore, we prefer to use qualifying phrases such as *having the appearance of* or *compatible with*, which connote the element of fallibility so often inherent in radiologic interpretation; in the final analysis, the demonstration of organisms by microbiologic or other means is the definitive indicator of activity in the majority of cases.

Several radiologic patterns can be identified in postprimary tuberculosis corresponding to the description of pathogenesis given earlier. In the past, we and others have used terms such as *exudative*, *fibroproductive*, *fibronodular*, and *fibrocalcific* to describe the radiologic patterns of the disease.[236, 255] These terms, however, make inferences about

activity and lack of activity of tuberculous lesions that are unwarranted and often misleading. Therefore, we now prefer to describe the radiologic findings simply in terms of the actual patterns of abnormality seen on radiography and CT, including air-space consolidation, nodular opacities, linear opacities, cavitation, lymphadenopathy, and airway abnormalities such as bronchiectasis and bronchostenosis. Any particular case may show one or more of these abnormalities. The pleural manifestations of tuberculosis are discussed in Chapter 69 *(see page 2743)*.

Anatomic Distribution

As indicated previously, a characteristic manifestation of postprimary tuberculosis is a tendency to localize in the apical and posterior segments of the upper lobes.[236, 254, 255, 302] For example, in one study of 423 adults with local pulmonary tuberculosis, the lesions were predominantly in the apical and posterior segments of an upper lobe in 85% and in the superior segment of one or the other lower lobe in 9.5%.[303] In about 70% to 90% of cases, the abnormalities involve more than one segment.[236, 255, 302] Although the anterior segment of the upper lobe is involved in 30% to 40% of cases,[236, 302] the findings are limited to this segment in a minority (about 2% to 7%).[236, 304, 305] Disease affects the lower lobes in 30% to 50% of patients;[236, 302] in approxi-

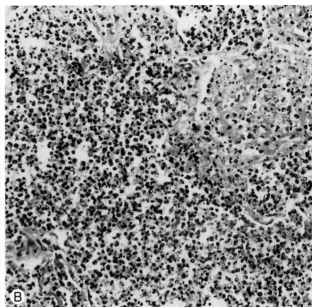

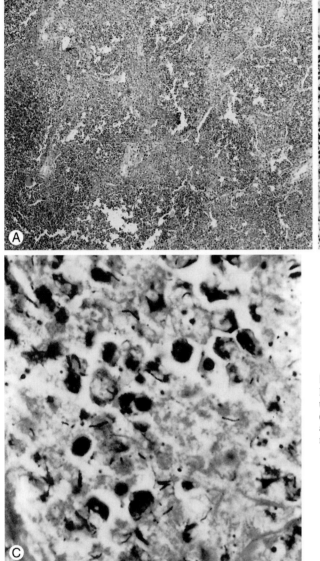

Figure 27–18. Tuberculous Pneumonia. Extensive destruction of lung parenchyma *(A)* is associated with a neutrophilic inflammatory reaction, resembling nontuberculous bacterial pneumonia. A magnified view *(B)* shows necrotic and viable polymorphonuclear leukocytes and the absence of granulomatous inflammation. Ziehl-Neelsen stain *(C)* reveals numerous acid-fast bacilli. *(A,* ×40; *B,* ×200; *C,* ×1000.)

mately 10% of cases, the abnormalities involve predominantly the superior segment of the lower lobe, and in about 2% to 7% they are limited to the basal segments.[236, 305] Although some investigators have found evidence that an atypical distribution of disease is seen more commonly in the elderly and in patients with diabetes,[272, 304, 306] others have failed to confirm this association.[111, 305]

Although the identification of parenchymal disease in apical and subapical areas of an upper lobe or the superior segment of a lower lobe supports a radiologic diagnosis of tuberculosis, definitive diagnosis requires culture of the organism. The radiologic pattern of postprimary tuberculosis may be highly suggestive, but is not diagnostic and is simulated by several mycotic infections (particularly histoplasmosis) and by infections of bacterial, viral, and parasitic origin.

Air-Space Consolidation

Focal areas of consolidation are seen on chest radiography and HRCT in approximately 50% to 70% of patients with active postprimary tuberculosis.[236, 255, 302] On the radiograph, the areas of consolidation have ill-defined margins (Fig. 27–24) and show a tendency to coalesce, often with small satellite foci being seen in the adjacent lung (Fig. 27–25). HRCT-pathologic correlations have shown that these areas of consolidation tend to be lobular in distribution; that is, they involve entire secondary lobules while sparing adjacent lobules (Fig. 27–26).[307, 308] There is also frequently an accentuation of the bronchovascular markings leading to the ipsilateral hilum. Associated hilar or mediastinal lymph node enlargement is relatively uncommon, being identified on chest radiographs in only 5% of 56 patients in one

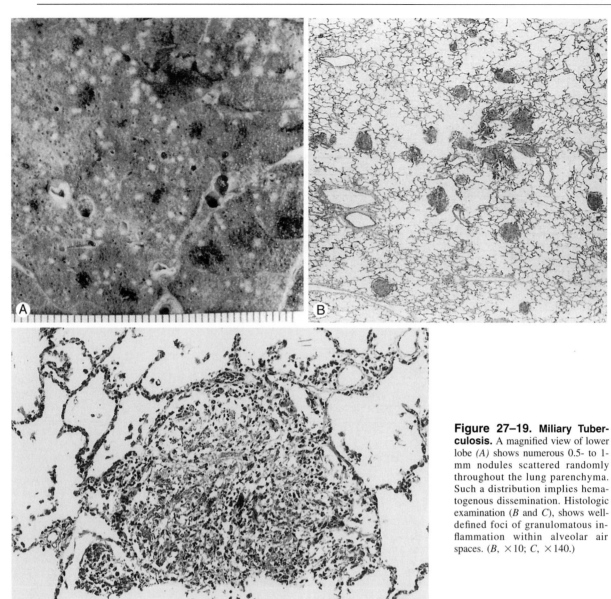

Figure 27–19. Miliary Tuberculosis. A magnified view of lower lobe *(A)* shows numerous 0.5- to 1-mm nodules scattered randomly throughout the lung parenchyma. Such a distribution implies hematogenous dissemination. Histologic examination *(B and C)*, shows well-defined foci of granulomatous inflammation within alveolar air spaces. *(B, ×10; C, ×140.)*

series[236] and in 9% of 158 in another.[255] On HRCT, mediastinal lymph node enlargement (defined as a lymph node > 10 mm in short-axis diameter) was identified in 7 (8%) of 89 patients in one series[302] and in 9 (31%) of 29 in a second.[307] As in primary disease, enlarged lymph nodes usually show inhomogeneous enhancement or low attenuation centers with rim enhancement after intravenous administration of contrast material.[237, 238]

In the majority of cases, the consolidation is limited to one segment or portions of several segments of a lobe.[310] Occasionally, disease evolves to affect an entire lobe (tuberculous lobar pneumonia) (Fig. 27–27) or, following endobronchial spread of disease, several lobes (tuberculous bronchopneumonia) (Fig. 27–28).[236, 310] Rarely, disease affects all lobes and leads to respiratory failure.[311]

Although not conclusive, the presence of consolidation is suggestive of active disease. In one study, the authors compared the HRCT findings in 32 patients with newly diagnosed active pulmonary tuberculosis and 34 patients with inactive disease.[312] (The diagnosis of active disease was based on positive cultures of sputum [$n = 21$] or bronchial washings [$n = 3$] or radiographic and clinical improvement after treatment with antituberculous drugs [$n = 8$]; the diagnosis of inactive disease was based on negative cultures and lack of progression on comparison of chest radiographs at recruitment with radiographs obtained 6 months previously or at follow-up.) Consolidation was seen on HRCT in 14 (44%) of 32 patients with active tuberculosis and in none of those with inactive disease. Another group of investigators reported seeing consolidation in 55 (62%) of 89 patients with active tuberculosis and in 20 (35%) of 57 patients with inactive disease.[302] In a third investigation of 27 patients who had active tuberculosis (confirmed by positive sputum culture), 17 (65%) had air-space consolidation and

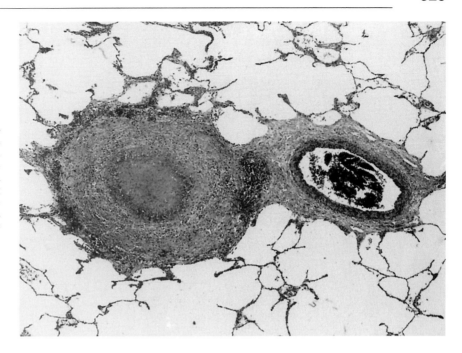

Figure 27–20. Tuberculous Bronchocentric Granulomatosis. The wall of a bronchiole adjacent to a medium-sized pulmonary artery is thickened by fibrous tissue and mononuclear inflammatory cells. The epithelium is destroyed and replaced by epithelioid histiocytes surrounding necrotic material. The adjacent parenchyma is entirely normal. This was an incidental finding in the left lower lobe of a patient who had chronic progressive tuberculosis in the right upper lobe.

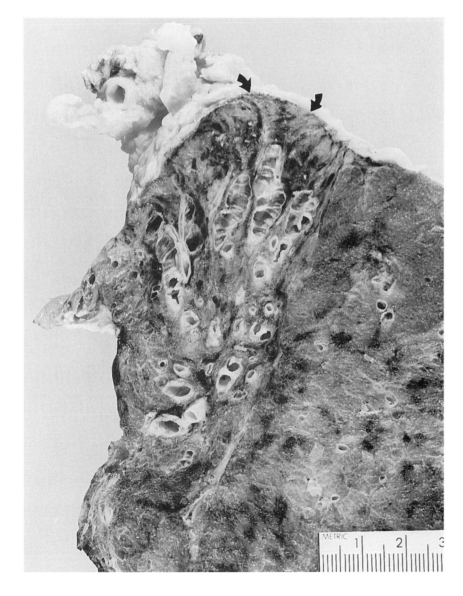

Figure 27–21. Tuberculous Bronchiectasis. Moderately severe cylindrical bronchiectasis is limited predominantly to the posterior segment of the right upper lobe. The apical parenchyma (arrows) is fibrotic and contains multiple minute white flecks, representing foci of calcified necrotic material. Thickened pleura and mediastinal adipose tissue are attached superiorly.

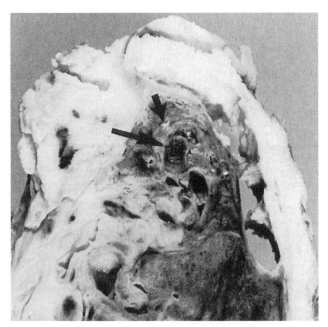

Figure 27–22. Remote Fibrocaseous Tuberculosis with Fungus Ball. A magnified view of the apex of the right lung shows pleural fibrosis, marked atelectasis and fibrosis of the upper lobe, and several foci of calcified necrotic material *(small arrow)*. These changes resulted from a remote episode of postprimary tuberculosis, treated by thoracoplasty. A 1-cm, somewhat lobulated fungus ball is also present within a bronchiectatic cavity *(large arrow)*.

26 (95%) had areas of ground-glass attenuation on HRCT;[312a] after 6 months of therapy, residual consolidation or ground-glass attenuation was seen in only 1 and 2 patients, respectively.

In the majority of cases, localized lobular areas of consolidation resolve within 1 month after the institution of chemotherapy,[308] whereas more extensive areas of consolidation usually improve gradually over several months (Fig. 27–29). In some cases, the disease worsens radiographically

after initiation of therapy but then subsequently clears.[312] In one study of 26 patients in whom follow-up HRCT scans were performed during 1 to 20 months of treatment, resolution of lobular consolidation was shown to start at the periphery of the lobule with eventual transformation into a poorly defined nodule, followed by appearance of a centrilobular nodule or branching linear opacities.[308] Even without treatment, localized areas of consolidation may regress and be replaced by small nodules and evidence of scarring with coarse linear opacities and loss of volume. Complete disappearance of tuberculous lesions with or without treatment is rare.[308]

Cavitation

Cavitation is identified on the chest radiograph in 20% to 45% of patients with active postprimary tuberculosis (Fig. 27–30).[236, 255, 308] It is seen more commonly on HRCT;[307–309] for example, in one study of 41 patients with active disease, it was identified in 58% of cases on HRCT scans compared to 22% of cases on chest radiographs.[308] Cavities may be single or multiple and thin or thick walled. Approximately 20% to 25% have an air-fluid level.[236, 255, 312a, 313]

With adequate therapy, a cavity may disappear; sometimes, its wall becomes paper thin, and it appears as an air-filled cystic space (Fig. 27–31). Such persistent cavitation after chemotherapy does not necessarily indicate active disease.[312, 312a] In a small percentage of these cases, the sputum culture becomes positive after chemotherapy is stopped.[314–317] In the study of 66 patients cited previously, cavitation was seen on HRCT in 16 (50%) of 32 patients with active disease and in 4 (12%) of 34 patients with inactive disease.[312] Rarely, a tuberculous cavity resembles a pneumatocele, increasing in size in its early stage and slowly decreasing in size thereafter.[317a]

Nodular Opacities

Nodular opacities can be classified into four types: (1) a single nodule usually greater than 1 cm in diameter

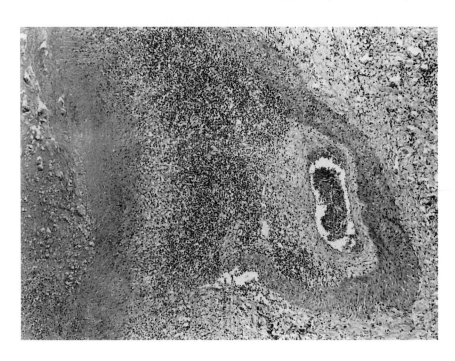

Figure 27–23. Tuberculous Vasculitis. The wall of a medium-sized pulmonary artery is focally disrupted by encroaching tuberculous inflammation. Although thrombosis and endarteritis obliterans result in vascular occlusion in most such instances, in some, aneurysm formation or rupture may occur. (×48.)

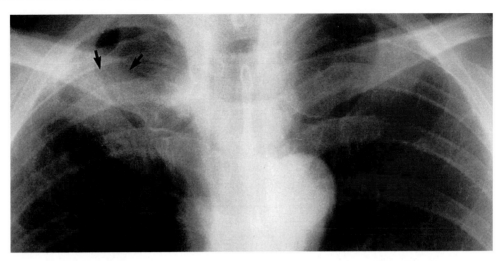

Figure 27–24. Air-Space Consolidation in Postprimary Tuberculosis. A view of the upper chest from a posteroanterior radiograph in a 66-year-old man demonstrates a poorly defined area of consolidation *(arrows)* in the right upper lobe. *Mycobacterium tuberculosis* was recovered from the sputum.

(tuberculoma), with or without adjacent smaller nodules; (2) multiple nodules usually less than 1 cm in diameter limited to one or two regions of the lung (focal nodular opacities), with or without associated branching linear opacities; (3) multiple nodules 2 to 10 mm in diameter involving several lobes usually in an asymmetric or patchy distribution (representing endobronchial spread of tuberculosis); and (4) innumerable nodules 1 to 3 mm in diameter diffusely throughout both lungs (miliary tuberculosis).

Tuberculoma. A tuberculoma may be a manifestation of either primary or postprimary tuberculosis; in the latter form, they have been described as the main or only abnormality seen on chest radiographs in approximately 5% of patients.[236, 255] The lesions are manifested by round or oval opacities situated most commonly in an upper lobe, the right more often than the left.[318] They usually measure between 1 and 4 cm in diameter and typically are smooth and sharply defined (Fig. 27–32);[318, 319] occasionally, they have indistinct, lobulated or spiculated margins (Figs. 27–33 and 27–34).[310, 320, 321] Small discrete nodules in the immediate vicinity of the main lesion—*satellite* lesions—can be identified in as many as 80% of cases.[318]

As with granulomas caused by other infectious organisms, tuberculomas often show little or no enhancement after intravenous administration of contrast material.[310, 322] In one study of 163 patients with solitary pulmonary nodules—including 111 malignant neoplasms, 43 granulomas (the authors did not specify how many of these were tuberculomas), and 9 benign neoplasms—the mean enhancement of granulomas was 11 HU compared with 42 HU for malignant neoplasms and 32 HU for benign neoplasms.[322] The authors excluded from the analysis nodules that had inhomogeneous attenuation or evidence of necrosis. These are common findings in tuberculomas and are more likely to be associated with enhancement. In another study of tuberculomas in 12 patients, 9 (75%) showed peripheral rim or central curvilinear enhancement with no enhancement of the remaining portions of the tuberculoma, 2 showed partial enhancement, and 1 showed homogeneous enhancement.[323] This pattern is similar to that of enlarged tuberculous mediastinal lymph nodes (*see* Fig. 27–7), the central low attenuation and the peripheral rim enhancement reflecting the presence of necrotic material surrounded by fibrous tissue and granulomatous inflammatory tissue.[237, 323] It has also been suggested that gadolinium diethylenetriaminepenta-acetic acid (DTPA)–enhanced magnetic resonance (MR) imaging may be helpful in distinguishing tuberculomas from pulmonary carcinomas. In one study in which this technique was used, two tuberculomas showed thin rim enhancement with no enhancement of the central portion of the lesion on T1-weighted images, a finding that was not seen in any of 20 carcinomas.[324] Although the presence of rim enhancement on CT or MR should suggest the possibility of a tuberculoma in the appropriate clinical setting, it should be remembered that a similar pattern may be seen with pulmonary carcinomas containing central areas of necrosis.[325]

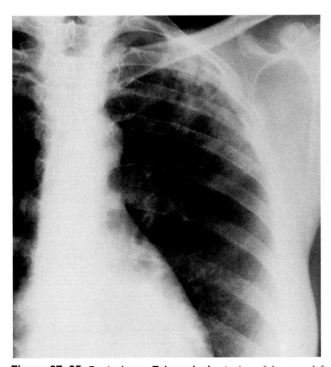

Figure 27–25. Postprimary Tuberculosis. A view of the upper left hemithorax from a posteroanterior radiograph in a 49-year-old woman reveals poorly defined focal areas of consolidation and small satellite foci in the left upper lobe. *Mycobacterium tuberculosis* was recovered from the sputum.

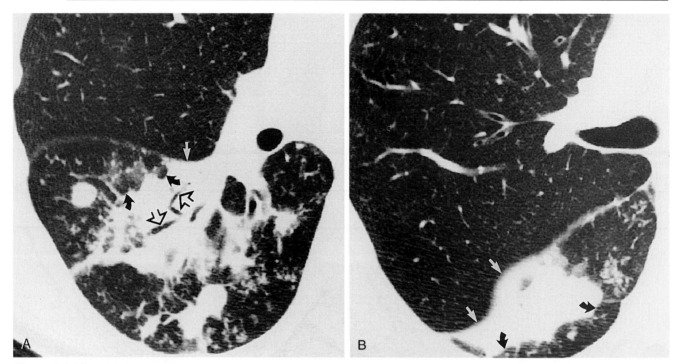

Figure 27–26. Air-Space Consolidation in Postprimary Tuberculosis. HRCT scans (*A* and *B*) in a 26-year-old woman demonstrate a focal area of consolidation with air bronchograms *(open arrows)* in the superior segment of the right lower lobe. The consolidation is marginated by the right major interlobar fissure *(straight arrows)* and by interlobular septa *(curved arrows)* with sparing of the adjacent secondary lobules. Several satellite nodules are also evident. Sputum cultures grew *Mycobacterium tuberculosis*.

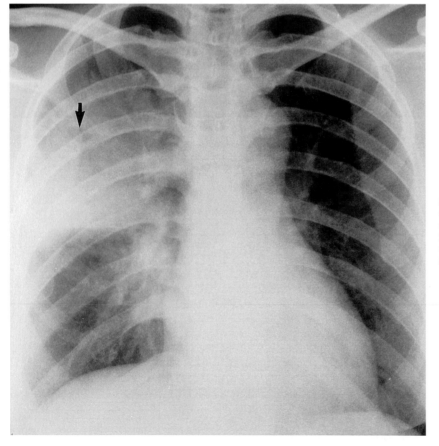

Figure 27–27. Tuberculous Lobar Pneumonia. A posteroanterior chest radiograph in a 34-year-old woman reveals right upper lobe consolidation and a small cavity *(arrow)*. The patient presented with a 2-week history of fever, chills, and malaise. Culture of bronchoalveolar lavage fluid grew *Mycobacterium tuberculosis*.

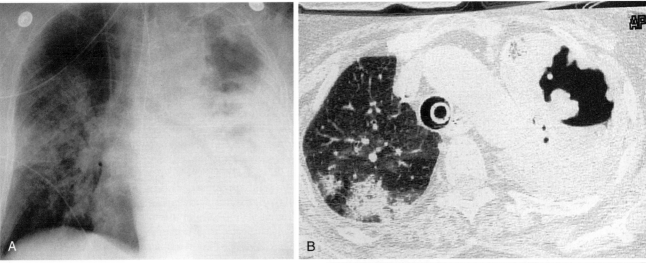

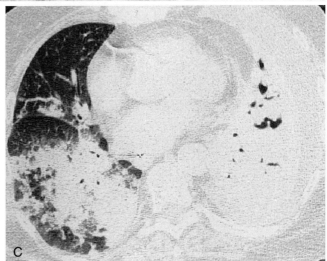

Figure 27–28. Tuberculous Bronchopneumonia. An anteroposterior chest radiograph *(A)* and HRCT scans *(B* and *C)* demonstrate a large cavity in the left upper lobe and extensive bilateral air-space consolidation. Evidence of cavitation is also present in the left lower lobe on HRCT. Also noted is a left pleural effusion. The patient was a 48-year-old alcoholic woman who presented with respiratory failure and died within 3 days of the radiograph and CT scan. Autopsy demonstrated tuberculous bronchopneumonia. Cultures grew *Mycobacterium tuberculosis.*

The majority of tuberculomas remain stable for a long time,[326] and many calcify. Calcification is usually diffuse, but may be central (Fig. 27–35) or punctate.[234, 320] CT is superior to radiography in the detection of any of these patterns.[327]

Focal Nodular Opacities. Nodular opacities measuring 2 to 10 mm in diameter and localized to one or two regions of the lungs, usually the apical or posterior segments of the upper lobes or the superior segment of the lower lobes, have been described as the main or only radiologic manifestation in 20% to 25% of patients with active postprimary tuberculosis (Fig. 27–36).[236, 255] More commonly, small nodular opacities are seen in association with focal areas of consolidation, a combination of findings that is seen on radiography and on HRCT in approximately 80% of patients.[236, 302]

On HRCT, the opacities have been shown to be centrilobular in distribution and often associated with branching linear opacities (Fig. 27–37),[302, 307] an appearance that has been likened to that of a *tree-in-bud.*[307] As indicated earlier, these abnormalities are common: centrilobular nodules measuring 2 to 5 mm in diameter or branching centrilobular linear opacities were identified on HRCT in 97% of 29 patients in one series[307] and in 92% of 89 patients in a second.[302] Pathologically, the nodules have been shown to reflect the presence of intrabronchiolar and peribronchiolar inflammatory exudate, whereas the branching linear opacities correlate with the presence of caseous material filling or surrounding terminal or respiratory bronchioles or alveolar ducts.[307, 308] The usefulness of the identification of centrilobular nodules in distinguishing between active and inactive disease is controversial. In one study of 66 patients, centrilobular nodules were seen in 29 (91%) of 32 with active disease and in none of 34 with inactive tuberculosis.[312] In another investigation, these abnormalities were identified in 92% of 89 patients with active tuberculosis and in 95% of 57 patients with inactive disease.[302] In a third study, centrilobular nodules were present in 17 (63%) of 27 patients who had active tuberculosis, but were absent in all after 6 months of therapy.[312a]

Localized nodular and branching linear opacities improve slowly with treatment, usually being replaced by changes reflecting the presence of fibrous tissue;[307] calcification develops in some cases (Fig. 27–38). In one follow-up study of 17 patients with newly diagnosed postprimary tuberculosis, residual centrilobular nodules and branching linear opacities were seen on HRCT in approximately 70% of patients 1 month after initiation of therapy, 40% at 3 months, and 25% at 12 months;[307] in all of these patients,

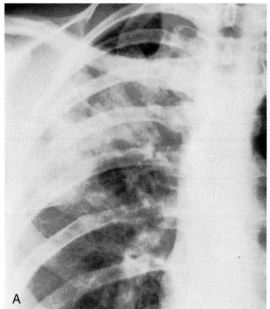

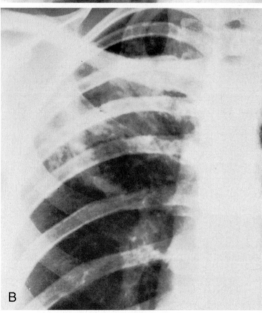

Figure 27–29. Postprimary Tuberculosis. A view of the upper half of the right hemithorax from a posteroanterior radiograph *(A)* shows inhomogeneous consolidation of much of the right upper lobe. This 28-year-old woman had had the abrupt onset of symptoms suggesting acute pneumonia approximately 1 week before these studies; *Mycobacterium tuberculosis* was isolated from the sputum, and she was placed on appropriate antituberculous therapy. Despite the extensive involvement, marked improvement had occurred within 4 weeks *(B)*.

follow-up HRCT scans showed evidence of fibrosis with irregular linear opacities, architectural distortion, and volume loss. In the study of 27 patients cited previously, linear opacities presented in 12 (45%), despite resolution of centrilobular and perivascular nodules.[312a]

Endobronchial Spread of Tuberculosis. Endobronchial spread of tuberculosis can be reasonably presumed to have occurred when multiple nodules measuring 2 to 10 mm in diameter are seen at a distance from a cavity or area of consolidation (Fig. 27–39) (the one exception being miliary

disease [*see* farther on]). Radiographic findings consistent with endobronchial spread of tuberculosis have been reported in 10% to 20% of patients with active postprimary disease.[236, 255] Studies using HRCT have shown a much higher prevalence; for example, HRCT findings consistent with endobronchial spread were seen in 34% of 89 patients in one study,[302] in 98% of 41 patients in a second series,[307] and in 97% of 31 patients in a third study.[312] The most common findings on HRCT consist of 2- to 4-mm diameter centrilobular nodules and branching linear opacities with sharply defined margins. Other abnormalities, in decreasing order of frequency, are 4- to 8-mm diameter nodules with poorly defined margins (also commonly located in a centrilobular distribution), lobular areas of consolidation, and thickening of the interlobular septa.[307, 308, 310] (Although nodules measuring 4 to 8 mm in diameter with poorly defined margins have been known as *acino-nodose lesions*, this term is inappropriate because these nodules do not represent acinar lesions but rather reflect the presence of inflammation and necrosis within and around bronchioles.[307, 308, 328])

Miliary Tuberculosis. The interval between dissemination and the development of radiographically discernible miliary tuberculosis is probably several weeks, during which time the foci of infection are too small for radiographic identification. When they have enlarged, their appearance is usually distinctive, consisting of discrete, pinpoint opacities usually evenly distributed throughout both lungs;[329, 330] sometimes, there is a slight basal predominance reflecting gravity-induced increased blood flow (Fig. 27–40). When first visible, the nodules measure 1 to 2 mm in diameter (hence the term *miliary*, which refers to the similarly sized millet seed); in the absence of adequate therapy, they may increase to 3 to 5 mm in diameter, a finding seen in approximately 10% of cases.[330] By this time, they may have become almost confluent, presenting a "snowstorm" appearance. The adult respiratory distress syndrome (ARDS) develops in some cases.[330] Pneumothorax or pneumomediastinum are rare complications.[331, 332]

Few patients die from miliary tuberculosis (proved pathologically) without demonstrable abnormality on the chest radiograph.[333, 335] Occasionally, the diagnosis is made after death in patients whose chest radiographs did not reveal the classic pattern;[333–335] usually, this occurs in older people with a clinically subacute form of the disease.[278, 335, 336]

The diagnostic accuracy in identifying the presence of miliary tuberculosis on the chest radiograph was assessed in a retrospective study that included radiographs of 71 patients with culture-proven, biopsy-proven, or autopsy-proven miliary disease; 44 patients who had normal chest radiographs and 22 who had radiographs showing localized tuberculosis were included as controls.[330] Three independent radiologists had a 60% to 70% sensitivity in identifying miliary tuberculosis and a 97% to 100% specificity in excluding it. In 30% of patients, nodules could not be seen on the radiograph at the time of diagnosis, even in retrospect.

HRCT can prove helpful in the diagnosis of miliary tuberculosis in patients with normal or nonspecific radiographic findings.[337, 338] Findings consist of nodules, usually sharply defined, measuring 1 to 4 mm in diameter and having a diffuse random distribution throughout both lungs (Fig. 27–41).[337–339, 366] Other abnormalities include nodular thickening of the interlobular septa and interlobar fissures,

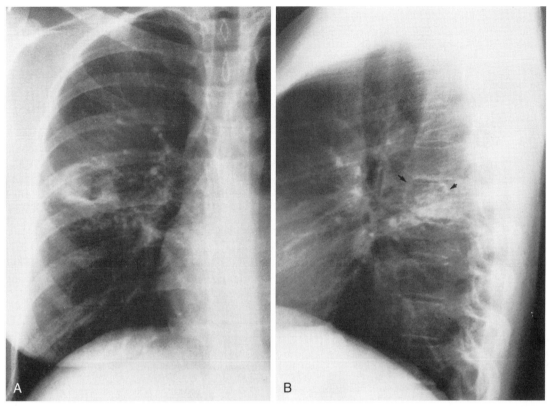

Figure 27–30. Cavitary Tuberculosis (Postprimary). Posteroanterior *(A)* and lateral *(B)* radiographs reveal a rather poorly defined, thin-walled cavity in the superior segment of the right lower lobe *(arrows in B)*. Both lungs were otherwise normal. *Mycobacterium tuberculosis* was recovered from the sputum.

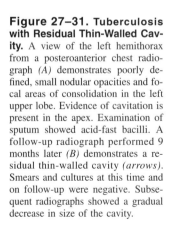

Figure 27–31. Tuberculosis with Residual Thin-Walled Cavity. A view of the left hemithorax from a posteroanterior chest radiograph *(A)* demonstrates poorly defined, small nodular opacities and focal areas of consolidation in the left upper lobe. Evidence of cavitation is present in the apex. Examination of sputum showed acid-fast bacilli. A follow-up radiograph performed 9 months later *(B)* demonstrates a residual thin-walled cavity *(arrows)*. Smears and cultures at this time and on follow-up were negative. Subsequent radiographs showed a gradual decrease in size of the cavity.

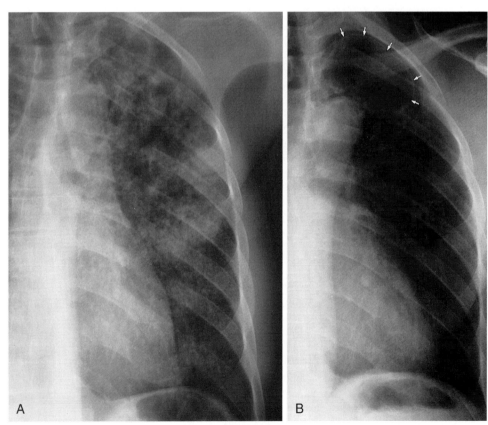

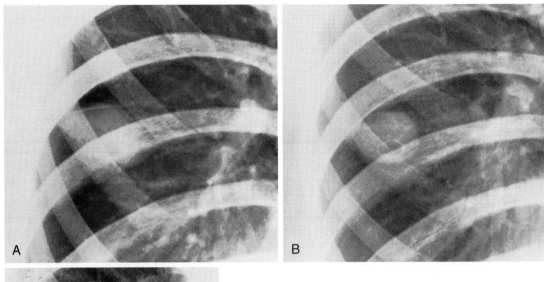

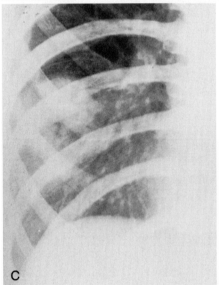

Figure 27–32. Tuberculoma with Reactivation. A view of the right midlung from a posteroanterior radiograph *(A)* reveals a sharply circumscribed, oval shadow measuring approximately 3 cm in diameter; a small, calcific ring shadow can be identified in the center of the lesion. The surrounding lung parenchyma is normal. Two years later *(B)*, the shadow is slightly smaller in size and the central ring calcification more evident. Two years later, the patient developed an abrupt onset of an acute respiratory illness; a radiograph at that time *(C)* revealed breakdown of the tuberculoma and the development of acute air-space disease in the surrounding parenchyma. Active tuberculosis was identified in the resected lobe.

nodular irregularity of vessels, and areas of ground-glass attenuation.[338, 339, 366] Although some nodules may be seen in relation to vessels, interlobular septa, or pleural surfaces, the vast majority have a random distribution in relation to the structures of the secondary pulmonary nodule.[338]

With appropriate treatment, clearing may be extremely rapid, usually faster than in nonhematogenous forms of tuberculosis.[340] Resolution is usually complete.[333, 341]

Bronchiectasis and Bronchostenosis

Bronchiectasis is seen on HRCT in 30% to 60% of patients with active postprimary tuberculosis.[302, 309, 312] The prevalence may be greater in patients with inactive disease; for example, in two studies, it was seen on HRCT in 56% of 32 patients and 63% of 89 patients with active tuberculosis compared with 71% of 34 and 86% of 57 patients with inactive disease.[302, 312] The bronchiectasis is bilateral in approximately 60% of cases and unilateral in the remainder.[309] It usually affects one or two lobes and involves mainly the upper lobes (Fig. 27–42).[309] In the majority of patients, the abnormality is not readily apparent on radiography.

As indicated previously, bronchitis is common in active tuberculosis; occasionally, associated granulation tissue is sufficient to cause a polypoid endobronchial mass that can result in atelectasis and obstructive pneumonitis.[342] Fibrosis and bronchostenosis as a result of healing can have the same effect, and both conditions may be misinterpreted as pulmonary carcinoma.[285, 343, 344] Tuberculous bronchitis also can be present in the absence of abnormalities on chest radiographs;[343] in such cases, mucosal ulceration can be a source for infection of other individuals and of sputum that yields positive culture results. The abnormality can usually be identified bronchoscopically.[344]

Several investigators have reviewed the CT findings in patients with tuberculous bronchostenosis.[345–348] In one series, the authors reviewed the CT images in 28 patients who had stenosis proved by bronchoscopy, including 18 with tuberculosis on bronchial biopsy and 10 with nonspecific biopsy findings but tuberculous lesions elsewhere in the thorax.[345] Twelve patients (43%) had CT findings of concentric bronchial stenosis, uniform thickening of the bronchial wall, and involvement of a long segment of one or more bronchi (Fig. 27–43). The stenoses were funnel-shaped or

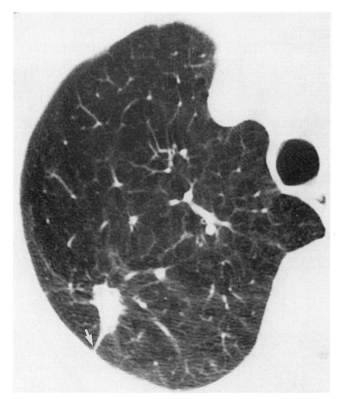

Figure 27–33. Tuberculoma. A view of the right upper lobe from an HRCT in a 59-year-old smoker demonstrates a 1.5-cm diameter nodule with spiculated margins and a pleural tag *(arrow)*. Emphysema is also present. The resected nodule was found to be a granuloma from which cultures grew *Mycobacterium tuberculosis.*

cough that has persisted since an upper respiratory tract infection and that is occasionally associated with hemoptysis.[8] The latter is usually minor and is of concern because it suggests active disease; however, it may also be related to bronchiectasis, broncholithiasis, or aspergilloma in cases of remote (inactive) disease. In fact, the first of these is a relatively common cause of hemoptysis in patients with inactive disease; in some studies, bronchiectasis has been shown to be twice as frequent in patients with hemoptysis as in patients with inactive pulmonary tuberculosis who do not have this symptom.[351] As might be expected, cough is particularly common and troublesome in patients with tracheobronchial disease.[352]

In some patients, the initial complaint is pleuritic chest pain, frequently associated with fever; this symptom is more common in young adults, a majority of whom are believed to have primary tuberculosis. Rarely, pleuritic chest pain is associated with spontaneous pneumothorax. As might be expected, hoarseness is usually a manifestation of laryngeal involvement and is associated with a positive sputum smear and culture. Shortness of breath is uncommon and usually indicates extensive disease, most often as a result of tuberculous bronchopneumonia or miliary disease complicated by ARDS.[353] Occasionally, there is acute onset of high fever, sweating, productive cough, pleuritic pain, and tachycardia suggestive of nontuberculous bacterial pneumonia.

Examination of the chest itself rarely provides information helpful in diagnosis. If an apical lesion is identified on the chest radiograph, post-tussive crackles on auscultation strongly suggest activity. In patients with recent bronchial dissemination of disease, crackles and rhonchi may be heard

diffuse and were located in the lobar bronchi with or without more proximal extension. In 14 patients (50%), CT showed obliteration of bronchial outlines by adjacent enlarged lymph nodes, parenchymal consolidation, and absence of intraluminal air. In two patients (17%), the abnormality was not visible on CT. Twenty-six of the 28 lobes supplied by diseased bronchi had evidence of atelectasis or consolidation.

In a more recent study of 17 patients with tuberculosis involving the trachea and main bronchi in whom spiral CT was performed, the findings consisted of irregular or smooth circumferential narrowing of the trachea or main bronchus with thickening of the airway wall.[347] Tracheal lesions were always associated with bronchial lesions. In none of the patients was the narrowing considered to be the result of enlarged mediastinal or hilar lymph nodes. Multiplanar and three-dimensional reconstruction images were considered to be helpful in distinguishing endobronchial from peribronchial abnormalities, in detecting subtle airway narrowing, and in evaluating the longitudinal extent of airway involvement (Fig. 27–44).

Clinical Manifestations

The most common symptoms of postprimary tuberculosis are nonspecific and may not direct the attention of the patient or the physician to the lungs; they include fatigue, weakness, anorexia, weight loss, and a low-grade fever (sometimes associated with rigors).[349, 350] Direct questioning often elicits a history of unproductive or mildly productive

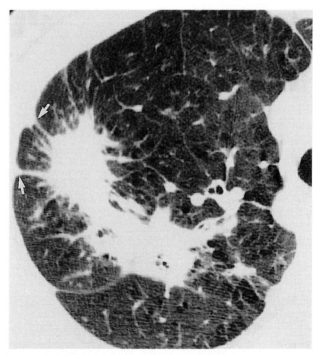

Figure 27–34. Tuberculoma. A view from an HRCT in a 48-year-old woman demonstrates a 3.5-cm diameter nodule with spiculated margins and pleural tags *(arrows)*. A focal area of consolidation is present posteromedial to the nodule. Bronchoscopic biopsy specimens demonstrated tissue necrosis; cultures grew *Mycobacterium tuberculosis.* At 3 months' follow-up, there had been marked improvement in the parenchymal abnormalities.

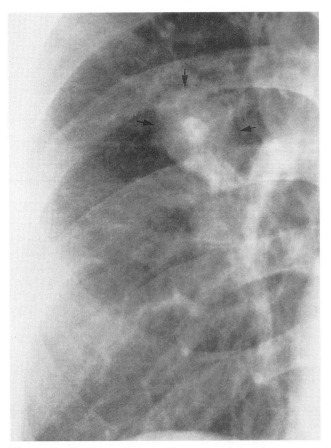

Figure 27–35. Tuberculoma. A view of the right lung from a postero-anterior chest radiograph in a 54-year-old man reveals a tuberculoma *(arrows)* with central calcification. The patient had been previously treated for postprimary tuberculosis.

over the affected areas; a localized wheeze should suggest the possibility of endobronchial disease.[344] Rarely, cavernous breathing is audible over a peripheral cavity. When onset of the disease is characterized by pain on respiration, a friction rub or signs of pleural effusion or pneumothorax may be heard. Sometimes, physical findings may suggest compression of mediastinal structures by enlarged lymph nodes.[354]

Miliary tuberculosis typically presents a different clinical picture from that of other types of pulmonary involvement. In North America, affected patients are usually elderly and often have concomitant chronic disease, such as alcoholism, diabetes mellitus, renal failure, or hematologic or solid malignancies;[111, 278, 355] another important risk factor is HIV infection. The vast majority of cases occur in adults; for example, in a population-based study that included consecutive cases of miliary tuberculosis in the Province of British Columbia, Canada, only 2 of 71 patients were younger than 18 years of age.[330] In another study in which the radiologic manifestations of tuberculosis were compared in younger adults (defined as those aged ≤ 64 years) and older patients (defined as those aged ≥ 65 years), miliary disease was identified on the chest radiograph in approximately 7% of older patients compared with 1% of younger adults.[111]

The onset of miliary disease is usually insidious; for example, in one review of 69 patients, the mean duration of symptoms until the time of diagnosis was almost 16 weeks, and more than half the patients had had symptoms for

more than 8 weeks.[119] Symptoms are usually nonspecific and include cough, weight loss, weakness, anorexia, and night sweats. Headache and abdominal pain should suggest involvement of the meninges and peritoneum. Funduscopic examination reveals choroidal tubercles in 30% to 60% of patients when a diligent search is made with mydriatic agents.[119, 356] Hepatomegaly with or without splenomegaly is not uncommon.[355] Although this form of disease can occur in patients with other types of pulmonary tuberculosis, in the majority of patients, there is no evidence of pulmonary disease other than miliary.[117, 119] When considering the diagnosis, it is important to remember that 10% to 30% of patients do not have miliary nodules on standard radiographs, even in retrospect.[330, 355] In addition, tuberculin testing with 5 tuberculin units (TU) is negative in at least 25% to 50% of patients.[329, 355, 357] Biopsy, particularly of the liver or bone marrow, may establish the diagnosis by demonstrating granulomatous inflammation.[358]

Active pulmonary tuberculosis, either miliary or other forms, is sometimes an incidental discovery at autopsy, particularly in the elderly. In many cases, the infection has been considered to be the main or an important contributing cause of death.[358–362] Premortem symptoms in these patients are often atypical and may be attributed to underlying nontuberculous disease; most groups stress the almost invariable finding of an unrelenting fever. Incidental discovery of tuberculosis in tissue specimens is not limited to the elderly,

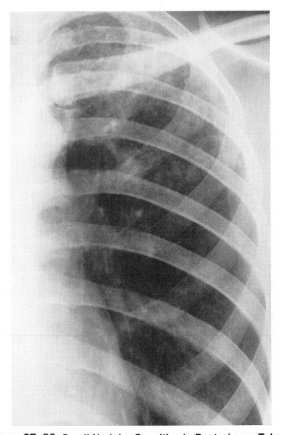

Figure 27–36. Small Nodular Opacities in Postprimary Tuberculosis. A view of the left upper chest from a posteroanterior radiograph in a 52-year-old woman demonstrates poorly defined small nodular opacities involving the apicoposterior segment of the left upper lobe. Sputum cultures grew *Mycobacterium tuberculosis*.

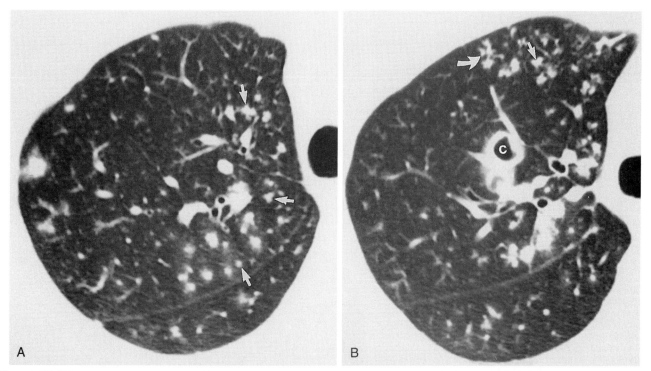

Figure 27–37. Small Nodular Opacities in Postprimary Tuberculosis. Views of the right upper lobe (*A* and *B*) from an HRCT scan in a 29-year-old woman demonstrate a cavity (C) and several nodular opacities measuring 2 to 7 mm in diameter. The majority of nodules are located near the center of the secondary lobule *(straight arrows)*. Also noted are centrilobular branching linear opacities. The combination of small nodules and branching centrilobular linear opacities gives an appearance that has been likened to a tree-in-bud *(curved arrow)*.

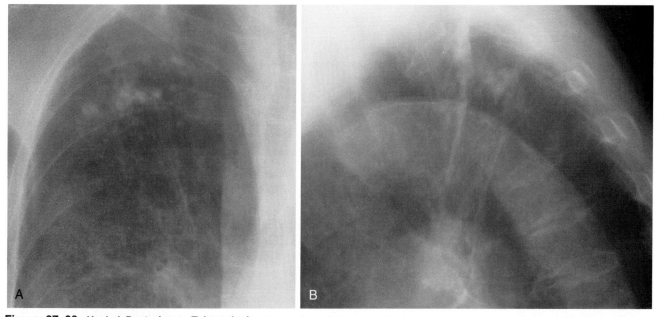

Figure 27–38. Healed Postprimary Tuberculosis. Views of the right upper lobe from posteroanterior *(A)* and lateral *(B)* chest radiographs demonstrate several small calcified nodular opacities. Also noted are coarse linear opacities consistent with fibrosis extending from the right hilum. The patient had been treated for postprimary tuberculosis 12 years previously.

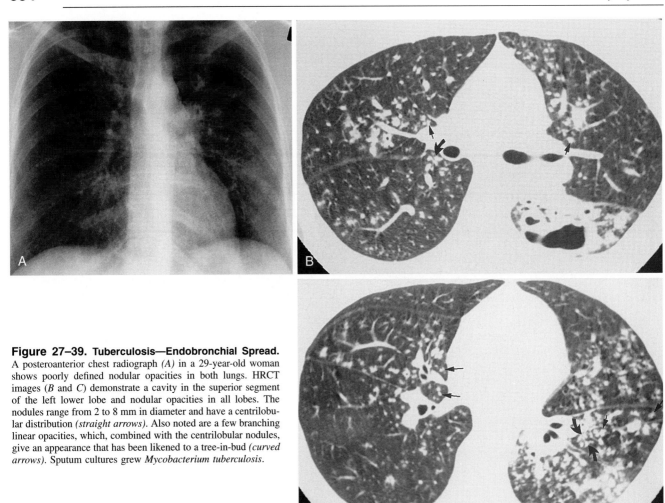

Figure 27–39. Tuberculosis—Endobronchial Spread.
A posteroanterior chest radiograph *(A)* in a 29-year-old woman shows poorly defined nodular opacities in both lungs. HRCT images *(B* and *C)* demonstrate a cavity in the superior segment of the left lower lobe and nodular opacities in all lobes. The nodules range from 2 to 8 mm in diameter and have a centrilobular distribution *(straight arrows)*. Also noted are a few branching linear opacities, which, combined with the centrilobular nodules, give an appearance that has been likened to a tree-in-bud *(curved arrows)*. Sputum cultures grew *Mycobacterium tuberculosis*.

however: it is an occasional finding in patients with solitary pulmonary nodules considered preoperatively to be carcinoma; in addition, in one investigation of explanted lungs from 183 patients undergoing pulmonary transplantation, unexpected tuberculosis was found in 8, in 4 of which the disease was considered to be active.[363]

Extrapulmonary Tuberculosis

Extrapulmonary tuberculosis can develop in several ways, perhaps the most common of which is by hematogenous dissemination during primary infection. Although the foci of infection established by such dissemination are usually inapparent at the time of the primary disease, as with postprimary pulmonary tuberculosis, they may reactivate and cause clinically evident disease months or years later. Such reactivation can occur in any tissue or organ in the body, but most often involves the lymph nodes, kidneys, adrenal glands, fallopian tubes and epididymis, and bones (particularly the thoracic spine). Extrapulmonary disease can also develop during either progressive primary or postprimary pulmonary tuberculosis (in both situations, particularly as miliary disease).

Before the onset of the AIDS epidemic, approximately 15% of cases of tuberculosis involved extrapulmonary sites in the absence of pulmonary disease.[364] Because the risk of developing extrapulmonary disease is much greater in patients with AIDS,[365] the incidence of this form of infection is increasing. Despite the annual reduction in the number of new cases of pulmonary tuberculosis in the United States before the 1980s, there was no corresponding decrease in the number of new cases of extrapulmonary tuberculosis.

Lymph Nodes

As indicated previously, pathologic involvement of regional hilar and mediastinal lymph nodes is almost invariable in primary tuberculosis, and the resulting nodal enlargement may lead to airway compression, pulmonary disease, and significant respiratory distress, particularly in children. Rarely, extranodal extension of infection causes additional complications, such as tracheoesophageal fistula.[368]

Although disease of extramediastinal lymph nodes is less common, it is still the most frequent form of extrapulmonary tuberculosis in the non-AIDS population (approximately 20% to 25% of cases).[364, 369] It appears to be more common in children and young adult immigrants from "underdeveloped" countries.[369, 370] Patients usually present with painless swelling, most often in the neck or supraclavic-

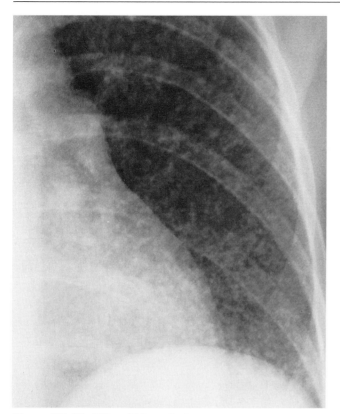

Figure 27–40. Miliary Tuberculosis. A view of the left lung from an anteroposterior chest radiograph in a 22-year-old woman demonstrates numerous sharply defined nodules measuring 1 to 3 mm in diameter. The diagnosis of miliary tuberculosis was proven by bone marrow biopsy.

Complications of tuberculous mediastinitis include erosion of the aorta,[376] paralysis of the phrenic nerve,[377] and superior vena cava syndrome.[377] Esophageal involvement usually occurs in the midthird and can result in stricture (owing to granulomatous inflammatory tissue in active disease and scar tissue after healing), tracheobronchial or mediastinal fistulas,[368, 378] and traction diverticuli.[379] Fibrosing mediastinitis may also result in narrowing of the trachea, bronchi, pulmonary arteries, pulmonary veins, or superior vena cava, with appropriate signs and symptoms (*see* page 2856).[380, 381]

Genitourinary Tract

Excluding the pleura (*see* page 2743) and lymph nodes, the most common site of extrapulmonary tuberculosis in adults is in the genitourinary tract; in fact, the discovery of sterile pyuria, hematuria, and albuminuria in a patient who has had pulmonary tuberculosis or who shows radiographic evidence of a healed pulmonary lesion should raise the possibility of the diagnosis. Local symptoms, including dysuria, polyuria, and flank pain, may be present and are more common than systemic symptoms.[382, 383] There is often extensive renal disease at the time of presentation.[384]

Because the disease is usually unilateral, there is typically no significant effect on renal function; however, both hypertension[385] and nephrolithiasis[386] have been reported as complications. As with cavitary pulmonary tuberculosis, rupture of a focus of disease into the renal pelvis may lead to dissemination of bacilli to and granulomatous inflammation of the ureter and urinary bladder; an ensuing ureteral stric-

ular region. Occasionally, tracheal impingement causes cough.[371] Although often localized to one side, concomitant involvement of both sides of the neck or of other lymph node groups is not uncommon.[372] Progression of disease may be followed by extension into the skin with the formation of a sinus tract. Rapid lymph node enlargement may occur; sometimes, this is seen during therapy, in which case it has been speculated to represent an immunologic reaction.[371] Chest radiographs often show no evidence of current or prior tuberculosis.[373] The diagnosis may be made by needle aspiration or by excisional lymph node biopsy, the latter sometimes in the setting of suspected metastatic carcinoma.

Mediastinum

Although mediastinal lymph node enlargement is relatively common in tuberculosis, extranodal extension of disease resulting in mediastinitis or fibrosing mediastinitis is rare.[374, 375] Tuberculous mediastinitis progresses insidiously and usually results in mild symptoms, including cough and low-grade fever.[374] The radiographic manifestations include mediastinal widening or a localized mass. Contrast-enhanced CT in two cases demonstrated inhomogeneous enhancement with localized areas of low attenuation;[374] T1-weighted and T2-weighted spin-echo MR images showed areas of low signal intensity as a result of fibrous tissue, and gadolinium-DTPA–enhanced T1-weighted MR images showed inhomogeneous enhancement with some areas remaining unenhanced.

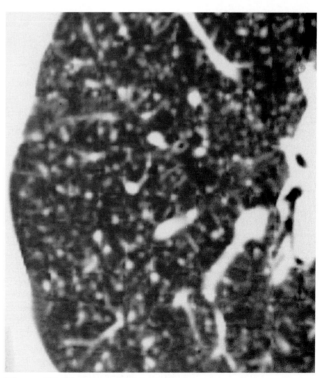

Figure 27–41. Miliary Tuberculosis. A view of the right lung from an HRCT scan in a 32-year-old man demonstrates multiple nodules measuring approximately 2 mm in diameter randomly distributed throughout the lung. The diagnosis of miliary tuberculosis was proven by open-lung biopsy.

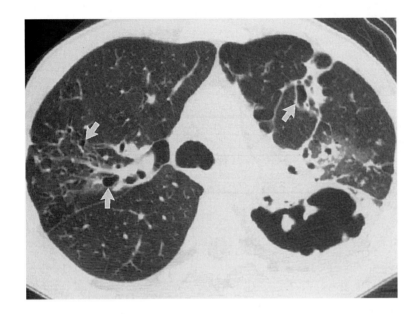

Figure 27–42. Postprimary Tuberculosis— Bronchiectasis. HRCT scan in a 39-year-old man demonstrates a large cavity in the superior segment of the left lower lobe and localized areas of bronchiectasis in the right upper and left upper lobes *(arrows)*. Sputum cultures grew *Mycobacterium tuberculosis.*

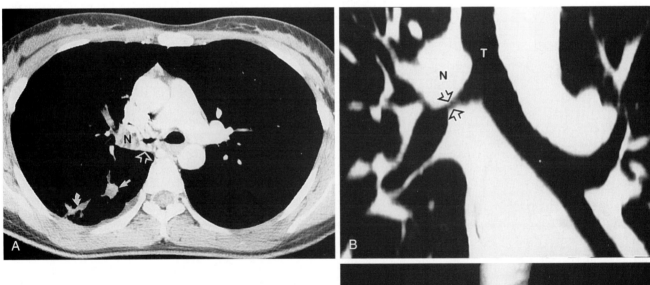

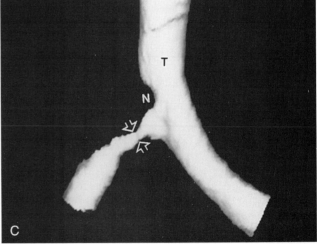

Figure 27–43. Postprimary Tuberculosis—Bronchial Stenosis. Contrast-enhanced spiral CT scan *(A)* in a 40-year-old woman demonstrates thickening of the wall of the right main bronchus *(open arrow)* with narrowing of the lumen. Also noted are a nodular opacity *(straight arrow)*, interlobular septal thickening *(curved arrow)*, right hilar lymphadenopathy (N), and a small right pleural effusion. Coronal reformation *(B)* and three-dimensional reconstruction *(C)* better demonstrate the localized narrowing of the bronchus *(open arrows)* as well as extrinsic compression of the distal trachea (T) and right bronchus by the enlarged right paratracheal and hilar nodes (N). The diagnosis of endobronchial tuberculosis was confirmed by bronchial biopsy. (Case courtesy of Dr. Kyung Soo Lee, Samsung Medical Center, Seoul, Korea.)

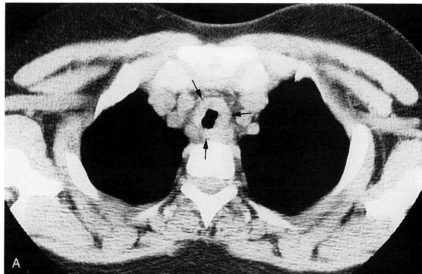

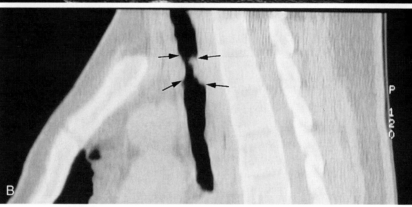

Figure 27–44. Tracheal Tuberculosis. A spiral CT scan *(A)* in a 27-year-old woman demonstrates circumferential thickening of the tracheal wall *(arrows)* resulting in narrowing of the lumen. The sagittal reconstruction *(B)* demonstrates the longitudinal extent of the tracheal involvement *(arrows)*. The diagnosis of tracheal tuberculosis was proven by bronchoscopic biopsy. (Case courtesy of Dr. Kyung Soo Lee, Samsung Medical Center, Seoul, Korea.)

ture may result in significant secondary effects on the kidney. Chest radiographic abnormalities consistent with prior tuberculosis are evident in 50% to 75% of patients.[382, 383] The diagnosis can be established by urine culture;[387] however, approximately 5% to 10% of patients with active pulmonary tuberculosis have positive urine cultures for *M. tuberculosis* in the absence of clinical and other laboratory findings of genitourinary disease.[8]

Tuberculosis of the female genital system usually occurs as salpingitis and oophoritis, manifested by pelvic pain, menstrual disturbance, or infertility; menstrual disorders, however, are frequent in women who have pulmonary tuberculosis without genital involvement, and their presence does not necessarily mean extension of the disease to the reproductive organs. In men, epididymitis, seminal vesiculitis, and prostatitis occur occasionally.

Bone and Joint

Involvement of the bones and joints occurs in about 10% of cases of non–AIDS-related extrapulmonary tuberculosis, most often in the elderly.[364] Infection can develop by hematogenous dissemination (usually to the metaphyseal region of the long bones)[388] or by direct extension from affected paravertebral lymph nodes to the thoracic and lumbosacral spine.[389] Typically, the disease is unifocal; occasionally, multiple sites are involved.[390] Joint involvement usually follows extension of disease from the adjacent bone.

Tuberculosis of the spine (Pott's disease) is the most common form of skeletal disease and usually affects the lower thoracic or upper lumbar vertebrae. Involvement of the cervical spine is rare and is usually associated with neck pain and stiffness;[391] disease may extend into the retropharynx, mediastinum, and posterior triangles. The early radiographic manifestations of spinal involvement consist of irregularity of the vertebral end plates, decreased height of the intervertebral disc space, and sclerosis of the adjacent bone; with progression of disease, there is a tendency to anterior wedging of the vertebral body, leading to kyphosis and development of paravertebral abscesses (the latter associated with displacement of the paraspinal interface[392]) (Fig. 27–45). CT is superior to the radiograph in demonstrating the extent of abnormalities, development of paraspinal abscesses, and involvement of the spinal canal.[393–395] With this technique, paravertebral abscesses show peripheral rim enhancement and low attenuation centers after intravenous administration of contrast material (*see* Fig. 27–45);[394, 395] in the majority of cases, amorphous calcification is also seen.[395] The extent of abnormalities is also well demonstrated on MR imaging.[396]

Tuberculosis occasionally involves the sternum, sternoclavicular joint, or a rib leading to osseous destruction and localized abscess formation (Fig. 27–46). Although these abnormalities are usually difficult to visualize on radiography, periosseous abscess formation can be readily detected on CT.[395, 397, 398] In one study of the CT findings in eight

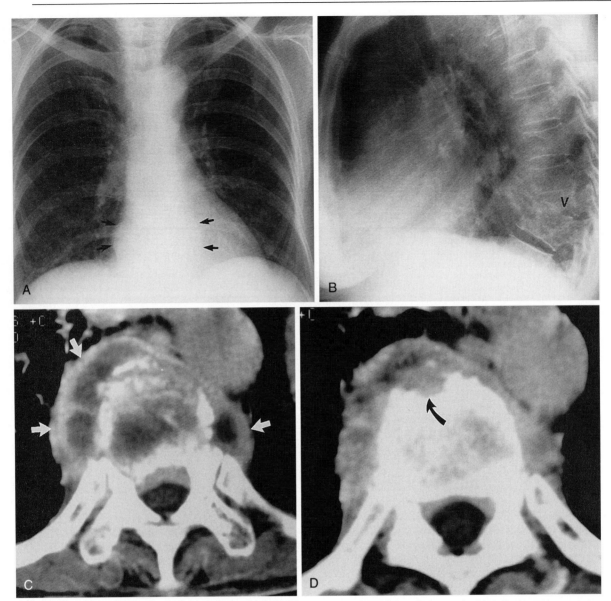

Figure 27–45. Tuberculous Spondylitis. A posteroanterior chest radiograph *(A)* in a 62-year-old man demonstrates miliary nodules and displacement of the paraspinal interfaces *(arrows)*. A lateral chest radiograph *(B)* shows destruction of the T-10 vertebral body (V) leading to localized kyphosis. Contrast-enhanced CT scans *(C* and *D)* demonstrate destruction of the T-10 vertebral body, paraspinal abscess formation with low attenuation centers and rim enhancement *(straight arrows)* as well as cortical erosion of the adjacent T-9 vertebral body *(curved arrow)*. Cultures of a needle biopsy specimen of the paraspinal abscess grew *Mycobacterium tuberculosis*.

patients with 13 surgically proven tuberculous rib lesions, contrast-enhanced CT demonstrated juxtacostal soft tissue masses with central low attenuation and peripheral rim enhancement in all cases;[397] 7 of the masses involved both sides of the ribs, and 6 involved only the inner aspect. Bone destruction was evident in only 4 of the 13 lesions: 2 were osteolytic and expansile with cortical destruction, and 2 demonstrated mild cortical irregularities. Tuberculosis may also lead to destruction of costal cartilages.[398] Rarely, rib or pleural tuberculosis is associated with the development of retromammary or intramammary tuberculous abscesses.[399]

Patients present with pain in the region of bone or articular disease. Compression of the spinal cord or associated nerves may lead to neurologic signs and symptoms. Patients with rib involvement may have a tender or non-tender mass on physical examination.[397] The diagnosis can

be confirmed by histologic examination of synovial or bone biopsy specimens or by acid-fast staining or culture of synovial fluid.

Central Nervous System

The most common manifestation of central nervous system tuberculosis is meningitis, a complication that is seen particularly in children in the setting of progressive primary or miliary disease and in patients with AIDS.[400] It is typically localized to the basal meninges but can spread to affect the entire brain or spinal cord; extension into the brain itself (encephalitis) occurs occasionally. Symptoms depend on the extent of such spread: most often, there is headache, irritability, fever, and neck stiffness; somnolence, vomiting, and convulsions occur in more severe cases.

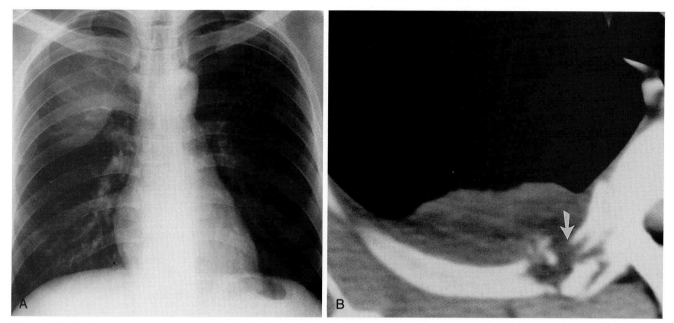

Figure 27–46. Tuberculosis of the Rib. A posteroanterior chest radiograph *(A)* in a 32-year-old man demonstrates a focal area of increased opacity in the right upper chest. The opacity has sharply defined margins medially and poorly defined margins superiorly and laterally, an appearance characteristic of an extrapulmonary lesion. A CT scan *(B)* demonstrates localized destruction of the posterior aspect of the right sixth rib *(arrow)* associated with a soft tissue mass. Repeated fine needle aspiration biopsies were nondiagnostic; the diagnosis of tuberculosis was proven at surgical resection.

The diagnosis is best made by culture of the tubercle bacillus from cerebrospinal fluid, which has been reported to be positive in about 50% to 80% of cases;[401] only 10% to 20% of CSF samples are smear positive. Although a low glucose and increased protein content and elevated white cell count (usually lymphocytes) in the cerebrospinal fluid are characteristic, these abnormalities may also be present in fungal meningitis.[402] Several groups have reported the diagnostic usefulness of enzyme-linked immunosorbent assay for the identification of mycobacterial antigen in cerebrospinal fluid.[403–405] Tuberculous meningitis is a serious complication; the mortality is high (30% to 40% in some series), and residual neurologic abnormalities are common in those who survive.[400, 406]

Central nervous system tuberculosis is also occasionally manifested by a localized intracerebral focus of granulomatous inflammation (tuberculoma). Paradoxically, these sometimes develop or increase in size during therapy.[407]

Skin

Cutaneous mycobacterial infection is most often caused by nontuberculous mycobacteria. However, in one review of 34 cases seen over a 10-year period, 20 were caused by *M. tuberculosis*.[408] Clinical manifestations may take several forms, including scrofuloderma, miliary tuberculosis (tuberculosis cutis miliaris disseminata),[409] lupus vulgaris, and tuberculous gumma.[410]

Cardiovascular System

The most common cardiac complication of tuberculosis is pericarditis. In areas of the world with a high prevalence of tuberculosis, the abnormality is relatively frequent.[411] However, tuberculosis is an uncommon cause of pericardial disease in "developed" countries; for example, in one study of 100 cases of acute pericarditis from Spain, it was the etiology in only 4.[412] The complication may occur by retrograde spread of organisms from involved mediastinal lymph nodes, by hematogenous dissemination, or by direct extension from the lung or mediastinum; the first mechanism is probably the most common.

The infection may result in the accumulation of fluid with relatively little pericardial thickening, leading to tamponade; extension of the inflammatory reaction into the myocardium or endarteritis of the coronary vessels occurs occasionally. In long-standing disease, there may be marked pericardial fibrosis, often with dystrophic calcification.[413, 414] This fibrosis is not uncommonly associated with clinical manifestations of constrictive pericarditis and is a particularly important cause of cardiac disease in some parts of the world in which the background prevalence of tuberculosis is high. Unilateral or bilateral pleural effusion is seen in some cases.

Organisms can be cultured from aspirated fluid in approximately 20% to 30% of cases;[411] as a result of this rather low incidence, the diagnosis is not uncommonly made histologically after excision of pericardium for relief of tamponade or constrictive pericarditis. Some investigators have documented high levels of adenosine deaminase in aspirated pericardial fluid, a finding that may prove to be diagnostically useful;[415] for example, in one study of 108 cases of pericardial effusion, of which 20 were tuberculous, 82 idiopathic, and the remainder the result of a variety of causes, the values for pericardial fluid adenosine deaminase were 126 ± 16 U/liter in the tuberculous group and approximately 25 to 30 ± 10 U/liter in the others.[416] Serologic diagnosis has also been reported by some investigators; for example, in one study of 51 African patients in which a 30-kDa *M. tuberculosis* antigen was used, the sensitivity for diagnosis was found to be 61% and the specificity 96%.[417] Unfortunately, with these degrees of sensitivity and specificity, these tests would not be useful in areas in which tuberculosis is an uncommon cause of pericarditis. Pericarditis has also been associated with a high level of antimycobacterial hsp60 antibody titer in pericardial fluid.[412]

Other cardiovascular complications of tuberculosis include aortic aneurysm (presumably related in most cases to local extension of mediastinal lymph node disease)[418] and myocardial tuberculomas.[419]

Gastrointestinal System

Involvement of the gastrointestinal tract is rarely seen nowadays in "developed" countries, but still has an appreciable incidence in some parts of the world in which tuberculosis is common. For example, in one review of the causes of lower gastrointestinal hemorrhage in 166 patients in India, tuberculosis was considered to be responsible in about 4%.[420] Although disease can be acquired by hematogenous dissemination during primary disease, it probably develops more frequently by swallowing organisms derived from a tuberculous cavity in the lung or (in the case of *M. bovis*) contaminated milk. Disease is most common in the ileocecal area or rectum, the latter sometimes being associated with perianal or ischiorectal abscesses.[421, 422] Clinical manifestations and complications include abdominal pain, bowel obstruction, fistula formation, perforation with peritonitis, hemorrhage, and a palpable mass.[423, 424]

Peritoneum

Tuberculous peritonitis can occur as part of disseminated disease or (rarely) after rupture of an intra-abdominal lymph node or bowel.[425] It is manifested clinically by abdominal pain and evidence of ascites;[426] systemic findings, such as fever and weight loss, are common. A "doughy" character may be noted on physical examination of the abdomen.[8] Some cases have been associated with the presence of a pelvic mass and an elevated serum CA 125, resulting in confusion with metastatic ovarian carcinoma.[427, 428] Although concomitant pleural effusion is common, radiographic evidence of pulmonary disease is usually absent.[8] Fluid derived from paracentesis yields organisms on culture in about 50% to 80% of cases.[425, 429] Laparoscopy enables biopsy of foci of granulomatous inflammation and has a high diagnostic yield.

Liver, Spleen, and Pancreas

Biopsy of the liver reveals granulomas in about 25% of patients with tuberculosis. Most often, this is the result of miliary disease; occasionally, there is localized hepatic infection without clinical or radiographic evidence of extrahepatic disease.[431] Although both forms of disease are uncommonly associated with clinical or biochemical evidence of hepatic dysfunction,[430] these may occur and are rarely accompanied by hepatic failure.[431] Although uncommonly seen because of its relative inaccessibility, splenic disease is also frequent in miliary tuberculosis; localized tuberculomas occur occasionally.[432]

Larynx

Although tuberculous laryngitis may be associated with advanced pulmonary tuberculosis, it occurs in the presence of minimal or apparently absent disease at this site in an appreciable number of cases. Because of the relatively easy access of organisms to the environment, this form of disease is associated with a particularly high degree of contagiousness; when combined with an absence of findings in the lungs, this can lead to a significant delay in diagnosis and serious outbreaks of infection. The incidence is highest in "developing" countries;[433] however, cases are also identified from time to time in "developed" nations.[434, 435]

Radiographic findings include swelling or focal masses involving the vocal cords, epiglottis, or aryepiglottic folds.[436] The most common finding on CT is diffuse thickening of the vocal cords and epiglottis without the presence of a focal mass;[437] even when a focal mass is seen, diffuse asymmetric thickening of the contralateral vocal cord, epiglottis, or paralaryngeal soft tissue is evident. As might be expected, cough is the most prominent symptom; a change in voice also may be noted. Patients are almost always smear positive.

Miscellaneous Sites

Tuberculous *otitis media* and *mastoiditis* are rare complications; typical manifestations include chronic tympanic membrane perforation and progressive hearing loss.[438] *Ocular* tuberculosis has been found to occur in about 1% to 2% of patients with tuberculosis in the pre-AIDS era.[439] In a review carried out between 1993 and 1994 of 100 patients with tuberculosis who were specifically evaluated for the presence of ophthalmic signs and symptoms, 18 patients with possible or probable ocular involvement were identified;[439] the most common finding was choroiditis. Risk factors for the presence of ocular disease included HIV infection and miliary disease. Many patients were asymptomatic.

Extensive *adrenal* disease may cause sufficient cortical destruction to result in biochemical and clinical manifestations of Addison's disease.[440] The presence of small, calcified glands on CT examination is a clue to the diagnosis in long-standing disease.[441] Although rarely seen in "developed" countries, tuberculous *mastitis* is still a problem in some areas of the world where there is a high background prevalence of tuberculosis;[442] the infection can be mistaken for carcinoma, particularly when axillary lymph nodes are also enlarged as a result of reactive changes or concomitant tuberculous infection. Involvement of the *thyroid gland* or *pancreas* is probably even more unusual, but may also result in a mistaken clinical impression of carcinoma.[443–445] Involvement of the pancreas has been associated with hyperamylasemia in some cases.[446] Extensive infection of *skeletal muscle* has been reported in a patient who had dermatomyositis.[447]

Laboratory Findings and Diagnosis

Techniques for the diagnosis of tuberculosis are numerous and possess varying degrees of complexity and expense as well as sensitivity and specificity;[448] not all are available to every physician or hospital laboratory, and a tiered system of diagnosis involving several levels of sophistication has been advocated.[449, 450] With the use of modern techniques, it has been suggested that identification of *M. tuberculosis* and reporting of drug sensibilities should be possible in at least 10 to 14 days and 15 to 30 days, respectively;[451] as molecular biologic techniques become more standardized and available, these times may be significantly shortened.

Tuberculin Skin Test

The tuberculin skin test is often helpful in the diagnosis of tuberculous infection. Over the years, numerous investigators have studied the indications for and limitations of its use;[452] summary reviews of their results and guidelines for the use and interpretation of the test have been reported by groups such as the American Thoracic Society and the Centers for Disease Control in Atlanta.[8, 453]

Technical Considerations

The material used for mycobacterial skin testing is a protein precipitate derived from filtrates of heat-killed cultures of bacilli grown in a synthetic medium.[454] The first material isolated for diagnostic purposes was known as *old tuberculin* (OT); a more purified and reliable form, purified protein derivative (PPD), was developed in the 1930s.[455] A specific lot of this substance, designated *PPD-S*, subsequently became the international standard for all tuberculins. Other PPD preparations have been developed for particular *Mycobacteria* species and have been designated by abbreviations such as *PPD-Y (M. kansasii)*, *PPD-B (M. intracellulare)*, and *PPD-F (M. fortuitum)*; however, these preparations have not been standardized and are not recommended for clinical use. Although additional purified mycobacterial substances, such as antigen complex A60,[456] have been investigated for diagnostic testing, PPD remains the standard throughout the world.

Diluted tuberculoprotein is adsorbed in varying amounts to the surface of glass or plastic containers,[457–459] a reaction that can result in the loss of most of its potency within hours to weeks after preparation.[459] This effect can be largely avoided by the addition of Tween 80, a detergent that stabilizes the tuberculin solution and that is always added nowadays.[460] Nevertheless, it is recommended that tuberculin should not be transferred from one container to another and that it should be administered promptly after filling of the injecting syringe.[8] Although tuberculin preparations are relatively stable, it is also recommended that they be kept refrigerated and out of contact with strong light.

PPD-S is available in several concentrations: 0.00002 mg/0.1 ml (1 TU, first strength), 0.00004 mg/0.1 ml (2 TU, RT-23), 0.0001 mg/0.1 ml (5 TU, intermediate strength), and 0.005 mg/0.1 ml (250 TU, second-test strength). Intermediate-strength PPD (5 TU) is the form that is employed for diagnostic skin testing and should be administered by the Mantoux method. The latter is carried out by injecting 0.1 ml of the solution intradermally in the forearm (usually the volar aspect) through a 26-gauge or 27-gauge short-beveled needle,[461] with the needle bevel pointing upward. A discrete 5- to 10-mm diameter wheal is produced with proper injection. In the case of improper injection, a second test dose can be administered immediately at a site several centimeters away from the first.

Tests should be read on the second or third day after injection, the diameter of induration being measured at a right angle to the line of injection (i.e., transversely to the long axis of the forearm) and recorded in millimeters. The degree of erythema is of no significance and need not be estimated, although its presence should suggest the possibility that injection was subcutaneous rather than intracutaneous.[462] The interpretation of a test as positive depends on the degree of induration as well as a number of clinical variables, such as likelihood of prior contact with *M. tuberculosis* and the presence of diseases or situations associated with an increased risk of tuberculosis. Thus, depending on the circumstance, a positive reaction may be considered to be as low as 5 mm or as high as 15 mm (Table 27–1).

Tuberculin can also be administered by jet injection or multiple puncture techniques, such as the Heaf and Disk tine test. In this method, tuberculin (either OT or PPD) is introduced into the skin via an applicator whose points are covered with dried tuberculin or by puncture through a film of liquid tuberculin. Because the amount of injected tuberculin cannot be precisely controlled, these techniques should not be used for diagnostic purposes.[8] They are useful, however, for epidemiologic surveys, particularly in children.[462, 463] Interpretation of the test should be done after 48 to 72 hours and depends on the reaction elicited: if this is one of discrete papules, the largest single papule is measured; if it is one of coalescent papules, the largest coalescent area is taken; if it is vesicular, it is noted as such and considered to be positive.[8] Individuals with a negative reaction to a multiple puncture test usually have a negative reaction to a Mantoux test; with the exception of vesicular reaction, it is recommended that those who show a positive reaction be

Table 27–1. CRITERIA FOR POSITIVE PURIFIED PROTEIN DERIVATIVE REACTIONS*

INDURATION	CLINICAL SETTING
≥5 mm	Individuals known to be HIV positive or to have risk factors associated with its presence
	Individuals having had recent close contact with a person known to have active tuberculosis
	Individuals whose chest radiographs are consistent with healed tuberculosis
≥10 mm	Individuals from areas of the world known to have a high prevalence of tuberculosis (e.g., "developing" countries and certain areas of large cities in "developed" countries)
	Intravenous drug users
	Residents of long-term care facilities (e.g., nursing homes, mental health institutions, prisons)
	Patients with conditions known to be associated with tuberculosis (e.g., silicosis, diabetes mellitus, gastrectomy, jejunoileal bypass, malignancy, chronic renal failure)
	Patients treated with high-dose corticosteroids and/or other immunosuppressive therapy
≥15 mm	All other individuals

HIV, human immunodeficiency virus.

Adapted from Diagnostic standards and classification of tuberculosis. Am Rev Respir Dis 142:725, 1990. Official Journal of the American Thoracic Society. © American Lung Association.

*Based on the administration of a single test dose of 5 TU.

further tested by the Mantoux method before decisions are made regarding therapy.[8]

Indications and Limitations

The Mantoux test to 5 TU is widely used to detect the presence of tuberculous infection and to aid in the establishment of priorities for follow-up and preventive therapy.[8] It is widely used in evaluating patients suspected of having tuberculosis on the basis of clinical and radiologic findings and patients in situations of high risk who have no evidence of disease.[464] A positive test is particularly useful in an individual known to be negative in a previous test (tuberculin converter). (Documentation by serial testing is important in these cases, because it has been shown that acceptance of a patient's recollection of a previous skin test is unreliable.[465]) Thus, individuals younger than 35 years of age whose previous reaction was negative and who show an increase in induration of more than 10 mm within a 2-year period should be considered to have been recently infected;[8] a similar conclusion would be reasonable in individuals over 35 years of age with a change of 15 mm or more. The results of several studies also indicate that the larger the size of the tuberculin reaction, the greater the risk of clinical tuberculosis in the future.[463, 466–468] Although the criteria for considering a test positive may be different in specific populations,[469] general indications for use of the test have been published (Table 27–2).[8]

Despite the diagnostic usefulness of a positive Mantoux reaction to 5 TU, it is important to remember that it does not necessarily signify active tuberculosis. Once a patient has been infected by M. tuberculosis and developed hypersensitivity, the reaction is generally positive, although it may decrease somewhat with time. Thus, interpretation of the test with respect to disease activity must always be made in the light of clinical and radiologic findings.

False-positive reactions to PPD may represent cross-reactions as a result of infection from nontuberculous mycobacteria. The latter are usually associated with foci of induration smaller than 10 mm in diameter and are unlikely to be involved if the induration is 15 mm or larger. Rarely, false-

Table 27–2. PERSONS IN WHOM TUBERCULIN TESTING IS INDICATED

Persons with signs (e.g., radiographic abnormality) and/or symptoms (e.g., cough, hemoptysis, weight loss) suggestive of current tuberculous disease

Recent contacts with known tuberculosis cases or persons suspected of having tuberculosis

Persons with abnormal chest radiographs compatible with past tuberculosis

Persons with medical conditions that increase the risk of tuberculosis (silicosis, gastrectomy, diabetes, immunosuppressive therapy, lymphoma)

Persons with HIV infection

Groups at high risk of recent infection with M. tuberculosis, such as immigrants from Asia, Africa, Latin America, and Oceania; some inner-city and skid row populations; personnel and long-term residents in some hospitals, nursing homes, mental institutions, and prisons

HIV, human immunodeficiency virus.
Adapted from Diagnostic standards and classification of tuberculosis. Am Rev Respir Dis 142:725, 1990.

positive reactions to PPD have been related to a specific PPD batch.[470] Previous vaccination with BCG is also a possible cause of a false-positive test interpretation. The age at which vaccination occurs is an important determinant of subsequent reactivity. Individuals vaccinated in infancy usually show induration less than 10 mm after the age of 2 years; however, those vaccinated at school age or older not uncommonly have induration greater than 10 mm. In one investigation of 2,424 subjects vaccinated 13 to 25 years previously, 1,489 (61%) showed a reaction greater than or equal to 5 mm (905 [29%] of a control group of 3,135 nonvaccinated individuals had a similar reaction).[471] Eleven per cent of vaccinated individuals showed a reaction greater than or equal to 15 mm (compared to 5% for the control group). Despite these findings, it has been recommended that a large reaction to 5 TU PPD be considered to indicate infection by M. tuberculosis, particularly in an individual from an area of high prevalence or with a high risk.[8]

Another drawback to the tuberculin test lies in false-negative reactions. Theoretically, such reactions may be related to several factors (Table 27–3), including (1) faulty technique of tuberculin administration; (2) faulty interpretation of the reaction;[471a] (3) inadequacy of the injected tuberculin;[472] and (4) diminished immunologic response to tuberculin.[473, 474] Possible errors in technique include the injection of too little antigen (e.g., as a result of leakage from the syringe) and subcutaneous rather than intradermal injection; however, there is evidence that these errors uncommonly lead to negative results.[475] Although errors in interpretation may be the result of inexperience, there is also a degree of interobserver and intraobserver disagreement in reading in experienced physicians.[474, 476] Problems with inadequate test specimens can usually be avoided by adhering to the principles of tuberculin preparation and handling described in the introductory part of this discussion.

Because the Mantoux test reaction to tuberculin is a measure of cell-mediated immunity, other indices of immunologic competence are also affected in patients infected by tubercle bacilli. For example, comparison of the in vitro lymphocyte response to tuberculin antigen from various mycobacterial species usually shows agreement with the results of skin tests.[477–479] An important clinical correlate of this general principle is the relatively high incidence of false-negative reactions to tuberculin in patients with a diminished or absent cell-mediated immunologic response. (Because a negative reaction is the expected situation in an individual recently infected with M. tuberculosis prior to the development of cell-mediated delayed hypersensitivity,[480] this is usually not considered a false-negative reaction.) A variety of underlying diseases are responsible for the lack of immune response. Various acute infections, particularly viral infections such as measles, but also many bacterial disorders, transiently depress the tuberculin reaction. A more permanent diminution or loss of delayed skin hypersensitivity also occurs in many other diseases, including sarcoidosis, chronic renal failure, malignancy, and (particularly) HIV infection (see page 1652).

A number of patients with active tuberculosis (particularly miliary[358] but also localized disease[481, 482]) are totally anergic. Testing with other antigens, such as Trichophyton, mumps, and Candida, to assess the possibility of a general deficiency of delayed hypersensitivity may be helpful in

Table 27–3. FACTORS CAUSING DECREASED ABILITY TO RESPOND TO TUBERCULIN

Factors related to the person being tested
   Infections
      Viral (measles, mumps, chickenpox)
      Bacterial (typhoid fever, brucellosis, typhus, leprosy, pertussis, overwhelming tuberculosis, tuberculous pleurisy)
      Fungal (South American blastomycosis)
   Live virus vaccinations (measles, mumps, polio)
   Metabolic derangements (chronic renal failure)
   Nutritional factors (severe protein depletion)
   Diseases affecting lymphoid organs (Hodgkin's disease, lymphoma, chronic lymphocytic leukemia, sarcoidosis)
   Drugs (corticosteroids and many other immunosuppressive agents)
   Age (newborns, elderly patients with *wanes* sensitivity)
   Recent or overwhelming infection with *M. tuberculosis*
   Stress (surgery, burns, mental illness, graft-versus-host reactions)
Factors related to the tuberculin used
   Improper storage (exposure to light and heat)
   Improper dilutions
   Chemical denaturation
   Contamination
   Adsorption (partially controlled by adding Tween 80)
Factors related to the method of administration
   Injection of too little antigen
   Delayed administration after drawing into syringe
   Injection prior to the development of delayed hypersensitivity
Factors related to reading the test and recording results
   Inexperienced reader
   Conscious or unconscious bias
   Error in recording

Adapted from Diagnostic standards and classification of tuberculosis. Am Rev Respir Dis 142:725, 1990.

identifying these patients.[483] *Selective anergy* to PPD also appears to occur in some patients.[484] A number of investigators have also shown that negative reactions to 5 TU occur in as many as 10% to 15% of patients who have relatively mild infection and a positive sputum culture;[473, 476, 480, 485] serial tuberculin testing, which would reveal whether true sensitivity was developing or the patients were truly anergic, has generally not been carried out.

Another important consideration in interpreting negative reactions is therapy, particularly immunosuppressive. For example, it is clear that corticosteroid therapy may render some previously positive reactors negative.[486] It is possible that a similar outcome may be seen after treatment for tuberculosis.[487] In addition to the well-documented diminution or disappearance of a positive reaction related to certain acute and chronic diseases and therapy, it is generally accepted that reaction to tuberculin tends to decrease with advancing age;[488, 489] there is evidence that such decrease is an all-or-none phenomenon rather than a gradual reduction, the proportion of patients with anergy increasing with each decade.[490]

In contrast to the loss of sensitivity to tuberculin that may occur with aging, treatment, or disease, some patients show an enhanced reaction with repeated testing. This *booster phenomenon* can be defined as an increase in tuberculin reaction size on repeated testing in the absence of new mycobacterial infection or BCG vaccination. In one investigation, such boosting occurred as early as 1 week after the initial tuberculin test;[491] the incidence increases with age and is most often seen in individuals older than 55.

The reaction is believed to occur in patients with remote tuberculous or nontuberculous mycobacterial infection or BCG vaccination in whom the immune stimulus of the administered tuberculoprotein results in an increased reaction on subsequent testing.[491a] As a result of these observations, it has been recommended that a second skin test be given 1 week after the first in patients in whom repeated monitoring of skin testing is anticipated, such as health care workers.[8, 491] If the second test is positive (booster effect), the patient should be considered to have had mycobacterial infection and be managed according to the results of other clinical, radiologic, and laboratory findings; if it is again negative, a positive reaction to a third test within the next few years likely represents new infection in the interval.[8]

Bacteriologic Investigation

Specimen Collection

Material for bacteriologic diagnosis can come from a variety of sources, including sputum; bronchial lavage, gastric, pleural, peritoneal or cerebrospinal fluid; and tissue specimens.

Sputum and Bronchopulmonary Washing Specimens. Sputum is the easiest and most valuable source of organisms in the setting of pulmonary disease. The patient should be instructed to cough up saliva-free material in appropriately labeled and clean specimen jars. Single, early morning specimens are preferred;[492] ideally, samples should be taken on 3 different days. In patients who do not expectorate spontaneously, inhalation of a warmed solution of hypertonic saline (3%) administered by ultrasonic nebulizer induces production of material sufficient for analysis in almost all patients; in one investigation of patients whose routine sputum specimens were smear negative, the number of cases diagnosed on samples of such induced sputum was approximately the same as that of samples obtained by bronchoscopy.[493] Specimens of sputum obtained immediately after bronchoscopy are also valuable because of the deep coughing that often ensues after the procedure. A pooled specimen collected over 12 to 48 hours may be helpful when other methods are not effective or appropriate.[494]

When a diagnosis of pulmonary tuberculosis is suspected and sputum is not available or is nondiagnostic, bronchoscopy may be indicated. The technique can be highly productive for both smear and culture diagnosis,[495–499] usually from brushings or lavage[500] and sometimes from biopsy specimens;[501] overall, the diagnostic yield in patients whose sputum specimens are smear negative is about 75% on culture.[493] In "developed" countries, it has been suggested that the yield from culture of material obtained on routine bronchoscopy of patients not considered to have tuberculosis is so low as to be ineffective on a cost-benefit basis;[502] however, this is not true in some areas of the world with high prevalence rates, where the incidence of positive smears and cultures in this type of patient has been fairly high.[496] As discussed farther on, the yield of granulomas on biopsy specimens is also high in selected cases. As might be expected, bronchoscopy is also helpful in diagnosing and following patients with tracheobronchial disease. Endoscopic findings include evidence of mucosal inflammation, polyps, ulceration, and stenosis.[352, 503–505]

Analyses of bronchoalveolar lavage (BAL) fluid cytology have been reported by several groups of investigators; although not useful diagnostically, most patients have been found to have an increase in the number of neutrophils and lymphocytes and a normal CD4-to-CD8 ratio.[500, 506, 507] A relatively prominent increase in the number of CD8 cells was found by one group in patients with miliary disease;[508] of some interest was the observation that the number of lavage CD8 cells was related to the time taken for radiographic clearing of the disease. The level of adenosine deaminase has been found to be elevated in lavage fluid from patients with tuberculosis;[509] however, it is also increased in those with other diseases, such as sarcoidosis.

Gastric Contents. Gastric contents may contain bacilli that have been carried up the tracheobronchial mucociliary escalator and swallowed. Although uncommonly performed nowadays, aspiration of this material is sometimes the only means of documenting the infection.[510] This is particularly the case in children or the elderly who cannot produce sputum, even after aerosol inhalation.[8] The technique involves the aspiration of about 50 ml of gastric contents early in the morning after an 8- to 10-hour fast, preferably with the patient still in bed.[8]

Body Fluids. Urine specimens are best obtained in the morning after rising, preferably during midstream; multiple samples are advised.[8] Pleural, pericardial, cerebrospinal, and peritoneal fluid should undergo biochemical and cytologic analysis in addition to smear and culture. The incidence of culture from these fluids is variable; in pleural fluid, it is approximately 15%,[511] in CSF 50% to 80%,[401] and pericardial fluid, about 20% to 30%.[411]

Tissue Fragments. Biopsy specimens from patients with suspected tuberculosis should be submitted for both pathologic and bacteriologic study; although necrotizing granulomatous inflammation strongly supports the diagnosis, fungal and some nonmycobacterial bacterial infections as well as some reactions to foreign material can show a similar histologic appearance. The finding of granulomas in pleural biopsy specimens almost always indicates tuberculosis; a positive culture of tissue containing acid-fast organisms is found in about 55% to 80% of proven cases of tuberculous effusion (*see* page 2746).[512, 513] The likelihood of a tuberculous cause is less for liver biopsy specimens showing granulomas because many other diseases also give rise to hepatic granulomas.[430]

Transbronchial, liver, and bone marrow biopsy specimens frequently show granulomatous inflammation in miliary tuberculosis, reported rates being about 45% to 75%,[514, 515] 75% to 100%,[516, 517] and 35% to 100%, respectively.[516] In one review of 10 reports of bone marrow biopsies, granulomas were identified in 78 (60%) of 128 cases;[516] necrosis was seen in about 30%. The identification of acid-fast organisms in tissue sections or marrow smears or a positive culture is achieved in only a small number of these cases (probably < 25%);[119, 355, 516, 518] nevertheless, in the appropriate clinical setting, the presence of granulomas alone is virtually diagnostic. Use of more sensitive techniques for the detection of mycobacteria, such as PCR, may increase the likelihood of a definite diagnosis.[518]

Although the diagnostic yield of transbronchial biopsy is probably highest in cases of miliary tuberculosis, there is evidence that it is also useful in patients with other forms of disease, particularly those who reside in areas with a high background prevalence of tuberculosis. For example, in one investigation of 170 patients from Taiwan who had solitary pulmonary nodules, of whom 120 had carcinoma, 40 tuberculosis, and 10 miscellaneous benign lesions, all underwent bronchoscopy with fluoroscopically guided transbronchial biopsy;[519] the diagnosis was confirmed in 84 (70%) of the cancer cases and 22 (55%) of the tuberculous cases (15 on biopsy specimens, 1 on a brushing smear, and 2 on postbronchoscopy sputum samples). As might be expected, the diagnostic yield was greater in larger nodules. Another group from Thailand studied 40 patients suspected to have tuberculosis but who had "minimal infiltration" on chest radiographs and negative sputum smears;[520] the diagnosis of tuberculosis was confirmed by bronchoscopy in 13 patients (33%; 3 on BAL smear, 6 on BAL culture, and 7 on biopsy specimens).

Identification of Mycobacteria

Many techniques have been used to identify and characterize mycobacteria in clinical specimens and to determine which particular species is present. The techniques vary considerably in sensitivity and specificity as well as availability and cost. Although routine culture remains the gold standard, the time involved for its completion (6 to 8 weeks in many cases) is an important limitation. In addition, sputum, body fluid, or tissue samples containing the organism are not always easily available for culture or other analysis. As a result, a variety of techniques have been investigated to identify the organism more rapidly in infected specimens and to assess its presence elsewhere by indirect means, such as serology.

Specimen Smears. Material from a variety of specimens can be smeared on a glass slide and stained by an acid-fast method, such as the Ziehl-Neelsen or Kinyoun technique, or with fluorescent dyes, such as auramine or rhodamine. The latter enable more rapid screening and are generally considered to be more sensitive; however, false-positive results are more frequent.[521] As a result, the procedure was thus used by only about half of the diagnostic laboratories in the United States in 1992.[522]

The sensitivity of organism detection in sputum samples is enhanced by digestion and centrifugation before smearing. The number of organisms required for identification on smears is usually substantial; in one study of 18 patients treated for tuberculosis, the number of organisms per milliliter of sputum at the time of conversion from smear positive to smear negative was estimated to range from 150 to 70,000 (mean, 9,500).[367] Although it has been estimated that with optimal laboratory conditions, positive smears can be documented with only 100 to 1,000 organisms per milliliter in most cases,[523] a more practical estimate is perhaps 5,000 to 9,500. Overall, approximately 50% to 80% of patients with active pulmonary tuberculosis have positive smears, depending on the population screened and the particular microbiology laboratory in which the smears are evaluated.[8]

A smear showing acid-fast organisms is virtually diagnostic of tuberculosis in a patient with clinical and radiographic findings suggestive of the disease. In the absence of such a setting, an acid-fast smear may be a false-positive finding,[524] particularly in a population with a low prevalence of tuberculosis. The identification of organisms on smears during the course of therapy may represent the presence of nonviable bacilli or contamination by NTM;[525] however, the possibility of noncompliance or drug-resistant organisms must also be considered.

Routine Culture. All clinical specimens, whether or not smear positive, should be inoculated onto culture media to definitively identify a mycobacterial species and to determine antibiotic sensitivity. The procedure is much more sensitive than microscopic examination of acid-fast stained smears; it has been estimated, for example, that culture can detect as few as 10 organisms per milliliter of digested and concentrated sputum.[8] Thus, it is not uncommon for a patient to have a negative result by microscopy and a positive one on culture. For example, in one investigation, positive smears were obtained in 57% and positive cultures in 96% of patients with cavitary disease and in 32% and 70% of those with noncavitary disease.[526] In another large series, 25% of patients were found to be smear negative/culture positive before treatment (some even with far advanced cavitary disease).[527]

The possibility of a false-positive culture for *M. tuberculosis* should be considered in a patient whose presentation or course of disease is atypical. Such false-positive cases have been documented in as many as 4% of isolates by some investigators.[527a] The most common cause appears to be cross-contamination of specimens in the laboratory during initial processing.[527a]

Three satisfactory sputum specimens should be obtained for smear and culture; when disease is minimal radiographically, six are necessary. It has been recommended that cultures be made on two media;[8] specimens showing no growth after 6 to 8 weeks' incubation are generally considered negative. Standard solid media include an egg yolk–potato mixture (e.g., Lowenstein-Jensen medium) and an agar-based medium, such as Middlebrook. In terms of isolation rate and time, the use of a biphasic liquid/solid culture media system has been found to be superior to standard culture on Lowenstein-Jensen medium and equivalent to that of the BACTEC system (*see* farther on).[528–530] It has been argued that the procedure is more suitable than the BACTEC system for laboratories that have a small number of specimens or in situations in which the disposal of radioactive waste is a problem.[529] In fact, using a liquid Middlebrook medium for culture and a particle counting immunoassay (latex particles coated with mycobacterial antigens), one group of investigators was able to detect mycobacteria several days earlier than with a BACTEC system.[531]

Radiometric Techniques. One of the earliest and most widely used methods to reduce the diagnostic time in cultured specimens is radiometry. In this technique, a decontaminated, concentrated specimen is inoculated in a liquid culture medium to which ^{14}C-labeled palmitic acid has been added. Mycobacteria metabolize this substance and produce $^{14}CO_2$ which can be detected in a BACTEC instrument and quantified as a growth index. Using this procedure, the organism can be detected in as few as 7 to 8 days in smear-positive patients and 16 to 20 days in smear-negative patients (times that are approximately twice as fast as those with conventional culture).[532, 533] With the BACTEC method as a base, *M. tuberculosis* can be distinguished from other mycobacterial species by either biochemical[534] or nucleic acid probe[535, 536] techniques. In addition to its rapidity, the

BACTEC method results in an increased sensitivity in mycobacterial detection (approximately 70% to 95% versus 60% to 80% for routine culture),[532, 533, 537, 538] an attribute that is particularly valuable in smear-negative patients.

Serology. As in other infectious diseases, the use of serology to diagnose tuberculosis has been extensively investigated.[539, 540] Tests have been conducted using a variety of standard serologic techniques[541, 542] and, more recently, enzyme-linked immunosorbent assay. Many antigens have been used as substrate, including crude filtrates or sonicates of tubercle bacilli, PPD, and various purified or partly purified antigens, such as *M. tuberculosis* antigens 5 and 6; mycobacterial glycolipids SAG A1, B1, and C; plasma membrane antigens;[539] cord factor; and a BCG cytoplasmic antigen.[540] The sensitivity of the tests varies with the antigen used and the specific diagnostic cutoff level;[539] overall, it is probably in the order of 70% to 85% and is greatest with more highly purified antigens. The authors of one review published in 1987 suggested that a specificity of 0.97 or greater would be possible with techniques available at that time.[539] Investigators in the 1990s have found similar values; for example, sensitivities and specificities in three studies ranged from 70% to 80% and 90% to 98%.[543–545]

The routine use of serology in the diagnosis of tuberculosis is somewhat limited by these findings, and the procedure likely has its greatest value in specific situations, such as extrapulmonary disease (particularly meningeal[403–405] or osteoarticular[546]) and (possibly) childhood disease.[8, 539] As might be expected, the value of the test is limited in patients who are immunosuppressed.[547]

Detection of Specific Mycobacterial Chemicals. Several groups of investigators have measured mycobacterial compounds, such as mycolic acid and tuberculostearic acid, by gas, high-performance, or capillary chromatography in an attempt to identify the presence of organisms rapidly in clinical specimens.[548–551] The technique has been used both to detect organisms in sputum and to identify particular mycobacterial species in culture isolates.[8] Although the latter can be accomplished in a matter of hours, it requires a relatively large number of organisms, somewhat limiting its usefulness.[6]

Molecular Biologic Techniques. Techniques such as DNA hybridization, restriction fragment length analysis, and PCR offer great promise for more rapid and reliable identification and characterization of mycobacteria.[552–554] DNA hybridization techniques using isotopically labeled probes have been used to identify various mycobacterial species in culture specimens;[536, 555, 556] however, the number of organisms necessary for a positive result is relatively high, hampering their use in diagnosis. The use of nonisotopically labeled probes and hybridization techniques in which specific probes are not necessary has also been described.[556, 557]

By amplifying the DNA present in clinical specimens, PCR can greatly increase the likelihood of detecting organisms.[558–561] In fact, some investigators have shown that the technique allows the identification of organisms in as many as one third of culture-negative specimens.[562, 563] In addition, because the DNA probe used can be highly specific for particular *Mycobacteria*, a negative test is useful for determining that acid-fast organisms identified on a smear are or are not *M. tuberculosis*. The attractiveness of PCR as a diagnostic tool is also enhanced by the rapidity with which it can be carried out, results usually being available the same day it is performed;[563a] a technique for quantification of organisms has been described.[564] The procedure has been most extensively investigated in specimens of sputum and BAL fluid; however, it can be used with paraffin-embedded tissue fragments,[565] blood,[566] and fluids such as pleural effusion and cerebrospinal fluid.[567, 567a]

Despite these advantages, PCR is not without limitations. False-positive results have been estimated by some workers to occur in as many as 1% to 2% of specimens.[552] Some investigators have also found marked variation in the results of different laboratories in the analysis of a test sample.[568] Moreover, the procedure is of limited value in distinguishing between active and recently treated or remote disease.[569, 570] For example, in one investigation of sputum or BAL fluid specimens from 65 patients, 37 were found to have a positive signal for *M. tuberculosis*;[569] of these, 15 had a history of prior disease and no evidence of activity at the time of the test. Perhaps the most important limitation in the routine use of PCR for diagnosis is that its sensitivity has been found to be relatively low (50% to 80%) in smear-negative cases, in which the procedure would theoretically have the greatest use.[571–575]

Further development of technical procedures and attention to quality control in the laboratory will likely increase the utility of PCR in the near future.[576] For example, in one investigation of 27 patients with suspected pulmonary tuberculosis in whom three sputum specimens were smear negative, mycobacterial DNA was specifically concentrated from BAL fluid samples before PCR analysis (sequence capture PCR);[577] in addition, several special precautions were taken to decrease the likelihood of specimen contamination. Of the 27 patients, active tuberculosis was confirmed in 9; PCR was positive in all of these, including 3 in whom all clinical specimens were culture negative. The test was negative in the remaining 18 patients as well as in 25 control patients with historical or radiographic evidence of prior tuberculosis. Despite these results, until these or other techniques are widely available and well standardized, PCR is likely to be of greatest value in specific clinical situations, such as immunodeficiency (particularly HIV infection), childhood infection, and disease in extrapulmonary locations or with atypical presentations.[569, 578] The procedure is also useful in confirming that organisms in a smear-positive patient are *M. tuberculosis* so that appropriate therapy and public health measures can be rapidy instituted.

Restriction fragment length polymorphism (RFLP) analysis (genetic fingerprinting) has become a particularly useful technique in epidemiologic investigation of tuberculosis.[552, 579] The procedure is based on the use of specific DNA insertion sequences (the most extensively investigated being IS6110) that occur in a variable number of copies and in different positions in different mycobacterial strains. By detecting different sequence patterns in clinical isolates, reliable information can be acquired concerning the origin of local outbreaks of disease.[580–582] Similar information can also be obtained by spoligotyping,[582a] a procedure in which spacer sequences within the *M. tuberculosis* genome are amplified by a PCR technique and then identified by using synthetic oligomeric DNA sequences. Although this technique has less discriminatory power compared with RFLP, it has the advantage of not requiring culture of the organism.

Cytopathologic Examination

A number of abnormal cytologic features suggestive of tuberculosis have been described in specimens of tracheobronchial secretions.[583–585] However, although cytologic examination of sputum or bronchial washings and brushings is useful occasionally when it directs clinical attention to the possibility of tuberculosis, it is unlikely to be rewarding as a primary diagnostic method. In particular, it is unlikely to provide additional information to that derived from acid-fast examination of a sputum smear.

In one study of sputum specimens from 40 patients with tuberculosis, multinucleated Langhans' giant cells and elongated, poorly defined, and finely vacuolated cells (interpreted as epithelioid cells) were the most frequently identified abnormalities (present in 60%);[584] however, the same cells were also found in a variety of other conditions. In a companion study, epithelioid cells were found more often in sputum samples from patients with proven tuberculosis (28%) than in those with chronic nonspecific inflammation (3%) or carcinoma (2%), and Langhans' giant cells were present only in patients with tuberculosis.[585] However, because Langhans' giant cells can be seen with granulomatous inflammation of widely varying causes,[586] their presence is clearly of little value in establishing a specific diagnosis. In addition, the number of cases of tuberculosis in which Langhans' giant cells are identified is small.[585, 587] In those cases in which cytologic appearances are suggestive of tuberculosis, restaining of the smeared material or of cell block preparations by the Ziehl-Neelsen method may permit identification of the organism.[588]

Specimens obtained by transthoracic needle aspiration are more useful than sputum or bronchial washings in the cytologic diagnosis of tuberculosis. In one study of 1,255 aspirates, a cytologic diagnosis suggestive of tuberculosis was made in 179 instances on the basis of the presence of finely granular necrotic material (occasionally with calcified fragments), epithelioid and Langhans' giant cells, and an increased number of lymphocytes.[589] Bacteriologic or histologic correlation (or both) was available in 57 of the 179 cases, and the diagnosis of tuberculosis was confirmed in 42; there were 9 definite false-positive results (including sarcoidosis, nonspecific inflammation, and cancer). Of the remaining patients in whom bacteriologic or histologic correlation was not obtained, the vast majority experienced a clinical and radiologic course consistent with the diagnosis of tuberculosis. Although this experience and that of others[590, 591] indicate the potential usefulness of transthoracic needle aspiration (especially in tuberculomas), it is clear that definitive diagnosis in these specimens should always rest with culture of organisms or their identification within tissue fragments. When interpreting the results of transthoracic needle aspiration, it must be remembered that one of the most frequent causes of false-positive diagnosis of malignancy in these specimens is tuberculosis.[592] Fine needle aspiration has also been used effectively in the diagnosis of extrapulmonary tuberculosis.[593, 594]

Hematologic and Biochemical Investigation

The white blood count in active pulmonary tuberculosis is usually within normal limits, but may be increased to

10,000 to 15,000/mm³. Despite this, there is evidence indicating that lymphokines from T lymphocytes suppress granulocytes in the bone marrow.[595, 596] Anemia is common in chronic pulmonary or miliary disease,[119] possibly related to lymphokine-induced blunting of erythropoietin response.[597] A variety of additional hematologic reactions occur in miliary tuberculosis. There is often a leukemoid reaction (sometimes in the absence of radiographic evidence of disease[358]) and lymphopenia.[119, 357, 598] Pancytopenia (with or without aplastic bone marrow) may be present.[599] Occasional cases of acquired failure of granulocytic nuclear segmentation (Pelger-Huët anomaly),[600] immune-related thrombocytopenic purpura,[601] hemophagocytic syndrome,[602, 603] and disseminated intravascular coagulation (sometimes associated with ARDS)[604, 605] have also been reported.

Hypercalcemia is fairly common in patients with active tuberculosis,[606–608] the incidence varying from about 5% to 50% in different reviews.[609] The likelihood of its development probably depends on several factors, including sun exposure, vitamin D intake, and form of tuberculous disease.[609] In one investigation, the complication was shown to be related to the production of 1,25-dihydroxyvitamin D by immune cells recovered by BAL.[610] The abnormality may be masked by accompanying hypoalbuminemia and may not be recognized until the patient shows improvement in nutritional status under treatment for the disease.[608, 611] Many patients have been receiving supplemental vitamin D. Hypercalcemia usually is relatively mild and reverts to normal levels with therapy directed toward the infection.[611] It may be associated with hypokalemia, presumably as the result of distal tubular damage caused by the excess of calcium permitting increased renal excretion of potassium.[606]

Hyponatremia develops in some cases of pulmonary tuberculosis,[119, 612, 613] but is more common in tuberculous meningitis;[119] it probably represents the effect of inappropriate antidiuretic hormone secretion, an explanation supported by the finding of elevated antidiuretic hormone activity in extracts from tuberculous lung tissue.[613] In one prospective study of 50 patients with advanced pulmonary tuberculosis, 92% were found to have evidence of sick euthyroid syndrome and 73% of males to have hypogonadotrophic hypogonadism;[614] by contrast, hypoadrenalism was uncommon. Other investigators have found evidence of hypoadrenalism in 0% to 55% of patients.[614]

Increased levels of the acute-phase reactants, serum amyloid A protein and C-reactive protein, have been found in pulmonary tuberculosis associated with lung destruction;[615] in some individuals with long-standing disease, amyloidosis develops. Measurements of these substances may be valuable as an indicator of response to treatment. An increase in the level of the intercellular adhesion molecule-1 (ICAM-1) has been documented in patients with miliary and "far advanced" disease;[616] this increase is generally not seen in patients with milder forms of disease and diminishes with therapy. A mild-to-moderate increase in the serum level of angiotensin-converting enzyme is also seen in many patients with miliary disease.[355, 617] As discussed elsewhere (*see* pages 839 and 2746), measurement of adenosine deaminase in aspirated fluid has been found by some investigators to have a high specificity and sensitivity in the diagnosis of pericardial and pleural tuberculosis.[415, 416] One group has used a panel of markers, including acute-phase reactants,

enzymes, and antituberculous antibodies, in an attempt to distinguish between patients with inactive and active disease (both untreated and treated);[617a] using discriminant analysis to identify the best variables, correct classification could be achieved in about 90% of patients. Measurement of lysozyme and interferon-gamma in both fluid and serum has also been investigated for potential diagnostic use (*see* page 2746).[617b, c]

Pulmonary Function Tests

In the absence of chronic bronchitis and emphysema, most patients with pulmonary tuberculosis show little impairment of respiratory function, even in the presence of advanced disease. This probably reflects sparing of the lower lobes and anterior segments of the upper lobes; in addition, because the disease interferes equally with ventilation and perfusion, $\dot{V}/\dot{Q}$ abnormalities do not develop.[619] An exception to this general rule is miliary tuberculosis, in which pulmonary function tests not uncommonly show a restrictive pattern and a reduction in the diffusing capacity. With treatment and restoration of the chest radiograph to normal, the diffusing capacity may remain considerably below predicted normal values.[620] Pulmonary function tests are useful to assess patients before surgery and to determine objectively the degree of disability in patients with diffuse chronic destructive tuberculosis.

Natural History and Prognosis

In "developed" countries in the pre-AIDS era, patients who died with active tuberculosis were often elderly and chronically ill from associated disease; they were equally likely to succumb from the tuberculosis (often not recognized) as from the underlying illness.[621, 622] After the appearance of AIDS, the demographics have changed somewhat, with a peak mortality in the 25- to 55-year-old age group in the United States, particularly among African Americans and Hispanic Americans;[623] although this change is largely related to HIV infection, the presence of alcohol or drug abuse in the absence of AIDS also appears to be an important risk factor for death.[623, 624] Delay in diagnosis and the presence of a drug-resistant organism have also been associated with a poorer prognosis.[624] Surgery—sometimes standard pneumonectomy but often extrapleural pneumonectomy—is being increasingly used in patients in the latter situation as well as in selected patients with recurrent or massive hemoptysis or bronchopleural fistulas uncontrolled by other means.[625–628]

The development of miliary tuberculosis is associated with a particularly poor prognosis. The reasons are complex and may be related to a combination of the relatively wide extent of disease; the frequent presence of concomitant conditions, such as AIDS, malnutrition, and alcoholism; and the fairly frequent delay in diagnosis. Not uncommonly, the abnormality is first identified at autopsy.[358, 360, 629] Even when the diagnosis is made during life, the prognosis must be guarded; for example, in one review of 109 patients, 26 (24%) died a median of 6 days after the initiation of treatment.[355] The cause of death in these patients is variable;

some develop complicating disease, such as ARDS or disseminated intravascular coagulation.

Overall, the 4- to 5-year mortality rate of untreated tuberculosis is said to be about 50%.[52] Timely diagnosis and adequate chemotherapy can reduce this dramatically (by at least 95%); in the United States, the rate has decreased progressively in the twentieth century from 12.4 per 100,000 in 1953, to 4.9 in 1963, 1.8 in 1973, 0.8 in 1983, and 0.6 in 1993.[22] The cause of death is variable. Some patients die suddenly of massive pulmonary hemorrhage or respiratory failure related to tuberculous pneumonia or ARDS (or both).[362, 621, 630] In others, a definite cause of death is not found, even at autopsy;[631] in this group, cardiac arrhythmias are a likely mechanism.[621, 631]

The coexistence of pulmonary tuberculosis and pulmonary carcinoma has been reported by several groups of investigators, and a pathogenetic relationship has been implied.[632–635] Although the basis of such a relationship is not certain, it has been speculated that it may be the result of "reactivation" of the pulmonary tuberculosis, either by direct erosion of a focus of encapsulated caseous material by carcinoma or secondary to the more general debilitation associated with malignancy.[636] In three series of approximately 300 cases of coexistent disease, it was concluded that the high incidence in males and the location, variety, and frequency of the various primary lung neoplasms were as would be expected in pulmonary carcinoma without coexisting tuberculosis.[637–639] In one study in which 54 patients with both diseases were compared with 41 patients with pulmonary carcinoma and no evidence of tuberculosis, the carcinoma was located in the same general area in both groups.

Whether or not the relationship between carcinoma and tuberculosis is coincidental, the recovery of acid-fast bacilli from patients with an upper-lobe lesion should not overly delay procedures aimed at detecting a neoplasm. Suspicion of coexistent disease should be raised when patients with proven tuberculosis who are receiving antituberculous therapy show progressive radiographic resolution of some opacities while others persist unchanged or enlarge.[640] There is evidence that patients with pulmonary carcinoma who develop tuberculosis have a shorter survival time than those who do not.[634]

BACILLE CALMETTE-GUÉRIN

BCG is an avirulent strain of *M. bovis* that has been widely used in the preparation of a prophylactic vaccine against *M. tuberculosis*. It has been estimated that approximately 3 billion doses of the vaccine have been given since the strain was developed.[641] Although its effectiveness is not uniform, it is still advocated as a means of prevention in some individuals and populations at high risk.[642, 643] In fact, on the basis of a meta-analysis of published reports in 1994, one group estimated that the vaccine reduces the risk of tuberculosis by approximately 50%.[644]

Of a wide variety of uncommon clinical complications associated with use of BCG, the most frequent are local abscess formation and regional lymphadenitis.[645, 646] Systemic complications and fatal disease as a result of disseminated BCG are uncommon but have been documented in a number of patients, especially children with immunodeficiency syndromes.[645, 647, 648] Pathologic findings in these cases are variable and may consist of poorly formed granulomas with or without necrosis, aggregates of macrophages filled with bacilli, or (rarely) spindle cell lesions.[648]

In contrast to the rarity of clinically manifest disease, histologic alterations are present in an appreciable number of individuals vaccinated with BCG. For example, in one autopsy study of 26 such individuals who died of causes unrelated to the vaccination itself, microscopic granulomatous inflammation was found at the vaccination site and in axillary lymph nodes in 17 patients and in a variety of visceral organs in 13 (including the lungs in 6).[649] No granulomas were identified in patients who had been vaccinated more than 40 months before death; tubercle bacilli were identified within granulomas only in axillary lymph nodes. Similar findings have been reported by other investigators.[650]

Preparations of both BCG vaccine and the methanol-extracted residue of killed bacilli have also been used as nonspecific immunostimulants in the treatment of neoplastic disease, most commonly carcinoma of the bladder[650a, b] and to a lesser extent breast carcinoma, leukemia, and melanoma.[651, 652] These preparations can be administered intravenously, intradermally, subcutaneously, intravesically, or (in the case of melanoma) directly into the lesions; rarely, oral vaccine has been used.[653] Although complications can occur with all routes of administration, it has been suggested that some modes of administration are more likely to result in disease than others.[654] Because these preparations are administered to patients who may have immunodeficiency related to either chemotherapy or neoplasia and because they are usually given repeatedly and in relatively large doses, the incidence of complications is significantly greater than that following antituberculous vaccination.[655]

The pathogenesis of therapy-related BCG pneumonitis may be related to two mechanisms. The most obvious is direct infection by the organism, a mechanism confirmed in some cases by the results of culture or histologic identification of acid-fast bacteria.[656–658] Moreover, BCG-related disease has occurred in some patients months or years after intravesical BCG instillation, sometimes after steroid therapy, suggesting reactivation of dormant organisms.[655] Despite these observations, identification of the organism is rare, and resolution of disease has been reported with corticosteroid therapy alone, leading some investigators to speculate that disease in some patients is the result of a hypersensitivity reaction.[659–661]

The spectrum of disease is variable.[662] Clinically and radiographically insignificant granulomas have been identified in individuals administered BCG by intravenous, intradermal, intravesical, and intralesional routes.[654, 662, 663, 663a] Similar histologic findings have also been demonstrated experimentally in dogs administered methanol-extracted residue intravenously, in the absence of apparent clinical or biochemical abnormality.[664] Both methanol-extracted residue and BCG therapy have also been associated with radiographic and HRCT changes indistinguishable from miliary tuberculosis, the latter by far the more common.[663, 663a, 665] Histologic examination of biopsy specimens from affected patients has shown necrotizing granulomas similar in all respects to miliary tuberculosis but in which organisms are rarely identified.[666] Clinical symptoms include fever, weight loss, fatigue, cough, and dyspnea. Some patients develop sepsis and shock.[667]

NONTUBERCULOUS MYCOBACTERIA

A small but increasing proportion of mycobacterial infection is caused by organisms other than *M. tuberculosis* or *M. bovis*; these have been referred to variously as *anonymous, atypical, chromogenic,* or *unclassified* mycobacteria, but are perhaps best designated *nontuberculous.*[668, 669] Features common to these organisms include ready growth of almost all strains on culture at 25 or 37° C (in contrast to *M. tuberculosis,* which grows only at 37° C) and nonpathogenicity for guinea pigs. Overall, approximately 20 species have been associated with human disease;[669] a number of these are rare, and some published reports may, in fact, represent examples of colonization or specimen contamination rather than true infection.[670] Of the several classification schemes developed to encompass these bacilli, that of Runyon[671] has come to be almost universally accepted. According to this scheme, organisms can be considered in four groups on the basis of cultural characteristics (principally, the presence or absence of pigment and the rate of growth).

Group I: The Photochromogens. Photochromogens include organisms that produce nonpigmented colonies when grown in the dark and pigmented ones (orange) after reincubation and exposure to light. The most important pathogen is *M. kansasii,* which is associated with pulmonary disease and, occasionally, cervical adenitis and disseminated disease. *M. marinum* causes principally skin and lymph node infection; *M. simiae* and *M. asiaticum*[672] have been shown to cause pulmonary disease occasionally (and in some centers have constituted a significant proportion of all NTM isolates.[672a])

Group II: The Scotochromogens. Scotochromogens produce yellow-to-orange pigmented colonies in either light or dark conditions; *M. szulgai* is scotochromogenic when grown at 37° C but photochromogenic at 25° C. The disease-producing organisms in this group are *M. scrofulaceum,* which characteristically produces a scrofula-like picture and rarely causes pulmonary disease; *M. szulgai,* which has been identified as the responsible agent in occasional cases of pulmonary infection; and *M. gordonae,* a common but usually nonpathogenic saprophyte that has rarely been associated with pulmonary disease.[673, 674, 674a]

Group III: The Nonphotochromogens. As expected from the name, colonies of nonphotochromogens are characteristically nonpigmented (white to beige) in both light and dark (with the exception of *M. xenopi,* which is scotochromogenic). This group contains the largest number of species of NTM pathogenic for humans, including the *M. avium* complex (*M. avium* and *M. intracellulare*), *M. xenopi,* the *M. terrae* complex (*M. nonchromogenicum, M. terrae,* and *M. trivale*),[675, 676] *M. malmoense, M. ulcerans, M. haemophilum,*[695] *M. shimoidei, M. genavense, M. celatum,* and *M. gastri.*[670]

By far the most important of these is the *M. avium* complex. Although initially designated as individual species because of their different pathogenicity for chickens, *M. avium* and *M. intracellulare* show some overlap of biologic characteristics and are not distinguishable by common labo-

ratory methods (although genetic probes can accomplish the task reliably and rapidly).[668] Consequently, the two organisms are frequently referred to as the *M. avium complex,* or *M. avium-intracellulare.* (Some observers have also included *M. scrofulaceum* in the group because of similar antigenic and biochemical properties and have referred to the whole group as the *MAIS complex* [*M. avium-intracellulare-scrofulaceum*]).[668] The organisms are particularly important as a cause of disease in patients with AIDS (*see* page 1654).

Group IV: The Rapid Growers. Rapid growers take only 3 to 5 days to reach full growth in culture. Human disease is caused by several species, including *M. fortuitum, M. chelonae, M. abscessus, M. peregrinum,* and *M. smegmatis;*[677] because of a number of similarities, these organisms are frequently grouped as the *M. fortuitum-chelonae* complex.[678, 679] The organisms produce skin and subcutaneous abscesses and pulmonary disease. In culture, coloring characteristically is identical to that of group III organisms, the two groups being most readily differentiated by their rate of growth.

Specific organisms within these four Runyon groups can be identified by biochemical analysis, serologic testing, chromatography, and genetic probes.[680] The majority of NTM pulmonary infections are caused by a few species, including *M. kansasii, M. chelonae* complex, and *M. avium-intracellulare;* however, new or previously nonpathogenic species are being seen more frequently, particularly in immunocompromised patients,[680, 681] and specific organisms may assume prominence in particular geographic regions. Most infections can be considered to fall in one of four clinical groups: pulmonary disease or cervical lymphadenitis in immunocompetent individuals, disseminated disease in immunocompromised patients, and local skin disease.[682]

Epidemiology

General Features

As with tuberculosis, the incidence of disease caused by NTM varies considerably throughout the world; in fact, there is evidence for a reciprocal relationship between the two diseases, the incidence of one being lower in areas in which the other is greater.[683] In the United States, it has been estimated that the overall incidence of NTM disease between 1981 and 1983 was 1.78 per 100,000.[682] The incidence per 100,000 for specific organisms was estimated as follows: *M. avium* complex, 1.28; *M. kansasii,* 0.33; *M. chelonae* complex, 0.19; and *M. scrofulaceum,* 0.11.[682] As a result of the AIDS epidemic, the proportion of tuberculous disease caused by NTM—particularly *M. avium* complex—has increased significantly in the last 15 years. There is also evidence that the number of cases is increasing in the non-AIDS population, at least in some areas of the world;[684–686] possible reasons include an aging population, improved methods for detecting organisms in clinical specimens, increased physician awareness of the disease, and increased exposure of patients to the source of the organism.[687]

When considering incidence figures, it must be remembered that there is considerable geographic variation: for example, in a study from Milwaukee published in 1979, 27% of all mycobacterial disease seen over a 3.5-year period was caused by nontuberculous organisms.[688] Similarly, a Veterans Administration Armed Forces study indicated a 21% incidence of NTM infection in the southern United States in 1965.[689] The incidence of infection by different species also shows marked geographic variation; for example, in southeast England between 1977 and 1984, the number of documented cases was greatest for *M. xenopi,* followed by *M. kansasii* and *M. avium* complex.[690] By contrast, *M. kansasii* infection is rare in Australia[691] and relatively common in parts of the southern United States.[692] Definite or probable *M. simiae* infection, which is generally rare, was found in 15 (15%) of 62 patients in whom the organism was isolated in San Antonio, Texas (the remaining isolates being considered saprophytes).[672a] The precise basis for this geographic variation in the incidence of species isolation is unknown but is presumably related, at least partly, to regional differences in mycobacterial habitat.

NTM pulmonary infection is rare in children.[693, 694] Most immunocompetent patients are men over the age of 50 years at the time of diagnosis.[683, 678, 692] Despite this, there is evidence that the disease is increasing in frequency in younger individuals and in women.[696, 697] Because the vast majority of immunocompromised patients who develop NTM infection have AIDS, the age and sex incidence for the disease in this group parallels that of AIDS itself.

NTM infection can be acquired by a variety of mechanisms,[678] including inhalation; ingestion; direct inoculation after trauma; and iatrogenically via syringe needles, medical instruments such as bronchoscopes and otoscopes,[698, 699] intravenous catheters,[700] and surgical skin incisions (e.g., after augmentation mammoplasty and median sternotomy[701, 702]). Although animal-to-human transmission may occur with some species (e.g., *M. simiae*), it is likely uncommon. Human-to-human transmission has not been convincingly documented; although familial clusters of disease have been reported occasionally, suggesting the possibility of person-to-person transmission, a common source of infection is more likely.[703, 704] The natural habitat of most NTM appears to be water, either natural as in rivers or ponds, or destined for human use (e.g., tap water, swimming pool, aquarium); depending on the species, the habitat can also be soil, dust, milk and milk products, and a variety of animal species.[668] Because many of the organisms are found in water, contamination of hospital water supplies can result in both true nosocomial infection and "pseudoinfection" (the latter sometimes related to bronchoscopy).[705, 706]

Although some patients diagnosed as having nontuberculous pulmonary disease are otherwise healthy,[688, 707] many have underlying lung disease. The most common associated conditions are chronic obstructive pulmonary disease (COPD), healed tuberculosis or fungal disease, bronchiectasis, alveolar proteinosis, pneumoconiosis (particularly silicosis), and cystic fibrosis (*see* farther on).[668, 708–711] Some investigators have found evidence of an association with pectus excavatum and scoliosis.[712] An increased risk of NTM infection has also been observed in patients with rheumatoid disease, diabetes mellitus, heart disease, alcoholism, and achalasia and in those who have had a partial gastrectomy.[668, 710, 713] It is also clear that immunocompromised patients are at increased risk for NTM infection; although this is particularly pertinent with respect to patients with AIDS (*see* page 1655), those with malignancy (particularly hairy cell

leukemia[714–716]), with organ transplants,[717, 718] and receiving corticosteroid or other immunosuppressive therapy are also at increased risk. One group of investigators found an association between neutropenia and *M. chelonae* infection in three patients.[719]

It has also become evident that patients with cystic fibrosis are at increased risk of NTM infection.[720–722] A review of the records from several institutions and of eight prospective investigations conducted from 1990 to 1995 revealed the presence of 84 positive NTM cultures from 644 patients (13%).[723] Approximately 50% of the cases with available material for examination (41 of 77) were smear positive. PPD reactions were positive (5 to 10 mm) in 23 of 73 patients (32%) tested. Most isolated species have been *M. avium* complex (55%) or *M. abscessus* (36%);[723] rarely, more than one species is identified in the same patient. Although many cases in which an NTM is isolated probably represent no more than airway colonization,[726] it is clear from the pathologic identification of granulomatous inflammation or the resolution of radiologic disease after therapy that some cases represent true, invasive disease.[724] The distinction between the two in the absence of histologic confirmation can be difficult (*see* farther on).

Specific Mycobacteria

Mycobacterium avium Complex

Organisms of the *M. avium* complex are widely distributed in water and soil throughout the world and have occasionally been isolated from dust, plants, raw milk, and even cigarettes.[697, 725, 727] They are particularly common in water, having been identified in such diverse sources as natural ponds, lakes, rivers, swamps, and bogs; public baths; and public drinking water systems. Pulmonary disease is believed to occur primarily by aerosol inhalation, and cervical lymphadenitis by ingestion of organisms derived from these sources.[668, 725, 728] As the name suggests, the organism also infects animals other than humans, particularly pigs and poultry; however, there is no evidence of significant animal-to-human transmission.

Overall, *M. avium-intracellulare* is the most common NTM to cause human disease. Moreover, with *M. kansasii* and *M. chelonae* complex, it comprises the vast majority of pulmonary infections in immunocompetent individuals. As with many other NTM, such infection is often associated with prior lung disease, such as COPD, pneumoconiosis, and bronchiectasis; a dusty environment, such as seen in some mines and farms, has also been identified as a risk factor.[668] The bacillus is also the most frequently identified organism in NTM-related lymphadenitis. Finally, it has become an important cause of disease in patients with AIDS, up to 50% of whom acquire the infection at some point during the course of their illness (*see* page 1654).

Mycobacterium kansasii

As indicated previously, *M. kansasii* is one of the more common pathogenic NTM in some parts of the world, such as the mid-southern United States, Wales, and southern England.[690, 692, 729, 730] In other geographic regions, such as Australia,[691] it is isolated relatively uncommonly. The bacillus has been detected by some investigators in water samples, including tap water,[731] in which it appears to be able to survive for long periods;[732] it has been suggested that infection occurs via aerosol dispersion from this source.[733] The organism has seldom been isolated from the soil.[725] In most immunocompetent individuals who acquire the infection, disease is confined to the lungs;[692] occasionally, the organism causes lymphadenitis.[734] Underlying lung disease, including pneumoconiosis and COPD, is common.[692, 730, 735, 736] A history of alcohol abuse has been noted by some investigators.[737] In immunocompromised individuals, underlying pulmonary disease is often absent, and the infection is not uncommonly disseminated.[692, 738]

Mycobacterium marinum

Infection with *M. marinum* is probably acquired by direct contact with contaminated fresh or salt water. As such, most reported cases have been in workers in the fishing industry[739] or individuals who come into contact with aquaria;[740, 741] as might be expected, skin cuts or abrasions appear to be an additional risk factor. Most infections are confined to the skin of the extremities; occasionally, there is extension into adjacent soft tissue or regional lymph nodes. Rarely, and typically in immunocompromised patients, the disease is disseminated.[742]

Mycobacterium simiae

As the name suggests, *M. simiae* was initially isolated from monkeys.[743] It can be transmitted from animal to animal and possibly from animal to human via aerosol or fecal-oral routes.[725] It has also been isolated from water. Overall, pulmonary disease is relatively uncommon;[744, 745] however, as indicated previously, the organism has been found to cause a high proportion of NTM disease in some regions.[672a] Disseminated infection occurs rarely.[746]

Mycobacterium scrofulaceum

M. scrofulaceum has been cultured from water in natural lakes and rivers[747] but appears to be rare or absent from drinking water (at least in the United States).[725] It has also been isolated from raw milk and other dairy products and can sometimes be found in the oropharynx of healthy subjects.[668] It is known particularly as a cause of cervical lymphadenitis in children.[668, 734] Pulmonary infection has also been documented in a number of reports, most often in adults with underlying lung disease, such as previous tuberculosis, pneumoconiosis, and COPD.[725] A particular association with arc welding has been noted.[725]

Mycobacterium szulgai

The source of *M. szulgai* is uncertain but is believed to be environmental.[725] There appears to be no particular geographic association with infection.[748] Most cases involve the lungs; however, bone, joint, bursa, and skin diseases are not uncommon. Dissemination occurs rarely.[749]

Mycobacterium xenopi

M. xenopi has been identified in tap water and shower heads[733, 750] and has been shown to be responsible for nosocomial outbreaks of disease traced to contaminated water systems.[751] The organism can grow at 45° C and has been isolated from both hot and cold water; in fact, it has been speculated that it proliferates in water heating systems.[725] Infection by *M. xenopi* is relatively common in some parts of the world; for example, in London, England,[752] and in Ontario,[753] it was considered to be the second most common NTM to cause disease in the 1970s. Pulmonary disease is the most frequent manifestation of infection.[753, 754]

Mycobacterium malmoense

M. malmoense has been isolated from soil, water, and both healthy and immunocompromised humans;[725] because of its isolation in the former individuals, it has been speculated that it might be a human commensal.[725] It is a relatively uncommon cause of infection, only about 200 cases having been documented by 1996.[725] The incidence of disease appears to be increasing,[756–758] however, and in some areas of the world, such as Sweden and Great Britain, it is a particularly important cause of NTM-related disease.[759] Most infections involve the lungs and cervical lymph nodes. One group documented the combination of *M. malmoense* and *Aspergillus* infection in three patients with COPD;[760] disease was progressive and led to death in all patients.

Mycobacterium haemophilum

The precise source of *M. haemophilum* is uncertain; possibilities include water, animal reservoirs such as frogs, and soil.[725] The organism does not grow at temperatures above 35° C, presumably explaining its predilection for cutaneous infection. Despite this, disseminated disease (including the lungs) can occur.[761, 762] The majority of infections have occurred in immunocompromised patients, particularly those with AIDS or who have received an organ transplant;[763, 764] a number of cases have also been documented in patients undergoing renal dialysis.[765]

Mycobacterium genavense

M. genavense is a relatively recently discovered mycobacterial species that has been particularly associated with infection in patients with AIDS.[766] The organism has been difficult to culture, failing to grow on standard solid media and, in some studies, taking up to 5 to 6 weeks to identify using a BACTEC system.[767] The source is unknown but has been speculated to be the human intestine.[725]

Mycobacterium chelonae Complex

The *M. chelonae* complex (comprising *M. chelonae*, *M. fortuitum*, and *M. abscessus*) is a particularly important cause of human disease among the NTM. Cases have been reported throughout the world, in some regions with a relatively high incidence.[768] The organisms are widely distributed in the environment and have been isolated from many water sources, including natural rivers, lakes, and seas and human drinking and waste water.[769] Strains of *M. fortuitum* (and possibly the other two species[725]) have also been isolated from soil and dust.[668]

Infections by these organisms are most common in the lungs and skin, the latter often related to trauma or surgical wound infection.[770] The organisms have been associated with nosocomial infection from several sources, including gentian violet solution,[771] bronchoscopes, and prostheses.[772] Some NTM have been shown experimentally to favor a lipid medium for growth,[773] an observation possibly relevant to the association of pulmonary infection by the *M. chelonae* complex with esophageal obstruction and mineral oil aspiration.[768, 773, 774] Underlying lung disease appears to be relatively uncommon compared to infection by other NTM; for example, in one investigation of 154 cases of pulmonary disease caused by rapid growers, previously treated mycobacterial disease was evident in 18% of patients and cystic

fibrosis in 6%.[768] Immunosuppression is evident in a minority of patients, but is more likely to be associated with dissemination.[775]

Pathologic Characteristics

In most cases, gross and histologic characteristics of pulmonary disease caused by NTM are identical to those of *M. tuberculosis* and are characterized by a variable degree fibrosis, cavitation, granulomatous inflammation, and caseation necrosis (Fig. 27–47).[776–778] Bronchial spread (resulting in bronchopneumonia or, sometimes, an endobronchial ulcer[779]) and miliary disease can occur, albeit less often than in tuberculosis. Because of the relatively frequent association with underlying chronic pulmonary disease, gross abnormali-

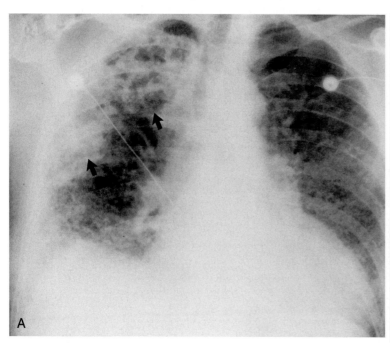

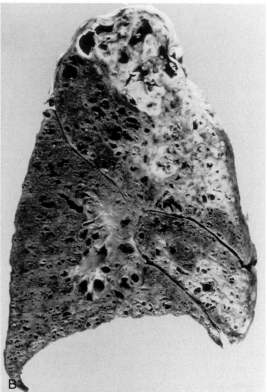

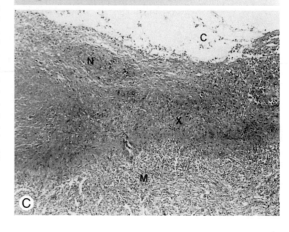

Figure 27–47. *Mycobacterium xenopi* **Pneumonia Superimposed on Idiopathic Pulmonary Fibrosis.** An anteroposterior chest radiograph *(A)* discloses inhomogeneous consolidation (superolateral to *arrows*) in the right upper lobe. Elsewhere in both lungs, there is a medium and coarse reticulonodular pattern consistent with diffuse interstitial fibrosis. The heart is moderately enlarged. The patient was a 69-year-old man who had complained of increasing dyspnea for 2 years, associated with nonproductive cough beginning 4 months previously. Prednisone therapy was instituted for a presumed diagnosis of idiopathic pulmonary fibrosis. The patient died shortly after this radiograph was obtained. A sagittal slice of the right lung *(B)* removed at autopsy shows typical features of idiopathic pulmonary fibrosis, with a "honeycomb" appearance in the basal aspect of the lower lobe. The upper and middle lobes also show extensive consolidation (white tissue in illustration). Spaces within the consolidated regions represent combined cavitation (evacuation of necrotic material) and cysts related to the underlying interstitial fibrosis. Histologically *(C)*, the appearance is indistinguishable from that caused by *Mycobacterium tuberculosis*, with cavity formation (C) and zones of necrotic material (N), epithelioid histiocytes (X), and mononuclear cells (M). Premortem culture of bronchial washings grew *Mycobacterium xenopi*. (*C*, ×60.)

ties caused by the organism may be difficult to identify, particularly in early infection (Fig. 27–48).

A definitive histologic diagnosis of the nontuberculous nature of the disease is usually not possible (with the possible exception of disseminated *M. avium-intracellulare* infection in AIDS [*see* farther on]). This was well illustrated in a study of 25 histopathologic slides of mycobacterial disease interpreted "blindly" by 27 pathologists as to their tuberculous or nontuberculous cause;[780] in 53% of judgments, the distinction was believed to be impossible, and in an additional 22% in which the "typical" or "atypical" nature was specified, the diagnosis was incorrect.

Lymph node biopsy specimens show a variety of patterns, including non-necrotizing granulomas (as in sarcoidosis), typical necrotizing (caseating) granulomas, and granulomas with abundant central polymorphonuclear leukocytes (similar to cat-scratch disease).[781] Some investigators have suggested that the presence of "atypical" features, such as ill-defined granulomas, irregular or serpiginous granulomas, predominantly sarcoid-like granulomas, lack of significant caseation, or a predominance of neutrophils in the center of areas of necrosis, is more likely with NTM than *M. tuberculosis* infection.[782]

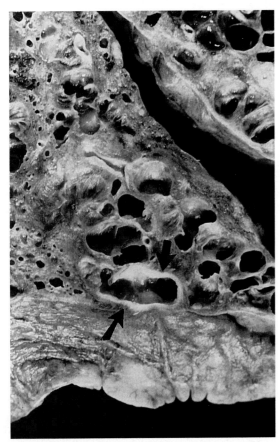

Figure 27–48. Bronchiectasis with Early *M. avium-intracellulare* Infection. A magnified view of a portion of the lower lobe and lingula shows patchy parenchymal fibrosis and prominent cylindric bronchiectasis. The wall of one bronchus *(arrow)* is thickened and white as a result of *Mycobacterium avium-intracellulare* infection (the organism was isolated from premortem specimens and sections of the airway wall showed necrotizing granulomatous inflammation). Such early disease can be easily overlooked on cursory examination.

The appearance of organisms in tissue specimens is also usually of no help in differentiating nontuberculous from tuberculous species. *M. kansasii* tends to be longer, thicker, and more coarsely beaded than *M. tuberculosis*, and the Ziehl-Neelsen stain may suggest the cause when such organisms are present.[668, 777] *M. avium-intracellulare* is smaller than most other mycobacteria and may be more difficult to recognize on smears; intracellular organisms within macrophages of patients with AIDS stain with periodic acid–Schiff.[592] The auramine-O fluorescent technique has been advocated as being superior to standard acid-fast stains in detecting nontuberculous organisms; however, although the technique probably has a higher sensitivity, it also has a lower specificity.[783] The advantages and limitations of these and other techniques for demonstrating NTM have been discussed in detail.[784] The use of PCR technology on paraffin-embedded tissue will undoubtedly greatly increase the rapidity, sensitivity, and specificity of pathologic diagnosis.[785]

The histologic characteristics of NTM infection may be altered in patients who are immunocompromised.[784, 786, 787] This is particularly noteworthy in some children and patients with AIDS infected with *M. avium-intracellulare*, in whom aggregates of macrophages stuffed with organisms may be associated with minimal or absent granulomatous reaction and necrosis (Fig. 27–49).[788, 789] This appearance seems to be characteristic of infection in these patient groups; disease caused by the organism in patients with other immunodeficient states (although itself often histologically atypical) often does not show the same pattern.[787] An abnormal reaction has also been well documented in patients with hairy cell leukemia, in whom infection by *M. kansasii*,[714] *M. scrofulaceum*, and *M. avium-intracellulare*[790] has been characterized histologically by the presence of necrotic, eosinophilic debris containing a polymorphonuclear infiltrate and a virtual absence of granulomatous response (Fig. 27–50).

Occasionally, lung biopsy specimens from patients who apparently are not immunocompromised reveal nonspecific chronic inflammation without a granulomatous component and yet grow an NTM species on culture;[776, 778] although the significance of this finding is not clear, it is probably best to consider the positive culture a result of colonization or contamination, while recognizing the possibility that the histologic reaction itself may be atypical.[776]

Radiologic Manifestations

As with the pathologic features, there is considerable overlap between the radiologic patterns of pulmonary disease caused by NTB and that caused by *M. tuberculosis*, precluding confident distinction between the two in any particular case (Fig. 27–51).[309, 791–795] Nevertheless, certain patterns are seen more commonly in NTB and may be helpful in suggesting the diagnosis in the appropriate clinical setting.[309, 796]

The radiographic findings of pulmonary disease caused by *M. avium* complex were initially assessed in a series of 114 nonimmunocompromised patients with at least two positive sputum cultures, no history of previous tuberculosis, and no other potential causative pathogen.[792] Six per cent of patients had normal radiographs, 10% had minimal disease, and 84% had moderately or far advanced disease. The abnor-

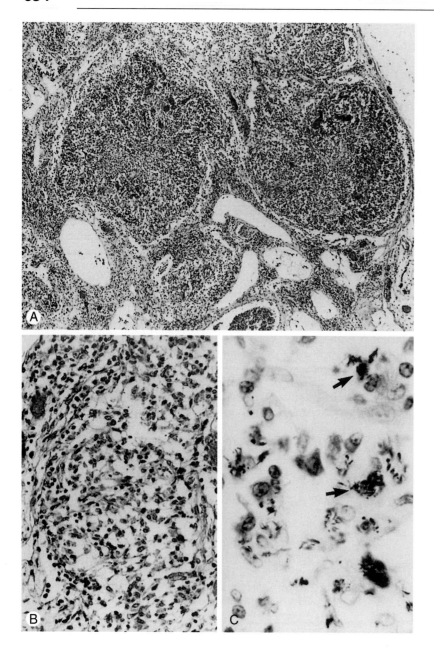

Figure 27–49. AIDS—*Mycobacterium avium-in-tracellulare* Infection. A portion of a mediastinal lymph node *(A)* taken from a patient with AIDS at autopsy shows lymphoid depletion and lack of germinal centers. Complete absence of granulomatous or other inflammatory reaction is noted. A magnified view *(B)* shows that many of the residual cells are histiocytes. Acid-fast stain *(C)* reveals the cells to contain numerous organisms *(arrows)*. (*A,* ×48; *B,* ×200; *C,* ×1000.)

malities involved the apical or posterior segments of the upper lobes in 92% of patients and were bilateral in 66% of cases. Seventy-seven per cent had cavitation, which was usually multiple; in the majority of cases, at least one of the cavities measured greater than 2 cm in diameter. Scarring and volume loss were common, occurring to some degree in 70% of upper-lobe foci. Evidence of endobronchial spread was seen in 81% of cases. Pleural effusions were uncommon (5% of cases) and usually small. Only 4% of patients had hilar or mediastinal lymphadenopathy. Subsequent investigators have found a lower prevalence of cavitation; for example, one or more cavities were identified on chest radiographs in 15 (43%) of 35[793] and 15 (38%) of 40[794] patients in two series and on HRCT scans in 8 (20%) of 40,[797] 9 (28%) of 32,[309] and 36 (65%) of 55[798] patients in three other investigations (Fig. 27–52). For unknown reasons, it appears that cavitation associated with *M. avium* complex disease is more

common in men than in women, particularly individuals in their sixties and seventies.[793, 794, 799]

A second radiographic pattern seen in patients with pulmonary disease caused by *M. avium* complex consists of bilateral small nodular opacities.[309, 794, 799, 800] The nodules usually are well circumscribed, measure less than 1 cm in diameter, and have a centrilobular distribution.[309, 797, 798] They have a tendency for a patchy distribution in all lobes,[309] although they occasionally involve predominantly the upper lobes (Fig. 27–53) or middle lobe and lingula.[794, 798, 799] This pattern occurs in 20% to 50% of cases of *M. avium* complex infection in nonimmunocompromised patients and is seen more commonly in women, who are affected in approximately 80% of cases.[309, 797, 799, 800] On HRCT, most of these patients have bronchiectasis (Fig. 27–53),[309, 798, 801] usually involving several lobes;[309, 801] occasionally, it involves only the middle lobe and lingular bronchi.[798] Pathologic correla-

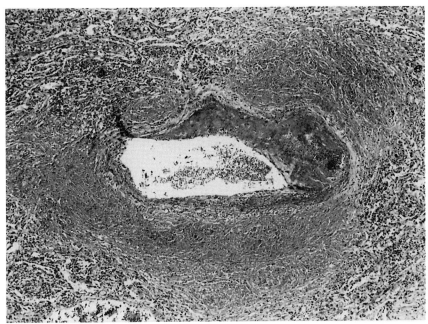

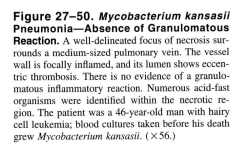

Figure 27–50. *Mycobacterium kansasii* **Pneumonia—Absence of Granulomatous Reaction.** A well-delineated focus of necrosis surrounds a medium-sized pulmonary vein. The vessel wall is focally inflamed, and its lumen shows eccentric thrombosis. There is no evidence of a granulomatous inflammatory reaction. Numerous acid-fast organisms were identified within the necrotic region. The patient was a 46-year-old man with hairy cell leukemia; blood cultures taken before his death grew *Mycobacterium kansasii*. (×56.)

tion shows that most of the nodules correspond to foci of granulomatous inflammation in lung parenchyma or peribronchial interstitial tissue.[797]

Both the incidence and the pattern of bronchiectasis differ in disease caused by *M. tuberculosis* and *M. avium* complex. In one study in which the HRCT findings were compared in 45 patients with pulmonary tuberculosis and 32 with *M. avium* complex, centrilobular nodules, consolidation, and cavity formation were seen with similar frequency in both infections.[309] Bronchiectasis, however, was identified on HRCT in 27% of patients with tuberculosis and 94% of patients with *M. avium* complex. When bronchiectasis was present, it involved a mean of 1.8 lobes in patients with tuberculosis and a mean of 4.6 lobes in patients with *M. avium* complex. In patients with tuberculosis, bronchiectasis most commonly involved the upper lobes, whereas in those with *M. avium* complex there was no lobar predominance.

The diagnostic significance of small nodules and the potential relationship with *M. avium* complex infection in patients with bronchiectasis was further assessed in a review of the HRCT scans and medical records of 100 patients with a CT diagnosis of bronchiectasis.[802] Twenty-four of the 100 patients had multiple nodules measuring 2 to 15 mm in diameter; in 19 of these, the nodules were in the same lobe as the bronchiectasis, and in the other 5 they were in different lobes. Mycobacterial cultures were performed on 63 of the 100 patients, including 15 of the 24 patients with lung nodules and 48 of the 76 patients without. Eight of the 15 patients with nodules (53%) had positive cultures for *M. avium* complex compared with only 3 (4%) of patients with no evidence of lung nodules. No other mycobacterial species were cultured in these patients. Although these observations suggest that the presence of multiple small nodules on CT in patients with bronchiectasis should prompt culture of tracheobronchial secretions, the implications of the subsequent identification of *M. avium* complex are controversial because it is not clear whether the presence of the organism is related to colonization or true infection.

This issue was addressed in another study of the HRCT findings in 40 patients with NTM, including 34 with *M. avium* complex. Bronchiectasis was identified on initial assessment in approximately 80% of cases, air-space consolidation in 70%, nodules in 70%, and cavities in 20%.[797] Ten patients had two to four serial CT scans with a follow-up ranging from 2 to 42 months. Each lung was divided into five zones: apical and posterior segments of upper lobe, anterior segment of upper lobe, middle lobe or lingula, superior segment of lower lobe, and basilar segments of lower lobe. Of the 100 lung zones, new disease developed in 12; bronchiectasis appeared in 10, preceded by nodules in the same 3 zones. New nodules appeared in 10 of the 100 zones, areas of consolidation in 9, and cavitation in 5. The bronchiectasis became more severe in six zones and less severe in one. These observations suggest that *M. avium* complex may, in fact, cause the bronchiectasis and that the presence of nodules in patients with bronchiectasis and positive culture is suggestive of pathogenic as opposed to saprophytic mycobacterial disease (Fig. 27–54).[797, 800]

An unusual pattern of clinical and radiologic findings has been reported in five patients who developed respiratory illness after use of hot tubs contaminated with *M. avium* complex.[803] The radiographs were reported as showing "interstitial infiltrates" or a miliary nodular pattern. HRCT showed patchy areas of ground-glass attenuation and ill-defined centrilobular nodules, findings consistent with a diagnosis of hypersensitivity pneumonitis.

The radiographic characteristics of *M. kansasii* pulmonary infection were reviewed in a study of 187 cases.[791] The chest radiograph was normal in 2% of patients, showed minimal abnormalities in 2%, and showed moderate or severe abnormalities in 96%. The abnormalities involved the upper lobes in all but one case; in every one, the upper-lobe disease began posterior to the trachea. The most frequent radiographic finding was cavitation, seen in 96% of patients with parenchymal abnormalities; 60% of patients had four or more cavities.[791] Evidence of endobronchial spread was

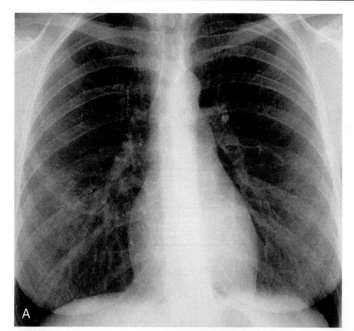

Figure 27–51. Pulmonary *Mycobacterium avium* Complex Infection. *A* posteroanterior chest radiograph *(A)* in a 28-year-old woman shows poorly defined small nodular opacities in the right lower lobe. Views of the right lung from an HRCT scan *(B* and *C)* demonstrate a cavity (C) in the right lower lobe associated with pleural tags *(open arrows)* and several centrilobular nodular opacities *(closed arrows)*. Three sputum cultures grew *M. avium* complex. The findings are indistinguishable from those of tuberculosis.

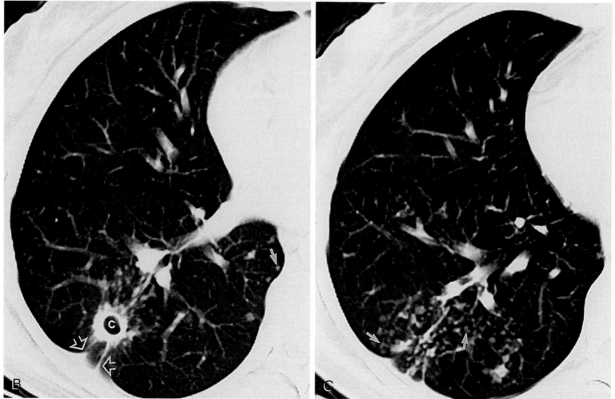

present in 63% of patients and bilateral parenchymal abnormalities in 41% (Fig. 27–55).[791] Scarring and volume loss were present in 68% of patients with upper-lobe foci. Blunting of the posterior or lateral costophrenic sulcus as a result of mild pleural thickening or small pleural effusion was uncommon (4%). In a subsequent study, the investigators compared the radiographic findings in 49 patients with *M. kansasii* infection and 27 with *M. tuberculosis*.[804] Solitary thin-walled cavities were seen in 39% of patients with *M. kansasii*, compared with only 4% of patients with *M. tuberculosis*; multiple thin-walled cavities were found in 45%

and 18% of patients, respectively. Patients with tuberculosis tended to show more extensive parenchymal disease than patients with *M. kansasii*. Given the greater prevalence of tuberculosis compared with nontuberculous disease in most populations, the findings have no predictive power in any individual case.

In another study in which the radiographic findings of 28 patients with pulmonary *M. kansasii* disease were compared with those of 56 patients with tuberculosis, no significant difference was seen in the prevalence, number, or size of cavities.[796] Areas of consolidation, however, were more

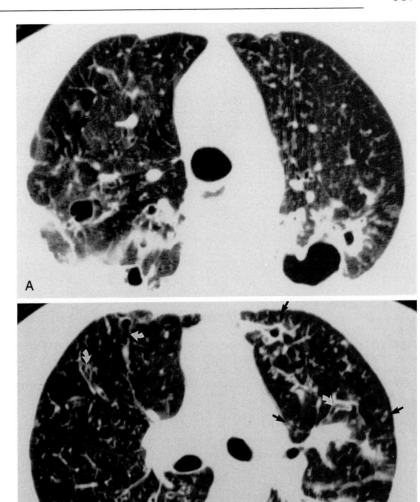

Figure 27–52. Pulmonary *Mycobacterium avium* Complex Infection. HRCT images (*A* and *B*) demonstrate cavities in the upper and lower lobes. Also noted are a few centrilobular nodules *(black arrows)* and evidence of bronchiectasis *(white arrows)*. Three consecutive sputum cultures grew *M. avium* complex. The patient was a 66-year-old woman.

common and larger in patients with tuberculosis than in those with *M. kansasii* infection. In addition, pleural effusion was present in 27% of patients with tuberculosis and in none of those with *M. kansasii* infection. The results of the various studies suggest that the radiographic findings of *M. kansasii* pulmonary infection are similar to those of *M. tuberculosis* except that pleural effusion is distinctly uncommon in patients with *M. kansasii*.

The radiographic findings of pulmonary infection caused by *M. malmoense* were reviewed in a study of 16 patients and compared with those of 32 age-matched, sex-matched, and race-matched patients with *M. tuberculosis*.[805] Findings seen more commonly in patients with *M. malmoense* included cavities larger than 6 cm in diameter (seen in 40% of cases), air-fluid levels (25% of cases), loss of lung volume (75% of cases), and coexistent pneumoconiosis (25% of cases). Air-space consolidation involving more than one segment was less common in *M. malmoense*, being seen in 20% of patients compared with 50% of patients with *M. tuberculosis*. The authors concluded that these differences were not sufficient to allow specific diagnosis.

Clinical Manifestations

The most common clinical presentation of NTM infection is similar to that of tuberculosis and, in a specific patient, is indistinguishable from that disease.[806, 807] Despite this, differences in presentation and clinical course have been documented between tuberculous and nontuberculous infection in some groups of patients. For example, in the previously cited review of 154 cases of pulmonary disease caused by rapid growers (approximately 80% *M. abscessus* and 15% *M. fortuitum*), the most common presenting symptom was cough (70% of cases);[768] sputum production and hemoptysis were documented in 10% to 15%. Systemic symptoms, such as fever and weight loss, were relatively uncommon at presentation (in approximately 10% to 20% of patients), but tended to develop as the disease progressed (in 40% to 60% during follow-up). A similar clinical picture has been described by other investigators.[685] A presentation of widespread pulmonary "infiltrates," high fever, and leukocytosis in excess of 20,000/mm³ has also been described.[768]

Clinical manifestations may differ somewhat in patients

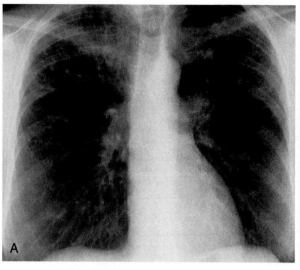

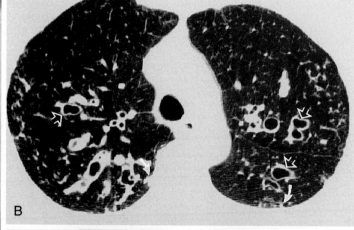

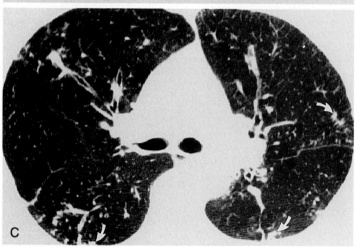

Figure 27–53. Pulmonary *Mycobacterium avium* Complex Infection. A posteroanterior chest radiograph *(A)* in a 52-year-old woman shows poorly defined small nodular opacities and evidence of bronchiectasis in the upper lung zones. HRCT images *(B* and *C)* demonstrate bilateral upper lobe and left lower lobe bronchiectasis *(open arrows)* and several centrilobular and subpleural nodules *(closed arrows).* Three separate sputum cultures grew *M. avium* complex.

with underlying lung disease, who are already likely to have pulmonary symptoms. For example, recovery of organisms in patients with cystic fibrosis has been associated with an increase in cough, sputum production, weight loss, and dyspnea and the presence of night sweats and pleuritic pain;[723] however, these findings are similar to those of nontuberculous bacterial infection and are of no help in differential diagnosis. Some patients have no evidence of previous pulmonary disease;[688] as described previously, many of these have been older women with a radiographic pattern of focal bronchiectasis and patchy nodules without cavitation.[808]

After the lung, lymph nodes are probably the most common site of NTM infection.[682, 755] The abnormality is usually seen in children under 5 years of age; adults are rarely affected in the absence of AIDS. In one review, the most common site of disease was unilateral submental and submaxillary lymph nodes, in contrast to tuberculous lymphadenitis, which usually affects the tonsillar and cervical nodes.[693] The onset of disease is usually insidious and relatively asymptomatic; nodes are typically unilateral and nontender. Rapid enlargement occurs occasionally. As disease progresses, sinus tracts may develop with the overlying skin. Rarely, infection has been documented in sites other than the neck; in one case, enlargement of a subcarinal lymph node resulted in symptomatic airway compression.[809] Identification of the causative organism has been documented in only about 50% of cases (the diagnosis in the others being

made on the basis of histologic examination). Approximately 75% to 80% of cases in which an organism is isolated are the result of *M. avium-intracellulare* infection; most of the remainder are caused by *M. scrofulaceum.*

Cutaneous disease is caused most often by *M. marinum,* the *M. chelonae* complex, and *M. ulcerans.*[682, 683, 810] Lesions related to *M. marinum* appear about 3 weeks after exposure to infected water as small papules or indurated nodules on the extremities that ulcerate and heal spontaneously within a few months. Skin and subcutaneous infection with *M. chelonae* or *M. fortuitum* often occurs after trauma or surgical procedures;[682] abscess formation is common. *M. ulcerans* infections occur after minor injury to an exposed body surface by a thorn, sharp instrument, or piece of wood; in tropical and subtropical climates, severe ulceration develops, which may cause deformities and contractures and necessitate amputation of a limb.[693] Skin, tendon, and synovial involvement is also a relatively common manifestation of NTM disease in transplant recipients.[718]

Apart from patients with AIDS—in whom the incidence of disseminated *M. avium* complex infection is as high as 15% to 25%—disseminated disease by NTM is rare. Virtually all affected patients are immunocompromised as a result of therapy or underlying disease.[678, 693, 811] In patients with *M. avium* complex, the presentation tends to be one of fever of unknown origin; disease related to *M. kansasii* and *M. chelonae* tends to present as subcutaneous nodules or draining

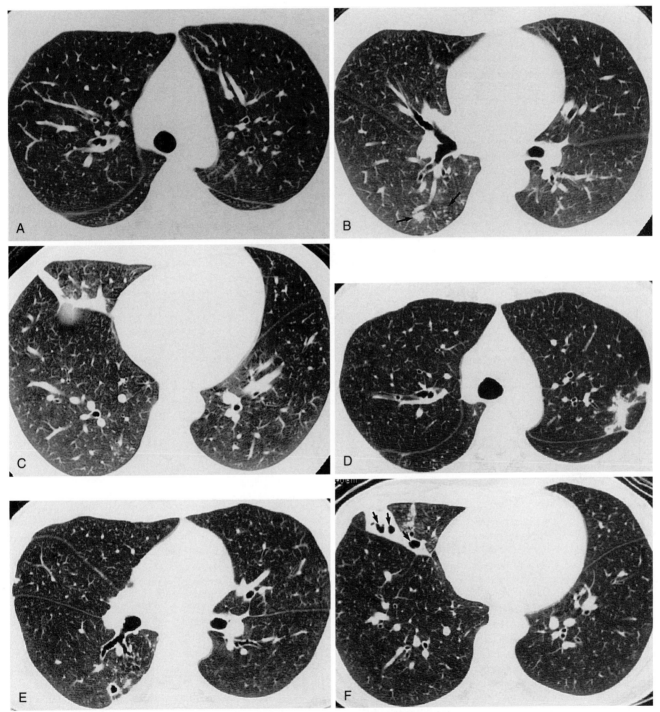

Figure 27–54. Pulmonary *Mycobacterium avium* Complex Infection—Progression Over Three Years. A 27-year-old woman presented with a history of chronic cough and recurrent pneumonia. HRCT scan through the upper lobes *(A)* is normal. A scan at the level of the right middle lobe bronchus *(B)* shows mild volume loss of the right middle lobe and anterior displacement of the major fissure. Several small nodules *(arrows)* are present in the superior segment of the right lower lobe. An image at a more caudad level *(C)* shows focal areas of consolidation in the atelectatic right middle lobe. Cultures grew *M. avium* complex. HRCT scans performed at corresponding levels *(D, E, F)* 3 years later demonstrate development of focal nodular opacities and interlobular septal thickening in the left upper lobe *(D)*, cavitation in the superior segment of the right lower lobe *(E)*, and bronchiectasis *(arrows)* in the right middle lobe *(F)*. Three sputum cultures again grew *M. avium* complex.

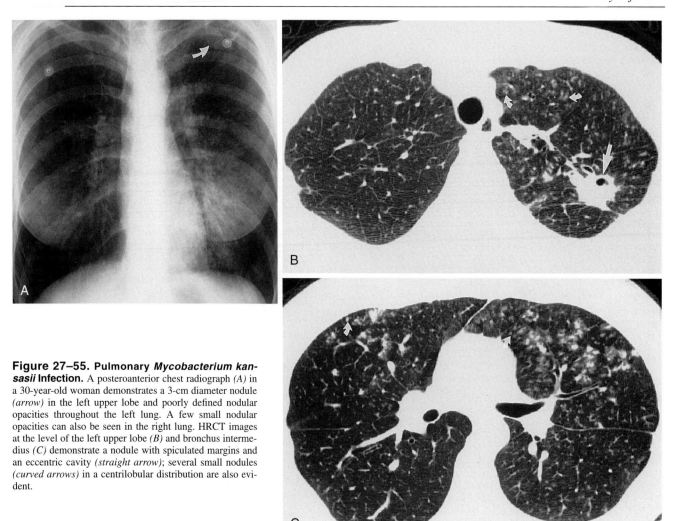

Figure 27–55. Pulmonary *Mycobacterium kansasii* Infection. A posteroanterior chest radiograph *(A)* in a 30-year-old woman demonstrates a 3-cm diameter nodule *(arrow)* in the left upper lobe and poorly defined nodular opacities throughout the left lung. A few small nodular opacities can also be seen in the right lung. HRCT images at the level of the left upper lobe *(B)* and bronchus intermedius *(C)* demonstrate a nodule with spiculated margins and an eccentric cavity *(straight arrow)*; several small nodules *(curved arrows)* in a centrilobular distribution are also evident.

abscesses.[755] Pulmonary involvement is common in disseminated disease, with a miliary radiographic pattern in most patients and parenchymal consolidation in roughly 25%.[811]

Diagnosis

Techniques of culture, staining, and identification of NTM are similar to those used for *M. tuberculosis*. One difference is the necessity of culture at two temperatures (35° C and 28 to 32° C) for samples suspected of harboring organisms such as *M. marinum*, *M. ulcerans*, *M. haemophilum*, and *M. chelonae*.[755] A radiometric culture system (BACTEC) in combination with NAP (*p*-nitro-α-acetylamino-β-hydroxypropiophenone) has been used to differentiate *M. tuberculosis* from NTM;[812] the compound selectively inhibits growth of the former organism and allows documentation of the presence of NTM in as few as 5 days. Analysis of mycolic acid profile by high-performance liquid chromatography[813] and of cell wall content by gas-liquid chromatography and thin-layer chromatography[814] has been used to differentiate individual NTM species. The use of genetic probes is even more rapid and specific and promises to facilitate diagnosis greatly.[680, 785, 815, 816]

In contrast to *M. tuberculosis*, whose identification signifies disease, isolation of NTM from sputum not uncommonly represents environmental contamination of culture material or colonization of the respiratory tract.[817] For example, in one study of 1,610 patients admitted to a Connecticut hospital, culture grew NTM considered to be saprophytes, commensals, and contaminants in 5% of hospital patients and 6% of clinic patients.[818] The diagnosis of disease is made even more difficult by the fact that both the diseased and the colonized states are commonly associated with underlying pulmonary disease.[708] As a result, interpretation of a positive smear or culture must be done carefully and in the light of underlying clinical and radiologic features. Guidelines for diagnosis have been published by the American Thoracic Society on the basis of three forms of clinical presentation (Table 27–4): (1) cavitary lung disease; (2) noncavitary lung disease; and (3) any form of lung disease whose sputum evaluation is considered nondiagnostic or in whom another disease cannot be excluded.[755] Using strict criteria such as these, a minority of NTM isolates are associated with clinically important disease. For example, in one study of 80 cases, only 17 and 23 (21% and 29%) were considered to represent definite and probable infection.[819]

Although some investigators have advocated the use of

Table 27–4. RECOMMENDED DIAGNOSTIC CRITERIA FOR PULMONARY DISEASE CAUSED BY NONTUBERCULOUS MYCOBACTERIA (NTM)

Patients with Cavitary Lung Disease

Presence of two or more sputum specimens (or sputum and a bronchial washing) that are acid-fast bacilli smear positive and/or result in moderate-to-heavy growth of NTM on culture

Other reasonable causes for the disease process have been excluded (e.g., tuberculosis, fungal disease)

Patients with Noncavitary Lung Disease

Presence of two or more sputum specimens (or sputum and a bronchial washing) that are acid-fast bacilli smear positive and/or produce moderate-to-heavy growth on culture

If the isolate is *Mycobacterium kansasii* or *Mycobacterium avium* complex, failure of the sputum cultures to clear with bronchial toilet or within 2 weeks of institution of specific mycobacterial drug therapy (although studied only for these two species, this criterion is probably valid for other species of NTM)

Other reasonable causes for the disease process have been excluded

Patients with cavitary or noncavitary lung disease whose sputum evaluation is nondiagnostic or in whom another disease cannot be excluded

A transbronchial or open-lung biopsy yields the organism and shows mycobacterial histopathologic features (i.e., granulomatous inflammation, with or without acid-fast bacilli). No other criteria needed

A transbronchial or open-lung biopsy that fails to reveal the organism but shows mycobacterial histopathologic features in the absence of a prior history of other granulomatous or mycobacterial disease plus (1) presence of two or more positive cultures of sputum or bronchial washings; (2) other reasonable causes for granulomatous disease have been excluded

Adapted from Wallace RJ Jr, O'Brien R, Glassroth J, et al: Diagnosis and treatment of disease caused by nontuberculous mycobacteria. Am Rev Respir Dis 142:940, 1990.

species-specific skin tests for screening patients at risk of infection,[820] cross-reactions between PPD-S and NTM antigens limit the usefulness of the test, and most investigators believe it is of little or no practical help in diagnosis.[755] An example of this limitation is provided by an investigation of 44 persons infected with *M. marinum* after exposure to the organism in a swimming pool;[821, 822] all 44 patients lived in an area where there was little reported tuberculosis, and none had received BCG vaccine. Twelve years after their illness, testing with PPD-*marinum* produced an induration 10 mm or more in diameter in 26 (59%); however, at least one of the other three antigens used (related to *M. tuberculosis*, *M. kansasii*, and *M. intracellulare*) produced reactions of similar size in almost an equal number of patients.

Natural History and Prognosis

Pulmonary disease caused by NTM tends to progress if untreated.[823] In the study of 154 patients with infection by rapid growers cited previously, 21 (14%) died as a direct result of the infection.[768] As might be expected, the prognosis varied with the presence of underlying lung disease: in the 11 patients without such disease, the average time to death was approximately 8 years; by contrast, in 4 patients with severe underlying lung disease, death occurred within 1 year of the diagnosis of infection. Similar observations have been made by other investigators.[710] The cause of death in these patients is variable; many, particularly those with obstructive airway disease, die of cor pulmonale. As indicated previously, dissemination is unusual in the absence of an immunocompromised state; however, when it occurs, it is often fatal.[678]

In view of the difficulty in determining when NTM are pathogenic in some cases, the clear-cut difference in prognosis after treatment between two groups of patients judged to have *M. avium-intracellulare* infection in one report[824] and between those considered to be "asymptomatic" and "symptomatic" in two others[825, 826] raises the possibility that at least some patients with a good prognosis were colonized only. Similarly, it would seem reasonable to question pathogenicity in favor of colonization in those patients who have repeated positive cultures despite treatment and whose clinical condition remains stable.[688, 707]

REFERENCES

1. Goodwin RA, Des Prez RM: Apical localization of pulmonary tuberculosis, chronic pulmonary histoplasmosis, and progressive massive fibrosis of the lung. Chest 83:801, 1983.
2. Smith DW: Mycobacteria. *In* Braude AI, Davis CE, Fierer J (eds): Medical Microbiology and Infectious Diseases. Philadelphia, WB Saunders, 1981, p 416.
3. Barksdale L, Kim K-S: *Mycobacterium.* Bact Rev 41:217, 1977.
4. Fisher JF, Ganapathy M, Edwards BH, et al: Utility of Gram's and Giemsa stains in the diagnosis of pulmonary tuberculosis. Am Rev Respir Dis 141:511, 1990.
5. Hinson JM Jr, Bradsher RW, Bodner SJ: Gram-stain neutrality of *Mycobacterium tuberculosis.* Am Rev Respir Dis 123:365, 1981.
6. Good RC, Mastro TD: The modern mycobacteriology laboratory: How it can help the clinician. Clin Chest Med 10:315, 1989.
7. Siddiqi SH, Hwangbo CC, Silcox V, et al: Rapid radiometric methods to detect and differentiate *Mycobacterium tuberculosis/M. bovis* from other mycobacterial species. Am Rev Respir Dis 130:634, 1984.
8. Bass JB Jr, Farer LS, Hopewell PC, et al: Diagnostic standards and classification of tuberculosis. Am Rev Respir Dis 142:725, 1990.
9. Humphrey DM, Weiner MH: Mycobacterial antigen detection by immunohistochemistry in pulmonary tuberculosis. Hum Pathol 18:701, 1987.
10. Coates ARM, Hewitt J, Allen BW, et al: Antigenic diversity of *Mycobacterium tuberculosis* and *Mycobacterium bovis* detected by means of monoclonal antibodies. Lancet 2:167, 1981.
11. Kubica GP: Phage typing of *Mycobacterium tuberculosis*: A time standardization. Am Rev Respir Dis 126:3, 1982.
12. Editorial: Bovine tuberculosis. BMJ 3:488, 1972.
13. Wilkins EG, Griffiths RJ, Roberts C: Pulmonary tuberculosis due to *Mycobacterium bovis.* Thorax 41:685, 1986.
14. Wilkins EG, Griffiths RJ, Roberts C: Bovine variants of *Mycobacterium tuberculosis* isolated in Liverpool during the period 1969 to 1983: An epidemiological survey. QJM 59:627, 1986.
15. Liss GM, Wong L, Kittle DC, et al: Occupational exposure to *Mycobacterium bovis* infection in deer and elk in Ontario. Can J Public Health 85:326, 1994.
16. Thompson PJ, Cousins DV, Gow BL, et al: Seals, seal trainers, and mycobacterial infection. Am Rev Respir Dis 147:164, 1993.
17. Sjögren I, Hillerdal O: Bovine tuberculosis in man—reinfection or endogenous exacerbation. Scand J Respir Dis 59:167, 1978.
18. Bates JH, Stead WW: The history of tuberculosis as a global epidemic. Med Clin North Am 77:1205, 1993.
19. Sudre P, ten Dam HG, Kochi A: Tuberculosis: A global overview of the situation today. Bull WHO 70:149, 1992.
20. Barnes PF, Barrows SA: Tuberculosis in the 1990s. Ann Intern Med 119:400, 1993.
21. Tuberculosis Programme, Division of Communicable Diseases, World Health Organization: Tuberculosis Notifications Update, July 1992. WHO/TB 9. Geneva, World Health Organization, 1992.
22. Centers for Disease Control and Prevention: Reported tuberculosis in the United States, 1995. Atlanta, Centers for Disease Control and Prevention, 1996, pp 5–7.
23. Rieder HL: Epidemiology of tuberculosis in Europe. Eur Respir J 8(Suppl 20):620s, 1995.
24. Statistics Canada, Health Statistics Division. Tuberculosis Statistics, Ottawa, 1994.
25. Riley RL: Disease transmission and contagion control. Am Rev Respir Dis 125(Suppl):16, 1982.
26. Canetti G: Present aspects of bacterial resistance in tuberculosis. Am Rev Respir Dis 92:687, 1965.
27. Leff A, Geppert EF: Public health and preventive aspects of pulmonary tuberculosis: Infectiousness, epidemiology, risk factors, classification, and preventive therapy. Arch Intern Med 139:1405, 1979.
28. Loudon RG, Brown LC: Cough frequency in patients with respiratory disease. Am Rev Respir Dis 96:1137, 1967.
29. Loudon RG, Spohn SK: Cough frequency and infectivity in patients with pulmonary tuberculosis. Am Rev Respir Dis 99:109, 1969.
30. Loudon RG, Roberts RM: Droplet expulsion from the respiratory tract. Am Rev Respir Dis 95:435, 1967.
31. Loudon RG, Bumgarner LR, Lacy J, et al: Aerial transmission of mycobacteria. Am Rev Respir Dis 100:165, 1969.
32. Liippo KK, Kulmala K, Tala EOJ: Focusing tuberculosis contact tracing by smear grading of index cases. Am Rev Respir Dis 148:235, 1993.
33. Brooks SM, Lassiter NL, Young EC: A pilot study concerning the infection risk of sputum-positive tuberculous patients on chemotherapy. Am Rev Respir Dis 108:799, 1973.
34. Gunnels JJ, Bates JH, Swindoll H: Infectivity of sputum-positive tuberculous patients on chemotherapy. Am Rev Respir Dis 109:323, 1974.
35. Yeager H Jr, Lacy J, Smith LR, et al: Quantitative studies of mycobacterial populations in sputum and saliva. Am Rev Respir Dis 95:998, 1967.
36. Menzies D: Effect of treatment on contagiousness of patients with active pulmonary tuberculosis. Infect Control Hosp Epidemiol 18:582, 1997.
37. O'Brien JK, Sandman LA, Kreiswirth BN, et al: DNA fingerprints from *Mycobacterium tuberculosis* isolates of patients confined for therapy noncompliance show frequent clustering. Chest 112:387, 1997.
38. Bloch AB, Rieder HL, Kelly GD, et al: The epidemiology of tuberculosis in the United States: Implications for diagnosis and treatment. Clin Chest Med 10:297, 1989.
39. Jochem K, Tannenbaum TN, Menzies D: Prevalence of tuberculin skin test reactions among prison workers. Can J Public Health 88:202, 1997.
40. Comstock GW, Livesay UT, Woolpert SF: The prognosis of a positive tuberculin reaction in childhood and adolescence. Am J Epidemiol 99:131, 1974.
41. Sacks JJ, Brenner ER, Breeden DC, et al: Epidemiology of a tuberculosis outbreak in a South Carolina junior high school. Am J Public Health 75:361, 1985.
42. Darney PD, Clenny ND: Tuberculosis outbreak in an Alabama high school. JAMA 216:2117, 1971.
43. Hoge CW, Fisher L, Donnell HD Jr, et al: Risk factors for transmission of *Mycobacterium tuberculosis* in a primary school outbreak: Lack of racial difference in susceptibility to infection. Am J Epidemiol 139:520, 1994.
44. Kaupas V: Tuberculosis in a family day-care home: Report of an outbreak and recommendations for prevention. JAMA 228:851, 1974.
45. Stead WW, Lofgren JP, Warren E, et al: Tuberculosis as an endemic and nosocomial infection among the elderly in nursing homes. N Engl J Med 312:1483, 1985.
46. Houk VN, Baker JH, Sorensen K, et al: The epidemiology of tuberculosis infection in a closed environment. Arch Environ Health 16:26, 1968.
47. Tuberculosis in a nursing care facility—Washington. MMWR 32:121, 1983.
48. Welty C, Burstin S, Muspratt S, et al: Epidemiology of tuberculous infection in a chronic care population. Am Rev Respir Dis 132:133, 1985.
49. Catanzaro A: Nosocomial tuberculosis. Am Rev Respir Dis 125:559, 1982.
50. Kline SE, Hedemark LL, Davies SF: Outbreak of tuberculosis among regular patrons of a neighborhood bar. N Engl J Med 333:222, 1995.
51. Dutt AK, Mehta JB, Whitaker BJ, et al: Outbreak of tuberculosis in a church. Chest 107:447, 1995.
51a. Mangura BT, Napolitano EC, Passannante MR, et al: *Mycobacterium tuberculosis* miniepidemic in a church gospel choir. Chest 113:234, 1998.
52. Medical Section of the American Lung Association: Control of tuberculosis in the United States. Am Rev Respir Dis 146:1623, 1992.
53. Belfield PW, Arnold AG, Williams SE, et al: Recent experience of tuberculosis in junior hospital doctors in Leeds and Bradford. Br J Dis Chest 78:313, 1984.
54. Burrill D, Enarson DA, Allen EA, et al: Tuberculosis in female nurses in British Columbia: Implications for control programs. Can Med Assoc J 132:137, 1985.
55. Pearson ML, Jereb JA, Frieden TR, et al: Nosocomial transmission of multidrug-resistant *Mycobacterium tuberculosis*: A risk to patients and health care workers. Ann Intern Med 117:191, 1992.
56. Wilkins D, Woolcock AJ, Cossart YE: Tuberculosis: Medical students at risk. Med J Aust 160:395, 1994.
57. Yoder KM: Tuberculosis: A reemerging hazard for oral healthcare workers. J Dent Hyg 67:208, 1993.
58. Stead WW: Management of health care workers after inadvertent exposure to tuberculosis: A guide for the use of preventive therapy. Ann Intern Med 122:906, 1995.
59. Sokolove PE, Mackey D, Wiles J, et al: Exposure of emergency department personnel to tuberculosis: PPD testing during an epidemic in the community. Ann Emerg Med 24:418, 1994.
60. Bailey TC, Fraser VJ, Spitznagel EL, et al: Risk factors for a positive tuberculin skin test among employees of an urban, midwestern teaching hospital. Ann Intern Med 122:580, 1995.
61. Richmond JY, Knudsen RC, Good RC: Biosafety in the clinical mycobacteriology laboratory. Clin Lab Med 16:527, 1996.
62. Lurie MB, Dannenberg AM Jr: Macrophage function in infectious disease with inbred rabbits. Bact Rev 29:466, 1965.
63. Apt AS, Avdienko VG, Nikonenko BV, et al: Distinct H-2 complex control of mortality and immune responses to tuberculosis infection in virgin and BCG-vaccinated mice. Clin Exp Immunol 94:322, 1993.
64. Forget A, Skamene E, Gros P, et al: Differences in response among inbred mouse strains to infection with small doses of *Mycobacterium bovis* BCG. Infect Immun 32:42, 1981.
65. Stead WW, Lofgren JP, Senner JW, et al: Racial differences in susceptibility to infection with *M. tuberculosis.* N Engl J Med 322:422, 1990.
66. Spach DH, Silverstein FE, Stamm WE: Transmission of infection by gastrointestinal endoscopy and bronchoscopy. Ann Intern Med 118:117, 1993.
67. Eastlund T: Infectious disease transmission through cell, tissue, and organ transplantation: Reducing the risk through donor selection. Cell Transplant 4:455, 1995.
68. Hutton MD, Stead WW, Cauthen GM, et al: Nosocomial transmission of tuberculosis associated with a draining abscess. J Infect Dis 161:286, 1990.
69. Snider WR, Cohen D, Reif JS, et al: Tuberculosis in canine and feline populations: Study of high risk populations in Pennsylvania, 1966–1968. Am Rev Respir Dis 104:866, 1971.
70. Snider WR: Tuberculosis in canine and feline populations: Review of the literature. Am Rev Respir Dis 104:877, 1971.
71. Cappucci DT Jr, O'Shea JL, Smith GD: An epidemiologic account of tuberculosis transmitted from man to monkey. Am Rev Respir Dis 106:819, 1972.
72. Renner M, Bartholomew WR: Mycobacteriologic data from two outbreaks of bovine tuberculosis in nonhuman primates. Am Rev Respir Dis 109:11, 1974.

73. Hoyt EM: Primary inoculation tuberculosis: Report of a case. JAMA 245:1556, 1981.
74. Duray PH, Flannery B, Brown S: Tuberculosis infection from preparation of frozen sections. N Engl J Med 305:167, 1981.
75. Glassroth J, Robbins AG, Snider DE Jr: Tuberculosis in the 1980s. N Engl J Med 302:1441, 1980.
76. Davies BH: Infectivity of tuberculosis. Thorax 35:481, 1980.
76a. Falk A, Fuchs GF: Prophylaxis with isoniazid in inactive tuberculosis: A Veterans Administration Cooperative Study XII. Chest 73:44, 1978.
77. Stead WW: Pathogenesis of the sporadic case of tuberculosis. N Engl J Med 277:1008, 1967.
78. Stead WW: Pathogenesis of a first episode of chronic pulmonary tuberculosis in man: Recrudescence of residua of the primary infection or exogenous reinfection? Am Rev Respir Dis 95:729, 1967.
79. Raleigh JW, Wichelhausen R: Exogenous reinfection with *Mycobacterium tuberculosis* confirmed by phage typing (case report). Am Rev Respir Dis 108:639, 1973.
80. Small PM, Shafer RW, Hopewell PC, et al: Exogenous reinfection with multidrug-resistant *Mycobacterium tuberculosis* in patients with advanced HIV infection. N Engl J Med 238:1137, 1993.
81. Nardell E, McInnis B, Thomas B, et al: Exogenous reinfection with tuberculosis in a shelter for the homeless. N Engl J Med 315:1570, 1986.
82. van Soolingen D, Hermans PW: Epidemiology of tuberculosis by DNA fingerprinting. Eur Respir J 20(Suppl):649s, 1995.
83. Buskin SE, Gale JL, Weiss NS, et al: Tuberculosis risk factors in adults in King County, Washington, 1988 through 1990. Am J Public Health 84:1750, 1994.
84. Friedman LN, Williams MT, Singh TP, et al: Tuberculosis, AIDS, and death among substance abusers on welfare in New York City. N Engl J Med 334:828, 1996.
85. Harries AD, Thomas J, Chugh KS: Malnutrition in African patients with pulmonary tuberculosis. Hum Nutr Clin Nutr 39:361, 1985.
85a. Heyderman RS, Goyal M, Roberts P, et al: Pulmonary tuberculosis in Harare, Zimbabwe: Analysis by spoligotyping. Thorax 53:346, 1998.
86. Arango L, Brewin AW, Murray JF: The spectrum of tuberculosis as currently seen in a metropolitan hospital. Am Rev Respir Dis 108:805, 1973.
87. McGowan JE Jr, Blumberg HM: Inner-city tuberculosis in the USA. J Hosp Infect 30:282, 1995.
88. Stead WW: Special problems in tuberculosis: Tuberculosis in the elderly and in residents of nursing homes, correctional facilities, long-term care hospitals, mental hospitals, shelters for the homeless, and jails. Clin Chest Med 10:397, 1989.
89. Schieffelbein CW Jr, Snider DE Jr: Tuberculosis control among homeless populations. JAMA 148:1843, 1988.
90. Torres RA, Mani S, Altholz J, et al: Human immunodeficiency virus infection among homeless men in a New York City shelter: Association with *Mycobacterium tuberculosis* infection. Arch Intern Med 150:2030, 1990.
91. McAdam JM, Brickner PW, Scharer LL, et al: The spectrum of tuberculosis in a New York City Men's Shelter Clinic (1982–1988). Chest 97:798, 1990.
92. Brudney K, Dobkin J: Resurgent tuberculosis in New York City. Am Rev Respir Dis 144:745, 1991.
93. Patek KR: Pulmonary tuberculosis in residents of lodging houses, night shelters and common hostels in Glasgow: A five year prospective study. Br J Dis Chest 79:60, 1985.
94. Bergmire-Sweat D, Barnett BJ, Harris SL, et al: Tuberculosis outbreak in a Texas prison. Epidemiol Infect 117:485, 1996.
95. Yamanaka K, Kondo T, Miyao M: Tuberculosis among the homeless people of Nagoya, Japan. Respir Med 88:763, 1994.
96. Barr RG, Menzies R: The effect of war on tuberculosis: Results of a tuberculin survey among displaced persons in El Salvador and a review of the literature. Tuber Lung Dis 75:251, 1994.
97. Geiseler PJ, Nelson KE, Crispen RG, et al: Tuberculosis in physicians: A continuing problem. Am Rev Respir Dis 133:773, 1986.
98. Teppo J, Ojajärvi J, Brander E: The tuberculosis morbidity among pathologists in Finland. Scand J Respir Dis 55:257, 1974.
99. Rao VR, Joanes RF, Kilbane P, et al: Outbreak of tuberculosis after minimal exposure to infection. BMJ 281:187, 1980.
100. Ward M, Poirier J, Lambert A, et al: Tuberculosis outbreak at a Canadian Forces Base—Ontario. Can Dis Week Rep 7:157, 1981.
101. Nelson S, Mason C, Bagby G, et al: Alcohol, tumor necrosis factor, and tuberculosis. Alcohol Clin Exp Res 19:17, 1995.
102. Perlman DC, Salomon N, Perkins MP, et al: Tuberculosis in drug users. Clin Infect Dis 21:1253, 1995.
103. Perlman DC, Salomon N, Perkins MP, et al: Tuberculosis in drug users. Clin Infect Dis 21:1253, 1995.
104. Sapira JD, Ball JC, Penn H: Causes of death among institutionalized narcotic addicts. J Chron Dis 22:733, 1970.
105. Leonhardt KK, Gentile F, Gibert BP, et al: A cluster of tuberculosis among crack house contacts in San Mateo County, California. Am J Public Health 84:1834, 1994.
106. Couser JI Jr, Glassroth J: Tuberculosis: An epidemic in older adults. Clin Chest Med 14:491, 1993.
107. Aktogu S, Yorgancioglu A, Cirak K, et al: Clinical spectrum of pulmonary and pleural tuberculosis: A report of 5,480 cases. Eur Respir J 9:2031, 1996.
108. Couser JI Jr, Glassroth J: Tuberculosis: An epidemic in older adults. Clin Chest Med 14:491, 1993.

109. Mackay AD, Cole RB: The problems of tuberculosis in the elderly. QJM 53:497, 1984.
110. Liaw YS, Yang PC, Yu CJ, et al: Clinical spectrum of tuberculosis in older patients. J Am Geriatr Soc 43:256, 1995.
111. Korzeniewska-Kosela M, Krysl J, Müller NL, et al: Tuberculosis in young adults and the elderly: A prospective comparison study. Chest 106:28, 1994.
112. Hamadeh MA, Glassroth JS: Tuberculosis in pregnancy. Chest 101:1114, 1992.
113. Davidson PT: Managing tuberculosis during pregnancy. Lancet 346:199, 1995.
114. Espinal MA, Reingold AL, Lavandera M: Effect of pregnancy on the risk of developing active tuberculosis. J Infect Dis 173:488, 1996.
115. Good S, Iseman M, Davidson P, et al: Tuberculosis in association with pregnancy. Am J Obstet Gynecol 140:492, 1981.
115a. Cantwell MF, McKenna MT, McCray E, et al: Tuberculosis and race/ethnicity in the United States: Impact of socioeconomic status. Am J Respir Crit Care Med 157:1016, 1997.
116. Stead WW: Genetics and resistance to tuberculosis: Could resistance be enhanced by genetic engineering? Ann Intern Med 116:937, 1992.
117. Biehl JP: Miliary tuberculosis: A review of sixty-eight adult patients admitted to a municipal general hospital. Am Rev Tuberc 77:605, 1958.
118. Falk A: U.S. Veterans Administration—Armed Forces cooperative study on the chemotherapy of tuberculosis: XII. Results of treatment in miliary tuberculosis: A follow-up study of 570 adult patients. Am Rev Respir Dis 91:6, 1965.
119. Munt PW: Miliary tuberculosis in the chemotherapy era: With a clinical review in 69 American adults. Medicine 51:139, 1972.
120. Ormerod LP, Horsfield N: Miliary tuberculosis in a high prevalence area of the U.K.: Blackburn 1978–1993. Respir Med 89:555, 1995.
120a. Griffith DE: The United States and worldwide tuberculosis control: A second change for Prince Prospero. Chest 113:1434, 1998.
121. Binkin NJ, Zuber PL, Wells CD, et al: Overseas screening for tuberculosis in immigrants and refugees to the United States: Current status. Clin Infect Dis 23:1226, 1996.
122. Nolan CM, Elarth AM: Tuberculosis in a cohort of Southeast Asian refugees. Am Rev Respir Dis 137:805, 1988.
123. Kent JH: The epidemiology of multidrug-resistant tuberculosis in the United States. Med Clin North Am 77:1391, 1993.
124. Minh V-D, Prendergast TJ, Engle P: Tuberculosis in refugees from Southeast Asia. Chest 82:133, 1982.
125. Scalcini M, Carre G, Jean-Baptiste M: Antituberculous drug resistance in central Haiti. Am Rev Respir Dis 142:508, 1990.
126. Iseman MD, Sbarbaro JA: The increasing prevalence of resistance to antituberculosis chemotherapeutic agents: Implications for global tuberculosis control. Curr Clin Top Infect Dis 12:188, 1992.
127. Lavy A, Mates A: A 10 year survey on *Mycobacterium tuberculosis* isolates in Israel and their drug resistance. Isr J Med Sci 30:805, 1994.
128. Vidal SM, Malo D, Vogan K, et al: Natural resistance to infection with intracellular parasites: Isolation of a candidate for Bcg. Cell 73:469, 1993.
128a. Skamene E: The *Bcg* gene story. Immunology 191:451, 1994.
129. Crowle AJ, Elkins N: Relative permissiveness of macrophages from black and white people for virulent tubercle bacilli. Infect Immun 58:632, 1990.
130. Comstock GW: Tuberculosis in twins: A re-analysis of the Prophit survey. Am Rev Respir Dis 117:621, 1978.
131. Comstock GW: Epidemiology of tuberculosis. Am Rev Respir Dis 125:8, 1982.
132. Singh SPN, Mehra NK, Dingley HB, et al: Human leukocyte antigen (HLA)-linked control of susceptibility to pulmonary tuberculosis and association with HLA-DR types. J Infect Dis 148:676, 1983.
133. Hafez M, El-Salab S, El-Shennawy F, et al: HLA-antigens and tuberculosis in the Egyptian population. Tubercle 66:35, 1985.
134. Teran L, Selman M, Mendoza M, et al: Increase of unidentified HLA antigens in pulmonary tuberculosis. Ann Clin Res 17:40, 1985.
135. Cox RA, Arnold DR, Cook D, et al: HLA phenotypes in Mexican Americans with tuberculosis. Am Rev Respir Dis 126:653, 1982.
136. Bothamley GH, Beck JS, Schreuder GM, et al: Association of tuberculosis and *M. tuberculosis*-specific antibody levels with HLA. J Infect Dis 159:549, 1989.
137. Sepulveda RL, Heiba IM, King A, et al: Evaluation of tuberculin reactivity in BCG-immunized siblings. Am J Respir Crit Care Med 149:620, 1994.
138. van Eden W, de Vries RRP, Stanford JL, et al: HLA-DR3-associated genetic control of response to multiple skin tests with new tuberculins. Clin Exp Immunol 52:287, 1983.
139. Leff A, Geppert EF: Public health and preventive aspects of pulmonary tuberculosis: Infectiousness, epidemiology, risk factors, classification, and preventive therapy. Arch Intern Med 139:1405, 1979.
140. Sasaki A, Kamado K, Uehara M: Changes in causes of death in diabetic patients based on death certificates during a 30-year period in Osaka District, Japan, with special reference to cancer mortality. Diabetes Res Clin Pract 24:103, 1994.
141. Koziel H, Koziel MJ: Pulmonary complications of diabetes mellitus: Pneumonia. Infect Dis Clin North Am 9:65, 1995.
142. Holden HM, Hiltz JE: The tuberculous diabetic. Can Med Assoc J 87:797, 1962.
143. Zack MB, Fulkerson LL, Stein E: Glucose intolerance in pulmonary tuberculosis. Am Rev Respir Dis 108:1164, 1973.
144. Pablos-Mendez A, Blustein J, Knirsch CA: The role of diabetes mellitus in the higher prevalence of tuberculosis among Hispanics. Am J Public Health 87:574, 1997.
145. Rosenman KD, Hall N: Occupational risk factors for developing tuberculosis. Am J Ind Med 30:148, 1996.
146. Mosquera JA, Rodrigo L, Gonzalvez F: The evolution of pulmonary tuberculosis

in coal miners in Asturias, northern Spain: An attempt to reduce the rate over a 15-year period, 1971–1985. Eur J Epidemiol 10:291, 1994.

147. Sluis-Cremer GK: Active pulmonary tuberculosis discovered at post-mortem examination of the lungs of black miners. Br J Dis Chest 74:374, 1980.

148. Morgan EJ: Silicosis and tuberculosis. Chest 75:202, 1979.

149. Becklake MR: The mineral dust diseases. Tuber Lung Dis 73:13, 1992.

150. Cowie RL: The epidemiology of tuberculosis in gold miners with silicosis. Am J Respir Crit Care Med 150:1460, 1994.

151. Brink GC, Grzybowski S, Lane GB: Silicotuberculosis. Can Med Assoc J 82:959, 1960.

152. Cheng SJ, Ma Y, Pan YX: A study on the diagnosis of pulmonary tuberculosis and silicotuberculosis by PCR. Chung Hua Chieh Ho Ho Hu Hsi Tsa Chih 16:221, 1993.

153. Buskin SE, Weiss NS, Gale JL, et al: Tuberculosis in relation to a history of peptic ulcer disease and treatment of gastric hyperacidity. Am J Epidemiol 141:218, 1995.

154. Steiger Z, Nickel WO, Shannon GJ, et al: Pulmonary tuberculosis after gastric resection. Am J Surg 131:668, 1976.

155. Lundegardh G, Helmick C, Zack M, et al: Mortality among patients with partial gastrectomy for benign ulcer disease. Dig Dis Sci 39:340, 1994.

156. Bruce RM, Wise L: Tuberculosis after jejunoileal bypass for obesity. Ann Intern Med 87:574, 1977.

157. Snider DE: Jejunoileal bypass for obesity: A risk factor for tuberculosis. Chest 81:531, 1982.

158. Rutsky EA, Rostand SG: Mycobacteriosis in patients with chronic renal failure. Arch Intern Med 140:57, 1980.

159. Pradhan RP, Katz LA, Nidus BD, et al: Tuberculosis in dialyzed patients. JAMA 229:798, 1974.

160. Andrew OT, Schoenfeld PY, Hopewell PC, et al: Tuberculosis in patients with end-stage renal disease. Am J Med 68:59, 1980.

161. Sasaki S, Akiba T, Suenaga M, et al: Ten years' survey of dialysis-associated tuberculosis. Nephron 24:141, 1979.

162. Leading article: Tuberculosis in patients having dialysis. BMJ 280:349, 1980.

163. Stead WW, Dutt AK: What's new in tuberculosis? Am J Med 71:1, 1981.

164. Reyes JM, Putong PB: Association of pulmonary alveolar lipoproteinosis with mycobacterial infection. Am J Clin Pathol 74:478, 1980.

165. Witty LA, Tapson VF, Piantadosi CA: Isolation of mycobacteria in patients with pulmonary alveolar proteinosis. Medicine 73:103, 1994.

166. Garcia Rio F, Alvarez-Sala R, Caballero P, et al: Six cases of pulmonary alveolar proteinosis: Presentation of unusual associations. Monaldi Arch Chest Dis 50:12, 1995.

167. Gaynor CD, McCormack FX, Voelker DR, et al: Pulmonary surfactant protein A mediates enhanced phagocytosis of *Mycobacterium tuberculosis* by a direct interaction with human macrophages. J Immunol 155:5343, 1995.

168. Steer A: Focal pulmonary alveolar proteinosis in pulmonary tuberculosis. Arch Pathol 87:347, 1969.

169. Scadding JG: *Mycobacterium tuberculosis* in the aetiology of sarcoidosis. BMJ 2:1617, 1960.

170. Victorio-Navarra ST, Dy EE, Arroyo CG, et al: Tuberculosis among Filipino patients with systemic lupus erythematosus. Semin Arthritis Rheum 26:628, 1996.

171. Shyam C, Malaviya AN: Infection-related morbidity in systemic lupus erythematosus: A clinico-epidemiological study from northern India. Rheumatol Int 16:1, 1996.

172. Janwityanuchit S, Totemchokchyakarn K, Krachangwongchai K, et al: Infection in systemic lupus erythematosus. J Med Assoc Thai 76:542, 1993.

173. Gordeuk VR, McLaren CE, MacPhail AP, et al: Associations of iron overload in Africa with hepatocellular carcinoma and tuberculosis: Strachan's 1929 thesis revisited. Blood 87:3470, 1996.

174. Abbott MR, Smith DD: Mycobacterial infections in immunosuppressed patients. Med J Aust 1:351, 1981.

175. Murray JF: Tuberculosis and HIV infection worldwide. Pneumologie 49(Suppl 3):653, 1995.

176. Castro KG: Tuberculosis as an opportunistic disease in persons infected with human immunodeficiency virus. Clin Infect Dis 21(Suppl 1):S66, 1995.

177. Barnes PF, Le HQ, Davidson PT: Tuberculosis in patients with HIV infection. Med Clin North Am 77:1369, 1993.

178. MacKinnon J: Tuberculosis occurring during steroid therapy. BMJ 2:1375, 1959.

179. Millar JW, Horne NW: Tuberculosis in immunosuppressed patients. Lancet 1:1176, 1979.

180. Cisneros JR, Murray KM: Corticosteroids in tuberculosis. Ann Pharmacother 30:1298, 1996.

181. Alzeer AH, FitzGerald JM: Corticosteroids and tuberculosis: Risks and use as adjunct therapy. Tuber Lung Dis 74:6, 1993.

182. Tomasson HO, Brennan M, Bass MJ: Tuberculosis and nonsteroidal anti-inflammatory drugs. Can Med Assoc J 130:275, 1984.

183. Korner MM, Hirata N, Tenderich G, et al: Tuberculosis in heart transplant recipients. Chest 111:365, 1997.

184. Munoz P, Palomo J, Munoz R, et al: Tuberculosis in heart transplant recipients. Clin Infect Dis 21:398, 1995.

185. Meyers BR, Halpern M, Sheiner P, et al: Tuberculosis in liver transplant patients. Transplantation 58:301, 1994.

186. Nishizaki T, Yanaga K, Soejima Y, et al: Tuberculosis following liver transplantation: Report of a case and review of the literature. Transpl Int 9:589, 1996.

187. Miller RA, Lanza LA, Kline JN, et al: *Mycobacterium tuberculosis* in lung transplant recipients. Am J Respir Crit Care Med 152:374, 1995.

188. Dromer C, Nashef SA, Velly JF, et al: Tuberculosis in transplanted lungs. J Heart Lung Transplant 12:924, 1993.

189. Lichtenstein IH, MacGregor RR: Mycobacterial infections in renal transplant recipients: Report of five cases and review of the literature. Rev Infect Dis 5:216, 1983.

190. Sakhuja V, Jha V, Varma PP, et al: The high incidence of tuberculosis among renal transplant recipients in India. Transplantation 61:211, 1996.

191. Edelstein CL, Jacobs JC, Moosa MR: Pulmonary complications in 110 consecutive renal transplant recipients. S Afr Med J 85:160, 1995.

192. Hall CM, Willcox PA, Swanepoel CR, et al: Mycobacterial infection in renal transplant recipients. Chest 106:435, 1994.

193. Ip MS, Yuen KY, Chiu EK, et al: Pulmonary infections in bone marrow transplantation: The Hong Kong experience. Respiration 62:80, 1995.

194. Torre-Cisneros J, de la Mata M, Rufian S, et al: Importance of surveillance mycobacterial cultures after liver transplantation. Transplantation 60:1054, 1995.

195. Kaplan MH, Armstrong D, Rosen P: Tuberculosis complicating neoplastic disease: A review of 201 cases. Cancer 33:850, 1974.

196. Rho R, Laddis T, McQuain C, et al: Miliary tuberculosis in a patient with Epstein-Barr virus-associated angioimmunoblastic lymphadenopathy. Ann Hematol 72:333, 1996.

197. Cole ST, Telenti A: Drug resistance in *Mycobacterium tuberculosis*. Eur Respir J 8(Suppl 20):701s, 1995.

198. Leading article: Drug-resistant tuberculosis. BMJ 283:336, 1981.

199. Ben-Dov I, Mason GR: Drug-resistant tuberculosis in a Southern California hospital: Trends from 1969 to 1984. Am Rev Respir Dis 135:1307, 1987.

200. Chawla PK, Klapper PJ, Kamholz SL, et al: Drug-resistant tuberculosis in an urban population including patients at risk for human immunodeficiency virus infection. Am Rev Respir Dis 146:280, 1992.

200a. Harrow EM, Rangel JM, Arriega JM, et al: Epidemiology and clinical consequences of drug-resistant tuberculosis in a Guatemalan hospital. Chest 113:1452, 1998.

201. Frieden TR, Sterling T, Pablo-Mendez A, et al: Multiple drug-resistant tuberculosis in New York City. N Engl J Med 328:521, 1993.

202. al Jarad N, Parastatides S, Paul EA, et al: Characteristics of patients with drug resistant and drug sensitive tuberculosis in East London between 1984 and 1992. Thorax 49:808, 1994.

203. Neville K, Bromberg A, Bromberg R, et al: The third epidemic—multidrug-resistant tuberculosis. Chest 105:45, 1994.

204. Beck-Sague C, Dooley SW, Hutton MD, et al: Hospital outbreak of multidrug-resistant *Mycobacterium tuberculosis* infections: Factors in transmission to staff and HIV-infected patients. JAMA 268:1280, 1992.

205. Edlin BR, Tokars JI, Grieco MH, et al: An outbreak of multidrug-resistant tuberculosis among hospitalized patients with the acquired immunodeficiency syndrome. N Engl J Med 326:1514, 1992.

206. Pearson ML, Jereb JA, Frieden TR, et al: Nosocomial transmission of multidrug-resistant *Mycobacterium tuberculosis*: A risk to patients and health care workers. Ann Intern Med 117:191, 1992.

207. Jones BE, Ryu R, Yang Z, et al: Chest radiographic findings in patients with tuberculosis with recent or remote infection. Am J Respir Crit Care Med 156:1270, 1997.

208. Colice GL: Pulmonary tuberculosis: Is resurgence due to reactivation or new infection? Postgrad Med 97:35, 1995.

208a. McDonough KA, Kress Y: Cytotoxicity for lung epithelial cells is a virulence-associated phenotype of *Mycobacterium tuberculosis*. Infect Immunol 63:4802, 1995.

209. Goren MB: Immunoreactive substances of *Mycobacteria*. Am Rev Respir Dis 125:50, 1982.

209a. Gordon AH, D'Arcy Hart P, Young MR: Ammonia inhibits phagosome-lysosome fusion in macrophages. Nature 286:79, 1980.

210. Myrvik QN, Leake ES, Wright MJ: Disruption of phagosomal membranes of normal alveolar macrophages by the H37Rv strain of *Mycobacterium tuberculosis*. Am Rev Respir Dis 129:322, 1984.

211. Middlebrook G: Isoniazid-resistance and catalase activity of tubercle bacilli: A preliminary report. Am Rev Tuberc 69:471, 1954.

212. Diaz GA, Wayne LG: Isolation and characterization of catalase produced by *Mycobacterium tuberculosis*. Am Rev Respir Dis 110:312, 1974.

213. Dunlap NE, Briles DE: Immunology of tuberculosis. Med Clin North Am 77:1235, 1993.

214. Munk ME, Emoto M: Functions of T-cell subsets and cytokines in mycobacterial infections. Eur Respir J 8(Suppl 20):668s, 1995.

214a. Schluger NW, Rom WN: The host immune responce to tuberculosis. Am J Respir Crit Care Med 157:679, 1998.

215. Yu CT, Wang CH, Huang TJ, et al: Relation of bronchoalveolar lavage T lymphocyte subpopulations to rate of regression of active pulmonary tuberculosis. Thorax 50:869, 1995.

216. Boom WH: The role of T-cell subsets in *Mycobacterium tuberculosis* infection. Infect Agents Dis 5:73, 1996.

216a. Condos R, Rom WM, Liu YM, et al: Local immune responses correlate with presentation and outcome in tuberculosis. Am J Respir Crit Care Med 157:729, 1998.

217. Ohmen JD, Barnes PF, Grisso CL, et al: Evidence for a superantigen in human tuberculosis. Immunity 1:35, 1994.

218. Pithie AD, Lammas DA, Fazal N, et al: CD4+ cytolytic T cells can destroy autologous and MHC-matched macrophages but fail to kill intracellular *Mycobacterium bovis*-BCG. FEMS Immunol Med Microbiol 11:145, 1995.

218a. Schlesinger LS: Role of mononuclear phagocytes in *M. tuberculosis* pathogenesis. J Invest Med 44:312, 1996.

218b. Gaynor CF, McCormack D, Voelker S, et al: Pulmonary surfactant protein A mediates enhanced phagocytosis of *Mycobacterium tuberculosis* by a direct interaction with human macrophages. J Immunol 155:5343, 1995.

219. Vorwald AJ: The early cellular reactions in the lungs of rabbits injected intravenously with human tubercle bacilli. Am Rev Tuberc 25:74, 1932.

220. Jones GS, Amirault HJ, Andersen BR: Killing of *Mycobacterium tuberculosis* by neutrophils: A nonoxidative process. J Infect Dis 162:700, 1990.

221. Van den Oord JJ, de Wolf-Peeters C, Fachetti F, et al: Cellular composition of hypersensitivity-type granulomas: Immunohistochemical analysis of tuberculous and sarcoid lymphadenitis. Hum Pathol 15:559, 1984.

222. Law K, Weiden M, Harkin T, et al: Increased release of interleukin-1 beta, interleukin-6, and tumor necrosis factor-alpha by bronchoalveolar cells lavaged from involved sites in pulmonary tuberculosis. Am J Respir Crit Care Med 153:799, 1996.

223. Toossi Z, Gogae P, Shiratsuchi H, et al: Enhanced production of TGF-beta by blood monocytes from patients with active tuberculosis and presence of TGF-beta in tuberculous granulomatous lung lesions. J Immunol 154:465, 1995.

224. Dannenberg AM Jr: Pathogenesis of pulmonary tuberculosis. Am Rev Respir Dis 125:25, 1982.

225. Weber AL, Bird KT, Janower ML: Primary tuberculosis in childhood with particular emphasis on changes affecting the tracheobronchial tree. Am J Roentgenol 103:123, 1968.

226. Medlar EM: The behavior of pulmonary tuberculous lesions: A pathological study. Am Rev Tuberc 71:1, 1955.

227. Alame T, Dierckx P, Carlier S, et al: Lymph node perforation into the airway in AIDS-associated tuberculosis. Eur Respir J 8:658, 1995.

228. Stead WW, Bates JH: Evidence of a "silent" bacillemia in primary tuberculosis. Ann Intern Med 74:559, 1971.

229. Stead WW, Kerby GR, Schlueter DP, et al: The clinical spectrum of primary tuberculosis in adults: Confusion with reinfection in the pathogenesis of chronic tuberculosis. Ann Intern Med 68:731, 1968.

230. Leung AN, Müller NL, Pineda PR, et al: Primary tuberculosis in childhood: Radiographic manifestations. Radiology 182:87, 1992.

231. Nagakura Y: Pathologic-anatomic studies on resected lungs of younger patients with pulmonary tuberculosis. Clin Respir Organs (Tokyo) 15:462, 1960.

232. Joffe N: Cavitating primary pulmonary tuberculosis in infancy. Br J Radiol 33:430, 1960.

233. Choyke PL, Sostman HD, Curtis AM, et al: Adult-onset tuberculosis. Radiology 48:357, 1983.

234. Lee KS, Im JG: CT in adults with tuberculosis of the chest: Characteristic findings and role in management. Am J Roentgenol 164:1361, 1995.

235. Derham RJ: Postprimary intrathoracic tuberculosis in childhood with special reference to its sequelae. Texas J Med 52:583, 1956.

236. Woodring JH, Vandiviere HM, Fried AM, et al: Update: The radiographic features of pulmonary tuberculosis. Am J Roentgenol 146:497, 1986.

237. Im JG, Song KS, Kang HS, et al: Mediastinal tuberculous lymphadenitis: CT manifestations. Radiology 164:115, 1987.

237a. Pombo F, Rodriguez E, Mato J, et al: Patterns of contrast enhancement of tuberculous lymph nodes demonstrated by computed tomography. Clin Radiol 46:13, 1992.

238. Pastores SM, Naidich DP, Aranda CP, et al: Intrathoracic adenopathy associated with pulmonary tuberculosis in patients with human immunodeficiency virus infection. Chest 103:1433, 1993.

239. Hartman TE, Primack SL, Müller NL, et al: Diagnosis of thoracic complications in AIDS: Accuracy of CT. Am J Roentgenol 162:547, 1994.

240. Landay MJ, Rollins NK: Mediastinal histoplasmosis granuloma: Evaluation with CT. Radiology 172:657, 1989.

241. Frostad S: Segmental atelectasis in children with primary tuberculosis. Am Rev Respir Dis 79:597, 1959.

242. Frostad S: Lymph node perforation through the bronchial tree in children with primary tuberculosis. Acta Tuberc Scand 47(Suppl):104, 1959.

243. Matthews JI, Matarese SL, Carpenter JL: Endobronchial tuberculosis simulating lung cancer. Chest 86:642, 1984.

244. Serviansky B, Schwarz J: Calcified intrathoracic lesions caused by histoplasmosis and tuberculosis. Am J Roentgenol 77:1034, 1957.

245. Choyke PL, Sostman HD, Curtis AM, et al: Adult-onset pulmonary tuberculosis. Radiology 148:357, 1983.

246. Festenstein F: Spread of tuberculosis within a family. Lancet 1:603, 1981.

247. Enarson DA, Dorken E, Grzybowski S: Tuberculous pleurisy. Can Med Assoc J 126:493, 1982.

248. Myers JA, Bearman JE, Dixon HG: The natural history of tuberculosis in the human body: V. Prognosis among tuberculin-reactor children from birth to five years of age. Am Rev Respir Dis 87:354, 1963.

249. Pineda PR, Leung A, Müller NL, et al: Intrathoracic paediatric tuberculosis: A report of 202 cases. Tuber Lung Dis 74:261, 1993.

250. Zarabi M, Sane S, Girdany BR: The chest roentgenogram in the early diagnosis of tuberculous meningitis in children. Am J Dis Child 121:389, 1971.

251. Steiner P, Portugaleza O: Tuberculous meningitis in children: A review of 25 cases observed between the years 1965 and 1970 at the Kings County Medical Center of Brooklyn with special reference to the problem of infection with primary drug-resistant strains of *M. tuberculosis*. Am Rev Respir Dis 107:22, 1973.

252. Alland D, Kalkut GE, Moss AR, et al: Transmission of tuberculosis in New York City: An analysis by DNA fingerprinting and conventional epidemiologic methods. N Engl J Med 330:1710, 1994.

253. Small PM, Hopewell PC, Singh SP, et al: The epidemiology of tuberculosis in San Francisco: A population-based study using conventional and molecular methods. N Engl J Med 330:1703, 1994.

254. Poppius H, Thomander K: Segmentary distribution of cavities: A radiologic study of 500 consecutive cases of cavernous pulmonary tuberculosis. Ann Med Int Fenn 46:113, 1957.

255. Krysl J, Korzeniewska-Kosela M, Müller NL, et al: Radiologic features of pulmonary tuberculosis: An assessment of 188 cases. Can Assoc Radiol J 45:101, 1994.

256. Riley RL: Apical localization of pulmonary tuberculosis. Bull Johns Hopkins Hosp 106:232, 1960.

257. West JB: Localization of disease: Pulmonary tuberculosis. *In* Regional Differences in the Lung. New York, Academic Press, 1977, p 236.

258. Sekosan M, Cleto M, Senseng C, et al: Spindle cell pseudotumors in the lungs due to *Mycobacterium tuberculosis* in a transplant patient. Am J Surg Pathol 18:1065, 1994.

259. Links TP, Karrenbeld A, Steensma JT, et al: Fatal respiratory failure caused by pulmonary infiltration by pseudo-Gaucher cells. Chest 101:265, 1992.

260. Yamamura Y, Ogawa Y, Maeda H, et al: Prevention of tuberculous cavity formation by desensitization with tuberculin-active peptide. Am Rev Respir Dis 109:594, 1974.

261. Dannenberg AM Jr, Sugimoto M: Liquefaction of caseous foci in tuberculosis. Am Rev Respir Dis 113:257, 1976.

262. Converse PJ, Dannenberg AM Jr, Estep JE, et al: Cavitary tuberculosis produced in rabbits by aerosolized virulent tubercle bacilli. Infect Immun 64:4776, 1996.

263. Chang JC, Wysocki A, Tchou-Wong KM, et al: Effect of *Mycobacterium tuberculosis* and its components on macrophages and the release of matrix metalloproteinases. Thorax 51:306, 1996.

264. Ishida T, Yokoyama H, Kaneko S, et al: Pulmonary tuberculoma and indications for surgery: Radiographic and clinicopathological analysis. Respir Med 86:431, 1992.

265. Macleod WM, Smith AT: Some observations on the historical appreciation, pathological development, and behaviour of round tuberculous foci. Thorax 7:334, 1952.

266. Wayne LG: The bacteriology of resected tuberculous pulmonary lesions: II. Observations on bacilli which are stainable but which cannot be cultured. Am Rev Respir Dis 82:370, 1960.

267. al-Majed SA: Replacement of one lung by a large bulla in active tuberculosis. Thorax 50:427, 1995.

268. Auerbach O: Pathology of tuberculosis as affected by antibiotics. Am J Surg 89:627, 1955.

269. Bobrowitz ID, Rodescu D, Marcus H, et al: The destroyed tuberculous lung. Scand J Respir Dis 55:82, 1974.

270. Ashour M, Pandya L, Mezraqji A, et al: Unilateral post-tuberculous lung destruction: The left bronchus syndrome. Thorax 45:210, 1990.

271. Segarra F, Sherman DS, Rodriguez-Aguero J: Lower lung field tuberculosis. Am Rev Respir Dis 87:37, 1963.

272. Berger HW, Granada MG: Lower lung field tuberculosis. Chest 65:522, 1974.

273. Doherty JG, Rankin R, Kerr F: Miliary tuberculosis presenting as infection of a pacemaker pulse-generator pocket. Scott Med J 41:20, 1996.

274. Henderson CE, Turk R, Dobkin J, et al: Miliary tuberculosis in pregnancy. J Natl Med Assoc 85:685, 1993.

275. Kabani AM, Yao JD, Jadusingh IH, et al: Tuberculous fasciitis and tenosynovitis: An unusual presentation of miliary tuberculosis. Diagn Microbiol Infect Dis 16:67, 1993.

276. Cluroe AD: Legionnaire's disease mimicking pulmonary miliary tuberculosis in the immunocompromised. Histopathology 22:73, 1993.

277. Auerbach O: Acute generalized miliary tuberculosis. Am J Pathol 20:121, 1944.

278. Slavin RE, Walsh TJ, Pollack AD: Late generalized tuberculosis: A clinical pathologic analysis and comparison of 100 cases in the preantibiotic and antibiotic eras. Medicine 59:352, 1980.

279. Federmann M, Kley HK: Miliary tuberculosis after extracorporeal shock-wave lithotripsy. N Engl J Med 323:1212, 1990.

280. O'Brien JR: Non-reactive tuberculosis. J Clin Pathol 7:216, 1954.

281. Singh R, Joshi RC, Christie J: Generalized nonreactive tuberculosis: A clinico-pathologic study of four patients. Thorax 44:952, 1989.

282. Campo E, Condom E, Miro MJ, et al: Tuberculosis-associated hemophagocytic syndrome. Cancer 58:2640, 1986.

283. Auerbach O: Tuberculosis of the trachea and major bronchi. Am Rev Tuberc 60:604, 1949.

284. Salkin D, Cadden AV, Edson RO: The natural history of tuberculous tracheobronchitis. Am Rev Tuberc 47:351, 1943.

285. Ip MSM, So SY, Lam WK, et al: Endobronchial tuberculosis revisited. Chest 89:727, 1986.

286. Cudkowicz L: The blood supply of the lung in pulmonary tuberculosis. Thorax 7:270, 1952.

287. Lorenz R, Kraman SS: Intracavitary mass in a patient with far-advanced tuberculosis. Chest 82:91, 1982.

288. Lopez-Contreras J, Ris J, Domingo P, et al: Tuberculous pulmonary gangrene: Report of a case and review. Clin Infect Dis 18:243, 1994.

289. Auerbach O: Pathology and pathogenesis of pulmonary arterial aneurysm in tuberculous cavities. Am Rev Tuberc 39:99, 1939.

290. Plessinger VA, Jolly PN: Rasmussen's aneurysms and fatal hemorrhage in pulmonary tuberculosis. Am Rev Tuberc 60:589, 1949.

291. Cohen AS, Beaconsfield T, al-Kutoubi A, et al: Pulmonary artery reconstruction for tuberculosis. Ann Thorac Surg 61:1257, 1996.

292. Schmid FG, De Haller R: Late exudative complications of collapse therapy for pulmonary tuberculosis. Chest 89:822, 1986.

293. McBurney RP, Jamplis RW, Hedberg G: Oil granuloma and lipoid pneumonitis: A complication of oleothorax. J Thorac Surg 29:271, 1955.

294. Case records of the Massachusetts General Hospital: Weekly clinicopathological exercises: Case 38-1983: Empyema 40 years after a thoracoplasty. N Engl J Med 309:715, 1983.

295. Molinie V, Pouchot J, Navratil E, et al: Primary Epstein-Barr virus-related non-Hodgkin's lymphoma of the pleural cavity following long-standing tuberculous empyema. Arch Pathol Lab Med 120:288, 1996.

296. Martin A, Capron F, Liguory-Brunaud MD, et al: Epstein-Barr virus-associated primary malignant lymphomas of the pleural cavity occurring in longstanding pleural chronic inflammation. Hum Pathol 25:1314, 1994.

297. Aozasa K, Ohsawa M, Iuchi K, et al: Artificial pneumothorax as a risk factor for development of pleural lymphoma. Jpn J Cancer Res 84:55, 1993.

298. Harland RW, Sharma M, Rosenzweig DY: Lung carcinoma in a patient with Lucite sphere plombage thoracoplasty. Chest 103:1295, 1993.

299. Friedenberg RM, Isaacs N, Elkin M: The changing roentgenologic picture in pulmonary tuberculosis under modern chemotherapy. Am J Roentgenol 81:196, 1959.

300. Roque FT: A new face of tuberculosis. Am J Med Sci 2401:17, 1960.

301. Steer A: A study of healing and repair of pulmonary tuberculous lesions with and without chemotherapy. Am Rev Respir Dis 95:209, 1967.

302. Lee KS, Hwang JW, Chung MP, et al: Utility of CT in the evaluation of pulmonary tuberculosis in patients without AIDS. Chest 110:977, 1996.

303. Adler H: Phthisiogenetic studies by means of tomography in cases of localized pulmonary tuberculosis in adults. Acta Tuberc Scand 47(Suppl):13, 1959.

304. Spencer D, Yagan R, Blinkhorn R, et al: Anterior segment upper lobe tuberculosis in the adult: Occurrence in primary and reactivation disease. Chest 97:384, 1990.

305. Ikezoe J, Takeuchi N, Johkoh T, et al: CT appearance of pulmonary tuberculosis in diabetic and immunocompromised patients: Comparison with patients who had no underlying disease. Am J Roentgenol 159:1175, 1992.

306. Weaver RA: Unusual radiographic presentation of pulmonary tuberculosis in diabetic patients. Am Rev Respir Dis 109:162, 1974.

307. Im JG, Itoh H, Shim YS, et al: Pulmonary tuberculosis: CT findings—early active disease and sequential change with antituberculous therapy. Radiology 186:653, 1993.

308. Im JG, Itoh H, Han MC: CT of pulmonary tuberculosis. Semin Ultrasound CT MRI 16:420, 1995.

309. Primack SL, Logan PM, Hartman TE, et al: Pulmonary tuberculosis and *Mycobacterium avium-intracellulare*: A comparison of CT findings. Radiology 194:413, 1995.

310. Lee KS, Song KS, Lim TH, et al: Adult-onset pulmonary tuberculosis: Findings on chest radiographs and CT scans. Am J Roentgenol 160:753, 1993.

311. Penner C, Roberts D, Kunimoto D, et al: Tuberculosis as a primary cause of respiratory failure requiring mechanical ventilation. Am J Respir Crit Care Med 151:867, 1995.

312. Hatipoğlu ON, Osma E, Manisali M, et al: High-resolution computed tomographic findings in pulmonary tuberculosis. Thorax 51:397, 1996.

312a. Poey C, Verhaegen F, Giron J, et al: High-resolution chest CT in tuberculosis: Evolutive patterns and signs of activity. J Comput Assist Tomogr 21:601, 1997.

313. Cohen JR, Amorosa JK, Smith PR: The air-fluid level in cavitary pulmonary tuberculosis. Radiology 127:315, 1978.

314. Corpe RF, Blalock FA: A continuing study of patients with "open negative" status at Battey State Hospital. Am Rev Respir Dis 98:954, 1968.

315. Wilson TM, Doyle L, Gardiner MP: Open healing of tuberculous cavities: Results in 40 patients treated conservatively. BMJ 2:87, 1958.

316. Ryder JB: Prognosis of persistent cavitation in sputum-negative cases of tuberculosis following long-term chemotherapy. Tubercle 39:113, 1958.

317. Minarik L, Mercir S, Urge L: The fate of negative (open-healed) cavities in tuberculous patients discharged from institutional treatment. Rozhl Tuberc 20:509, 1960.

317a. Long R, Maycher B: Check-valve pneumatocele formation following fully treated tuberculosis: Case report. Can Assoc Radiol J 43:197, 1998.

318. Sochocky S: Tuberculoma of the lung. Am Rev Tuberc 78:403, 1958.

319. Bleyer JM, Marks JH: Tuberculomas and hamartomas of the lung: Comparative study of 66 proved cases. Am J Roentgenol 77:1013, 1957.

320. Winer-Muram HT, Rubin SA: Thoracic complications of tuberculosis. J Thorac Imaging 5:46, 1990.

321. Zwirewich CV, Vedal S, Miller RR, et al: Solitary pulmonary nodule: High-resolution CT and radiologic-pathologic correlation. Radiology 179:469, 1991.

322. Swensen SJ, Brown LR, Colby TV, et al: Pulmonary nodules: CT evaluation of enhancement with iodinated contrast material. Radiology 194:393, 1995.

323. Murayama S, Murakami J, Hashimoto S, et al: Noncalcified pulmonary tuberculomas: CT enhancement patterns with histologic correlation. J Thorac Imaging 10:91, 1995.

324. Sakai F, Sone S, Maruyama A, et al: Thin-rim enhancement in Gd-DTPA-enhanced magnetic resonance images of tuberculoma: A new finding of potential differential diagnostic importance. J Thorac Imaging 7:64, 1992.

325. Yamashita K, Matsunobe S, Tsuda T, et al: Intratumoral necrosis of lung carcinoma: A potential diagnostic pitfall in incremental dynamic computed tomography analysis of solitary pulmonary nodules? J Thorac Imaging 12:181, 1997.

326. Hoffmann L, Neumann P, Naegele E, et al: Tuberculous round foci of the lungs from the viewpoint of tuberculosis care and chest surgery [German]. Beitr Klin Tuberk 124:558, 1962.

327. Siegelman SS, Khouri NF, Leo FP, et al: Solitary pulmonary nodules: CT assessment. Radiology 160:307, 1986.

328. Itoh H, Tokunaga S, Todo G, et al: Radiologic-pathologic correlation of small lung nodules with special reference to peribronchial nodules. Am J Roentgenol 130:223, 1978.

329. Gelb AF, Leffler C, Brewin A, et al: Miliary tuberculosis. Am Rev Respir Dis 108:1327, 1973.

330. Kwong JS, Carignan S, Kang EY, et al: Miliary tuberculosis: Diagnostic accuracy of chest radiography. Chest 110:339, 1996.

331. Peiken AS, Lamberta F, Seriff NS: Bilateral recurrent pneumothoraces: A rare complication of miliary tuberculosis. Am Rev Respir Dis 110:512, 1974.

332. Narang RK, Kumar S, Gupta A: Pneumothorax and pneumomediastinum complicating acute miliary tuberculosis. Tubercle 58:79, 1977.

333. Biehl JP: Miliary tuberculosis: A review of sixty-eight adult patients admitted to a municipal general hospital. Am Rev Tuberc 77:605, 1958.

334. Campbell IG: Miliary tuberculosis in British Columbia. Can Med Assoc J 108:1517, 1973.

335. Grieco MH, Chmel H: Acute disseminated tuberculosis as a diagnostic problem: A clinical study based on twenty-eight cases. Am Rev Respir Dis 109:554, 1974.

336. Prout S, Benatar SR: Disseminated tuberculosis: A study of 62 cases. S Afr Med J 58:835, 1980.

337. Optican RJ, Ost A, Ravin CE: High-resolution computed tomography in the diagnosis of miliary tuberculosis. Chest 102:941, 1992.

338. Oh YW, Kim YH, Lee NJ, et al: High-resolution CT appearance of miliary tuberculosis. J Comput Assist Tomogr 18:862, 1994.

339. McGuinness G, Naidich DP, Jagirdar J, et al: High resolution CT findings in miliary lung disease. J Comput Assist Tomogr 16:384, 1992.

340. Massaro D, Katz S: Rapid clearing in hematogenous pulmonary tuberculosis. Arch Intern Med 113:573, 1964.

341. Bonstein H, Vullièmoz P, Michetti F, et al: Étude de la fonction pulmonaire chez 14 sujets guéris d'une tuberculose pulmonaire miliare. [A study of pulmonary function in 14 subjects recovered from miliary pulmonary tuberculosis.] Schweiz Z Tuberk 18:83, 1961.

342. Lynch JP, Ravikrishnan KP: Endobronchial mass caused by tuberculosis. Arch Intern Med 140:1090, 1980.

343. Mariotta S, Guidi L, Aquilini M, et al: Airway stenosis after tracheo-bronchial tuberculosis. Respir Med 91:107, 1997.

344. Hoheisel G, Chan BK, Chan CH, et al: Endobronchial tuberculosis: Diagnostic features and therapeutic outcome. Respir Med 88:593, 1994.

345. Choe KO, Jeong HJ, Sohn HY: Tuberculous bronchial stenosis: CT findings in 28 cases. Am J Roentgenol 155:971, 1990.

346. Lee KS, Kim YH, Kim WS, et al: Endobronchial tuberculosis: CT features. J Comput Assist Tomogr 15:424, 1991.

347. Kim Y, Lee KS, Yoon JH, et al: Tuberculosis of the trachea and main bronchi: CT findings in 17 patients. Am J Roentgenol 168:1051, 1997.

348. Moon WK, Im JG, Yeon KM, et al: Tuberculosis of the central airways: CT findings of active and fibrotic disease. Am J Roentgenol 169:649, 1997.

349. Eykyn S, Davidson C: Rigors in tuberculosis. Postgrad Med J 69:724, 1993.

350. Holmes P, Faulks L: Presentation of pulmonary tuberculosis. Aust NZ J Med 11:651, 1981.

351. Stinghe RV, Mangiulea VG: Hemoptysis of bronchial origin occurring in patients with arrested tuberculosis. Am Rev Respir Dis 101:84, 1970.

352. Mariotta S, Masullo M, Guidi L, et al: Tracheobronchial involvement in 84 cases of pulmonary tuberculosis. Monaldi Arch Chest Dis 50:356, 1995.

353. Penner C, Roberts D, Kunimoto D, et al: Tuberculosis as a primary cause of respiratory failure requiring mechanical ventilation. Am J Respir Crit Care Med 151:867, 1995.

354. Le Roux BT: Unusual presentations of tuberculosis. Thorax 26:343, 1971.

355. Maartens G, Willcox PA, Benatar SR: Miliary tuberculosis: Rapid diagnosis, hematologic abnormalities, and outcome in 109 treated adults. Am J Med 89:291, 1990.

356. Massaro D, Katz S, Sachs M: Choroidal tubercles: A clue to hematogenous tuberculosis. Ann Intern Med 60:231, 1964.

357. Sahn SA, Neff TA: Miliary tuberculosis. Am J Med 56:495, 1974.

358. Katz I, Rosenthal T, Michaeli D: Undiagnosed tuberculosis in hospitalized patients. Chest 87:770, 1985.

359. Edlin GP: Active tuberculosis unrecognized until necropsy. Lancet 1:650, 1978.

360. Bobrowitz ID: Active tuberculosis undiagnosed until autopsy. Am J Med 72:650, 1982.

361. Humphries MJ, Byfield SP, Darbyshire JH, et al: Deaths occurring in newly notified patients with pulmonary tuberculosis in England and Wales. Br J Dis Chest 78:149, 1984.

362. Chapman RC, Claydon SM: *Mycobacterium tuberculosis*: A continuing cause of sudden and unexpected death in west London. J Clin Pathol 45:713, 1992.

363. Stewart S, McNeil K, Nashef SA, et al: Audit of referral and explant diagnoses in lung transplantation: A pathologic study of lungs removed for parenchymal disease. J Heart Lung Transplant 14:1173, 1995.

364. Farer LS, Lowell LM, Meador MP: Extrapulmonary tuberculosis in the United States. Am J Epidemiol 109:205, 1979.

365. Small PM, Schecter GF, Goodman PC, et al: Treatment of tuberculosis in patients with advanced human immunodeficiency virus infection. N Engl J Med 324:289, 1991.

366. Hong SH, Im J-G, Lee JS, et al: High-resolution CT findings of miliary tuberculosis. J Comput Assist Tomogr 22:220, 1998.
367. Yeager H Jr, Lacy J, Smith LR, et al: Quantitative studies of mycobacterial populations in sputum and saliva. Am Rev Respir Dis 95:998, 1967.
368. Macchiarini P, Delamare N, Beuzeboc P, et al: Tracheoesophageal fistula caused by mycobacterial tuberculosis adenopathy. Ann Thorac Surg 55:1561, 1993.
369. Summers GD, McNicol MW: Tuberculosis of superficial lymph nodes. Br J Dis Chest 74:369, 1980.
370. Wilkins EGL, Roberts C: Superficial tuberculous lymphadenitis in Merseyside: 1969–1984. J Hyg 95:115, 1985.
371. Carter EJ, Mates S: Sudden enlargement of a deep cervical lymph node during and after treatment for pulmonary tuberculosis. Chest 106:1896, 1994.
372. Kent DC: Tuberculous lymphadenitis: Not a localized disease process. Am J Med Sci 254:866, 1967.
373. Manolidis S, Frenkiel S, Yoskovitch A, et al: Mycobacterial infections of the head and neck. Otolaryngol Head Neck Surg 109:427, 1993.
374. Kushihashi T, Munechika H, Motoya H, et al: CT and MR findings in tuberculous mediastinitis. J Comput Assist Tomogr 19:379, 1995.
375. Ramakantan R, Shah P: Dysphagia due to mediastinal fibrosis in advanced pulmonary tuberculosis. Am J Roentgenol 154:61, 1990.
376. Volini FL, Oldfield RC Jr, Thompson JR, et al: Tuberculosis of the aorta. JAMA 181:78, 1962.
377. Gupta SK: Spontaneous paralysis of the phrenic nerve: With a special reference to chronic pulmonary tuberculosis. Br J Dis Chest 54:283, 1960.
378. Bashi SA, Laajam MB, Joharjy IA, et al: Tuberculous oesophagopulmonary communication: Effectiveness of antituberculous chemotherapy: A case report and review of literature. Digestion 32:145, 1985.
379. Monig SP, Schmidt R, Wolters U, et al: Esophageal tuberculosis: A differential diagnostic challenge. Am J Gastroenterol 90:153, 1995.
380. Goodwin RA, Nickell JA, Des Prez RM: Mediastinal fibrosis complicating healed primary histoplasmosis and tuberculosis. Medicine 51:227, 1972.
381. Lee JY, Kim Y, Lee KS, et al: Tuberculous fibrosing mediastinitis: Radiologic findings. Am J Roentgenol 167:1598, 1996.
382. Christensen WI: Genitourinary tuberculosis: Review of 102 cases. Medicine 53:377, 1974.
383. Simon HB, Weinstein AJ, Pasternak MS, et al: Genitourinary tuberculosis: Clinical features in a general hospital. Am J Med 63:410, 1977.
384. Lattimer JK: Renal tuberculosis. N Engl J Med 273:208, 1965.
385. Marks LS, Poutasse EF: Hypertension from renal tuberculosis: Operative cure predicted by renal vein renin. J Urol 109:149, 1973.
386. Kollins SA, Hartman GW, Carr DT, et al: Roentgenographic findings in urinary tract tuberculosis. Am J Roentgenol 121:487, 1974.
387. Kenney M, Loechel AB, Lovelock FJ: Urine cultures in tuberculosis. Am Rev Respir Dis 82:564, 1960.
388. Berney S, Goldstein M, Bishko F: Clinical and diagnostic features of tuberculous arthritis. Am J Med 53:36, 1972.
389. Burke HE: The pathogenesis of certain forms of extrapulmonary tuberculosis. Am Rev Tuberc 62:48, 1950.
390. McTammany JR, Moser KM, Hook VN: Disseminated bone tuberculosis: Review of the literature and presentation of an unusual case. Am Rev Respir Dis 87:888, 1963.
391. Wurtz R, Quader Z, Simon D, et al: Cervical tuberculous vertebral osteomyelitis: Case report and discussion of the literature. Clin Infect Dis 16:806, 1993.
392. Weaver P, Lifeso RM: The radiological diagnosis of tuberculosis of the adult spine. Skeletal Radiol 12:178, 1984.
393. Maritz NGJ, De Villiers JFK, Van Castricum OQS: Computed tomography in tuberculosis of the spine. Comp Radiol 6:1, 1982.
394. Whelan MA, Naidich DP, Post JD, et al: Computed tomography of spinal tuberculosis. J Comput Assist Tomogr 7:25, 1983.
395. Coppola J, Müller NL, Connell DG: Computed tomography of musculoskeletal tuberculosis. J Can Assoc Radiol 38:199, 1987.
396. de Roos A, van Persijn van Meerten EL, Bloem JL, et al: MRI of tuberculous spondylitis. Am J Roentgenol 146:79, 1986.
397. Lee G, Im JG, Kim JS, et al: Tuberculosis of the ribs: CT appearance. J Comput Assist Tomogr 17:363, 1993.
398. Adler BD, Padley SPG, Müller NL: Tuberculosis of the chest wall: CT findings. J Comput Assist Tomogr 17:217, 1993.
399. Chung SY, Yang I, Bae SH, et al: Tuberculous abscess in retromammary region: CT findings. J Comput Assist Tomogr 20:766, 1996.
400. Shandera WX, Rodriguez P, Cate TR: Tuberculous meningitis among adults with and without HIV infection: Experience in an urban public hospital. Arch Intern Med 156:1710, 1996.
401. Weir MR, Thornton GF: Extrapulmonary tuberculosis: Experience of a community hospital and review of the literature. Am J Med 79:467, 1985.
402. Gierson HW, Owens GJ: Chloride content of the cerebrospinal fluid. Calif Med 94:77, 1961.
403. Sada E, Ruiz-Palacios GM, Lopez-Vidal Y, et al: Detection of mycobacterial antigen in cerebrospinal fluid of patients with tuberculous meningitis by enzyme linked immunoabsorbent assay. Lancet 2:651, 1983.
404. Baig SM: Anti-purified protein derivative cell-enzyme-linked immunosorbent assay, a sensitive method for early diagnosis of tuberculous meningitis. J Clin Microbiol 33:3040, 1995.
405. Park SC, Lee BI, Cho SN, et al: Diagnosis of tuberculous meningitis by detection of immunoglobulin G antibodies to purified protein derivative and lipoarabinomannan antigen in cerebrospinal fluid. Tuber Lung Dis 74:317, 1993.
406. Lorber J: Long-term follow-up of 100 children who recovered from tuberculous meningitis. Pediatrics 28:778, 1961.
407. Afghani B, Lieberman JM: Paradoxical enlargement or development of intracranial tuberculomas during therapy: Case report and review. Clin Infect Dis 19:1092, 1994.
408. Beyt BE Jr, Ortbals DW, Santa Cruz DJ, et al: Cutaneous mycobacteriosis: Analysis of 34 cases with a new classification of the disease. Medicine 60:95, 1981.
409. Libraty DH, Byrd TF: Cutaneous miliary tuberculosis in the AIDS era: Case report and review. Clin Infect Dis 23:706, 1996.
410. Farina MC, Gegundez MI, Pique E, et al: Cutaneous tuberculosis: A clinical, histopathologic, and bacteriologic study. J Am Acad Dermatol 33:433, 1995.
411. Hugo-Hamman CT, Scher H, De Moor MM: Tuberculous pericarditis in children: A review of 44 cases. Pediatr Infect Dis J 13:13, 1994.
412. Zayas R, Anguita M, Torres F, et al: Incidence of specific etiology and role of methods for specific etiologic diagnosis of primary acute pericarditis. Am J Cardiol 75:378, 1995.
413. Hageman JH, D'Esopo ND, Glenn WWL: Tuberculosis of the pericardium: A long-term analysis of forty-four proved cases. N Engl J Med 270:327, 1964.
414. Harvey AM, Whitehill MR: Tuberculous pericarditis. Medicine 16:45, 1937.
415. Koh KK, Kim EJ, Cho CH, et al: Adenosine deaminase and carcinoembryonic antigen in pericardial effusion diagnosis, especially in suspected tuberculous pericarditis. Circulation 89:2728, 1994.
416. Komsuoglu B, Goldeli O, Kulan K, et al: The diagnostic and prognostic value of adenosine deaminase in tuberculous pericarditis. Eur Heart J 16:1126, 1995.
417. Ng TT, Strang JI, Wilkins EG: Serodiagnosis of pericardial tuberculosis. QJM 88:317, 1995.
418. Ikezawa T, Iwatsuka Y, Naiki K, et al: Tuberculous pseudoaneurysm of the descending thoracic aorta: A case report and literature review of surgically treated cases. J Vasc Surg 24:693, 1996.
419. Baretti R, Eckel L, Beyersdorf F: Submitral left ventricular tuberculoma. Ann Thorac Surg 60:181, 1995.
420. Goenka MK, Kochhar R, Mehta SK: Spectrum of lower gastrointestinal hemorrhage: An endoscopic study of 166 patients. Indian J Gastroenterol 12:129, 1993.
421. Carrera GF, Young S, Lewiki AM: Intestinal tuberculosis. Gastrointest Radiol 1:147, 1976.
422. Bhansali SK: Abdominal tuberculosis: Experiences with 300 cases. Am J Gastroenterol 67:324, 1977.
423. Sherman S, Rohwedder JJ, Ravikrishnan KP, et al: Tuberculous enteritis and peritonitis: Report of 36 general hospital cases. Arch Intern Med 140:506, 1980.
424. Seabra J, Coelho H, Barros H, et al: Acute tuberculous perforation of the small bowel during antituberculosis therapy. J Clin Gastroenterol 16:320, 1993.
425. Singh MM, Bhargova AM, Jain KP: Tuberculous peritonitis: An evaluation of pathogenetic mechanisms, diagnostic procedures and therapeutic measures. N Engl J Med 281:1091, 1968.
426. Borhanmanesh F, Hekmat K, Vaezzadeh K, et al: Tuberculous peritonitis: Prospective study of 32 cases in Iran. Ann Intern Med 76:567, 1972.
427. Penna L, Manyonda I, Amias A: Intra-abdominal miliary tuberculosis presenting as disseminated ovarian carcinoma with ascites and raised CA125. Br J Obstet Gynaecol 100:1051, 1993.
428. Nistal de Paz F, Herrero Fernandez B, Perez Simon R, et al: Pelvic-peritoneal tuberculosis simulating ovarian carcinoma: Report of three cases with elevation of the CA 125. Am J Gastroenterol 91:1660, 1996.
429. Burack WR, Hollister RM: Tuberculous peritonitis: A study of forty-seven proved cases encountered by a general medical unit in twenty-five years. Am J Med 28:510, 1960.
430. Bowry S, Chan CH, Weiss H, et al: Hepatic involvement in pulmonary tuberculosis: Histologic and functional characteristics. Am Rev Respir Dis 101:941, 1970.
431. Hussain W, Mutimer D, Harrison R, et al: Fulminant hepatic failure caused by tuberculosis. Gut 36:792, 1995.
432. Sheen-Chen SM, Chou FF, Wan YL, et al: Tuberculosis presenting as a solitary splenic tumour. Tuber Lung Dis 76:80, 1995.
433. Beg MHA, Marfani S: The larynx in pulmonary tuberculosis. J Laryngol Otol 99:201, 1985.
434. Levenson MJ, Ingerman M, Grimes C, et al: Laryngeal tuberculosis: Review of twenty cases. Laryngoscope 94:1094, 1984.
435. Gertler R, Ramages L: Tuberculous laryngitis: A one year harvest. J Laryngol Otol 99:1119, 1985.
436. Lindell MM, Jing BS, Wallace S: Laryngeal tuberculosis. Am J Roentgenol 129:677, 1977.
437. Moon WK, Han MH, Chang KH, et al: Laryngeal tuberculosis: CT findings. Am J Roentgenol 166:445, 1996.
438. Kirsch CM, Wehner JH, Jensen WA, et al: Tuberculous otitis media. South Med J 88:363, 1995.
439. Bouza E, Merino P, Munoz P, et al: Ocular tuberculosis: A prospective study in a general hospital. Medicine 76:53, 1997.
440. Braidy J, Pothel C, Amra S: Miliary tuberculosis presenting as adrenal failure. Can Med Assoc J 124:748, 1981.
441. Villabona CM, Sahun M, Ricart W, et al: Tuberculous Addison's disease: Utility of CT in diagnosis and follow-up. Eur J Radiol 17:210, 1993.
442. Shinde SR, Chandawarkar RY, Deshmukh SP: Tuberculosis of the breast masquerading as carcinoma: A study of 100 patients. World J Surg 19:379, 1995.
443. Winkler S, Wiesinger E, Graninger W: Extrapulmonary tuberculosis with paravertebral abscess formation and thyroid involvement. Infection 22:420, 1994.
444. Wu CS, Wang SH, Kuo TT: Pancreatic tuberculosis mimicking pancreatic head carcinoma: A case report and review of the literature. Infection 22:287, 1994.

445. Tan KK: Tuberculosis of the thyroid gland—a review. Ann Acad Med Singapore 22:580, 1993.

446. Brusko G, Melvin WS, Fromkes JJ, et al: Pancreatic tuberculosis. Am Surg 61:513, 1995.

447. Davidson GS, Voorneveld CR, Krishnan N: Tuberculous infection of skeletal muscle in a case of dermatomyositis. Muscle Nerve 17:730, 1994.

448. Crawford JT: New technologies in the diagnosis of tuberculosis. Semin Respir Infect 9:62, 1994.

449. Wallace RJ Jr, O'Brien R, Glassroth J, et al: Diagnosis and treatment of disease caused by nontuberculous mycobacteria. Am Rev Respir Dis 142:940, 1990.

450. Laszlo A: Tuberculosis bacteriology laboratory services and incremental protocols for developing countries. Clin Lab Med 16:697, 1996.

451. Shinnick TM, Good RC: Diagnostic mycobacteriology laboratory practices. Clin Infect Dis 21:291, 1995.

452. Sepkowitz KA: Tuberculin skin testing and the health care worker: Lessons of the Prophit Survey. Tuber Lung Dis 77:81, 1996.

453. American Thoracic Society: The tuberculin skin test. Am Rev Respir Dis 124:356, 1981.

454. Huebner RE, Schein MF, Bass JB Jr: The tuberculin skin test. Clin Infect Dis 17:968, 1993.

455. Seibert FB, Glenn JT: Tuberculin purified derivative: Preparation and analysis of a large quantity for standard. Am Rev Tuberc 44:9, 1941.

456. Zou YL, Zhang JD, Chen MH, et al: Comparative cutaneous testing with purified protein derivative and the antigen complex A60 in vaccinated subjects and tuberculosis patients. Med Microbiol Immunol 184:9, 1995.

457. Marks J: Adsorption of tuberculin as a source of error in Mantoux tests. Tubercle 45:62, 1964.

458. Landi S, Held HR, Tseng MC: Disparity of potency between stabilized and nonstabilized dilute tuberculin solutions. Am Rev Respir Dis 104:385, 1971.

459. Wijsmuller G, Termini J: The tuberculin test: Effects of storage and method of delivery on reaction size. Am Rev Respir Dis 107:267, 1973.

460. Magnusson M, Guld J, Magnus K, et al: Diluents for stabilization of tuberculin. Bull WHO 19:799, 1958.

461. Flynn PM, Shenep JL, Mao L, et al: Influence of needle gauge in Mantoux skin testing. Chest 106:1463, 1994.

462. Comstock GW, Furcolow ML, Greenberg RL, et al: The tuberculin skin test: A statement by the Committee on Diagnostic Skin Testing, American Thoracic Society. Am Rev Respir Dis 104:769, 1971.

463. Browder AA, Griffon AL: Tuberculin tine tests on medical wards. Am Rev Respir Dis 105:299, 1972.

464. Woeltje KF, Kilo CM, Johnson K, et al: Tuberculin skin testing of hospitalized patients. Infect Control Hosp Epidemiol 18:561, 1997.

465. Reichman LB, O'Day R: The influence of a history of a previous test on the prevalence and size of reactions to tuberculin. Am Rev Respir Dis 119:587, 1979.

466. Egsmose T: The effect of an exorbitant intracutaneous dose of 200 micrograms PPD tuberculin compared with 0.02 micrograms PPD tuberculin. Am Rev Respir Dis 102:35, 1970.

467. Fine MH, Furcolow ML, Chick EW, et al: Tuberculin skin test reactions: Effects of revised classification on comparative evaluations. Am Rev Respir Dis 106:752, 1972.

468. Edwards LB, Acquaviva FA, Livesay VT: Identification of tuberculous infected: Dual tests and density of reaction. Am Rev Respir Dis 108:1334, 1973.

469. Muder RR, Brennen C, Yu KT: Choosing appropriate criteria for tuberculin positivity and conversion in a long-term care facility. Infect Control Hosp Epidemiol 14:523, 1993.

470. Shands JW Jr, Boeff D, Fauerbach L, et al: Tuberculin testing in a tertiary hospital: Product variability. Infect Control Hosp Epidemiol 15:758, 1994.

471. Miret-Cuadras P, Pina-Gutierrez JM, Juncosa S: Tuberculin reactivity in Bacillus Calmette-Guérin vaccinated subjects. Tuber Lung Dis 77:52, 1996.

471a. Kendig EL Jr, Kirkpatrick BV, Carter WH, et al: Underreading of the tuberculin skin test reaction. Chest 113:1175, 1998.

472. Zack MB, Fulkerson LL, Stein E: Clinical evaluation of persons positive to stabilized tuberculin but negative to nonstabilized tuberculin. Chest 60:437, 1971.

473. Schachter EN: Tuberculin negative tuberculosis. Am Rev Respir Dis 106:587, 1972.

474. Erdtmann FJ, Dixon KE, Llewellyn CH: Skin testing for tuberculosis: Antigen and observer variability. JAMA 28:479, 1974.

475. Rhoades ER, Bryant RE: The influence of local factors on the reaction to tuberculin. Chest 77:190, 1980.

476. Hyde L: Clinical significance of the tuberculin skin test. Am Rev Respir Dis 105:453, 1972.

477. Nilsson BS, Magnusson M: Comparison of the biologic activity of tuberculins by the use of lymphocyte cultures. Am Rev Respir Dis 108:565, 1973.

478. Heilman DH, Thornton C, Baetz B: A method for quantitating blastogenesis by tuberculins in cultures of human blood lymphocytes. Am Rev Respir Dis 101:569, 1970.

479. Chaparas SD, Sheagren JN, DeMeo A, et al: Correlation of human skin reactivity with lymphocyte transformation induced by mycobacterial antigens and histoplasmin. Am Rev Respir Dis 101:67, 1970.

480. Nash DR, Douglass JE: Anergy in active tuberculosis: A comparison between positive and negative, and an evaluation of 5 TU and 250 TU skin test doses. Chest 77:32, 1980.

481. Woodruff CE, Chapman PT, Howard WL, et al: Quantitative tests with old tuberculin in sanatorium practice. Am Rev Respir Dis 98:270, 1968.

482. Howard WL, Klopfenstein MD, Steininger WJ, et al: The loss of tuberculin sensitivity in certain patients with active pulmonary tuberculosis. Chest 57:530, 1970.

483. Wright PW, Crutcher JE, Holiday DB: Selection of skin test antigens to evaluate PPD anergy. J Fam Pract 41:59, 1995.

484. Montecalvo MA, Wormser GP: Selective tuberculin anergy: Case report and review. Mt Sinai J Med 61:363, 1994.

485. Holden M, Dubin MR, Diamond PH: Frequency of negative intermediate-strength tuberculin sensitivity in patients with active tuberculosis. N Engl J Med 285:1506, 1971.

486. Bovornkitti P, Kangsadl P, Sutherapat P, et al: Reversion and reconversion of tuberculin skin reactions in correlation with the use of prednisone. Dis Chest 38:51, 1960.

487. Atuk NO, Hunt EH: Serial tuberculin testing and isoniazid therapy in general hospital employees. JAMA 218:1795, 1971.

488. Woodruff CE, Chapman PT: Tuberculin sensitivity in elderly patients. Am Rev Respir Dis 104:261, 1971.

489. Slutkin G, Perez-Stable EJ, Hopewell PC: Time course and boosting of tuberculin reactions in nursing home residents. Am Rev Respir Dis 134:1048, 1986.

490. Battershill JH: Cutaneous testing in the elderly patient with tuberculosis. Chest 77:188, 1980.

491. Thompson NJ, Glassroth JL, Snider DE Jr, et al: The booster phenomenon in serial tuberculin testing. Am Rev Respir Dis 119:587, 1979.

491a. Miret-Cuadras P, Pina-Gutierrez JM, Juncosa S: Tuberculin reactivity in bacillus Calmette-Guérin vaccinated subjects. Tuber Lung Dis 77:52, 1996.

492. Kubica GP, Gross WM, Hawkins JE, et al: Laboratory services for mycobacterial diseases. Am Rev Respir Dis 112:773, 1975.

493. Anderson C, Inhaber N, Menzies D: Comparison of sputum induction with fibreoptic bronchoscopy in the diagnosis of tuberculosis. Am J Respir Crit Care Med 152:1570, 1995.

494. Diagnostic Standards and Classification of Tuberculosis and Other Mycobacterial Diseases. New York, American Lung Association, 1974.

495. Wilcox PA, Benatar SR, Potgieter PD: Use of the flexible fibre optic bronchoscope in diagnosis of sputum-negative pulmonary tuberculosis. Thorax 37:598, 1982.

496. Sarkar SK, Sharma TN, Purohit SD, et al: The diagnostic value of routine culture of bronchial washings in tuberculosis. Br J Dis Chest 76:358, 1982.

497. Mohan A, Pande JN, Sharma SK, et al: Bronchoalveolar lavage in pulmonary tuberculosis: A decision analysis approach. QJM 88:269, 1995.

498. Jayasundera CI, Attapattu M, Kumarasinghe MP: Atypical presentations of pulmonary tuberculosis diagnosed by fibreoptic bronchoscopy. Postgrad Med J 69:621, 1993.

499. Fujii H, Ishihara J, Fukaura A, et al: Early diagnosis of tuberculosis by fibreoptic bronchoscopy. Tuber Lung Dis 73:167, 1992.

500. Drent M, Wagenaar SS, Mulder PH, et al: Bronchoalveolar lavage fluid profiles in sarcoidosis, tuberculosis, and nonHodgkin's and Hodgkin's disease: An evaluation of differences. Chest 105:514, 1994.

501. Wallace JM, Deutsch AL, Harrell JH, et al: Bronchoscopy and transbronchial biopsy in evaluation of patients with suspected active tuberculosis. Am J Med 70:1189, 1981.

502. Kvale PA, Johnson MC, Wroblewski DA: Diagnosis of tuberculosis: Routine cultures of bronchial washings are not indicated. Chest 76:140, 1979.

503. Masotti A, Rodella L, Inaspettato G, et al: Clinical and bronchoscopic features of endobronchial tuberculosis. Monaldi Arch Chest Dis 50:89, 1995.

504. Rikimaru T, Tanaka Y, Ichikawa Y, et al: Endoscopic classification of tracheobronchial tuberculosis with healing processes. Chest 105:318, 1994.

505. Lee JH, Park SS, Lee DH, et al: Endobronchial tuberculosis: Clinical and bronchoscopic features in 121 cases. Chest 102:990, 1992.

506. Hoheisel GB, Tabak L, Teschler H, et al: Bronchoalveolar lavage cytology and immunocytology in pulmonary tuberculosis. Am J Respir Crit Care Med 149:460, 1994.

507. Ozaki T, Nakahira S, Tani K, et al: Differential cell analysis in bronchoalveolar lavage fluid from pulmonary lesions of patients with tuberculosis. Chest 102:54, 1992.

508. Ainslie GM, Solomon JA, Bateman ED: Lymphocyte and lymphocyte subset numbers in blood and in bronchoalveolar lavage and pleural fluid in various forms of human pulmonary tuberculosis at presentation and during recovery. Thorax 47:513, 1992.

509. Albera C, Mabritto I, Ghio P, et al: Adenosine deaminase activity and fibronectin levels in bronchoalveolar lavage fluid in sarcoidosis and tuberculosis. Sarcoidosis 10:18, 1993.

510. Jones FL Jr: The relative efficacy of spontaneous sputa, aerosol-induced sputa and gastric aspirates in the bacteriologic diagnosis of pulmonary tuberculosis. Dis Chest 50:403, 1966.

511. Light RW: Pleural diseases. Dis Mon 38:261, 1992.

512. Levine H, Metzger W, Lacera D, et al: Diagnosis of tuberculous pleurisy by culture of pleural biopsy specimen. Arch Intern Med 126:269, 1970.

513. Kumar S, Seshadri MS, Koshi G, et al: Diagnosing tuberculous pleural effusion: Comparative sensitivity of mycobacterial culture and histopathology. BMJ 283:20, 1981.

514. Pant K, Chawla R, Mann PS, et al: Fiberbronchoscopy in smear-negative miliary tuberculosis. Chest 95:1151, 1989.

515. Willcox PA, Potgieter PD, Bateman ED, et al: Rapid diagnosis of sputum-negative miliary tuberculosis using the flexible fibreoptic bronchoscope. Thorax 41:681, 1986.

516. Kinoshita M, Ichikawa Y, Koga H, et al: Re-evaluation of bone marrow aspiration in the diagnosis of miliary tuberculosis. Chest 106:690, 1994.

517. Berger HW, Samortin TG: Miliary tuberculosis: Diagnostic methods with emphasis on the chest roentgenogram. Chest 58:586, 1970.

518. Lombard EH, Victor T, Jordaan A, et al: The detection of *Mycobacterium tuberculosis* in bone marrow aspirate using the polymerase chain reaction. Tuber Lung Dis 75:65, 1994.

519. Lai RS, Lee SS, Ting YM, et al: Diagnostic value of transbronchial lung biopsy under fluoroscopic guidance in solitary pulmonary nodule in an endemic area of tuberculosis. Respir Med 90:139, 1996.

520. Charoenratanakul S, Dejsomritrutai W, Chaiprasert A: Diagnostic role of fiberoptic bronchoscopy in suspected smear negative pulmonary tuberculosis. Respir Med 89:621, 1995.

521. Banner AS: Tuberculosis: Clinical aspects and diagnosis. Arch Intern Med 139:1387, 1979.

522. Woods GL, Witebsky FG: Current status of mycobacterial testing in clinical laboratories: Results of a questionnaire completed by participants in the College of American Pathologists Mycobacteriology E Survey. Arch Pathol Lab Med 117:876, 1993.

523. Wolinsky E: Conventional diagnostic methods for tuberculosis. Clin Infect Dis 19:396, 1994.

524. Boyd JC, Marr JJ: Decreasing reliability of acid-fast smear techniques for detection of tuberculosis. Ann Intern Med 82:489, 1975.

525. Vidal R, Martin-Casabona N, Juan A, et al: Incidence and significance of acid-fast bacilli in sputum smears at the end of antituberculous treatment. Chest 109:1562, 1996.

526. Greenbaum M, Beyt BE Jr, Murray PR: The accuracy of diagnosing pulmonary tuberculosis at a teaching hospital. Am Rev Respir Dis 121:477, 1980.

527. Kim TC, Blackman RS, Heatwole KM, et al: Acid-fast bacilli in sputum smears of patients with pulmonary tuberculosis: Prevalence and significance of negative smears pretreatment and positive smears post-treatment. Am Rev Respir Dis 129:264, 1984.

527a. Burman WJ, Stone BL, Reves RR, et al: The incidence of false-positive cultures for *Mycobacterium tuberculosis*. Am J Respir Crit Care Med 155:321, 1997.

528. Sewell DL, Rashad AL, Rourke WJ Jr, et al: Comparison of the septi-Chek AFB and BACTEC systems and conventional culture for recovery of mycobacteria. J Clin Microbiol 31:2689, 1993.

529. Luquin M, Gamboa F, Barcelo MG, et al: Comparison of a biphasic nonradiometric system with Lowenstein-Jensen and Bactec-460 system for recovery of mycobacteria from clinical specimens. Tuber Lung Dis 77:449, 1996.

530. Pfyffer GE, Welscher HM, Kissling P, et al: Comparison of the Mycobacteria Growth Indicator Tube (MGIT) with radiometric and solid culture for recovery of acid-fast bacilli. J Clin Microbiol 35:364, 1997.

531. Drowart A, Cambiaso CL, Huygen K, et al: Detection of mycobacterial antigens present in short-term culture media using particle counting immunoassay. Am Rev Respir Dis 147:1401, 1993.

532. Kirihara JM, Hillier SL, Coyle MB: Improved detection times for *Mycobacterium avium* complex and *Mycobacterium tuberculosis* with the BACTEC radiometric system. J Clin Microbiol 22:841, 1985.

533. Park CH, Hixon DL, Ferguson CB, et al: Rapid recovery of mycobacteria from clinical specimens using automated radiometric technic. Am J Clin Pathol 81:341, 1984.

534. Siddiqi SH, Hwangbo CC, Silcox V, et al: Rapid radiometric methods to detect and differentiate *Mycobacterium tuberculosis/M. bovis* from other mycobacterial species. Am Rev Respir Dis 130:634, 1984.

535. Ellner PD, Kiehn TE, Cammarata R, et al: Rapid detection and identification of pathogenic mycobacteria by combining radiometric and nucleic acid probe methods. J Clin Microbiol 26:1349, 1988.

536. Lumb R, Lanser JA, Lim IS: Rapid identification of mycobacteria by the Gen-Probe Accuprobe system. Pathology 25:313, 1993.

537. Damato JJ, Collins MT, Rothlauf MV, et al: Detection of mycobacteria by radiometric and standard plate procedures. J Clin Microbiol 17:1066, 1983.

538. Morgan MA, Horstmeier CD, DeYoung DR, et al: Comparison of a radiometric method (BACTEC) and conventional culture media for recovery of mycobacteria from smear-negative specimens. J Clin Microbiol 18:384, 1983.

539. Daniel TM, Debanne SM: The serodiagnosis of tuberculosis and other mycobacterial diseases by enzyme-linked immunosorbent assay. Am Rev Respir Dis 135:1137, 1987.

540. Bothamley GH: Serological diagnosis of tuberculosis. Eur Respir J Suppl 20:676s, 1995.

541. Winters WD, Cox RA: Serodiagnosis of tuberculosis by radioimmunoassay. Am Rev Respir Dis 124:582, 1981.

542. Reggiardo Z, Aber VR, Mitchison DA, et al: Hemagglutination tests for tuberculosis with mycobacterial glycolipid antigens: Results in patients with active pulmonary tuberculosis before and during chemotherapy and in healthy tuberculosis contacts. Am Rev Respir Dis 124:21, 1981.

543. Maekura R, Nakagawa M, Nakamura Y, et al: Clinical evaluation of rapid serodiagnosis of pulmonary tuberculosis by ELISA with cord factor (trehalose-6, 6′-dimycolate) as antigen purified from *Mycobacterium tuberculosis*. Am Rev Respir Dis 148:997, 1993.

544. Charpin D, Herbault H, Gevaudan MJ, et al: Value of ELISA using A60 antigen in the diagnosis of active pulmonary tuberculosis. Am Rev Respir Dis 142:380, 1990.

545. Sada E, Brennan PJ, Herrera T, et al: Evaluation of lipoarabinomannan for the serological diagnosis of tuberculosis. J Clin Microbiol 28:2587, 1990.

546. Stroebel AB, Daniel TM, Lau JHK, et al: Serologic diagnosis of bone and joint tuberculosis by an enzyme-linked immunosorbent assay. J Infect Dis 146:280, 1982.

547. Pouthier F, Perriens JH, Mukadi Y, et al: Anti-A60 immunoglobulin G in the serodiagnosis of tuberculosis in HIV-seropositive and seronegative patients. AIDS 8:1277, 1994.

548. Minnikin DE, Minnikin SM, Parlett JH, et al: Mycolic acid patterns of some species of *Mycobacterium*. Arch Microbiol 139:225, 1984.

549. Lambert MA, Moss CW, Silcox VA, et al: Analysis of mycolic acid cleavage products and cellular fatty acids of *Mycobacterium* species by capillary gas chromatography. J Clin Microbiol 23:731, 1986.

550. Larsson L, Odham G, Westerdahl G, et al: Diagnosis of pulmonary tuberculosis by selected-ion monitoring: Improved analysis of tuberculostearate in sputum using negative-ion mass spectrometry. J Clin Microbol 25:893, 1987.

551. Alugupalli S, Olsson B, Larsson L: Detection of 2-eicosanol by gas chromatography-mass spectrometry in sputa from patients with pulmonary mycobacterial infections. J Clin Microbiol 31:1575, 1993.

552. Drobniewski FA, Kent RJ, Stoker NG, et al: Molecular biology in the diagnosis and epidemiology of tuberculosis. J Hosp Infect 28:249, 1994.

553. Shelhamer JH, Gill VJ, Quinn TC, et al: The laboratory evaluation of opportunistic pulmonary infections. Ann Intern Med 124:585, 1996.

554. Richeldi L, Barnini S, Saltini C: Molecular diagnosis of tuberculosis. Eur Respir J 20(Suppl):689s, 1995.

555. Shoemaker SA, Fisher JH, Scoggin CH: Techniques of DNA hybridization detect small numbers of mycobacteria with no cross-hybridization with non-mycobacterial respiratory organisms. Am Rev Respir Dis 131:760, 1985.

556. Peterson EM, Lu R, Floyd C, et al: Direct identification of *Mycobacterium tuberculosis*, *Mycobacterium avium*, and *Mycobacterium intracellulare* from amplified primary cultures in BACTEC media using DNA probes. J Clin Microbiol 27:1543, 1989.

557. Goto M, Oka S, Okuzumi K, et al: Evaluation of acridinium-ester-labeled DNA probes for identification of *Mycobacterium tuberculosis* and *Mycobacterium intracellulare* complex in culture. J Clin Microbiol 29:2473, 1992.

558. Hermans PWM, Schuitma ARJ, Van Soolingen D, et al: Specific detection of *Mycobacterium tuberculosis* complex strains by polymerase chain reaction. J Clin Microbiol 28:1204, 1990.

559. Del Portillo P, Thomas MC, Martinez E, et al: Multiprimer PCR system for differential identification of mycobacteria in clinical samples. J Clin Microbiol 34:324, 1996.

560. De Beenhouwer H, Liang Z, De Rijk P, et al: Detection and identification of mycobacteria by DNA amplification and oligonucleotide-specific capture plate hybridization. J Clin Microbiol 33:2994, 1995.

561. Schluger NW, Rom WN: The polymerase chain reaction in the diagnosis and evaluation of pulmonary infections. Am J Respir Crit Care Med 152:11, 1995.

562. Pierre C, Lecossier D, Boussougant Y, et al: Use of a reamplification protocol improves the sensitivity of detection of *Mycobacterium tuberculosis* in clinical samples by amplification of DNA. J Clin Microbiol 29:712, 1991.

563. Brisson-Noel A, Aznar C, Chureau C, et al: Diagnosis of tuberculosis by DNA amplification in clinical practice evaluation. Lancet 338:364, 1991.

563a. Cohen RA, Muzaffar S, Schwartz D, et al: Diagnosis of pulmonary tuberculosis using PCR assays on sputum collected within 24 hours of hospital admission. Am J Respir Crit Care Med 157:156, 1998.

564. Sweet-Cordero EA, Chambers HF, Cicero-Sabido R, et al: Burden of *Mycobacterium tuberculosis* in sputum samples can be reliably determined using a quantitative, non-radioactive polymerase chain reaction assay. Tuber Lung Dis 77:496, 1996.

565. Osaki M, Adachi H, Gomyo Y, et al: Detection of Mycobacterial DNA in formalin-fixed, paraffin-embedded tissue specimens by duplex polymerase chain reaction: Application to histologic diagnosis. Mod Pathol 10:78, 1997.

566. Condos R, McClune A, Rom WN, et al: Peripheral-blood-based PCR assay to identify patients with active pulmonary tuberculosis. Lancet 347:1082, 1996.

567. Querol JM, Minguez J, Garcia-Sanchez E, et al: Rapid diagnosis of pleural tuberculosis by polymerase chain reaction. Am J Respir Crit Care Med 152:1977, 1995.

567a. Shah S, Miller A, Mastellone A, et al: Rapid diagnosis of tuberculosis in various biopsy and body fluid specimens by the AMPLICOR *Mycobacterium tuberculosis* polymerase chain reaction test. Chest 113:1190, 1998.

568. Noordhoek GT, Kolk AHJ, Bjune G, et al: Sensitivity and specificity of PCR for detection of *Mycobacterium tuberculosis*: A blind comparison study among seven laboratories. J Clin Microbiol 32:277, 1994.

569. Schluger NW, Kinney D, Harkin TJ, et al: Clinical utility of the polymerase chain reaction in the diagnosis of infections due to *Mycobacterium tuberculosis*. Chest 105:1116, 1994.

570. Young JC, Yuan H, Mahmood A: Clinical significance of a polymerase chain reaction assay for the detection of *Mycobacterium tuberculosis*. Am J Clin Pathol 105:200, 1996.

571. Clarridge JE III, Shawer RM, Shinnick TM, et al: Large-scale use of polymerase chain reaction for detection of *Mycobacterium tuberculosis* in a routine mycobacteriology laboratory. J Clin Microbiol 31:2049, 1993.

572. Bergmann JS, Woods GL: Clinical evaluation of the Roche AMPLICOR PCR *Mycobacterium tuberculosis* test for detection of *M. tuberculosis* in respiratory specimens. J Clin Microbiol 34:1083, 1996.

573. Miller N, Hernandez SG, Cleary TJ: Evaluation of Gen-Probe amplified *Mycobacterium tuberculosis* direct test and PCR for direct detection of *Mycobacterium tuberculosis* in clinical specimens. J Clin Microbiol 32:393, 1994.

574. Chin DP, Yajko DM, Hadley WK, et al: Clinical utility of a commercial test based on the polymerase chain rection for detecting *Mycobacterium tuberculosis* in respiratory specimens. Am J Respir Crit Care Med 151:1872, 1995.

575. Lebrun L, Mathieu D, Saulnier C, et al: Limits of commercial molecular tests for diagnosis of pulmonary tuberculosis. Eur Respir J 10:1874, 1997.

576. Rodriguez JC, Fuentes E, Royo G: Comparison of two different PCR detection methods: Application to the diagnosis of pulmonary tuberculosis. APMIS 105:612, 1997.

577. Brugiere O, Vokurka M, Lecossier D, et al: Diagnosis of smear-negative pulmonary tuberculosis using sequence capture polymerase chain reaction. Am J Respir Crit Care Med 155:1478, 1997.

578. Pierre C, Olivier C, Lecossier D, et al: Diagnosis of primary tuberculosis in children by amplification and detection of mycobacterial DNA. Am Rev Respir Dis 147:420, 1993.

579. van Soolingen D, Hermans PWM: Epidemiology of tuberculosis by DNA fingerprinting. Eur Respir J 8(Suppl 20):649s, 1995.

580. Jereb JA, Burwen DR, Dooley SW, et al: Nosocomial outbreak of tuberculosis in a renal unit: Application of a new technique for restriction fragment length polymorphism analysis of *Mycobacterium tuberculosis* isolates. J Infect Dis 168:1219, 1993.

581. Dooley SW, Jarvis WR, Marlone WJ, et al: Multidrug-resistant tuberculosis. Ann Intern Med 117:257, 1992.

582. Genewein A, Telenti A, Bernasconi C, et al: Molecular approach to identifying route of transmission of tuberculosis in the community. Lancet 342:841, 1993.

582a. Hayward AC, Watson JM: Typing of mycobacteria using spoligotyping. Thorax 53:329, 1998.

583. Fang X, Ma B, Yang X: Bronchial tuberculosis: Cytologic diagnosis of fiberoptic bronchoscopic brushings. Acta Cytol 41:1463, 1997.

584. Nasiell MJ, Roger V, Nasiell K, et al: Cytologic findings indicating pulmonary tuberculosis: I. The diagnostic significance of epithelioid cells and Langerhans' giant cells found in sputum and bronchial secretions. Acta Cytol 16:146, 1972.

585. Roger V, Nasiell M, Nasiell K, et al: Cytologic findings indicating pulmonary tuberculosis: II. The occurrence in sputum of epithelioid cells and multinucleated giant cells in pulmonary tuberculosis, chronic nontuberculous inflammatory lung disease and bronchogenic carcinoma. Acta Cytol 16:538, 1972.

586. Tani EM, Schmitt FCL, Oliveira MLS, et al: Pulmonary cytology in tuberculosis. Acta Cytol 31:460, 1987.

587. Palva T, Saloheimo M: Observations on the cytologic pattern of bronchial aspirates in pulmonary tuberculosis. Acta Tuberc Scand 31:278, 1955.

588. Johnston WW, Frable WJ: Diagnostic Respiratory Cytopathology. New York, Masson Publishing, USA, 1979.

589. Dahlgren SE, Ekström P: Aspiration cytology in the diagnosis of pulmonary tuberculosis. Scand J Respir Dis 53:196, 1972.

590. Robicheaus G, Moinuddin SM, Lee LH: The role of aspiration biopsy cytology in the diagnosis of pulmonary tuberculosis. Am J Clin Pathol 83:719, 1985.

591. Bailey TM, Akhtar M, Ali MA: Fine needle aspiration biopsy in the diagnosis of tuberculosis. Acta Cytol 29:732, 1985.

592. Pappolla MA, Mehta VT: PAS reaction stains phagocytosed atypical *Mycobacteria* in paraffin sections. Arch Pathol Lab Med 108:372, 1984.

593. Mondal A, Patra DK: Efficacy of fine needle aspiration cytology in the diagnosis of tuberculosis of the thyroid gland: A study of 18 cases. J Laryngol Otol 109:36, 1995.

594. Penne D, Oyen R, Demedts M, et al: Tuberculosis of the adrenal glands: Diagnosis by CT-guided fine needle biopsy. J Belge Radiol 76:324, 1993.

595. Editorial: Mycobacterial infections and leucopenia. Lancet 2:184, 1981.

596. Agarwal MK, Muthuswamy PP, Banner AS, et al: Septicemia: Occurrence with bacteriologically positive pulmonary tuberculosis. JAMA 238:2297, 1977.

597. Ebrahim O, Folb PI, Robson SC, et al: Blunted erythropoietin response to anaemia in tuberculosis. Eur J Haematol 55:251, 1995.

598. Lombard EH, Mansvelt EP: Haematological changes associated with miliary tuberculosis of the bone marrow. Tuber Lung Dis 74:131, 1993.

599. Demiroglu H, Ozcebe OI, Ozdemir L, et al: Pancytopenia with hypocellular bone marrow due to miliary tuberculosis: An unusual presentation. Acta Haematol 91:49, 1994.

600. Shenkenberg TD, Rice L, Waddell CC: Acquired Pelger-Huet nuclear anomaly with tuberculosis. Arch Intern Med 142:153, 1982.

601. al-Majed SA, al-Momen AK, al-Kassimi FA, et al: Tuberculosis presenting as immune thrombocytopenic purpura. Acta Haematol 94:135, 1995.

602. Barnes N, Bellamy D, Ireland R, et al: Pulmonary tuberculosis complicated by haemophagocytic syndrome and rifampicin-induced tubulointerstitial nephritis. Br J Dis Chest 78:395, 1984.

603. Cassim KM, Gathiram V, Jogessar VB: Pancytopaenia associated with disseminated tuberculosis, reactive histiocytic haemophagocytic syndrome and tuberculous hypersplenism. Tuber Lung Dis 74:208, 1993.

604. Goldfine ID, Schachter H, Barclay WR, et al: Consumption coagulopathy in miliary tuberculosis. Ann Intern Med 71:775, 1969.

605. Mavligit GM, Binder RA, Crosby WH: Disseminated intravascular coagulation in miliary tuberculosis. Arch Intern Med 130:388, 1972.

606. Bradley GW, Sterling GM: Hypercalcaemia and hypokalaemia in tuberculosis. Thorax 33:464, 1978.

607. Johnson NM, Shneerson G: Hypercalcaemia and hypercalciuria associated with pulmonary tuberculosis. Br J Dis Chest 74:201, 1980.

608. Need AG, Phillips, PJ, Chiu FTS, et al: Hypercalcaemia associated with tuberculosis. BMJ 280:831, 1980.

609. Chan TY, Chan CH, Shek CC: The prevalence of hypercalcaemia in pulmonary and miliary tuberculosis—a longitudinal study. Singapore Med J 35:613, 1994.

610. Cadranel JL, Garabedian M, Milleron B, et al: Vitamin D metabolism by alveolar immune cells in tuberculosis: Correlation with calcium metabolism and clinical manifestations. Eur Respir J 7:1103, 1994.

611. Sullivan JN, Salmon WD Jr: Hypercalcemia in active pulmonary tuberculosis. South Med J 80:572, 1987.

612. Shalhoub RJ, Antoniou LD: The mechanism of hyponatremia in pulmonary tuberculosis. Ann Intern Med 70:943, 1969.

613. Vorherr H, Massry SG, Fallet R, et al: Antidiuretic principle in tuberculous lung tissue of a patient with pulmonary tuberculosis and hyponatremia. Ann Intern Med 72:383, 1970.

614. Post FA, Soule SG, Willcox PA, et al: The spectrum of endocrine dysfunction in active pulmonary tuberculosis. Clin Endocrinol 40:367, 1994.

615. de Beer FC, Nel AE, Gie RP, et al: Serum amyloid A protein and C-reactive protein levels in pulmonary tuberculosis: Relationship to amyloidosis. Thorax 39:196, 1984.

616. Shijubo N, Imai K, Nakanishi F, et al: Elevated concentrations of circulating ICAM-1 in far advanced and miliary tuberculosis. Am Rev Respir Dis 148:1298, 1993.

617. Brice EA, Friedlander W, Bateman ED, et al: Serum angiotensin-converting enzyme activity, concentration, and specific activity in granulomatous interstitial lung disease, tuberculosis, and COPD. Chest 107:706, 1995.

617a. Ameglio F, Giannarelli D, Cordiali-Fei P, et al: Use of discriminant analysis to assess disease activity in pulmonary tuberculosis with a panel of specific and nonspecific serum markers. Am J Clin Pathol 101:719, 1994.

617b. Valdes L, San Jose E, Alvarez D, et al: Diagnosis of tuberculous pleurisy using the biologic parameters adenosine deaminase, lysozyme, and interferon gamma. Chest 103:458, 1993.

617c. Villena V, Lopez-Encuentra A, Echave-Sustaeta J, et al: Interferon-gamma in 388 immunocompromised and immunocompetent patients for diagnosing pleural tuberculosis. Eur Respir J 9:2635, 1996.

618. Ameglio F, Giannarelli D, Cordiali-Fei P, et al: Use of discriminant analysis to assess disease activity in pulmonary tuberculosis with a panel of specific and nonspecific serum markers. Am J Clin Pathol 101:719, 1994.

619. Simpson DG, Kuschner M, McClement J: Respiratory function in pulmonary tuberculosis. Am Rev Respir Dis 87:1, 1963.

620. Williams MH Jr, Yoo OH, Kane C: Pulmonary function in miliary tuberculosis. Am Rev Respir Dis 107:858, 1973.

621. Davis CE Jr, Carpenter JL, McAllister CK, et al: Tuberculosis: Cause of death in antibiotic era. Chest 88:726, 1985.

622. Teale C, Goldman JM, Pearson SB: The association of age with the presentation and outcome of tuberculosis: A five-year survey. Age Ageing 22:289, 1993.

623. Friedman LN, Williams MT, Singh TP, et al: Tuberculosis, AIDS, and death among substance abusers on welfare in New York City. N Engl J Med 334:828, 1996.

624. Zafran N, Heldal E, Pavlovic S, et al: Why do our patients die of active tuberculosis in the era of effective therapy? Tuber Lung Dis 75:329, 1994.

625. Brown J, Pomerantz M: Extrapleural pneumonectomy for tuberculosis. Chest Surg Clin North Am 5:289, 1995.

626. Conlan AA, Lukanich JM, Shutz J: Elective pneumonectomy for benign lung disease: Modern-day mortality and morbidity. J Thorac Cardiovasc Surg 110:1118, 1995.

627. Treasure RL, Seaworth BJ: Current role of surgery in *Mycobacterium tuberculosis*. Ann Thorac Surg 59:1405, 1995.

628. Ashour M: Pneumonectomy for tuberculosis. Eur J Cardiothorac Surg 12:209, 1997.

629. Selby C, Thomson D, Leitch AG: Death in notified cases of tuberculosis in Edinburgh: 1983–1992. Respir Med 89:369, 1995.

630. Penner C, Roberts D, Kunimoto D, et al: Tuberculosis as a primary cause of respiratory failure requiring mechanical ventilation. Am J Respir Crit Care Med 151:867, 1995.

631. Ellis ME, Webb AK: Cause of death in patients admitted to hospital for pulmonary tuberculosis. Lancet 1:665, 1983.

632. White FC, Beck F, Pecora DV: Coexisting primary lung carcinoma and pulmonary tuberculosis: A report of fifteen cases discovered through a chest clinic and hospital. Am Rev Tuberc 79:134, 1959.

633. Mody KM, Poole G: Coexistent lung carcinoma and tuberculosis. Br J Dis Chest 57:200, 1963.

634. Chen YM, Chao JY, Tsai CM, et al: Shortened survival of lung cancer patients initially presenting with pulmonary tuberculosis. Jpn J Clin Oncol 26:322, 1996.

635. Aoki K: Excess incidence of lung cancer among pulmonary tuberculosis patients. Jpn J Clin Oncol 23:205, 1993.

636. Snider GL, Placik B: The relationship between pulmonary tuberculosis and bronchogenic carcinoma: A topographic study. Am Rev Respir Dis 99:229, 1969.

637. Carey JM, Geer AE: Bronchogenic carcinoma complicating pulmonary tuberculosis: A report of eight cases and a review of 140 cases since 1932. Ann Intern Med 49:161, 1958.

638. Meyer EC, Scatliff JH, Lindskog GE: The relation of antecedent tuberculosis to bronchogenic carcinoma: A study of the tuberculin test, radiologic and pathologic evidences. J Thorac Cardiovasc Surg 38:384, 1959.

639. Mok CK, Nandi P, Ong GB: Coexistent bronchogenic carcinoma and active pulmonary tuberculosis. J Thorac Cardiovasc Surg 76:469, 1978.

640. Ting YM, Church WR, Ravikrishnan KP: Lung carcinoma superimposed on pulmonary tuberculosis. Radiology 119:307, 1976.

641. Roche PW, Triccas JA, Winter N: BCG vaccination against tuberculosis: Past disappointments and future hopes. Trends Microbiol 3:397, 1995.

642. Brewer TF, Colditz GA: Bacille Calmette-Guérin vaccination for the prevention of tuberculosis in health care workers. Clin Infect Dis 20:136, 1995.

643. American Thoracic Society: Control of tuberculosis in the United States. Am Rev Respir Dis 146:1623, 1992.

644. Colditz GA, Brewer TF, Berkey CS, et al: Efficacy of BCG vaccine in the prevention of tuberculosis: Meta-analysis of the published literature. JAMA 271:698, 1994.

645. Sparks FC: Hazards and complications of BCG immunotherapy. Med Clin North Am 60:499, 1976.

646. Gupta K, Singh N, Bhatia A: Cytomorphologic patterns in Calmette Guérin bacillus lymphadenitis. Acta Cytol 41:348, 1997.

647. Casanova JL, Blanche S, Emile JF, et al: Idiopathic disseminated bacillus Calmette-Guérin infection: A French national retrospective study. Pediatrics 98:774, 1996.

648. Abramowsky C, Gonzalez B, Sorensen RU: Disseminated bacillus Calmette-Guérin infections in patients with primary immunodeficiencies. Am J Clin Pathol 100:52, 1993.

649. Gormsen H: On the occurrence of epithelioid cell granulomas in the organs of BCG-vaccinated human beings. Acta Pathol Microbiol Scand 111(Suppl):117, 1955.

650. Trevenen CL, Pagtakhan RD: Disseminated tuberculoid lesions in infants following BCG vaccinations. Can Med Assoc J 127:502, 1982.

650a. O'Donnell MA, DeWolf WC: Bacillus Calmette-Guérin immunotherapy for superficial bladder cancer: New prospects for an old warhorse. Surg Oncol Clin North Am 4:189, 1995.

650b. Crawford ED: Diagnosis and treatment of superficial bladder cancer: An update. Semin Urol Oncol 14:1, 1996.

651. Wiseman CL: Inflammatory breast cancer: 10-year follow-up of a trial of surgery, chemotherapy, and allogeneic tumor cell/BCG immunotherapy. Cancer Invest 13:267, 1995.

652. Mastrangelo MJ, Maguire HC Jr, Sato T, et al: Active specific immunization in the treatment of patients with melanoma. Semin Oncol 23:773, 1996.

653. Schapira DV, McPherson TA: Pneumonitis with oral BCG. N Engl J Med 296:397, 1977.

654. Hatzitheofilou C, Obenchain DF, Porter DD, et al: Granulomas in melanoma patients treated with BCG immunotherapy. Cancer 49:55, 1982.

655. Izes JK, Bihrle W 3d, Thomas CB: Corticosteroid-associated fatal mycobacterial sepsis occurring 3 years after instillation of intravesical bacillus Calmette-Guérin. J Urol 150:1498, 1993.

656. Rawls WH, Lamm DL, Lowe BA, et al: Fatal sepsis following intravesical bacillus Calmette-Guérin administration for bladder cancer. J Urol 144:1328, 1990.

657. Hoffler D, Niemeyer R, Strack G, et al: Sputum-positive lung tuberculosis after instillation of BCG for bladder cancer. Clin Nephrol 36:307, 1991.

658. Palayew M, Briedis D, Libman M, et al: Disseminated infection after intravesical BCG immunotherapy: Detection of organisms in pulmonary tissue. Chest 104:307, 1993.

659. Israel-Biet D, Venet A, Sandron D, et al: Pulmonary complications of intravesical Bacille Calmette-Guérin immunotherapy. Am Rev Respir Dis 135:761, 1987.

660. LeMense GP, Strange C: Granulomatous pneumonitis following intravesical BCG: What therapy is needed? Chest 106:1624, 1994.

661. Reinert KU, Sybrecht GW: T-helper cells alveolitis after bacillus Calmette-Guérin immunotherapy for superficial bladder tumor. J Urol 151:1634, 1994.

662. Whittaker JA, Bentley DP, Melville-Jones GR, et al: Granuloma formation in patients receiving BCG immunotherapy. J Clin Pathol 29:693, 1976.

663. Au FC, Webber B, Rosenberg SA: Pulmonary granulomas induced by BCG. Cancer 41:2209, 1978.

663a. Jasmer RM, McCowin MJ, Webb WR: Miliary lung disease after intravesical bacillus Calmette-Guérin immunotherapy. Radiology 201:43, 1996.

664. Hart IR, Fidler IJ, Hanna MG Jr, et al: The effects of intravenous administration of methanol extraction residue (MER) of tubercle bacilli in the dog. Cancer Immunol Immunother 3:229, 1978.

665. Hill CA: Thoracic tuberculosis, mycobacteriosis, MERosis, and BCGosis in a cancer treatment center. Radiology 153:311, 1984.

666. Sampson MG, Colman NC: Pulmonary complications of oral BCG. Chest 80:655, 1981.

667. Garyfallou GT: Mycobacterial sepsis following intravesical instillation of bacillus Calmette-Guérin. Acad Emerg Med 3:157, 1996.

668. Wolinsky E: Nontuberculous mycobacteria and associated disease. Am Rev Respir Dis 119:107, 1979.

669. Gangadharam PRJ: Microbiology of nontuberculosis mycobacteria. Semin Respir Infect 11:231, 1996.

670. Wayne L, Sramek H: Agents of newly recognized or infrequently encountered mycobacterial diseases. Clin Microbiol Rev 5:1, 1992.

671. Runyon EH: Anonymous mycobacteria in pulmonary disease. Med Clin North Am 43:273, 1959.

672. Blacklock ZM, Dawson DJ, Kane DW, et al: *Mycobacterium asiaticum* as a potential pulmonary pathogen for humans: A clinical and bacteriologic review of five cases. Am Rev Respir Dis 127:241, 1983.

672a. Valero G, Peters J, Jorgensen JH, et al: Clinical isolates of *Mycobacterium simiae* in San Antonio, Texas: An 11-yr review. Am J Respir Crit Care Med 152:1555, 1995.

673. Douglas JG, Calder MA, Choo-Kang YF, et al: *Mycobacterium gordonae*: A new pathogen? Thorax 41:152, 1986.

674. Clague H, Hopkins CA, Roberts C, et al: Pulmonary infection with *Mycobacterium gordonae* in the presence of bronchial carcinoma. Tubercle 66:61, 1985.

674a. Resch B, Eber E, Beitzke A, et al: Pulmonary infection due to *Mycobacterium gordonae* in an adolescent immunocompetent patient. Respiration 64:300, 1997.

675. Tsukamura M, Kita N, Otsuka W, et al: A study of the taxonomy of the *Mycobacterium nonchromogenicum* complex and report of six cases of lung infection due to *Mycobacterium nonchromogenicum*. Microbiol Immunol 27:219, 1983.

676. Kuze F, Mitsuoka A, Chiba W, et al: Chronic pulmonary infection caused by *Mycobacterium terrae* complex: A resected case. Am Rev Respir Dis 128:561, 1983.

677. Wallace RJ Jr, Nash DR, Tsukamur M, et al: Human disease due to *Mycobacterium smegmatis*. J Infect Dis 158:52, 1988.

678. Wallace RJ Jr, Swenson JM, Silcox VA, et al: Spectrum of disease due to rapidly growing *Mycobacteria*. Rev Infect Dis 5:657, 1983.

679. Rolston KV, Jones PG, Fainstein V, et al: Pulmonary disease caused by rapidly growing mycobacteria in patients with cancer. Chest 87:503, 1985.

680. Tortoli E, Piersimoni C, Kirschner P, et al: Characterization of mycobacterial isolates phylogenetically related to, but different from *Mycobacterium simiae*. J Clin Microbiol 35:697, 1997.

681. Liu F, Andrews D, Wright DN: *Mycobacterium thermoresistibile* infection in an immunocompromised host. J Clin Microbiol 19:546, 1984.

682. Horsburgh CR Jr: Epidemiology of disease caused by nontuberculous mycobacteria. Semin Respir Infect 11:244, 1996.

683. O'Brien RJ, Geiter LJ, Snider DE: The epidemiology of nontuberculous mycobacterial diseases in the United States: Results from a national survey. Am Rev Respir Dis 135:1007, 1987.

684. Tala E, Viljanen M: Mycobacterial infections in Finland. Scand J Infect Dis 98(Suppl):7, 1995.

685. Romanus V: Mycobacterial infections in Sweden. Scand J Infect Dis 98(Suppl):15, 1995.

686. Myrvang B: Mycobacterial infections in Norway. Scand J Infect Dis 98(Suppl):12, 1995.

687. Rosenzweig DY: Nontuberculous mycobacterial disease in the immunocompetent adult. Semin Respir Infect 11:252, 1996.

688. Rosenzweig DY: Pulmonary mycobacterial infections due to *Mycobacterium intracellulare-avium* complex: Clinical features and course in 100 consecutive cases. Chest 75:115, 1979.

689. Veterans Administration: Armed Forces Study on the Chemotherapy of Tuberculosis. Q Prog Rep 21:8, 1965.

690. Yates MD, Grange JM, Collins CH: The nature of mycobacterial disease in south east England, 1977–84. J Epidemiol Commun Health 40:295, 1986.

691. Dawson DJ, Reznikov M, Blacklock ZM, et al: Atypical mycobacteria isolated from clinical material in south-eastern Queensland. Pathology 6:153, 1974.

692. Ahn CH, Lowell JR, Onstad GD, et al: A demographic study of disease due to *Mycobacterium kansasii* or *M. intracellulare-avium* in Texas. Chest 75:120, 1979.

693. Lincoln EM, Gilbert LA: Disease in children due to mycobacteria other than *Mycobacterium tuberculosis*. Am Rev Respir Dis 105:683, 1972.

694. Correa AG, Starke JR: Nontuberculous mycobacterial disease in children. Semin Respir Infect 11:262, 1996.

695. Saubolle MA, Kiehn TE, White MH, et al: *Mycobacterium haemophilum*: Microbiology and expanding clinical and geographic spectra of disease in humans. Clin Microbiol Rev 9:435, 1996.

696. Prince DS, Peterson DD, Steiner RM, et al: Infection with *Mycobacterium avium* complex in patients without predisposing conditions. N Engl J Med 321:863, 1989.

697. Reich JM, Johnson RE: *Mycobacterium avium* complex pulmonary disease: Incidence, presentation, and response to therapy in a community setting. Am Rev Respir Dis 143:1381, 1991.

698. Wheeler PW, Lancaster D, Kaiser AB: Bronchopulmonary cross-colonization and infection related to mycobacterial contamination of suction valves of bronchoscopes. J Infect Dis 159:954, 1989.

699. Lowry PW, Jarvis WR, Oberle AD, et al: *Mycobacterium chelonae* causing otitis media in an ear-nose-and-throat practice. N Engl J Med 319:978, 1988.

700. Hoy JF, Rolston KVI, Hopfer RL, et al: *Mycobacterium fortuitum* bacteremia in patients with cancer and long-term venous catheters. Am J Med 83:213, 1987.

701. Hoffman PC, Fraser DW, Robicsek F, et al: Two outbreaks of sternal wound infections due to organisms of the *Mycobacterium fortuitum* complex. J Infect Dis 143:533, 1981.

702. Clegg HW, Foster MT, Sanders WE Jr, et al: Infection due to organisms of the *Mycobacterium fortuitum* complex after augmentation mammaplasty: Clinical and epidemiologic features. J Infect Dis 147:427, 1983.

703. Onstad GD: Familial aggregations of Group I atypical mycobacterial disease. Am Rev Respir Dis 99:426, 1969.

704. Penny ME, Cole RB, Gray J: Two cases of *Mycobacterium kansasii* infection occurring in the same household. Tubercle 63:129, 1982.

705. Bennett SN, Peterson DE, Johnson DR, et al: Bronchoscopy-associated *Mycobacterium xenopi* pseudoinfections. Am J Respir Crit Care Med 150:245, 1994.

706. Maloney S, Welbel S, Daves B, et al: *Mycobacterium abscessus* pseudoinfection traced to an automated endoscope washer: Utility of epidemiologic and laboratory investigation. J Infect Dis 169:1166, 1994.

707. Dutt AK, Stead WW: Long-term results of medical treatment in *Mycobacterium intracellulare* infection. Am J Med 67:449, 1979.

708. Iseman MD, Corpe RF, O'Brien RJ, et al: Disease due to *Mycobacterium avium-intracellulare*. Chest 87(Suppl):1398, 1985.

709. Yeager H Jr, Raleigh JW: Pulmonary disease due to *Mycobacterium intracellulare*. Am Rev Respir Dis 108:547, 1973.

710. Johanson WG Jr, Nicholson DP: Pulmonary disease due to *Mycobacterium kansasii*: An analysis of some factors affecting prognosis. Am Rev Respir Dis 99:73, 1969.

711. Witty LA, Tapson VF, Piantadosi CA: Isolation of mycobacteria in patients with pulmonary alveolar proteinosis. Medicine 73:103, 1994.

712. Iseman MD, Buschmann DL, Ackerson LM: Pectus excavatum and scoliosis: Thoracic abnormalities associated with pulmonary disease caused by *Mycobacterium avium* complex. Am Rev Respir Dis 144:914, 1991.

713. Karsell PR: Achalasia, aspiration, and atypical mycobacteria. Mayo Clin Proc 68:1025, 1993.

714. Rice L, Shenkenberg T, Lynch EC, et al: Granulomatous infections complicating hairy cell leukemia. Cancer 49:1924, 1982.

715. Weinstein RA, Golomb HM, Grumet G, et al: Hairy cell leukemia: Association with disseminated atypical mycobacterial infection. Cancer 48:380, 1981.

716. Castor B, Juhlin I, Henriques B: Septic cutaneous lesions caused by *Mycobacterium malmoense* in a patient with hairy cell leukemia. Eur J Clin Microbiol Infect Dis 13:145, 1994.

717. LeMense GP, VanBakel AB, Crumbley AJ 3rd, et al: *Mycobacterium scrofulaceum* infection presenting as lung nodules in a heart transplant recipient. Chest 106:1918, 1994.

718. Patel R, Roberts GD, Keating MR, et al: Infections due to nontuberculous mycobacteria in kidney, heart, and liver transplant recipients. Clin Infect Dis 19:263, 1994.

719. McWhinney PH, Yates M, Prentice HG, et al: Infection caused by *Mycobacterium chelonae*: A diagnostic and therapeutic problem in the neutropenic patient. Clin Infect Dis 14:1208, 1992.

720. Hjelt K, Hojlyng N, Howitz P, et al: The role of Mycobacteria Other Than Tuberculosis (MOTT) in patients with cystic fibrosis. Scand J Infect Dis 26:569, 1994.

721. Kilby JM, Gilligan PH, Yankaskas JR, et al: Nontuberculous mycobacteria in adult patients with cystic fibrosis. Chest 102:70, 1992.

722. Aitken ML, Burke W, McDonald G, et al: Nontuberculosis mycobacterial disease in adult cystic fibrosis patients. Chest 103:1096, 1993.

723. Olivier KN, Yankaskas JR, Knowles MR: Nontuberculous mycobacterial pulmonary disease in cystic fibrosis. Semin Respir Infect 11:272, 1996.

724. Tomashefski JF Jr, Stern RC, Demko CA, et al: Nontuberculous mycobacteria in cystic fibrosis: An autopsy study. Am J Respir Crit Care Med 154:523, 1996.

725. Falkinham JO 3rd: Epidemiology of infection by nontuberculous mycobacteria. Clin Microbiol Rev 9:177, 1996.

726. Torrens JK, Dawkins P, Conway SP, et al: Non-tuberculous mycobacteria in cystic fibrosis. Thorax 53:182, 1998.

727. Eaton T, Falkinham JO III, von Reyn CF: Recovery of *Mycobacterium avium* from cigarettes. J Clin Microbiol 33:2757, 1995.

728. Wendt SL, George KL, Parker BC, et al: Epidemiology of nontuberculous mycobacteria: III. Isolation of potentially pathogenic mycobacteria in aerosols. Am Rev Respir Dis 122:259, 1980.

729. Ahn CH, Lowell JR, Onstad GD, et al: A demographic study of disease due to *Mycobacterium kansasii* or *M. intracellulare-avium* in Texas. Chest 75:120, 1979.

730. Jenkins PA: The epidemiology of opportunist mycobacterial infections in Wales, 1952–1978. Rev Infect Dis 3:1021, 1981.

731. Engel HWB, Berwald LG, Havelaar AH: The occurrence of *Mycobacterium kansasii* in tap water. Tubercle 61:21, 1980.

732. Joynson DHM: Water: The natural habitat of *Mycobacterium kansasii*. Tubercle 60:77, 1979.

733. Collins CH, Yates MD: Infection and colonisation by *Mycobacterium kansasii* and *Mycobacterium xenopi*: Aerosols as a possible source? J Infect 8:178, 1984.

734. Colville A: Retrospective review of culture-positive mycobacterial lymphadenitis cases in children in Nottingham, 1979–1990. Eur J Clin Microbiol Infect Dis 12:192, 1993.

735. Johanson WG Jr, Nicholson DP: Pulmonary disease due to *Mycobacterium kansasii*: An analysis of some factors influencing prognosis. Am Rev Respir Dis 99:73, 1969.

736. Owens MW, Kinasewitz GT, Gonzalez E: Sandblaster's lung with mycobacterial infection. Am J Med Sci 295:554, 1988.

737. Contreras MA, Cheung OT, Sanders DE, et al: Pulmonary infection with nontuberculous mycobacteria. Am Rev Respir Dis 137:149, 1988.

738. Levine B, Chaisson RE: *Mycobacterium kansasii*: A cause of treatable pulmonary disease associated with advanced human immunodeficiency virus (HIV) infection. Ann Intern Med 114:861, 1991.

739. Zeligman I: *Mycobacterium marinum* granuloma: A disease acquired in the tributaries of Chesapeake Bay. Arch Dermatol 106:26, 1972.

740. Barrow GI, Hewitt M: Skin infection with *Mycobacterium marinum* from a tropical fish tank. BMJ 2:505, 1971.

741. Ries KM, White GL Jr, Murdock RT: Atypical mycobacterial infection caused by *Mycobacterium marinum*. N Engl J Med 322:633, 1990.

742. Gombert M, Goldstein E, Corrado M, et al: Disseminated *Mycobacterium marinum* infection after renal transplantation. Ann Intern Med 94:486, 1981.

743. Weiszfeiler JG, Karasseva V, Karczag E: *Mycobacterium simiae* and related mycobacteria. Rev Infect Dis 3:1040, 1981.

744. Bell RC, Higuchi JH, Donovan WN, et al: *Mycobacterium simiae* clinical features and follow up of twenty-four patients. Am Rev Respir Dis 127:35, 1983.

745. Lavy A, Yoshpe-Purer Y: Isolation of *Mycobacterium simiae* from clinical specimens in Israel. Tubercle 63:279, 1982.

746. Rose HD, Dorff GI, Lauwasser M, et al: Pulmonary and disseminated *Mycobacterium simiae* infection in humans. Am Rev Respir Dis 126:1110, 1982.

747. Falkinham JO III, Parker BC, Gruft H: Epidemiology of nontuberculous mycobacteria: I. Geographic distribution in the eastern United States. Am Rev Respir Dis 121:931, 1980.

748. Maloney JM, Gregg CR, Stephens DS, et al: Infections caused by *Mycobacterium szulgai* in humans. Rev Infect Dis 9:1120, 1987.

749. Gur H, Porat S, Haas H, et al: Disseminated mycobacterial disease caused by *Mycobacterium szulgai*. Arch Intern Med 144:1861, 1984.

750. Gross WM, Hawkins JE, Murphy DB: Origin and significance of *Mycobacterium xenopi* in clinical specimens: I. Water as a source of contamination. Bull Int Union Tuberc 51:267, 1976.

751. Costrini AM, Mahler DA, Gross WM, et al: Clinical and roentgenographic features of nosocomial pulmonary disease due to *Mycobacterium xenopi*. Am Rev Respir Dis 123:104, 1981.

752. Smith MJ, Citron KM: Clinical review of pulmonary disease caused by *Mycobacterium xenopi*. Thorax 38:373, 1983.

753. Simor AE, Salit IE, Vellend H: The role of *Mycobacterium xenopi* in human disease. Am Rev Respir Dis 129:435, 1984.

754. Koizumi JH, Summers HM: *Mycobacterium xenopi* and pulmonary disease. Am J Clin Pathol 73:826, 1980.

755. Wallace RJ Jr, O'Brien R, Glassroth J, et al: Diagnosis and treatment of disease caused by nontuberculous mycobacteria. Am Rev Respir Dis 142:940, 1990.

756. Connolly MJ, Magee JG, Hendrick DJ: *Mycobacterium malmoense* in the northeast of England. Tubercle 66:211, 1985.

757. France AJ, McLeod DT, Calder MA, et al: *Mycobacterium malmoense* infections in Scotland: An increasing problem. Thorax 42:593, 1987.

758. Katila M-L, Brander E, Viljanen T: Difficulty with *Mycobacterium malmoense*. Lancet 2:510, 1989.

759. Hoffner SE, Henriques B, Petrini B, et al: *Mycobacterium malmoense*: An easily missed pathogen. J Clin Microbiol 29:2673, 1991.

760. Bollert FG, Sime PJ, MacNee W, et al: Pulmonary *Mycobacterium malmoense* and aspergillus infection: A fatal combination? Thorax 49:521, 1994.

761. Rogers PL, Walker RE, Lane HC, et al: Disseminated *Mycobacterium* infection in two patients with the acquired immunodeficiency syndrome. Am J Med 84:640, 1988.

762. Becherer P, Hopfer RL: Infection with *Mycobacterium haemophilum*. Clin Infect Dis 14:793, 1992.

763. Dever LL, Martin JW, Seaworth B, et al: Varied presentations and responses to treatment of infections caused by *Mycobacterium haemophilum* in patients with AIDS. Clin Infect Dis 14:1195, 1992.

764. Higgins RM, Chan AP, Porter D, et al: Mycobacterial infections after renal transplantation. QJM 78:145, 1991.

765. Gouby A, Branger B, Oules R, et al: Two cases of *Mycobacterium haemophilum* infection in a renal-dialysis unit. J Med Microbiol 25:299, 1988.

766. Nadal DR, Caduff R, Kraft M, et al: Invasive infection with *Mycobacterium genavense* in three children with the acquired immunodeficiency syndrome. Eur J Clin Microbiol Infect Dis 12:37, 1993.

767. Coyle MB, Carlson LDC, Wallis CK, et al: Laboratory aspects of "*Mycobacterium genavense*," a proposed species isolated from AIDS patients. J Clin Microbiol 30:3206, 1992.

768. Griffith DE, Girard WM, Wallace RJ Jr: Clinical features of pulmonary disease caused by rapidly growing mycobacteria: An analysis of 154 patients. Am Rev Respir Dis 147:1271, 1993.

769. Collins CH, Grange JM, Yates MD: A review: Mycobacteria in water. J Appl Bacteriol 57:193, 1984.

770. Wallace RJ Jr, Swenson JM, Silcox VA, et al: Spectrum of disease due to rapidly growing mycobacteria. Rev Infect Dis 5:657, 1983.

771. Safraneck TJ, Jarvis WR, Carson LA: *Mycobacterium chelonae* wound infections after plastic surgery employing contaminated gentian violet skin-marking solution. N Engl J Med 317:197, 1987.

772. Repath F, Seabury JH, Sanders CV, et al: Prosthetic valve endocarditis due to *Mycobacterium chelonei*. South Med J 69:1244, 1976.

773. Hutchins GM, Boitnott JK: Atypical mycobacterial infection complicating mineral oil pneumonia. JAMA 240:539, 1978.

774. Aronchick JM, Miller WT, Epstein DM, et al: Association of achalasia and pulmonary *Mycobacterium fortuitum* infection. Radiology 160:85, 1986.

775. Ingram CW, Tanner DC, Durack DT, et al: Disseminated infection with rapidly growing mycobacteria. Clin Infect Dis 16:463, 1993.

776. Marchevsky A, Damsker B, Gribetz A, et al: The spectrum of pathology of nontuberculous mycobacterial infections in open-lung biopsy specimens. Am J Clin Pathol 78:695, 1982.

777. Snijder J: Histopathology of pulmonary lesions caused by atypical mycobacteria. J Pathol Bacteriol 90:65, 1965.

778. Merchx JJ, Soule EH, Karlson AG: The histopathology of lesions caused by infection with unclassified acid-fast bacteria in man: Report of 25 cases. Am J Clin Pathol 41:244, 1964.

779. Connolly MG Jr, Baughman RP, Dohn MN: *Mycobacterium kansasii* presenting as an endobronchial lesion. Am Rev Respir Dis 148:1405, 1993.

780. Is the histopathology of nonphotochromogenic mycobacterial infections distinguishable from that caused by *Mycobacterium tuberculosis*? Am Rev Respir Dis 87:289, 1963.

781. Reid JD, Wolinsky E: Histopathology of lymphadenitis caused by atypical *Mycobacteria*. Am Rev Respir Dis 99:8, 1969.

782. Pinder SE, Colville A: Mycobacterial cervical lymphadenitis in children: Can histological assessment help differentiate infections caused by nontuberculous mycobacteria from *Mycobacterium tuberculosis*? Histopathology 22:59, 1993.

783. Kommareddi S, Abramowsky CR, Swinehart GL, et al: Nontuberculous mycobacterial infections: Comparison of the fluorescent auramine-O and Ziehl-Neelsen techniques in tissue diagnosis. Hum Pathol 15:1085, 1984.

784. Chester AC, Winn WC: Unusual and newly recognized patterns of nontuberculous mycobacterial infection with emphasis on the immunocompromised host. *In* Sommers SC, Rosen PP, Fechner RE (eds): Pathology Annual, Part I. Vol 21. Norwalk, CT, Appleton-Century-Crofts, 1986.

785. Cook SM, Bartos RE, Pierson CL, et al: Detection and characterization of atypical mycobacteria by the polymerase chain reaction. Diagn Mol Pathol 3:53, 1994.

786. Fraser DW, Buxton AE, Naji A, et al: Disseminated *Mycobacterium kansasii* infection presenting as cellulitis in a recipient of a renal homograft. Am Rev Respir Dis 112:125, 1975.

787. Farhi DC, Mason UG III, Horsburgh CR: Pathologic findings in disseminated *Mycobacterium avium-intracellulare* infection. Am J Clin Pathol 85:67, 1986.

788. Greene JB, Sidhu GS, Lewin S, et al: *Mycobacterium avium-intracellulare*: A cause of disseminated life-threatening infection in homosexuals and drug abusers. Ann Intern Med 97:539, 1982.

789. Niedt GW, Schinella RA: Acquired immunodeficiency syndrome. Arch Pathol Lab Med 109:727, 1985.

790. Gallo JH, Young GAR, Forrest PR, et al: Disseminated atypical mycobacterial infection in hairy cell leukemia. Pathology 15:241, 1983.

791. Christensen EE, Dietz GW, Ahn CH, et al: Radiographic manifestations of pulmonary *Mycobacterium kansasii* infections. Am J Roentgenol 131:985, 1978.

792. Christensen EE, Dietz GW, Ahn CH, et al: Pulmonary manifestations of *Mycobacterium intracellulare*. Am J Roentgenol 133:59, 1979.

793. Albelda SM, Kern JA, Marinelli DL, et al: Expanding spectrum of pulmonary disease caused by nontuberculous mycobacteria. Radiology 157:289, 1985.

794. Woodring JH, Mac Vandiviere H, Melvin IG: Roentgenographic features of pulmonary disease caused by atypical mycobacteria. South Med J 80:1488, 1987.

795. Scully RE, Mark EJ, McNeely WF, et al: Case records of the Massachusetts General Hospital, Case 17-1989. N Engl J Med 320:1130, 1989.

796. Evans AJ, Crisp AJ, Hubbard RB, et al: Pulmonary *Mycobacterium kansasii* infection: Comparison of radiological appearances with pulmonary tuberculosis. Thorax 51:1243, 1996.

797. Moore EH: Atypical mycobacterial infection in the lung: CT appearance. Radiology 187:777, 1993.

798. Lynch DA, Simone PM, Fox MA, et al: CT features of pulmonary *Mycobacterium avium* complex infection. J Comput Assist Tomogr 19:353, 1995.

799. Miller WT Jr: Spectrum of pulmonary nontuberculous mycobacterial infection. Radiology 191:343, 1994.

800. Prince DS, Peterson DD, Steiner RM, et al: Infection with *Mycobacterium avium* complex in patients without predisposing conditions. N Engl J Med 321:863, 1989.

801. Hartman TE, Swensen SJ, Williams DE: *Mycobacterium avium-intracellulare* complex: Evaluation with CT. Radiology 187:23, 1993.

802. Swensen SJ, Hartman TE, Williams DE: Computed tomographic diagnosis of *Mycobacterium avium-intracellulare* complex in patients with bronchiectasis. Chest 105:49, 1994.

803. Embil J, Warren P, Yakrus M, et al: Pulmonary illness associated with exposure to *Mycobacterium avium* complex in hot tub water. Chest 111:813, 1997.

804. Zvetina JR, Demos TC, Maliwan N, et al: Pulmonary cavitations in *Mycobacterium kansasii*: Distinctions from *M. tuberculosis*. Am J Roentgenol 143:127, 1984.

805. Evans AJ, Crisp AJ, Colville A, et al: Pulmonary infections caused by *Mycobacterium malmoense* and *Mycobacterium tuberculosis*: Comparison of radiographic features. Am J Roentgenol 161:733, 1993.

806. Curry FJ: Atypical acid-fast mycobacteria. N Engl J Med 272:415, 1965.

807. Christianson LC, Dewlett HJ: Pulmonary disease in adults associated with unclassified mycobacteria. Am J Med 29:980, 1960.

808. Prince DA, Peterson DD, Steiner RM, et al: Infection with *Mycobacterium avium* complex in patients without predisposing conditions. N Engl J Med 321:863, 1989.

809. Souid AK, Mortelliti AJ, Anwer F, et al: Nontuberculous Mycobacteria subcarinal lymphadenitis and severe airway obstruction. Clin Pediatr 34:657, 1995.

810. Dalovisio JR, Pankey GA: Dermatologic manifestations of nontuberculous mycobacterial diseases. Infect Dis Clin North Am 8:677, 1994.

811. Saito H, Tasaka H, Osasa S, et al: Disseminated *Mycobacterium intracellulare* infection. Am Rev Respir Dis 109:572, 1974.

812. Lazlo A, Siddiqi SH: Evaluation of a rapid radiometric differentiation test for the *Mycobacterium tuberculosis*-complex by selective inhibition with p-nitro-α-acetylamino-β-hydroxypropiophenone. J Clin Microbiol 19:694, 1984.

813. Ritter D, Carlson LD, Logan BK, et al: Differentiation of *Mycobacterium genavense* and *Mycobacterium simiae* by automated mycolic acid analysis with high-performance liquid chromatography. J Clin Microbiol 34:2004, 1996.

814. Parez JJ, Fauville-Dufaux M, Dossogne JL, et al: Faster identification of mycobacteria using gas liquid and thin layer chromatography. Eur J Clin Microbiol Infect Dis 13:717, 1994.

815. Del Portillo P, Thomas MC, Martinez E, et al: Multiprimer PCR system for differential identification of mycobacteria in clinical samples. J Clin Microbiol 34:324, 1996.

816. Takewaki S, Okuzumi K, Ishiko H, et al: Genus-specific polymerase chain reaction for the mycobacterial DNA J gene and species-specific oligonucleotide probes. J Clin Microbiol 31:446, 1993.

817. Ahn CH, Lowell JR, Onstad GD, et al: Elimination of *Mycobacterium intracellulare* from sputum after bronchial hygiene. Chest 76:480, 1979.

818. Warring FC Jr: Mycobacteria in a New England hospital: A study of mycobacterial species occurring in the sputum of patients with chronic pulmonary disease. Am Rev Respir Dis 98:965, 1968.

819. Choudhri S, Manfreda J, Wolfe J, et al: Clinical significance of nontuberculous mycobacteria isolates in a Canadian tertiary care center. Clin Infect Dis 21:128, 1995.

820. Pinto-Powell R, Olivier KN, Marsh BJ, et al: Skin testing with *Mycobacterium avium* sensitin to identify infection with *M. avium* complex in patients with cystic fibrosis. Clin Infect Dis 22:560, 1996.

821. Schaeter WB, Davis CL: A bacteriologic and histopathologic study of skin granuloma due to *Mycobacterium balnei*. Am Rev Respir Dis 84:837, 1961.

822. Judson FN, Feldman RA: Mycobacterial skin tests in humans 12 years after infection with *Mycobacterium marinum*. Am Rev Respir Dis 109:544, 1974.

823. Francis PB, Jay SJ, Johanson WG Jr: The course of untreated *Mycobacterium kansasii* disease. Am Rev Respir Dis 111:477, 1975.

824. Engbaek HC, Vergmann B, Bentzon MW: A prospective study of lung disease caused by *Mycobacterium avium*/*Mycobacterium intracellulare*. Eur J Respir Dis 65:411, 1984.

825. Schraufnagel DE, Leech JA, Pollak B: *Mycobacterium kansasii*: Colonization and disease. Br J Dis Chest 80:131, 1986.

826. Hunter AM, Campbell IA, Jenkins PA, et al: Treatment of pulmonary infections caused by *Mycobacteria* of the *Mycobacterium avium-intracellulare* complex. Thorax 36:326, 1981.

CHAPTER 28

Fungi and Actinomyces

Fungi can be discussed in two major groups according to the pathogenesis of the disease they cause. Some organisms (such as *Histoplasma capsulatum*, *Coccidioides immitis*, *Paracoccidioides brasiliensis*, and *Blastomyces dermatitidis*) are primary pathogens that most frequently infect healthy individuals. They are found in specific geographic areas—hence the term *endemic* that is often used to describe the infections—and typically dwell in the soil as saprophytes. In appropriate climatic conditions, they germinate and produce spores, which, when inhaled by a susceptible host, change form (a process known as *dimorphism*) and proliferate. In the individual who has an intact inflammatory response and adequate cell-mediated immunity, such proliferation is almost invariably limited, the resulting disease being subclinical or mild and evidenced only by the development of a positive skin test result. In a few apparently "normal" individuals, however, fulminant primary infection or chronic pulmonary disease, with or without systemic dissemination, can cause significant morbidity and is occasionally fatal. Such complications are much more common in patients who have an underlying immune deficiency, such as acquired immunodeficiency syndrome (AIDS).[1]

A second group of organisms (including *Aspergillus* and *Candida* species and the species that cause mucormycosis) are opportunistic invaders that chiefly affect immunocompromised hosts or grow in the presence of underlying pulmonary disease. In contrast to members of the previous group, these organisms are not dimorphic, can be found throughout the world, and are usually ubiquitous in the environment. Intact mucosal barriers and adequate phagocytic function (including polymorphonuclear leukocytes, macrophages, or both) are the major host factors that determine whether or not colonization progresses to clinically important disease. In the latter situation, the fungi may be present as saprophytes (e.g., a mycetoma) or, more commonly, as invasive organisms that cause tissue destruction. Because of underlying immunosuppression, infection by more than one organism sometimes occurs.[2–4]

In addition to saprophytic and invasive infection, some fungi (particularly *Aspergillus* species, but also possibly *H. capsulatum*) can cause disease by an exaggerated hypersensitivity reaction without actually invading tissue. Inhalation of massive amounts of fungi can itself provoke a toxic, nonallergic pulmonary reaction. Such pulmonary *mycotoxicosis* (organic dust toxic syndrome) has been reported in workers exposed to extremely moldy silage;[5–7] typically, it is transitory, and testing fails to indicate sensitization (*see* page 2379).

The identification of a fungus as the cause of pleuropulmonary disease can be difficult, particularly in those cases in which the clinical presentation simulates more common

bacterial or viral infection.[8] The responsible organism can be identified by a variety of means, including skin testing, serology, culture of body fluid or tissue, immunochemical reactions, and molecular biologic techniques; use of more than one method and multiple samples increases the likelihood of a positive diagnosis.[9, 10]

When considering infections caused by organisms that are often colonists of the oropharynx or respiratory tract (such as *Candida albicans*), it is necessary to demonstrate the organism in tissue to be certain that a particular radiographic abnormality is truly caused by the fungus. Although many fungi can be identified with routine tissue stains, such as hematoxylin and eosin (H & E), special procedures that more clearly outline the cell wall are usually performed to confirm their presence. The most useful of these are the periodic acid–Schiff (PAS) and silver methenamine stains (especially Grocott's modification of Gomori's method); Gram, mucicarmine, and acid-fast stains can also be helpful in certain situations. The use of calcofluor white, a cotton whitener that is taken up by many fungi and that fluoresces on exposure to ultraviolet light, has been advocated as a more rapid method of confirming the presence of these organisms;[11] this agent can be used on frozen sections[11] and in combination with Papanicolaou's stain.[12] A number of fungi, including *C. immitis*, *Aspergillus* and *Candida* species, *B. dermatitidis*, and *Cryptococcus neoformans*, are naturally autofluorescent and have been identified within tissues by ultraviolet illumination alone.[13, 14] When making a diagnosis of a fungal infection on tissue sections, it is important to remember that altered tissue components or cells sometimes closely resemble hyphae or yeasts.[15, 16]

In addition to indicating the presence of fungi, examination of tissue or cytology specimens can also be helpful in identifying a particular species. Ideally, this should be correlated with laboratory culture; however, the histologic appearance alone may be highly suggestive or even diagnostic of a specific organism (e.g., encapsulated forms of *C. neoformans*).[17] A more specific and sensitive means of identification is the use of fluorescein-labeled antibody directed against individual fungi; although a number of technical problems may limit the application of this technique,[17] it could theoretically be used for virtually any species.[18] Immunohistochemical examination of paraffin-embedded tissue and molecular biologic techniques are also sensitive and specific techniques for identification.

The Actinomycetaceae, which include microorganisms such as *Actinomyces israelii* and *Nocardia* species, are presently classified as bacteria. Because many of their clinical and pathologic characteristics are similar to those of the fungi, however, they can be conveniently considered along with true mycotic infections.

HISTOPLASMOSIS

Histoplasmosis is an endemic fungal disease of quite varied clinical and radiographic manifestations caused by the dimorphic organisms *Histoplasma capsulatum* and *H. duboisii*.[19–24] The former is the more important organism with respect to the number of cases. It exists as a saprophyte in soil in its mycelial form and in infected animals and humans as an oval, 2- to 5-μm yeast. Various strains of the organism have been identified using sequence-specific DNA probes.[25]

Epidemiology

The natural habitat of *H. capsulatum* is soil that contains a high nitrogen content, usually derived from the guano of birds or bats. Thus, areas such as chicken houses, blackbird and pigeon roosts, bat-infested caves or attics, and other sites where bird guano accumulates are the most common sources for outbreaks of infection.[19, 26, 27] Situations in which clouds of dust are raised, such as bulldozing of roosting sites, are particularly likely to be associated with disease because of aerosolization of the spores. Infection, however, can occur without such an obvious source; striking increases in positive skin reactions to *H. capsulatum* have been detected in individuals living in proximity to recognized roost sites, even in the absence of any incident that might disturb the terrain.[28–30]

Because of their high body temperature, fowl are not believed to be infected, although they can carry the organism in their feathers.[19] By contrast, the organism has been isolated from the viscera of a variety of bats, whose body temperatures are relatively low,[31] and it is possible that these animals are able to spread the disease to each other. Animal-to-human and person-to-person transmission are not known to occur. Laboratory workers who come into contact with contaminated material have an increased risk of infection, usually by inhalation;[32] occasionally, infection is acquired by direct intracutaneous inoculation.[33] This route may also be the means for infection in the rare example of peritoneal disease associated with dialysis.[34] Rare cases have been acquired by organ transplantation.[35]

Although the organism is of worldwide distribution, most reports of disease have come from North America, particularly the central and eastern portions and notably in the Ohio, Mississippi, and St. Lawrence river valleys, where the organism is considered endemic. Occasional reports of infection have originated in South and Central America.[34, 36, 37] Rarely, "primary" infection has been reported in India,[38, 39] Africa,[40] Southeast Asia,[41] and parts of Europe.[42–44] Because infection by *H. capsulatum* can occur during only a brief stay in an endemic area, it is likely that some cases recognized in these regions are acquired elsewhere.[25, 45–49] For example, in a study of histoplasmin sensitivity tests of 575 individuals in Pakistan, all six positive reactors had been in known endemic areas in other countries.[50] Despite this, some cases have developed in patients who have not left their native land,[39, 42] and lack of travel history to recognized endemic areas should not exclude the diagnosis.

In endemic areas, infection by *H. capsulatum* is common. For example, in epidemiologic investigations, a positive histoplasmin skin test has been found in as many as 70% to 80% of the population in endemic areas.[51, 52] Similarly, serial postmortem examinations have revealed splenic calcification—representing remote granulomas derived from hematogenous dissemination during primary infection[53]—in many individuals.[54] In a radiographic autopsy study of three populations, for example, typical punctate calcifications were found in only 2% and 3% of 102 and 108 specimens of spleen from the two nonendemic areas (Rotterdam and New York City), but in 53 (44%) of 120 specimens from the endemic Cincinnati area.[55]

Even in highly endemic areas, infection is unevenly distributed, probably reflecting point sources of heavily contaminated soil.[56–59] These point sources are believed to be responsible for the miniepidemics that occasionally develop in endemic areas, such as occurred in the city of Montreal during the years preceding the 1967 world exposition;[55] the latter outbreak was undoubtedly related to the extensive earth moving required to create the subway and new islands in the St. Lawrence River. Similar outbreaks have been described in individuals associated with a wagon train,[60] in employees of a pulp and paper factory exposed to a high level of bird guano,[27] and in cave explorers (spelunkers) who enter caves containing bat guano.[61, 62]

In endemic areas, the frequency and number of pulmonary and mediastinal calcifications observed radiographically and at autopsy increase with advancing age, possibly as a result of repeated infections.[20] Although persons of any age may develop clinically evident disease,[63] this is more common and of greater significance in infants,[64] the elderly, and the immunosuppressed.[65–68] Rare cases have been reported in individuals with long-standing sarcoidosis.[68a]

Pathogenesis and Pathologic Characteristics

In appropriate environmental conditions, the mycelia of *H. capsulatum* produce microconidia measuring 2 to 5 μm in diameter that are inhaled and deposited in transitional airways and alveolar air spaces. The earliest host response, observed both experimentally in previously uninfected animals[69, 70] and in humans,[71] is an infiltrate of polymorphonuclear leukocytes. These cells are unable to kill the organism effectively and are soon replaced by lymphocytes and macrophages, which destroy the conidia and spores but not before some have been transformed into budding yeasts. The yeasts are phagocytosed by macrophages in which they appear on H & E–stained sections as small dots surrounded by a clear halo (Fig. 28–1).[72] In contrast to infection with *H. duboisii* (*see* farther on), multinucleated giant cells typically are few in number. The ability of macrophages to phagocytose and kill the yeasts effectively is of prime importance in controlling the disease at this point.[73–75]

About 1 to 2 weeks after the initial infection, this nonspecific neutrophil and macrophage inflammatory reaction is succeeded by the development of lymphocyte-mediated cellular immunity[76] accompanied by granulomatous inflammation, necrosis, and fibrosis (Fig. 28–2). The appearance at this stage is identical, both macroscopically and histologically, to primary tuberculosis. In many cases, the ensuing focus of parenchymal disease is too small to be detected radiographically and occasionally, individual foci of necrosis coalesce and enlarge, resulting in one or more foci of disease large enough to be identifiable.

Regional lymph node involvement in primary histoplasmosis is invariable, resulting in enlargement that often is more prominent than that observed in primary tuberculosis.[77] Complications related to nodal disease are also similar to those of primary tuberculosis and include atelectasis and obstructive pneumonitis caused by airway compression (Fig.

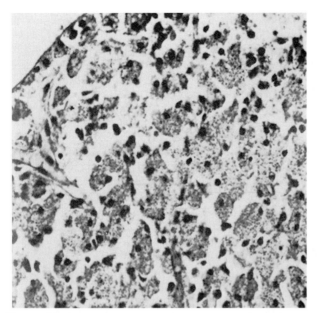

Figure 28–1. Histoplasmosis—Phagocytosis of Organisms.
Greatly swollen histiocytes are evident in the mucosa of the appendix, with innumerable phagocytosed yeasts of *Histoplasma capsulatum* appearing as small black dots. Similar cells are found in the early stages of pulmonary infection (×400). (From Schwarz J: Hum Pathol 13:519, 1982.)

28–3) and broncholithiasis;[78] rarely, a lymph node containing a focus of healed disease serves as a source of reactivation.

Blood-borne dissemination of organisms occurs early in the course of disease,[71] in the vast majority of cases resulting in small extrapulmonary foci of granulomatous inflammation, particularly in the liver and spleen.[53] These foci can subsequently undergo necrosis and calcification, becoming visible morphologically and radiographically as markers of prior disease. As in primary tuberculosis, such hematogenous spread is seldom clinically significant. When it is, organisms can be seen within macrophages as small, oval dots distending the cytoplasm in a fashion identical to that of early primary infection (*see* Fig. 28–1).[19, 79] Such infection is usually most prominent in the spleen, liver, bone marrow, lymph nodes, gastrointestinal tract, and adrenal glands; sometimes, the alveolar interstitium itself is infiltrated by yeast-containing macrophages as part of the generalized infection.[19] The inflammatory reaction in these cases is variable, consisting of well-formed granulomas in cases in which there are relatively few organisms and a protracted course and a virtual absence of granulomatous response in cases associated with numerous yeast forms and a rapid course.[19]

In most cases of primary *Histoplasma* infection, healing is rapid and progressive, leaving only small areas of encapsulated necrotic parenchyma as residua. The morphology of the healed foci of infection is again similar to that of tuberculosis, except that both parenchymal and nodal sites tend to be larger.[80] Lesions in both areas may be single or multiple; two to four primary parenchymal foci are present in about 10% of patients.[80] Healed lesions possess a well-defined fibrous capsule that surrounds caseous necrotic material; occasionally, prominent concentric laminations are evident, particularly in larger nodules (Fig. 28–4). Calcification is frequent. Microscopic examination shows amorphous debris

enveloped by fibrous tissue that contains a variable number of mononuclear inflammatory cells.

In tissue sections, organisms usually cannot be identifed with H & E stain except when they are within macrophages as part of disseminated or early local disease. When lying free in necrotic tissue, they are best seen with Gomori's or Grocott's methenamine silver stain, both of which are taken up by the cell wall.[72] Some organisms are acid-fast.[81] Organisms have also been identified as unstained refractile particles on fine needle aspiration specimens.[82] The yeasts are typically fairly uniform in size (3 to 5 μm) and oval in shape (Fig. 28–5), although they can assume a crescentic form as a result of collapse of cell walls and loss of cytoplasm.[83] Hyphal forms have been identified rarely, usually in association with endocarditis.[84] The yeast may be confused with a variety of other fungi, including *Pneumocystis carinii*, *Toxoplasma gondii*, yeast forms of *Candida* species, capsule-deficient forms of *C. neoformans*, and microforms of *B. dermatiditis*.[17, 85]

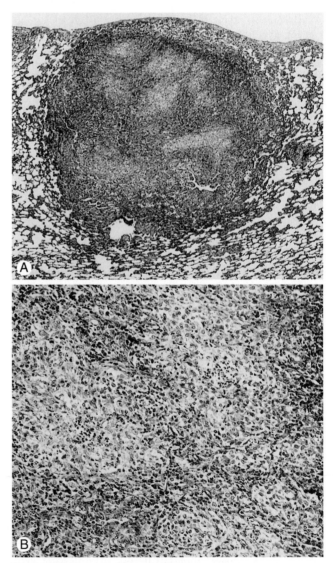

Figure 28–2. Acute Histoplasmosis. A well-defined focus of subpleural granulomatous inflammation is seen in *A*. A magnified view *(B)* shows two discrete granulomas with early central necrosis. Incidental finding in a dog sacrificed for experimental purposes; although seldom seen, this appearance is undoubtedly similar in human infection. (*A*, ×32; *B*, ×160.)

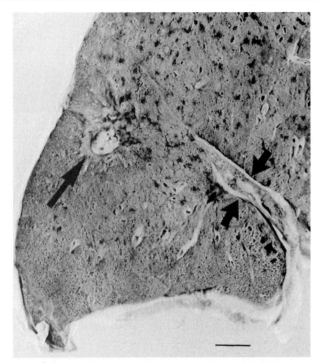

Figure 28–3. Chronic (Inactive) Histoplasmosis with Middle Lobe Collapse. A slice of right lung shows a focus of necrotic tissue surrounded by irregular strands of fibrous tissue in the superior segment of the lower lobe *(long arrow)*. This represents the initial site of infection (analogous to the Ghon focus of tuberculosis). The right middle lobe *(short arrows)* shows marked atelectasis and fibrosis as a result of spread of infection to peribronchial lymph nodes and obstruction of the middle lobe bronchus. (Bar = 1 cm.)

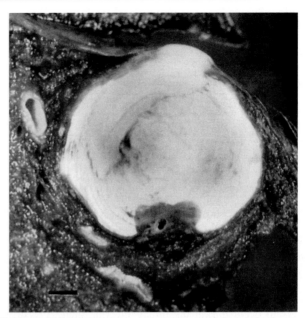

Figure 28–4. Histoplasmoma. A well-circumscribed subpleural nodule shows prominent laminations. Although this appearance has been described in tuberculosis, in our experience it is much more common in histoplasmosis. (Bar = 5 mm.)

Organisms can be identified histologically in many cases of histoplasmosis: in one series of unselected autopsies, they were detected in 70 of 94 cases (74%) with remote granulomatous disease;[77] in another series of surgically resected granulomas that had no evidence of other infectious organisms, they were found in 68 of 79 cases (86%).[86] (Both polymerase chain reaction [PCR] analysis[87] and culture,[88] however, may reveal the presence of the organisms in granulomas in which they are not seen by routine histochemical staining.) Despite the high frequency of histologic identification, culture of organisms from these lesions appears to be uncommon; in the studies cited previously, culture was positive in only 1 of 109 cases. In endemic areas, the likelihood that pulmonary granulomas are the result of histoplasmosis is high. For example, in one autopsy study, parenchymal calcifications larger than 4 mm and lymph node calcifications larger than 10 mm had an 80% probability of being caused by histoplasmosis.[77]

Although there are many similarities in the pathogenesis and pathology of tuberculosis and histoplasmosis, there are also fundamental differences.[20] Histoplasmosis is a relatively benign condition compared with tuberculosis; although many individuals are infected, clinically detected disease is rare. As in tuberculosis, the initial infection results in the development of cell-mediated immunity, reflected in the acquisition by macrophages of fungicidal properties. In contrast to tuberculosis, however, there is evidence that this immunity is more ephemeral. For example, in one investigation of histoplasmin-positive individuals, 15% to 20% reverted to nega-

tive when re-examined 2 years after the initial test;[89] of equal significance was the observation that most of these individuals subsequently become positive once again, presumably as a result of reinfection. In view of these findings, the terms *primary* and *postprimary* (*secondary*) as applied to tuberculosis may not be suitable to a classification of histoplasmosis. Moreover, in contrast to the endogenous reactivation of disease in postprimary tuberculosis, recurrent pneumonia caused by *H. capsulatum* has been hypothesized to be related most commonly to infection from an exogenous source.[20]

The nomenclature that has been proposed for types of disease caused by *H. capsulatum* is variable.[19, 90] We use a simple division into asymptomatic and symptomatic; the

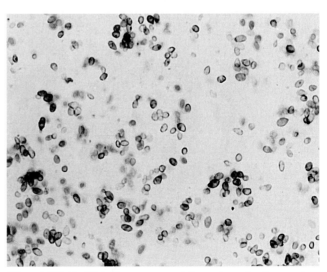

Figure 28–5. *Histoplasma capsulatum.* Grocott's silver methenamine stain showing round-to-oval yeasts of uniform size. (×800.)

latter can, in turn, be subdivided into acute, chronic, and disseminated histoplasmosis. It is likely that these clinical categories are dependent on a combination of the size and virulence of the initial inoculum and on the state of the host's immunity.[19, 20] The degree of immunity also appears to determine the length of the incubation period; nonimmunized individuals develop symptoms about 2 weeks after exposure, whereas those who are immune become symptomatic in as short a period as 3 days.

Asymptomatic Histoplasmosis

Estimates from endemic areas indicate that 95% to 99% of infections are not associated with symptoms, even with retrospective enquiry of histoplasmin converters.[20, 91] Despite the lack of complaints, chest radiographs of such converters have revealed pulmonary parenchymal opacities, with or without hilar lymph node enlargement, in as many as 10% to 25% of cases. It is believed that symptoms are more likely to occur during the initial infection than in recurrent ones. The lack of symptoms may reflect a low exposure dose in a nonimmunized person or a moderate-sized inoculum in one who is immunized.

Acute Histoplasmosis

The abrupt onset of symptoms in a patient with clinical and laboratory evidence of *H. capsulatum* infection is best designated *acute histoplasmosis*. Under this diagnostic umbrella are a variety of syndromes, in some of which the diagnosis can be suspected in the absence of an abnormal chest radiograph and without isolation of the organism.

Clinical Manifestations

Symptoms of flulike disease are perhaps the most common clinical manifestation of acute histoplasmosis. They consist of fever, headache, chills, cough, and retrosternal discomfort, the last-named probably being related to mediastinal node involvement;[20, 92] anorexia and nausea occur in some individuals.[93] In most of these cases, physical examination of the chest is normal. Hepatosplenomegaly may develop, usually in children. Erythema nodosum or erythema multiforme is occasionally present, usually in young women, and is sometimes associated with arthralgia;[20, 94, 95] in such cases, the diagnosis becomes evident through awareness of an ongoing miniepidemic.

Even with the relatively high levels of exposure that may occur in miniepidemics, symptoms may be mild; in fact, such exposure may not be recognized until many years later when calcific nodules are seen radiologically in the lungs.[40, 96, 97] Despite this observation, a high level of exposure is probably more likely to result in symptoms and may lead to severe illness and death.[36, 98] In this situation, symptoms may include cough with mucopurulent sputum, hemoptysis, and musculoskeletal pain. Crackles, a friction rub, and signs of consolidation may be evident. Pericarditis develops occasionally. The differential diagnosis in these cases includes acute viral or bacterial pneumonia;[40, 64, 92, 99] however, because hilar lymph node enlargement is uncommon in these

infections, this finding should suggest acute histoplasmosis in endemic areas. In rare cases, there is complicating adult respiratory distress syndrome.[98]

Radiologic Manifestations

The chest radiograph is normal in the majority of patients.[100, 101] The most common radiographic abnormalities consist of single or multiple poorly defined areas of airspace consolidation.[101] Severe disease is characterized by homogeneous parenchymal consolidation of nonsegmental anatomic distribution, simulating acute bacterial air-space pneumonia (Fig. 28–6). In contrast to the latter, the disease tends to clear in one area and appear in another. Some authorities cite the results of experimental work in monkeys and dogs and rare reported cases in humans as evidence that acute cavitation may occur.[102] Hilar lymph node enlargement is common;[40, 64, 92] pleural effusion is rare.

After heavy exposure, the radiograph may show widely disseminated, fairly discrete nodular shadows throughout the lungs, individual lesions measuring up to 3 or 4 mm in diameter;[104] such abnormalities may not be apparent for a week or more, despite the presence of symptoms. Hilar lymph node enlargement is present in the majority of cases.[40, 105–107] The parenchymal shadows may clear completely in 2 to 8 months or may fibrose and persist; as indicated previously, the chest radiograph 1 to several years later not uncommonly, reveals widely disseminated punctate calcifications (Fig. 28–7).[36, 96, 106]

A variant of acute histoplasmosis has been described in which affected patients are presumed to be heavily exposed

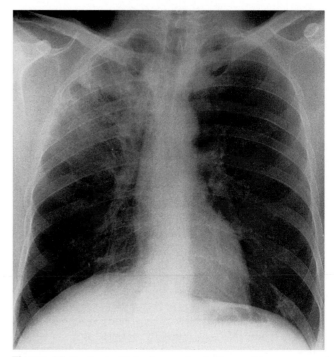

Figure 28–6. Acute Histoplasmosis. A 48-year-old man presented with a 3-week history of right-sided pleuritic chest pain. A posteroanterior chest radiograph demonstrates extensive consolidation in the right upper lobe and small areas of consolidation in the left lung apex. Sputum cultures grew *Histoplasma capsulatum*. (Courtesy of Dr. Thomas Hartman, Mayo Clinic, Rochester, MN.)

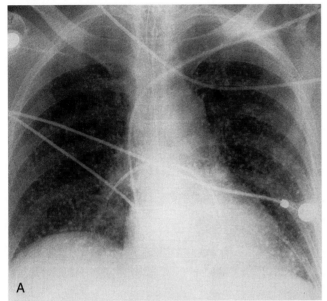

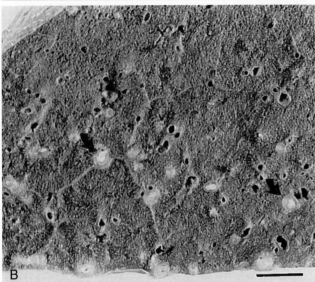

Figure 28–7. Histoplasmosis—Calcified Nodules. An anteroposterior chest radiograph *(A)* demonstrates numerous bilateral calcified nodules. This pattern may be seen after inhalation of a large number of organisms or with miliary disease. A magnified view of the corresponding gross specimen *(B)* shows well-defined nodules *(arrows)* with central necrotic material (white) surrounded by a fibrous capsule (gray). The nodules were an incidental finding at autopsy; the patient had no respiratory symptoms. (Bar = 1 cm.)

and to mount a vigorous immune response.[20] In these patients, acquired resistance appears to limit the tissue response to minute foci of granulomatous inflammation, which are seen on chest radiographs as miliary lesions unassociated with hilar node enlargement. These lesions usually clear completely without loss of pulmonary function. It has been suggested that this process may be the result of an exaggerated immunologic reaction.[20]

Histoplasmosis can also be manifested by unilateral or bilateral enlargement of hilar or mediastinal lymph nodes in the absence of other radiographic abnormalities. Of 269 patients in one series, 25 (9%) presented in this fashion, 20 of whom were asymptomatic.[108] This form of disease appears

to be particularly common in children,[64] in whom it may produce significant tracheal or bronchial obstruction.[109, 110] Extrinsic pressure from fibrotic nodes may also cause airway obstruction, particularly of the middle lobe bronchus, with resulting atelectasis and obstructive pneumonitis.[64, 92, 99] Calcification of lymph nodes, usually of the bronchopulmonary group, may be associated with broncholithiasis (Fig. 28–8);[111] in many such cases, CT reveals parabronchial calcification and thereby indicates the nature of the abnormality (*see* page 2287).

Histoplasmoma

Histoplasmoma is a relatively common form of pulmonary histoplasmosis that may or may not be associated with a history of previous symptomatic disease.[112, 113] The abnormality typically appears as a sharply defined nodule between 0.5 and 3 cm in diameter, in most cases in a lower lobe.[92, 114, 115] Although the lesion may be solitary, smaller satellite lesions are often seen.[116] The nodules may have a central focus of calcification, producing a characteristic "target" lesion (Fig. 28–9) or be diffusely calcified; such calcification is frequently identified on CT even when it is not apparent on the radiograph (Fig. 28–10).[117, 118] Hilar lymph node calcification is also common, although node enlargement is unusual. Pleural effusion or thickening is rare. An unusual case has been reported of a patient who had a 3-cm diameter cavitated and calcified nodule in which adjacent pleural thickening resulted in round atelectasis.[119]

When multiple, histoplasmomas seldom exceed four or five in number and often differ considerably in size (Fig. 28–11). Serial radiographs over months or years may reveal moderate growth, even to a point where neoplasia may be considered.[120] Even the presence of calcification does not necessarily mean that a histoplasmoma is "healed": such lesions may also increase in size, and histologic examination has shown apparently active fibrosis 10 years or more after they are first discovered. Although the pathogenesis of this phenomenon is not certain, it has been postulated to represent a reaction similar to that seen in fibrosing mediastinitis (*see* farther on).[114, 120]

The presence of central or diffuse calcification in a nodule 3 cm or less in diameter is virtually diagnostic of a granuloma. In an area endemic for histoplasmosis, *H. capsulatum* is the most likely cause; however, in the absence of calcification, the differential diagnosis must include all other causes of solitary or multiple nodules.

Chronic Histoplasmosis

In contrast to most individuals who have acute disease, which typically subsides clinically and radiographically without treatment in weeks to months, rare cases of histoplasmosis progress and become chronic, either in the lungs or in the mediastinum.

Chronic Pulmonary Histoplasmosis

Some cases of chronic pulmonary histoplasmosis are virtually identical to chronic active tuberculosis, both patho-

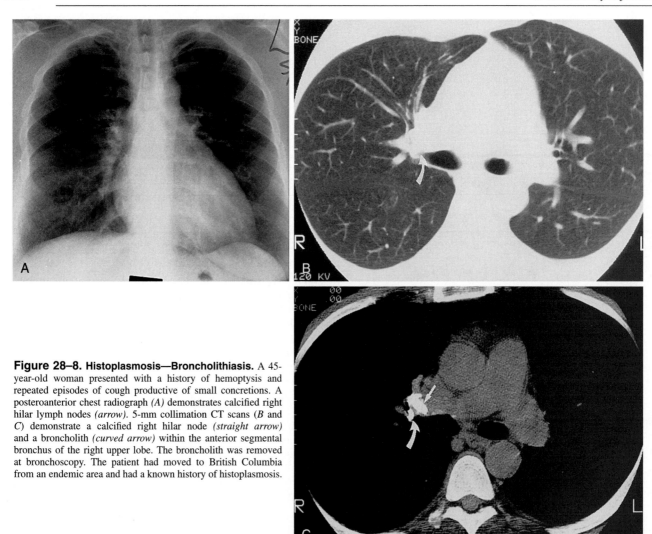

Figure 28–8. Histoplasmosis—Broncholithiasis. A 45-year-old woman presented with a history of hemoptysis and repeated episodes of cough productive of small concretions. A posteroanterior chest radiograph *(A)* demonstrates calcified right hilar lymph nodes *(arrow)*. 5-mm collimation CT scans *(B* and *C)* demonstrate a calcified right hilar node *(straight arrow)* and a broncholith *(curved arrow)* within the anterior segmental bronchus of the right upper lobe. The broncholith was removed at bronchoscopy. The patient had moved to British Columbia from an endemic area and had a known history of histoplasmosis.

logically and radiologically (Fig. 28–12). Affected patients have progressive, predominantly upper lobe disease characterized by fibrosis, necrosis, cavitation, and granulomatous inflammation. A background of pulmonary emphysema may or may not be present, and the infection may spread to involve the mediastinum or sites outside the thorax, in a fashion similar to the chronic disseminated form of disease.

It has been suggested that some cases of chronic pulmonary histoplasmosis represent an altogether different form of disease.[19] According to this view, the organism (which is usually present in small numbers) is best regarded as a colonist or at most as minimally invasive, the surrounding parenchymal inflammation, necrosis, and fibrosis representing an immune response of the host to the organism. The process is believed to begin when spores of *H. capsulatum* are inhaled and enter emphysematous spaces. An inflammatory exudate (which is predominantly fluid) develops within the spaces; endobronchial spread of the antigen-rich fluid then produces transient upper lobe segmental areas of consolidation characteristic of this form of the disease.[22, 121]

Pathologically, the consolidated areas are composed of interstitial aggregates of macrophages, lymphocytes, and plasma cells.[19] Foci of necrosis can be identified within the area of pneumonia and are believed to be the result of

ischemia, at least in part. Cavities may also form and can increase in size; their lining is necrotic tissue containing sparse organisms. In severe, chronic histoplasmosis (as in other fungal diseases), serum factors have been described that interfere with lymphocyte transformation following exposure to autologous antigen[122] and that inhibit the adherence of polymorphonuclear leukocytes and alveolar macrophages;[122a] however, the role (if any) that these play in the pathogenesis of this form of disease is uncertain.

The radiographic appearance simulates postprimary tuberculosis,[124–126] the earliest manifestations consisting of segmental or subsegmental areas of consolidation in the apices of the lungs, frequently outlining spaces of centrilobular emphysema. Thick-walled bullae sometimes contain fluid levels; with time, they can disappear completely or can gradually increase in size. In some patients, there is an increase in the wall thickness of bullae. Serial chest radiographs tend to show progressive loss of volume associated with increased prominence of linear opacities.

Chronic pulmonary histoplasmosis tends to be associated with cough and expectoration, which in some cases are likely the result of underlying chronic obstructive pulmonary disease rather than the infection itself. Spillage from infected cavities or bullae may be accompanied by fever. Patients

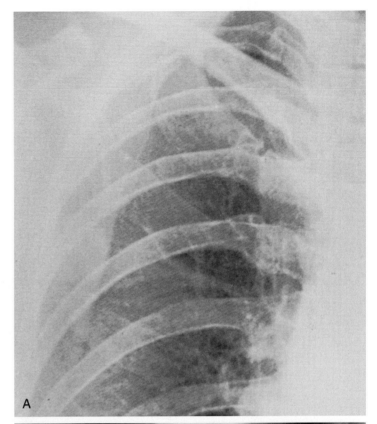

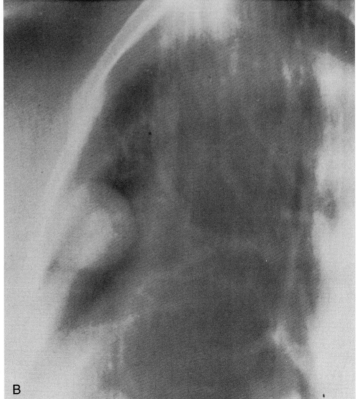

Figure 28–9. Histoplasmoma. Views of the upper half of the right lung from a posteroanterior radiograph *(A)* and an anteroposterior tomogram *(B)* show a sharply demarcated, circular shadow measuring 2.8 cm in diameter situated just deep to the visceral pleura. The density is homogeneous except for a central, punctate deposit of calcium. Such central calcification represents the characteristic appearance of chronic granulomatous infection (the *target* lesion). The patient was a 51-year-old asymptomatic woman whose chest radiograph was normal 1 year earlier. (Courtesy of Dr. Max J. Palayew, Jewish General Hospital, Montreal.)

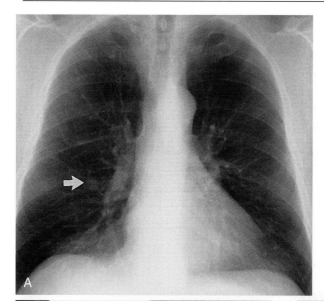

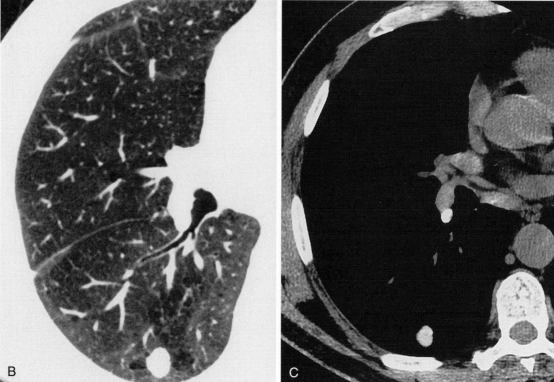

Figure 28–10. Calcified Histoplasmoma. A posteroanterior chest radiograph *(A)* demonstrates a 1.5-cm diameter nodule in the right lower lobe *(arrow)*; calcification is not apparent. HRCT (*B* and *C*) demonstrates diffuse calcification of the nodule as well as calcified right hilar and subcarinal nodes. The patient was an asymptomatic 54-year-old man.

who develop cavitary disease may complain of weight loss, deep-seated chest pain, hemoptysis, and general malaise; however, they can also remain asymptomatic.[19] The prognosis in patients with chronic cavitary disease is difficult to predict. The infection is progressive in some patients,[128] and prognosis may be poor if adequate treatment is not instituted;[129, 130] dissemination is rare.[19, 91]

Chronic Mediastinal Histoplasmosis

A variety of clinical and radiologic abnormalities can result from involvement of the mediastinum by histoplasmosis. Sometimes, they are related to one or more enlarged mediastinal lymph nodes.[131] Rarely, direct spread outside the capsule of such nodes or from pulmonary lesions leads to an ill-defined, matted mass of necrotic and fibrotic tissue. Perhaps more frequently (although still rarely), the process is secondary to an exuberant fibrous reaction that has been hypothesized to be caused by chronic immunologic stimulation by histoplasmin antigens similar to that seen in histoplasmomas (fibrosing mediastinitis; *see* page 2856).[20, 132]

CT scans of the mediastinum are essential for elucidation of the abnormalities. The most common findings are mediastinal or hilar masses, calcification within the mediastinal mass or associated lymph nodes, superior vena cava obstruction, pulmonary artery narrowing, and bronchial nar-

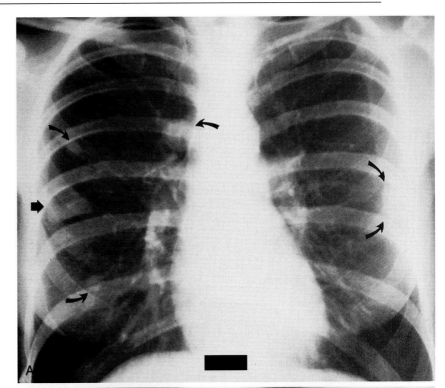

Figure 28–11. Multiple Nodules Caused by Histoplasmosis—Little Change Over 7 Years. A screening chest radiograph *(A)* of this 41-year-old asymptomatic woman shows multiple, well-defined nodules ranging from 1 to 3 cm in diameter throughout both lungs *(arrows)*. The nodule in the right axillary zone indicated by the *fat arrow* contains a central area of radiolucency, suggesting either cavitation or replacement of its center by lipid. Seven years later *(B)*, the only change that had occurred was that the solitary nodule projected above the right hilum either had disappeared or had undergone cavitation, leaving a thin wall. The radiolucent center of the nodule indicated by the *arrow* was still present, lending support to its lipid nature.

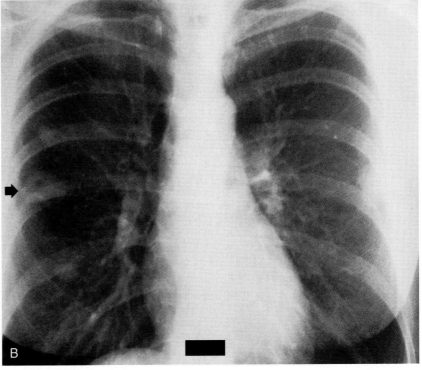

rowing.[133, 134] The presence of a localized calcified mediastinal soft tissue mass is the most frequent of these abnormalities; in a patient with an appropriate clinical history, this finding strongly suggests a diagnosis of *H. capsulatum*–induced fibrosing mediastinitis and precludes need for biopsy.[133, 134] For example, in one review of 33 patients (14 with pathologically proven histoplasmosis, 9 with presumed histoplasmosis, and 10 with idiopathic fibrosing mediastinitis), all patients who had disease secondary to proven or presumed histoplasmosis had localized soft tissue hilar and mediastinal masses (approximately two thirds of which were calcified), whereas the majority of patients who had idiopathic disease had diffuse soft tissue infiltration of the mediastinum without evidence of calcification.[134] In patients without calcification or with progressive radiographic findings, tissue should be obtained for definitive diagnosis.[134] MR imaging is comparable to CT in defining the extent of lymphadenopathy and allows diagnosis of vascular obstruc-

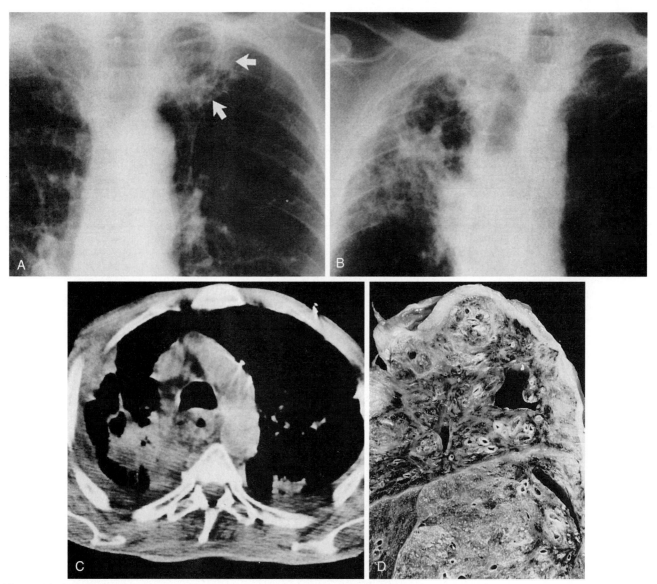

Figure 28–12. Chronic Progressive Histoplasmosis. A view of the upper half of the left lung *(A)* reveals a poorly defined, inhomogeneous opacity *(arrows)* containing a central radiolucency representing a cavity. The right lung was clear at that time. Approximately 1 year later *(B)*, the left apical lesion had almost completely resolved, but there was now extensive disease throughout the right upper lobe, associated with considerable loss of volume (note the tracheal shift to the right). CT scan at the level of the aortic arch *(C)* shows a large homogeneous opacity abutting the posterior mediastinum and containing a well-defined cavity in its anterior portion. A slice of right lung at autopsy *(D)* shows extensive fibrosis of the upper lobe and superior segment of the lower lobe, each of which has an irregularly shaped cavity. The appearance is similar to that of chronic tuberculosis; however, *H. capsulatum* was identified by culture and in tissue sections.

tion without the need for intravenous contrast material.[135, 136] CT is superior to MR imaging, however, at demonstrating calcification.[135]

Superior Vena Cava Obstruction. Encroachment on the superior vena cava by enlarged mediastinal nodes may result in the classic picture of the superior vena cava syndrome.[137–141] Obstruction is readily recognized on contrast-enhanced CT, MR imaging, or angiography (Fig. 28–13).

Pulmonary Arterial and Venous Obstruction. In a few cases, severe mediastinitis results in obstruction of pulmonary arteries or veins (or both) as they leave and enter the mediastinum. The effects on the lungs, more commonly local than general, include oligemia and the manifestations of pulmonary venous hypertension.

Tracheal and Major Airway Encroachment. The trachea and major bronchi may be narrowed by lymph nodes involved by granulomatous inflammation (particularly those in the right paratracheal and subcarinal chains) or by local or diffuse mediastinal fibrosis. Because the cartilaginous rings offer some support, obstruction is seldom complete; in most cases, it is associated with one or more other manifestations of mediastinal involvement.

Esophageal Obstruction. During either the active or the healed stage, enlarged posterior mediastinal lymph nodes may encroach on the esophagus and displace or partially obstruct it causing dysphagia. Healing of the affected lymph nodes may result in traction diverticula.[64, 138] Endoscopic ultrasonography may be helpful in confirming the diagnosis.

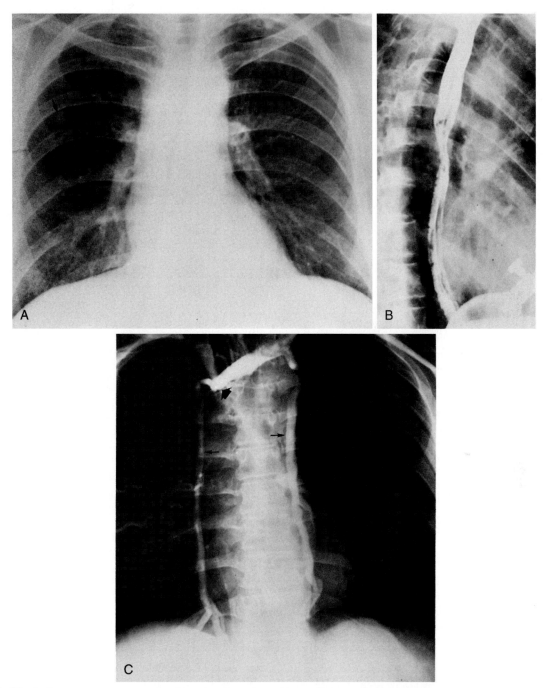

Figure 28–13. Mediastinal Histoplasmosis—Superior Vena Cava Obstruction. A posteroanterior radiograph *(A)* shows a somewhat widened upper mediastinum possessing a smooth contour. A partly calcified nodule can be identified in the upper portion of the right lung *(arrow)*. This 51-year-old man presented with a typical picture of obstruction of the superior vena cava. In addition to the symptoms and signs referable to the head and neck and upper extremities, the patient complained of "hemoptysis," which on further questioning and examination was found to arise from the esophagus rather than the lungs and to be caused by "downhill" esophageal varices *(B)*. A radiograph of the thorax after rapid injection of contrast medium into an antecubital vein *(C)* reveals complete obstruction of the superior vena cava just proximal to the junction of the right and left innominate veins *(thick arrow)*. Filling of the internal mammary veins can be identified on both sides *(thin arrows)*, representing part of the extensive collateral circulation. Note the multiple small foci of calcification in the spleen; this finding, in addition to a strongly positive histoplasmin skin test, constituted highly suggestive evidence for the diagnosis of mediastinal histoplasmosis.

(Esophageal mucosal nodules or ulcers may also be seen in disseminated histoplasmosis, in which case the diagnosis may be made by biopsy.[142])

Pericarditis. This complication can be the result of direct rupture of a focus of necrotic tissue into the pericardial cavity or of an immunologic response to *H. capsulatum*.[137, 143, 144] Pericardial effusion may be apparent radiologically as enlargement of the cardiovascular silhouette. Associated mediastinal lymph node enlargement is common. Tamponade, calcification of the pericardium, or constrictive pericarditis may develop.[91, 145] These complications usually occur in young adults and, in the acute phase, are often associated with pleural effusion, usually left-sided.[20, 91]

Disseminated Histoplasmosis

Clinically apparent disseminated histoplasmosis is an extremely rare occurrence; its incidence has been estimated to range from 1 per 100,000 to 1 per 500,000 infected people per year[21] (although these figures are likely higher now because of the AIDS epidemic). Affected patients usually have active or healed foci of granulomatous inflammation in the lungs.

In contrast to the fungicidal capability of macrophages that is acquired by most persons infected with *H. capsulatum*, those with symptomatic disseminated disease develop a parasitization of their macrophages, manifested by increased intracellular survival and multiplication of the organism. Approximately one third of patients are infants under 2 years of age; another 20% are adults who are immunosuppressed.[146–148] Although no obvious host defect can be found in the remainder, the rarity of this form of infection and the pathologic findings suggest an unrecognized deficiency in host defense.[19, 21] In some patients, this defect appears to be transitory, since those who survive the infection with treatment do not necessarily continue to exhibit increased susceptibility. Symptomatic disseminated histoplasmosis has been subdivided into three types based on clinical and pathologic features: acute, subacute, and chronic.[19, 21]

Acute Disseminated Histoplasmosis

Acute disseminated histoplasmosis is characterized pathologically by massive accumulation of parasitized mononuclear phagocytes accompanied by little tissue reaction. Lymph nodes, liver, spleen, bone marrow, and adrenal glands are predominantly affected. This is the most severe type of disseminated infection and occurs most frequently in infants and young children and in patients who are immunocompromised by conditions such as AIDS or organ transplantation. Its course is often measured in weeks. Clinical findings include high persistent fever, prominent hepatosplenomegaly, anemia, leukopenia, and thrombocytopenia; some patients also develop interstitial pneumonia. The radiographic and HRCT findings are usually similar to those of miliary tuberculosis,[149] consisting of 1- to 3-mm diameter nodules randomly distributed throughout both lungs (Fig. 28–14).

Subacute Disseminated Histoplasmosis

This form of disease is characterized by a moderate degree of macrophage parasitization. Focal aggregates of macrophages, often with central necrosis, are found most commonly in the gastrointestinal tract, the adrenal glands, the adventitia of meningeal vessels, and the cardiac valves, particularly the aortic.[150] The disease occurs in both children and adults. Typically the clinical course runs for months. Symptoms and signs include moderate fever, mild-to-moderate hepatosplenomegaly, and abdominal pain (caused by gastrointestinal ulceration); sometimes there is evidence of Addison's disease, meningitis, focal cerebritis, or endocarditis. Anemia, leukopenia and/or thrombocytopenia may be present.

Chronic Disseminated Histoplasmosis

Chronic disseminated histoplasmosis is a relatively mild form of disseminated disease that is associated with little or no fever, absence of hepatosplenomegaly, and no evidence of bone marrow suppression. Patients are almost invariably adult, and the time course is months to years. Parasitization of mononuclear phagocytes is relatively mild; although focal aggregates of infected macrophages with central necrosis are seen, they are not nearly as common as in the subacute form. Instead, true granulomas and multinucleated giant cells are often identified, presumably reflecting more adequate host defense. The reason for the protracted course of the disease is unclear. There is experimental evidence that relatively avirulent strains of the organism can persist in host epithelial cells, where they are presumably protected from macrophages and other immune mediator cells;[151] it has been speculated that such organisms may provide a reservoir for recurrent disease long after the initial infection has occurred.

The diagnosis is often made after the discovery and biopsy of an oropharyngeal ulcer, a presentation that appears to be particularly common in some parts of the world.[39] Oropharyngeal disease can also be the presenting feature of disseminated histoplasmosis in patients with AIDS.[152] Specific organ involvement may result in Addison's disease, meningitis, endocarditis, or laryngitis.[153] Individual cases of disseminated histoplasmosis associated with infection-associated hemophagocytic syndrome[154] and glomerulonephritis (the latter mimicking Wegener's granulomatosis)[155] have also been reported.

Laboratory Findings

Mycology

Examination of smears of expectorated material, pleural fluid, or bone marrow for the presence of organisms is seldom useful in patients who have acute histoplasmosis. Culture is more reliable, and in suspected cases the body fluids, bone marrow, or tissue should be appropriately inoculated; growth usually takes 2 to 4 weeks. Cultures are seldom positive in asymptomatic individuals or in the presence of self-limited disease, even in patients who are acutely ill from exposure to a heavy inoculum;[19] during more severe disease or in the presence of thin-walled cavities, growth is successful in no more than a third of patients. In the presence of thick-walled cavities, positive sputum culture has been reported in 50% to 70% of cases (provided that multiple specimens are collected).[19, 157] The use of *Histoplasma*-spe-

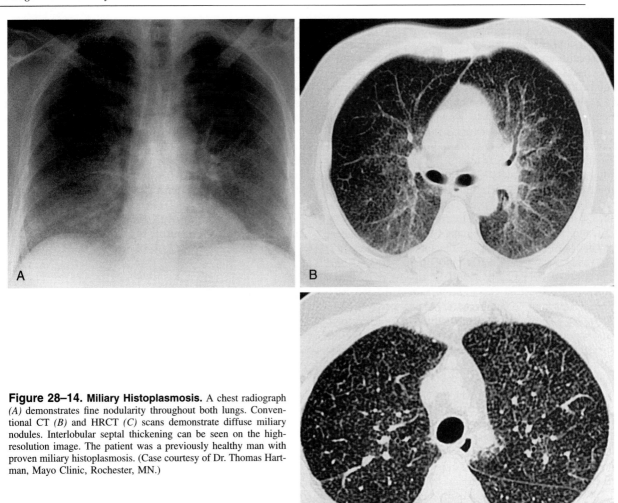

Figure 28–14. Miliary Histoplasmosis. A chest radiograph *(A)* demonstrates fine nodularity throughout both lungs. Conventional CT *(B)* and HRCT *(C)* scans demonstrate diffuse miliary nodules. Interlobular septal thickening can be seen on the high-resolution image. The patient was a previously healthy man with proven miliary histoplasmosis. (Case courtesy of Dr. Thomas Hartman, Mayo Clinic, Rochester, MN.)

cific DNA probes promises to be more sensitve than culture in many of these situations.[158]

Positive results on smear and culture in symptomatic disseminated histoplasmosis vary with the severity of the disease. In the acute, relatively severe form, blood and bone marrow smears, appropriately stained, are usually diagnostic; the frequency of positive cases decreases to 50% in moderate and 20% in mild forms of the disease. Culture results are generally better, and blood, bone marrow, liver, and even urine should be sampled for this purpose when disseminated disease is suspected.

Hematology

The white cell count is usually normal, but may increase to 15,000/mm³ in patients with the acute epidemic form[36] and to 20,000/mm³ in those who have cavitary disease.[128] Leukopenia, anemia, and thrombocytopenia develop in approximately 50% of patients with symptomatic disseminated disease, but rarely in those with other varieties.

Skin Tests

The skin test is performed intradermally with 0.1 ml of a solution of 1:100 histoplasmin, a positive result consisting of an area of induration measuring 5 mm or more that is read within 48 hours. The test becomes positive 2 to 4 weeks after infection and usually remains so for 10 years or more after the initial exposure.[19, 90] Such cutaneous hypersensitivity is seen in almost all patients with asymptomatic or self-limited acute infection, in 75% to 80% of those with chronic pulmonary histoplasmosis, and in 30% to 50% of patients with symptomatic disseminated disease.[19, 159] Although useful in epidemiologic studies, the test serves little or no purpose in the diagnosis of disease in the individual patient because a positive reaction does not prove the presence of active infection.

Serology

There are a number of different methods for detecting serum antibodies in histoplasmosis, and most experts agree that using multiple tests, with both mycelial and yeast antigens, increases diagnostic accuracy.[160] The latex agglutination (LA) test is a simple screening test that may become positive earlier than the complement-fixation (CF) test.[90] Although it is positive in most patients with self-limited infections, however, it is present in only 50% of patients with chronic disease.[160, 161] The CF test may be performed using either mycelial or yeast antigen and is more sensitive but less specific than the immunodiffusion (ID) test, since a positive CF for histoplasmosis may be found in patients who have coccidioidomycosis, blastomycosis, or cryptococcosis.[156, 162] The ID test uses concentrated histoplasmin as antigen and produces an M band during early infection or recovery and an H band in the presence of active disease.[90] A radioimmunoassay appears to be more sensitive (but less specific) than either CF or ID tests.[163]

Most authorities accept a fourfold rise in titer in serial determinations or a single determination of greater than 1:32 as being strong evidence of recent infection. Titers of 1:8 to 1:32 have been found as anamnestic responses in the general population in areas of high endemicity.[19] In regions where the prevalence of positive skin test reactors is relatively low, some investigators accept yeast-phase titers of 1:32 and mycelial titers of 1:8 or more as highly suggestive evidence of active disease;[156] yeast titers of 1:8 and 1:16 have been regarded as presumptive evidence of the diagnosis.

There are two major problems with the use of serologic tests in diagnosis of histoplasmosis. One is the delay in the development of appropriate antibodies, the results of most tests becoming available several weeks after the onset of clinically evident infection. The second is related to sensitivity and specificity, which vary between individual tests as well as the different forms of the disease. For example, although a rise in titer is detectable in about 95% of mild subclinical or symptomatic cases,[19, 121] only 25% of patients with chronic pulmonary histoplasmosis have titers 1:32 or greater.[19, 164] Lower titers are found in patients with disseminated disease, titers above 1:8 being present in 60% to 70%.[128, 165, 166] Only 10% of patients with residual histoplasmomas have yeast-phase antigen titers of 1:32 or more.[116, 164] As might be expected, serologic tests are of little value in immunosuppressed patients;[146] however, detection of *Histoplasma* polysaccharide antigen in bronchoalveolar lavage (BAL) specimens has been found by some investigators to be both sensitive and specific in diagnosing the disease in patients with AIDS.[167]

Miscellaneous Findings

Levels of serum angiotensin-converting enzyme activity have been reported to be elevated in patients with acute pulmonary histoplasmosis, making this test of little value in the differentiation from sarcoidosis.[168] Strongly positive precipitins against farmer's lung antigens have also been described in cases of acute epidemic histoplasmosis.[169]

Histoplasmosis Caused by *Histoplasma duboisii*

Histoplasmosis caused by *H. duboisii* is uncommon relative to disease caused by its North American cousin. Although the organism has been designated a separate species, it has also been speculated to represent only a variety of *H. capsulatum* and thus is known by some observers as *H. capsulatum* var. *duboisii*.[37] Although the disease occurs primarily in Central Africa, cases have been identified elsewhere (e.g., the United States and Chile) after residence in edemic areas.[170, 171] Occasional cases have been associated

with AIDS.[172] The yeasts are double walled and measure 12 to 15 μm in diameter, appreciably larger than those of *H. capsulatum*. The natural reservoir of the organism is unclear; however, as with *H. capsulatum*, it has been isolated from soil mixed with bat guano.[173] As with *H. capsulatum*, asymptomatic infection of individuals in regions endemic for *H. duboisii* is probably common.[174]

The disease typically involves the skin, subcutaneous tissues, and bone, but occasionally is widely disseminated. Pulmonary involvement is uncommon,[170, 175] even in the presence of dissemination; however, occasional cases of predominant lung disease have been reported.[176] Histologically, lesions are characterized by aggregates of multinucleated, yeast-containing giant cells associated with a variety of mononuclear and polymorphonuclear inflammatory cells; necrosis is variable.

COCCIDIOIDOMYCOSIS

Coccidioidomycosis is a highly infectious disease caused by the dimorphic fungus *Coccidioides immitis*.[177–182] In its natural habitat (soil) and on artificial media, it grows as a mycelium of septate hyphae that produces numerous 2- to 5-μm arthrospores when mature. The latter are freed as the mycelium fragments, are quite resistant to drying and are highly virulent: experimental primate infection has resulted from as few as 10 organisms.[183] Within tissue, the organisms exist as spherules measuring from 10 to greater than 100 μm in diameter.[177] These reproduce by endosporulation (i.e., the cytoplasm of the spherule undergoes cleavage to produce spores, the latter developing, in turn, into mature spherules); there is no budding.

Epidemiology

Coccidioidomycosis is almost exclusively a disease of the Western Hemisphere and is found principally in its endemic areas in the southwestern United States, northern Mexico, and portions of Central and South America (primarily Venezuela, Paraguay, Argentina, Colombia, Guatemala, and Honduras).[184] Within the United States, the disease is found mostly in California, central and southern Arizona, western Texas, southern New Mexico, southwestern Utah, and the southern tip of Nevada. In California, endemicity is greatest in the San Joaquin Valley, although cases have been documented from San Francisco to the Mexican border.[185, 186] Some infections that develop outside of the usual areas may be related to airborne dispersal of arthrospores by strong winds.[187] Even in endemic regions, there are local pockets where arthrospores of *C. immitis* are concentrated, as has been shown by differences in skin test reactivity of men in adjacent work camps.[185]

In endemic areas, the incidence of infection is high: approximately 25% of newly arrived persons can be expected to have positive skin tests at the end of 1 year and 50% at the end of 4 years. Most conversions are unassociated with symptoms. It has been estimated that in the United States there are 100,000 new infections per year.[177] In some regions (e.g., Arizona), the incidence of the disease increased substantially between 1990 and 1995, possibly as a result of an older population and an increased number of patients with AIDS.[188] The incubation period ranges from 1 to 4 weeks.

Proliferation of the mycelial form of the fungus requires an alkaline soil free from severe frost and a dry season that follows a wet one. As might be expected, the risk of acquiring the infection is greatest during dry and windy conditions in which soil is disturbed. Local outbreaks have occurred after the formation of dust clouds generated by an earthquake[189] or by earth moving during construction[190] or archeology digs;[186] the latter outbreaks can be kept to a minimum by dust control. More serious miniepidemics, such as the one that occurred in the southern San Joaquin Valley between 1991 and 1993, are less common and may be related to both climatic factors (such as prolonged drought) and social factors (such as increased immigration of susceptible individuals).[192]

Although coccidioidomycosis commonly affects a variety of domestic animals, including swine, sheep, and cattle, these animals seldom show clinical evidence of disease. Animal-to-animal and animal-to-human spread are generally not believed to occur; however, one group has documented the aquisition of disease by a veterinarian during the course of an autopsy.[193] The disease is also probably not transmitted from person to person (although six individuals have been reported to acquire the disease after exposure to a patient with a draining sinus whose plaster cast and surgical dressings served as culture media for the proliferation of arthrospores).[191]

The majority of infections that appear outside the endemic zone are believed to be related to travel within it;[194] although most examples of such travel are recent, cases have been documented of reactivation of quiescent disease acquired many years earlier.[195] Several cases have also been reported in which the source of infection was contaminated soil, food, cotton, or wool shipped from an endemic area.[196, 197] In addition, laboratory workers exposed to arthrospores in the course of handling contaminated material are at increased risk.[198] Rare cases of primary cutaneous inoculation have been documented in individuals in a variety of occupations, including agricultural workers, morticians, and laboratory technicians;[199] in these cases, the disease usually follows a benign course and remains localized to the inoculated skin and regional lymph nodes.[177]

Approximately 20% to 40% of patients who acquire the infection have clinical manifestations, of whom about 2% to 3% have illness lasting weeks or months;[188] clinical evidence of disseminated disease occurs in less than 0.1%. There is evidence that disseminated disease is more likely to occur in Filipinos and African Americans than in whites,[187] although the epidemiologic data supporting such a hypothesis have been questioned.[178] An increased risk of infection in native Americans has been documented.[177] Individuals who are immunocompromised, with conditions such as AIDS[202] or organ transplants,[203] also have an increased susceptibility to both pulmonary and disseminated disease.

Skin reactivity to *C. immitis* is long-lived but does wane with time,[177] suggesting the possibility of exogenous reinfection in endemic areas. Reactivation of quiescent disease in nonendemic areas has been documented,[177] however, and it is likely that some cases of late-onset, disseminated disease in endemic areas are the result of a loss of immunocompetence in individuals who experienced asymptomatic

dissemination during primary infection. Patients can also develop acute or chronic progressive disease after a period of remission following their primary infection, possibly as a consequence of an impairment in their host defenses.[90, 204] The natural history of coccidioidomycosis is characterized by a variety of pathologic, radiographic, and clinical patterns that can be considered under the headings of primary, persistent primary, chronic progressive, and disseminated disease.

Primary Coccidioidomycosis

Within the lung, inhaled arthrospores develop into sporangia (spherules) that rapidly induce an exudate of edema and polymorphonuclear leukocytes in a pattern of typical bronchopneumonia.[205] Although this reaction often persists, with time granulomatous inflammation also develops, consisting of both true granulomas and scattered multinucleated giant cells containing spherules (Fig. 28–15). The combination of exudative and granulomatous inflammation is also seen in other forms of coccidioidomycosis and is characteristic of the disease.[206, 207] It has been suggested that the exudative reaction occurs in response to the released endospores and the granulomatous one to intact spherules.[177] As might be expected, the development of a granulomatous reaction in immunocompromised individuals (e.g., with AIDS) is often deficient.[208]

In the majority of cases, the pneumonic focus remains relatively small and undergoes resolution, leaving small scars as residua. In some, however, disease progresses to involve a whole lobe or lung in a pattern resembling confluent bacterial bronchopneumonia. In these cases, necrosis may be extensive and can be associated with cavitation. Ulcerative bronchitis and bronchiolitis are often prominent, and bronchiectasis may develop if the patient survives.[206] Hilar and mediastinal lymph nodes may be enlarged and may contain a substantial amount of necrotic tissue and organisms; erosion of the capsule and spread of infected material into adjacent structures, such as bronchi or mediastinum, can result in the dissemination of disease in a fashion similar to tuberculosis.[206]

In tissue sections stained with H & E or silver and in cytologic preparations, the organisms appear as round spherules measuring 10 to greater than 100 μm in diameter; most are between 20 and 40 μm.[209] They typically have thick, refractile walls and can appear empty or can contain numerous endospores ranging in diameter from 2 to 5 μm (*see* Fig. 28–15). Released endospores may be confused with a number of other organisms, including *H. capsulatum, C. neoformans,* and small forms of *B. dermatitidis.* Hyphae and a variety of architecturally unusual forms have also been described,[210, 211] usually in association with solid or cavitary coccidioidal nodules.

The radiographic findings in primary disease vary from no abnormalities to areas of patchy air-space consolidation. The latter is usually unilateral; involves mainly the lower lobes; and may be homogeneous or mottled, segmental or nonsegmental (Fig. 28–16).[212] In one series of 59 cases, such air-space consolidation was observed in 27 patients (46%) and was the most common mode of radiographic presentation.[213] There is a tendency for the areas of consolidation to resolve in one region, while new ones develop in another.[214]

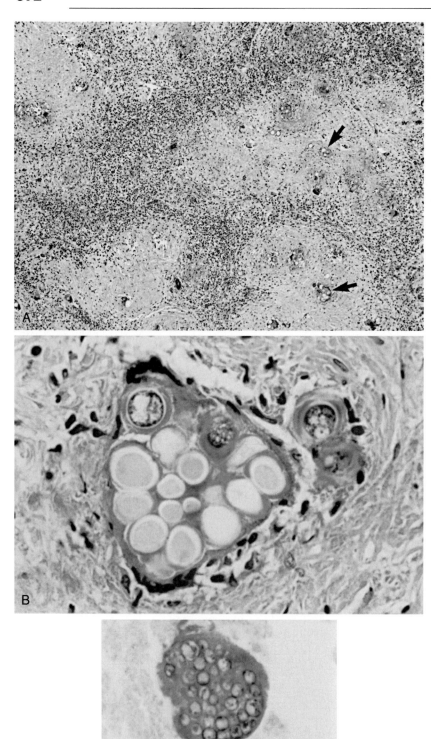

Figure 28–15. Coccidioidomycosis. A large focus of parenchymal consolidation *(A)* shows fibrosis, mononuclear inflammatory cells, and numerous multinucleated giant cells with phagocytosed spherules *(arrows)*. A magnified view of a giant cell *(B)* shows intracytoplasmic spherules with prominent capsules. An individual spherule *(C)* shows numerous endospores. *(A, ×56; B, ×600; C, ×1000.)*

Sometimes, the foci of consolidation are transformed into thin-walled cavities, which may resolve spontaneously.[215] Small pleural effusions occur in approximately 20% of cases;[213, 216] large effusions are rare.

Lymph node enlargement occurs in approximately 20% of cases, seldom in the absence of parenchymal involvement. In the series of 59 patients cited previously, enlarged hilar nodes were detected in 11 (19%) and enlarged mediastinal nodes in 5 (8.5%);[213] node enlargement was the sole radiographic abnormality in only one individual. In the majority of patients, enlarged nodes do not result in symptoms; rarely the tracheal lumen is compromised, particularly in children.[217, 218] Involvement of paratracheal nodes may indicate imminent dissemination of the infection,[219] although even the scalene nodes may be affected without clinical or serologic evidence of such progression.[220]

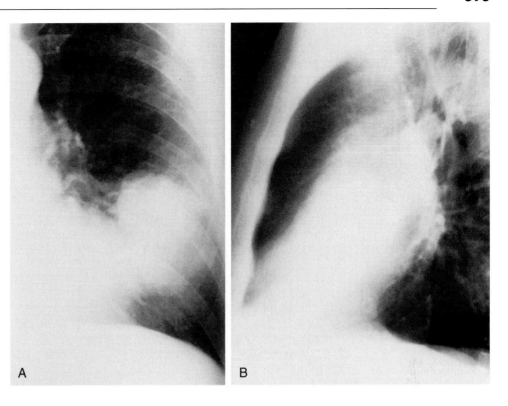

Figure 28–16. Primary Coccidioidomycosis. Views of the left lung from posteroanterior *(A)* and lateral *(B)* radiographs reveal homogeneous consolidation of much of the lingular segment of the left upper lobe. A faint air bronchogram could be identified on the original radiographs but does not reproduce well. The upper border of the consolidation is sharply circumscribed, resembling a mass. On surgical excision, it proved to be coccidioidomycosis.

The frequency with which primary coccidioidomycosis is recognized clinically probably depends on how closely it is looked for as well as on the degree of exposure. Overall, it has been estimated that about 60% to 80% of patients are asymptomatic.[221] When present, symptoms that accompany primary infection are often nonspecific and flu-like, consisting of fever, cough (usually nonproductive), chest pain, headache, and (sometimes) a generalized erythematous rash.[222] On physical examination, crackles and wheezes may be heard; signs of consolidation are rare. More severe disease may be manifested by expectoration and hemoptysis; prostration and death occur rarely.[223] Diabetic ketoacidosis has been documented in some patients.[224]

A more specific syndrome, commonly known as *valley fever*, occurs in 5% to 20% of patients with symptomatic coccidioidomycosis. It may be seen in isolated cases or in miniepidemics[186, 190, 225] and consists of erythema nodosum or erythema multiforme, arthralgia, and (sometimes) eosinophilia. This combination of findings may be associated with flu-like symptoms and should suggest the diagnosis in an endemic area. Because the findings are noted at the onset of skin test reactivity and affected patients are usually sensitive to coccidioidin, it has been suggested that the pathogenesis of this form of disease is related to an immunologic mechanism, such as deposition of immune complexes in subcutaneous tissues.[177] However, we are aware of only one study of immune complexes in coccidioidomycosis in which serum levels correlated with the severity of the disease;[226] in this study, there were no patients with erythema nodosum.

Persistent Primary Coccidioidomycosis

Primary disease that persists longer than 6 weeks is designated *persistent primary coccidioidomycosis*[178] and is associated with several pulmonary manifestations. The most serious is progressive pneumonia that can spread to involve large portions of the lungs and may prove fatal. More commonly, one or more nodules develop; these may persist indefinitely[227] and occasionally serve as a focus for reactivated disease.[195] Cavitation can occur either within areas of pneumonia or as a result of the "shelling out" of presumed stable nodules. Hematogenous dissemination of the organism may result in miliary disease.[178, 221]

Nodular lesions (coccidioidomas) represent localized foci of completely or partially resolved pneumonia. Pathologically, they are similar to the nodular lesions of histoplasmosis and tuberculosis, consisting of a central zone of necrotic tissue surrounded by a variably well-developed fibrous capsule and a chronic inflammatory infiltrate.[228] Small satellite granulomas can often be identified at the periphery of the nodule.

Radiographically a nodule develops over a period of approximately 5 to 6 weeks,[216] as a focus of consolidation becomes smaller, denser, and better defined. Occasionally, nodular opacities result from filling in of a cavity.[214] The nodules range in diameter from 0.5 to 5 cm and are located in the lung periphery in more than 90% of cases.[214] Although usually single, they are occasionally multiple (Fig. 28–17).[213, 216] They tend to occur in the mid and upper lung zones and, in contrast to tuberculosis, may develop in the anterior segment of an upper lobe.[215] Calcification is uncommon, but may occur as soon as 1 year after discovery.[229] On CT, the necrotic central zone may be identifiable, and the nodule may show marked enhancement after intravenous administration of contrast material.[230] In one study of 17 patients who had coccidioidomas, 10 of the nodules showed homogeneous attenuation, 2 had central areas of low attenuation related to necrosis, 2 were cavitated, 2 had foci of calcification, and 1 had focal bubble-like lucencies.[230a]

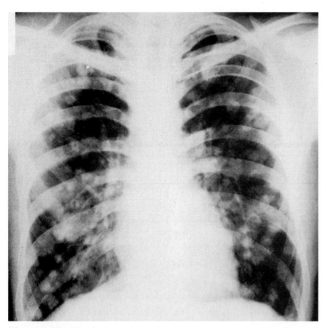

Figure 28–17. Coccidioidomycosis. A posteroanterior radiograph reveals multiple sharply circumscribed nodules distributed randomly throughout both lungs and ranging from 3 to 15 mm in diameter. There is no evidence of calcification or cavitation. The patient was a 25-year-old asymptomatic man living in Arizona. (Courtesy of Dr. Paul Capp, University of Arizona Medical Center, Tucson.)

Cavities have been reported to occur in 10% to 15% of patients who have pulmonary disease.[213, 231] They are usually single and located in the upper lobes[22, 232] and may be thin or thick walled (Figs. 28–18 and 28–19); thin-walled ("grape-skin") cavities have a tendency to change size,[229, 233] possibly reflecting a variable check-valve communication with the proximal bronchial tree.

Almost all patients with nodular coccidioidomycosis are asymptomatic, even in the presence of cavitation. In fact,

nodules may not be discovered for months or years after the patient has left an endemic area.[232, 233] They are most often found incidentally and investigated to exclude the possibility of malignancy. Transthoracic needle aspiration may provide the diagnosis by revealing the spherules on Papanicolaou-stained specimens.[209, 234, 235] Occasionally, mycetomas develop and lead to hemoptysis.[236, 237] Rarely, a localized nodule is associated with hemoptysis secondary to the development of a bronchoarterial fistula (Fig. 28–20).[238] A case has also been reported in which an endobronchial coccidioidoma developed in the right main bronchus, resulting in dyspnea and wheezing.[239] Rarely, coccidioidal and tuberculous infection coexists, creating obvious problems in diagnosis and management, particularly if both diseases are located in the same lobe.[229]

In contrast to the nodular form of disease, persistent coccidioidal pneumonia is commonly accompanied by hemoptysis, fever, cough, and expectoration, especially when cavitation occurs.[22] Hemoptysis is rarely fatal.[207] Pneumothorax and empyema develop in about 2% of patients with acute cavitary disease (Fig. 28–21)[227, 240] and usually require surgical intervention.[241, 242]

Chronic Progressive Coccidioidomycosis

Chronic progressive coccidioidomycosis (chronic progressive coccidioidal pneumonia and chronic pulmonary coccidioidomycosis) comprises less than 1% of cases of coccidioidal pulmonary disease.[178, 243] Some investigators have recognized two varieties—chronic progressive fibronodular disease and chronic progressive necrotizing disease, the latter associated with cavitation.[221]

Chronic progressive coccidioidal pneumonia can occur either in temporal continuity with primary coccidioidomycosis or after a variable time interval during which the infection has apparently been stable and unaccompanied by clinical

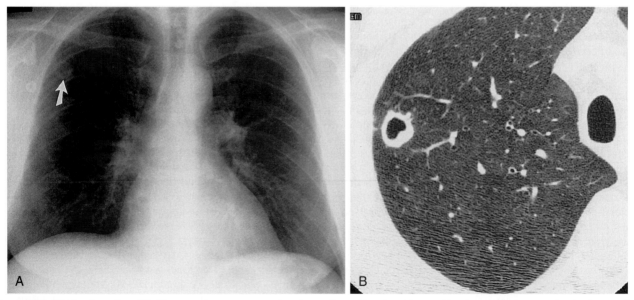

Figure 28–18. Cavitary Coccidioidomycosis. A posteroanterior chest radiograph *(A)* in a 44-year-old patient demonstrates a sharply circumscribed, 2-cm diameter cavitated nodule *(arrow)* in the right upper lobe. HRCT *(B)* demonstrates uneven wall thickness and smooth outer margins. Coccidioidomycosis was proven by surgical resection.

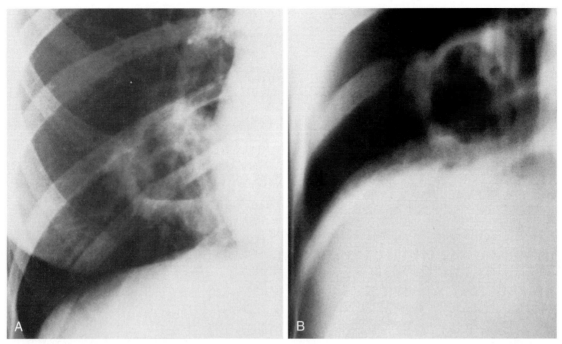

Figure 28–19. Cavitary Coccidioidomycosis. A detail view of the lower half of the right lung from a posteroanterior radiograph *(A)* reveals a thick-walled cavity measuring 5 cm in diameter and containing a prominent air-fluid level. A tomogram in anteroposterior *(B)* projection reveals to better advantage the thick irregular wall and the rather shaggy inner lining. *Coccidioides immitis* was recovered by bronchial brushing. The patient was a 22-year-old woman living in Arizona. (Courtesy of Dr. Paul Capp, University of Arizona Medical Center, Tucson.)

evidence of activity. In the latter situation, it is believed that there is reactivation of quiescent disease, presumably as a result of some alteration in host defense. Because reactivation may occur outside endemic areas, it is essential that an appropriate travel history be obtained as a clue to the correct diagnosis.

Disease usually develops insidiously and has a prolonged course of up to 15 years (average, 5 years[178]). Symptoms include cough, weight loss, fever, hemoptysis, chest pain, and dyspnea. Individuals of Philippine extraction, African Americans,[179, 243] and patients with insulin-dependent diabetes mellitus[244] appear to be at increased risk of developing this type of disease, although they appear to respond well to treatment. About 85% of the fatalities occur in patients who are immunocompromised.[179, 245] Although dissemination can occur,[180] the disease remains confined to the lungs in most cases.[243] Radiographic changes resemble those of chronic cavitary tuberculosis, consisting of small nodular or irregular linear opacities, single or multiple cavities, and volume loss.[214] These abnormalities usually involve the upper lobes and may be unilateral or bilateral.

Disseminated Coccidioidomycosis

Disseminated coccidioidomycosis is a rare manifestation of the disease, with an incidence of approximately 1 in 6,000 cases.[212] It may occur as a complication of the primary illness or after reactivation of latent disease in susceptible individuals. The course may be chronic and insidious or rapidly fatal, the latter usually in association with primary disease. Dissemination shows considerable male predominance and a predilection for African Americans and Filipinos. Pregnant women are also susceptible, especially during

the third trimester,[246] although some have speculated that the risk in the groups of women that have been studied is related to low socioeconomic status rather than pregnancy itself.[247] As might be expected, patients with immunodeficiency diseases[248] (particularly AIDS[249–251]) or receiving immunosuppressive therapy (including corticosteroids[252]) are at increased risk; withdrawal of immunosuppressive agents may improve host defense and permit survival.[253]

Although disseminated disease can affect any organ of the body, either alone or in combination, the principal sites of involvement are the skin, bones, joints, kidneys, and central nervous system.[178] Involvement of the last-named tissue is particularly common and concerning because it is frequently fatal.[221] The complication occurs in 30% to 50% of patients with disseminated coccidioidomycosis, sometimes as the sole extrapulmonary site of disease and occasionally without radiologic or pathologic evidence of pulmonary involvement.[206] Complications include meningitis (the most common), meningoencephalitis, and meningomyelitis.[254] In most cases, the interval between primary infection and the development of meningitis is less than 3 months,[255] although it may be as long as 14 years.[256] Skin involvement occurs in most patients and consists of a variety of lesions, often involving the nasolabial folds. Osteomyelitis occurs in 10% to 50% of cases, most commonly in vertebrae and usually as a single lesion;[178] it is best detected by bone scintigraphy.[257, 258]

In patients who die of disseminated disease, pulmonary involvement is the rule and is usually extensive.[206, 207] Pathologic characteristics are essentially the same as those observed in severe primary disease.[206] Hematogenous dissemination resulting in miliary disease occurs occasionally (Fig. 28–22); it usually appears early in the course of the infection and seldom more than 2 months after onset.[219, 259] Miliary

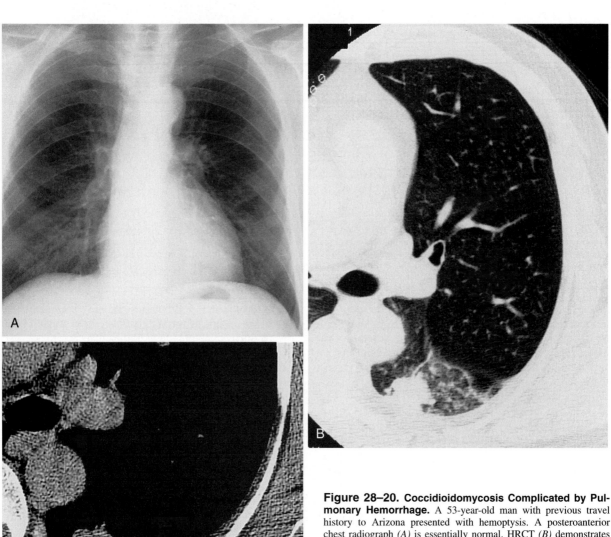

Figure 28–20. Coccidioidomycosis Complicated by Pulmonary Hemorrhage. A 53-year-old man with previous travel history to Arizona presented with hemoptysis. A posteroanterior chest radiograph (A) is essentially normal. HRCT (B) demonstrates an irregularly marginated nodule in the superior segment of the left lower lobe. The area of ground-glass attenuation surrounding the nodule was due to pulmonary hemorrhage. Soft tissue windows (C) better demonstrate the irregular margins of the nodule as well as a focal eccentric area of calcification (arrow). Surgical resection demonstrated coccidioidomycosis. The pulmonary hemorrhage was the result of a bronchoarterial fistula.

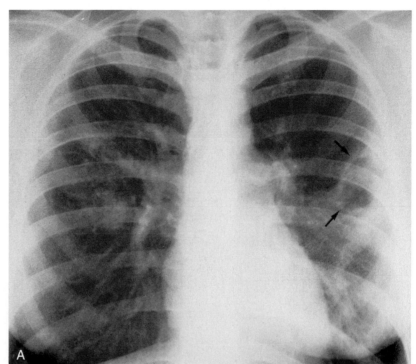

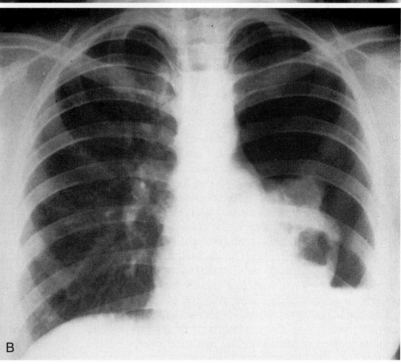

Figure 28–21. Cavitary Coccidioidomycosis with Perforation into Pleural Space. A posteroanterior radiograph *(A)* reveals a solitary, thin-walled cavity in the axillary portion of the left lung *(arrows)*, its lateral aspect abutting the visceral pleura. Patchy consolidation is noted in the midportion of the right lung as well. Eight days later, shortly after the onset of severe left chest pain and dyspnea, another radiograph *(B)* reveals a massive hydropneumothorax associated with total collapse of the left lung. The air-containing cavity is well seen within the collapsed lung. Culture of pleural fluid grew *Coccidioides immitis*. (Courtesy of Dr. Paul Capp, University of Arizona Medical Center, Tucson.)

involvement of the lungs may or may not be associated with systemic miliary spread and rarely occurs without evidence of extrapulmonary disease.[178] The miliary-like radiographic pattern seen in acute histoplasmosis in response to the inhalation of large numbers of organisms does not occur. In two cases of disseminated coccidioidomycosis, however, the lesions calcified in much the same manner as they do in widely disseminated histoplasmosis.[263] In patients with AIDS, disseminated coccidioidomycosis may be seen as a diffuse reticular nodular pattern on the chest radiograph.[216, 264]

Symptoms are usually minimal, consisting of mild fe-ver, dyspnea, and weight loss. Sputum cultures and skin tests are usually negative, although the CF test may be weakly positive.[221] Rare instances of adult respiratory distress syndrome have been associated with miliary disease.[265]

Laboratory Findings

Mycology

Wet mounts of sputum, urine, pus, gastric washings, or exudates from cutaneous lesions treated with 10% potassium

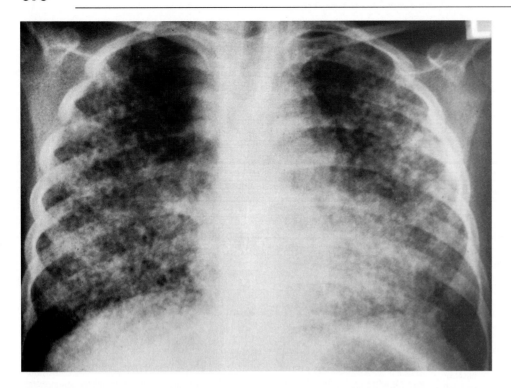

Figure 28–22. Disseminated Coccidioidomycosis. Multiple punctate opacities measuring up to 2 mm in diameter are scattered widely throughout both lungs, in some areas being so numerous as to be almost confluent. This represents miliary spread of the disease. This child had acute leukemia and was receiving antineoplastic therapy; on appropriate therapy, he recovered from acute coccidioidomycosis but subsequently died from the primary disease. (Courtesy of Dr. Paul Capp, University of Arizona Medical Center, Tucson.)

hydroxide may reveal spherules.[266] Some observers have found the yield from Papanicolaou-stained cytologic preparations to be greater.[266] When sputum is unavailable or examination is not diagnostic, bronchoscopy has proved to be a valuable procedure for obtaining material.[267] In one investigation comparing the yield of different methods in detecting the organism, cytologic examination of BAL or bronchial wash specimens was found to be positive in 8 of 19 patients with AIDS and 11 of 35 without; transbronchial biopsy showed organisms in all eight cases in which it was performed.[268] Culture of BAL fluid yielded the fungus in all 54 patients. However, in another investigation of 250 core needle biopsy specimens of pulmonary nodules, in which spherules of *C. immitis* were seen in 54, culture was positive in only 5 of the 52 instances in which it was performed.[269]

Culture of the organism is not difficult; however, proper methods are important to prevent laboratory acquisition of the disease, for which there is a significant risk. Although positive urine culture provides evidence of dissemination, such a finding does not invariably indicate clinically significant disease; in one study in which 7 of 29 patients had positive urine cultures, more than half manifested no other evidence of extrathoracic spread, and two underwent spontaneous cure of their illness.[270]

Hematology

The hemoglobin value is decreased in many patients who have disseminated disease. The white cell count is normal or moderately elevated in most patients, often with a significant degree of eosinophilia,[271] particularly in those with erythema nodosum.

Serology and Skin Tests

IgM antibodies against *C. immitis* have been measured with three serologic tests: tube precipitation (TP), latex particle agglutination (LPA), and immunodiffusion (ID) using heated coccidioidin (IDTP). All three are invaluable tests for screening sera, becoming positive 1 to 3 weeks after exposure; the LPA test is more sensitive but less specific than TP, and neither provides positive results in cerebrospinal fluid of patients with meningitis.[177] Because of ease of performance, the ID test is probably more widely used.

IgG can be detected using CF, LA, ID, and radioimmunoassay tests.[272] An enzyme-linked immunosorbent assay (ELISA) that gives results comparable to these methods has also been developed.[273, 274] The CF test is costly and time-consuming; it is also unreliable for comparing results from different laboratories because of variations in the techniques employed.[177] It becomes positive in serum some 3 weeks or more after exposure, but in a large percentage of patients with primary infection in whom precipitin reactions are positive, the CF test never becomes positive.[161] The CF reaction becomes positive in the cerebrospinal fluid in most patients who develop meningitis and is diagnostic of dissemination; seropositivity occurs in 50% of patients within 4 weeks and in 90% within 8 weeks.[179] Serum CF titers sustained above 1:16 to 1:32 are unusual in uncomplicated primary coccidioidomycosis and indicate a high risk for progressive primary or hematogenously disseminated infection.[179] A modified test using a coccidioidal CF antigen that was cloned and affinity purified has shown some promise (sensitivity of 97% and specificity of 100% when evaluated with sera from 43 infected patients).[275] The LA test is useful in detecting early disease; however, a false-positive rate of about 5% has been reported, and it is recommended that the reaction be confirmed by ID testing.[10]

Skin testing can be done with either spherulin (antigen prepared from the sporangium of *C. immitis*) or coccidioidin (antigen from mycelial filtrate), the former being the more sensitive.[276–278] One-tenth milliliter of a 1:100 solution, is used, and the reaction is read at 24 and 48 hours. In the relatively benign nondisseminated form of disease, the skin test is positive in virtually all patients within 3 weeks of the onset of infection; it may revert to negative within 2 years, but can remain positive for as long as 10 years. Patients with disseminated disease are often anergic, and the skin test reaction may be negative. A combination of a negative skin test and a CF titer greater than 1:16 is practically pathognomonic of disseminated disease.

NORTH AMERICAN BLASTOMYCOSIS

North American blastomycosis is caused by the dimorphic fungus *Blastomyces dermatitidis*, an organism that occurs as a mycelium in culture and presumably in its natural habitat and as a yeast at 37° C.[279, 280] In the latter form, it reproduces by buds that show a characteristic broad-necked attachment to the parent cell. In tissue, the yeasts are round or oval in shape and possess thick walls that have a diameter that ranges from 2 to 30 μm (commonly 8 to 15 μm) (Fig. 28–23).[17] Intracellular nuclei of the larger forms frequently stain with hematoxylin, permitting identification of the fungus on routine histologic preparations in many cases.

Epidemiology

The term *North American blastomycosis* is actually a misnomer because the disease is considered to be endemic to several regions of Africa,[281, 282] and a number of cases have been reported from Central and South America. Nevertheless, the disease occurs most commonly in the Western Hemisphere, mainly the central and southeastern United States (where endemic areas include the Ohio, Mississippi, and Missouri river valleys [particularly in Wisconsin])[284–286] and southern Canada (principally Quebec, Ontario, and Manitoba).[283, 287, 288]

The relative lack of sensitivity and specificity of skin tests and serology in the detection *B. dermatitidis* has hampered determination of the incidence of the infection. There is evidence from *in vitro* lymphocyte studies that the likelihood of developing subclinical infection is significantly greater than that of contracting symptomatic disease.[289] Judging by the number of patients detected and the brevity of the period of exposure in several recognized miniepidemics, it appears that the risk of symptomatic disease is high compared with that associated with *H. capsulatum* or *C. immitis*.[290–293] Despite this, there is little doubt that symptomatic blastomycosis is much less common than clinically detected histoplasmosis or coccidioidomycosis. In Wisconsin, where the disease is a reportable condition, 670 cases were identified between 1986 and 1995 (mean annual incidence of 1.4 per 100,000).[294] Men are most commonly affected, the male predominance being 3:2 in Wisconsin between 1986 and 1990[294] and varying from about 5:1 to 15:1 in different series.[284, 295, 296] Most patients are middle-aged (mean age in the Wisconsin data, 46 years). Although the disease is uncommon in children, a 1979 review of the literature documented 110 cases in patients under the age of 20 years.[297] There appears to be no racial predominance.[295]

Reports of individual patients and of clusters of cases clearly implicate wooded areas as a source of many infections.[290–293, 298] It is possible that the male predominance in these cases is at least partly attributable to the fact that hunters are usually men; additional support for this hypothesis is provided by the tendency for hunting dogs to acquire the disease.[299] *B. dermatitidis* can be found in soil, although it is fastidious with respect to its growth in this substance;[279] most isolations have been from samples with a high organic content and a restricted pH range.[290] Despite these observations, some cases of disease occur in urban settings without an obvious association with wooded country.[300]

Acquisition of the infection is believed to be by inhalation of airborne spores. Laboratory workers also may acquire the disease by this route,[301] although infection in this population appears to be more common by direct inoculation through the skin.[302] Accidental inoculation can result in disseminated disease in immunocompromised individuals.[303] There is evidence that occasional cases develop by reactivation of endogenous organisms acquired during a primary infection.[304]

The disease involves the genitourinary tract in up to 20% of cases, and organisms may be seen in urine and genitourinary secretions;[305] several instances of sexually transmitted disease have been reported.[305, 306] Apart from these examples, person-to-person transmission is not known to occur. The disease is as common in dogs as in humans;[295] however, with the exception of one case report of a human acquiring the disease after a dog bite,[307] there is no evidence of transmission from one to the other.[308] Nevertheless, the diagnosis of blastomycosis in dogs has been made at the same time as that in human patients, sometimes providing the first clue to the nature of the infecting agent and presumably reflecting a common source of exposure.[299]

Most reported cases of blastomycosis have been in otherwise healthy individuals, indicating that it acts as a primary pathogen.[279] Nevertheless, underlying illness,[284, 309] particularly immunodeficiency,[310–313] is clearly associated with an increased risk of the disease. There is evidence that the proportion of such cases may be increasing.[314] Corticosteroid therapy has also been identified as a risk factor.[279, 315, 316] In one series, the clinical presentation was found to be similar in immunocompromised hosts and individuals with

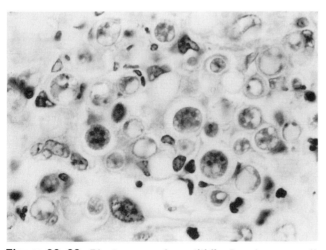

Figure 28–23. *Blastomyces dermatitidis.* Organisms are easily identifiable with hematoxylin and eosin stain and show well-developed capsules and, in some, prominent nuclear material. (×1000.)

normal host defenses;[310] in other studies, disseminated and aggressive disease has been found to be more likely in immunodeficient patients.[314, 316–318]

Pathogenesis

As might be expected from the previous discussion, cell-mediated immunity has an important role in preventing the development of blastomycosis. Based on T-cell ratios in blood and BAL fluid, the results *in vitro* studies indicate impairment of T-cell helper activity at the time of infection;[319, 320] recovery after therapy reflects the development of specific immunity. *In vitro* transformation of lymphocytes in response to blastomycin has been reported to be a sensitive procedure in the diagnosis of acute blastomycosis.[290, 321] There is evidence that such transformation may be related

to the presence of the WI-1 cell wall antigen.[322] It is also likely that neutrophils have a role to play in killing the organism, at least in some strains.[323]

Pathologic Characteristics

The gross appearance of acute blastomycosis is usually that of bronchopneumonia. The initial exudative inflammatory reaction is followed rapidly by a mononuclear cell infiltrate and, in many instances, by granuloma formation. As in coccidioidomycosis, both suppurative and granulomatous forms of inflammation frequently coexist, although in individual cases either may be the exclusive or predominant type (Fig. 28–24).[324, 325] The relative proportion of each pattern is quite variable, both among individual patients and at different sites in the same patient at the same time.[326]

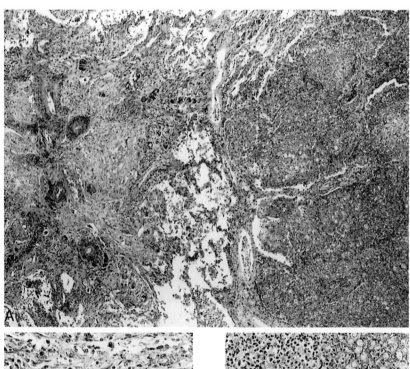

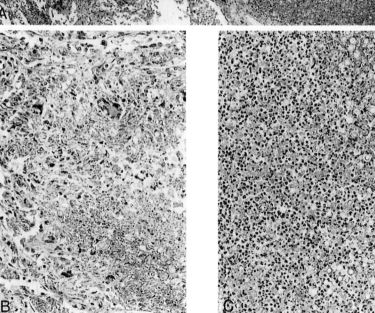

Figure 28–24. North American Blastomycosis. Extensive parenchymal inflammation *(A)* showing a granulomatous reaction on the left (seen at higher magnification in *B*) and a necrotizing suppurative one on the right (illustrated in *C*). Fungi are more easily identified in the latter site. (*A*, ×40; *B* and *C*, ×180.)

Organisms tend to be more abundant in areas of suppurative inflammation. Granulomas are usually composed of epithelioid and multinucleated giant cells surrounding a focus of suppurative necrosis; non-necrotizing granulomas are less common, and caseation necrosis is rare.

Progression of disease is manifested initially by coalescence of separate areas of pneumonia and, eventually, by perforation of an airway; resultant drainage of liquefied, necrotic material leads to cavity formation.[327] Airway involvement in the form of ulcerative bronchitis is fairly common,[324] being observed in 13 of 37 patients in one study in which airways were not specifically selected for examination.[327] Tracheal involvement has been documented rarely.[328] In one unusual case, the organism caused recurrent airway obstruction at a tracheostomy site.[329] Fibrotic or calcified parenchymal nodules representing foci of healed infection are found infrequently.

The organisms are usually easily identifiable with H & E stain and characteristically have intracellular nuclei and a single broad-based bud.[17] Small forms can be confused with *H. capsulatum* and larger forms with *C. neoformans* and *C. immitis*.[330] Hyphae are rarely seen in tissue or sputum samples.[315, 331] Some organisms are acid-fast.[81]

Radiologic Manifestations

The radiographic findings are nonspecific.[284, 332] The most common pattern—reported in 25% to 75% of patients—is one of acute air-space consolidation.[333–335] This may be patchy or confluent and subsegmental, segmental, or nonsegmental (Fig. 28–25).[284, 285, 335–337] In adults, the upper lobes are affected more frequently than the lower lobes in a ratio of approximately 2:1;[284, 337, 338] however, in one review of the radiographic findings in 18 children, consolidation most commonly involved the lower lobes.[339] The next most common radiographic presentation—seen in up to 30% of cases[334]—is a mass, either single or multiple;[290, 338, 340] when solitary, it can mimic primary carcinoma, especially when associated with unilateral lymph node enlargement or bone destruction.[341, 342] Cavitation occurs in approximately 15% to 20% of cases.[284, 285, 337, 338] Interstitial nodular or micronodular disease is uncommon.[290, 338, 340] Overwhelming infection (Fig. 28–26) is usually accompanied by a radiographic pattern of miliary dissemination[317, 343] and can be associated with the adult respiratory distress syndrome.[318, 344, 345] One case has been reported in which there was right middle lobe syndrome.[346]

Hilar and mediastinal lymph node enlargement is uncommon, even on CT.[347] Pleural effusion has been identified on chest radiographs in 10% to 15% of cases and is almost invariably associated with parenchymal disease.[337, 348] Pleural thickening without free effusion is a more common radiographic finding.[349] Radiographic evidence of calcification of parenchymal lesions or lymph nodes is extremely rare.[338, 340] Osteolytic lesions in the thoracic skeleton usually are associated with superficial abscesses.[284] Occasionally, mediastinal involvement leads to superior vena cava obstruction or brachial plexopathy.[350]

The CT findings of pulmonary blastomycosis have been described in a review of 16 patients.[347] The most common abnormalities were a localized mass (seen in 14 [88%]

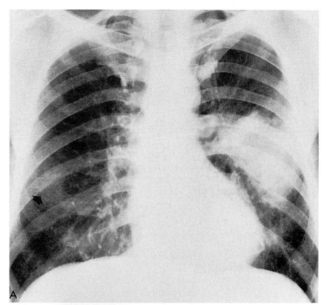

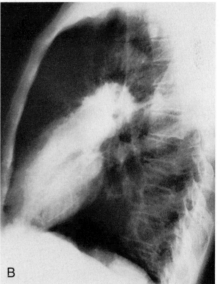

Figure 28–25. North American Blastomycosis. This 55-year-old male immigrant was well until 2 months before admission, at which time he developed an abrupt onset of pleuritic pain in the left side of the chest. He had experienced a 9-kg weight loss during the previous year. One month before admission, a right lower molar tooth had been extracted, followed by the development of swelling below the right eye. Two weeks before admission, he developed a painful swelling of the right side of the chest in the anterior axillary line. On admission, posteroanterior (PA) *(A)* and lateral *(B)* chest radiographs demonstrated a large, poorly defined shadow of homogeneous density in the lingula; the consolidation is nonsegmental and shows no evidence of an air bronchogram. In addition, the PA radiograph reveals destruction of the anterior portion of the right fifth rib *(arrow)*. *Blastomyces dermatitidis* was cultured from a 24-hour sputum collection, from pus aspirated from the swelling under the right eye, and from fluid aspirated from the swelling over the right fifth rib.

patients) and consolidation (in 9 [56%]). The masses ranged from 3 to 16 cm in diameter (mean, 8 cm), and most (12 of 14 [86%]) contained air bronchograms. In 11 patients, the abnormalities were unilateral, and in 5 they involved both lungs. There was no lobar predominance. Cavitation was seen in two patients, calcified hilar nodes in seven (44%), and enlarged noncalcified nodes in one.

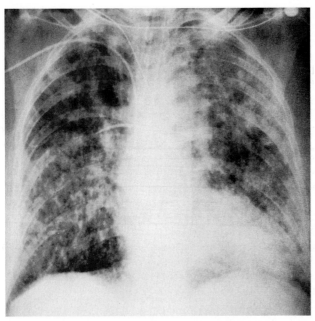

Figure 28–26. Disseminated Pulmonary Blastomycosis. A chest radiograph in anteroposterior projection, supine position, reveals widespread disease of both lungs in a pattern suggesting patchy air-space consolidation and interstitial disease. *B. dermatitidis* was recovered from the sputum. The patient was a 62-year-old woman. (Courtesy of St. Boniface Hospital, Winnipeg.)

Clinical Manifestations

Although infection in miniepidemics may be associated with flu-like symptoms only, it is more commonly manifested by symptoms of acute pneumonia, including the abrupt onset of fever, chills, productive cough, and pleuritic chest pain.[290–293] Arthralgias and myalgias are not uncommon, and erythema nodosum develops occasionally.[279, 351] Crackles and rhonchi may be heard in some patients, but signs of parenchymal consolidation are seldom apparent.[296]

Pulmonary disease may be rapidly progressive and complicated by miliary spread, the adult respiratory distress syndrome, or both.[345, 352] A more indolent variant resembling tuberculosis sometimes follows the initial pulmonary infection and is occasionally the first manifestation.[353] Such disease can remain confined to the lungs or can spread locally in the thorax or elsewhere.[345, 355] Uncommonly, the initial presentation is related to an extrapulmonary site; in one account of three such patients, episodes of pneumonia had occurred 33, 32, and 4 months earlier, and re-examination of postbronchoscopy sputum specimens revealed *B. dermatitidis* in all three.[351] Fibrosing mediastinitis has also been reported.[356]

Dissemination most commonly occurs to skin, bone, and the genitourinary tract. Bone lesions develop in about 25% of sporadic cases,[252, 284] sometimes by direct extension from the pleura to the ribs.[296, 357] Involvement of the vertebrae can lead to spinal cord compression.[354] Skin lesions are as common as those in the lung and tend to resemble neoplasms, both clinicaly and pathologically, as a result of prominent epidermal hyperplasia;[284, 285] a similar hyperplastic epithelial reaction was documented in one case of tracheal disease.[329] Chronic draining sinuses may develop into the

subcutaneous tissue.[298] The genitourinary system is involved in about 10% of male patients.[285] Other rare sites of involvement include the eye,[358] paranasal sinuses,[359] peritoneum,[360] and larynx.[361]

Although overwhelming pulmonary infection is serious and can lead to respiratory failure and death, there is evidence that prompt diagnosis and intensive antifungal therapy can result in recovery with preservation of good respiratory funcion.[345] The case fatality rate in the patients reported to the Wisconsin Department of Health between 1986 and 1995 was 4.3% (29 of 670 patients).[294] As might be expected, the disease appears to be more aggressive in the immunocompromised; in one series of such patients, the mortality rate was about 30%.[314]

Laboratory Findings

Mycology

B. dermatitidis can be identified by microscopic examination of sputum or of secretions obtained from dermal, subcutaneous, or other lesions after digestion in 10% potassium hydroxide.[90, 279] Organisms may also be seen in Papanicolaou-stained specimens submitted for cytologic study;[362–364] perhaps because of the frequency of airway involvement, they are particularly likely to be identified in sputum specimens.[362] Growth may take from 1 to several weeks.

Hematology

The leukocyte count is normal or only moderately raised in most patients,[284, 348] but may exceed 30,000/mm³ when disease is extensive.[309] Anemia may develop in patients who have chronic disease.[284]

Serology and Skin Tests

Skin tests, using either mycelial or yeast antigens, have no practical value in diagnosis.[161, 284] Standard serologic tests include a CF test, a double ID assay,[365] an enzyme immunoassay,[366] and a radioimmunoassay.[367] Although positive results support the diagnosis in the appropriate situation, the low sensitivity (varying from about 40% to 85%[10]) and cross-reactivity with other fungi (particularly *H. capsulatum*)[24] significantly limit their usefulness. The use of the antigen WI-1, a protein found in the outer wall of the organism, may prove to be more useful.[367] An immunoblot test using another cell wall antigen also shows some promise.[367a]

SOUTH AMERICAN BLASTOMYCOSIS

South American blastomycosis (paracoccidioidomycosis) is caused by the dimorphic fungus *Paracoccidioides brasiliensis*. The organism grows as a mycelium at 30°C; however, both in culture at 37°C and in tissue, yeasts are predominant. The latter are round to oval in shape and quite variable in diameter, ranging from 2 or 3 μm for recently separated buds up to 30 μm (and occasionally 60 μm) for mature mother cells. Characteristically, reproduction is by multiple, narrow-necked buds that appear around the perimeter of the mother cells (*pilot wheel* arrangement).[371]

Epidemiology

The disease is found principally in South and Central America, most commonly in Brazil, Colombia, Venezuela, Peru, Ecuador, and Paraguay. Patients whose disease is recognized in North America or Europe have invariably had prior travel to endemic areas.[368–370] Clinical disease shows a striking male predominance, the reported male-to-female incidence ranging from 12:1 to 27:1;[371] in three series of 142 patients, 140 were male.[372–374] This remarkable male predominance of disease is in sharp contrast to the results of epidemiologic studies in which testing with paracoccidioidin antigen has revealed a 50:50 distribution between the sexes.[90] Although the reasons for this discrepancy are unclear, it is possible that it is the result of a larger exposure dose in men than in women. Disease is seen most commonly in individuals between 25 and 45 years of age.

The natural habitat of the organism is believed to be the soil, from which it has occasionally been recovered.[375] This hypothesis is supported by the observation that farmers, manual laborers, and other workers engaged in rural occupations are particularly susceptible to the disease.[371, 374, 376] Despite this observation, many cases have been reported in city dwellers who have not had obvious contact with soil.[368]

Although it was formerly thought that the disease was initially acquired via the oropharynx or gastrointestinal tract, the results clinical,[374] experimental,[377] and pathologic[373] studies have shown that the majority of infections are probably acquired by inhalation, resulting in primary pneumonia and secondary systemic dissemination. It is perhaps not surprising that occasional cases of oropharyngeal or visceral disease are recognized in the absence of clinical or radiographic evidence of pulmonary involvement; as in other visceral mycoses, this presumably represents slow progression or reactivation of extrapulmonary disease that has originated from pulmonary foci that have healed.[378] Animal-to-human and person-to-person transmission have not been documented. Despite this, the incidence of dermal sensitivity to paracoccidioidin is higher in households of patients with proven South American blastomycosis than in control subjects;[379] it has been suggested that this may be related to common exposure (possibly to the microenvironment of the infected individual himself).[379]

Pathogenesis

As in most other mycotic infections, experimental evidence indicates that the major mechanism of host defense in South American blastomycosis is cell-mediated immunity. Some patients have depression of delayed skin hypersensitivity and of *in vitro* tests of cell-mediated immunity, which return to normal with clinical improvement after treatment. Healthy mice survive intraperitoneal and intratracheal injection of the yeast form of *P. brasiliensis*, although athymic mice die; in the latter animals, thymic transplant heightens resistance.[380]

Pathologic Characteristics

Pathologically, pulmonary South American blastomycosis can take a variety of forms:[371–373] (1) multiple smooth or lobulated nodules that may become confluent and resemble fibrocaseous tuberculosis, with or without cavitation; (2) solitary paracoccidioidomas; (3) occasionally, rapidly progressive necrosis and inflammation similar to acute bacterial pneumonia, usually in patients receiving corticosteroid[371] or immunosuppressive[381] therapy; (4) interstitial fibrosis, occasionally complicated by cor pulmonale and usually unassociated with either nodules or cavities; and (5) miliary nodules representing hematogenous spread. Histologic findings consist of a combination of granulomatous and exudative inflammation. Granulomas vary considerably in appearance, from non-necrotic forms that resemble those seen in sarcoidosis to those with central necrosis similar to that of North American blastomycosis or tuberculosis.[371]

Organisms can be seen with H & E stain, but are usually identified in greater numbers with silver preparations. Mature yeast forms may appear empty or may contain a contracted protoplasmic body; pseudohyphae, representing elongated mature yeasts, may be identified.[17] The presence of multiple, narrow-necked buds is required for confident identification. Small forms can be confused with *H. capsulatum*, medium-sized forms with *C. neoformans* and *B. dermatitidis*, and large forms with *C. immitis*.[17]

Radiologic Manifestations

The radiographic patterns of pulmonary disease are indistinguishable from those of other mycotic infections. In the primary form of the disease, transient air-space opacities may appear in midlung zones.[90] In immunosuppressed patients, an acute progressive pneumonia may develop whose course is sometimes fulminant and fatal. Paracoccidioidomas—single or multiple, solid or cavitary—represent a more benign but sometimes persistent abnormality.[302, 303] Progressive pulmonary paracoccidioidomycosis is perhaps the most commonly recognized form of disease.[384, 385] Although this variety is sometimes confused with tuberculosis, the lower lobes are more frequently involved than the upper, and cavitation is less commonly seen radiographically (Fig. 28–27).[90] Hilar lymph node enlargement can occur by itself or in association with any form of pulmonary disease (Fig. 28–28).

Clinical Manifestations

The results of skin test studies indicate that infection is often asymptomatic or associated with mild, nonspecific complaints;[379, 386] support for this observation has been provided by the occasional incidental finding of an inactive focus of disease at autopsy.[378] Most clinically important disease occurs in patients in whom dissemination has occurred, typically to the skin or oral or nasal mucosa. In one series of 41 laborers, 29 had ulcers, either in the mouth or (occasionally) on the skin;[376] 28 of these had pulmonary involvement. Symptoms and physical signs were scanty,

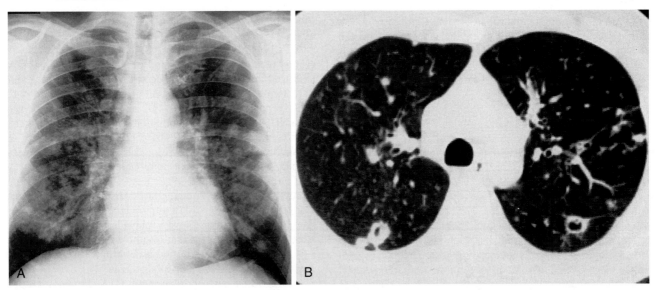

Figure 28–27. South American Blastomycosis. A 52-year-old man presented with fever and severe headache. He had no respiratory symptoms. CT demonstrated intracerebral granulomas. An admission posteroanterior chest radiograph *(A)* shows numerous bilateral nodules measuring 0.5 to 2 cm in diameter as well as paratracheal and right hilar lymphadenopathy. CT scan *(B)* demonstrates that some of the nodules are cavitated. Fine-needle aspiration biopsy of one of the nodules demonstrated *Paracoccidioide brasiliensis.* (Case courtesy of Dr. Arthur Soares Souza, Jr, Instituto de Radiodiagnostico Rio Preto, Sao Paulo, Brazil.)

and pulmonary disease was not generally suspected. In the remaining 12 patients, the disease was restricted to the lung.

Dissemination also occurs not uncommonly to the regional lymph nodes and liver and spleen, sometimes resulting in hepatosplenomegaly or cervical lymphadenopathy; less often, other organs, such as the adrenal glands, central nervous system, and intestine, are affected.[90] Clinically sig-

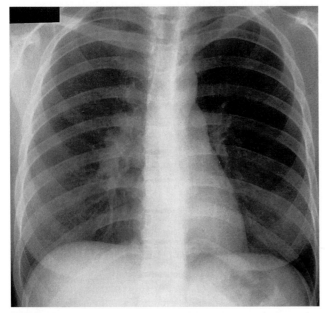

Figure 28–28. South American Blastomycosis. A 28-year-old woman presented with epigastric pain and weakness. She had had cervical lymphadenopathy for 3 years but no respiratory symptoms. A chest radiograph demonstrates right hilar lymphadenopathy. A diagnosis of South American blastomycosis was confirmed by biopsy of a cervical lymph node. (Case courtesy of Dr. Arthur Soares Souza, Jr, Instituto de Radiodiagnostico Rio Preto, Sao Paulo, Brazil.)

nificant pulmonary infection is present in 80% to 90% of patients who have chronic disseminated disease.[371]

Laboratory Findings

The organism can be identified in sputum or contaminated secretions after digestion with 10% potassium hydroxide. Microscopic examination of smears of oral ulcers has been found by some investigators to be particularly helpful in diagnosis.[387] Although useful in epidemiologic studies, the skin test is of limited value in a specific case. Of greater importance are serologic tests, of which the CF and ID tests are both sensitve and specific.

CRYPTOCOCCOSIS

In the vast majority of cases, cryptococcosis is caused by *C. neoformans,* a unimorphic fungus that exists in yeast form both in its natural habitat and in animals and humans. Although rather pleomorphic, the organisms are usually round to oval in shape and from 2 to 20 μm in diameter in tissue (most commonly, 5 to 10 μm). The majority of strains possess a well-defined capsule that becomes visible as a pericellular halo with India ink preparations and standard tissue mucin stains. Reproduction is by formation of a bud that characteristically is solitary and possesses a narrow base.

Two varieties of the organism—*C. neoformans* var. *neoformans* and *C. neoformans* var. *gattii*—have been described.[388] Rare cases of cryptococcosis caused by *Cryptococcus albidus* have been reported in an otherwise healthy individual[389] and in a patient with chronic renal failure.[390] A case caused by *Cryptococcus laurentii* has also been documented in a patient with dermatomyositis who was receiving corticosteroid therapy.[391]

Epidemiology

Although cryptococcosis is found throughout the world, there is evidence that the two varieties *C. neoformans* var. *neoformans* and *C. neoformans* var. *gattii* may have different sources and epidemiologic characteristics, the latter having been identified predominantly in tropical regions.[388] In one investigation, disease caused by *C. neoformans* var. *gattii* was seen almost exclusively in young, otherwise healthy individuals, suggesting a pattern of endogenous infection similar to that of histoplasmosis or coccidioidomycosis.[388]

Although *C. neoformans* var. *neoformans* has been found in a variety of environmental sites, the most important natural habitat is dried pigeon excreta, from which it has been isolated in many locations throughout the world.[392] In one study, cultures from a vacant tower yielded 10 million cells of *C. neoformans* per gram of pigeon droppings;[393] the undisturbed air in the tower contained an average of 45 cells per 100 liters of air, and it was estimated that exposure of a person to this air for 1 hour would result in the deposition of approximately 40 cells within the lung.

Despite the association of the organism with pigeon droppings, repeated exposure to pigeons has uncommonly been found to be associated with an increased risk of cryptococcosis.[394, 395] In one survey of cryptococcal infections in southern California, 25 of 49 were associated with serotypes B and C; however, in no case was serotype B and in only two instances was serotype C isolated from local samples of pigeon excreta, so that the source of infection in these cases was undetermined.[396] The author of this report also noted regional differences in infection by different strains, most cases in the United States (except southern California) being caused by serotype A and most in Denmark and Italy by serotype D. There is no evidence of transmission from animal-to-human or person-to-person. The disease can affect persons of any age and either sex; however, some workers have documented a male predominance[397] and a peak incidence in middle age.[388]

Although *C. neoformans* can cause pulmonary or disseminated disease in otherwise normal individuals, it is seen most frequently as an opportunistic invader in compromised hosts, particularly patients with AIDS or lymphoma (especially Hodgkin's disease);[398–401] patients with chronic pulmonary disease also have an increased risk.[402–405] An unusual degree of susceptibility appears to be associated with corticosteroid therapy;[398, 406–408] in rare instances, increased cortisol levels have been caused by Cushing's syndrome.[409, 410]

Pathogenesis

Although usually found in tissues as an encapsulated organism measuring 5 to 10 μm in diameter, such forms have been observed infrequently in nature,[411] and there is evidence that many naturally occurring organisms are considerably smaller than this; for example, in one study conducted in a contaminated tower, 60% of airborne cells were less than 4.7 μm in diameter.[393] In addition, when organisms are experimentally inoculated into soil, they rapidly lose their capsules and decrease in size to an average of 3 μm in diameter.[412]

These observations have two important implications. First, the small size of naturally occurring organisms is appropriate for the production of disease by inhalation, a feature that would be less likely to occur with larger forms. Second, it has been shown that the cryptococcal capsule is capable of reducing neutrophil phagocytosis to an appreciable extent and that virulence can be correlated with the presence of capsular material.[413] Encapsulation has been shown to occur when capsule-deficient forms are incubated with human lung tissue in vitro.[412] On the basis of these findings, it has been suggested that inhaled capsule-deficient forms are normally rapidly destroyed by host leukocytes, resulting in no infection. In cases in which leukocyte or macrophage function is impaired, there may be sufficient time for encapsulated forms to be produced locally; because these are more resistant to phagocytosis, proliferation and disease ensue. Because cryptococcosis is occasionally caused by capsule-deficient forms,[414–416] however, it is likely that other considerations, such as inoculum size or unidentified virulence factors, are also important in pathogenesis.

Pathologic Characteristics

Grossly, pulmonary cryptococcosis can have several forms:[392, 398]

1. Relatively well-defined, solitary or multiple nodules that may be solid and rubbery or necrotic and occasionally cavitated. Some nodules have a mucoid or gelatinous appearance caused by the presence of large numbers of heavily encapsulated organisms.[392] Well-developed primary complexes similar to those seen in tuberculosis or histoplasmosis are uncommon;[417] however, they are rarely a source for endogenous reinfection.

2. Ill-defined areas of parenchymal consolidation that may involve part or all of the lobe. Similar to the nodular form, these can possess a gelatinous appearance that can be confused with mucin-secreting bronchioloalveolar carcinoma or pneumococcal pneumonia.

3. Widely disseminated parenchymal nodules measuring 1 to 2 mm, representing miliary hematogenous spread.

4. In immunocompromised patients, particularly those with AIDS, predominantly interstitial proliferation of organisms accompanied by minimal cellular inflammation and no granuloma formation.[401]

As with other fungal infections, the inflammatory reaction to *Cryptococcus* is quite variable (Fig. 28–29).[392, 398, 418, 419] The gelatinous forms described previously are composed of numerous heavily encapsulated organisms that appear to spread within alveolar spaces with minimal cellular reaction. Although clusters of organisms may be necrotic, tissue necrosis usually is absent. In other cases, there is granulomatous inflammation, consisting mostly of poorly organized aggregates of epithelioid cells and multinucleated giant cells; well-defined granulomas, with or without necrosis, are usually sparse. Still other lesions are characterized by a predominantly polymorphonuclear infiltrate, sometimes with microabscess formation. Occasionally, organisms are confined mostly or entirely to alveolar capillaries, with or without infiltration of the adjacent interstitium.[398]

The organisms stain poorly but are recognizable with H & E; they are best identified with Grocott's methenamine

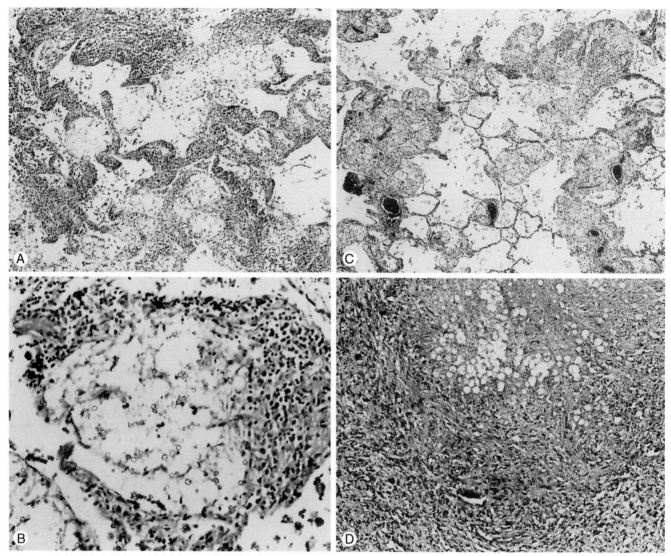

Figure 28–29. Cryptococcosis—Variable Inflammatory Reaction. In *A,* intra-alveolar clusters (seen in magnified view in *B*) of *Cryptococcus neoformans* are surrounded by thickened alveolar septa containing a mononuclear inflammatory infiltrate. Similar clusters *(C)* from another patient are associated with virtual absence of host reaction. A section from a hilar lymph node *(D)* in a third patient shows granulomatous inflammation. (*A,* ×46; *B,* ×200; *C,* ×40; *D,* ×100.)

silver, PAS, or mucicarmine stains (Fig. 28–30). The last-named is taken up by the capsule and is specific for *Cryptococcus*; however, well-developed capsules are not present in all organisms. Cases of infection with capsule-deficient strains have occasionally been confused with histoplasmosis and North American blastomycosis.[414–416]

Radiologic Manifestations

The most common radiographic manifestation of cryptococcal infection consists of single or multiple nodules, usually subpleural in location and ranging from 0.5 to 4 cm in diameter.[420–422] An alternative presentation is in the form of a localized area of less well-defined air-space consolidation,[420–423] segmental or nonsegmental in distribution but usually confined to one lobe (Fig. 28–31). Cavitation is relatively uncommon compared with its incidence in other mycoses (Fig. 28–32); it was observed in 16 of 101 cases in one series[397] and in 3 of 26 in another.[405]

These findings are less frequently seen in patients with AIDS, in whom the most common manifestation is perihilar or diffuse nodular or reticulonodular interstitial infiltrates.[424, 425] Similar widely disseminated disease can also occur in patients without AIDS and gives rise to a miliary pattern or to multiple, diffuse, ill-defined opacities.[405, 426] Calcification is extremely rare.[427] Hilar and mediastinal lymph node enlargement is unusual (Fig. 28–33), but may be massive.[427] Pleural effusion is uncommon and usually connotes dissemination of the organism in a patient with underlying disease.[428–430] As with other infectious diseases, fulminating cryptococcosis may be associated with the adult respiratory distress syndrome.[406, 431]

Several authors have commented on the ability of pulmonary cryptococcosis to mimic primary pulmonary carcinoma.[404, 432, 433] Most often, this occurs as a well-circumscribed mass; occasionally, it appears as lobar or segmental consolidation with loss of volume as a result of bronchial occlusion. In such cases, concomitant fungal involvement of

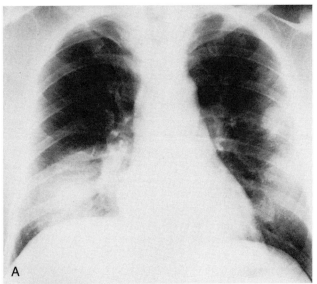
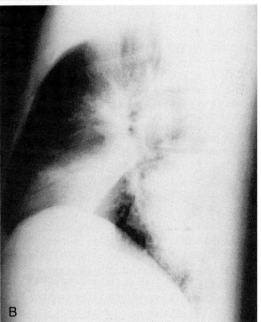

Figure 28–31. Acute Cryptococcal Pneumonia. Posteroanterior *(A)* and lateral *(B)* radiographs reveal nonsegmental homogeneous consolidation of both lower lobes and the right middle lobe. *C. neoformans* was recovered from the sputum.

the central nervous system is easily mistaken for metastatic disease. The CT findings of cryptococcal pneumonia, similar to those on radiography, are nonspecific, the diagnosis seldom being suspected radiologically.[434]

Clinical Manifestations

Most patients who acquire cryptococcosis are immunocompromised; in the non-AIDS population, about 20% to 30% are otherwise healthy.[399, 420] In the latter individuals, disease is usually confined to the lungs. In immunocompromised patients, dissemination is common and usually occurs weeks to months after the onset of pneumonia; few patients survive without fungicidal therapy.[431]

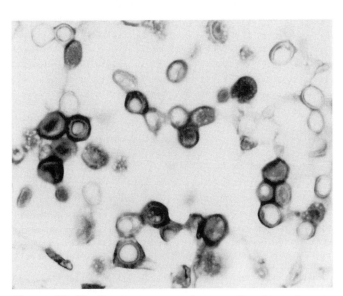

Figure 28–30. *Cryptococcus neoformans.* Round-to-oval yeasts with thick, darkly staining capsules. (Mucicarmine, ×1000.)

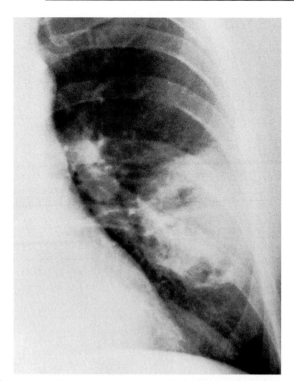

Figure 28–32. Pulmonary Cryptococcosis. A view of the left hemithorax from a posteroanterior radiograph demonstrates a well-circumscribed mass situated in the axillary portion of the left lower lobe; its lateral aspect abuts against the visceral pleura. Several irregular areas of radiolucency are present throughout the mass, representing multiple foci of cavitation. *C. neoformans* was cultured from the sputum.

The initial lung infection often does not result in symptoms and is probably recognized infrequently.[388] When disease confined to the lungs causes symptoms, these are usually mild and include cough, scanty mucoid or (rarely) bloody sputum, chest pain, and low-grade fever.[388, 397, 403] A history of exposure to pigeon excreta may suggest the diagnosis; however, as indicated previously, this is uncommon. Physical examination of the chest occasionally reveals crackles and rhonchi but seldom signs of consolidation.

The organism has a particular affinity for the central nervous system, a common clinical presentation being low-grade meningitis. Less frequently, the neurologic picture is of an expanding intracranial lesion[426] or a psychiatric problem.[434] Although the lung is almost invariably the portal of entry in these cases, there is little doubt that the pulmonary lesion can resolve even in the presence of dissemination,[90, 399] and in immunocompromised patients.[400] Dissemination also occurs to the skin (causing acneiform lesions), bones (typically resulting in osteolytic lesions), and, less commonly, the viscera;[407, 436] spread to lymph nodes, liver, and spleen may produce a clinical picture simulating sarcoidosis.[437]

Laboratory Findings

Mycology

The organism can be identifed by the presence of a characteristic halo in specimens of sputum, cerebrospinal fluid, or urine that have been mixed with a drop of India ink and examined wet under a coverslip; as might be expected, diligent search enhances the yield of positive diagnoses.[399, 438, 439] The organism also may be seen in routinely stained sputum or other cytology specimens;[440, 441] however, as in tissue, it is better identified by mucicarmine or silver stain.

Although the organism is not a common saprophyte in humans, positive culture cannot be definitely considered to indicate disease.[439, 442] Colonization occurs most frequently in patients with chronic pulmonary disease,[439, 442, 443] including lipid pneumonia.[444] Identification on cytologic examina-

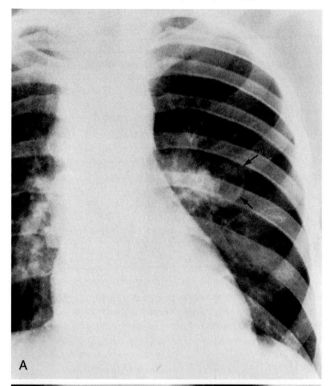

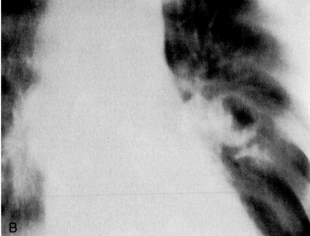

Figure 28–33. Cryptococcosis—Pulmonary and Lymph Node Involvement. Selected views from a posteroanterior radiograph *(A)* and an anteroposterior tomogram *(B)* demonstrate a sharply circumscribed cavity in the parahilar area of the left lung *(arrows in A)*; the wall of the cavity is fairly thick and its inner surface somewhat irregular and shaggy. An irregular nodular contour of the upper half of the mediastinum, particularly on the right, indicates enlarged mediastinal nodes. Both the cavitation and the node enlargement are unusual manifestations of the disease.

tion of deep cough specimens of sputum[445] or needle aspirates[446, 447] increases the likelihood of the organism being pathogenic, particularly when there is a radiographic opacity or cryptococcal antigenemia. Positive spinal fluid or blood culture is confirmative.[438] Cultures of lesions removed during surgery may fail to produce growth despite a characteristic appearance on tissue staining, presumably the result of nonviable organisms.[399]

Serology and Skin Tests

The various serologic tests used to detect antibody to *C. neoformans* are neither 100% specific nor sensitive; however, the CF test appears to be more sensitive than either a modified latex fixation or a slide agglutination test.[435, 448] An LA test for antigen is fairly specific, especially when controlled for the presence of rheumatoid factor,[449] although its sensitivity appears to vary considerably;[399, 449] it appears to be particularly useful in patients with AIDS[400] and meningitis.[450] Skin tests are not helpful because of cross-reactivity with other fungi.[451]

PNEUMOCYSTIS CARINII

Although *P. carinii* has historically been considered to be a protozoan, morphologic, biochemical, and genetic studies have revealed a much closer relationship with fungi,[452–455] and it is now considered by most authorities to be properly classified with these organisms.[456] *In vivo*, the organism can be identified in two forms:[457–459] (1) a thick-walled, round or crescent-shaped cyst measuring 3 to 6 μm in diameter that may contain up to eight intracystic bodies believed to represent developing trophozoites (sporozoites); the cyst wall takes up silver, rendering it visible by light microscopy and providing the basis for the diagnosis of infection in the majority of cases; and (2) extracystic trophozoites that range in diameter from 1 to 5 μm, are pleomorphic in shape, and often show pseudopod-like surface projections. It has been proposed that the life cycle of the organism begins with trophozoites, which enlarge extracellularly, become mature, and encyst (Fig. 28–34).[457] Individual cysts then undergo maturation by developing intracystic sporozoites that are eventually liberated; the collapsed cysts correspond to the crescentic forms seen by light microscopy (*see* farther on). The possibility that trophozoites can reproduce by binary fission has also been suggested.[455, 457]

Some success has been achieved growing the organism in cell cultures;[460, 461] however, routine laboratory culture methods are insufficient for diagnosis. The entire topic of *Pneumocystis* pneumonia has been the subject of several reviews;[462, 463] features particular to the infection in patients with AIDS are discussed on page 1656.

Epidemiology

Although *P. carinii* infection is common in humans,[464] it results in clinically significant pneumonia almost uniquely in individuals with underlying disease. Despite this, there is serologic evidence that some cases of "atypical" pneumonia

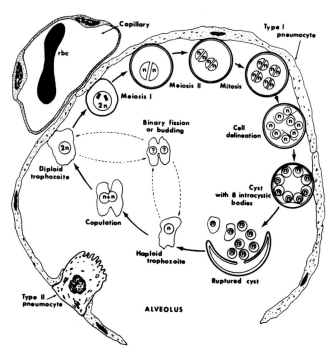

Figure 28–34. *Pneumocystis carinii*—**Hypothesized Reproductive Cycle.** Diagrammatic representation of an alveolus illustrating potential mechanisms of cyst development and organism reproduction. (From Gutierrez Y: The biology of *Pneumocystis carinii*. Semin Diagn Pathol 6:203, 1989.)

in apparently healthy individuals may be caused by the organism.[464]

Pneumonia has been described in two clinicopathologic forms: an *infantile type* that often occurs in miniepidemics and a sporadic form that occurs in immunocompromised children and adults. The former variety was originally reported in Europe during and immediately after World War II as a disease termed *interstitial plasma cell pneumonitis*. The abnormality tended to occur in epidemics, frequently in crowded nurseries harboring undernourished, marasmic infants between the ages of 2 and 5 months. With the postwar improvement in socioeconomic status, this form of disease largely disappeared from Europe; however, outbreaks have been observed more recently in Vietnam in similar circumstances.[465]

The second form of pneumocystosis occurs sporadically in children and adults whose immune status is compromised. This variety is particularly prevalent and virulent in patients with AIDS, in whom it has been estimated that at least one episode of pneumonia occurs at some point during the course of the disease in the absence of prophylaxis and antiviral therapy.[466] A second important group at risk is immunosuppressed organ transplant recipients;[467] some investigators have found the risk in this group to be related to the particular type of immunosuppression.[468] In patients with malignancy, infection is manifested most often in patients with lymphoreticular neoplasms (usually associated with concomitant cytotoxic therapy);[469–472] individuals with solid tumors (including lung carcinoma) are affected less often.[473] Pneumonia is also seen in patients with systemic vasculitis or connective tissue disorders (usually in association with corticosteroid and cytotoxic therapy),[474–477] congenital immunodeficiency diseases, and (rarely) adrenocorticotropic hormone-producing neoplasms.[478, 479] In one investigation of patients with systemic lupus erythematosus or polymyositis/dermatomyositis, risk factors in addition to corticosteroid therapy included the presence of interstitial pulmonary fibrosis and a low blood lymphocyte count.[480] A common feature associated with many of these conditions is therapy with corticosteroids.[477, 481] Symptoms or a radiographic abnormality may become apparent for the first time in patients in whom corticosteroid therapy is being reduced while other immunosuppressive therapy is being maintained;[471, 482, 483] the same sequence of events has been noted in experimental animals.[484]

P. carinii is an organism of global distribution that is found in the lungs of many animals, including the rat, mouse, rabbit, and dog. Immunologic and genetic investigations have shown that at least some of the organisms found in these animals are closely related to the agent that infects humans.[486, 487] There are significant differences between them,[488] however, and the results of some experimental studies suggest that transmission of organisms between different animal species is not possible;[489] thus, although it remains conceivable that organisms that infect animals can also infect humans (the animals serving as a natural reservoir of disease),[487] this is by no means certain. Some investigators have found that the organism that infects humans shows little genetic variation in different parts of the world.[490] Because *P. carinii* appears to be a fungus, it is possible that an environmental source of the organism may eventually be identified.

The mode of transmission has not been conclusively demonstrated; however, because of the universal presence of the organism within the lungs, it is presumed to be by inhalation. Supporting this concept are experimental studies in which infection has been transmitted to otherwise isolated rats exposed to an air supply derived from the environment of affected animals;[491, 492] it has been impossible to transmit disease with food and water.[493] Studies of health care workers have not implicated them as a source.[485] Whatever its origin, infection is undoubtedly common, as evidenced by the presence of antibodies to the organism in a high proportion of healthy individuals at an early age.[494] In one investigation of more than 400 immunocompetent individuals, the percentage of persons who had IgG antibodies to the surface antigen gp95 (as measured by ELISA) was 30 in those 1 to 9 years old and 56 in those 10 to 19 years old.[464]

The results of some serologic[495] and molecular[496] studies as well as the documentation of occasional clusters of pneumocystosis[497-499] have suggested that infection may be transmitted directly from person-to-person. Most investigators have failed to find evidence for such spread,[500, 501] however, and it is generally considered that the majority of cases of clinical disease result from reactivation of latent infection acquired previously in the life of a patient who has subsequently become immunocompromised. In support of this hypothesis are experimental studies in which isolated animals treated with corticosteroids have developed the disease;[502] in addition, clinical evidence of infection in humans appears to be related to the intensity of immunosuppression.[503, 504] Despite these observations, there is experimental evidence suggesting transmission of infection between animals,[492] and it has generally been difficult or impossible to

identify the organism in the lungs of healthy individuals;[505] as a result, there has been speculation that an exogenous source of infection may be more important than is generally believed.[495, 504, 507]

Pathogenesis

The factors involved in the transformation from a state of symbiosis to one of pathogenicity and the mechanisms by which *P. carinii* produces tissue damage and clinical disease are incompletely understood.[508, 509] It is clear, however, that alterations in host immune function are of prime importance. As indicated previously, both clinical and experimental observations indicate that immunosuppression is capable of inducing disease. This effect is most closely associated with T-cell function, particularly of CD4+ cells,[510] an observation most dramatically demonstrated in patients with AIDS. In such individuals, a CD4+ count of less than 200 cells × 10⁶/liter is not uncommonly associated with *P. carinii* pneumonia;[504, 511] moreover, there is a more or less linear relationship between the CD4+ blood count and the risk of developing the disease.[512]

Although a deficiency in CD4+ cells is the cellular abnormality most closely associated with pneumocystosis, other immune and inflammatory cells, particularly CD8+ T cells and alveolar macrophages, are also involved in the process.[510] For example, there is experimental evidence that CD8+ lymphocytes are recruited into the lung during the infection, where they provide a supportive role in defense.[513] Alveolar macrophages bind and phagocytose organisms, following which they are stimulated to release a variety of proinflammatory substances;[513a] of these, tumor necrosis factor-α appears to be particularly important.[513a, 514, 515] The effect of alveolar macrophages in defense is illustrated by animal experiments in which enhancement of their function by colony-stimulating factor was associated with a reduction in the intensity of pneumonia[516] and decrease in their number with an increased susceptibility to infection.[506] A protective role for polymorphonuclear leukocytes has also been suggested by several observations. Experimental studies in rats have shown that *Pseudomonas*-induced pulmonary leukocytosis appears to aid the prevention of *P. carinii* pneumonia.[517] In addition, there is evidence for abnormal neutrophil function in patients with AIDS who have had *Pneumocystis* pneumonia.[518] It is also possible that humoral factors play a role in pathogenesis;[509, 519] for example, in one investigation, a relative deficiency of IgG antibodies in BAL fluid was found in patients with AIDS and *P. carinii* pneumonia compared to AIDS patients without the infection.[520]

Both quantitative and qualitative abnormalities of surfactant have been documented in the BAL fluid of patients with AIDS before the development of *Pneumocystis* pneumonia,[509, 521] and it has been speculated that such alterations may be related to the saprophyte-pathogen transformation of the organism.

The precise location in the lung in which the organisms reside in the absence of disease is uncertain. In animals without evidence of disease by standard light microscopy, ultrastructural examination shows the trophozoites to be intimately associated with type I pneumocytes, apparently anchored to them via shallow cytoplasmic invaginations (Fig.

28–35).[522] Such attachment is likely mediated by a variety of substances, including fibronectin,[523] vitronectin,[524] and specific glycoproteins on the organism's surface.[525] It is possible that the components of surfactant with which the organism must be in contact in this location act to inhibit binding and phagocytosis by alveolar macrophages.[532] Experiments with animals that have active pneumonitis have also shown close apposition of trophozoites to alveolar type I cells,[526] with subsequent epithelial degeneration and necrosis.[527, 528] The results of studies with infected cell cultures have shown that attachment of the organism to epithelial cells also promotes its proliferation and inhibits growth of the epithelial cells.[526] It has also been shown that trophozoites have slender filopodia that extend to the epithelial surface and to adjacent organisms;[460, 530] although some have considered these to be attachment organs that may be related to epithelial damage, many filopodia appear to be free in the alveolar space unattached to the epithelium, and it has been suggested that they may instead be a means of increasing the absorptive surface of the organism.[530]

In most cases of active disease, the organisms are found predominantly within alveolar air spaces; they are seldom identified in the alveolar interstitium or elsewhere in the body,[533-535] suggesting limited invasive capability. The trophozoites produce no known toxins.

Pathologic Characteristics

Gross specimens of lung affected by *Pneumocystis* pneumonia are uncommonly seen in an untreated stage because the vast majority of infections are identified before they are seen by the pathologist. When untreated infection is encountered, it is usually diffuse, all lobes possessing a firm, rubbery consistency. Occasionally, disease is focal and

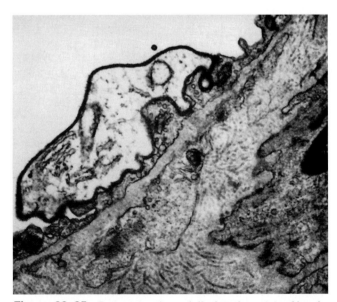

Figure 28–35. *Pneumocystis carinii*—**Attachment to Alveolar Epithelium.** A transmission electron micrograph shows a trophozoite of *P. carinii* intimately associated with a rat alveolar epithelial cell; extensive cell membrane interdigitation is evident. (From Limper AH, Thomas CF Jr, Anders RA, et al: Interactions of parasite and host epithelial cell cycle regulation during *Pneumocystis carinii* pneumonia. J Lab Clin Med 130:138, 1997.)

limited predominantly to one lobe in either a diffuse or nodular fashion;[482] the latter situation is more common in individuals with AIDS.

There is considerable variation in the type and severity of histologic changes seen in *P. carinii* infection. The organism has sometimes been seen in touch imprints of lungs that show no histologic features of infection (although the results of these studies have been questioned[506]); for example, in one investigation of 200 consecutive autopsies, 7 such cases were identified, all affected patients having recently received radiation therapy or chemotherapy for underlying malignancy.[536] These cases presumably represent an early stage of the disease in which the patient has died before appreciable pathologic changes of infection have had a chance to develop. Such early infection is rarely seen histologically as single or minute clusters of cysts intimately associated with the alveolar epithelial surface (*see* page 1721).

In the typical case of clinically evident pneumonia, histologic examination shows alveolar interstitial inflammation, proliferation of type II alveolar epithelial cells, and a finely vacuolated ("foamy"), eosinophilic intra-alveolar exudate (Fig. 28–36).[537] The latter consists of cysts and trophozoites admixed with host-derived material, including surfactant, fibrin, immunoglobulins, and adhesive matrix proteins such as fibronectin and vitronectin.[454, 529] This exudate is highly characteristic of *Pneumocystis* infection and can be identified in tissue sections and in bronchial lavage specimens stained by the Papanicolaou method;[538, 539] its presence should prompt the use of special stains or immunohistochemical techniques for definitive identification of the organism (*see* farther on). Although highly suggestive of *Pneumocystis* infection when present, the absence of exudate does not exclude the diagnosis: of 53 cases in two studies, only 27 (50%) showed this feature.[540, 541]

The alveolar interstitium typically contains a mixed infiltrate of lymphocytes and plasma cells. Sporadic infection in immunocompromised patients tends to be associated with relatively mild inflammation, predominantly lymphocytic; in patients with AIDS, such inflammation may be absent altogether. By contrast, in the epidemic infantile form of disease, an interstitial plasma cell infiltrate is usually prominent.[482]

Although the features just described are characteristic of *Pneumocystis* pneumonia, other pathologic abnormalities are found in addition or by themselves in a significant number of cases.[542, 543] One of the most common is diffuse alveolar damage (hyaline membranes, type II cell hyperplasia, alveolar air-space proteinaceous exudate, and interstitial thickening by edema fluid and mononuclear inflammatory cells).[541] Cysts tend to be less numerous in this histologic variant. In some cases, they can be identified within both alveolar exudate and hyaline membranes, implying that the reaction is a direct effect of the organisms on the tissue. In others, the hyaline membranes are free of cysts, suggesting that the diffuse alveolar damage is a secondary phenomenon analogous to adult respiratory distress syndrome that is sometimes encountered in pneumonia caused by other organisms.

Other pathologic changes that may be seen either alone or in association with the typical features include granulomatous inflammation (in which organisms may be few in number and difficult to identify in BAL fluid[544]),[545, 546] vascular

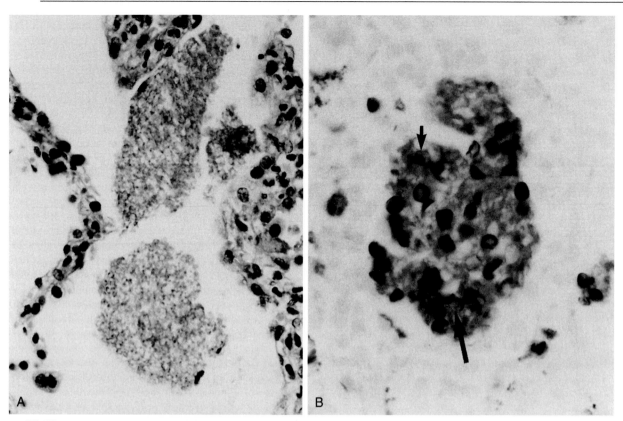

Figure 28–36. *Pneumocystis carinii* **Pneumonia.** A magnified view *(A)* of a transbronchial biopsy specimen from a 42-year-old man with AIDS shows mild interstitial thickening resulting from edema and a mononuclear inflammatory cell infiltrate; two clusters of finely vacuolated proteinaceous material are present within alveolar air spaces. Silver stain *(B)* of one of these clusters shows it to contain multiple more or less round or sickle-shaped *(long arrow)* cysts. One cyst contains a characteristic central dot *(short arrow)*, representing focal thickening of the capsule seen *en face*. *(A,* ×440; *B,* Grocott's silver methenamine, ×1000.)

invasion (sometimes with vasculitis),[547] parenchymal calcification (usually associated with prior treatment),[548] necrosis, and cyst formation.[533, 542, 549, 550] Pathologic findings in the last-named complication are variable: some cases consist of blebs and others of parenchymal cyst–like spaces lined by either a thin layer of fibrous tissue or by lung parenchyma consolidated by the foamy exudate of typical *Pneumocystis* infection. There is evidence that the pathogenesis of at least some of these lesions is related to tissue invasion by trophozoites.[533] All these atypical pathologic manifestations are more common in patients with AIDS, particularly those who have received prophylactic therapy for the infection.

Fibrosis is variable in occurrence and severity and can be present in a focal or diffuse distribution and within the alveolar interstitium, air spaces, or both.[551] It can be evident at the time of the initial diagnosis, but usually is more prominent in patients who have been treated. In one study, some degree of interstitial fibrosis was identified in biopsy specimens in 12 (33%) of 36 patients;[540] in another investigation in which follow-up biopsy specimens were obtained 19 to 60 days after the initial diagnosis, it was present in all 16 cases.[552] Occasionally, the fibrosis is severe enough to be manifested by residual restrictive lung disease.[553]

Cysts of *P. carinii* can be identified, albeit with great difficulty, by routine H & E and Papanicolaou staining;[554] however, they are much more easily seen after processing by Gomori's or Grocott's methenamine silver technique.[537]

The silver is taken up by the cyst wall, resulting in a round, oval, or crescent-shaped appearance (the last-named representing an effete cyst that has discharged its sporozoites). A small black dot caused by focal thickening of the wall is identifiable in the central portion of some cysts.[555] Several variations of the methenamine silver staining method have been reported that substantially reduce total staining time;[556, 557] the toluidine blue,[558] modified Gridley,[559] and Diff-Quik[560, 561] stains are also efficient and rapid. Calcofluor white has also been found to be useful and, in a small number of cases, to be positive when standard silver stains are negative.[550, 562] Intracystic sporozoites and free trophozoites can be identified with Giemsa's and Wright's stains.[563] Some authorities have advocated the use of plastic-embedded specimens[564] or combined Giemsa and silver stains[565] for simultaneous demonstration of both cysts and trophozoites. Although not autofluorescent, the organisms can be detected in cytologic specimens stained by Papanicolaou's method and examined in ultraviolet light.[566] Organisms have also been identified in formalin-fixed, paraffin-embedded material by in situ hybridization.[567] Details of the results of these and other special staining procedures have been discussed in several reviews.[554, 568]

When present in BAL fluid in clusters of 10 to 30 cysts, as in the typical case, differentiation of *P. carinii* from other organisms usually is not difficult if the size and shape characteristics described previously are fulfilled. If few in number, however, distinction from other fungi, such as *H. capsulatum*, *Penicillium marneffei*, *C. neoformans*, *P. brasiliensis*, and *Candida* species, may be difficult.[569, 570]

Cysts can disappear in tissue sections rapidly after therapy. In one autopsy study of nine patients in whom the diagnosis of *Pneumocystis* pneumonia had been made 2 to 21 days before death—all patients had received trimethoprim-sulfamethoxazole therapy—cysts were identified in only two cases, and these were in patients who had died only 2 and 5 days after the onset of therapy.[571] Other investigators have documented less rapid histologic clearing, particularly in patients with AIDS.[572] In fact, in the latter group, clearing may be absent altogether.[573] When they are identified in these circumstances, cysts often show morphologic evidence of degeneration.[551]

Radiologic Manifestations

In the early stage of *Pneumocystis* pneumonia, a granular pattern or hazy opacity (ground-glass pattern) is apparent, particularly in the perihilar areas (Fig. 28–37).[574–576] In later stages, the pattern is usually one of air-space consolidation (although a granular or reticulogranular pattern may still be present at the periphery of the consolidated area).[577] Terminally the lungs may be massively consolidated, to a point of almost complete airlessness: in some patients, the acute onset and diffuse involvement are characteristic of the adult respiratory distress syndrome.[578, 579]

Pneumonia is usually bilateral and most prominent in the lower lobes. Less commonly, it involves the upper lobes predominantly or exclusively. Although this distribution is seen most frequently in patients with AIDS who are receiving prophylactic aerosolized pentamidine,[580, 581] it may also occur in those not receiving prophylaxis. Rarely, there is lobar consolidation;[577, 582] in one patient in whom this was the initial radiographic finding, autopsy revealed many more organisms in the consolidated lobe than elsewhere.[582] An atypical radiographic distribution may also be seen in patients whose thorax has been irradiated; in two such cases, lung zones within the irradiation fields were spared *Pneumocystis* involvement, suggesting that tissue thus damaged may not support the growth of the organism.[582]

Another uncommon presentation of *P. carinii* pneumonia is as solitary or multiple, solid or cavitary nodular opacities.[583–586] Although most commonly seen in patients with AIDS, such nodules have also been described in patients with lymphoma.[546, 583] A relatively common radiographic manifestation in patients with AIDS is cystic lung disease (*see* page 1660). Unusual extrapulmonary features of *P. carinii* infection include pleural effusion;[587, 588] enlarged non-calcified[588, 589] or calcified[590, 591] hilar and mediastinal lymph nodes; and calcification of the spleen, liver, kidney, adrenal glands, and abdominal lymph nodes.[587, 591]

Although the majority of patients have radiologic findings, patients can present with dyspnea and fever, later proved to be caused by *P. carinii* pneumonia, with a normal chest radiograph and without hypoxemia;[592] in fact, as many as 10% of patients with AIDS with proven *P. carinii* pneumonia have normal chest radiographs.[593, 594] The organism can also be found in the lungs of patients who have died as a result of malignancy or transplant rejection in the absence of clinically or radiographically apparent pulmonary disease. This was demonstrated in a radiologic-pathologic correlative study in which the incidence of *P. carinii* infection of the lung was determined in 100 consecutive autopsies of patients with hematologic malignancies and a control group of 50 patients with either acute myocardial infarcts (25 patients) or chronic obstructive pulmonary disease (25 patients).[595] In this study, 13 instances of *P. carinii* infection were found in the study group and 1 in the control group: of these 14 patients, 5 were classified as having "uncomplicated" pneumonia (with a histologically typical response to the organism) and 5 as manifesting no evidence of host response; the remaining 4 cases could not be assessed because of complicating bacterial, viral, or fungal infection. All five patients with the typical histologic response had hematologic malignancy and showed radiographic evidence of diffuse pulmonary disease; by contrast, the five without pathologic evidence of host response showed no evidence of parenchymal disease on their chest radiographs. From this study, it might be concluded that the chest radiograph constitutes an efficient means of establishing when *P. carinii* infestation is significant; however, it could also be interpreted as reflecting the stage of infestation and perhaps the degree of immunoincompetence.

The predominant CT finding in *P. carinii* pneumonia is areas of ground-glass attenuation. This attenuation may be diffuse or have a distinct mosaic pattern, areas of normal lung intervening between the foci of ground-glass attenuation (Fig. 28–38).[596–598] Associated thickening of interlobular septa is seen in 20% to 50% of cases[596, 598] and parenchymal consolidation in approximately 40%.[598] With time, the areas of ground-glass attenuation progress to consolidation; eventually, interstitial abnormalities become evident and may predominate.[594] The interstitial findings may consist of thickened interlobular septa or irregular lines of attenuation (Fig. 28–39).[594–598] Occasionally, patients develop a CT pattern of diffuse fibrosis[594] or mild, peripheral bronchiectasis and bronchiolectasis.[599]

Clinical Manifestations

In infants, the clinical course is often one of rapid progression associated with severe dyspnea, tachypnea, and cyanosis.[600] Death can occur within hours or days and has been estimated to be the outcome in 20% to 50% of cases.[465] In the *child-adult* form of *P. carinii* pneumonia, the onset is usually insidious. There are significant differences in the clinical course of patients with and without AIDS. In the latter, the duration of prodromal symptoms tends to be shorter, often with a relatively acute presentation of fever and hypoxemia.[601–603] In patients with AIDS, there is often a prodrome of fever, malaise, cough, and breathlessness, which may be of several weeks' duration before recognition of the infection (*see* page 1667).

Dyspnea is the most common symptom; in some patients, a dry hacking cough is also present. Physical signs are usually minimal and include a few scattered crackles and wheezes. In severe infection, patients may show a hemodynamic profile similar to that of patients with bacterial sepsis, including the presence of tachycardia, increased cardiac index, and low systemic vascular resistance index.[604] In pa-

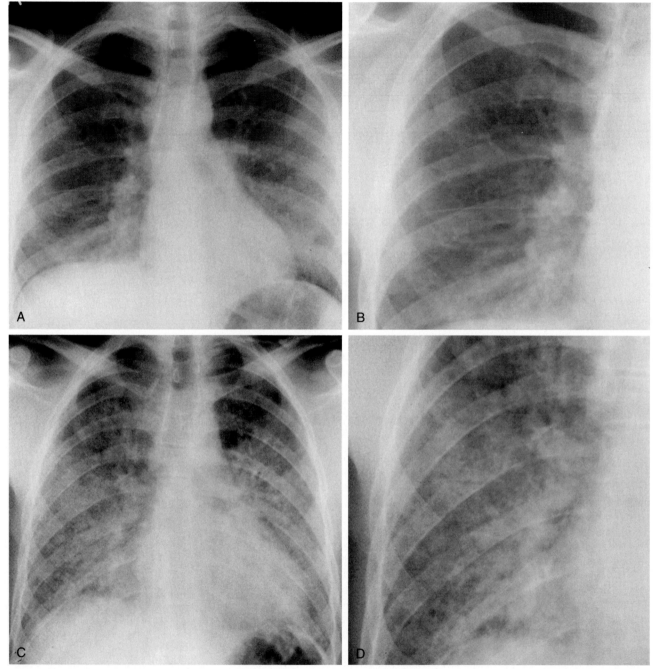

Figure 28–37. *Pneumocystis carinii* **Pneumonia in AIDS.** A posteroanterior chest radiograph *(A)* and a close-up view of the right lung *(B)* show a diffuse hazy increase in lung opacity (ground-glass opacity) throughout both lungs, worse in the lower lobes. The appearance in this clinical setting is suggestive of early *P. carinii* pneumonia. Several days later, the disease had progressed to consolidation *(C, D)*. An open-lung biopsy disclosed classic histopathology of *P. carinii* pneumonia.

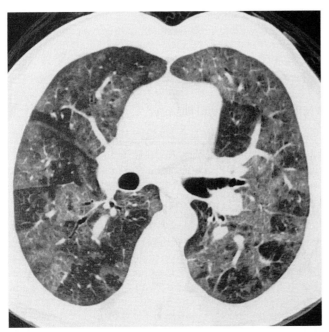

Figure 28–38. *Pneumocystis carinii* **Pneumonia.** HRCT demonstrates characteristic appearance consisting of bilateral areas of ground-glass attenuation and areas of normal-appearing lung causing a mosaic pattern. The patient was a 46-year-old man with AIDS.

tients with AIDS, the clinical picture may be complicated by the presence of other infectious[605, 606] or neoplastic disease or by disseminated pneumocystosis; in the latter situation, signs and symptoms of infection relate to the specific organ or tissue affected.[607, 608] Unusual clinical manifestations include hemoptysis,[609] asthma,[610] and hypertrophic osteoarthropathy.[611] Some patients with previous infection have evidence of bronchial hyper-responsiveness.[612]

The development of sudden onset of shortness of breath in a patient with AIDS should raise the possibilty of *Pneu-*

mocystis-related pneumothorax. The complication is usually associated with parenchymal air cysts radiologically. Thoracoscopy has revealed the presence of white-yellow nodules on the visceral or parietal pleura in some patients;[613] histologic examination of biopsy or brush specimens of these lesions may reveal the presence of *P. carinii.* Although usually unilateral, pneumothorax may be bilateral and fatal.[614] Pneumomediastinum may also develop.[615]

Laboratory Findings and Diagnosis

In most patients with *Pneumocystis* pneumonia, the white blood cell count is slightly to moderately increased, with polymorphonuclear leukocytes predominating. Leukopenia may occur, however, in which case the prognosis is worse (*see* farther on). Lymphopenia is found in approximately 50% of patients.[616] Immunosuppressed patients, both transplant recipients and those with AIDS, usually show a reversal of T-cell helper-to-suppressor ratio.

The serum lactate dehydrogenase (LDH) is frequently elevated in patients with active *Pneumocystis* pneumonia,[617, 618] including those with AIDS who have been treated prophylactically.[619] However, the diagnostic utility of this finding is limited, since the enzyme is also elevated in patients who have other infections, particularly disseminated tuberculosis but also tuberculous and other bacterial pneumonia.[618] Moreover, in one investigation of 93 patients with human immunodeficiency virus (HIV) infection and pneumonia, an elevated LDH was shown to be more a marker of the extent of radiographic disease than an indicator of *Pneumocystis* infection.[620] Many patients also have an elevation of other serum enzymes, such as aspartate aminotransferase (AST), alanine aminotransferase (ALT), and alkaline phosphatase.[618] Analysis of *Pneumocystis*-related pleural effusion has shown the LDH to be greater than 400 (with a ratio to serum LDH > 1), the pH greater than 7.3, and the glucose normal.[621] Hypercalcemia (hypothesized to be re-

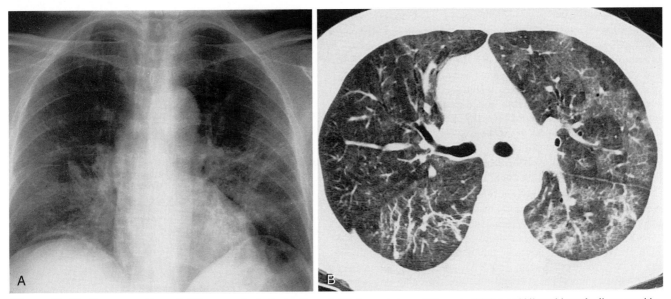

Figure 28–39. *Pneumocystis carinii* **Pneumonia.** A chest radiograph *(A)* demonstrates perihilar consolidation and bilateral irregular linear opacities. HRCT *(B)* shows bilateral areas of ground-glass attenuation and irregular linear opacities involving mainly the lower lobes. The patient was a 56-year-old woman who developed *P. carinii* pneumonia after renal transplantation.

lated to macrophage dysfunction) has been described rarely.[622]

A variety of serologic tests for antigen and antibody have been used in cases of suspected *P. carinii* pneumonia, with variable results.[623–625] In one investigation using indirect immunofluorescence, seroconversion or a fourfold increase in antibody titer was identified in only 3% of patients with AIDS-related pneumonia but in 45% of patients with other causes of immunosuppression.[626] In a second study in which an ELISA technique was used, almost 45% of a group of AIDS patients were found to mount an antibody response on serial testing.[627]

Patients with *Pneumocystis* pneumonia almost always have a reduced DLco (< 70% of predicted in 72 of 78 patients in one investigation.[628] A significant increase in the A-a gradient for oxygen is also typical of active infection.

Although pneumocystosis may be strongly suspected from a combination of radiologic and clinical findings and the results of the laboratory tests described above, definitive diagnosis requires demonstration of *P. carinii* in tissue or respiratory secretions. Several techniques have been used to obtain material for analysis, the most common being BAL and aerosol-induced sputum production. Although these techniques almost always suffice in patients with AIDS (in whom the burden of organisms tends to be high), transbronchial or open biopsy is sometimes required, particularly in patients with other causes of immunosuppression.[574] Other techniques, such as cutting-needle biopsy, tracheal aspiration, and transthoracic needle aspiration, may also yield diagnostic material[629–631] but have been rarely used. Analysis of serum for the presence of organism-specific DNA or β-glucan (a component of the cyst wall) has also been performed, some investigators finding the procedure to be diagnostically useful[632, 633] and others not.[634] Rarely, organisms are identified in foci of extrapulmonary disease, including pleural fluid.[621] The pros and cons of these techniques have been most studied in patients with AIDS (*see* page 911).

The traditional method by which organisms have been identified is microscopic examination of specimens stained with silver; as discussed previously (*see* page 911), a variety of other stains have also been used, in many cases with comparable results. In an attempt to increase both sensitivity and rapidity of diagnosis, many laboratories now use either immunologic[635, 636, 636a] or molecular biologic techniques.[544, 637, 638] Numerous investigations have been conducted to identify the relative benefits of one technique over another. The results are somewhat variable and depend, in part, on the underlying disease (particularly AIDS versus other immunocompromised states) and the technique by which organisms are obtained from the patient (e.g., induced sputum versus biopsy). In general, however, the following conclusions can be made with a reasonable degree of confidence:

1. In tissue specimens from patients with clinically evident pneumonia, immunofluoresence and PCR have little to offer over standard histochemical stains.[639]

2. Immunofluorescent techniques[504, 631, 640–643] and PCR[644] are more sensitive than standard histochemical staining in both induced sputum and BAL specimens; however, some investigators have found the positive and negative predictive values for PCR tests to be significantly less in patients who are immunocompromised as a result of leukemia or lymphoma rather than AIDS.[645]

3. PCR is more sensitive and at least as specific as immunofluorescence, again in both induced sputum and BAL specimens;[646–651] some investigators have found that positive test results rapidly revert to negative after the onset of therapy.[648]

Prognosis and Natural History

Pneumocystis pneumonia is a serious disease, the overall mortality rate varying from 10% to 60% in different reported series.[652] This rather large range reflects several factors, including the presence or absence of AIDS, the prevalence of other AIDS-related diseases in specific geographic regions,[653] and the effect of therapy.[654] The results of some epidemiologic studies suggest that the prognosis improved significantly in patients with AIDS between the 1980s and early 1990s,[655–657] a finding attributed by some to the use of new therapy such as steroids, overall improved care in the intensive care unit,[657] and earlier recognition and presentation of disease. There is evidence from a number of investigations that the prognosis is worse in patients with non–AIDS-related pneumonia.[477, 481, 658]

An important predictor of poor prognosis in patients with AIDS-related pneumonia is acute respiratory failure.[657, 659] Other factors that have been associated with increased mortality include an increase in interleukin-8 in BAL fluid,[660] a high Acute Physiology and Chronic Health Evaluation (APACHE) score, an elevated serum LDH on admission to the hospital[661] (although some investigators have found no association between LDH and prognosis[662, 663]), and leukopenia. Studies in which the relationship between the severity of disease has been related to the number of cysts identified in tissue or BAL fluid specimens have yielded conflicting results;[663–665] however, some workers have found low numbers of cysts to be associated with a relatively poor outcome (possibly reflecting a greater number of free trophozoites).[666] Attempts to predict prognosis on the basis of a clinical staging system have also been devised.[652, 662] According to one of these, the A-a oxygen gradient, total lymphocyte count, and body mass index are combined to give four stages;[652] in a review of approximately 575 patients with *Pneumocystis* pneumonia at more than 50 hospitals, the mortality rates for the four groups were 1%, 8%, 23%, and 48%.

The use of prophylactic therapy, in both patients with AIDS and those without, has been clearly shown to reduce the incidence of pneumonia. In one investigation, the risk of developing the disease in this setting was closely related to a decrease in T-helper level to less than 75×10^6/liter.[511] One group of investigators found no difference in the number of cysts in BAL fluid specimens between patients treated prophylactically with pentamidine and those without such treatment.[667] In our experience, most individuals who survive a single episode of *Pneumocystis* pneumonia have little evidence of residual clinical disability. Pneumonia may recur, however, particularly in patients with AIDS (*see* page 1669).

CANDIDIASIS

Candidiasis is caused by a dimorphic fungus whose yeast forms are 2 to 4 μm in diameter and possess a thin wall that stains with PAS and Grocott's methenamine silver and is weakly gram-positive. Hyphae and pseudohyphae may be produced. The organism can secrete an aspartic proteinase that may be important in disease pathogenesis and useful in diagnosis.[668]

Although *C. albicans* is the most important pathogen, a variety of other species have been implicated, particularly in the immunocompromised host in one study of 136 episodes of fungemia over a 4-year period, *Candida* species were the responsible organisms in 90%; of these, 59% were caused by species other than *C. albicans*.[531] The proportion of forms other than *C. albicans* increased from 42% to 70% over the time span of the study.

Epidemiology

Candida organisms are common human saprophytes, *C. albicans* being found normally in the gastrointestinal tract and mucocutaneous regions and a variety of non-*albicans* species being found on the skin. Their numbers are held in check naturally by saprophytic bacteria. Conditions in which the composition of the normal flora is altered are thus likely to lead to overgrowth of *Candida* species and an increased risk of infection. Such conditions exist in the oral cavity of neonates before the establishment of a normal resident population of bacteria and of adults receiving antibiotic therapy; the latter group has a high yield of positive culture results[669] that may remain positive for up to 2 weeks after discontinuation of the therapy.[670] Inhaled corticosteroids are also an important factor in overgrowth of the fungus in the upper airways.

Other conditions that are associated with increased colonization include diabetes mellitus,[671] chronic debilitating disease, use of indwelling urinary and intravenous catheters,[672] and a prolonged hospital stay.[673] In such situations, the development of candidiasis is not infrequent, much more often in the form of local mucocutaneous infection (oropharynx, vagina, and skin) than of clinically significant visceral or disseminated disease.[674] Pulmonary infection is relatively uncommon; in one series of 125 pulmonary complications seen in immunocompromised patients, it was documented in only six cases (5%).[675]

Whether confined to the lungs or widely disseminated, candidiasis seldom occurs in otherwise healthy individuals; when it does, it is probable that some impairment of host defense has not been recognized.[676] Specific conditions that favor the development of visceral infection include malignancy (usually in association with immunosuppressive chemotherapy or the granulocytopenia occasioned by acute leukemia or lymphoma),[677, 678] extensive burns, major abdominal or open heart surgery,[678, 678a] intravenous drug abuse in addicts (with a propensity for the development of endocarditis),[680] organ transplantation,[681, 682] parenteral hyperalimentation, central venous catheters,[672] and extended antibiotic therapy. The importance of cell-mediated immunity and normal phagocytic activity as defense mechanisms is reflected in the numerous inherited and acquired disorders that are complicated by chronic mucocutaneous and invasive candidiasis, including a variety of congenital thymic deficiencies, chronic granulomatous disease of childhood, endocrine deficiencies, thymoma, and AIDS.[683, 684]

Pathologic Characteristics

Several pathologic forms of pulmonary candidiasis can be seen. The most common occurs as part of a systemic hematogenous (miliary) infection associated with multiorgan involvement and a primary extrapulmonary site (usually the gastrointestinal tract). Grossly, the lungs contain multiple, randomly distributed, white nodules ranging in diameter from barely visible to several centimeters and surrounded by a hemorrhagic rim.[685] Histologically, these are composed of a central zone of necrotic parenchyma with admixed *Candida* organisms, often surrounded by intra-alveolar hemorrhage (Fig. 28–40).[685, 686] The inflammatory cellular response is related to the integrity of host defenses, there being little or none in granulocytopenic patients and a variably intense polymorphonuclear infiltrate in other individuals. Granulomas are rarely seen.[687] Although small vessels may show intraluminal fungi, invasion and occlusion of large pulmonary arteries as in mucormycosis and aspergillosis are usu-

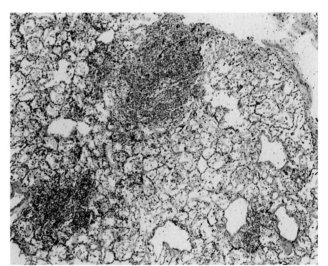

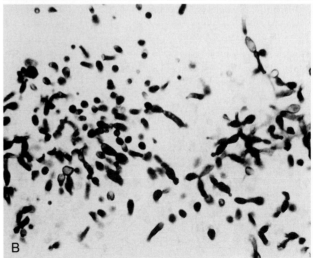

Figure 28–40. *Candida albicans* Pneumonia. A section of lung parenchyma *(A)* shows three foci of acute inflammation, the two largest associated with necrosis. These represent septicemic seeding, probably from the esophagus, in a 48-year-old man with disseminated large cell lymphoma. Organisms appear as pseudohyphae and round or oval yeasts *(B)*. (A, ×40; B, Grocott's methenamine silver, ×600.)

ally absent. In addition to the lungs, other viscera are commonly involved, including the heart, kidneys, liver, and spleen (the last two especially in patients with leukemia).[678]

Pulmonary candidiasis can also occur as a primary infection that in many cases is probably acquired by aspiration of organisms from the oral cavity. Pathologically the pattern is that of a bronchopneumonia associated with a variably intense neutrophil infiltrate.[685, 688, 689] The infection may remain limited to the lungs[676] or may disseminate.[689] Rarely, *Candida* infection is manifested by an intracavitary fungus ball (mycetoma).[690]

Radiologic Manifestations

One of the most reliable descriptions of the radiographic manifestations of pulmonary candidiasis has come from a study of 20 patients in whom *C. albicans* was the sole organism found in the lung on postmortem culture or identified histologically as being invasive into lung parenchyma.[691] All patients had air-space consolidation, and 11 had an interstitial component. Eight patients had bilateral lobar consolidation, eight had patchy bilateral areas of consolidation, and four had unilateral lobar or segmental consolidation. Pleural effusion was present in five patients; evidence of cavitation or hilar or mediastinal lymph node enlargement was seen in none. Although a diffuse nodular or miliary pattern was not observed in this series, it has been described by others (Fig. 28–41).[692, 692a] Nodules may range from a few millimeters to 3 cm in diameter.[675] Unusual manifestations include cavitation in consolidated lung and formation of an acute "mycetoma."[693, 694]

The HRCT findings of *Candida* pneumonia have been reported in a small number of cases.[695, 696] In one review of nine patients, seven had a bilateral, predominantly nodular pattern, and two had bilateral areas of ground-glass attenua-

tion and consolidation (Fig. 28–42).[695] The nodules ranged from 3 to 30 mm in diameter. Halos of ground-glass attenuation surrounding the nodules were seen in four patients. Less commonly, the nodules are sharply circumscribed and surrounded by normal parenchyma (Fig. 28–43). Pathologic correlation shows the nodules may represent foci of acute inflammation with or without abscess formation, foci of granulomatous inflammation, or infarction.[238, 697] The halo of ground-glass attenuation that surrounds some of the nodules results from hemorrhage adjacent to an area of necrosis.[238]

Because CT is superior to chest radiography in the detection of nodular opacities in *Candida* pneumonia,[695] it may allow suspicion of the diagnosis when the radiographic findings are nonspecific. For example, in one study comparing the differential diagnostic ability of HRCT and chest radiography, two independent radiologists correctly suggested the diagnosis of *Candida* pneumonia among their three diagnostic choices in 56% of cases on CT compared to 22% on chest radiography of patients who were immunocompromised.[695]

Clinical Manifestations

The symptoms of pulmonary candidiasis are nonspecific and include cough, purulent expectoration, and hemoptysis. Many patients have evidence of involvement of other organs or tissues; such disseminated disease is often a terminal event in debilitated and immunocompromised patients, many of whom are receiving antibiotic, corticosteroid, or immunosuppressive therapy. Although any organ or tissue may be involved clinically, the heart, genitourinary tract, meninges, and eyes are most frequently affected.[90] An uncommon form of candidiasis manifested by asthma and transient pulmonary opacities similar to allergic bronchopulmonary aspergillosis has also been described.[698]

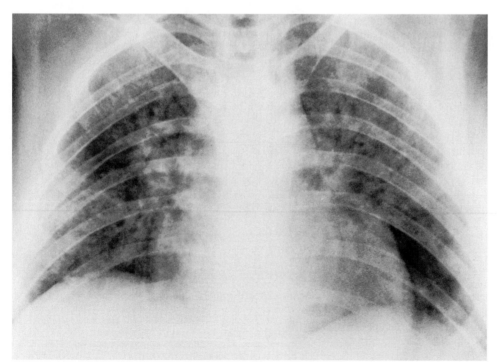

Figure 28–41. Disseminated Candidiasis. This 19-year-old man had acute leukemia, for which he was receiving high doses of antineoplastic drugs and corticosteroids. During the course of therapy, he developed clinical evidence of diffuse pneumonia. This anteroposterior radiograph reveals widespread involvement of both lungs by patchy and confluent areas of air-space consolidation. At autopsy, there was widespread organ involvement by *C. albicans.*

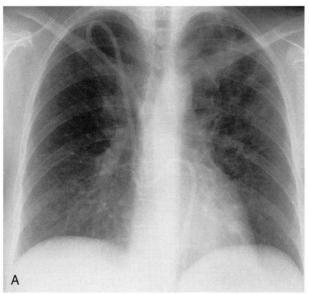

A

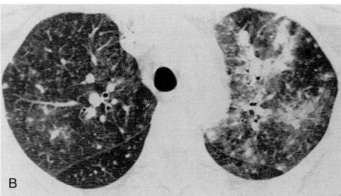

B

Figure 28–42. *Candida* **Pneumonia.** A posteroanterior chest radiograph *(A)* demonstrates poorly defined areas of consolidation and a few nodular opacities in the upper lobes. HRCT *(B)* demonstrates nodules of various sizes, focal areas of consolidation, and ground-glass attenuation. The patient was a 27-year-old woman who developed *Candida* pneumonia after bone marrow transplantion.

Laboratory Findings

The diagnosis of invasive candidiasis should be considered in patients with radiographic evidence of pulmonary disease who have repeated, heavy growth of *C. albicans* in sputum that is otherwise pathogen-free. Because the organism is commonly a saprophyte of the oropharynx and occasionaly of the lower respiratory tract, conclusive diagnosis usually requires its demonstration in tissue.[699] Suspicion should be increased when the patient is known to be a compromised host and has a positive blood culture; however, because transient candidemia can occur without tissue dissemination, this is also not an absolute criterion of disease. The innocuousness of transient fungemia and funguria in

Figure 28–43. *Candida* **Granulomas.** A 28-year-old patient with acute leukemia presented with fever and a chest radiograph that showed questionable abnormalities. HRCT scan demonstrates smoothly marginated nodules measuring 2 to 5 mm in diameter situated mainly in the subpleural regions, suggesting hematogenous dissemination. On open-lung biopsy, the nodules were shown to represent well-defined granulomas containing *C. albicans.*

the healthy individual was dramatically illustrated in an experiment invoving ingestion of 10^{12} cells of *C. albicans*;[700] although a transient toxic reaction lasted from 2 to 9 hours after ingestion and *Candida* organisms were cultured from the blood and urine at 3 and 6 hours, no other untoward effects were identified.

A variety of serologic tests using agglutinating and precipitating antibodies as well as *Candida* antigen have been developed in an attempt to aid in the diagnosis of invasive candidiasis.[679, 701–703] None, however, is sufficiently sensitive or specific to warrant routine use.

ASPERGILLOSIS

Although approximately 300 species of *Aspergillus* have been described,[704] only a small number have been associated with human disease. By far the most important is *Aspergillus fumigatus*;[705] *Aspergillus niger, Aspergillus flavus,* and *Aspergillus glaucis*[705, 706] are occasionally pathogenic and infection is rarely caused by a variety of other forms.[704, 706–712] The various species are structurally similar and difficult to differentiate without culture. An exception is *A. niger,* whose spores contain a black pigment that can be observed sometimes in tissue or expectorated material; in fact, the diagnosis of pleuropulmonary disease caused by this organism has been made by detecting a combination of black expectoration and a pleural fluid pH less than 5.9 (as a result of oxalic acid [*see* farther on]).[713] Although the organisms are present throughout the world, certain species can assume prominence in a specific geographic area; for example, one report from the Sudan suggests *A. flavus* is responsible for the majority of infections in this region.[714] Occasionally, more than one species is isolated from one specimen or different specimens in the same patient.

In the mycelial phase, the organisms occur as septate, rather uniform hyphae, 2 to 4 μm in diameter, with characteristic dichotomous branching at an angle of 45 degrees (Fig. 28–44). In tissue, the hyphae are frequently oriented roughly in the same direction and appear to radiate from a

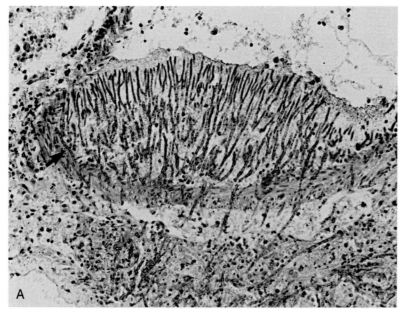

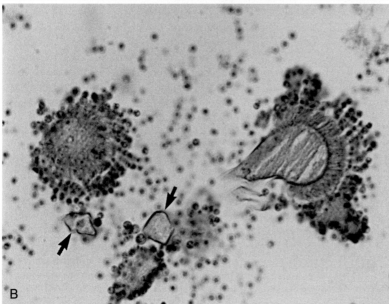

Figure 28–44. *Aspergillus* Species. Fan-shaped mass of septate hyphae *(A)* branching at an angle of approximately 45 degrees *(arrow)*. Note how the fungi traverse the pulmonary artery wall with absence of inflammatory reaction or necrosis. Conidiophores *(B)*, showing fruiting heads and minute spores. Several calcium exalate crystals are also evident *(arrows)*. (*A*, periodic acid–Schiff, ×150; *B*, Grocott's methenamine silver, ×720.)

common point, resulting in a fan-like appearance. They are usually visible with H & E stain, but are particularly well seen with PAS and Grocott's methenamine stains. Although the organisms are typically quite uniform in size and shape, degenerated forms may be swollen and somewhat variable in appearance, superficially resembling the Phycomycetes. In addition, fungi such as *Chaetomium globosum* or *Pseudallescheria boydii* can resemble healthy *Aspergillus* organisms;[715] as a result, definite identification of a particular fungus as *Aspergillus* usually requires cultural, immunohistochemical, or molecular confirmation, particularly if only small amounts of tissue are available. Reproduction is characterized by the formation of conidiophores that have terminal expanded vesicles, which produce chains of spores; although usually not encountered in tissue, both conidiophores

and spores may be seen in cavities that communicate with the atmosphere and are diagnostic of the fungus.

Aspergillus organisms are extremely hardy and ubiquitous in the environment, having been found in soil, water, and decaying organic material of many types. In most instances, infection is believed to occur by inhalation of airborne conidia from a variety of contaminated areas. Colonization of the nasal mucosa not uncommonly precedes either disseminated or pulmonary infection;[716] occasionally, such infections occur by way of the gastrointestinal or genitourinary tract. There is no evidence of transmission from animal-to-human or from person-to-person. An unusual source of exposure is marijuana, from which a number of *Aspergillus* species have been isolated;[717] smoking this substance has been implicated in the development of both invasive pulmonary disease[718, 719] and allergic bronchopulmonary aspergillosis.[720]

Pathogenesis

The pathogenesis of the various types of *Aspergillus* infection is complex and incompletely understood.[721] As might be expected, the quantity and virulence of inhaled organisms[722–726] and the adequacy of host defense are important factors. A brief overview of some of the features common to the various types of disease is given here; more details related to specific forms are presented in the appropriate sections.

Although *Aspergillus* species produce a variety of enzymes and toxins,[704] the precise mechanisms by which any of these may be involved in the production of disease are unclear. Intravenous injection of mycelial extracts from *A. fumigatus* and *A. flavus* is lethal in several animals and is capable of producing lung hemorrhage in dogs.[727] Similar extracts are capable of depleting serum complement by activation of both classic and alternative pathways.[728] Several proteases are produced by *Aspergillus* organisms;[729, 730] although the results of some investigations provide evidence that they are involved in tissue invasion,[731, 732] those of others suggest that they have little, if any, role.[733–735] *Aspergillus* organisms also produce a variety of aflatoxins, which are known carcinogens and hepatotoxins; whether these play any part in the production of pulmonary disease is not known.

The presence of intact host defense, particularly that related to macrophages and neutrophils, is clearly important in limiting the proliferation and spread of *Aspergillus* organisms. Experimental studies suggest that alveolar macrophages may prevent germination of conidia by phagocytosing and killing them and that defense against invasion is dependent on this mechanism, at least initially.[736, 737] In addition, neutrophils are capable of killing conidia in a pregerminative stage.[738] There is evidence that surfactant proteins A and D may have an important facilitatory role in these processes[739] and that a variety of inflammatory cytokines are involved.[740] *Aspergillus* organisms produce several substances that appear to be able to decrease the effectiveness of these inflammatory cellular reactions. For example, there is evidence that spores of *A. fumigatus* secrete chemicals that inhibit phagocytosis,[741] the production of reactive oxygen intermediates,[742] and the development of T-cell cytotoxicity.[743] In addition, several species produce a compound that appears to interfere with complement activity, thus inhibiting conidial opsonization and, possibly, the production of chemotactic factors.[744]

Certain *Aspergillus* species, notably *A. niger*, are sometimes associated with local tissue deposition of crystals of calcium oxalate (*see* Fig. 28–44).[745, 746] These are believed to be derived from a combination of calcium derived from the host and oxalate produced by the organisms themselves.[747] They have been identified in fungus balls,[745, 746] invasive pulmonary aspergillosis,[745] and *Aspergillus* empyema.[748] Although the crystals are usually found in the vicinity of the fungus itself, some authors have reported cases of invasive aspergillosis associated with both disseminated pulmonary and renal oxalosis;[745, 749] in one of these, the presence of renal failure and antineutrophil cytoplasmic antibodies (c-ANCA) in the patients' serum resulted in a misdiagnosis of Wegener's granulomatosis.[749] It has been speculated that the oxalic acid may cause local tissue damage—possibly via an association with ferric ion and subsequent oxidant generation[750]—and result in intracavitary hemorrhage in patients with fungus balls.[746, 751] The crystals may be seen in respiratory tract secretions examined cytologically and may precede the development of radiologic abnormalities.[752] Determination of oxalic acid levels in BAL fluid has also been advocated as a means of diagnosing invasive disease.[753]

Disease caused by *Aspergillus* species can be manifested in three ways, each with distinctive clinical, radiologic, and pathologic features: (1) *saprophytic infestation*, in which the fungus colonizes airways, cavities (aspergilloma), or necrotic tissue; (2) *allergic disease*, characterized by such entities as allergic bronchopulmonary aspergillosis (ABPA) and extrinsic allergic alveolitis; and (3) *invasive disease*, a form that is usually acute in onset and rapidly fatal and rarely insidious and associated with a relatively good prognosis. Although these three varieties are not mutually exclusive—for example, occasional cases of saprophytic or allergic disease progress to invasive aspergillosis (Fig. 28–45)—as a rule, crossover does not occur.

Saprophytic Aspergillosis

Saprophytic aspergillosis is characterized by mycelial growth and sometimes conidiophore production unassociated with invasion of viable tissue. Within the lungs, it may take three forms: (1) colonization of the tracheobronchial tree without the formation of macroscopically visible colonies; (2) the development of a grossly identifiable colony within a pre-existing cavity or ectatic bronchus (fungus ball, aspergilloma); and (3) invasion of necrotic tissue. Although usually unassociated with clinical consequences, saprophytic growth occasionally leads to tissue damage and symptoms (particularly hemoptysis). In addition, the colonies can serve as a source for the development of invasive disease when local or systemic defenses become compromised.

Airway Colonization

Airway colonization usually occurs in patients with underlying airway disease, such as asthma, bronchiectasis, or chronic bronchitis. In these abnormalities, the organism has been cultured in 2% to 3% of patients in some series.[754] Evidence of colonization has also been found by PCR analysis of BAL fluid in about 10% to 20% of patients who are apparently immunocompetent and have clinical or radiologic findings of pulmonary disease other than those usually associated with *Aspergillus* infection.[755, 756] Colonization is particularly common in patients with cystic fibrosis, in whom positive sputum cultures have been reported in as many as 50% to 55% of individuals;[757, 758] the finding appears to be more common in older individuals.[759] Although some of these patients have APBA, in others there is no evidence of a hypersensitivity reaction to the fungus. In the latter individuals, minute fungal colonies appear to be able to survive in mucopurulent exudate within the airway lumen and, possibly, the alveolar air spaces.[760] In one investigation

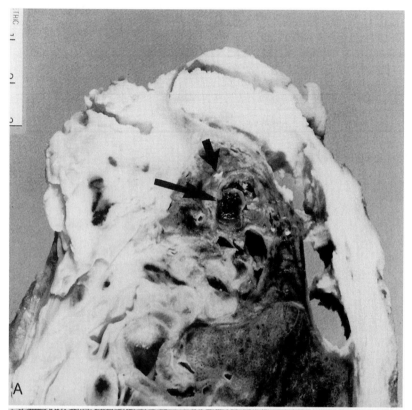

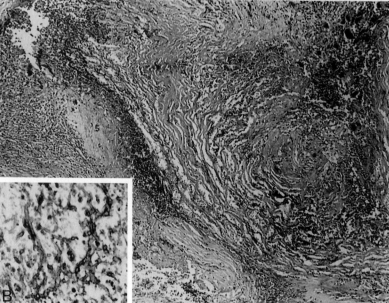

Figure 28–45. Remote Fibrocaseous Tuberculosis with Mycetoma and Invasive Aspergillosis. The upper portion of the right lung *(A)* shows pleural fibrosis, marked atelectasis and fibrosis of the upper lobe, and several foci of calcified necrotic material *(small arrow)*. These changes resulted from a remote episode of postprimary tuberculosis, treated by thoracoplasty. A 1-cm, somewhat lobulated fungus ball is also present within a bronchiectatic cavity *(large arrow)*. A section *(B)* through the region of pleural fibrosis shows necrosis and poorly defined granulomatous inflammation in relation to fungal hyphae *(magnified in inset)*. Similar foci were found in the lung and represent direct invasion from the intracavitary fungus ball presumed *Aspergillus* species. The fungus ball was not identifiable on conventional chest radiographs. (Periodic acid–Schiff, ×56; *inset*, ×250.)

of 65 patients with cystic fibrosis who underwent lung transplantation, the presence of *Aspergillus* colonization before transplantation was not associated with the development of invasive disease in the post-transplant period.[758] The factors that aid *Aspergillus* organisms to colonize the airways are not clear; however, there is experimental evidence that they produce several substances that cause epithelial damage and inhibit ciliary function.[761]

Fungus Ball

A *fungus ball* (mycetoma, aspergilloma*) can be defined as a conglomeration of intertwined fungal hyphae admixed with mucus and cellular debris within a pulmonary cavity or ectatic bronchus. Historically, the most common underlying cause has been tuberculosis, approximately 25% to 55% of patients having a history of this disease.[762, 762a] In fact, the likelihood of developing the complication in tuberculosis is appreciable: in one long-term study of 544 patients with healed open tuberculous cavities, 59 (11%) had radiographic evidence of aspergilloma formation;[763] in a follow-up report 3 years later, the prevalence had increased to 17%.[764] The authors of this study also recorded the development of aspergillomas in many patients who had a positive precipitin test to aspergillin but initially no radiographic evidence of an intracavitary fungus ball. Despite these observations, it is likely that as the prevalence of chronic (inactive) tuberculosis decreases in the population, the proportion of cases of aspergilloma associated with this underlying cause will decrease.[762a] The second most common underlying disease associated with aspergilloma is sarcoidosis;[762, 765] in one prospective evaluation of 100 patients with this disease, 10 developed aspergillomas.[766]

Other predisposing conditions associated less often with aspergilloma formation include bronchiectasis of any cause (including cystic fibrosis),[767, 768] chronic fungal cavities,[769–771] bronchogenic cysts, acute and chronic bacterial abscesses,[772] cavities related to *P. carinii* in patients with AIDS,[773] cavitary carcinoma,[774] radiation fibrosis,[775] apical fibrobullous changes of rheumatoid disease,[776] ankylosing spondylitis,[777, 778] and pulmonary sequestration.[779] Of a somewhat analogous nature is the conglomeration of *Aspergillus* hyphae that can develop in the bronchial stump remaining after pneumonectomy, especially in association with the use of silk sutures.[780, 781] Intrapleural aspergillomas have also been described.[782] The common factor in all these conditions is the presence of an enlarged cystic space in which the normal clearance mechanisms are impaired. Although many fungal conidia inhaled within such spaces are probably killed by host inflammatory cells, defective clearance presumably favors the establishment of colonies, which can then enlarge and form the grossly visible fungus ball. There is also evidence that proteases produced by the fungus may induce the detachment of epithelial cells from the mucosa.[783]

Although most aspergillomas exist as purely saprophytic growths, occasional examples are associated with allergic or invasive disease (*see* farther on). In fact, it is not uncommon to find evidence of hypersensitivity to *Aspergillus* in the presence of an aspergilloma.[784, 785] Moreover, occasional patients have all the immunologic criteria in keeping with a diagnosis of ABPA in the absence of asthma or radiographic evidence of mucoid impaction.[786] Because aspergillomas can also develop as a complication of ABPA,[787–790] it may be impossible to establish whether ABPA preceded or followed the development of the aspergilloma.[791]

As indicated previously, the vast majority of fungus balls are caused by *Aspergillus* species. However, clinically and radiologically identical infections have also been reported with many other organisms, including *Candida* species,[690] *Streptomyces* species, *Nocardia* species,[694, 792] *Phycomycetes* species,[793] *Sporothrix schenckii*,[794] *Trichophyton* species,[795] *C. immitis*,[796] *P. boydii*,[797, 798] *Syncephalastrum* species,[799] and *Cladosporium cladosporioides*.[800]

Pathologic Characteristics

Pathologically an aspergilloma characteristically consists of a round-to-oval-shaped mass of greenish or brown, somewhat friable material situated within a cavity having a fibrous wall of variable thickness (Fig. 28–46). Histologically, the wall is composed of mature fibrous tissue containing a variable number of chronic inflammatory cells and blood vessels; the latter, which mostly represent branches of the bronchial arteries and veins, may be abundant and undoubtedly are the source of hemoptysis in most cases.[801] An epithelial lining may be absent or may consist of normal-appearing respiratory epithelium or metaplastic squamous cells. An acute inflammatory or (rarely) granulomatous reaction can be present at the junction of the wall and the fungus ball; however, invasion of tissue by the organism is usually not seen.

Radiologic Manifestations

Radiographically a fungus ball consists of a solid, more or less round mass of soft tissue density within a spherical or ovoid cavity, usually in an upper lobe.[802, 803] Typically, the mass is separated from the wall of the cavity by an air space of variable size and shape, resulting in the distinctive air-crescent sign (Fig. 28–47). A fluid level is seldom present within the cavity.[804] Occasionally, the mycelial mass grows to fill a cavity completely, effectively obliterating the air space necessary for its radiographic identification (the abnormality being recognized as a result of hemoptysis or as an incidental finding at autopsy). Most cavities are thin walled; in one series, they averaged 5.5 × 3.5 cm in diameter.[802] They are often contiguous with a pleural surface, which itself may be thickened.[805] In fact, thickening of the walls of tuberculous cavities or of the adjacent pleura has been described as an early radiographic sign of *Aspergillus* colonization, antedating the detection of the fungus ball.[806]

The fungus ball usually moves when the patient changes position;[807, 808] however, some are irregular in shape, conforming, for example, to an elongated bronchiectatic cavity, in which case change in the position of the patient may not be accompanied by a concomitant movement of the fungus ball. The size of the ball can also change,[809] or it

---

*Because a variety of fungi other than *Aspergillus* species can produce the complication (*see* farther on), use of the term *aspergilloma* synonymously with fungus ball is, strictly speaking, inappropriate without ancillary serologic or cultural confirmation; however, because of common usage and because *Aspergillus* is by far the most frequent etiologic agent of a fungus ball, we and most others use the designation in the absence of definitive proof.

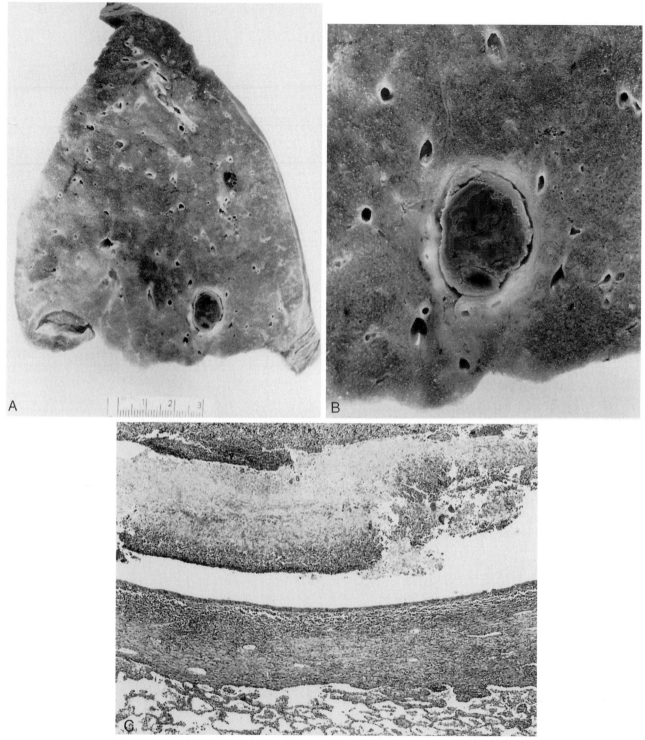

Figure 28–46. Aspergilloma. A slice of left lower lobe *(A)* shows a somewhat laminated mass that resembles a thrombus within a thin-walled cavity (shown magnified in *B*). Note that the mass conforms to the contours of the cavity and virtually fills it, making movement impossible. A section through the cavity wall *(C)* shows fibrosis, chronic inflammation, and an intact epithelial lining. The fungus ball itself consists of scattered polymorphonuclear leukocytes and numerous hyphae (barely visible at this magnification). The patient was a 26-year-old woman with hemoptysis; the cause of the cavity was not determined. *(C, ×40.)*

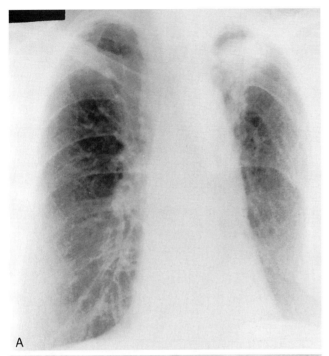

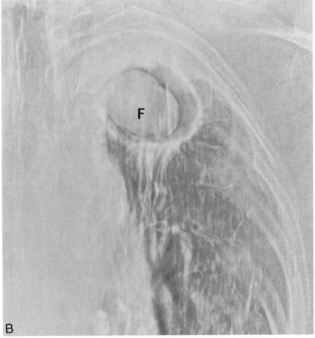

Figure 28–47. Aspergilloma in a Tuberculous Cavity. A postero-anterior chest radiograph *(A)* and a xerotomogram *(B)* demonstrate a left apical opacity consisting of a well-defined homogeneous mass almost completely surrounded by an air crescent; portions of a thin-walled cavity are visible inferiorly and laterally. The left hilum is elevated as a result of upper lobe fibrosis secondary to long-standing tuberculosis. The sixth and eighth left ribs and part of the lower lobe were surgically excised many years previously for bronchiectasis. A prominent apical fibrotic cap is also seen. F, fungus ball.

can remain constant for many years.[804] Calcification of the mycelial ball occurs in some cases; this may be apparent as scattered small nodules, as a fine rim around the periphery of the mass, or as an extensive process involving the greater part of the mycetoma.[802, 804, 810] The radiologic differential

diagnosis should include a fragment of tissue in a carcinoma that has undergone necrosis, a mass of necrotic lung in an abscess, a degenerated hydatid cyst, and an intracavitary blood clot. In one exceptional case, the intracavitary mass was a retained surgical sponge.[811]

As on the radiograph, the most characteristic finding of aspergilloma on CT consists of an ovoid or round soft tissue intracavity mass that usually moves when the patient is turned from the supine to the prone position (Fig. 28–48).[812, 813] Areas of increased attenuation, presumably representing calcium deposits, are relatively common.[812] CT may also allow visualization of aspergillomas not apparent on the radiograph.[812, 813] In one review of 25 cases in which abnormalities consistent with an aspergilloma were identified by HRCT, irregular fungal strands could be seen between the fungus ball and the surrounding cavity wall in cases in which an air crescent was not visible on the radiograph.[812] CT may also demonstrate fungal fronds situated on the cavity wall that intersect with each other and form an irregular sponge-like network, before the development of the mature fungus ball (Fig. 28–49).[812]

The characteristic air-crescent sign has also been described on MR imaging in a case of an aspergilloma originating within a cavitary pulmonary carcinoma.[813a] The procedure also demonstrated a difference in signal intensity between the cavity wall and the intracavitary mass, indicating different tissue characteristics.

Clinical Manifestations and Diagnosis

Cough and expectoration are common;[767] hemoptysis has been reported in 50% to 95% of cases.[814–816] The latter varies from relatively minor streaking of the sputum to life-threatening hemorrhage. There is evidence that serious bleeding may be more frequent in patients with AIDS.[773] An appreciable number of patients have alcoholic cirrhosis or impaired respiratory function.[817, 818] Rarely, the fungus extends through the cavity wall into the adjacent tissue (*see* Fig. 28–45);[819] in this situation, complications such as pleural effusion[820] and vertebral destruction and cord compression[821, 822] have been reported.

Most often, the presence of an aspergilloma is readily apparent from the typical radiologic features; in the few patients in whom confirmation is necessary, the diagnosis usually can be corroborated by transthoracic needle aspiration for culture or cytologic examination, or bronchial washings of the affected lobe. The diagnosis is supported by the finding of a positive precipitin test to fungal antigen[823, 824] or by an elevated level of *Aspergillus*-specific IgE.[785] After resection, the precipitin test reaction becomes weaker, but rarely reverts to negative.[764] IgG-ELISA serology and immunoblotting may also be useful, both in confirming the disease and in following its activity.[825]

Prognosis

The prognosis of patients with aspergillomas is generally good. In the long-term study reported by the British Thoracic and Tuberculosis Association in 1970, patients with the abnormality fared no worse than those with open, healed tuberculous cavities without a fungus ball.[764] The lesions undergo spontaneous lysis in 5% to 10% of cases,[764, 816–818]

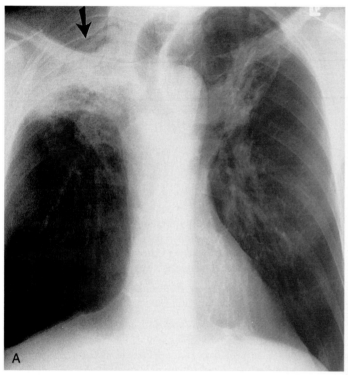

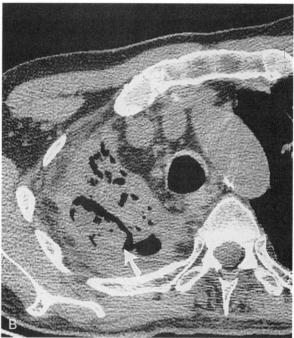

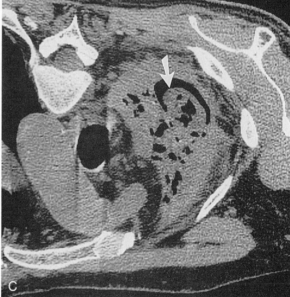

Figure 28–48. Aspergilloma with Air Crescent Sign and Change in Position. A 65-year-old man with previous tuberculosis presented with hemoptysis. A posteroanterior chest radiograph *(A)* demonstrates extensive scarring in the upper lobes. A large aspergilloma in the right upper lobe shows a characteristic crescent of air between it and the cavity wall *(arrow)*. Note the marked pleural thickening surrounding the cavity containing the aspergilloma. HRCT with the patient supine *(B)* and prone *(C)* shows a change in position of the aspergilloma *(arrows)* despite its large size. Also evident are extensive bronchiectasis and marked pleural thickening. *A. fumigatus* was recovered at bronchoscopy.

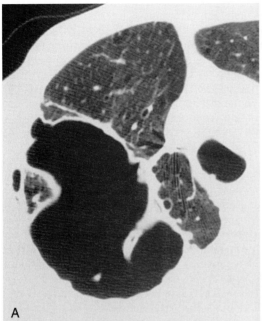

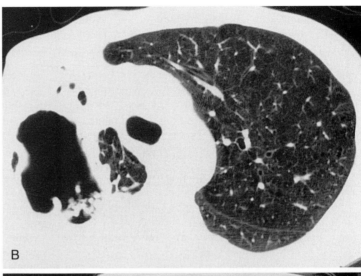

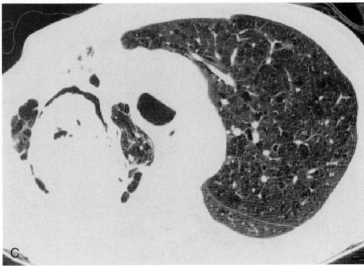

Figure 28–49. Aspergilloma—Development and Growth Over Time. A 59-year-old woman with previous right mastectomy and right upper lobectomy presented with cough and weight loss. HRCT scan targeted to the right lung *(A)* demonstrates a large cystic lesion in the superior segment of the right lower lobe; evidence of bronchiectasis is also noted. No other abnormality was found. All cultures were negative. HRCT scan 18 months later *(B)* shows a small mount of soft tissue in the dependent portion of the cystic lesion; increased thickness of the wall of the cyst is evident. The patient also has evidence of more extensive bronchiectasis and scarring in the right lung. Four years later, the patient developed hemoptysis. HRCT scan *(C)* demonstrates a large fungus ball within the cavity. *Aspergillus fumigatus* was recovered at bronchoscopy.

and some disappear when bacterial infection develops within the cavity.[823] The exception to these general statements is the occasional patient who presents with massive hemoptysis, in whom death may occur. In addition, as indicated previously, some aspergillomas are complicated by local pulmonary invasion[819] or disseminated disease.[791, 828]

Invasion of Necrotic Tissue

Invasion of necrotic tissue is the least common variety of saprophytic aspergillosis and consists of fungal invasion and colonization of dead tissue, the latter usually the result of infarction,[829] acute bacterial infection,[830] or a necrotic neoplasm.[774] Because the underlying tissue is already necrotic, the presence of the fungus does not have any pathogenic significance. Provided that the patient is not immunocompromised, extension of the fungus outside the colonized tissue is most unlikely.

Allergic Aspergillosis

Hypersensitivity reactions to *Aspergillus* organisms can take three forms: (1) *extrinsic allergic alveolitis*, most likely the result of hypersensitivity to inhaled conidia and usually seen in an occupational setting,[831] such as the production of malt;[832–835] (2) a *Loeffler-like* syndrome;[762] and (3) *ABPA*.* The last-named is by far the most common of the three and is the subject of the remainder of the discussion in this section.

The diagnosis of ABPA can be difficult and depends on the demonstration of several abnormalities;[836] in a particular patient, confidence in diagnosis depends on the number and type that are identified. These abnormalities include (in approximate order of diagnostic importance)

1. Radiographic or CT manifestations of mucoid impaction or ectasia of proximal bronchi.[837, 838, 838a]

2. Asthma (an almost invariable finding in the United States but not in the United Kingdom[839, 840] or some parts of Australia[841]).

---

*The vast majority of cases with the clinical, radiologic, and immunologic characteristics of ABPA are, in fact, caused by *Aspergillus* organisms. As with saprophytic fungus balls, however, some patients manifest the same characteristics in association with other organisms (the immunologic and cultural findings, of course, being specific for the causative fungus); such organisms include *Stemphylium lanuginosum*, *Helminthosporium* species, *Curvularia* species, *Candida* species, *Schizophyllum commune*, *Fusarium vasinfectum*, and *Drechslera hawaiiensis*.[839, 851–855]

3. Eosinophilia of blood (> 1,000/mm³) and sputum (common in adults but often absent in children[839] and not necessarily present in every acute attack).[842]

4. An elevated level of total serum IgE.[843] This measurement has been used both as an indicator of acute exacerbations of disease[844, 845] and as a means of confirming the diagnosis after a therapeutic trial of corticosteroids;[846] in fact, it has been suggested that failure to achieve a reduction in IgE levels greater than 35% by 2 months after the institution of corticosteroid therapy should make one question the diagnosis.[846]

5. Characteristic histologic findings on specimens obtained by bronchoscopy.[846a]

6. An elevated level of serum IgE antibody to *Aspergillus* (compared with asthmatic patients who have immediate cutaneous reactivity to *Aspergillus* but do not have ABPA).[839, 844, 847]

7. An immediate cutaneous reaction to *Aspergillus* antigen.

8. Precipitating antibodies against *Aspergillus* antigen. Such antibodies can be demonstrated in more than 90% of patients;[848] some investigators have found the level of serum IgG antibodies to *A. fumigatus* (measured by ELISA) to be as useful an indicator of activity as IgE determinations.[849]

9. Positive sputum culture for *Aspergillus* species.[850]

10. Positive delayed skin reaction to intracutaneous injection of *Aspergillus* antigen.

Pathogenesis

The pathogenesis of ABPA is not entirely clear. The fungus is clearly able to proliferate in the airway lumen, theoretically resulting in the production of a continual supply of antigen that may lead to chronic inflammation of the airway wall, precipitating antibodies in the blood, skin sensitivity, and tissue and blood eosinophilia. Why some individuals develop the condition and others do not, however, remains a mystery. There is experimental evidence that spores of *A. fumigatus* show enhanced binding to activated epithelial cells and basement membrane components, a feature that may be related to the colonization of the airways of patients with asthma, in whom such mucosal abnormalities are not uncommon.[856] ABPA sometimes occurs in identical twins[857] and in families,[858, 859] raising the possibility of a genetic factor; however, these associations are uncommon, and other studies, such as determination of HLA antigen profiles,[860] have failed to support a hereditary link.

Attempts to correlate attacks of ABPA with a heavy exposure to spores have usually proved unsuccessful,[861] although environmental point sources have been identified occasionally.[862, 863] Despite this, it is generally accepted that episodes of ABPA are more common during periods of high atmospheric *Aspergillus* spore counts, which tend to occur during the winter months.[861, 862, 864]

In most cases of ABPA, mucous plugging and ectasia occur in one or more orders of bronchi distal to a lobar bronchus. The formation of plugs of inspissated mucus within proximal bronchi also occurs occasionally in patients without other criteria for ABPA. The pathogenesis of this abnormality—which has been termed *mucoid impaction*[865] or *plastic bronchitis*[866]—and the part, if any, played by fungi in pathogenesis are unknown. To complicate matters, both simple mucous plugging and typical ABPA also occur in patients with cystic fibrosis.[867–869] In fact, ABPA has been estimated to develop in approximately 10% of patients with this disease[870, 871] and may be a factor in the clinical deterioration with which it is commonly associated.[870] A positive correlation also has been described between impaired pulmonary function in patients with cystic fibrosis and the presence of serum antibodies to *A. fumigatus*.[872]

Pathologic Characteristics

Pathologically, segmental and proximal subsegmental airways are dilated and filled with plugs of inspissated mucus containing scattered macrophages, numerous eosinophils, and Charcot-Leyden crystals.[873–875] Bronchial walls adjacent to the mucous plugs contain an inflammatory infiltrate composed of eosinophils, lymphocytes, and plasma cells. Although fungal invasion is typically absent, chondritis and cartilage destruction are occasionally seen.[876, 877] The diagnosis can be suspected on examination of expectorated mucous plugs or intraluminal material removed by bronchoscopy or in bronchial washings.[846a] A "geometric" arrangement of layers of eosinophils alternating with layers of mucus is characteristic of the material (Fig. 28–50);[878] the diagnosis can be confirmed by identifying fragments of hyphae within the mucus by special stains.

In some cases, the histologic pattern of bronchocentric granulomatosis can also be seen in smaller airways (Fig. 28–51).[873, 875, 878–880] As the name suggests, the characteristic feature of this abnormality is necrotizing granulomatous inflammation centered about bronchioles and small bronchi. Early in the course of the disease, residual airway epithelium can often be identified on one portion of the wall, clearly establishing the bronchocentric nature of the process; in later stages, the mucosa may be completely destroyed and replaced by a zone of palisaded epithelioid histiocytes that surrounds necrotic intraluminal debris. The bronchocentric pattern may be recognized at this point only indirectly by one or more of three features—the apparent absence of small airways in tissue sections, the presence of pulmonary arteries adjacent to the necrotic foci, or the demonstration of the residua of the airway elastic tissue framework by appropriate stains (*see* Fig. 28–51).

The intraluminal necrotic material associated with bronchocentric granulomatosis typically contains numerous eosinophils, scattered Charcot-Leyden crystals, and fragmented fungal hyphae. An infiltrate of plasma cells, lymphocytes, histiocytes, and eosinophils surrounds the layer of palisaded histiocytes and frequently extends into the adventitia of the adjacent pulmonary artery. Because there is no evidence of necrosis or thrombosis, this vascular inflammation is best interpreted as a secondary rather than primary vasculitis. Although the histologic pattern of bronchocentric granulomatosis can be caused by other conditions (e.g., infections such as tuberculosis[881] [*see* page 823], ruptured hydatid cyst,[882] and immunologic abnormalities such as rheumatoid disease[873, 883] and ankylosing spondylitis[885]), it is probably most commonly associated with ABPA. Occasionally, a pattern of follicular or xanthomatous bronchiolitis is present instead of the more typical granulomatosis.[884]

The lung parenchyma in ABPA has a variable appearance. In some cases, it is more or less normal. In others,

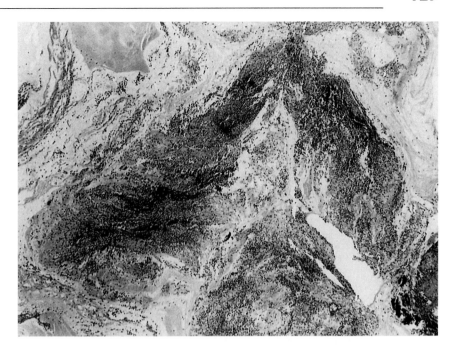

Figure 28–50. Mucous Plug in Allergic Bronchopulmonary Aspergillosis. The section shows a fragment of a mucous plug removed at bronchoscopy in a patient with typical allergic bronchopulmonary aspergillosis. A "Christmas tree" pattern of alternating bands of mucus and eosinophils is evident. Minute fragments of fungal hyphae were identified within the mucus by silver stain. (×40.)

alveolar air spaces are filled with foamy lipid-laden macrophages surrounded by a mild interstitial mononuclear inflammatory infiltrate, representing a nonspecific reaction to bronchiolar plugging (obstructive pneumonitis). Collections of intra-alveolar eosinophils and mononuclear cells in a pattern histologically identical to idiopathic eosinophilic pneumonia are seen occasionally.[873, 886]

Radiologic Manifestations

The radiographic pattern of ABPA is identical to that of mucoid impaction.[789, 887] Homogeneous, finger-like shadows of unit density lie in a precise bronchial distribution, usually involving the upper lobes and almost always in the more central segmental bronchi rather than peripheral branches (Fig. 28–52).[789] These bifurcating opacities have been variously described, according to their orientation on the radiograph, as having a *gloved-finger, inverted Y or V,* or *cluster-of-grapes* appearance. Although involvement of main and lobar bronchi is uncommon, cases have been described in which an entire lung has been collapsed distal to a huge mucous plug.[840, 888, 889] Occasionally, isolated lobar or segmental collapse also occurs, sometimes coincident with clinical exacerbation.[802] The shadows tend to be transient but may persist unchanged for weeks or even months or may enlarge (Fig. 28–53).

After expectoration of a mucous plug, residual bronchial dilation may be evident (Fig. 28–54);[767, 890] when severely dilated, such bronchi may contain a fluid level[838, 891] or an aspergilloma (Fig. 28–55). Occasionally, mucous plugs calcify (Fig. 28–56). Mucoid impaction tends to recur in the same segmental bronchi, suggesting that bronchial damage predisposes to further episodes.[789] Pleural disease is uncommon in ABPA; however, both effusion[892] and spontaneous pneumothorax[893] have been reported.

As with radiographs, the CT findings of ABPA consist principally of mucoid impaction and bronchiectasis involving predominantly the segmental and subsegmental airways

(Fig. 28–57).[894–896] High attenuation of the mucous plugs, presumably related to the presence of calcium, was evident on HRCT in 4 (28%) of 14 patients in one study.[897] Other abnormalities include atelectasis and areas of consolidation. Several groups have compared the findings on CT with those on radiography in asthmatic patients with and without ABPA. In one study in which CT scans were performed with 3-mm-thick sections, bronchiectasis was identified on CT in 14 (82%) of 17 patients with ABPA compared to 10 (59%) of cases on radiography.[896] Evidence of bronchiectasis was seen on CT and on radiography in 2 of 11 (18%) patients without ABPA. In the majority of patients with ABPA, the bronchiectasis involved only the medial two thirds of the lungs. Other findings in patients with ABPA included "parenchymal shadowing" in 14 of 17 (82%) patients, pleural thickening in 14, and atelectasis in 9. Another group compared the HRCT findings in eight asthmatic patients with ABPA to the findings in eight without;[895] bronchiectasis was identified in six patients with ABPA and in three without. These studies indicate that bronchiectasis is seen in the majority of patients with ABPA, but that it may also occur in uncomplicated asthma. Furthermore, bronchiectasis is not always present in patients with ABPA. Focal areas of mucoid impaction and bronchiectasis may mimic a nodule or mass lesion on CT.[898]

Although the bronchiectasis seen in patients with ABPA most commonly involves the upper lobes and affects predominantly the segmental and subsegmental bronchi, it may be widespread and involve more peripheral bronchi.[896, 899] In one review of the CT scans of 146 patients with bronchiectasis (including patients with idiopathic bronchiectasis, ABPA, hypogammaglobulinemia, impaired mucociliary clearance, and cystic fibrosis diagnosed in adult life), 11 of 15 (73%) patients with ABPA had widespread bronchiectasis; in only 2 patients was it limited to the upper lobes.[899] Six of 15 patients had only central bronchiectasis, 1 had only peripheral bronchiectasis, and 8 had both central and peripheral disease. There was a slightly greater prevalence of central

Text continued on page 935

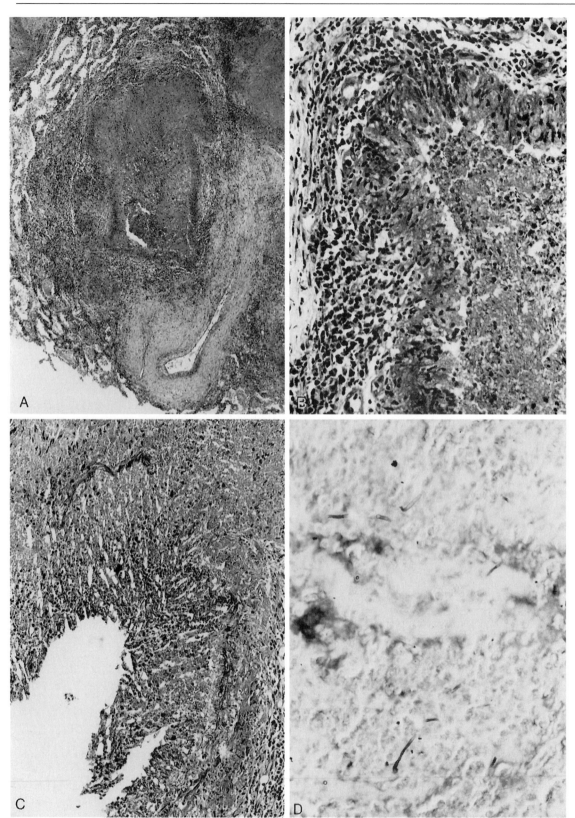

Figure 28–51. Allergic Bronchopulmonary Aspergillosis—Bronchocentric Granulomatosis. This section *(A)* from an open-lung biopsy from a 27-year-old asthmatic patient with ill-defined bilateral upper lobe opacification shows a large focus of necrotic material situated adjacent to a thick-walled pulmonary artery; no residual airway structure is apparent. Magnified view *(B)* shows palisaded epithelioid histiocytes adjacent to the necrotic material and surrounded by abundant mononuclear inflammatory cells. An elastic stain *(C)* shows fragmented elastic tissue surrounding the necrotic focus, confirming that the lesion is centered on a bronchiole. Small fragments of degenerated fungal hyphae *(D)* consistent with *Aspergillus* species are present within the necrotic material. *(A,* ×40; *B,* ×250; *C,* Verhoeff–Van Gieson ×150; *D,* Grocott's silver methenamine ×300.)

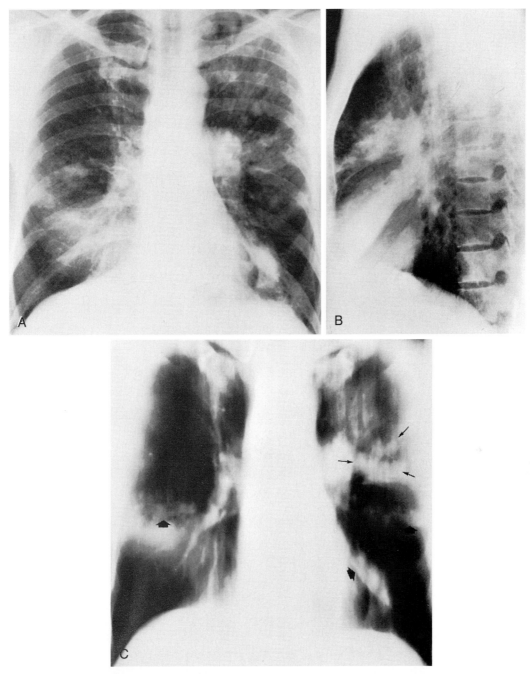

Figure 28–52. Allergic Bronchopulmonary Aspergillosis. Posteroanterior *(A)* and lateral *(B)* radiographs reveal extensive bilateral disease, all lobes of the lung being affected by a process possessing an unusual mixed pattern. In the left upper lobe, the pattern appears to be one of air-space consolidation, confluent shadows of homogeneous density being associated with an air bronchogram; the medial segment of the right middle lobe shows a combination of atelectasis and consolidation; broad areas of consolidation extend into the anterior basal segment of the left lower lobe and the anterior segment of the left upper lobe. A full lung tomogram in anteroposterior projection *(C)* shows numerous broad-band shadows bilaterally, each measuring approximately 1 cm in diameter and extending in a distribution compatible with the bronchovascular bundles *(thick arrows)*. In the midportion of the left lung, one of these shadows possesses a Y configuration *(thin arrows)*. These band shadows are caused by inspissated mucus within markedly dilated bronchi; the Y-shaped shadow in the left midlung represents one that is bifurcating. With the exception of the right middle lobe, all impacted bronchi are unassociated with consolidation or atelectasis of the lung distal to them, presumably as a result of effective collateral ventilation.

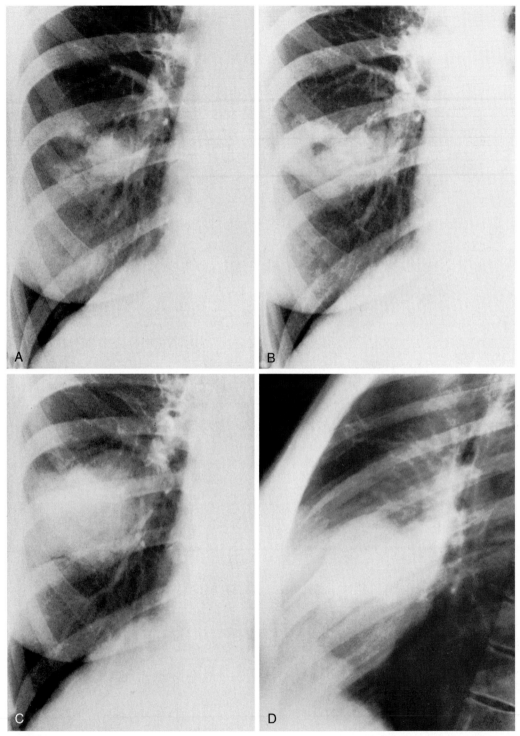

Figure 28–53. Allergic Bronchopulmonary Aspergillosis. A detail view of the lower half of the right lung *(A)* of a 29-year-old asthmatic woman reveals a roughly circular opacity measuring about 3 cm in diameter; the lesion was situated in the middle lobe. Two years later *(B)*, the opacity had increased considerably in size and possessed a prominent Y configuration, the two prongs facing laterally. The peripheral parenchyma is air containing despite the total obstruction that must be present in the affected airways. One month later *(C* and *D)*, a rather abrupt enlargement of the mucoid impaction occurred. Corticosteroid therapy was instituted at this time, and 2 weeks later the opacity had almost completely resolved, leaving markedly dilated segmental bronchi.

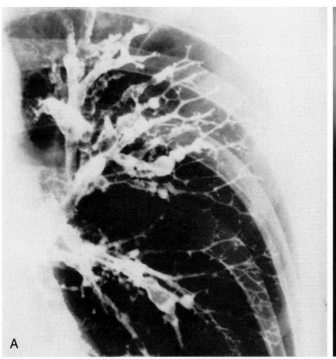

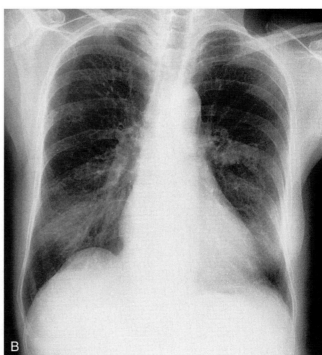

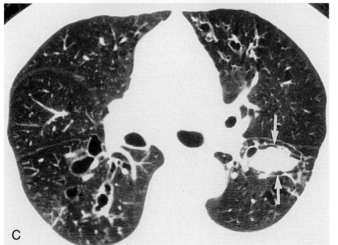

Figure 28–54. Allergic Bronchopulmonary Aspergillosis. A bronchogram *(A)* of the left lung in a patient with established mucoid impaction reveals irregular dilation of the segmental and subsegmental branches of the left upper lobe bronchus. Contrast medium that has passed beyond the bronchiectatic segments has opacified airways of normal appearance. This proximal bronchiectasis is characteristic of mucoid impaction, with or without hypersensitivity bronchopulmonary aspergillosis. A postero-anterior chest radiograph *(B)* from another patient reveals focal nodular opacities in the superior segment of the left lower lobe; HRCT *(C)* demonstrates mucoid impaction in this segment *(arrows)* as well as extensive bronchiectasis.

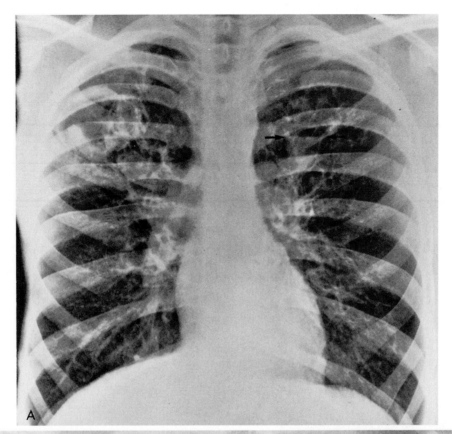

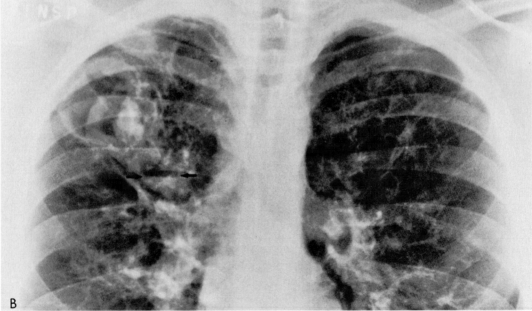

Figure 28–55. Allergic Bronchopulmonary Aspergillosis Associated with Aspergilloma. This 19-year-old man had a long-standing history of asthma accompanied by frequent pulmonary infections. A radiograph *(A)* reveals a large, shaggy cavity in the right upper lobe associated with a broad, finger-like opacity extending inferomedially to the upper portion of the right hilum (probably representing mucoid impaction). In the left upper lobe, there is evidence of severe bronchiectasis, one of the markedly dilated bronchi possessing a prominent air-fluid level *(arrows)*. A number of bronchi viewed end-on in the parahilar zones show thickening of their walls. Two weeks later *(B)*, the fluid level has disappeared from the bronchiectatic segment on the left; however, the cavity in the right upper lobe now shows evidence of a large intracavitary foreign body. Note the prominent air-fluid level in the markedly dilated bronchus extending from the cavity to the right hilum *(arrows in B)*. *A. fumigatus* was recovered from the sputum, and precipitins to the organism were found in the serum. Skin tests for *A. fumigatus* were positive.

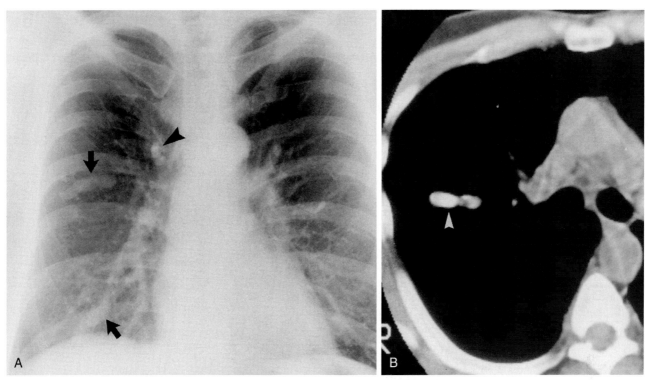

Figure 28–56. Allergic Bronchopulmonary Aspergillosis with Partly Calcified Bronchoceles. A posteroanterior chest radiograph *(A)* reveals branching, band-like opacities in the right lower lobe *(oblique arrow)* and the right upper lobe *(vertical arrow)*; an end-on round opacity *(arrowhead)* is seen in the upper hilum. CT scan *(B)* shows calcific material *(white arrowhead)* within the bronchocele. The patient was a 42-year-old man with a history of asthma and peripheral blood eosinophilia.

bronchiectasis in ABPA compared to other diseases, but exclusively central bronchiectasis was also seen in 7% of patients with idiopathic bronchiectasis and 10% of patients with impaired mucociliary clearance.[899] The authors concluded that although there are differences in distribution of bronchiectasis in groups of patients with different causes, the CT findings are of limited value in distinguishing various causes of bronchiectasis in the individual patient.[899]

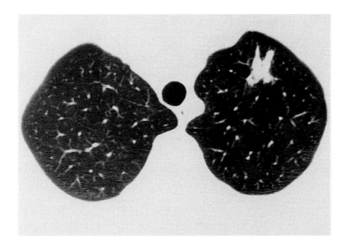

Figure 28–57. Allergic Bronchopulmonary Aspergillosis with Mucoid Impaction. HRCT scan targeted to the left upper lobe demonstrates branching opacities characteristic of mucoid impaction in the left upper lobe. The patient was a 73-year-old woman with asthma.

Clinical Manifestations

Studies in the United States have shown that most patients with ABPA are more than 30 years of age and often have a variety of allergic manifestations, including rhinitis, conjunctivitis, asthma, eczema, urticaria, drug allergy, and food allergy.[900] Chronic sinusitis also may be present and have similar pathologic features as the pulmonary disease.[884] Acute episodes of ABPA are sometimes associated with increased cough, hemoptysis, fever, pleuritic pain, wheezing, and dyspnea;[842, 901] however, perhaps just as often there is little change in the clinical state of the patient, and the incident is not recognized unless a chest radiograph is obtained or serum IgE levels are monitored.[902, 903] Most patients with ABPA whose disease remits on steroid therapy show subsequent exacerbations.[842] Even those with relatively advanced disease characterized by bronchiectasis, fibrosis, and functional obstruction unresponsive to corticosteroids may still have acute episodes accompanied by a rise in precipitins and IgE.[847] With recurrent attacks, almost half the patients expectorate mucous plugs,[864, 901] and a slightly lesser number produce sufficient sputum to suggest the development of bronchiectasis.[864]

Prognosis

The long-term prognosis of ABPA is usually good; although it has been well established that unrecognized episodes of disease can result in irreversible airway obstruction, severe bronchiectasis, pulmonary fibrosis, and even death,[127] follow-up studies have shown little clinical deterioration in the majority of cases.[682] Functional disability has been shown to be related to the chronicity of the disease;[864] in one investigation of 17 patients with bronchiectasis and pulmonary fibrosis who survived for 5 years, respiratory impairment was mild to moderate in 7 and severe in 4.[847] The necessity of monitoring patients with periodic serum sampling for IgE has been emphasized,[902] an increase usually occurring before radiographic evidence of mucous plugging.

Invasive Aspergillosis

Invasive aspergillosis is characterized by extension of *Aspergillus* organisms into viable tissue, usually associated with tissue destruction. Although such invasion can be seen in association with a fungus ball or ABPA, this is rare and almost always focal and minimal; conceptually, therefore, these cases are not included under this heading. Despite this, it should be remembered that both aspergilloma[905] and the mucous plugs of ABPA[906] can serve as sources of fungus in clinically significant invasive disease.

Epidemiology

Invasive aspergillosis almost invariably develops in patients whose host defenses are impaired, often as a result of cancer and its therapy.[762, 907] In one retrospective study of 98 patients published in 1970, almost 90% had underlying neoplastic disease, almost all of which was lymphoreticular or hematologic in nature.[908] Patients with acute myelogenous leukemia are particularly susceptible;[907, 909, 910] a significant risk for patients with chronic myelogenous leukemia has also been documented in some studies.[911] A major predisposing factor in these patients is granulocytopenia.[910, 912] Other conditions that are associated with an increased risk of invasive aspergillosis include organ transplantation,[913–915] viral infection (particularly by influenza virus),[916, 917] renal or hepatic failure,[919, 920] and diabetes.[921] In contrast to the situation with bacterial infection, alcoholism per se is rarely associated with the complication.[922, 923] Similarly the disease is relatively infrequent in patients with AIDS,[924] although it certainly can occur, particularly when associated with risk factors such as corticosteroid therapy or neutropenia.[925]

Occasional patients with chronic obstructive pulmonary disease (including emphysema, asthma, and cystic fibrosis)[926–928] and chronic interstitial fibrosis[928] also develop invasive aspergillosis; corticosteroid therapy seems to be important in the pathogenesis of disease in some of these cases.[928] Rare cases have been described in apparently healthy hosts, either after surgery[710] or de novo.[929–932, 932a] The disease has also been described in patients with Cushing's syndrome[933] and after near-drowning.[934]

Because many patients who acquire invasive aspergillosis are already hospitalized, nosocomial sources of infection are important to identify. Such sources have included central venous catheters,[935] bird excreta adjacent to a ventilation system,[936] and dust created during hospital renovation.[911, 937, 938] Controlled studies have shown fewer *Aspergillus* spores in hospital rooms ventilated with filtered air and as a consequence a reduction in the incidence of invasive disease[939, 940] (however, replacement of such air filter systems has itself been associated with the development of disease).[941] Isolation of *A. fumigatus* and several other species has also been documented in opened parenteral medications and cracked dialysis bags and has occasionally been associated with outbreaks of clinically significant invasive disease.[704]

Pathogenesis

That alteration of host defenses is important in the development of invasive aspergillosis has also been documented experimentally. The administration of cytotoxic drugs, radiotherapy, or a deficient diet or the transplantation of leukemia renders mice more susceptible than control animals to fatal pulmonary disease after inhalation of *Aspergillus* spores; moreover, episodes of pneumonia are more frequent and severe.[942] There is evidence, at least in steroid-treated animals, that one important deficiency is decreased lysosomal killing of macrophage-ingested spores, permitting their intracellular germination and subsequent proliferation.[943, 944]

The lungs are involved in the vast majority of cases of invasive aspergillosis.[907, 908] In many of these, infection remains confined to this site, although direct extension into the pleural cavity[945] or pericardium[946, 947] has occasionally been reported. Spread of organisms outside the thorax occurs in 25% to 50% of patients.[907, 908, 948] Dissemination occurs chiefly to the gastrointestinal tract, brain, liver, kidneys, and heart, although virtually any organ may be affected;[907, 908] rarely, disseminated disease occurs in the absence of lung involvement.[907, 908]

Invasive pulmonary aspergillosis is manifested by four major clinicopathologic forms of disease that are useful to consider separately: acute bronchopneumonia, angioinvasive aspergillosis, acute tracheobronchitis, and chronic necrotizing aspergillosis.[949] The first two comprise the majority of cases; in one review of 84 cases, they accounted for 30 and 29 cases, respectively.[950] Other uncommon clinical and pathologic forms of invasive aspergillosis within the thorax include bronchiolitis and bronchiolitis obliterans,[951] miliary disease[950] fibrosing mediastinitis (in one case associated with an ABPA-like syndrome),[952] and pleural infiltration with or without effusion (sometimes as a consequence of rupture[820] or resection of a fungus ball[828, 953] and, in one series, in patients who had been treated for tuberculosis with artificial pneumothorax[820]).

Acute Bronchopneumonia

Acute bronchopneumonia may develop secondary to bronchitis, as described farther on, or, more commonly, in a fashion analogous to bacterial bronchopneumonia. Pathologically, the inflammatory reaction is patchy in distribution and centered about terminal airways (Fig. 28–58).[949] Areas of pneumonia may be sharply circumscribed and show small (1 to 2 mm) foci of central cavitation. Microscopically, the lesions are composed of a central zone of necrotic tissue containing hyphae surrounded by edema, hemorrhage, and an inflammatory infiltrate of polymorphonuclear leukocytes.[954] Vascular permeation can occur, but often is not apparent.[908] In some cases, the process becomes confluent (simulating acute air-space pneumonia; Fig. 28–59[955]) or

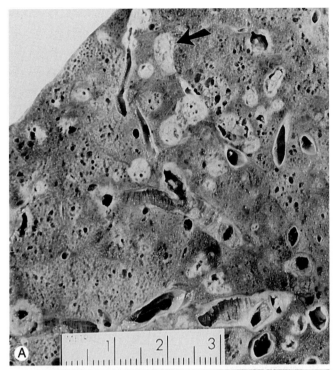

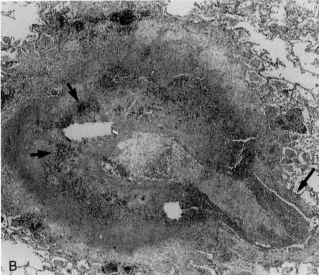

Figure 28–58. *Aspergillus* **Bronchopneumonia.** A magnified view of a slice of an upper lobe *(A)* shows multiple, well-defined white nodules, some clearly necrotic *(arrow)*. A section of a small (early) lesion *(B)* shows it to be clearly centered on a membranous bronchiole *(large arrow)*. Fungal hyphae are barely identifiable *(small arrows)* in the central necrotic region. *(B, ×25.)* *(A from Fraser RS: Pulmonary aspergillosis: Pathologic and pathogenetic features. In Rosen PP, Fechner RE [eds]: Pathology Annual, Part 1. Norwalk, CT, Appleton & Lange, 1993, p 231.)*

present also in the patient with normal radiograph, consisted of bilateral, predominantly peribronchial consolidation (Fig. 28–61). Sometimes the predominant finding on CT consists of poorly defined centrilobular nodular opacities measuring 2 to 5 mm in diameter, shown pathologically to be bronchiolitis (Fig. 28–62).[957] As might be expected, patients who have CT findings consistent with bronchitis or bronchopneumonia (centrilobular nodules and peribronchial consolidation) are more likely to have a diagnostic BAL than those who have CT findings consistent with angioinvasive aspergillosis (nodules > 1 cm diameter, segmental consolidation); in one study of 21 patients who had proven *Aspergillus* infection, the procedure yielded fungus in 8 of 10 patients who had CT evidence of bronchitis or bronchopneumonia and only 2 of 11 who had angioinvasive disease.[957a]

Clinically, patients characteristically present with unremitting fever that responds poorly or not at all to antibiotic therapy; sometimes, there is an initial response and then failure. Dyspnea and tachypnea occur in cases of more extensive disease.[908]

nodular (resembling an abscess or angioinvasive disease; Fig. 28–60[908, 955, 956]).

The radiographic pattern is one of patchy or homogeneous air-space consolidation without specific features.[908] In one review of nine patients, the findings included bilateral air-space consolidation in five, unilateral consolidation in one, small ill-defined nodules in two, and a normal chest radiograph in one.[957] The most common findings on CT,

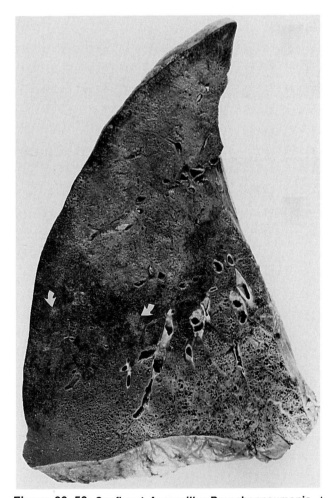

Figure 28–59. Confluent *Aspergillus* Bronchopneumonia. A slice of lower lobe shows fairly homogeneous hemorrhagic consolidation of the superior segment, resembling a pattern of air-space pneumonia. In contrast to this disease, however, the consolidation does not extend to the pleura and is associated with additional small foci of disease elsewhere *(arrows)*, indicating that it most likely represents confluence of multiple foci of bronchopneumonia.

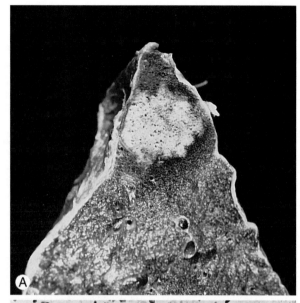

Figure 28–60. Aspergillosis—Nodular Air-Space Pneumonia. A magnified view of the superior segment of a lower lobe *(A)* shows a somewhat lobulated but well-circumscribed focus of consolidation in which the underlying lung architecture can be appreciated. Histologic sections show a partially necrotic neutrophilic exudate *(B)* containing fragmented hyphae (the latter evident only with silver stain *[C]*).

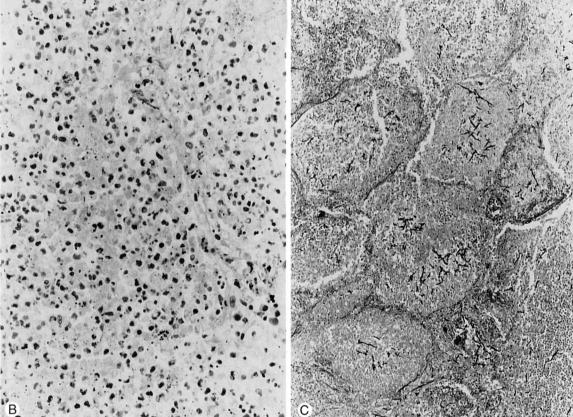

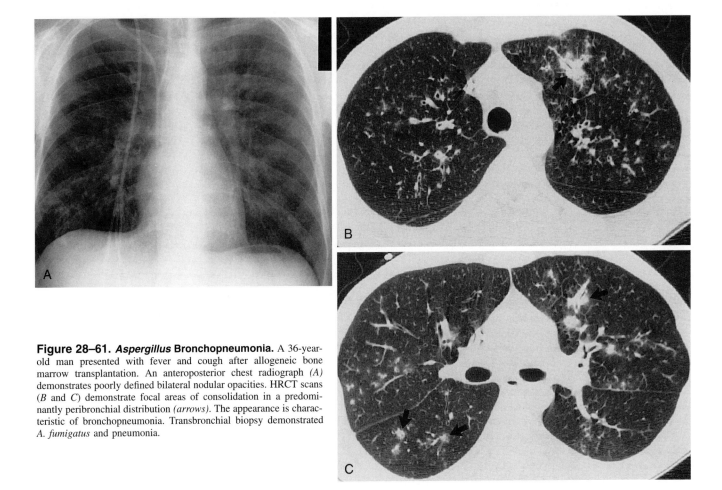

Figure 28–61. *Aspergillus* **Bronchopneumonia.** A 36-year-old man presented with fever and cough after allogeneic bone marrow transplantation. An anteroposterior chest radiograph *(A)* demonstrates poorly defined bilateral nodular opacities. HRCT scans *(B* and *C)* demonstrate focal areas of consolidation in a predominantly peribronchial distribution *(arrows).* The appearance is characteristic of bronchopneumonia. Transbronchial biopsy demonstrated *A. fumigatus* and pneumonia.

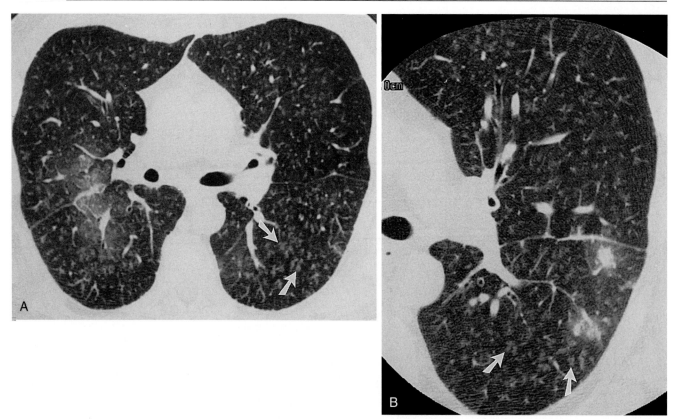

Figure 28–62. *Aspergillus* **Bronchiolitis and Bronchopneumonia.** HRCT *(A)* demonstrates a localized area of ground-glass attenuation in the right lung and bilateral poorly defined small nodular opacities. HRCT targeted to the left lung *(B)* better delineates the opacities *(arrows)* and shows them to have a centrilobular distribution characteristic of bronchiolitis. Focal areas of consolidation in the left lower lobe are also evident. Open-lung biopsy demonstrated *Aspergillus* bronchiolitis and bronchopneumonia. The patient was a 52-year-old man who had undergone bone marrow transplantation.

Angioinvasive Aspergillosis

Angioinvasive aspergillosis is probably the most common manifestation of invasive pulmonary aspergillosis. Although it can be seen in association with any of the other forms, it is frequently the sole abnormality. There are two pathologic patterns:[949, 958] (1) a relatively well-defined nodule with a pale or yellowish center and hemorrhagic rim (Fig. 28–63); and (2) a less well-defined, roughly wedge-shaped, pleural-based hemorrhagic area resembling a typical thromboembolic infarct (Fig. 28–64). Although the latter appearance probably reflects vascular occlusion and air-space hemorrhage with or without ischemic necrosis, it is likely that the former is the result of locally produced toxins diffusing into the adjacent lung parenchyma.[949] Histologic examination of the central (pale) portion of the nodules shows necrotic lung parenchyma infiltrated by numerous fungal hyphae (Fig. 28–63); the adjacent parenchyma shows intra-alveolar hemorrhage. Characteristically, there is also extensive vascular permeation and apparent occlusion of small to medium arteries by fungal hyphae (Fig. 28–44); thrombus may or may not be present. An inflammatory reaction is often absent or minimal (probably reflecting the granulocytopenia present in many patients); vasculitis is seen occasionally.

Fragments of necrotic lung infiltrated by fungus (pulmonary sequestra*) may become separated from viable parenchyma (Fig. 28–65), the space between the two representing the air crescents seen radiologically (*see* farther on). It has been speculated that the development of these seques-

tra is related to enzymatic liquefaction of pulmonary tissue at the junction of tissue invaded and not invaded by fungus.[959, 960] This hypothesis is supported by the observations that neutrophils are frequently prominent at this site and that the formation of sequestra in leukemic patients often occurs during bone marrow recovery and a rising neutrophil count. Despite this, neutrophils do not appear to be present in all cases,[961] and it is possible that additional mechanisms are involved.

The radiographic pattern consists of nodules or single or multiple areas of homogeneous consolidation (Fig. 28–66).[956, 962, 963] Cavitation is common[907, 964] and is sometimes manifested by an air crescent partly or completely surrounding a central homogeneous mass (Fig. 28–66).[965] This air-crescent sign can develop from 1 day to 3 weeks after the appearance of the initial radiographic abnormality.[909, 966–968] Occasionally, the characteristically patchy consolidation extends to involve an entire lobe, radiographically simulating acute bacterial pneumonia.[969] Pleural involvement is rare but may result in effusion or pneumothorax owing to a bronchopleural fistula.[970] Pneumopericardium occurs rarely.[947, 971]

---

*Although these intracavitary fragments of lung tissue have been termed *fungus balls* or *mycetomas* because of their resemblance radiologically to the saprophytic form of aspergillosis, it is clear that they are different with respect to pathogenesis, pathologic appearance, and clinical implication. As a result, these terms are inappropriate, and we advocate instead use of the term *pulmonary sequestrum*.[959]

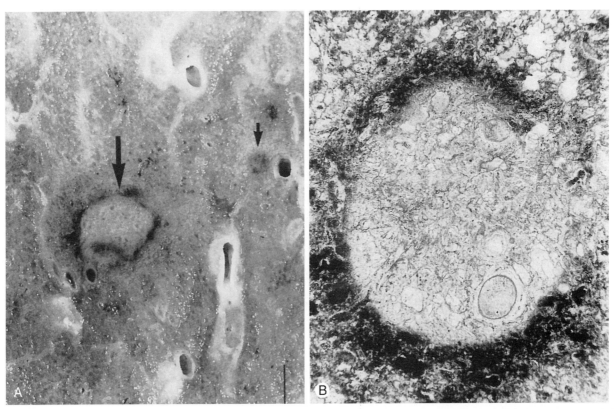

Figure 28–63. Angioinvasive Aspergillosis. A magnified view *(A)* of lung parenchyma shows a roughly circular focus of necrosis surrounded by a well-defined hemorrhagic rim *(long arrow)*. The underlying lung architecture is easily distinguished, implying coagulative necrosis. A smaller focus is present at the right *(short arrow)*. (Bar = 5 mm.) Corresponding histologic appearance *(B)* confirms that central pallor corresponds to necrotic lung parenchyma. *(B, ×16.)*

CT may demonstrate a characteristic finding in early angioinvasive aspergillosis, consisting of a halo of ground-glass attenuation surrounding a soft tissue nodule (Fig. 28–67).[968] This "halo sign" is related to the presence of hemorrhage surrounding the central necrotic nodule.[238, 972] With time, these lesions may develop air crescents or progress to frank cavitation (Fig. 28–68).[968] In the appropriate clinical setting, the presence of a soft tissue nodule with a halo sign is highly suggestive of angioinvasive aspergillosis.[968, 972] One prospective study involved 30 patients with granulocytopenia, nodular lesions on the chest radiograph, and clinical suspicion of invasive aspergillosis;[973] 22 patients had early invasive aspergillosis with clinical symptoms and signs for fewer than 10 days, and 8 had *Pseudomonas* or *Staphylococcus* infection. HRCT demonstrated a halo sign in 16 of the 22 patients with angioinvasive aspergillosis (sensitivity, 73%), but in none of 8 patients with nodular opacities related to bacterial infection (specificity, 100%). MR imaging had a similar sensitivity (73%), but zero specificity in the early diagnosis of aspergillosis; however, later in the course of the infection (clinical symptoms and signs > 10 days), it showed target-like lesions with increased signal intensity in the rim of the nodule and decreased signal intensity centrally. This was most evident using intravenous contrast enhancement with gadolinium diethylenetriaminepentaacetic acid (Gd-DTPA).

Despite the diagnostic usefulness of the halo sign,

not all patients with early angioinvasive aspergillosis have nodules surrounded by a halo of ground-glass attenuation.[238, 695, 974] Furthermore, a halo sign may be seen in association with nodules of other causes, including infection by *Candida* species, *Mucorales* species, cytomegalovirus, and herpes simplex; Wegener's granulomatosis; metastatic angiosarcoma; and Kaposi's sarcoma.[238, 695, 974a]

Patients with angioinvasive aspergillosis commonly present with fever, dyspnea, and nonproductive cough. Pleuritic chest pain is also frequent;[908] the combination of such pain with sinus tenderness, epistaxis, and nasal discharge has been stressed as a useful clue to the diagnosis.[975] Vascular infiltration by the fungus can result in several complications. Hemoptysis is the most frequent; when massive, it tends to occur during cavity formation,[966, 976] often shortly after recovery from chemotherapy-induced neutropenia.[977] *In situ* thrombosis of large pulmonary arteries may suggest a diagnosis of acute thromboembolic disease.[978] Mediastinal and chest wall vessels are also affected occasionally, resulting in the superior vena cava syndrome or an absent peripheral pulse from subclavian artery occlusion.[979] Invasion of the pleura[980] or chest wall[981] can result in effusion, fistulas, or osteomyelitis, with corresponding signs and symptoms. In the 25% to 50% of patients in whom dissemination occurs, involvement of the gastrointestinal tract (often associated with hemorrhage), central nervous system, or both is frequently a terminal event.[956]

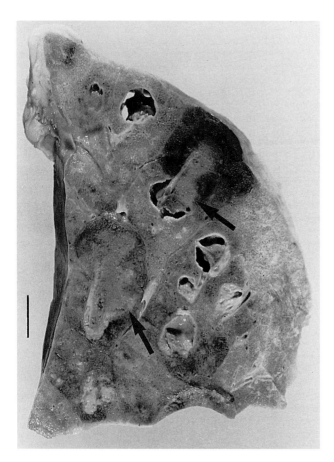

Figure 28–64. Invasive Aspergillosis—Parenchymal Hemorrhage. A small portion of lung shows several foci of necrosis *(arrows)* related to *Aspergillus* bronchopneumonia. One lobule has an additional hemorrhagic appearance in a pattern suggestive of infarction. Histologic examination showed extension of fungus into the pulmonary arteries adjacent to the inflamed airways; the lung parenchyma showed air-space hemorrhage without necrosis. (Bar = 0.5 cm.) (From Fraser RS: Pulmonary aspergillosis: Pathologic and pathogenetic features. *In* Rosen PP, Fechner RE [eds]: Pathology Annual, Part 1. Norwalk, CT, Appleton & Lange, 1993, p 231.)

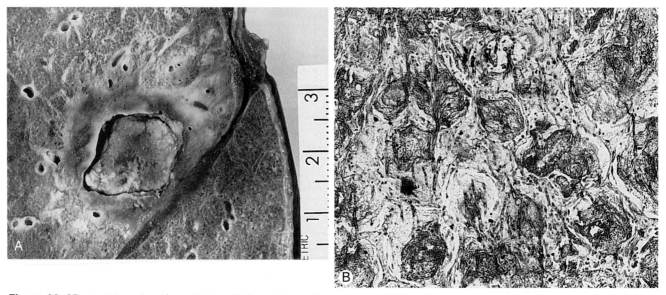

Figure 28–65. Angioinvasive Aspergillosis with Lung Sequestrum. A magnified view of an upper lobe and superior segment of lower lobe *(A)* shows a poorly defined focus of consolidation within which is a cavity containing a fragment of granular material resembling lung parenchyma. Histologic examination *(B)* shows the latter to consist of necrotic lung infiltrated by fungal hyphae. The patient had been treated for acute myelogenous leukemia (the thickening of the perivascular tissue above the cavity represents leukemic infiltration of the interstitium). (B, ×100.) (From Fraser RS: Pulmonary aspergillosis: Pathologic and pathogenetic features. *In* Rosen PP, Fechner RE [eds]: Pathology Annual, Part 1. Norwalk, CT, Appleton & Lange, 1993, p 231.)

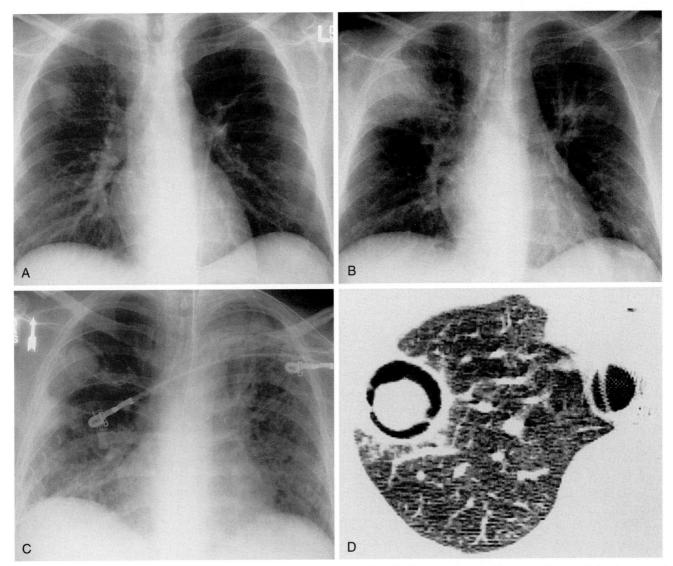

Figure 28–66. Angioinvasive Aspergillosis—Progression of Radiographic Findings. A 23-year-old patient with acute leukemia presented with fever and cough. An anteroposterior (AP) chest radiograph *(A)* demonstrates a rounded area of consolidation in the right upper lobe, which, 1 week later *(B)*, has shown considerable progression. The following day, the patient underwent open-lung biopsy that demonstrated pulmonary hemorrhage but failed to identify any organisms. An AP chest radiograph 2 weeks after biopsy *(C)* and HRCT *(D)* demonstrate a smoothly marginated cavity in the right upper lobe containing a soft tissue mass. Repeat biopsy performed under CT guidance confirmed the diagnosis of invasive aspergillosis, the soft tissue mass within the cavity representing necrotic lung (sequestrum).

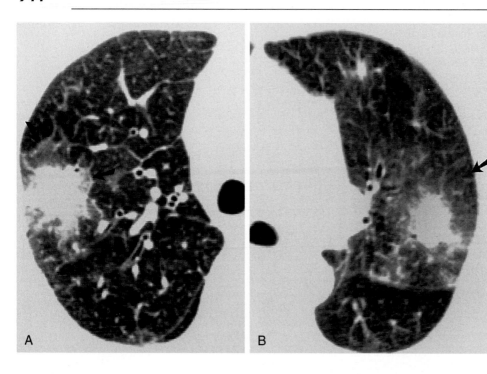

Figure 28–67. Angioinvasive Aspergillosis—CT Halo Sign. HRCT of the right upper *(A)* and left upper *(B)* lobes demonstrates nodules that are surrounded by a halo of ground-glass attenuation *(arrows)* (halo sign). The patient was a 72-year-old woman with severe neutropenia undergoing chemotherapy for leukemia. Diagnosis was proven by bronchoalveolar lavage.

Acute Tracheobronchitis

Acute tracheobronchitis is a relatively uncommon manifestation of invasive aspergillosis in which infection is limited principally to the larger airways with little, if any, extension of organisms into surrounding pulmonary parenchyma or blood vessels.[949, 982] The abnormality accounts for about 5% of cases of invasive disease. Although it can be seen in any immunocompromised patient,[983–985] there seems to be a particular predilection for patients with lung or heart-lung transplants,[914, 986] possibly related to increased airway susceptibility as a result of trauma at the anastomotic site or interruption of the bronchial vascular supply.

The reason why these cases are predominantly intraluminal with minimal tissue invasion is unclear. In one report, the degree and duration of neutropenia and the history of immunosuppressive therapy were less in patients with tracheobronchitis than in patients with other forms of invasive disease, suggesting that a lesser degree of host defense impairment might be responsible.[950] However, this speculation has not been supported by other investigations.

Pathologic findings consist of focal[914, 984] or diffuse[982] mucosal ulceration, often associated with pseudomembranes or occlusive plugs composed of mucus, sloughed epithelial cells, and hyphae (Fig. 28–69).[982] Microscopically, the surface epithelium is ulcerated, and there is usually an intense acute inflammatory reaction in the submucosa (Fig. 28–69). Typically, hyphae are seen only within the superficial portion of the bronchial wall; conidiophores are rather frequently identified.[907, 987] Rarely, bronchial aspergillosis is manifested pathologically as bronchocentric granulomatosis.[918, 929] Some of these cases have been associated with the chronic necrotizing form of disease (*see* farther on). Unless there is associated parenchymal disease, there may be little abnormality on the chest radiograph; patchy areas of atelectasis related to the mixed mucous/mycelial plugs may be the only radiographic clue to the diagnosis.[813]

Clinically, patients manifest dyspnea, cough, and hemoptysis; sputum production was scanty in seven of eight patients in one series,[908] possibly as a result of the extensive epithelial ulceration that resulted in deficient mucociliary clearance. Localized or generalized wheezing may be apparent.[988] If extensive enough or if located in a strategic site such as the trachea, the intraluminal mucous or hyphal plugs can lead to respiratory failure.[908] Occasionally, fungi extend through the airway wall; depending on their initial location and the direction in which they spread, they may then cause bronchoesophageal or bronchopleural fistulas[989] or sudden massive hemorrhage (as a result of infiltration of a major pulmonary artery).

Chronic Necrotizing Aspergillosis

Chronic necrotizing aspergillosis ("semi-invasive" aspergillosis) is a rare form of invasive aspergillosis characterized by slowly progressive upper-lobe disease that may spread to the contralateral lung, mediastinum, pleural space, or chest wall.[990, 991] Many patients have underlying chronic pulmonary disease, including remote infarction, inactive tuberculosis, chronic obstructive pulmonary disease, or fibrosis related to previous resectional surgery, radiation therapy, or pneumoconiosis. Although abnormalities of host defense may be apparent, they are typically relatively mild compared with those associated with more virulent forms of invasive disease (e.g., diabetes, poor nutrition, connective tissue disorders). A history of intensive immunosuppressive therapy is usually absent; however, some patients have been taking low doses of corticosteroids.

Pathologic findings have been described infrequently.[992] In most patients, there is a combination of necrosis, fibrosis, and granulomatous inflammation resembling that seen with fibrocaseous tuberculosis;[990, 992] coagulative necrosis and vascular invasion by fungal hyphae similar to the angioinvasive

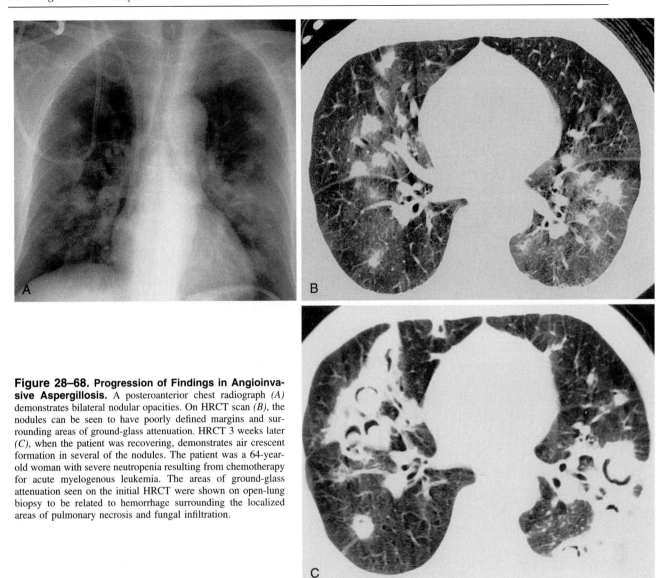

Figure 28–68. Progression of Findings in Angioinvasive Aspergillosis. A posteroanterior chest radiograph *(A)* demonstrates bilateral nodular opacities. On HRCT scan *(B)*, the nodules can be seen to have poorly defined margins and surrounding areas of ground-glass attenuation. HRCT 3 weeks later *(C)*, when the patient was recovering, demonstrates air crescent formation in several of the nodules. The patient was a 64-year-old woman with severe neutropenia resulting from chemotherapy for acute myelogenous leukemia. The areas of ground-glass attenuation seen on the initial HRCT were shown on open-lung biopsy to be related to hemorrhage surrounding the localized areas of pulmonary necrosis and fungal infiltration.

form of disease may also be seen. A less common manifestation is the presence of a a large ectatic airway containing abundant fungal hyphae similar in appearance to a fungus ball; in contrast to the latter, however, focal necrosis of the airway wall is associated with invasive hyphae. Occasional cases have also been described in which there was massive parenchymal necrosis and relatively little fibrosis[993] or bronchocentric granulomatosis.[992, 994]

Radiographic manifestations usually consist initially of an area of consolidation in the upper lobe, which develops progressive cavitation over several weeks or months.[813] The cavitation may be associated with an intracavitary soft tissue opacity. Adjacent pleural thickening is common. The process may extend to involve the chest wall and mediastinum.[813]

Clinically, the disease has an indolent course (typically months and sometimes years); in one series of 10 patients, the duration of signs and symptoms from onset to time of diagnosis ranged from 2 to 24 months (mean, 8.6 months).[992] Cough, expectoration (sometimes bloody), fever, and weight loss are the usual features. An increased white blood cell count is not infrequent. Spread of the infection outside the thorax is uncommon; however, in some cases, it has been successfully controlled.[992]

Diagnosis

The diagnosis of invasive aspergillosis should be suspected in any patient who is immunocompromised or has acute leukemia or other lymphoreticular or hematologic disease associated with granulocytopenia when fever does not respond to broad-spectrum antibiotics. It may be difficult to prove. Sputum is unavailable for culture in many cases; even when present, the sensitivity of such culture (which depends on the number of specimens and on the nature of the underlying disease) is probably in the order of 50% to 60%.[995, 996] Similar values have been found for culture of respiratory tract secretions sampled by BAL or bronchial washing or brushing. To compound matters, a positive culture may reflect simple colonization. Nevertheless, in the appropriate clinical setting, repeated positive sputum or BAL fluid cultures have been found to be a reliable method of diagnosis,[996–998] particularly when accompanied by protected brush

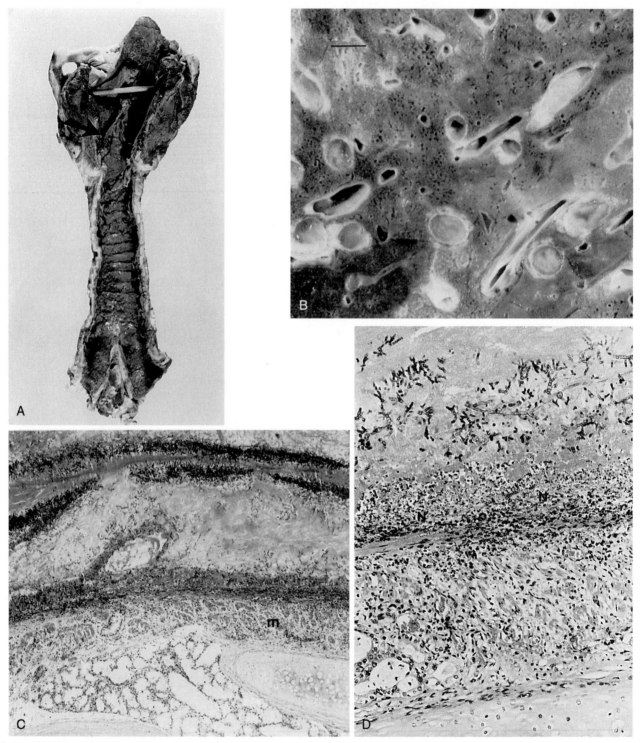

Figure 28–69. *Aspergillus* **Tracheobronchitis.** The anterior mucosa of the larynx and trachea from a patient with acute leukemia *(A)* shows a pseudomembrane in the upper portion *(arrow)* and diffuse fine granularity in the lower. Close-up view of an upper lobe removed at autopsy from a 23-year-old woman who died of respiratory failure 6 weeks after bone marrow transplantation *(B)* shows most airways to be completely occluded by mucous plugs. (The parenchyma shows changes indicative of organizing diffuse alveolar damage, consistent with the respiratory distress syndrome.) Other lobes were similar. (Bar = 5 mm.) Sections from one of the affected bronchi *(C, D)* show mucus permeated by numerous fungal hyphae within the bronchial lumen. The epithelium is destroyed and replaced by a layer of neutrophils (mostly necrotic) (N); there is no fungal invasion beneath the muscularis mucosa (m). *(C,* ×40; *D,* ×250.)

and transbronchial biopsy specimens obtained at bronchoscopy.[913, 999] Surveillance nasal cultures may also help in decision making,[1000, 1001] but negative results do not exclude the diagnosis. Blood cultures are infrequently positive.[814] Culture and histochemical staining of cytocentrifuged material obtained by BAL have been reported to have a high diagnostic yield.[998]

Serologic diagnosis has not been widely used; however, one group of investigators found measuring of *A. fumigatus*–specific IgG to be useful in following patients who had undergone lung transplantation.[1002] An LA test based on the identification of serum galactomannan (a cell wall component of *Aspergillus*) has been found to have a sensitivity ranging from about 15% to 95% in different series;[995] some, albeit not all,[1002a] investigators have found that identification of this substance in serum or BAL fluid by an ELISA technique may be diagnostically useful.[1003, 1004]

The use of PCR[755, 1005, 1006] or radioimmunoassay[1007] in specimens of blood or BAL fluid is also likely to prove valuable in diagnosis, particularly in neutropenic patients before the onset of radiographic abnormalities. For example, in one investigation of 601 blood samples from four groups (control patients [35], patients with febrile neutropenia either with [36] or without [29] evidence of fungal colonization, and patients with documented invasive fungal infection [21]), detection of *Aspergillus* by PCR of blood was associated with most of the clinically relevant infections (sensitivity of 100% if two specimens were tested and specificity of 98%).[1006]

Prognosis

The prognosis of invasive aspergillosis is generally poor. Recovery is associated with early diagnosis, appropriate therapy, and reversal of the underlying immunosuppression.[909, 1008, 1009] For these reasons, there seems to be general agreement that when the diagnosis is strongly suspected, empiric treatment with fungicide(s) should be initiated promptly and continued aggressively until resolution of disease.[1010] Resectional surgery also may be required for cure in some cases.[909, 913, 913a]

ZYGOMYCOSIS

Zygomycosis (mucormycosis, phycomycosis) is caused by fungi of the orders Entomophthorales and Mucorales, which includes a variety of species in the genera *Conidiobolus*,[1011] *Basidiobolus*, *Rhizopus*, *Rhizomucor*, *Mucor*, *Absidia*,[1012] *Saksenaea*,[1013] and *Cunninghamella*.[1014–1017] In tissue, the organisms appear as broad (5 to 20 μm), frequently irregular, nonseptate hyphae that generally branch at a 90-degree angle. *Rhizopus* species are responsible for the acute rhinocerebral form of the disease, whereas a variety of species of other genera, as well as *Rhizopus*, are the cause of pulmonary disease.[90] The pathologic and radiographic features of thoracic disease caused by all species are similar. *Rhizopus* species have also been implicated occasionally as a cause of extrinsic allergic alveolitis.[1018]

Epidemiology

The fungi are ubiquitous and worldwide in distribution. They are commonly found in decaying organic material, such as fruit or bread, and are frequent laboratory contaminants. In culture and in nature, hyphae produce large sporangia that liberate sporangiospores into the air; inhalation of the latter is believed to cause most cases of human infection. Uncommonly, the disease occurs by direct cutaneous invasion from contaminated material such as surgical dressings.[1019]

Infection occurs almost invariably in patients with underlying disease, particularly during treatment with corticosteroids or antibiotics. The most common primary diseases are diabetes (especially when associated with ketoacidosis), chronic (and rarely acute[1020]) renal failure, lymphoma, and leukemia.[1021] In one autopsy series of patients with leukemia, it was identified in 2% of cases.[1022] *Rhizopus* species, in particular, appear to have a predilection for patients with acidosis; many cases of rhinocerebral involvement occur in diabetics with ketoacidosis.[1023] Patients with an acidotic state from diarrhea, uremia,[90] and even chronic salicylate poisoning[1024] are also at risk. Infection has only rarely been reported in apparently normal hosts.[1025, 1026] As with aspergillosis, neutropenia is also an important predisposing factor.[1027]

Pathologic Characteristics

Histologically, the inflammatory reaction to the fungus is variable, ranging from none to an intense neutrophil infiltrate. Multinucleated giant cells are sometimes present, apparently in relationship to fragments of dead or degenerating hyphae;[1019, 1027] true granuloma formation is rare.[1019, 1028] Fungal hyphae are often seen within vascular lumens and extending through their walls into the adjacent pulmonary parenchyma (Fig. 28–70); concomitant necrosis and hemorrhage are common.[793, 1019, 1027]

The organisms are broad and nonseptate and stain well with H & E and Grocott's methenamine silver. Sporangia[1024] and chlamydoconidia[1029] can occasionally be seen. The most important fungus with which *Mucor* species can be confused histologically is *Aspergillus*. The fact that *Aspergillus* organisms are septate, are usually relatively thin, and show regular dichotomous branching at a 45-degree angle aids in differentiation; however, some varieties of *Aspergillus* closely resemble *Mucor* species (and vice versa), and culture is desirable for definitive identification.

Radiologic Manifestations

The most common radiographic findings consist of unilateral or bilateral air-space consolidation.[1030] Lung involvement is frequently segmental and homogeneous, reflecting the vascular obstruction.[1031–1033] The consolidation may also be round and rapidly progressive (Fig. 28–71);[1034] occasionally, there is lobar expansion.[1030] Another common presentation consists of solitary or multiple, small or large nodules;[1030] in one case, a nodular opacity was found to be a thrombosed vessel subtending a pulmonary infarct.[1035] As with angioinvasive aspergillosis, CT may show a halo of ground-glass attenuation surrounding the nodule (halo sign).[974a] Occlusion of a major pulmonary artery has been demonstrated angiographically.[1036] Cavitation is frequent, and

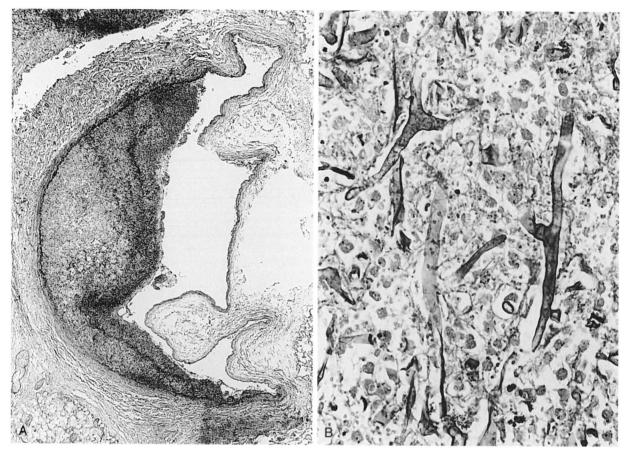

Figure 28–70. Mucormycosis. A large pulmonary vein is partly occluded by a mass of fungus *(A)* associated with minimal thrombus or inflammatory reaction. High magnification *(B)*, shows broad, nonseptate hyphae, some with a folded or wrinkled appearance. *(A, ×18; B, ×500.)*

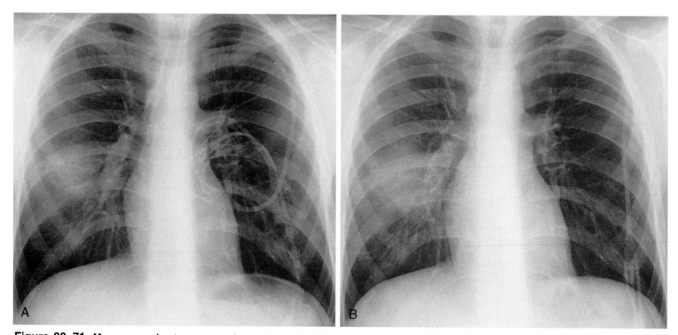

Figure 28–71. Mucormycosis. A posteroanterior *(A)* chest radiograph demonstrates a rounded area of consolidation in the superior segment of the right lower lobe. A follow-up radiograph obtained the next day *(B)* shows considerable increase in size of the consolidation. Because of the patient's severe clinical findings, a right lower lobectomy was performed. This demonstrated hemorrhagic necrosis with extensive angioinvasive mucormycosis. The patient was a 15-year-old boy with severe neutropenia secondary to chemotherapy for acute leukemia. (Case courtesy of Dr. James Barrie, University of Alberta Hospital, Edmonton, Canada.)

the chest radiograph may show a crescent sign identical to that in angioinvasive aspergillosis;[1037–1039] as with the latter disease, this often occurs at the same time as chemotherapy-induced remission.[1022] Associated findings seen in a small percentage of patients include hilar and mediastinal lymph node enlargement and unilateral or bilateral pleural effusion.[1030] Because mucormycosis can be a rapidly progressive disease, it is perhaps not surprising that the chest radiograph is sometimes interpreted as normal shortly before death even when extensive pneumonia is found at autopsy.[1040]

Clinical Manifestations

Mucormycosis can be divided into several clinicopathologic varieties, of which the main forms are rhinocerebral, pulmonary, cutaneous and subcutaneous (including sternotomy wound sites[1041]), and gastrointestinal. Usually there is only local progression of disease at these sites, although dissemination occasionally results in multiorgan involvement.[1019, 1027] Rhinocerebral mucormycosis is a fulminant disease that involves the nose and paranasal sinuses and frequently extends into the orbits and cranium;[1023] occasionally, it extends to the lungs, presumably by aspiration, or elsewhere in the body through the bloodstream. As indicated previously, the infection often occurs in a patient with uncontrolled diabetes.

Primary pulmonary mucormycosis occurs most often in individuals with lymphoproliferative or hematologic disorders; transplant recipients[1042, 1043] or diabetics are less frequently affected.[1044] Patients are usually ill with fever, chest pain, and bloody sputum. Massive pulmonary hemorrhage, commonly fatal, can occur as a result of erosion of a pulmonary artery.[977, 1045–1047] In most instances, this complication is preceded by radiographic opacities, often with cavitation or air crescents; rarely, it is a presenting feature in a patient without radiologically evident disease.[1048] Infrequent complications include pulmonary artery aneurysm,[1049, 1050] pulmonary vein thrombosis with pulmonary infarction,[1051] bronchopleural fistula,[1052] superior vena caval obstruction,[1053] empyema,[1054] mediastinitis,[1028] peripheral neurologic symptoms following extension to the vertebral column and spinal cord,[1055] tracheal destruction,[1056] and tracheal or bronchial obstruction caused by an intraluminal fungal mass.[1057–1059] The diagnosis in any of these situations can be difficult to make and usually requires histologic confirmation.

The prognosis is grave; in one review of the literature published in 1994, the mortality rate for patients with isolated pulmonary disease was 65% and for those with disseminated disease approximately 95%.[1021] Some therapeutic success can be achieved with control of diabetes and reduction or cessation of immunosuppressive therapy; however, aggressive antifungal medication, surgery, or both are usually required.

GEOTRICHOSIS

Geotrichosis is a rare infection caused by *Geotrichum candidum*, a ubiquitous yeast-like fungus that in nature is found in soil, sewage, animal excreta, and a variety of dairy and other spoiled food products. It can also be a normal inhabitant of the human gastrointestinal tract[1060] and is sometimes isolated from the sputum of healthy subjects.[1061] There are no known endemic areas; occupational associations; or age, sex, or racial predispositions. In the majority of cases, the disease is believed to be caused by infection by endogenous saprophytic organisms. In sputum stained with Gram or PAS stain, the fungi appear as fragments of septate hyphae associated with large rectangular arthrospores measuring 4 to 12 μm in diameter; in tissue, these are frequently rounded.[1061]

G. candidum is detected most frequently as a saprophyte in the sputum of patients who have chronic pulmonary disease. Disease is rare and has been divided into bronchial and bronchopulmonary forms. The former is characterized by symptoms of bronchitis or asthma, sometimes associated with eosinophilia.[1062, 1063] Bronchoscopic or gross pathologic examination reveals yellow-white plaques similar to those of oral candidiasis adherent to the airway mucosa.[1061] Invasion of underlying parenchyma does not occur. By contrast, in the bronchopulmonary form, tissue invasion is characteristic and may be extensive. Fever and hemoptysis are present in most cases, and crackles, rhonchi, and signs of consolidation may be detected. In both bronchial and bronchopulmonary forms, purulent expectoration may be copious, and the sputum may be gelatinous.[1060] Pathologic features in fatal cases have been those of bronchopneumonia associated with an acute inflammatory reaction.[1060, 1061] Rarely, the lungs have been reported to be involved as part of a hematogenous systemic infection derived from an extrapulmonary source.[1064] In one patient, fungemia was reported to occur after bronchoscopy; at autopsy, there was no evidence of tissue invasion.[1065]

Radiographic findings are not distinctive. The bronchial form of the disease may show no abnormalities[1062] or merely an accentuation of basal pulmonary markings.[1063] The bronchopulmonary form usually is manifested by parenchymal consolidation, predominantly in the upper lobes and frequently associated with thin-walled cavities.[1066]

A positive skin test or agglutination test is useful in confirming the presence of the fungus;[1063] however, false-positive reactions have been described in normal subjects and in patients with fungal disease of other cause.[1060] Because colonization is relatively more common than infection, tissue confirmation of the presence of fungus and an inflammatory reaction to it are desirable before the disease is definitively diagnosed.

SPOROTRICHOSIS

Sporotrichosis is caused by *S. schenckii*, a dimorphic fungus that is a common saprophyte of worldwide distribution. The organism has been isolated from soil, sphagnum moss, peat moss, decaying vegetable matter, thorns, and a variety of other substances; rarely, it can be isolated from secretions derived from the normal human respiratory tract.[794, 1067–1069] The disease is usually acquired by direct inoculation of organisms into the skin through a scratch from thorns, splinters, grasses, or other contaminated objects. In many cases, this can be considered an occupational hazard, individuals such as farmers, laborers, florists, and horticulturalists being especially vulnerable.[1070, 1071] The organism is also occasionally transmitted by animal or insect bites or by contact with infected animals or (rarely) humans.[1070] Respiratory disease is usually primary and presumably results from inhalation of airborne spores; occasionally, it represents dissemination from cutaneous lesions.

Most affected individuals have no evidence of immunodeficiency, particularly when the infection is confined to the skin; however, alcoholics appear to be unusually susceptible to both cutaneous and pulmonary disease.[1072–1076] Despite these observations, immunologic studies have shown cell-mediated immunity to be normal in patients who have cutaneous disease but abnormal in those with the disseminated form;[1077] moreover, there is evidence that immunocompromised patients are at increased risk.[1078] Disease is most frequently seen in Central and South America (especially Mexico, Brazil, and Uruguay), South Africa, Japan, and the United States.[1070] The incubation period in the cutaneous form averages about 3 weeks. Repeated exposure in endemic areas is said to confer immunity.[90]

Pathologic characteristics of pulmonary lesions resemble those of postprimary tuberculosis and usually consist of solitary or multiple thin-walled cavities of variable size surrounded by patchy areas of ill-defined parenchymal consolidation;[1070, 1079] occasionally, solitary peripheral nodules (sporotrichomas) have been identified.[1080] Although neutrophils appear to be important in the host reaction to the fungus,[1081, 1082] the typical histologic appearance consists of multifocal areas of liquefactive or coagulative necrosis surrounded by a granulomatous inflammatory infiltrate containing numerous giant cells;[1070, 1079, 1080] well-defined granulomas tend to be sparse.[1083] Fibrosis is frequently present and may be prominent. Organisms stain with PAS and Grocott's methenamine stains but can be rather scanty and difficult to identify with certainty.[17] They may assume several forms, including cigar shapes (gram-positive spindle-shaped rods up to 10 μm in length), round or oval budding yeasts 3 to 5 μm in diameter, hyphae, or "asteroid bodies" (consisting of a central 3- to 5-μm yeast form from which emanate numerous eosinophilic projections—the Splendore-Hoeppli phenomenon). Immunohistochemical reactions are considerably more sensitive in detecting the organisms than routine histochemical stains.[1084]

Radiographically the disease also closely resembles postprimary tuberculosis and as a result is probably frequently misdiagnosed.[1072] Findings include isolated nodular masses that may cavitate and leave thin-walled cavities[1072, 1085–1087] and a diffuse reticulonodular pattern.[1076] Hilar lymph node enlargement occurs in many cases and may cause bronchial obstruction;[1088] bronchopulmonary and mediastinal lymph node enlargement can be present in the absence of parenchymal disease.[90, 1089] In some cases, pulmonary disease spreads through the pleura into the chest wall, creating a sinus tract.[1088] Pulmonary manifestations depend on whether the lung is the only site of involvement:[1090] if no other organ systems are affected (skin, bone, joints), lung changes are indistinguishable from those of postprimary tuberculosis; however, if the skin or joints are also involved, chest radiographs tend to show multiple small nodules that are seldom cavitary.

Sporotrichosis has a variety of clinical forms, including lymphocutaneous (by far the most frequent), mucocutaneous, extracutaneous (usually musculoskeletal and occasionally pulmonary), and disseminated. A review of the medical records of the Mayo Clinic covering a 45-year period disclosed 58 cases, 11 of which were associated with extracutaneous infection; in 7 of these, the joints were affected.[1091] Clinical manifestations in the cutaneous form consist of a pustule on the hand or arm accompanied by enlargement of regional lymph nodes. Pulmonary involvement may be associated with severe malaise, cough, and fever. In disseminated disease, the joints may be tender and swollen; anemia and polymorphonuclear leukocytosis may develop. The diagnosis should be considered in any case of chronic cavitary disease suspected of being tuberculosis in which acid-fast organisms are not found. Such disease may progress slowly over several years.[1092]

The organism can readily be isolated from the sputum[1088] and may be seen in sputum specimens submitted for cytologic examination.[1092, 1093] However, as indicated previously, it can exist as a simple saprophyte, and its presence in these specimens does not necessarily indicate disease.[1094] In addition, isolated laryngeal involvement may be a source of organisms in the absence of lower respiratory tract infection.[1095] Serologic investigation using the direct fluorescent antibody technique appears to be highly specific.[1096] Skin test reactions to sporotrichin also may be helpful in some cases; however, in two studies of prison inmates and hospital patients without a history of sporotrichosis, approximately 10% of 552 individuals were positive reactors.[1097, 1098]

ADIASPIROMYCOSIS

Adiaspiromycosis is a disease of worldwide distribution that is found in many animals but only rarely in humans.[1099, 1100] It is caused by the dimorphic fungus *Chrysosporium parvum* (*Emmonsia crescens*). Infection is believed to be acquired by inhalation of spores (aleuriospores) measuring 3 to 4 μm in diameter that are produced by mycelial organisms in the soil.[1101] Within the lungs, individual spores grow into large (200 to 600 μm), thick-walled adiaspores that apparently do not proliferate by either endosporulation or budding. In the natural infection, systemic spread is believed not to occur outside the lung, the life cycle being completed when the infected animal dies and liberates the adiaspores. Infection in humans results in variably severe disease, ranging from solitary granulomas discovered as an incidental finding at autopsy[1099] to extensive bilateral pneumonia.[1102] The latter is believed to be caused by the inhalation of an unusually large number of aleuriospores, although endogenous spread of infection has also been considered a possibility.[1102]

Pathologically, the lungs show a variable number of firm white nodules usually ranging in diameter from 1 to 2 mm.[1101, 1103, 1104] Histologically, the nodules are composed of one to five adiaspores associated with either a granulomatous or suppurative reaction; necrosis may or may not be present. In older lesions, concentric layers of thick collagen are present at the periphery. The adiaspores are spherical, measure between 200 and 300 μm in diameter, and possess a thick (20 to 70 μm) wall that stains with PAS and Grocott's silver methenamine. Occasionally, the spores collapse, resulting in a variety of shapes and sizes that may obscure the diagnosis.[1103]

The characteristic radiographic finding is diffuse reticulonodular disease suggestive of miliary tuberculosis.[1102–1104] Patients may be asymptomatic or complain of low-grade fever, cough, and dyspnea.[1102, 1104] In one unusual case, numerous adiaspores were identified in association with chronic left lower lobe bronchiectasis, although it was not established that the two were pathogenetically related.[1105] Follow-up of the occasional patient in whom the diagnosis has been made during life has shown the disease to be generally self-limited and without significant sequelae;[1100] however, progression can occur and require surgical intervention.[1104]

PSEUDALLESCHERIASIS

Pseudallescheriasis (allescheriasis, monosporidiosis, petriellidiosis) is caused by a ubiquitous soil-inhabiting and sewage-inhabiting fungus that in its perfect form is known as *P. boydii* (*Allescheria boydii, Petriellidium boydii*) and in its imperfect form as *Scedosporium apiospermum* (*Monosporium apiospermum*).[798] In tissue, the organism appears as septate hyphae similar to *Aspergillus* species, from which it usually cannot be confidently distinguished by morphology alone.

Although the most common clinical manifestation of infection is a subcutaneous mycetoma, the organism has also been found in a variety of other locations.[1106] In the lungs, it occurs most frequently as a colonizer in association with immunosuppressive or corticosteroid therapy and with chronic fibrotic disease, such as tuberculosis,[797, 1107] sarcoidosis,[1108] or ankylosing spondylitis.[1109, 1110] Allergic bronchopulmonary disease similar to that caused by *Aspergillus* has also been documented.[1111] Occasionally, the organism is isolated from the sputum of patients who show no radiographic evidence of disease.[1106] Rare cases of apparently primary pneumonia have also been reported, sometimes associated with widespread dissemination.[1112–1114] These usually occur in patients with cancer or connective tissue or other systemic or immunocompromising disease;[1115, 1116] however, they have also been reported in otherwise healthy individuals.[1115, 1117, 1118]

Pathologically, the infection can be manifested as a typical fungus ball[797, 798, 1107, 1119] or as hyphae lining the wall of a pre-existing cavity without significant intracavitary growth.[1108] In most cases in which there has been histologic examination, lung tissue surrounding the fungal hyphae has shown only fibrosis and chronic inflammation accompanied by a variable amount of granulation tissue. Occasionally, an acute inflammatory or chronic granulomatous reaction has been identified,[1117, 1120] in some cases associated with tissue or vascular invasion.[1121, 1122] Cavitation and sequestrum formation identical to invasive aspergillosis have also been described.[1123]

The radiographic patterns are also similar to those of aspergillosis, consisting of a fungus ball, bronchiectasis (in patients with allergic disease), or nodules with or without cavitation, sometimes accompanied by a pulmonary sequestrum.[1107, 1108, 1119, 1124]

Clinically, affected patients may be asymptomatic or may suffer repeated episodes of hemoptysis; sometimes, the only symptoms and signs are those of the underlying disease.

Many of the reported cases have involved farmers or other individuals from rural areas.[797, 1110, 1117] Extension from the lungs to contiguous thoracic spine has been reported.[1118] Symptoms of asthma associated with peripheral eosinophilia and an elevated serum IgE are seen in patients with allergic disease.[1111]

The fungus can be cultured from sputum or blood, and precipitating antibodies are found in the serum.[797, 1107] Confident identification is usually not possible by histologic examination alone, and the organism must be cultured for certain diagnosis. In several cases, *Aspergillus* species and *P. boydii* have coexisted in the same lesion.[1109, 1112]

PENICILLIOSIS

Penicillium species are ubiquitous inhabitants of soil and decomposing organic matter. Although more than 300 have been described, the most frequent to be implicated in human infection is *P. marneffei*;[1125–1127] rare examples of invasive disease caused by other species have been reported.[1127a, 1130] The organisms are common airborne contaminants of culture media, and care must be exercised in interpreting a positive culture result as definitive evidence of disease. Despite this, the organism is clearly a potential pathogen in a variety of sites, including the lungs[1128, 1129] and pleura.[1130] One review of the literature published in 1996 documented 155 cases.[1131] Most have been in individuals residing in Southeast Asia;[1131] approximately 1,300 cases are said to have occurred in Thailand in 1995.[1132] Although the disease can also develop elsewhere, most often there is a history of residence in or travel to an endemic region.[1125]

Approximately 80% of patients have evidence of underlying immunodeficiency;[1131] in fact, in endemic areas, the organism has been found to be the third most common cause of opportunistic infection in patients with AIDS.[1131] Occasional patients are otherwise healthy.[1128] As might be expected, an experimental animal model of disease has shown cell-mediated immunity to be important in pathogenesis.[1133]

In one series, pathologic findings consisted of randomly distributed ''abscesses'' composed of necrotic tissue surrounded by numerous macrophages.[1128] Although true granulomas were not evident in this review, they have been documented by other investigators.[1125] Organisms stain well with PAS and Grocott's methenamine silver stains and can be present in both necrotic foci and in macrophage cytoplasm. They can be confused in both tissue and cytologic specimens with *P. carinii* and *H. capsulatum*.[1126, 1127] Identification of the organism in formalin-fixed tissue has been carried out with a monclonal antibody directed to galactomannan.[1134]

Clinical features include fever, weight loss, anemia, and leukocytosis.[1131] Skin lesions (usually papules with or without central necrosis) occur in about two thirds of patients.[1134] Hepatomegaly and lymph node enlargement can be present. Pleural effusion has been reported with absence of disease elsewhere.[1130] Cough is the principal manifestation of pulmonary involvement. An unusual case of upper airway obstruction caused by a *Penicillium*-related retropharyngeal abscess has been described.[1135] Preliminary studies using ID and LA tests to identify *P. marneffei* antigens[1136] and a fluorescent-antibody test for the tissue form of the organism[1136a] have shown some promise.

MISCELLANEOUS FUNGI

Malassezia furfur (*Pityrosporum orbiculare* and *Pityrosporum ovale*) is a fungus that is found normally on the skin and is responsible for several relatively innocuous dermatitides. Growth requires a high concentration of free fatty acids, a feature possibly related to the occasional instances of pulmonary and other visceral infections in patients receiving intravenous lipid therapy. It has been suggested that the organisms originate on the skin of the affected patient and subsequently migrate along the outside of the intravascular catheter;[1137] however, there is also evidence that they can be introduced in contaminated fat emulsion, intravenous fluids, or the tubing itself.[1137] Two groups appear to be at risk for the disease—neonates who have underlying cardiopulmonary disease and adults who have severe gastrointestinal disease and immunosuppression. Pathologically, small to medium-sized pulmonary arteries contain intravascular lipid, in some cases harboring *Malassezia* organisms; vasculitis is frequently present.[1138] The fungus can be identified by silver and Gram stains as a 2- to 4-μm, round-to-elliptical budding yeast. Radiographic findings have been reported to consist predominantly of streaky bilateral infiltrates (sic) and lobar consolidation.[1138] Clinically, all reported patients have received intravenous lipid therapy through a central venous catheter, typically for a prolonged period of time.

A variety of fungal organisms that are usually considered nonpathogenic for humans can cause disease in a host whose immune status is compromised. With the increasing use of anticancer chemotherapy and the improved treatment and prolonged survival of many immunodeficient individuals, such organisms will probably be recognized with increasing frequency. Pulmonary infection is often part of a systemic mycosis, but may be an isolated finding. Clinical and radiographic features are nonspecific, and identification of the organisms requires culture.

Examples of unusual fungi that have been identified as the causative agent of pneumonia include *Fusarium* species,[1139] *Chaetomium* species,[715] *Trichosporon* species (most often *T. beigelii* [*T. cutaneum*] and rarely *T. capitatum*),[1140–1142] and *Kluyveromyces fragilis*.[1143] *Hansenula polymorpha* was cultured from a child with chronic granulomatous disease who developed mediastinal lymphadenitis.[1144] *Curvularia lunata* has been reported to be associated with fungus ball formation[852] and disseminated infection in an alcoholic patient with chronic obstructive pulmonary disease.[1145] One case has been reported in which inhalation of *Trichosporon terrestre*, which was found in the house dust of the affected patient, might have caused acute eosinophilic pneumonia.[1146] Organisms of the genera *Bipolaris* and *Exserohilum* can also cause pulmonary disease whose manifestations are believed to be related to a hypersensitivity reaction.[1147]

Alternaria species are common soil saprophytes that are frequent laboratory contaminants. Their inhaled conidia have been implicated as a cause of extrinsic allergic alveolitis and asthma.[1148] In addition, one exceptional case has been described of a young, apparently immunocompetent man whose chest radiograph revealed nodular opacities and who presented with weight loss, fatigue, and dyspnea; the resected specimen revealed necrotizing granulomas that contained stainable and culturable *Alternaria* macroconidia.[1149]

ACTINOMYCETOUS INFECTION

The order Actinomycetales contains a number of species that can cause human disease. Although some of these have fairly typical bacterial features (such as the mycobacteria), other families show a number of fungal characteristics, including the formation of mycelia, extensive branching in a fungal pattern in tissue, and frequent production of chronic necrotizing and fibrosing disease. For these reasons, these species are often categorized with the true fungi for purposes of discussion, and this custom is followed here. Despite this categorization, their ultrastructural characteristics, the presence of muramic acid within the cell wall, and their sensitivity to "ordinary" antibiotics and insensitivity to antifungal agents all indicate that they are bacteria, not fungi.

Organisms responsible for human disease derive from two families, the Actinomycetaceae and the Nocardiaceae. By far the most important genera are *Actinomyces* and *Nocardia*; cases have also been reported of pneumonia in immunocompromised patients caused by *Rhodococcus equi* (*see* page 1645) and by *Rothia dentocariosa*.[1150] Rare infections that histologically resemble actinomycosis but are caused by other bacteria (bacterial pseudomycosis, botryomycosis) are also discussed in this section.

ACTINOMYCOSIS

Actinomycosis is caused by members of the family Actinomycetaceae, of which the most important genus is *Actinomyces*. This contains several species, including *A. israelii*, which has traditionally been regarded as the most important cause of disease in humans, and *A. bovis*, which produces lumpy jaw disease in cattle and rare instances of human infection. Other species known to cause human actinomycosis are *A. odontolyticus*,[1151] *A. naeslundi*,[1153, 1154] *A. viscosus*,[1152, 1153, 1155, 1156] *A. meyeri*,[1157] *A. neuii*,[1158] *A. pyogenes*,[1159] *Bifidobacterium eriksonii* (*Actinomyces eriksonii*),[1160] and *Arachnia propionica* (*Actinomyces propionicus*).[1161] Clinical, pathologic, and radiographic features of disease are similar with all species.

The organisms are nonmotile and non–spore-forming and consist of branching filaments about 0.2 to 0.3 μm in diameter that are pleomorphic in shape. They are anaerobic or microaerophilic and form mycelia that fragment into bacillary or coccobacillary forms. Within tissue, mycelia are characteristically aggregated in clusters called *sulfur granules* because of their yellow color (although their sulfur content is minimal).[1160] The granules range in diameter from 40 to greater than 400 μm, the larger ones being visible with the naked eye in pus or tissue. Microscopically, they are round-to-oval, slightly lobulated, basophilic masses that often possess a series of radiating, eosinophilic, club-shaped enlargements at their periphery (Fig. 28–72). In the center of the granules, organisms can usually be identified as gram-positive and silver-positive filaments, although they occa-

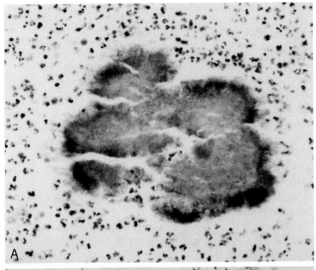

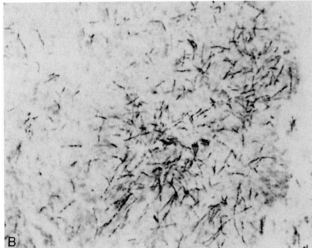

Figure 28–72. Sulfur Granule in Actinomycosis. A view of a transthoracic needle aspirate *(A)* shows a typical sulfur granule surrounded by numerous polymorphonuclear leukocytes. Silver stain *(B)* of the granule shows thin, branching filaments. *(A,* ×400; *B,* Grocott's methenamine silver, ×800.)

sionally stain only weakly and at intervals, giving the appearance of chains or masses of cocci.[1160, 1162] In contrast to *Nocardia* species, they are usually not acid-fast, although some strains may show this quality if weak decolorizing solutions are used.[1163] Although granules can develop in other bacterial infections[1160] and may may be absent in cases of culture-proven actinomycosis,[1162] they are present in the majority of *Actinomyces* infections, and their presence in the sputum or in exudate from sinus tracts is highly suggestive of the diagnosis; they are rarely seen in nocardiosis.

Epidemiology

The organisms are normal inhabitants of the human oropharynx and are frequently found in the crypts of surgically excised tonsils[1162] and in dental caries and at gingival margins of persons with poor oral hygiene.[1153] In the majority of cases, disease is believed to be acquired by the spread of endogenous organisms from these sites,[1157] usually directly

from the oropharynx into the lungs by aspiration or into the gastrointestinal tract by swallowing. Occasional cases have been reported in which the organism appeared to be carried into the lung along with aspirated foreign material, such as a chicken bone.[1164, 1165] Rare examples of exogenous transmission by human or animal bites or by other cutaneous trauma have also been reported.[90] Exceptionally, pulmonary disease occurs secondary to that in the liver, either by direct extension across the diaphragm[1166] or by hematogenous spread via the hepatic veins.[1167]

The disease is of worldwide distribution, and no age or race is immune; however, men acquire the disease slightly more often than women, and children are uncommonly affected.[1168] There is no occupational predilection or seasonal variation. Although most infections occur in individuals who are not immunocompromised, occasional cases have been reported in persons with impaired host defenses,[1151, 1169] sometimes with unusual species of relatively low-grade pathogenicity.

Before the advent of antibiotics, actinomycosis was the most commonly diagnosed "fungal" disease of the lungs, presenting a fairly typical clinical picture of empyema and sinus tracts in the chest wall. Although in some parts of the world such infection is still fairly common,[1170, 1171] this advanced stage is rarely seen now in "developed" countries. In fact, the clinical presentation of actinomycosis has changed greatly, and the incidence of thoracic involvement has declined markedly. For example, in one review of 85 cases of thoracic actinomycosis in 1957, the chest lesions were considered to be primary in 70 and secondary to either cervicofacial or abdominal disease in the other 15;[1172] by contrast, the chest was involved in only 1 of 36 cases reported in 1970[1173] and in 3 of 43 cases in another series in 1976.[1174] The pattern of thoracic disease also appears to have changed; although chest wall involvement was identified in almost half of affected patients in older series,[1175] more recent reports have found it in only 10% to 20%,[1177] a decrease possibly related to earlier diagnosis and more effective treatment.

Actinomycosis occurs most commonly as a disease of the cervicofacial region after dental extraction, usually in the form of osteomyelitis of the mandible or as a soft tissue abscess that often drains spontaneously through the skin. Acute upper airway obstruction has been reported to complicate the latter form of disease.[1178] Gastrointestinal infection is next in frequency followed by thoracopulmonary disease. Female genital infection related to the use of contraceptive intrauterine devices is also well described[1179] and has occasionally been complicated by thoracic disease.[1180]

Pathogenesis and Pathologic Characteristics

The pathogenesis of actinomycosis is not well understood. The organism does not appear to produce toxins, and the presence of granules has not been shown to inhibit phagocytosis or other host defense mechanisms.[1160] In cultures of tissue specimens, the organism is frequently associated with other bacteria,[1156] particularly *Actinobacillus actinomycetemcomitans*.[1181–1183] Although the role, if any, of these organisms in the production of disease is unclear,[1160] it has been hypothesized that they may enhance the pathogenicity of *Actinomyces* by lowering oxygen tension or inhibiting phagocytosis.[1157] The reason for the greater pathogenicity of *A. israelii* compared with other *Actinomyces* species is also unclear. Differences in the inflammatory reaction to these organisms in experimental animals have suggested that such features as rough versus smooth growth and variable cell surface structures may be involved.[1184]

Grossly, chronic pulmonary actinomycosis is characterized by multiple abscesses interconnected by sinus tracts and surrounded by a variable amount of fibrous tissue.[1162, 1185] Individual abscesses range in size from microscopic to many centimeters, with an average of 3.5 cm in one series.[1162] Pleural fibrosis and adhesions are common. Consolidation occasionally occurs without obvious abscess formation.[1162] Rare cases have been reported to present as an endobronchial mass.[1186]

Histologically, the abscesses are composed of an outer rim of granulation tissue surrounding masses of polymorphonuclear leukocytes that often contain typical sulfur granules (Fig. 28–73).[1171] The surrounding lung parenchyma shows a variable degree of fibrosis and chronic inflammation. Occasional multinucleated giant cells may be seen, but true granuloma formation is rare.[1162, 1185] Organisms can be identified within the granules by their Gram and silver stain positivity, lack of acid-fastness, and fine filamentous branching pattern; they are usually not present outside granules. Granules may be seen in sputum[1187] and in specimens obtained by needle aspiration.[1188, 1189]

Radiologic Manifestations

The typical pattern of acute pulmonary actinomycosis consists of air-space consolidation, without recognizable segmental distribution, commonly in the periphery of the lung and with a predilection for the lower lobes. Once the pneumonia has developed, the course of events depends largely on whether antibiotic therapy is instituted. With appropriate therapy, most cases resolve without complications. If therapy is not instituted, an abscess may develop, and the infection may extend into the pleura and thence into the chest wall, with abscess formation in these areas. Extension across the interlobar fissures is also common but is not unique to this disease—it may also occur in blastomycosis, cryptococcosis, and tuberculosis.

Although the previous description is perhaps the most common radiographic manifestation of actinomycosis, other abnormalities are not infrequent. In our experience and that of others, the infection not uncommonly presents radiographically as a mass, sometimes cavitated,[1190] that simulates pulmonary carcinoma.[1191–1194] In fact, surgical excision of such a mass because of a suspicion of malignancy is not a rare mode of diagnosis. Because prolonged antibiotic therapy is usually required for cure, a pulmonary lesion may undergo initial remission after institution of therapy, only to exacerbate when therapy has been withdrawn too early.[1170] In those patients in whom the pleuropulmonary disease becomes chronic, extensive fibrosis in and about the lung can become

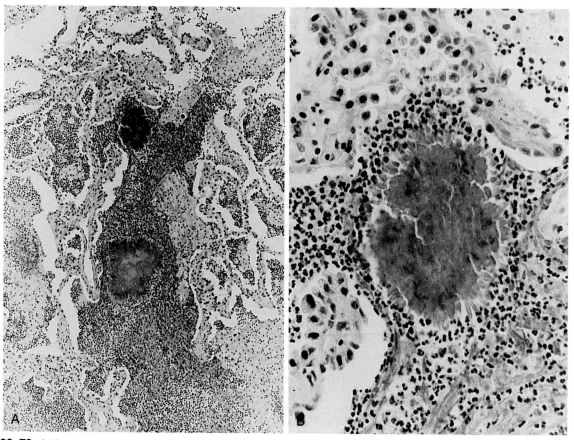

Figure 28–73. Actinomycosis. A section of lung parenchyma *(A)* shows a mild degree of alveolar interstitial fibrosis and extensive air-space filling by alveolar macrophages. A darker neutrophilic exudate is also evident, probably in a respiratory bronchiole; it contains two small actinomycotic colonies (one of which is magnified in *B*). (*A*, ×150; *B*, ×250.)

a prominent radiographic feature, the result of severe distortion of normal anatomic structures (Fig. 28–74).[1195] Pleural effusion is occasionally the only radiographic manifestation;[1196] whether an isolated finding such as this or associated with parenchymal disease, its development almost invariably indicates empyema.[1197, 1198] Lobar atelectasis or segmental opacities, sometimes associated with hemoptysis, can also occur as a result of localized endobronchial actinomycosis.[1169, 1199] Radiographic patterns of miliary disease, multiple nodules, and bilateral apical disease simulating tuberculosis have also been described.[1167, 1200] Mediastinal and pericardial involvement may occur, but are uncommon.[1201]

The manifestations of chest wall involvement include a soft tissue mass and rib abnormalities, sometimes without evidence of pulmonary disease.[1066, 1202, 1203] Periosteal proliferation along the ribs may have a peculiar wavy configuration;[1190] in fact, such involvement of several adjacent ribs in the absence of empyema is suggestive of the disease.[1172] Frank rib and, occasionally, vertebral destruction may occur.[1190] Both CT[1177, 1204] and ultrasonography[1205] have been advocated as useful procedures to determine the presence and extent of chest wall involvement.

In one investigation of eight patients, central low-attenuation regions were identified in three (38%) in the areas of

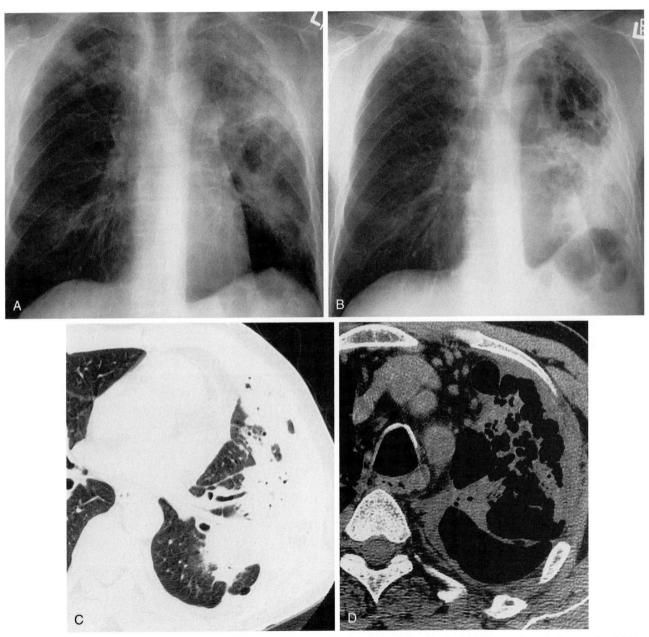

Figure 28–74. Pleuropulmonary Actinomycosis. A 55-year-old alcoholic man presented with a 6-month history of cough, fever, and weight loss. A posteroanterior (PA) chest radiograph *(A)* demonstrates bilateral areas of consolidation involving the upper lobes. Cultures, bronchoscopy, and open-lung biopsy failed to yield a definitive diagnosis, and the patient was treated empirically with antibiotics. A PA chest radiograph performed 4 months later *(B)* shows fibrosis in the left upper lobe and adjacent pleural thickening. Note volume loss of the left lung because of the fibrosis. Consolidation has also developed in the lingula and in the left lower lobe. HRCT *(C, D)* confirms the lingular and left lower lobe consolidation as well as marked pleural thickening, particularly adjacent to the anterolateral aspect of the upper lobe. A small left pleural effusion is also evident. Repeat pleural and open-lung biopsy demonstrated *Actinomyces israelii.*

consolidation on CT, corresponding to abscess formation pathologically (Fig. 28–75).[1177] Pleural thickening was identified on radiography in four cases and pleural effusion in three. Pleural thickening localized to the pleura abutting an area of consolidation was seen on CT in all patients. Small pleural effusions were identified in five patients (62%); in only two of these was the effusion an empyema. Invasion through the chest wall was present in only one case; there was no associated rib destruction or periosteal reaction. Hilar or mediastinal lymphadenopathy was seen on CT in six cases (75%).

Clinical Manifestations

The initial clinical manifestations of pulmonary involvement are nonproductive cough and low-grade fever. With time, the cough becomes productive of purulent and, in many cases, blood-streaked sputum. As the disease progresses, weight loss, anemia, and finger clubbing may occur.[1203, 1206] Pain on breathing commonly develops as the infection spreads to the pleura and chest wall. Physical examination may reveal signs of consolidation and, occasionally, a soft tissue mass in the chest wall.[1190]

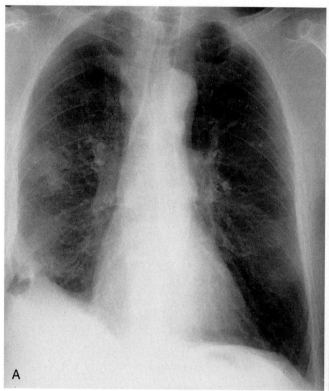

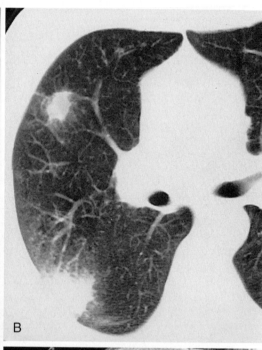

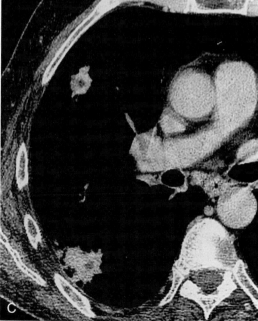

Figure 28–75. Pleuropulmonary Actinomycosis. A posteroanterior chest radiograph *(A)* reveals patchy areas of consolidation in the right upper and lower lobes and associated right pleural thickening. A 10-mm collimation CT scan *(B)* better demonstrates the focal areas of consolidation in the right lung and also shows a localized area of consolidation in the left upper lobe. HRCT *(C)* performed after intravenous administration of contrast material and targeted to the area of consolidation in the right lung demonstrates localized areas of low attenuation within the consolidation consistent with abscess formation. The patient was a 59-year-old alcoholic man with surgically confirmed pleuropulmonary actinomycosis.

Further progression of infection may result in sinus tracts through the skin or, rarely, bronchocutaneous fistulas. Infection may also extend through the diaphragm into the liver creating intercostal fistulas along the way;[1195] into the soft tissues of the neck causing Pancoast's syndrome;[1207] or into the mediastinum, causing such complications as pericarditis (sometimes constrictive)[1208, 1209] and systemic–pulmonary artery fistulas.[1210] Amyloidosis has been described as a complication of long-standing disease.[1211] Dissemination of actinomycosis to extrapulmonary sites is not uncommon[1212–1214] and may simulate metastatic pulmonary carcinoma.[1182] The rare case of predominantly endobronchial actinomycosis also may be confused with carcinoma.[1215] In these cases, the process appears endoscopically as an exophytic, yellow-white mass within the airway lumen;[1169] cytologic or histologic examination or culture should establish the diagnosis.

The prognosis is generally good, provided that the infection is recognized and appropriate antibiotic therapy is instituted. Rarely, the course is complicated by massive hemoptysis.[1216]

NOCARDIOSIS

Nocardiosis is caused by species of the family Nocardiaceae, of which the most important with respect to human pulmonary disease is *Nocardia asteroides*.[1217] *N. brasiliensis* is the next most common species to be isolated;[1218] *N. caviae*,[792] *N. nova*,[1219] *N. transvalensis*,[1220] and *N. farcinica*[1221] also cause pulmonary disease occasionally, but are more commonly associated with cutaneous and subcutaneous infection.

The organisms are aerobic, nonmotile, and non–spore-forming and in tissue show delicate branching filamentous hyphae. They are gram-positive and usually acid-fast, although many show this property only with weak decolorizing agents;[1163] some strains are non–acid-fast. Sulfur granules are rarely found and then almost invariably in association with cutaneous and subcutaneous disease.[1222] The organism may be identified on smears or cultures of exudate from the lung and extrathoracic abscesses; however, prolonged culture using selective media may be necessary for successful isolation.[1223] Culture of blood and cerebrospinal fluid is rarely positive.[1224, 1225]

Epidemiology

Nocardia species are common natural inhabitants of soil throughout the world. In some tropical and subtropical regions, they are the principal cause of mycetoma of the foot (maduromycosis), in which case they are introduced into the skin by direct inoculation. Most cases of pulmonary disease are believed to be acquired by inhalation of organisms from contaminated soil. Person-to-person transmission is rare, but there is little doubt that it happens: miniepidemics have occurred in renal transplant units,[1226, 1227] and there has been one report of a cluster of three cases in which one patient had laryngeal involvement.[1228] A case of catheter-associated bacteremia with pulmonary involvement has also been reported.[1219]

Instances in which the organism has been identified in the sputum of apparently healthy individuals with normal chest radiographs and no subsequent disease have suggested that it may exist as a saprophyte.[1229, 1230] Such colonization may not be rare: in one investigation of 36 hospitalized patients from whom *Nocardia* organisms were isolated, 19 (53%) were judged to be free of disease;[1231] most of these patients had underlying pulmonary disease, usually obstructive in nature.

Although *Nocardia* formerly was seen almost exclusively as a primary pulmonary pathogen, it is now more frequently recognized as an opportunistic invader in patients with underlying disease.[1217, 1231–1234] Patients with lymphoma,[1235, 1236] organ transplants,[1237, 1238] and, for reasons not well understood, alveolar proteinosis appear to be most susceptible.[1239–1241] Patients who have systemic lupus erythematosus,[1242] who are receiving low-dose methotrexate[1243] or corticosteroid therapy,[1233] or who have an endogenous cause for increased glucocorticoids[1244] are also vulnerable.[1217, 1243] It is a relatively uncommon cause of opportunistic infection in patients who have AIDS.[1223]

Pathologic Characteristics

Morphologically, nocardiosis is most commonly manifested either by homogeneous, gray-white consolidation of part or all of a lobe or by relatively well-circumscribed solitary or multiple nodules.[1245] Expansion and confluence of the nodules can result in the formation of a large multiloculated abscess, and cavitation may ensue. Small miliary nodules can be present as a result of hematogenous dissemination.[1246] Microscopically, there is an infiltrate of polymorphonuclear leukocytes located in microabscesses or macroabscesses within which organisms can usually be identified with appropriate stains (Fig. 28–76). Granulomatous inflammation is rare.[1245]

Radiologic Manifestations

The most frequent radiographic abnormality is air-space consolidation, usually homogeneous and nonsegmental[1247, 1248] but sometimes patchy and inhomogeneous (Fig. 28–77).[1249] In one review of 21 patients, multilobar consolidation was present in the majority.[1250] In contrast to actinomycosis, nocardiosis shows no predilection for the lower lobes.[1250] Cavitation is frequent;[1249, 1250] in one series of 12 cases, it was the most common radiographic manifestation, in a consolidated lobe in 3 patients and in a solitary mass in 4.[1251] As with actinomycosis, infection may extend into the pleural space and cause effusion or empyema; the former was identified in 10 of 21 patients in one series.[1250] Evidence of chest wall involvement is rare.[1252] Rare manifestations include a solitary pulmonary nodule,[1247, 1250] broncholithiasis following hilar lymph node involvement,[1253] and "fungus" ball formation.[1234] Extension to the pericardium or mediastinum occurs occasionally.[1250, 1254, 1255]

CT may be helpful in assessing the extent of disease and as a guide to obtain material for a definitive diagnosis.[1255, 1256] In one review of the CT findings in five patients, the predominant abnormality consisted of multifocal areas

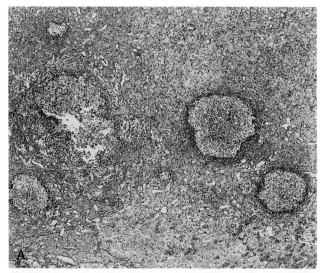

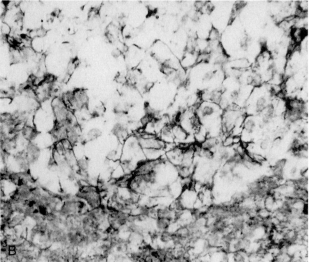

Figure 28–76. Nocardiosis. A section through a focus of subpleural consolidation *(A)* shows obliteration of lung tissue by fibrovascular tissue, within which are multiple well-defined microabscesses. The organism itself *(B)* consists of finely branching filaments. (*A*, ×48; *B*, Grocott's silver methenamine, ×800.)

of consolidation.[1256] Localized areas of low attenuation with rim enhancement suggestive of abscess formation were present within the areas of consolidation in three patients and cavitation in one. Variable-sized pulmonary nodules were identified in three patients (Fig. 28–78). Pleural involvement was present in all cases, including effusion in four, empyema in one, and thickening in four. Chest wall extension was identified in three patients.

Clinical Manifestations

Cough, purulent sputum, pleural pain, and night sweats are the usual symptoms; hemoptysis occurs occasionally.[1257] Physical examination may reveal crackles, signs of consolidation, or pleural effusion.[1234, 1247] The course is usually chronic; however, acute fulminating pneumonia may develop in patients with impaired resistance.[1252] The infection can

spread to other areas of the body, most often the brain or subcutaneous tissue.[1237, 1239, 1247] Empyema and rib osteomyelitis develop in a small number of cases.[1234] Superior vena cava obstruction is a rare complication.[1258] Because the infection is superimposed on another disease in many cases, the signs and symptoms of the primary abnormality may confuse the clinical picture.

The white cell count usually is moderately elevated, with neutrophilia; lymphocytosis or leukopenia develops in a few cases.[1234] Animal inoculation and serologic tests do not aid diagnosis. The organism can be identified in fine needle aspirates and bronchial wash specimens, but may be easily missed during screening if not specifically looked for.[1259]

The prognosis of pulmonary nocardiosis is not good. In one review of 35 patients, the case fatality rate was 40%.[1217] In another analysis of 147 case reports, the mortality of patients with serious underlying disease not treated with corticosteroids or antineoplastic agents was no higher than for those acutely ill with only nocardial infection.[1243] The recovery rate was only 15% to 20% for patients with one or more of the following findings: symptoms of less than 3 weeks' duration, disseminated infection, prior corticosteroid therapy, or prior antineoplastic therapy. Once dissemination has occurred, usually manifested by a brain abscess, the prognosis is worsened considerably.[1260–1262]

BOTRYOMYCOSIS (BACTERIAL PSEUDOMYCOSIS)

Botryomycosis is a rare chronic infectious disease whose clinical course and histopathologic features resemble those of actinomycosis but which is caused by nonactinomycotic bacteria. In the majority of cases, the disease is located in the skin and subcutaneous tissues, where it grossly resembles a mycetoma.[1263] Visceral involvement is seen less commonly and usually affects multiple organs, especially the genitourinary tract; in these circumstances, the lungs may be involved as part of the systemic disease. Rare cases have also been reported of primary pulmonary[1194, 1264] or tracheal[1264a] disease; patients with cystic fibrosis appear to be at increased risk.[1265] The abnormality has also been reported in occasional patients with AIDS.[1266] The disease has been thought by some to occur as a result of an unusual symbiotic relationship between the organism and the host,[1267] although the details of this relationship are far from clear. An immunodeficiency state is not usually apparent.

The majority of cases have been associated with *Staphylococcus aureus*,[1263] although a variety of other species have also been implicated, including *Escherichia coli*, *Proteus* species, *Actinobacillus*,[1263] nonhemolytic *Streptococcus*,[1264] and *Pseudomonas aeruginosa*.[1265, 1267] Experimental disease has been produced in animals with both *S. aureus*[1268] and *P. aeruginosa*.[1269]

Pathologically, the lungs contain from one to many nodules that range in diameter from a few millimeters to several centimeters. Histologically, there is a polymorphonuclear leukocytic infiltrate, often with microabscess formation, associated with well-defined, irregularly lobulated, basophilic masses 50 to 200 μm in diameter that resemble the granules of actinomycosis. The surrounding tissue shows a

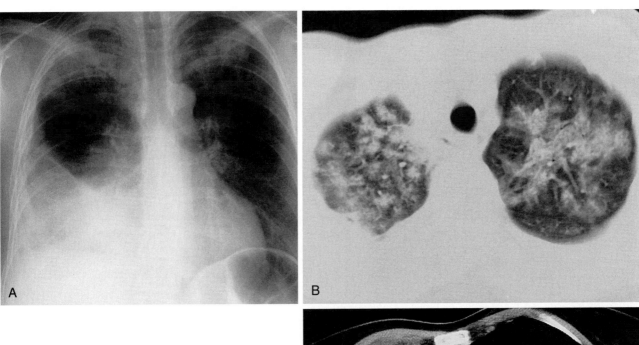

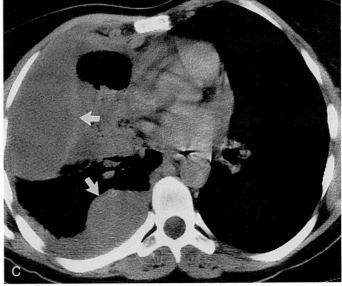

Figure 28–77. Pleuropulmonary Nocardiosis. A 36-year-old previously healthy man presented with severe pleuritic chest pain. A posteroanterior chest radiograph *(A)* demonstrates areas of consolidation in the upper lobes and right middle lobe and a right pleural effusion. CT scan *(B)* shows extensive consolidation in the upper lobes. CT scan photographed using soft tissue windows *(C)* demonstrates a large right pleural effusion with evidence of loculation anterolaterally and posteromedially *(arrows)*. Consolidation in the right middle lobe is also evident. *Nocardia asteroides* was recovered from both bronchoalveolar lavage and pleural fluid.

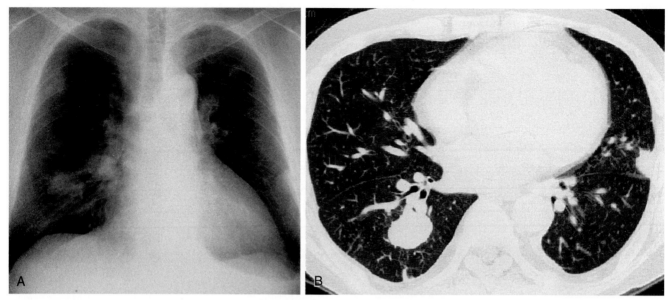

Figure 28–78. *Nocardia* **Pneumonia After Renal Transplantation.** A 41-year-old man on immunosuppressive therapy after renal transplantation presented with fever and cough. A Posteroanterior chest radiograph *(A)* demonstrates bilateral nodular opacities. HRCT *(B)* demonstrates nodules in lingula and right lower lobe. *N. asteroides* was recovered on bronchoalveolar lavage.

variable degree of fibrosis and nonspecific chronic inflammation. Multinucleated giant cells, often apparently in relation to fragmented granules, are occasionally seen, although well-formed granulomas are rare.[1263] The true nature of the granules usually can be appreciated only with Gram and silver methenamine stains that show gram-negative rods or gram-positive cocci and the absence of typical *Actinomyces* filaments.

Radiographically, the cases of primary pneumonia described in one series of patients with cystic fibrosis showed homogeneous consolidation and atelectasis, usually involv-

ing an entire upper lobe.[1265] The appearance can also be in the form of a fairly well-defined mass.[1194, 1264] We have seen one case with multiple nodules, some cavitated, simulating Wegener's granulomatosis.

Clinical features are nonspecific; in patients with cystic fibrosis, they may be dominated by the underlying disease.[1265] One patient has been described who presented with hemoptysis.[1194] Extension of infection to involve the thoracic spine and the development of chronic draining sinuses in postoperative incision sites in the skin have been described.[1265]

REFERENCES

1. Stansell JD: Pulmonary fungal infections in HIV-infected persons. Semin Respir Infect 8:116, 1993.
2. Papasian CJ, Zarabi CM, Dall LH, et al: Invasive polymycotic pneumonia in an uncontrolled diabetic. Arch Pathol Lab Med 115:517, 1991.
3. Reed AE, Body BA, Austin MB, et al: *Cunninghamella bertholletiae* and *Pneumocystis carinii* pneumonia as a fatal complication of chronic lymphocytic leukemia. Hum Pathol 19:1470, 1988.
4. Ramirez-Ortiz R, Rodriguez J, Soto Z, et al: Synchronous pulmonary cryptococcosis and histoplasmosis. South Med J 90:729, 1997.
5. May JJ, Stallones L, Darrow D, et al: Organic dust toxicity (pulmonary mycotoxicosis) associated with silo unloading. Thorax 41:919, 1986.
6. Lecours R, Laviolette M, Cormier Y: Bronchoalveolar lavage in pulmonary mycotoxicosis (organic dust toxic syndrome). Thorax 41:924, 1986.
7. Emanuel DA, Wenzel FJ, Lawton BR: Pulmonary mycotoxicosis. Chest 67:293, 1975.
8. Davies SF: Fungal pneumonia. Med Clin North Am 78:1049, 1994.
9. Kaufman L: Laboratory methods for the diagnosis and confirmation of systemic mycoses. Clin Infect Dis 14:S23, 1992.
10. Maxson S, Jacobs RF: Community-acquired fungal pneumonia in children. Semin Respir Infect 11:196, 1996.
11. Monheit JE, Cowan DF, Moore DG: Rapid detection of fungi in tissues using calcofluor white and fluorescence microscopy. Arch Pathol Lab Med 108:616, 1984.
12. Monheit JG, Brown G, Kott MM, et al: Calcofluor white detection of fungi in cytopathology. Am J Clin Pathol 85:222, 1986.
13. Graham AR: Fungal autofluorescence with ultraviolet illumination. Am J Clin Pathol 79:231, 1983.
14. Mann JL: Autofluorescence of fungi: An aid to detection in tissue sections. Am J Clin Pathol 79:587, 1983.
15. Teague MD, Tham KT: Hyphalike pseudofungus in a lymph node. Arch Pathol Lab Med 118:95, 1994.
16. Wasdahl DA, Goellner JR, Scheithauer BW: Red blood cell "ghosts" as look-alikes for infectious organisms: A report of two cases. Acta Cytol 37:100, 1993.
17. Schwarz J: The diagnosis of deep mycoses by morphologic methods. Hum Pathol 13:519, 1982.
18. Jensen HE, Schonheyder HC, Hotchi M, et al: Diagnosis of systemic mycoses by specific immunohistochemical tests. APMIS 104:241, 1996.
19. Goodwin RA Jr, Des Prez RM: Histoplasmosis. Am Rev Respir Dis 117:929, 1978.
20. Goodwin RA Jr, Loyd JE, Des Prez RM: Histoplasmosis in normal hosts. Medicine 60:231, 1981.
21. Goodwin RA Jr, Shapiro JL, Thurman GH, et al: Disseminated histoplasmosis: Clinical and pathologic correlations. Medicine 59:1, 1980.
22. Goodwin RA Jr, Owens FT, Snell JD, et al: Chronic pulmonary histoplasmosis. Medicine 55:413, 1976.
23. Schwarz J: Histoplasmosis. New York, Praeger Special Studies, 1981.
24. Bradsher RW: Histoplasmosis and blastomycosis. Clin Infect Dis 22(Suppl 2):S102, 1996.
25. Keath EJ, Kobayashi GS, Medoff G: Typing of *Histoplasma capsulatum* by restriction fragment length polymorphisms in a nuclear gene. J Clin Microbiol 30:2104, 1992.
26. Taylor ML, Granados J, Toriello C: Biological and sociocultural approaches of histoplasmosis in the state of Guerrero, Mexico. Mycoses 39:375, 1996.
27. Stobierski MG, Hospedales CJ, Hall WN, et al: Outbreak of histoplasmosis among employees in a paper factory—Michigan, 1993. J Clin Microbiol 34:1220, 1996.
28. Tosh FE, Doto IL, Beecher SB, et al: Relationship of starling-blackbird roosts and endemic histoplasmosis. Am Rev Respir Dis 101:283, 1970.
29. Chick EW, Flanigan C, Compton SB, et al: Blackbird roosts and histoplasmosis: An increasing medical problem. Chest 77:584, 1980.
30. Chick EW, Compton SB, Pass T III, et al: Hitchcock's birds, or the increased rate of exposure to *Histoplasma* from blackbird roost sites. Chest 80:434, 1981.
31. Ajello L, Hosty TS, Palmer J: Bat histoplasmosis in Alabama. Am J Trop Med Hyg 16:329, 1967.
32. Furcolow ML, Guntheroth WG, Willis MJ: The frequency of laboratory infections with *Histoplasma capsulatum*: Their clinical and x-ray characteristics. J Lab Clin Med 40:182, 1952.
33. Tesh RB, Schneidau JD Jr: Primary cutaneous histoplasmosis. N Engl J Med 275:597, 1966.
34. Lopes JO, Alves SH, Benevenga JP, et al: The second case of peritonitis due to *Histoplasma capsulatum* during continuous ambulatory peritoneal dialysis in Brazil. Mycoses 37:161, 1994.
35. Wong SY, Allen DM: Transmission of disseminated histoplasmosis via cadaveric renal transplantation: Case report. Clin Infect Dis 14:232, 1992.
36. Houston S: Histoplasmosis and pulmonary involvement in the tropics. Thorax 49:598, 1994.
37. Del Valle J, Pedroza S, Alcantara R, et al: Pulmonary histoplasmosis in Mexico. Rev Mex Tuberc 18:521, 1957.
38. Randhawa HS, Khan ZU: Histoplasmosis in India: Current status. Indian J Chest Dis Allied Sci 36:193, 1994.
39. Padhye AA, Pathak AA, Katkar VJ, et al: Oral histoplasmosis in India: A case report and an overview of cases reported during 1968–92. J Med Vet Mycol 32:93, 1994.
40. Murray JF, Lurie HI, Kaye J, et al: Benign pulmonary histoplasmosis (cave disease) in South Africa. S Afr Med J 31:245, 1957.
41. Wang TL, Cheah JS, Holmberg K: Case report and review of disseminated histoplasmosis in Southeast Asia: Clinical and epidemiological implications. Trop Med Int Health 1:35, 1996.
42. Earle JHO, Highman JH, Lockey E: A case of disseminated histoplasmosis. BMJ 1:607, 1960.
43. Confalonieri M, Gandola L, Aiolfi S, et al: Histoplasmin sensitivity among a student population in Crema, PO Valley, Italy. Microbiologica 17:151, 1994.
44. Arab HC, Yilmaz H, Ucar AI, et al: A chronic cavitary pulmonary histoplasmosis case from Turkey. J Trop Med Hyg 98:190, 1995.
45. Keath EJ, Kobayashi GS, Medoff G: Typing of *Histoplasma capsulatum* by restriction fragment length polymorphisms in a nuclear gene. J Clin Microbiol 30:2104, 1992.
46. Sakula A: Calcified pulmonary histoplasmosis. Tubercle 42:241, 1961.
47. Edge JR: Pulmonary histoplasmosis. Br J Tuberc 52:45, 1958.
48. Reid JD, Cable JV, Laurenson GR: Histoplasmosis: A report of cases in New Zealand. N Z Med J 57:325, 1958.
49. Madden M, Kennedy JD, Hitchcock HT, et al: Chronic pulmonary histoplasmosis in an Irishman. Thorax 36:705, 1981.
50. Siddiqi SH, Stauffer JC: Prevalence of histoplasmin sensitivity in Pakistan. Am J Trop Med Hyg 29:109, 1980.
51. Furcolow ML: Environmental aspects of histoplasmosis. Arch Environ Health 10:4, 1965.
52. Leggiadro RJ, Luedtke GS, Convey A, et al: Prevalence of histoplasmosis in a midsouthern population. South Med J 84:1360, 1991.
53. Okudaira M, Straub M, Schwarz J: The etiology of discrete splenic and hepatic calcifications in an endemic area of histoplasmosis. Am J Pathol 39:599, 1961.
54. Baker RD: Histoplasmosis in routine autopsies. Am J Clin Pathol 41:457, 1964.
55. Schwarz J, Baum GL: Pulmonary histoplasmosis. Semin Roentgenol 5:13, 1970.
56. Dodge HJ, Ajello L, Engelke OK: The association of a bird-roosting site with infection of school children by *H. capsulatum*. Am J Public Health 55:1203, 1965.
57. Emmons CW: Isolation of *Histoplasma capsulatum* from soil in Washington, DC. Public Health Rep 76:591, 1961.
58. Emmons CW: Association of bats with histoplasmosis. Public Health Rep 73:590, 1958.
59. Storch G, Burford JG, George RB, et al: Acute histoplasmosis: Description of an outbreak in northern Louisiana. Chest 77:38, 1980.
60. Gustafson TL, Kaufman L, Weeks R, et al: Outbreak of acute pulmonary histoplasmosis in members of a wagon train. Am J Med 71:759, 1981.
61. Johnson JE III, Radimer G, DiSalvo AF, et al: Histoplasmosis in Florida: 1. Report of a case and epidemiologic studies. Am Rev Respir Dis 101:299, 1970.
62. Lottenberg R, Waldman RH, Ajello L, et al: Pulmonary histoplasmosis associated with exploration of a bat cave. Am J Epidemiol 110:156, 1979.
63. Butler JC, Heller R, Wright PF: Histoplasmosis during childhood. South Med J 87:476, 1994.
64. Riggs W Jr, Nelson P: The roentgenographic findings in infantile and childhood histoplasmosis. Am J Roentgenol 97:181, 1966.
65. Peterson MW, Pratt AD, Nugent KM: Pneumonia due to *H. capsulatum* in a bone marrow transplant recipient. Thorax 42:698, 1987.
66. Tomita T, Chiga M: Disseminated histoplasmosis in acquired immunodeficiency syndrome: Light and electron microscopic observations. Hum Pathol 19:438, 1988.
67. Wheat J: Endemic mycoses in AIDS: A clinical review. Clin Microbiol Rev 8:146, 1995.
68. Wheat J: Histoplasmosis and coccidioidomycosis in individuals with AIDS: A clinical review. Infect Dis Clin North Am 8:467, 1994.
68a. Yaseen Z, Havlichek D, Mathes B, et al: Disseminated histoplasmosis in a patient with sarcoidosis: A controversial relationship and a diagnostic dilemma. Am J Med Sci 313:187, 1997.
69. Procknow JJ, Page MI, Loosli CG: Early pathogenesis of experimental histoplasmosis. Arch Pathol 69:65, 1960.
70. Baughman RP, Kim CK, Vinegar A, et al: The pathogenesis of experimental pulmonary histoplasmosis. Am Rev Respir Dis 134:771, 1986.
71. Case report: Tissue morphology of *Histoplasma capsulatum* in acute histoplasmosis. Am Rev Respir Dis 130:317, 1984.
72. Dumont A, Piché C: Electron microscopic study of human histoplasmosis. Arch Pathol 87:168, 1969.
73. Wu-Hsieh BA: Resistance mechanisms in murine experimental histoplasmosis. Arch Med Res 24:233, 1993.
74. Newman SL, Gootee L: Colony-stimulating factors activate human macrophages to inhibit intracellular growth of *Histoplasma capsulatum* yeasts. Infect Immun 60:4593, 1992.
75. Wu-Hsieh BA, Lee GS, Franco M, et al: Early activation of splenic macrophages by tumor necrosis factor alpha is important in determining the outcome of experimental histoplasmosis in mice. Infect Immun 60:4230, 1992.
76. Allendoerfer R, Magee DM, Deepe GS Jr, et al: Transfer of protective immunity in murine histoplasmosis by a CD4+ T-cell clone. Infect Immun 61:714, 1993.

77. Straub M, Schwarz J: The healed primary complex in histoplasmosis. Am J Clin Pathol 25:727, 1955.

78. Bhagavan BS, Rao DRG, Weinberg T: Histoplasmosis producing broncholithias. Arch Pathol 91:577, 1971.

79. Binford CH: Histoplasmosis: Tissue reactions and morphologic variations of the fungus. Am J Clin Pathol 25:25, 1955.

80. Straub M, Schwarz J: The healed primary complex in histoplasmosis. Am J Clin Pathol 25:727, 1955.

81. Wages DS, Wear DJ: Acid-fastness of fungi in blastomycosis and histoplasmosis. Arch Pathol Lab Med 106:440, 1982.

82. Stong GC, Raval HB, Martin JW, et al: Nodular subcutaneous histoplasmosis: A case report with diagnosis by fine needle aspiration biopsy. Acta Cytol 38:777, 1994.

83. Kirk ME, Lough J, Warner HA: *Histoplasma* colitis: An electron microscopic study. Gastroenterology 61:46, 1971.

84. Hutton JP, Durham JB, Miller DP, et al: Hyphal forms of *H. capsulatum*: A common manifestation of intravascular infections. Arch Pathol Lab Med 109:330, 1985.

85. Macher A: Histoplasmosis and blastomycosis. Med Clin North Am 64:447, 1980.

86. Segal EL, Starr GF, Weed LA: Study of surgically excised pulmonary granulomas. JAMA 170:515, 1959.

87. Collins MH, Jiang B, Croffie JM, et al: Hepatic granulomas in children: A clinicopathologic analysis of 23 cases including polymerase chain reaction for histoplasma. Am J Surg Pathol 20:332, 1996.

88. Hsu RM, Connors AF Jr, Tomashefski JF Jr: Histologic, microbiologic, and clinical correlates of the diagnosis of sarcoidosis by transbronchial biopsy. Arch Pathol Lab Med 120:364, 1996.

89. Zeidberg LD, Dillon A, Gass RS: Some factors in the epidemiology of histoplasmin sensitivity in Williamson County, Tennessee. Am J Public Health 41:80, 1951.

90. Rippon SW: Medical Mycology: The Pathogenic Fungi and the Pathogenic Actinomycetes. 3rd ed. Philadelphia, WB Saunders, 1988.

91. Wheat LJ, Wass J, Norton J, et al: Cavitary histoplasmosis occurring during two large urban outbreaks: Analysis of clinical, epidemiologic, roentgenographic, and laboratory features. Medicine 63:201, 1984.

92. Curry FJ, Wier JA: Histoplasmosis: A review of one hundred consecutively hospitalized patients. Am Rev Tuberc 77:749, 1958.

93. Brodsky AL, Gregg MB, Loewenstein MS, et al: Outbreak of histoplasmosis associated with the 1970 Earth Day activities. Am J Med 54:333, 1973.

94. Saslaw S, Beman FM: Erythema nodosum as a manifestation of histoplasmosis. JAMA 170:1178, 1959.

95. Medeiros AA, Marty SD, Tosh FE, et al: Erythema nodosum and erythema multiforme as clinical manifestations of histoplasmosis in a community outbreak. N Engl J Med 274:415, 1966.

96. Procknow JJ: Pulmonary histoplasmosis in a farm family—fifteen years later. Am Rev Respir Dis 95:171, 1967.

97. Seward CW, Mohr JA, Rhoades ER: An outbreak of histoplasmosis in Oklahoma. Am Rev Respir Dis 102:950, 1970.

98. Wynne JW, Olsen GN: Acute histoplasmosis presenting as the adult respiratory distress syndrome. Chest 66:158, 1974.

99. Palayew MJ, Frank H, Sedlezky I: Our experience with histoplasmosis: An analysis of seventy cases with follow-up study. J Can Assoc Radiol 17:142, 1966.

100. Goodwin RA, Loyd JE, Des Prez RM: Histoplasmosis in normal hosts. Medicine 60:231, 1981.

101. Conces DJ Jr: Histoplasmosis. Semin Roentgenol 1:14, 1996.

102. Chick EW, Bauman DS: Acute cavitary histoplasmosis—fact or fiction? Chest 65:479, 1974.

103. Murray JF, Howard D: Laboratory-acquired histoplasmosis. Am Rev Respir Dis 89:631, 1964.

104. Furcolow ML, Grayston JT: Occurrence of histoplasmosis in epidemics: Etiologic studies. Am Rev Tuberc 68:307, 1953.

105. Babbitt DP, Waisbren BA: Epidemic pulmonary histoplasmosis: Roentgenographic findings. Am J Roentgenol 83:236, 1960.

106. Wolopitz A, Van Eeden J: Histoplasmosis—cave disease. S Afr Med J 37:1002, 1963.

107. Fissel GE: Acute fulminating histoplasmosis. Am J Roentgenol 76:60, 1956.

108. Connell JV Jr, Muhm JR: Radiographic manifestations of pulmonary histoplasmosis: A 10-year review. Am J Roentgenol 121:281, 1976.

109. Greenwood MF, Holland P: Tracheal obstruction secondary to *Histoplasma* mediastinal granuloma. Chest 62:642, 1972.

110. Woods LP: Mediastinal *Histoplasma* granuloma causing tracheal compression in a 4-year-old child. Surgery 58:448, 1965.

111. Baum GL, Bernstein IL, Schwarz J: Broncholithiasis: Produced by histoplasmosis. Am Rev Tuberc 77:162, 1968.

112. Prager RL, Burney DP, Waterhouse G, et al: Pulmonary, mediastinal, and cardiac presentations of histoplasmosis. Ann Thorac Surg 30:385, 1980.

113. Straus SE, Jacobson ES: The spectrum of histoplasmosis in a general hospital: A review of 55 cases diagnosed at Barnes Hospital between 1966 and 1977. Am J Med Sci 279:147, 1980.

114. Goodwin RA Jr, Snell JD Jr: The enlarging histoplasmoma: Concept of a tumor-like phenomenon encompassing the tuberculoma and coccidioidoma. Am Rev Respir Dis 100:1, 1969.

115. Connell JV Jr, Muhm JR: Radiographic manifestations of pulmonary histoplasmosis: A 10-year review. Radiology 121:281, 1976.

116. Richert JH, Campbell CC: The significance of skin and serologic tests in the diagnosis of pulmonary residuals of histoplasmosis: A review of 123 cases. Am Rev Respir Dis 86:381, 1962.

117. Siegelman SS, Khouri NF, Leo FP, et al: Solitary pulmonary nodules: CT assessment. Radiology 160:307, 1986.

118. Zerhouni EA, Stitik FP, Siegelman SS, et al: CT of the pulmonary nodule: A cooperative study. Radiology 160:319, 1986.

119. Stancato-Pasik A, Mendelson DS, Marom Z: Rounded atelectasis caused by histoplasmosis. Am J Roentgenol 165:275, 1990.

120. Palayew MJ, Frank H: Benign progressive multinodular pulmonary histoplasmosis: A radiological and clinical entity. Radiology 111:311, 1974.

121. Goodwin RA Jr, Snell JD, Hubbard WW, et al: Early chronic pulmonary histoplasmosis. Am Rev Respir Dis 93:47, 1966.

122. Cox RA: Immunologic studies of patients with histoplasmosis. Am Rev Respir Dis 120:143, 1979.

122a. Rasp FL, Sarosi GA, Repine JE: Serum from patients with invasive fungal infections inhibits the adherence of polymorphonuclear leukocytes and alveolar macrophages. Am Rev Resp Dis 123:636, 1981.

123. Rasp FL, Sarosi GA, Repine JE: Serum from patients with invasive fungal infections inhibits the adherence of polymorphonuclear leukocytes and alveolar macrophages. Am Rev Respir Dis 123:636, 1981.

124. Loewen DF, Procknow JJ, Loosli CG: Chronic active pulmonary histoplasmosis with cavitation: A clinical and laboratory study of thirteen cases. Am J Med 28:252, 1960.

125. Pugsley HE, Brown AS, Cheung OT: Chronic cavitary histoplasmosis of the lung. Can Med Assoc J 88:646, 1963.

126. Baum GL: Cavitation in histoplasmosis: Some further comments. Chest 67:625, 1975.

127. Davies SF, Sarosi GA: Acute cavitary histoplasmosis. Chest 73:103, 1978.

128. Rubin HMD, Furcolow ML, Yates JL, et al: The course and prognosis of histoplasmosis. Am J Med 27:278, 1959.

129. Baum GL, Schwartz J: Chronic pulmonary histoplasmosis. Am J Med 33:873, 1962.

130. Veterans Administration—Armed Forces Cooperative Study on Histoplasmosis: Histoplasmosis cooperative study: II. Chronic pulmonary histoplasmosis treated with and without amphotericin B. Am Rev Respir Dis 89:641, 1964.

131. Savides TJ, Gress FG, Wheat LJ, et al: Dysphagia due to mediastinal granulomas: Diagnosis with endoscopic ultrasonography. Gastroenterology 109:366, 1995.

132. Mathisen DJ, Grillo HC: Clinical manifestation of mediastinal fibrosis and histoplasmosis. Ann Thorac Surg 54:1053, 1992.

133. Weinstein JB, Aronberg DJ, Sagel SS: CT of fibrosing mediastinitis: Findings and their utility. Am J Roentgenol 141:247, 1983.

134. Sherrick AD, Brown LR, Harms GF, et al: The radiographic findings of fibrosing mediastinitis. Chest 106:484, 1994.

135. Farmer DW, Moore E, Amparo E, et al: Calcific fibrosing mediastinitis: Demonstration of pulmonary vascular obstruction by magnetic resonance imaging. Am J Roentgenol 143:1189, 1984.

136. Rholl KS, Levitt RG, Glazer HS: Magnetic resonance imaging of fibrosing mediastinitis. Am J Roentgenol 145:255, 1985.

137. Owen GE, Scherr SN, Segre EJ: Histoplasmosis involving the heart and great vessels. Am J Med 32:552, 1962.

138. Felson B: Some less familiar roentgen manifestations of intrathoracic histoplasmosis. Arch Intern Med 103:54, 1959.

139. Marshall RJ, Edmundowicz AC, Andrews CE: Chronic obstruction of the superior vena cava due to histoplasmosis. Circulation 29:604, 1964.

140. Miller DB, Allen ST Jr, Amidon EL: Obstruction of the superior vena cava presumably due to histoplasmosis. Am Rev Tuberc 77:848, 1958.

141. Lull GF Jr, Winn DF Jr: Chronic fibrous mediastinitis due to *Histoplasma capsulatum* (histoplasmal mediastinitis): Report of three cases with different presenting symptoms. Radiology 73:367, 1959.

142. Marshall JB, Singh R, Demmy TL, et al: Mediastinal histoplasmosis presenting with esophageal involvement and dysphagia: Case study. Dysphagia 10:53, 1995.

143. Friedman JL, Baum GL, Schwartz J: Primary pulmonary histoplasmosis: Associated pericardial and mediastinal manifestations. Am J Dis Child 109:298, 1965.

144. Kilburn CD, McKinsey DS: Recurrent massive pleural effusion due to pleural, pericardial, and epicardial fibrosis in histoplasmosis. Chest 100:1715, 1991.

145. Hurwitz JK, Pastor BH: Pericardial calcification associated with histoplasmosis. N Engl J Med 260:543, 1959.

146. Kauffman CA, Israel KS, Smith JW, et al: Histoplasmosis in immunosuppressed patients. Am J Med 64:923, 1978.

147. Weeks E, Jones CM, Guinee V, et al: Histoplasmosis in hairy cell leukemia: Case report and review of the literature. Ann Hematol 65:138, 1992.

148. Witty LA, Steiner F, Curfman M, et al: Disseminated histoplasmosis in patients receiving low-dose methotrexate therapy for psoriasis. Arch Dermatol 128:91, 1992.

149. McGuinness G, Naidich DP, Jagirdar J, et al: High resolution CT findings in miliary lung disease. J Comput Assist Tomogr 16:384, 1992.

150. Blair T, Raymond L: *Histoplasma capsulatum* endocarditis. Chest 79:620, 1981.

151. Eissenberg LG, West JL, Woods JP, et al: Infection of P388D1 macrophages and respiratory epithelial cells by *Histoplasma capsulatum*: Selection of avirulent variants and their potential role in persistent histoplasmosis. Infect Immun 59:1639, 1991

152. Cole MC, Grossman ME: Disseminated histoplasmosis presenting as tongue nodules in a patient infected with human immunodeficiency virus. Cutis 55:104, 1995.

153. Sataloff RT, Wilborn A, Prestipino A, et al: Histoplasmosis of the larynx. Am J Otolaryngol 14:199, 1993.

154. Keller FG, Kurtzberg J: Disseminated histoplasmosis: A cause of infection-associated hemophagocytic syndrome. Am J Pediatr Hematol Oncol 16:368, 1994.

155. Le TH, Godeau P: Disseminated histoplasmosis with glomerulonephritis mimicking Wegener's granulomatosis. Am J Kidney Dis 21:542, 1993.

156. Wheat J, French MLV, Kohler RB, et al: The diagnostic laboratory tests for histoplasmosis: Analysis of experience in a large urban outbreak. Ann Intern Med 97:680, 1982.

157. Littman ML: The systemic mycoses. Am J Med 27:1, 1959.

158. Huffnagle KE, Gander RM: Evaluation of gen-probe's *Histoplasma capsulatum* and *Cryptococcus neoformans* accuprobes. J Clin Microbiol 31:419, 1993.

159. Goodwin RA, Alcorn GL: Histoplasmosis with symptomatic lymphadenopathy. Chest 77:213, 1980.

160. Jacobson ES, Straus SE: Reevaluation of diagnostic *Histoplasma* serologies. Am J Med Sci 281:143, 1981.

161. Campbell CC: Use and interpretation of serologic and skin tests in the respiratory mycoses: Current considerations. Dis Chest 54(Suppl):305, 1968.

162. George RB, Lambert RS, Bruce MJ, et al: Radioimmunoassay: A sensitive screening test for histoplasmosis and blastomycosis. Am Rev Respir Dis 124:407, 1981.

163. Davies SF: Serodiagnosis of histoplasmosis. Semin Respir Infect 1:9, 1986.

164. Veterans Administration—Armed Forces Cooperative Study on Histoplasmosis: Histoplasmosis cooperative study: I. Frequency of histoplasmosis among adult hospitalized males. Am Rev Respir Dis 84:663, 1961.

165. Reddy P, Gorelick DF, Brasher CA, et al: Progressive disseminated histoplasmosis as seen in adults. Am J Med 48:629, 1970.

166. Sarosi GA, Voth DW, Dahl BA, et al: Disseminated histoplasmosis: Results of long-term follow-up: A center for disease control cooperative mycoses study. Ann Intern Med 75:511, 1971.

167. Wheat LJ, Connolly-Stringfield P, Williams B, et al: Diagnosis of histoplasmosis in patients with the acquired immunodeficiency syndrome by detection of *Histoplasma capsulatum* polysaccharide antigen in bronchoalveolar lavage fluid. Am Rev Respir Dis 145:1421, 1992.

168. Davies SF, Rohrbach MS, Thelen V, et al: Elevated serum angiotensin-converting enzyme (SACE) activity in acute pulmonary histoplasmosis. Chest 85:307, 1984.

169. Starr JC, Hahn HH, Wheat LJ: Farmer's lung serologies: An early manifestation of acute histoplasmosis. Chest 86:269, 1984.

170. Lanceley JL, Lunn HF, Wilson AMM: Histoplasmosis in an African child. J Pediatr 59:756, 1961.

171. Oddo D, Etchart M, Thompson L: *Histoplasmosis duboisii* (African histoplasmosis): An African case reported from Chile with ultrastructural study. Pathol Res Pract 186:514, 1990.

172. Arendt V, Coremans-Pelseneer J, Gottlob R, et al: African histoplasmosis in a Belgian AIDS patient. Mycoses 34:59, 1991.

173. Gugnani HC, Muotoe-Okafor FA, Kaufman L, et al: A natural focus of *Histoplasma capsulatum var. duboisii* is a bat cave. Mycopathologia 127:151, 1994.

174. Muotoe-Okafor FA, Gugnani HC, Gugnani A: Skin and serum reactivity among humans to histoplasmin in the vicinity of a natural focus of *Histoplasma capsulatum var. duboisii*. Mycopathologia 134:71, 1996.

175. Clark BM, Greenwood BM: Pulmonary lesions in African histoplasmosis. J Trop Med Hyg 71:4, 1968.

176. Gentilini M, Desportes M, Danis M, et al: Histoplasmose pulmonaire africaine a *Histoplasma duboisii*. Ann Intern Med 128:32, 1977.

177. Drutz DJ, Catanzaro A: Coccidioidomycosis: Part I. Am Rev Respir Dis 117:559, 1978.

178. Drutz DJ, Catanzaro A: Coccidioidomycosis: Part II. Am Rev Respir Dis 117:727, 1978.

179. Bayer AS: Fungal pneumonias: Pulmonary coccidioidal syndromes (Part I). Primary and progressive primary coccidioidal pneumonias—diagnostic, therapeutic, and prognostic considerations. Chest 79:575, 1981.

180. Bayer AS: Fungal pneumonias: Pulmonary coccidioidal syndromes (Part 2). Miliary, nodular, and cavitary pulmonary coccidioidomycosis—chemotherapeutic and surgical considerations. Chest 79:686, 1981.

181. Stevens DA: Coccidioidomycosis. N Engl J Med 332:1077, 1995.

182. Galgiani JN: Coccidioidomycosis. Curr Clin Top Infect Dis 17:188, 1997.

183. Converse JL, Reed RE, Kuller HW, et al: Experimental epidemiology of coccidioidomycosis: I. Epizootiology of naturally exposed monkeys and dogs. *In* Ajello L (ed): Coccidiodomycosis. Tucson, University of Arizona Press, 1965, p 397.

184. Ajello L: Coccidioidomycosis and histoplasmosis: A review of their epidemiology and geographical distribution. Mycopathol Mycol Appl 45:221, 1971.

185. Rao S, Biddle M, Balchum OJ, et al: Focal endemic coccidioidomycosis in Los Angeles County. Am Rev Respir Dis 105:410, 1972.

186. Werner SB, Pappagianis D, Heindl L, et al: An epidemic of coccidioidomycosis among archeology students in northern California. N Engl J Med 286:507, 1972.

187. Flynn NM, Hoeprich PD, Kawachi MM, et al: An unusual outbreak of windborne coccidioidomycosis. N Engl J Med 301:358, 1979.

188. Centers for Disease Control and Prevention: Coccidioidomycosis—Arizona, 1990–1995. JAMA 277:104, 1997.

189. Schneider E, Hajjeh RA, Spiegel RA, et al: A coccidioidomycosis outbreak following the Northridge, Calif, earthquake. JAMA 277:904, 1997.

190. Joffe B: An epidemic of coccidioidomycosis probably related to soil. N Engl J Med 262:720, 1960.

191. Eckmann BH, Schaefer GL, Huppert M: Bedside interhuman transmission of coccidioidomycosis via growth on fomites: An epidemic involving six persons. Am Rev Respir Dis 89:175, 1964.

192. Pappagianis D: Marked increase in cases of coccidioidomycosis in California: 1991, 1992, and 1993. Clin Infect Dis 19:S14, 1994.

193. Kohn GJ, Linne SR, Smith CM, et al: Acquisition of coccidioidomycosis at necropsy by inhalation of coccidioidal endospores. Diagn Microbiol Infect Dis 15:527, 1992.

194. Standaert SM, Schaffner W, Galgiani JN, et al: Coccidioidomycosis among visitors to a *Coccidioides immitis*-endemic area: An outbreak in a military reserve unit. J Infect Dis 171:1672, 1995.

195. Small MJ: Late progression of pulmonary coccidioidomycosis. Arch Intern Med 104:68, 1959.

196. Albert BL, Sellers TF Jr: Coccidioidomycosis from fomites: Report of a case and review of the literature. Arch Intern Med 112:253, 1963.

197. Gehlbach SH, Hamilton JD, Conant NF: Coccidioidomycosis: An occupational disease in cotton mill workers. Arch Intern Med 131:254, 1973.

198. Johnson JE II, Perry JE, Fekety FR, et al: Laboratory-acquired coccidioidomycosis: A report of 210 cases. Ann Intern Med 60:941, 1964.

199. Levan NE, Huntington RW Jr: Primary cutaneous coccidioidomycosis in agricultural workers. Arch Dermatol 92:215, 1965.

200. Sievers ML: Disseminated coccidioidomycosis among Southwestern American Indians. Am Rev Respir Dis 109:602, 1974.

201. Geller RD, Maynard JE, Jones V: Coccidioidin sensitivity among Southwestern American Indians. Am Rev Respir Dis 107:301, 1973.

202. Ampel NM, Dols CL, Galgiani JN: Coccidioidomycosis during human immunodeficiency virus infection: Results of a prospective study in a coccidioidal endemic area. Am J Med 94:235, 1993.

203. Holt CD, Winston DJ, Kubak B, et al: Coccidioidomycosis in liver transplant patients. Clin Infect Dis 24:216, 1997.

204. Walker MP, Brody CZ, Resnik R: Reactivation of coccidioidomycosis in pregnancy. Obstet Gynecol 79:815, 1992.

205. Huppert M, Sun SH, Gleason-Jordan I, et al: Lung weight parallels disease severity in experimental coccidioidomycosis. Infect Immun 14:1356, 1976.

206. Forbus WD: Coccidioidomycosis: A study of 95 cases of the disseminated type with special reference to the pathogenesis of the disease. Milit Surg 99:653, 1946.

207. Huntington RW Jr, Waldmann WJ, Sargent JA, et al: Pathologic and clinical observations on 142 cases of fatal coccidioidomycosis with necropsy. *In* Ajello L (ed): Coccidioidomycosis. Tucson, University of Arizona Press, 1965, p 143.

208. Graham AR, Sobonya RE, Bronnimann DA, et al: Quantitative pathology of coccidioidomycosis in acquired immunodeficiency syndrome. Hum Pathol 19:800, 1988.

209. Raab SS, Silverman JF, Zimmerman KG: Fine-needle aspiration biopsy of pulmonary coccidioidomycosis: Spectrum of cytologic findings in 73 patients. Am J Clin Pathol 99:582, 1993.

210. Smith AG, Gillotte JP: Aberrant forms of *Coccidioides immitis* in a coccidioidoma. Am J Clin Pathol 34:477, 1960.

211. Winn RE, Johnson R, Galgiani JN, et al: Cavitary coccidioidomycosis with fungus ball formation: Diagnosis by fiberoptic bronchoscopy with coexistence of hyphae and spherules. Chest 105:412, 1994.

212. Hinshaw HC, Garland LH: Diseases of the Chest. 3rd ed. Philadelphia, WB Saunders, 1969.

213. Greendyke WH, Resnick DL, Harvey WC: The varied roentgen manifestations of primary coccidioidomycosis. Am J Roentgenol 109:491, 1970.

214. Batra P, Batra RS: Thoracic coccidioidomycosis. Semin Roentgenol 1:28, 1996.

215. Klein EW, Griffin JP: Coccidioidomycosis (diagnosis outside the Sonoran Zone): The roentgen features of acute multiple pulmonary cavities. Am J Roentgenol 94:653, 1965.

216. Batra P: Pulmonary coccidioidomycosis. J Thorac Imaging 7:29, 1992.

217. Winter B, Villaveces J, Spector M: Coccidioidomycosis accompanied by acute tracheal obstruction in a child. JAMA 195:1001, 1966.

218. Moskowitz PS, Sue JY, Gooding CA: Tracheal coccidioidomycosis causing upper airway obstruction in children. Am J Roentgenol 139:596, 1982.

219. Colwell JA, Tillman SP: Early recognition and therapy of disseminated coccidioidomycosis. Am J Med 31:676, 1961.

220. Coburn JW: Scalene lymph node involvement in primary and disseminated coccidioidomycosis: Evidence of extrapulmonary spread in primary infection. Ann Intern Med 56:911, 1962.

221. Cantanzaro A: Pulmonary coccidioidomycosis. Med Clin North Am 64:461, 1980.

222. Bayer AS, Yoshikawa TT, Galpin JE: Unusual syndromes of coccidioidomycosis—diagnostic and therapeutic considerations. Medicine 55:131, 1976.

223. Lopez AM, Williams PL, Ampel NM: Acute pulmonary coccidioidomycosis mimicking bacterial pneumonia and septic shock: A report of two cases. Am J Med 95:236, 1993.

224. Westphal SA, Sarosi GA: Diabetic ketoacidosis associated with pulmonary coccidioidomycosis. Clin Infect Dis 18:974, 1994.

225. Ramras DG, Walch HA, Murray JP, et al: An epidemic of coccidioidomycosis in the Pacific beach area of San Diego. Am Rev Respir Dis 101:975, 1970.

226. Cox RA, Pope RM, Stevens DA: Immune complexes in coccidioidomycosis: Correlation with disease involvement. Am Rev Respir Dis 126:439, 1982.

227. Winn WA: Coccidioidomycosis: The need for careful evaluation of the clinical pattern and anatomical lesions. Arch Intern Med 106:463, 1960.

228. Deppisch LM, Donowho EM: Pulmonary coccidioidomycosis. Am J Clin Pathol 58:489, 1972.

229. Schwarz J, Baum GL: Coccidioidomycosis. Semin Roentgenol 5:29, 1970.

230. Stark P, Wong V, Gold P: Solitary pulmonary granuloma with marked enhancement on dynamic CT scanning. Radiology 28:489, 1988.

230a. Kim K-I, Leung AN, Flint JDA, Müller NL: Chronic pulmonary coccidioidomycosis: Computed tomographic and pathologic findings in 18 patients. Can Assoc Radiol J 49:in press, 1998.

231. Salkin D, Birsner TW, Tarr AD, et al: Roentgen analysis of coccidioidomycosis in pediatric cases in private practice. In Ajello L (ed): Coccidioidomycosis. Tucson, University of Arizona Press, 1967, p 63.

232. Winn WA: A long-term study of 300 patients with cavitary-abscess lesions of the lung of coccidioidal origin: An analytical study with special reference to treatment. Dis Chest 54(Suppl I):268, 1968.

233. Spivey CG Jr, Jones FL, Bopp RK: Cavitary coccidioidomycosis: Experience in a tuberculosis hospital outside the endemic area. Dis Chest 56:13, 1969.

234. Freedman SI, Ang EP, Haley RS: Identification of coccidioidomycosis of the lung by fine needle aspiration biopsy. Acta Cytol 30:420, 1986.

235. Raab SS, Silverman JF, Zimmerman KG: Fine-needle aspiration biopsy of pulmonary coccidioidomycosis: Spectrum of cytologic findings in 73 patients. Am J Clin Pathol 99:582, 1993.

236. Rohatgi PK, Schmitt RG: Pulmonary coccidioidal mycetoma. Am J Med Sci 287:27, 1984.

237. Winn RE, Johnson R, Galgiani JN, et al: Cavitary coccidioidomycosis with fungus ball formation: Diagnosis by fiberoptic bronchoscopy with coexistence of hyphae and spherules. Chest 105:412, 1994.

238. Primack SL, Hartman TE, Lee KS, et al: Pulmonary nodules and the CT halo sign. Radiology 190:513, 1994.

239. Beller TA, Mitchell DM, Sobonya RE, et al: Large airway obstruction secondary to endobronchial coccidioidomycosis. Am Rev Respir Dis 120:939, 1979.

240. University of California, School of Medicine: Chest conference. Am Rev Respir Dis 82:400, 1960.

241. Cunningham RT, Einstein H: Coccidioidal pulmonary cavities with rupture. J Thorac Cardiovasc Surg 84:172, 1982.

242. Edelstein G, Levitt RG: Cavitary coccidioidomycosis presenting as spontaneous pneumothorax. Am J Roentgenol 141:533, 1983.

243. Bayer AS, Yoshikawa TT, Guze LB: Chronic progressive coccidioidal pneumonitis: Report of six cases with clinical, roentgenographic, serologic, and therapeutic features. Arch Intern Med 139:536, 1979.

244. Baker EJ, Hawkins JA, Waskow EA: Surgery for coccidioidomycosis in 52 diabetic patients with special reference to related immunologic factors. J Thorac Cardiovasc Surg 75:680, 1978.

245. Roberts CJ: Coccidioidomycosis in acquired immune deficiency syndrome: Depressed humoral as well as cellular immunity. Am J Med 76:734, 1984.

246. Peterson CM, Schuppert K, Kelly PC, et al: Coccidioidomycosis and pregnancy. Obstet Gynecol Surv 48:149, 1993.

247. Catanzaro A: Pulmonary mycosis in pregnant women. Chest 86:145, 1984.

248. Rutala PJ, Smith JW: Coccidioidomycosis in potentially compromised hosts: The effect of immunosuppressive therapy in dissemination. Am J Med Sci 275:283, 1978.

249. Bronnimann DA, Adam RD, Galgiani JN, et al: Coccidioidomycosis in the acquired immunodeficiency syndrome. Ann Intern Med 106:372, 1987.

250. Fish DG, Mapel NM, Galgiani JN, et al: Coccidioidomycosis during human immunodeficiency virus infection: A review of 77 patients. Medicine 69:384, 1990.

251. Jones JL, Fleming PL, Ciesielski CA, et al: Coccidioidomycosis among persons with AIDS in the United States. J Infect Dis 171:961, 1995.

252. Castellot JJ, Creveling RL, Pitts FW: Fatal miliary coccidioidomycosis complicating prolonged prednisone therapy in a patient with myelofibrosis. Ann Intern Med 52:254, 1960.

253. Kaplan JE, Zoschke D, Kisch AL: Withdrawal of immunosuppressive agents in the treatment of disseminated coccidioidomycosis. Am J Med 68:624, 1980.

254. Mischel PS, Vinters HV: Coccidioidomycosis of the central nervous system: Neuropathological and vasculopathic manifestations and clinical correlates. Clin Infect Dis 20:400, 1995.

255. Bouza E, Dreyer JS, Hewitt WL, et al: Coccidioidal meningitis: An analysis of thirty-one cases and review of the literature. Medicine 60:139, 1981.

256. Danoff D, Munk ZM, Case B, et al: Disseminated coccidioidomycosis: Clinical, immunologic and therapeutic aspects. Can Med Assoc J 118:390, 1978.

257. Boddicker JH, Fong D, Walsh TE, et al: Bone and gallium scanning in the evaluation of disseminated coccidioidomycosis. Am Rev Respir Dis 122:279, 1980.

258. Stadalnik RC, Goldstein E, Hoeprich PD, et al: Diagnostic value of gallium and bone scans in evaluation of extrapulmonary coccidioidal lesions. Am Rev Respir Dis 121:673, 1980.

259. Goldstein E: Miliary and disseminated coccidioidomycosis. Ann Intern Med 89:365, 1978.

260. DePaula A: Microepidemic of histoplasmosis. Rev Serv Nac Tuberc 3:11, 1959.

261. Ponnampalam JT: Histoplasmosis in Malaya. Br J Dis Chest 58:49, 1964.

262. Gelfand M: Cave disease: A report of three cases from Southern Rhodesia. Cent Afr J Med 8:461, 1962.

263. Sargent EN, Balchum E, Freed AL, et al: Multiple pulmonary calcifications due to coccidioidomycosis. Am J Roentgenol 109:500, 1970.

264. Galgiani JN, Ampel NM: C. immitis in patients with human immunodeficiency virus infections. Semin Respir Infect 5:151, 1990.

265. Larsen RA, Jacobson JA, Morris AH, et al: Acute respiratory failure caused by primary pulmonary coccidioidomycosis: Two case reports and a review of the literature. Am Rev Respir Dis 131:797, 1985.

266. Warlick MA, Quan SF, Sobonya RE: Rapid diagnosis of pulmonary coccidioidomycosis: Cytologic vs. potassium hydroxide preparations. Arch Intern Med 143:723, 1983.

267. Wallace JM, Catanzaro A, Moser KM, et al: Flexible fiberoptic bronchoscopy for diagnosing pulmonary coccidioidomycosis. Am Rev Respir Dis 123:286, 1981.

268. DiTomasso JP, Ampel NM, Sobonya RE, et al: Bronchoscopic diagnosis of pulmonary coccidioidomycosis: Comparison of cytology, culture, and transbronchial biopsy. Diagn Microbiol Infect Dis 18:83, 1994.

269. Chitkara YK: Evaluation of cultures of percutaneous core needle biopsy specimens in the diagnosis of pulmonary nodules. Am J Clin Pathol 107:224, 1997.

270. Defelice R, Wieden MA, Galgiani JN: The incidence and implications of coccidioidouria. Am Rev Respir Dis 125:49, 1982.

271. Harley WB, Blaser MJ: Disseminated coccidioidomycosis associated with extreme eosinophilia. Clin Infect Dis 18:627, 1994.

272. Catanzaro A, Flatauer F: Detection of serum antibodies in coccidioidomycosis by solid-phase radioimmunoassay. J Infect Dis 147:32, 1983.

273. Martins TB, Jaskowski TD, Mouritsen CL, et al: Comparison of commercially available enzyme immunoassay with traditional serological tests for detection of antibodies to Coccidioides immitis. J Clin Microbiol 33:940, 1995.

274. Standaert SM, Schaffner W, Galgiani JN, et al: Coccidioidomycosis among visitors to a Coccidioides immitis–endemic area: An outbreak in a military reserve unit. J Infect Dis 171:1672, 1995.

275. Johnson SM, Zimmermann CR, Pappagianis D: Use of a recombinant Coccidioides immitis complement fixation antigen-chitinase in conventional serological assays. J Clin Microbiol 34:3160, 1996.

276. Scalarone GM, Levine HB, Pappagianis D, et al: Spherulin as a complement-fixing antigen in human coccidioidomycosis. Am Rev Respir Dis 110:324, 1974.

277. Stevens DA, Levine HB, TenEyck DR: Dermal sensitivity to different doses of spherulin and coccidioidin. Chest 65:530, 1974.

278. Levine HB, Gonzalez-Ochoa A, TenEyck DR: Dermal sensitivity to Coccidioides immitis: A comparison of responses elicited in man by spherulin and coccidioidin. Am Rev Respir Dis 107:379, 1973.

279. Sarosi GA, Davies SF: Blastomycosis. Am Rev Respir Dis 120:911, 1979.

280. Bradsher RW: Blastomycosis. Clin Infect Dis 14(Suppl 1):S82, 1992.

281. Jerray M, Hayouni A, Benzarti M, et al: Blastomycosis in Africa: A new case from Tunisia. Eur Respir J 5:365, 1992.

282. Baily GG, Robertson VJ, Neill P, et al: Blastomycosis in Africa: Clinical features, diagnosis, and treatment. Rev Infect Dis 13:1005, 1991.

283. Sekhon AS, Bogorus MS, Sims HV: Blastomycosis: Report of three cases from Alberta with a review of Canadian cases. Mycopathologia 68:53, 1979.

284. Witorsch P, Utz JP: North American blastomycosis: A study of 40 patients. Medicine 47:169, 1968.

285. Veterans Administration—Blastomycosis Cooperative Study of the Veterans Administration: Blastomycosis. I. A review of 198 collected cases in Veterans Administration hospitals. Am Rev Respir Dis 89:659, 1964.

286. Furcolow ML, Chick EW, Busey JF, et al: Prevalence and incidence studies of human and canine blastomycosis: I. Cases in the United States. 1885–1968. Am Rev Respir Dis 102:60, 1970.

287. Kane J, Righter J, Krajden S, et al: Blastomycosis: A new endemic focus in Canada. Can Med Assoc J 129:728, 1983.

288. St-Germain G, Murray G, Duperval R: Blastomycosis in Quebec (1981–90): Report of 23 cases and review of published cases from Quebec. Can J Infect Dis 4:89, 1993.

289. Vaaler AK, Bradsher RW, Davies SF: Evidence of subclinical blastomycosis in forestry workers in northern Minnesota and northern Wisconsin. Am J Med 89:470, 1990.

290. Klein BS, Vergeront JM, Weeks RJ, et al: Isolation of Blastomyces dermatitidis in soil associated with a large outbreak of blastomycosis in Wisconsin. N Engl J Med 314:529, 1986.

291. Tosh FE, Hammerman KJ, Weeks RJ, et al: A common source epidemic of North American blastomycosis. Am Rev Respir Dis 109:525, 1974.

292. Sarosi GA, Hammerman KJ, Tosh FE, et al: Clinical features of acute pulmonary blastomycosis. N Engl J Med 290:540, 1974.

293. Cockerill FR III, Roberts GD, Rosenblatt JE, et al: Epidemic of pulmonary blastomycosis (Namekagon fever) in Wisconsin canoeists. Chest 86:688, 1984.

294. Centers for Disease Control and Prevention: Blastomycosis—Wisconsin, 1986–1995. JAMA 276:444, 1996.

295. Furcolow ML, Balows A, Menges RW, et al: Blastomycosis: An important medical problem in the central United States. JAMA 198:529, 1966.

296. Abernathy RS: Clinical manifestations of pulmonary blastomycosis. Ann Intern Med 51:707, 1959.

297. Yogev R, Davis AT: Blastomycosis in children: A review of the literature. Mycopathologia 68:139, 1979.

298. Smith JG Jr, Harris JS, Conant NF, et al: An epidemic of North American blastomycosis. JAMA 158:641, 1955.

299. Sarosi GA, Eckman MR, Davies SF, et al: Canine blastomycosis as a harbinger of human disease. Ann Intern Med 91:733, 1979.

300. Manetti AC: Hyperendemic urban blastomycosis. Am J Public Health 81:633, 1991.

301. Baum GL, Lerner PI: Primary pulmonary blastomycosis: A laboratory-acquired infection. Ann Intern Med 73:263, 1970.
302. Denton JF, DiSalvo AF, Hirsch ML: Laboratory-acquired North American blastomycosis. JAMA 199:935, 1967.
303. Case report: Disseminated inoculation blastomycosis in a renal transplant recipient. Am Rev Respir Dis 130:1180, 1984.
304. Kravitz GR, Davies SF, Eckman MR, et al: Chronic blastomycotic meningitis. Am J Med 71:501, 1981.
305. Eickenberg H-U, Amin M, Lich R Jr: Blastomycosis of the genitourinary tract. J Urol 113:650, 1975.
306. Craig MW, Davey WN, Green RA: Conjugal blastomycosis. Am Rev Respir Dis 102:86, 1970.
307. Gnann JW Jr, Bressler GS, Bodet CA III, et al: Human blastomycosis after a dog bite. Ann Intern Med 98:48, 1983.
308. Menges RW, Furcolow ML, Selby LA, et al: Clinical and epidemiologic studies on seventy-nine canine blastomycosis cases in Arkansas. Am J Epidemiol 81:164, 1965.
309. Guha PK, Thompson JR: Acute pulmonary blastomycosis: A diagnostic challenge in a tuberculosis sanatorium. Am Rev Respir Dis 86:640, 1962.
310. Recht LD, Davies SF, Eckman MR, et al: Blastomycosis in immunosuppressed patients. Am Rev Respir Dis 125:359, 1982.
311. Pappas PG, Pottage JC, Powderly WG, et al: Blastomycosis in patients with the acquired immunodeficiency syndrome. Ann Intern Med 116:847, 1992.
312. Winquist EW, Walmsley SL, Berinstein NL: Reactivation and dissemination of blastomycosis complicating Hodgkin's disease: A case report and review of the literature. Am J Hematol 43:129, 1993.
313. Serody JS, Mill MR, Detterbeck FC, et al: Blastomycosis in transplant recipients: Report of a case and review. Clin Infect Dis 16:54, 1993.
314. Pappas PG, Threlkeld MG, Bedsole GD, et al: Blastomycosis in immunocompromised patients. Medicine 72:311, 1993.
315. Atkinson JB, McCurley TL: Pulmonary blastomycosis: Filamentous forms in an immunocompromised patient with fulminating respiratory failure. Hum Pathol 14:186, 1983.
316. Berger R, Kraman S: Acute miliary blastomycosis after "short-course" corticosteroid treatment. Arch Intern Med 141:1223, 1981.
317. Stelling CB, Woodring JH, Rehm SR, et al: Miliary pulmonary blastomycosis. Radiology 150:7, 1984.
318. Skillrud DM, Douglas WW: Survival in adult respiratory distress syndrome caused by blastomycosis infection. Mayo Clin Proc 60:266, 1985.
319. Bradsher RW: Development of specific immunity in patients with pulmonary or extrapulmonary blastomycosis. Am Rev Respir Dis 129:430, 1984.
320. Jacobs RF, Marmer DJ, Balk RA, et al: Lymphocyte subpopulations of blood and alveolar lavage in blastomycosis. Chest 88:579, 1985.
321. Dismukes WE: Blastomycosis: Leave it to beaver. N Engl J Med 314:575, 1986.
322. Klein BS, Sondel PM, Jones JM: WI-1, a novel 120-kilodalton surface protein on Blastomyces dermatitidis yeast cells, is a target antigen of cell-mediated immunity in human blastomycosis. Infect Immun 60:4291, 1992.
323. Morrison CJ, Stevens DA: Mechanisms of fungal pathogenicity: Correlation of virulence in vivo, susceptibility to killing by polymorphonuclear neutrophils in vitro, and neutrophil superoxide anion induction among Blastomyces dermatitidis isolates. Infect Immun 59:2744, 1991.
324. Schwarz J, Baum GL: Blastomycosis. Am J Clin Pathol 21:999, 1951.
325. Williams JE, Moser SA, Turner SH, et al: Development of pulmonary infection in mice inoculated with Blastomyces dermatitidis conidia. Am J Respir Crit Care Med 149:500, 1994.
326. Vanek J, Schwarz J, Hakim S: North American blastomycosis: A study of ten cases. Am J Clin Pathol 54:384, 1970.
327. Schwarz J, Salfelder K: Blastomycosis: A review of 152 cases. Curr Top Pathol 65:166, 1977.
328. Kaufman J: Tracheal blastomycosis. Chest 93:424, 1988.
329. Christie AJ, Binns PM, Kredo KR: Long-standing indolent blastomycosis at internal opening of tracheostomy. Chest 95:932, 1989.
330. Watts JC, Chandler FW, Mihalov ML, et al: Giant forms of Blastomyces dermatitidis in the pulmonary lesions of blastomycosis: Potential confusion with coccidioides immitis. Am J Clin Pathol 93:575, 1990.
331. Hardin HF, Scott DI: Blastomycosis: Occurrence of filamentous forms in vivo. Am J Clin Pathol 62:104, 1974.
332. Larson RE, Bernatz PE, Geraci JE: Results of surgical and nonoperative treatment for pulmonary North American blastomycosis. J Thorac Cardiovasc Surg 51:714, 1966.
333. Sheflin JR, Campbell JA, Thompson GP: Pulmonary blastomycosis: Findings on chest radiographs in 63 patients. Am J Roentgenol 154:117, 1990.
334. Brown LR, Swensen SJ, Van Scoy RE, et al: Roentgenologic features of pulmonary blastomycosis. Mayo Clin Proc 66:29, 1991.
335. Kuzo RS, Goodman LR: Blastomycosis. Semin Roentgenol 1:45, 1996.
336. Pfister AK, Goodwin AW, Squire EW, et al: Pulmonary blastomycosis: Roentgenographic clues to the diagnosis. South Med J 59:1441, 1966.
337. Sheflin JR, Campbell JA, Thompson GP: Pulmonary blastomycosis: Findings on chest radiographs in 63 patients. Am J Roentgenol 154:1177, 1990.
338. Halvorsen RA, Duncan JD, Merten DF, et al: Pulmonary blastomycosis: Radiologic manifestations. Radiology 150:1, 1984.
339. Alkrinawi S, Reed MH, Pasterkamp H: Pulmonary blastomycosis in children: Findings on chest radiographs. Am J Roentgenol 165:651, 1995.
340. Rabinowitz JG, Busch J, Buttram WR: Pulmonary manifestations of blastomycosis: Radiological support of a new concept. Radiology 120:25, 1976.
341. Kepron MW, Schoemperlen CB, Hershfield ES, et al: North American blastomycosis in Central Canada: A review of 36 cases. Can Med Assoc J 106:243, 1972.
342. Poe RH, Vassallo CL, Plessinger VA, et al: Pulmonary blastomycosis versus carcinoma—a challenging differential. Am J Med Sci 263:145, 1972.
343. Griffith JE, Campbell GD: Acute miliary blastomycosis presenting as fulminating respiratory failure. Chest 75:630, 1979.
344. Evans ME, Haynes JB, Atkinson JB, et al: Blastomyces dermatitidis and the adult respiratory distress syndrome: Case reports and review of the literature. Am Rev Respir Dis 126:1099, 1982.
345. Meyer KC, McManus EJ, Maki DG: Overwhelming pulmonary blastomycosis associated with the adult respiratory distress syndrome. N Engl J Med 329:1231, 1993.
346. Kinzy JD, Powers WP, Baddour LM: Case report: Blastomyces dermatitidis as a cause of middle lobe syndrome. Am J Med Sci 312:191, 1996.
347. Winer-Muram HT, Beals DH, Cole Jr FH: Blastomycosis of the lung: CT features. Radiology 182:829, 1992.
348. Kinasewitz GT, Penn RL, George RB: The spectrum and significance of pleural disease in blastomycosis. Chest 86:580, 1984.
349. Jay SJ, O'Neill RP, Goodman N, et al: Pleural effusion: A rare manifestation of acute pulmonary blastomycosis. Am J Med Sci 274:325, 1977.
350. Neuzil KM, Mitchell HC, Loyd JE, et al: Extrapulmonary thoracic disease caused by Blastomyces dermatitidis. Chest 106:1885, 1994.
351. Laskey W, Sarosi GA: Endogenous activation in blastomycosis. Ann Intern Med 88:50, 1978.
352. Renston JP, Morgan J, DiMarco AF: Disseminated miliary blastomycosis leading to acute respiratory failure in an urban setting. Chest 101:1463, 1992.
353. Frean J, Blumberg L, Woolf M: Disseminated blastomycosis masquerading as tuberculosis. J Infect 26:203, 1993.
354. Lagging LM, Breland CM, Kennedy DJ, et al: Delayed treatment of pulmonary blastomycosis causing vertebral osteomyelitis, paraspinal abscess, and spinal cord compression. Scand J Infect Dis 26:111, 1994.
355. Neuzil KM, Mitchell HC, Loyd JE, et al: Extrapulmonary thoracic disease caused by Blastomyces dermatitidis. Chest 106:1885, 1994.
356. Lagerstrom CF, Mitchell HG, Graham BS, et al: Chronic fibrosing mediastinitis and superior vena caval obstruction from blastomycosis. Ann Thorac Surg 54:764, 1992.
357. Hawley C, Felson B: Roentgen aspects of intrathoracic blastomycosis. Am J Roentgenol 75:751, 1956.
358. Lopez R, Mason JO, Parker JS, et al: Intraocular blastomycosis: Case report and review. Clin Infect Dis 18:805, 1994.
359. Day TA, Stucker FJ: Blastomycosis of the paranasal sinuses. Otolaryngol Head Neck Surg 110:437, 1994.
360. Perez-Lasala G, Nolan RL, Chapman SW, et al: Peritoneal blastomycosis. Am J Gastroenterol 86:357, 1991.
361. Reder PA, Neel HB 3d: Blastomycosis in otolaryngology: Review of a large series. Laryngoscope 103:53, 1993.
362. Sutliff WD, Cruthirds TP: Blastomyces dermatitidis in cytologic preparations. Am Rev Respir Dis 108:149, 1973.
363. Covell JL, Lowry EH Jr, Feldman PS: Cytologic diagnosis of blastomycosis in pleural fluid. Acta Cytol 26:833, 1982.
364. Sanders JS, Sarosi GA, Nollet DJ, et al: Exfoliative cytology in the rapid diagnosis of pulmonary blastomycosis. Chest 72:193, 1977.
365. Williams JE, Murphy R, Standard PG, et al: Serologic response in blastomycosis: Diagnostic value of double ID assay. Am Rev Respir Dis 123:209, 1981.
366. Klein BS, Kuritsky JN, Chappell WA, et al: Comparison of the enzyme immunoassay, ID and complement fixation tests in detecting antibody in human serum to the A antigen of Blastomyces dermatitidis. Am Rev Respir Dis 133:144, 1986.
367. Soufleris AJ, Klein BS, Courtney BT, et al: Utility of anti-WI-1 serological testing in the diagnosis of blastomycosis in Wisconsin residents. Clin Infect Dis 19:87, 1994.
367a. Hurst SF, Kaufman L: Western immunoblot analysis and serologic characterization of Blastomyces dermatitidis yeast form extracellular antigens. J Clin Microbiol 30:3043, 1992.
368. Murray HW, Littman ML, Roberts RB: Disseminated paracoccidioidomycosis (South American blastomycosis) in the United States. Am J Med 56:209, 1974.
369. Fountain FF, Sutliff WD: Paracoccidioidomycosis in the United States. Am Rev Respir Dis 99:89, 1969.
370. Bouza E, Winston DJ, Rhodes J, et al: Paracoccidioidomycosis (South American blastomycosis) in the United States. Chest 72:100, 1977.
371. Angulo-Ortega A, Pollak L: Paracoccidioidomycosis. In Baker RD (ed): Human Infection with Fungi, Actinomycetes and Algae. New York, Springer-Verlag, 1971.
372. Pena CE: Deep mycotic infections in Colombia: A clinicopathologic study of 162 cases. Am J Clin Pathol 47:505, 1967.
373. Salfelder K, Doehnert G, Doehnert H-R: Paracoccidioidomycosis: Anatomic study with complete autopsies. Virchows Arch Abt Path Anat 348:51, 1969.
374. Restrepo A, Robledo M, Gutierrez F, et al: Paracoccidioidomycosis (South American blastomycosis): A study of 39 cases observed in Medellin, Colombia. Am J Trop Med Hyg 19:68, 1970.
375. de Albornoz MB: Isolation of Paracoccidioides brasiliensis from rural soil in Venezuela. Sabouraudia 9:248, 1971.
376. Londero AT, Ramos CD: Paracoccidioidomycosis: A clinical and mycologic study of forty-one cases observed in Santa Maria, RS, Brazil. Am J Med 52:771, 1972.

377. Mackinnon JE: Pathogenesis of South American blastomycosis. Trans Trop Med Hyg 53:487, 1959.

378. Angulo-Ortega A: Calcifications in paracoccidioidomycosis—are they the morphological manifestation of subclinical infections? In: Paracoccidioidomycosis, Pan American Symposium on Paracoccidioidomycosis, 1st, Medellin, Colombia, 1971, p 129.

379. Greer DL, De Estrada DD, De Trejos LA: Dermal reactions to paracoccidioidin among family members of patients with paracoccidioidomycosis. In: Paracoccidioidomycosis, Pan American Symposium on Paracoccidioidomycosis, 1st, Medellin, Colombia, 1971, p 76.

380. Robledo MA, Graybill JR, Ahrens J, et al: Host defense against experimental paracoccidioidomycosis. Am Rev Respir Dis 125:563, 1982.

381. Severo LC, Londero AT, Geyer GR, et al: Acute pulmonary paracoccidioidomycosis in an immunosuppressed patient. Mycopathologia 68:171, 1979.

382. Severo LC, Porto NS, Camargo JJ, et al: Multiple paracoccidioidomas simulating Wegener's granulomatosis. Mycopathologia 91:117, 1985.

383. Agia GA, Hurst DJ, Rogers WA: Paracoccidioidomycosis presenting as a cavitating pulmonary mass. Chest 78:650, 1980.

384. Londero AT, Ramos CD, Lopes JOS: Progressive pulmonary paracoccidioidomycosis: A study of 34 cases observed in Rio Grande do Sul (Brazil). Mycopathologia 63:53, 1978.

385. Tani EM, Franco M: Pulmonary cytology in paracoccidioidomycosis. Acta Cytol 28:571, 1984.

386. Restrepo A, Cano LE, Tabares AM: A comparison of mycelial filtrate—a yeast lysate-paracoccidioidin in patients with paracoccidioidomycosis. Mycopathologia 84:49, 1983.

387. Sposto MR, Mendes-Giannini MJ, Moraes RA, et al: Paracoccidioidomycosis manifesting as oral lesions: Clinical, cytological and serological investigation. J Oral Pathol Med 23:85, 1994.

388. Rozenbaum R, Goncalves AJ: Clinical epidemiological study of 171 cases of cryptococcosis. Clin Infect Dis 18:369, 1994.

389. Krumholz RA: Pulmonary cryptococcosis: A case due to *Cryptococcus albidus*. Am Rev Respir Dis 105:421, 1972.

390. Horowitz ID, Blumberg EA, Krevolin L: *Cryptococcus albidus* and mucormycosis empyema in a patient receiving hemodialysis. South Med J 86:1070, 1993.

391. Lynch JP III, Schaberg DR, Kissner DG, et al: *Cryptococcus laurentii* lung abscess. Am Rev Respir Dis 123:135, 1981.

392. Salfelder K: Cryptococcosis. In: Baker RD (ed): Human Infection with Fungi, Actinomycetes and Algae. New York, Springer-Verlag, 1971, p 383.

393. Ruiz A, Bulmer GS: Particle size of airborne *Cryptococcus neoformans* in a tower. Appl Environ Microbiol 41:1225, 1981.

394. Pathmanathan R, Soon ST: Cryptococcosis in the University Hospital, Kuala Lumpur and review of published cases. Trans Trop Med Hyg 76:21, 1982.

395. Bisseru B, Bajaj A, Carruthers RH, et al: Pulmonary and bilateral retinochoroidal cryptococcosis. Br J Opthalmol 67:157, 1983.

396. Bennett JE, Kwon-Chung KJ, Howard DH: Epidemiologic differences among serotypes of *Cryptococcus neoformans*. Am J Epidemiol 105:582, 1977.

397. Campbell GD: Primary pulmonary cryptococcosis. Am Rev Respir Dis 94:236, 1966.

398. McDonnell JM, Hutchins GM: Pulmonary cryptococcosis. Hum Pathol 16:121, 1985.

399. Kerkering TM, Duma RJ, Shadomy S: The evolution of pulmonary cryptococcosis: Clinical implications from a study of 41 patients with and without compromising host factors. Ann Intern Med 94:611, 1981.

400. Zuger A, Louie E, Holzman RS, et al: Cryptococcal disease in patients with the acquired immunodeficiency syndrome: Diagnostic features and outcome of treatment. Ann Intern Med 104:234, 1986.

401. Gal AA, Koss MN, Hawkins J, et al: The pathology of pulmonary cryptococcal infections in the acquired immunodeficiency syndrome. Arch Pathol Lab Med 110:502, 1986.

402. Kaplan MH, Rosen PP, Armstrong D: Cryptococcosis in a cancer hospital: Clinical and pathological correlates in forty-six patients. Cancer 39:2265, 1977.

403. Lewis JL, Rabinovich S: The wide spectrum of cryptococcal infections. Am J Med 53:315, 1972.

404. Schwarz J, Baum GL: Cryptococcosis. Semin Roentgenol 5:49, 1970.

405. Gordonson J, Birnbaum W, Jacobson G, et al: Pulmonary cryptococcosis. Radiology 112:557, 1974.

406. Henson DJ, Hill AR: Cryptococcal pneumonia: A fulminant presentation. Am J Med Sci 288:221, 1984.

407. Nottebart HC, McGehee RF, Utz JP: Cryptococcosis complicating sarcoidosis. Am Rev Respir Dis 107:1060, 1973.

408. Bernstein B, Flomenberg P, Letzer D: Disseminated cryptococcal disease complicating steroid therapy for *Pneumocystis carinii* pneumonia in a patient with AIDS. South Med J 87:537, 1994.

409. Ferguson RP: Cryptococcosis and Cushing's syndrome. Ann Intern Med 87:65, 1977.

410. Kramer M, Corrado ML, Bacci V, et al: Pulmonary cryptococcosis and Cushing's syndrome. Arch Intern Med 143:2179, 1983.

411. Emmons CW: Natural occurrence of opportunistic fungi. Lab Invest 11:1026, 1962.

412. Farhi F, Bulmer GS, Tacker JR: *Cryptococcus neoformans*: IV. The not-so-encapsulated yeast. Infect Immun 1:526, 1970.

413. Bulmer GS, Sans MD: *Cryptococcus neoformans*: III. Inhibition of phagocytosis. J Bacteriol 95:5, 1968.

414. Farmer SG, Komorowski RA: Histologic response to capsule-deficient *Cryptococcus neoformans*. Arch Pathol 96:383, 1973.

415. Gutierrez F, Fu YS, Lurie HI: Cryptococcosis histologically resembling histoplasmosis: A light and electron microscopical study. Arch Pathol 99:347, 1975.

416. Harding SA, Scheld WM, Feldman PS, et al: Pulmonary infection with capsule-deficient *Cryptococcus neoformans*. Virchow Arch Path Anat Histol 382:113, 1979.

417. Baker RD: The primary pulmonary lymph node complex of cryptococcosis. Am J Clin Pathol 65:83, 1976.

418. Fisher BD, Armstrong D: Cryptococcal interstitial pneumonia: Value of antigen determination. N Engl J Med 297:1440, 1977.

419. Baker RD, Haugen RK: Tissue changes and tissue diagnosis in cryptococcosis: A study of 26 cases. Am J Clin Pathol 25:14, 1955.

420. Khoury MB, Godwin JD, Ravin CE, et al: Thoracic cryptococcosis: Immunologic competence and radiologic appearance. Am J Roentgenol 142:893, 1984.

421. Patz EF Jr, Goodman PC: Pulmonary cryptococcosis. J Thorac Imaging 7:51, 1992.

422. Woodring JH, Ciporkin G, Lee C, et al: Pulmonary cryptococcosis. Semin Roentgenol 1:67, 1996.

423. Feigin DS: Pulmonary cryptococcosis: Radiologic-pathologic correlates of its three forms. Am J Roentgenol 141:1263, 1983.

424. Miller Jr WT, Edelman JM, Miller WT: Cryptococcal pulmonary infection in patients with AIDS: Radiographic appearance. Radiology 175:725, 1990.

425. Sider L, Westcott MA: Pulmonary manifestations of cryptococcosis in patients with AIDS: CT features. J Thorac Imaging 9:78, 1994

426. Werner WA: Pulmonary and cerebral cryptococcosis without meningitis. Am Rev Respir Dis 92:476, 1965.

427. Geraci JE, Donoghue FE, Ellis FH Jr, et al: Focal pulmonary cryptococcosis: Evaluation of necessity of amphotericin B therapy. Mayo Clin Proc 40:552, 1965.

428. Salyer WR, Salyer DC: Pleural involvement in cryptococcosis. Chest 66:139, 1974.

429. Smilack JD, Bellet RE, Talman WT Jr: Cryptococcal pleural effusion. JAMA 232:639, 1975.

430. Young EJ, Hirsh DD, Fainstein V, et al: Pleural effusions due to *Cryptococcus neoformans*: A review of the literature and report of two cases with cryptococcal antigen determinations. Am Rev Respir Dis 121:743, 1980.

431. Perla EN, Maayan S, Miller SN, et al: Disseminated cryptococcosis presenting as the adult respiratory distress syndrome. N Y State J Med 85:704, 1985.

432. Long RF, Berens SV, Shambhag GR: An unusual manifestation of pulmonary cryptococcosis (case report). Br J Radiol 45:757, 1972.

433. Meighan JW: Pulmonary cryptococcosis mimicking carcinoma of the lung. Radiology 103:61, 1972.

434. Littman ML: Cryptococcosis (torulosis): Current concepts and therapy. Am J Med 27:976, 1959.

435. Gordon MA, Vedder DK: Serologic tests in diagnosis and prognosis of cryptococcosis. JAMA 197:961, 1966.

436. Burch KH, Fine G, Quinn EL, et al: *Cryptococcus neoformans* as a cause of lytic bone lesions. JAMA 231:1057, 1975.

437. Coodley EL: Cryptococcosis—revisited: Report of a case. Dis Chest 52:558, 1967.

438. Tynes B, Mason KN, Jennings AE, et al: Variant forms of pulmonary cryptococcosis. Ann Intern Med 69:1117, 1968.

439. Warr W, Bates JH, Stone A: The spectrum of pulmonary cryptococcosis. Ann Intern Med 69:1109, 1968.

440. Gleason TH, Hammar SP, Barthas M, et al: Cytological diagnosis of pulmonary cryptococcosis. Arch Pathol Lab Med 104:384, 1980

441. Kanjanavirojkul N, Puapairoj A: Cytologic diagnosis of *Cryptococcus neoformans* in HIV-positive patients. Acta Cytol 41:493, 1997.

442. Hammerman KJ, Powell KE, Christianson CS, et al: Pulmonary cryptococcosis: Clinical forms and treatment. A Center for Disease Control cooperative mycoses study. Ann Rev Respir Dis 108:1116, 1973.

443. Duperval R, Hermans, PE, Brewer NS, et al: Cryptococcosis, with emphasis on the significance of isolation of *Cryptococcus neoformans* from the respiratory tract. Chest 72:13, 1977.

444. Subramanian S, Kherdekar SS, Babu PGV, et al: Lipoid pneumonia with *Cryptococcus neoformans* colonization. Thorax 37:319, 1982.

445. Guptka RK: Diagnosis of unsuspected pulmonary cryptococcosis with sputum cytology. Acta Cytol 29:154, 1985.

446. Walts AE: Localized pulmonary cryptococcosis: Diagnosis by fine needle aspiration. Acta Cytol 27:457, 1983.

447. Silverman JF, Johnsrude IS: Fine needle aspiration cytology of granulomatous cryptococcosis of the lung. Acta Cytol 29:157, 1985.

448. Walter JE, Jones RD: Serodiagnosis of clinical cryptococcosis. Am Rev Respir Dis 97:275, 1968.

449. Jensen WA, Rose RM, Hammer SM, et al: Serologic diagnosis of focal pneumonia caused by *Cryptococcus neoformans*. Am Rev Respir Dis 132:189, 1985.

450. Bloomfield N, Gordon MA, Elmendorf DF Jr: Detection of *Cryptococcus neoformans* in body fluids by latex particle agglutination. Proc Soc Exp Biol Med 114:64, 1963.

451. Atkinson AJ, Bennett JE: Experience with a new skin test antigen prepared from *Cryptococcus neoformans*. Am Rev Respir Dis 97:637, 1968.

452. Allegra CJ, Kovacs JA, Drake JC, et al: Activity of antifolates against *Pneumocystis carinii* dihydrofolate reductase and identification of a potent new agent. J Exp Med 165:926, 1987.

453. Edman JC, Kovacs JA, Masur H, et al: Ribosomal RNA sequence shows *Pneumocystis carinii* to be a member of the fungi. Nature 33:519, 1988.

454. Bedrossian CWM: Ultrastructure of *Pneumocystis carinii*: A review of internal and surface characteristics. Semin Diagn Pathol 6:212, 1989.

455. Haque A, Plattner SB, Cook RT, et al: *Pneumocystis carinii*: Taxonomy as viewed by electron microscopy. Am J Clin Pathol 87:504, 1987.

456. Smulian AG, Walzer PD: The biology of *Pneumocystis carinii*. Crit Rev Microbiol 18:191, 1992.

457. Hasleton PS, Curry A, Rankin EM: *Pneumocystis carinii* pneumonia: A light microscopical and ultrastructural study. J Clin Pathol 34:1138, 1981.

458. Ishida T, Matsui Y, Matsumura Y, et al: Ultrastructural observation of *Pneumocystis carinii* in bronchoalveolar lavage fluid from non-AIDS patients with *P. carinii* pneumonia. Chest 105:1342, 1994.

459. Cushion MT, Ruffolo JJ, Walzer PD: Analysis of the developmental stages of *Pneumocystis carinii*, in vitro. Lab Invest 58:324, 1988.

460. Pifer LL, Hughes WT, Murphy MJ: Propagation of *Pneumocystis carinii* in vitro. Pediatr Res 11:305, 1977.

461. Beck JM, Newbury RL, Palmer BE: *Pneumocystis carinii* pneumonia in scid mice induced by viable organisms propagated in vitro. Infect Immun 64:4643, 1996

462. Santamauro JT, Stover DE: *Pneumocystis carinii* pneumonia. Med Clin North Am 81:299, 1997.

463. Levine SJ: *Pneumocystis carinii*. Clin Chest Med 17:665, 1996.

464. Lundgren B, Lebech M, Lind K, et al: Antibody response to a major human *Pneumocystis carinii* surface antigen in patients without evidence of immunosuppression and in patients with suspected atypical pneumonia. Eur J Clin Microbiol Infect Dis 12:105, 1993.

465. Hughes WT: *Pneumocystis carinii* pneumonia. N Engl J Med 297:1381, 1977.

466. Kovacs JA: Diagnosis, treatment and prevention of *Pneumocystis carinii* pneumonia in HIV-infected patients. AIDS Updates 2:1, 1989.

467. Ballardie FW, Winearis CG, Cohen J, et al: *Pneumocystis carinii* pneumonia in renal transplant recipients: Clinical and radiographic features, diagnosis and complications of treatment. QJM 57:729, 1985.

468. Lufft V, Kliem V, Behrend M, et al: Incidence of *Pneumocystis carinii* pneumonia after renal transplantation: Impact of immunosuppression. Transplantation 62:421, 1996.

469. Varthalitis I, Aoun M, Daneau D, et al: *Pneumocystis carinii* pneumonia in patients with cancer: An increasing incidence. Cancer 71:481, 1993.

470. Sepkowitz KA, Brown AE, Telzak EE, et al: *Pneumocystis carinii* pneumonia among patients without AIDS at a cancer hospital. JAMA 267:832, 1992.

471. van der Lelie J, Venema D, Kuijper EJ, et al: *Pneumocystis carinii* pneumonia in HIV-negative patients with haematologic disease. Infection 25:78, 1997.

472. Robert NJ, Pifer LL, Niell HB, et al: Incidence of *Pneumocystis carinii* antigenemia in ambulatory cancer patients. Cancer 53:1878, 1984.

473. Fossieck BE, Spagnolo SV: *Pneumocystis carinii* pneumonitis in patients with lung cancer. Chest 78:721, 1980.

474. Godeau B, Coutant-Perronne V, Le Thi Huong D, et al: *Pneumocystis carinii* pneumonia in the course of connective tissue disease: Report of 34 cases. J Rheumatol 21:246, 1994.

475. Stenger AA, Houtman PM, Bruyn GA, et al: *Pneumocystis carinii* pneumonia associated with low dose methotrexate treatment for rheumatoid arthritis. Scand J Rheumatol 23:51, 1994.

476. Ognibene FP, Shelhamer JH, Hoffman GS, et al: *Pneumocystis carinii* pneumonia: A major complication of immunosuppressive therapy in patients with Wegener's granulomatosis. Am J Respir Crit Care Med 151:795, 1995.

477. Godeau B, Coutant-Perronne V, Le Thi Huong D, et al: *Pneumocystis carinii* pneumonia in the course of connective tissue disease: Report of 34 cases. J Rheumatol 21:246, 1994.

478. Natale RB, Yagoda A, Brown A, et al: Combined *Pneumocystis carinii* and *Nocardia asteroides* pneumonitis in a patient with an ACTH-producing carcinoid. Cancer 47:2933, 1981.

479. Fulkerson WJ, Newman JH: Endogenous Cushing's syndrome complicated by *Pneumocystis carinii* pneumonia. Am Rev Respir Dis 59:188, 1984.

480. Kadoya A, Okada J, Iikuni Y, et al: Risk factors for *Pneumocystis carinii* pneumonia in patients with polymyositis/dermatomyositis or systemic lupus erythematosus. J Rheumatol 23:1186, 1996.

481. Gerrard JG: *Pneumocystis carinii* pneumonia in HIV-negative immunocompromised adults. Med J Aust 162:233, 1995.

482. Burke BA, Good RA: *Pneumocystis carinii* infection. Medicine 52:23, 1973.

483. Doak PB, Becroft DMO, Harris EA, et al: *Pneumocystis carinii* pneumonia—transplant lung. QJM 42:59, 1973.

484. Frenkel JK, Good JT, Shultz JA: Latent *Pneumocystis* infection of rats, relapse and chemotherapy. Lab Invest 15:1559, 1966.

485. Lidman C, Olsson M, Bjorkman A, et al: No evidence of nosocomial *Pneumocystis carinii* infection via health care personnel. Scand J Infect Dis 29:63, 1997.

486. Kovacs JA, Halpern JL, Lundgren B, et al: Monoclonal antibodies in *Pneumocystis carinii*: Identification of specific antigens and characterization of antigenic differences between rat and human isolates. J Infect Dis 159:60, 1989.

487. Lee C-H, Lu J-J, Bartlett MS, et al: Nucleotide sequence variation in *Pneumocystis carinii* strains that infect humans. J Clin Microbiol 31:754, 1993.

488. Gutierrez Y: The biology of *Pneumocystis carinii*. Semin Diagn Pathol 6:203, 1989.

489. Gigliotti F, Harmsen AG, Haidaris CG, et al: *Pneumocystis carinii* is not universally transmissible between mammalian species. Infect Immun 61:2886, 1993.

490. Wakefield AE, Fritscher CC, Malin AS, et al: Genetic diversity in human-derived *Pneumocystis carinii* isolates from four geographic locations shown by analysis of mitochondrial rRNA gene sequences. J Clin Microbiol 32:2959, 1994.

491. Hendley JO, Weller TH: Activation and transmission in rats of infection with *Pneumocystis*. Proc Soc Exp Biol Med 137:1401, 1971.

492. Sepkowitz K, Schluger N, Godwin T, et al: DNA amplification in experimental pneumocystosis: Characterization of serum *Pneumocystis carinii* DNA and potential *P. carinii* carrier states. J Infect Dis 168:421, 1993.

493. Hughes WT: Natural mode of acquisition for de novo infection with *Pneumocystis carinii*. J Infect Dis 145:842, 1982.

494. Tauber MI, Beckers ML, Sieben M: Parasitologic and serologic observations of infection with *Pneumocystis* in humans. J Infect Dis 136:43, 1977.

495. Leigh TR, Millett MJ, Jameson B, et al: Serum titres of *Pneumocystis carinii* antibody in health care workers caring for patients with AIDS. Thorax 48:619, 1993.

496. Latouche S, Poirot JL, Bernard C, et al: Study of internal transcribed spacer and mitochondrial large-subunit genes of *Pneumocystis carinii* hominis isolated by repeated bronchoalveolar lavage from human immunodeficiency virus-infected patients during one or several episodes of pneumonia. J Clin Microbiol 35:1687, 1997.

497. Singer C, Armstrong D, Rosen PP, et al: *Pneumocystis carinii* pneumonia: A cluster of eleven cases. Ann Intern Med 82:772, 1975.

498. Chave JP, David S, Wauters JP, et al: Transmission of *Pneumocystis carinii* from AIDS patients to other immunosuppressed patients: A cluster of *Pneumocystis carinii* pneumonia in renal transplant recipients. AIDS 5:927, 1991.

499. Hennequin C, Page B, Roux P, et al: Outbreak of *Pneumocystis carinii* pneumonia in a renal transplant unit. Eur J Clin Microbiol Infect Dis 14:122, 1995.

500. Hardy AM, Wajszczuk CP, Suffredini AF, et al: *Pneumocystis carinii* pneumonia in renal-transplant recipients treated with cyclosporine and steroids. J Infect Dis 149:143, 1984.

501. Latouche S, Poirot JL, Maury E, et al: *Pneumocystis carinii* hominis sequencing to study hypothetical person-to-person transmission. AIDS 11:549, 1997.

502. Frenkel JK, Good JT, Schultz JA: Latent *Pneumocystis* infection in rat relapse and chemotherapy. Lab Invest 15:1559, 1966.

503. Hughes WT, Feldman S, Aur RJA, et al: Intensity of immunosuppressive therapy and the incidence of *Pneumocystis carinii* pneumonitis. Cancer 36:2004, 1975.

504. Elvin K, Lidman C, Tynell E, et al: Natural history of asymptomatic and symptomatic *Pneumocystis carinii* infection in HIV infected patients. Scand J Infect Dis 26:643, 1994.

505. Peters SE, Wakefield AE, Sinclair K, et al: A search for *P. carinii* in postmortem lungs by DNA amplification. J Pathol 166:195, 1992.

506. Limper AH, Hoyte JS, Standing JE: The role of alveolar macrophages in *Pneumocystis carinii* degradation and clearance from the lung. J Clin Invest 99:2110, 1997.

507. Millard PR, Heryet AR: Observations favouring *Pneumocystis carinii* pneumonia as a primary infection: A monoclonal antibody study on paraffin sections. J Pathol 154:365, 1988.

508. Martin WJ II: Pathogenesis of *Pneumocystis carinii* pneumonia. Am J Respir Cell Mol Biol 8:356, 1993.

509. Balzer PD: *Pneumocystis carinii*: Recent advances in basic biology and their clinical application. AIDS 7:1293, 1993.

510. Shellito JE: Host defense against *Pneumocystis carinii*: More than the CD4+ lymphocyte. J Lab Clin Med 128:448, 1996.

511. Saah AJ, Hoover DR, Peng Y, et al: Predictors for failure of *Pneumocystis carinii* pneumonia prophylaxis. Multicenter AIDS Cohort Study. JAMA 273:1197, 1995.

512. Masur H, Ognibene FP, Yarchoan R, et al: CD4 counts as predictors of opportunistic pneumonias in human immunodeficiency virus (HIV) infection. Ann Intern Med 111:223, 1989.

513. Beck JM, Newbury RL, Palmer BE, et al: Role of CD8+ lymphocytes in host defense against *Pneumocystis carinii* in mice. J Lab Clin Med 128:477, 1996.

513a. Limper AH: Tumor necrosis factor-alpha–mediated host defense against *Pneumocystis carinii*. Am J Respir Cell Mol Biol 16:110, 1997.

514. Kolls JK, Beck JM, Nelson S, et al: Alveolar macrophage release of tumor necrosis factor during murine *Pneumocystis carinii* pneumonia. Am J Respir Cell Mol Biol 8:370, 1993.

515. Kolls JK, Lei D, Vazquez C, et al: Exacerbation of murine *Pneumocystis carinii* infection by adenoviral-mediated gene transfer of a TNF inhibitor. Am J Respir Cell Mol Biol 16:112, 1997.

516. Mandujano JF, D'Souza NB, Nelson S, et al: Granulocyte-macrophage colony stimulating factor and *Pneumocystis carinii* pneumonia in mice. Am J Respir Crit Care Med 151:1233, 1995.

517. Pesanti EL: Effects of bacterial pneumonitis on development of pneumocystosis in rats. Am Rev Respir Dis 125:723, 1982.

518. Laursen AL, Rungby J, Andersen PL: Decreased activation of the respiratory burst in neutrophils from AIDS patients with previous *Pneumocystis carinii* pneumonia. J Infect Dis 172:497, 1995.

519. Hofmann BO, Odum N, Platz P, et al: Humoral responses to *Pneumocystis carinii* in patients with acquired immunodeficiency syndrome and in immunocompromised homosexual men. J Infect Dis 152:838, 1985.

520. Laursen AL, Jensen BN, Andersen PL: Local antibodies against *Pneumocystis carinii* in bronchoalveolar lavage fluid. Eur Respir J 7:679, 1994.

521. Escamilla R, Prevost MC, Hermant C, et al: Surfactant analysis during *Pneumocystis carinii* pneumonia in HIV-infected patients. Chest 101:1558, 1992.

522. Long EG, Smith JS, Meier JL: Attachment of *Pneumocystis carinii* to rat pneumocytes. Lab Invest 54:609, 1986.

523. Wisniowski P, Pasula R, Martin WJ II: Isolation of *Pneumocystis carinii* gp120 by fibronectin affinity: Evidence for manganese dependence. Am J Respir Cell Mol Biol 11:262, 1994.

524. Limper AH, Standing JE, Hoffman OA, et al: Vitronectin binds to *Pneumocystis carinii* and mediates organism attachment to cultured lung epithelial cells. Infect Immun 61:4302, 1993.

525. Pottratz ST, Paulsrud J, Smith JS, et al: *Pneumocystis carinii* attachment to cultured lung cells by pneumocystis gp120, a fibronectin binding protein. J Clin Invest 88:403, 1991.

526. Long EG, Smith JS, Meier JL: Attachment of *Pneumocystis carinii* to rat pneumocytes. Lab Invest 54:609, 1986.

527. Lank PN, Minda M, Pietra GG, et al: Alveolar response to experimental *Pneumocystis carinii* pneumonia in the rat. Am J Pathol 99:561, 1980.

528. Yoneda K, Walzer PD: Mechanism of pulmonary alveolar injury in experimental *Pneumocystis carinii* pneumonia in the rat. Br J Exp Pathol 62:339, 1981.

529. Limper AH, Thomas CF Jr, Anders RA, et al: Interactions of parasite and host epithelial cell cycle regulation during *Pneumocystis carinii* pneumonia. J Lab Clin Med 130:132, 1997.

530. Murphy MJ, Pifer LL, Hughes WT: *Pneumocystis carinii* in vitro: A study by scanning electron microscopy. Am J Pathol 86:387, 1977.

531. Meunier-Carpentier F, Kiehn TE, Armstrong D: Fungemia in the immunocompromised host: Changing patterns, antigenemia, high mortality. Am J Med 71:363, 1981.

532. Koziel H, Phelps DS, Fishman JA, et al: Surfactant protein A reduces binding and phagocytosis of *Pneumocystis carinii* by alveolar macrophages *in vitro*. Am J Respir Cell Mol Biol 18:834, 1998.

533. Murry CE, Schmidt RA: Tissue invasion by *Pneumocystis carinii*: A possible cause of cavitary pneumonia and pneumothorax. Hum Pathol 23:1380, 1992.

534. Grimes MM, LaPook JD, Bar MH, et al: Disseminated *Pneumocystis carinii* infection in a patient with acquired immunodeficiency syndrome. Hum Pathol 18:307, 1987.

535. Heyman MR, Rasmussen P: *Pneumocystis carinii* involvement of the bone marrow in acquired immunodeficiency syndrome. Am J Clin Pathol 87:780, 1987.

536. Esterly JA: *Pneumocystis carinii* in lungs of adults at autopsy. Am Rev Respir Dis 97:935, 1968.

537. Watts JC, Chandler FW: Evolving concepts of infection by *Pneumocystis carinii*. *In* Rosen PP, Fechner RE (eds): Pathology Annual Part 1. Vol 26. Norwalk, CT, Appleton & Lange, 1991, p 93.

538. Schumann GB, Swensen JJ: Comparison of Papanicolaou's stain with the Gomori methenamine silver (GMS) stain for the cytodiagnosis of *Pneumocystis carinii* in bronchoalveolar lavage (BAL) fluid. Am J Clin Pathol 95:583, 1991.

539. Tregnago R, Xavier RG, Pereira RP, et al: The diagnosis of *Pneumocystis carinii* pneumonia by cytologic evaluation of Papanicolaou and Leishman-stained bronchoalveolar specimens in patients with the acquired immunodeficiency syndrome. Cytopathology 4:77, 1993.

540. Weber WR, Asken FB, Dehner LP: Lung biopsy in *Pneumocystis carinii* pneumonia: A histopathologic study of typical and atypical features. Am J Clin Pathol 67:11, 1977.

541. Askin FB, Katzenstein ALA: *Pneumocystis* infection masquerading as diffuse alveolar damage: A potential source of diagnostic error. Chest 79:420, 1981.

542. Travis WD, Pittaluga S, Lipschik GY, et al: Atypical pathologic manifestations of *Pneumocystis carinii* pneumonia in the acquired immune deficiency syndrome: Review of 123 lung biopsies from 76 patients with emphasis on cysts, vascular invasion, and granulomas. Am J Surg Pathol 14:615, 1990.

543. Foley NM, Griffiths MH, Miller RF: Histologically atypical *Pneumocystis carinii* pneumonia. Thorax 48:996, 1993.

544. Wakefield AE, Miller RF, Guiver LA, et al: Granulomatous *Pneumocystis carinii* pneumonia: DNA amplification studies on bronchoscopic alveolar lavage samples. J Clin Pathol 47:664, 1994.

545. Cruickshank B: Pulmonary granulomatous pneumocystosis following renal transplantation: Report of a case. Am J Clin Pathol 63:384, 1975.

546. Hartz JW, Geisinger KR, Scharyj M, et al: Granulomatous pneumocystosis presenting as a solitary pulmonary nodule. Arch Pathol Lab Med 109:466, 1985.

547. Liu YC, Tomashefski JF Jr, Tomford JW, et al: Necrotizing *Pneumocystis carinii* vasculitis associated with lung necrosis and cavitation in a patient with acquired immunodeficiency syndrome. Arch Pathol Lab Med 113:494, 1989.

548. Lee MM, Schinella RA: Pulmonary calcification caused by *Pneumocystis carinii* pneumonia: A clinicopathological study of 13 cases in acquired immune deficiency syndrome patients. Am J Surg Pathol 15:376, 1991.

549. Feuerstein IM, Archer A, Pluda JM, et al: Thin-walled cavities, cysts, and pneumothorax in *Pneumocystis carinii* pneumonia: Further observations with histopathologic correlation. Radiology 174:697, 1990.

550. Fraire AE, Kemp B, Greenberg SD, et al: Calcofluor white stain for the detection of *Pneumocystis carinii* in transbronchial lung biopsy specimens: A study of 68 cases. Mod Pathol 9:861, 1996.

551. Saldana MJ, Mones JM, Martinez GR: The pathology of treated *Pneumocystis carinii* pneumonia. Semin Diagn Pathol 6:300, 1989.

552. DeLorenzo LJ, Maguire GP, Wormser GP, et al: Persistence of *Pneumocystis carinii* pneumonia in the acquired immunodeficiency syndrome. Chest 88:79, 1985.

553. Suffredini AF, Owens GR, Tobin MJ, et al: Long-term prognosis of survivors of *Pneumocystis carinii* pneumonia: Structural and functional correlates. Chest 89:229, 1986.

554. Pintozzi RL, Blecka LJ, Nanos S: The morphologic identification of *Pneumocystis carinii*. Acta Cytol 23:35, 1979.

555. Watts JC, Chandler FW: *Pneumocystis carinii* pneumonitis: The nature and diagnostic significance of the methenamine silver-positive "intracystic bodies." Am J Surg Pathol 9:744, 1985.

556. Pintozzi RL: Technical methods: Modified Grocott's methenamine silver nitrate method for quick staining of *Pneumocystis carinii*. J Clin Pathol 31:803, 1978.

557. Musto L, Flanigan M, Elbadawi A: Ten-minute silver stain for *Pneumocystis carinii* and fungi in tissue sections. Arch Pathol Lab Med 106:292, 1982.

558. Paradis IL, Ross C, Dekker A, et al: A comparison of modified methenamine silver and toluidine blue stains for the detection of *Pneumocystis carinii* in bronchoalveolar lavage specimens from immunosuppressed patients. Acta Cytol 34:511, 1990.

559. Lindley RP, Mooney P: A rapid stain for *Pneumocystis*. J Clin Pathol 40:811, 1987.

560. Blumenfeld W, McLeod GJ: *Pneumocystis carinii* in sputum: Comparable efficacy of screening stains and determination of cyst density. Arch Pathol Lab Med 112:816, 1988.

561. Chandra P, Delaney MD, Tuazon CU: Role of special stains in the diagnosis of *Pneumocystis carinii* infection from bronchial washing specimens in patients with the acquired immune deficiency syndrome. Acta Cytol 32:105, 1988.

562. Aslanzadeh J, Stelmach PS: Detection of *Pneumocystis carinii* with direct fluorescence antibody and calcofluor white stain. Infection 24:248, 1996.

563. Domingo J, Waksal HW: Wright's stain in rapid diagnosis of *Pneumocystis carinii*. Am J Clin Pathol 81:511, 1984.

564. Schwartz DA, Munger RG, Katz SM: Plastic embedding evaluation of *Pneumocystis carinii* pneumonia in AIDS. Am J Surg Pathol 11:304, 1987.

565. Shota T: Simultaneous demonstration of cyst walls and intracystic bodies of *Pneumocystis carinii* in paraffin embedded lung sections using Gomori's methenamine silver nitrate and Giemsa stain. J Clin Pathol 39:1269, 1986.

566. Ghali VS, Garcia RL, Skolom J: Fluorescence of *Pneumocystis carinii* in Papanicolaou smears. Hum Pathol 15:907, 1984.

567. Kobayashi M, Urata T, Ikezoe T, et al: Simple detection of the 5S ribosomal RNA of *Pneumocystis carinii* using in situ hybridisation. J Clin Pathol 49:712, 1996.

568. Kim HK, Hughes WT: Comparison of methods for identification of *Pneumocystis carinii* in pulmonary aspirates. Am J Clin Pathol 60:462, 1973.

569. Chan JKC, Tsang DNC, Wong DKK: *Penicillium marneffei* in bronchoalveolar lavage fluid. Acta Cytol 33:523, 1989.

570. Silletti RP, Glezerov V, Schwartz IS: Pulmonary paracoccidioidomycosis misdiagnosed as *Pneumocystis* pneumonia in an immunocompromised host. J Clin Microbiol 34:2328, 1996.

571. Sattler FR, Remington JS: Intravenous trimethoprim-sulfamethoxazole therapy for *Pneumocystis carinii* pneumonia. Am J Med 70:1215, 1981.

572. Shelhamer JH, Ognibene FP, Macher AM, et al: Persistence of *Pneumocystis carinii* in lung tissue of acquired immunodeficiency syndrome patients treated for *Pneumocystis* pneumonia. Am Rev Respir Dis 130:1161, 1984.

573. DeLorenzo LJ, Maguire GP, Wormser GP, et al: Persistence of *Pneumocystis carinii* pneumonia in the acquired immunodeficiency syndrome. Chest 88:79, 1985.

574. Peters SG, Prakash UB: *Pneumocystis carinii* pneumonia: Review of 53 cases. Am J Med 82:73, 1987.

575. Cohen BA, Pomeranz S, Rabinowitz JG, et al: Pulmonary complications of AIDS: Radiologic features. Am J Roentgenol 143:115, 1984.

576. DeLorenzo LJ, Huang CT, Maguire GP, et al: Roentgenographic patterns of *Pneumocystis carinii* pneumonia in 104 patients with AIDS. Chest 91:323, 1987.

577. Goodman PC: *Pneumocystis carinii* pneumonia. J Thorac Imaging 6:16, 1991.

578. Suffredini AF, Tobin MJ, Wajszczuk CP, et al: Acute respiratory failure due to *Pneumocystis carinii* pneumonia: Clinical, radiographic, and pathologic course. Crit Care Med 13:237, 1985.

579. Maxfield RA, Sorkin IB, Fazzini EP, et al: Respiratory failure in patients with acquired immunodeficiency syndrome and *Pneumocystis carinii* pneumonia. Crit Care Med 14:443, 1986.

580. Chaffey MH, Klein JS, Gamsu G, et al: Radiographic distribution of *Pneumocystis carinii* pneumonia in patients with AIDS treated with prophylactic inhaled pentamidine. Radiology 175:715, 1990.

581. Milligan SA, Stulbarg MS, Gamsu G, et al: *Pneumocystis carinii* pneumonia radiographically simulating tuberculosis. Am Rev Respir Dis 132:1124, 1985.

582. Forrest JV: Radiographic findings in *Pneumocystis carinii* pneumonia. Radiology 103:539, 1972.

583. Cross AS, Steigbigel RT: *Pneumocystis carinii* pneumonia presenting as localized nodular densities. N Engl J Med 291:831, 1974.

584. Barrio JL, Suarez M, Rodriguez JL, et al: *Pneumocystis carinii* pneumonia presenting as cavitating and noncavitating solitary pulmonary nodules in patients with the acquired immunodeficiency syndrome. Am Rev Respir Dis 134:1094, 1986.

585. Bleiweiss IJ, Jagirdar JS, Klein MJ, et al: Granulomatous *Pneumocystis carinii* pneumonia in three patients with the acquired immune deficiency syndrome. Chest 94:580, 1988.

586. Chechani V, Zaman MK, Finch PJP: Chronic cavitary *Pneumocystis carinii* pneumonia in a patient with AIDS. Chest 95:1347, 1989.

587. Lubat E, Megibow AJ, Balthazar EJ, et al: Extrapulmonary *Pneumocystis carinii* infection in AIDS: CT findings. Radiology 174:157, 1990.

588. Eagar GM, Friedland JA, Sagel SS: Tumefactive *Pneumocystis carinii* infection in AIDS: Report of three cases. Am J Roentgenol 160:1197, 1993.

589. Mayor B, Schnyder P, Giron J, et al: Mediastinal and hilar lymphadenopathy due to *Pneumocystis carinii* infection in AIDS patients: CT features. J Comput Assist Tomogr 18:408, 1994.

590. Groskin SA, Massi AF, Randall PA: Calcified hilar and mediastinal lymph nodes in an AIDS patient with *Pneumocystis carinii* infection. Radiology 175:345, 1990.

591. Radin DR, Baker EL, Klatt EC, et al: Visceral and nodal calcification in patients with AIDS-related *Pneumocystis carinii* infection. Am J Roentgenol 154:27, 1990.

592. Goodman JL, Tashkin DP: *Pneumocystis* with normal chest X-ray film and arterial oxygen tension: Early diagnosis in a patient with the acquired immune deficiency syndrome. Arch Intern Med 143:1981, 1983.

593. Murray JF, Mills J: Pulmonary infectious complications of human immunodeficiency virus infection. Am Rev Respir Dis 141:1356, 1990.

594. Naidich DP, McGuinness G: Pulmonary manifestations of AIDS: CT and radiographic correlations. Radiol Clin North Am 29:999, 1991.

595. Dee P, Winn W, McKee K: *Pneumocystis carinii* infection of the lung: Radiologic and pathologic correlation. Am J Roentgenol 132:741, 1979.

596. Bergin CJ, Wirth RL, Berry GJ, et al: *Pneumocystis carinii* pneumonia: CT and HRCT observations. J Comput Assist Tomogr 14:756, 1990.

597. Kuhlman JE, Kavuru M, Fishman EK, et al: *Pneumocystis carinii* pneumonia: Spectrum of parenchymal CT findings. Radiology 175:711, 1990.

598. Hartman TE, Primack SL, Müller NL, et al: Diagnosis of thoracic complications in AIDS: Accuracy of CT. Am J Roentgenol 162:547, 1994.

599. McGuinness G, Naidich DP, Garcy SM, et al: AIDS associated bronchiectasis: CT features. J Comput Assist Tomogr 17:260, 1993.

600. Falkenbach KH, Bachmann KD, O'Loughlin BJ: *Pneumocystis carinii* pneumonia. Am J Roentgenol 85:706, 1961.

601. Kovacs JA, Hiemenz JW, Macher AM, et al: *Pneumocystis carinii* pneumonia: A comparison between patients with the acquired immunodeficiency syndrome and patients with other immunodeficiencies. Ann Intern Med 100:663, 1984.

602. Engelberg LA, Lerner CW, Tapper ML: Clinical features of *Pneumocystis* pneumonia in the acquired immune deficiency syndrome. Am Rev Respir Dis 130:689, 1984.

603. Sterling RP, Bradley BB, Khalil KG, et al: Comparison of biopsy-proven *Pneumocystis carinii* pneumonia in acquired immune deficiency syndrome patients and renal allograft recipients. Ann Thorac Surg 38:494, 1984.

604. Parker MM, Ognibene FP, Rogers P, et al: Severe *Pneumocystis carinii* pneumonia produces a hyperdynamic profile similar to bacterial pneumonia with sepsis. Crit Care Med 22:50, 1994.

605. Lehner PJ, Rawal B, Hoyle C, et al: Dual infection with *Pneumocystis carinii* and respiratory viruses complicating bone marrow transplantation. Bone Marrow Transplant 9:213, 1992.

606. Mahaffey KW, Hippenmeyer CL, Mandel R, et al: Unrecognized coccidioidomycosis complicating *Pneumocystis carinii* pneumonia in patients infected with the human immunodeficiency virus and treated with corticosteroids: A report of two cases. Arch Intern Med 153:1496, 1993.

607. Ragni MV, Dekker A, DeRubertis FR, et al: *Pneumocystis carinii* infection presenting as necrotizing thyroiditis and hypothyroidism. Am J Clin Pathol 95:489, 1991.

608. Carter TR, Cooper PH, Petri WA Jr, et al: *Pneumocystis carinii* infection of the small intestine in a patient with acquired immune deficiency syndrome. Am J Clin Pathol 89:679, 1988.

609. Mascarenhas DA, Vasudevan VP, Vaidya KP: *Pneumocystis carinii* pneumonia: Rare cause of hemoptysis. Chest 99:251, 1991.

610. Schnippere S, Small CB, Lehach J, et al: *Pneumocystis carinii* pneumonia presenting as asthma: Increased bronchial hyperresponsiveness in *Pneumocystis carinii* pneumonia. Ann Allergy 70:141, 1993.

611. May T, Rabaud C, Amiel C, et al: Hypertrophic pulmonary osteoarthropathy associated with granulomatous *Pneumocystis carinii* pneumonia in AIDS. Scand J Infect Dis 25:771, 1993.

612. Ong EL, Hanley SP, Mandal BK: Bronchial responsiveness in AIDS patients with *Pneumocystis carinii* pneumonia. AIDS 6:1331, 1992.

613. Slabbynck H, Kovitz KL, Vialette JP, et al: Thoracoscopic findings in spontaneous pneumothorax in AIDS. Chest 106:1582, 1994.

614. Lazard T, Guidet B, Meynard JL, et al: Generalized air cysts complicated by fatal bilateral pneumothoraces in a patient with AIDS-related *Pneumocystis carinii* pneumonia. Chest 106:1271, 1994.

615. Rumbak MJ, Winer-Muram HT, Beals DH, et al: Tension pneumomediastinum complicating *Pneumocystis carinii* pneumonia in acquired immunodeficiency syndrome. Crit Care Med 20:1492, 1992.

616. Bradshaw M, Myerowitz RL, Schneerson R, et al: *Pneumocystis* pneumonitis. Ann Intern Med 73:775, 1970.

617. Grover SA, Coupal L, Suissa S, et al: The clinical utility of serum lactate dehydrogenase in diagnosing *Pneumocystis carinii* pneumonia among hospitalized AIDS patients. Clin Invest Med 15:309, 1992.

618. Quist J, Hill AR: Serum lactate dehydrogenase (LDH) in *Pneumocystis carinii* pneumonia, tuberculosis, and bacterial pneumonia. Chest 108:415, 1995.

619. Meeker DP, Matysik GA, Stelmach K, et al: Diagnostic utility of lactate dehydrogenase levels in patients receiving aerosolized pentamidine. Chest 104:386, 1993.

620. Boldt MJ, Bai TR: Utility of lactate dehydrogenase vs radiographic severity in the differential diagnosis of *Pneumocystis carinii* pneumonia. Chest 111:1187, 1997.

621. Horowitz ML, Schiff M, Samuels J, et al: *Pneumocystis carinii* pleural effusion: Pathogenesis of pleural fluid analysis. Am Rev Respir Dis 148:232, 1993.

622. Ahmed B, Jaspan JB: Case report: Hypercalcemia in a patient with AIDS and *Pneumocystis carinii* pneumonia. Am J Med Sci 306:313, 1993.

623. Leggiadro RJ, Yolken RH, Simkins JH, et al: Measurement of *Pneumocystis carinii* antigen by enzyme immunoassay. J Infect Dis 144:484, 1981.

624. Meyers JD, Pifer LL, Sale GE, et al: The value of *Pneumocystis carinii* antibody and antigen detection for diagnosis of *Pneumocystis* pneumonia after marrow transplantation. Am Rev Respir Dis 120:1283, 1979.

625. Tanabe K, Furuta T, Ueda K, et al: Serological observations of *Pneumocystis carinii* infection in humans. J Clin Microbiol 22:1058, 1985.

626. Elvin K, Bjorkman A, Heurlin N, et al: Seroreactivity to *Pneumocystis carinii* in patients with AIDS versus other immunosuppressed patients. Scand J Infect Dis 26:33, 1994.

627. Lundgren B, Lundgren JD, Nielsen T, et al: Antibody responses to a major *Pneumocystis carinii* antigen in human immunodeficiency virus-infected patients with and without *P. carinii* pneumonia. J Infect Dis 165:1151, 1992.

628. Mitchell DM, Fleming J, Harris JR, et al: Serial pulmonary function tests in the diagnosis of *P. carinii* pneumonia. Eur Respir J 6:823, 1993.

629. Walzer PD, Perl DP, Krogstad DJ, et al: *Pneumocystis carinii* pneumonia in the United States: Epidemiologic, diagnostic, and clinical features. Ann Intern Med 80:83, 1974.

630. Johnson HD, Johnson WW: *Pneumocystis carinii* pneumonia in children with cancer: Diagnosis and treatment. JAMA 214:1067, 1970.

631. Alvarez F, Bandi V, Stager C, et al: Detection of *Pneumocystis carinii* in tracheal aspirates of intubated patients using calcofluor-white (Fungi-Fluor) and immunofluorescence antibody (Genetic Systems) stains. Crit Care Med 25:948, 1997.

632. Wagner D, Koniger J, Kern WV, et al: Serum PCR of *Pneumocystis carinii* DNA in immunocompromised patients. Scand J Infect Dis 29:159, 1997.

633. Yasuoka A, Tachikawa N, Shimada K, et al: (1–>3) beta-D-glucan as a quantitative serological marker for *Pneumocystis carinii* pneumonia. Clin Diagn Lab Immunol 3:197, 1996.

634. Tamburrini E, Mencarini P, Visconti E, et al: Detection of *Pneumocystis carinii* DNA in blood by PCR is not of value for diagnosis of *P. carinii* pneumonia. J Clin Microbiol 34:1586, 1996.

635. Midgley J, Parsons PA, Shanson DC, et al: Monoclonal immunofluorescence compared with silver stain for investigating *Pneumocystis carinii* pneumonia. J Clin Pathol 44:75, 1991.

636. Homer KS, Wiley EL, Smith AL, et al: Monoclonal antibody to *Pneumocystis carinii*: Comparison with silver stain in bronchial lavage specimens. Am J Clin Pathol 97:619, 1992.

636a. Metersky ML, Aslenzadeh J, Stelmach P: A comparison of induced and expectorated sputum for the diagnosis of *Pneumocystis carinii* pneumonia. Chest 113:1555, 1998.

637. Leigh TR, Wakefield AE, Peters SE, et al: Comparison of DNA amplification and immunofluorescence for detecting *Pneumocystis carinii* in patients receiving immunosuppressive therapy. Transplantation 54:468, 1992.

638. Sethi KK: Application of immunoblotting to detect soluble *Pneumocystis carinii* antigen(s) in bronchoalveolar lavage of patients with *Pneumocystis* pneumonia and AIDS. J Clin Pathol 43:584, 1990.

639. Amin MB, Mezger E, Zarbo RJ: Detection of *Pneumocystis carinii*: Comparative study of monoclonal antibody and silver staining. Am J Clin Pathol 98:13, 1992.

640. Halford JA, Shield PW, Wright RG: The value of direct fluorescent antibody (DFA) testing for the detection of *Pneumocystis carinii* in cytological specimens. Cytopathology 5:234, 1994.

641. Wazir JF, Macrorie SG, Coleman DV: Evaluation of the sensitivity, specificity, and predictive value of monoclonal antibody 3F6 for the detection of *Pneumocystis carinii* pneumonia in bronchoalveolar lavage specimens and induced sputum. Cytopathology 5:82, 1994.

642. Fortun J, Navas E, Marti-Belda P, et al: *Pneumocystis carinii* pneumonia in HIV-infected patients: Diagnostic yield of induced sputum and immunofluorescent stain with monoclonal antibodies. Eur Respir J 5:665, 1992.

643. Fraser JL, Lilly C, Israel E, et al: Diagnostic yield of bronchoalveolar lavage and bronchoscopic lung biopsy for detection of *Pneumocystis carinii*. Mayo Clin Proc 71:1025, 1996.

644. Chouaid C, Roux P, Lavard I, et al: Use of the polymerase chain reaction technique on induced-sputum samples for the diagnosis of *Pneumocystis carinii* pneumonia in HIV-infected patients: A clinical and cost-analysis study. Am J Clin Pathol 104:72, 1995.

645. Weig M, Klinker H, Bogner BH, et al: Usefulness of PCR for diagnosis of *Pneumocystis carinii* pneumonia in different patient groups. J Clin Microbiol 35:1445, 1997.

646. Eisen D, Ross BC, Fairbairn J, et al: Comparison of *Pneumocystis carinii* detection by toluidine blue O staining, direct immunofluorescence and DNA amplification in sputum specimens from HIV positive patients. Pathology 26:198, 1994.

647. Tamburrini E, Mencarini P, De Luca A, et al: Diagnosis of *Pneumocystis carinii* pneumonia: Specificity and sensitivity of polymerase chain reaction in comparison with immunofluorescence in bronchoalveolar lavage specimens. J Med Microbiol 38:449, 1993.

648. Leigh TR, Gazzard BG, Rowbottom A, et al: Quantitative and qualitative comparison of DNA amplification by PCR with immunofluorescence staining for diagnosis of *Pneumocystis carinii* pneumonia. J Clin Pathol 46:140, 1993.

649. Weber R, Kuster H, Speich R: Simplified sample processing combined with a sensitive one-tube nested PCR assay for detection of *Pneumocystis carinii* in respiratory specimens. J Clin Microbiol 35:1691, 1997.

650. Ortona E, Margutti P, Tamburrini E, et al: Detection of *Pneumocystis carinii* in respiratory specimens by PCR-solution hybridization enzyme-linked immunoassay. J Clin Microbiol 35:1589, 1997.

651. Graves DC, Chary-Reddy S, Becker-Hapak M: Detection of *Pneumocystis carinii* in induced sputa from immunocompromised patients using a repetitive DNA probe. Mol Cell Probes 11:1, 1997.

652. Bennett CL, Weinstein RA, Shapiro MF, et al: A rapid preadmission method for predicting inpatient course of disease for patients with HIV-related *Pneumocystis carinii* pneumonia. Am J Respir Crit Care Med 150:1503, 1994.

653. Abouya YL, Beaumel A, Lucas S, et al: *Pneumocystis carinii* pneumonia: An uncommon cause of death in African patients with acquired immunodeficiency syndrome. Am Rev Respir Dis 145:617, 1992.

654. Bennett CL, Adams J, Bennett RL, et al: The learning curve for AIDS-related *Pneumocystis carinii* pneumonia: Experience from 3,981 cases in Veterans Affairs Hospitals 1987–1991. J Acquir Immune Defic Syndr Hum Retrovirol 8:373, 1995.

655. Lundgren JD, Barton SE, Katlama C, et al: Changes in survival over time after a first episode of *Pneumocystis carinii* pneumonia for European patients with acquired immunodeficiency syndrome. Multicentre Study Group on AIDS in Europe. Arch Intern Med 155:822, 1995.

656. Jacobson LP, Kirby AJ, Polk S, et al: Changes in survival after acquired immunodeficiency syndrome (AIDS): 1984–1991. Am J Epidemiol 138:952, 1993.

657. Bennett RL, Gilman SC, George L, et al: Improved outcomes in intensive care units for AIDS-related *Pneumocystis carinii* pneumonia: 1987–1991. J Acquir Immune Defic Syndr 6:1319, 1993.

658. Sepkowitz KA: *Pneumocystis carinii* pneumonia among patients with neoplastic disease. Semin Respir Infect 7:114, 1992.

659. Fernandez P, Torres A, Miro JM, et al: Prognostic factors influencing the outcome in *Pneumocystis carinii* pneumonia in patients with AIDS. Thorax 50:668, 1995.

660. Benfield TL, Vestbo J, Junge J, et al: Prognostic value of interleukin-8 in AIDS-associated *Pneumocystis carinii* pneumonia. Am J Respir Crit Care Med 151:1058, 1995.

661. Benson CA, Spear J, Hines D, et al: Combined APACHE II score and serum lactate dehydrogenase as predictors of in-hospital mortality caused by first episode *Pneumocystis carinii* pneumonia in patients with acquired immunodeficiency syndrome. Am Rev Respir Dis 144:319, 1991.

662. Vanhems P, Toma E: Evaluation of a prognostic score: *Pneumocystis carinii* pneumonia in HIV-infected patients. Chest 107:107, 1995.

663. Vestbo J, Nielsen TL, Junge J, et al: Amount of *Pneumocystis carinii* and degree of acute lung inflammation in HIV-associated *P. carinii* pneumonia. Chest 104:109, 1993.

664. Blumenfeld W, Miller CN, Chew KL, et al: Correlation of *Pneumocystis carinii* cyst density with mortality in patients with acquired immunodeficiency syndrome and pneumocystis pneumonia. Hum Pathol 23:612, 1992.

665. Orholm M, Nielsen TL, Holten-Andersen W, et al: *Pneumocystis carinii* pneumonia in AIDS patients: Clinical course in relation to the parasite number found in routine specimens obtained by fiberoptic bronchoscopy. Scand J Infect Dis 24:301, 1992.

666. Blumenfeld W, Miller CN, Chew KL, et al: Correlation of *Pneumocystis carinii* cyst density with mortality in patients with acquired immunodeficiency syndrome and *Pneumocystis pneumonia*. Hum Pathol 23:612, 1992.

667. Ng VL, Geaghan SM, Leoung G, et al: Lack of effect of prophylactic aerosolized pentamidine on the detection of *Pneumocystis carinii* in induced sputum or bronchoalveolar lavage specimens. Arch Pathol Lab Med 117:493, 1993.

668. Ruchel R, Zimmermann F, Boning-Stutzer B, et al: Candidiasis visualised by proteinase-directed immunofluorescence. Virchows Arch (A) 419:199, 1991.

669. Seelig MS: The role of antibiotics in the pathogenesis of *Candida* infections. Am J Med 40:887, 1966.

670. Chakravarty SC: Bronchopulmonary candidiasis: Clinical aspect. Dis Chest 51:608, 1967.

671. Odds FC, Evans EGV, Taylor MAR, et al: Prevalence of pathogenic yeasts and humoral antibodies to *Candida* in diabetic patients. J Clin Pathol 31:840, 1978.

672. Chakravarty SC, Sandhu RS: Incidence of bronchopulmonary candidiasis in patients treated with antibiotics. Acta Tuberc Scand 44:152, 1964.

673. Toala P, Schroeder SA, Daly AK, et al: *Candida* at Boston City Hospital: Clinical and epidemiological characteristics and susceptibility to eight antimicrobial agents. Arch Intern Med 126:983, 1970.

674. Kirkpatrick CH, Smith TK: Chronic mucocutaneous candidiasis: Immunologic and antibiotic therapy. Ann Intern Med 80:310, 1974.

675. Logan PM, Primack SL, Staples C, et al: Acute lung disease in the immunocompromised host: Diagnostic accuracy of the chest radiograph. Chest 108:1283, 1995.

676. Worthington M: Fatal *Candida* pneumonia in a nonimmunosuppressed host. J Infect 7:159, 1983.

677. Meunier-Carpentier F, Kiehn TE, Armstrong D: Fungemia in the immunocompromised host: Changing patterns, antigenemia, high mortality. Am J Med 71:363, 1981.

678. Myerowitz RL, Pazin GJ, Allen CM: Disseminated candidiasis: Changes in incidence, underlying diseases, and pathology. Am J Clin Pathol 68:29, 1977.

678a. Hogevik H, Alestig K: Fungal endocarditis. A report on seven cases and a brief review. Infection 24:17, 1996.

679. Gaines JD, Remington JS: Diagnosis of deep infection with *Candida*: A study of *Candida* precipitins. Arch Intern Med 132:699, 1973.

680. Wikler A, Williams EG, Douglass ED, et al: Mycotic endocarditis: Report of a case. JAMA 119:333, 1942.

681. Rifkind D, Marchioro TL, Schneck SA, et al: Systemic fungal infections complicating renal transplantation and immunosuppressive therapy: Clinical, microbiologic, neurologic and pathologic features. Am J Med 43:28, 1967.

682. Howard RJ, Simmons RL, Najarian JS: Fungal infections in renal transplant recipients. Ann Surg 188:598, 1978.

683. Kauffman CA, Shea MJ, Frame PT: Invasive fungal infections in patients with chronic mucocutaneous candidiasis. Arch Intern Med 141:1076, 1981.

684. Whimbey E, Gold JWM, Polsky B, et al: Bacteremia and fungemia in patients with the acquired immunodeficiency syndrome. Ann Intern Med 104:511, 1986.

685. Dubois PJ, Myerowitz RL, Allen CM: Pathoradiologic correlation of pulmonary candidiasis in immunosuppressed patients. Cancer 40:1026, 1977.

686. Kassner EG, Kauffman SL, Yoon JJ, et al: Pulmonary candidiasis in infants: Clinical, radiologic, and pathologic features. Am J Roentgenol 137:707, 1981.

687. Parker JC Jr, McCloskey JJ, Knauer KA: Pathobiologic features of human candidiasis: A common deep mycosis of the brain, heart and kidney in the altered host. Am J Clin Pathol 65:991, 1976.

688. Linhartova A, Chung W: Bronchopulmonary moniliasis in the newborn. J Clin Pathol 16:56, 1963.

689. Rose HD, Sheth NK: Pulmonary candidiasis: A clinical and pathological correlation. Arch Intern Med 138:964, 1978.

690. Shelly MA, Poe RH, Kapner LB: Pulmonary mycetoma due to *Candida albicans*: Case report and review. Clin Infect Dis 22:133, 1996.

691. Buff SJ, McLelland R, Gallis HA, et al: *Candida albicans* pneumonia: Radiographic appearance. Am J Roentgenol 138:645, 1982.

692. Ramirez G, Shuster M, Kozub W, et al: Fatal acute *C. albicans* bronchopneumonia: Report of a case. JAMA 199:340, 1967.

692a. Pagani JJ, Libshitz HI: Opportunistic fungal pneumonia in cancer patients. Am J Roentgenol 137:1033, 1981.

693. Watanakunakorn C: Acute pulmonary mycetoma due to *C. albicans* with complete resolution. J Infect Dis 148:1131, 1983.

694. Schwarz J, Baum GL, Straub M: Cavitary histoplasmosis complicated by fungus ball. Am J Med 31:692, 1961.

695. Janzen DL, Padley SPG, Adler BD, et al: Acute pulmonary complications in immunocompromised non-AIDS patients: Comparison of diagnostic accuracy of CT and chest radiography. Clin Radiol 47:159, 1993.

696. Primack SL, Müller NL: High-resolution computed tomography in acute diffuse lung disease in the immunocompromised patient. Radiol Clin North Am 32:731, 1994.

697. Brown MJ, Miller RR, Müller NL: Acute lung disease in the immunocompromised host: CT and pathologic examination findings. Radiology 190:247, 1994.

698. Akiyama K, Mathison DA, Riker JB, et al: Allergic bronchopulmonary candidiasis. Chest 85:699, 1984.

699. Ellis CA, Spivack ML: The significance of candidemia. Ann Intern Med 67:511, 1967.

700. Krause W, Matheis H, Wulf K: Fungaemia and funguria after oral administration of *Candida albicans*. Lancet 1:598, 1969.

701. Taschdjian CL, Kozinn PJ, Cuesta MB, et al: Serodiagnosis of candidal infections. Am J Clin Pathol 57:195, 1972.

702. MacDonald F, Odds FC: Purified *Candida albicans* proteinase in the serological diagnosis of candidosis. JAMA 243:2409, 1980.

703. Meckstroth KL, Reiss E, Keller JW, et al: Detection of antibodies and antigenemia in leukemic patients with candidiasis by enzyme-linked immunosorbent assay. J Infect Dis 144:24, 1981.

704. Bardana EJ Jr: The clinical spectrum of aspergillosis: Part I. Epidemiology, pathogenicity, infection in animals and immunology of *Aspergillus*. CRC Crit Rev Clin Lab Sci 13:21, 1981.

705. Young RC, Jennings A, Bennett J: Species identification of invasive aspergillosis in man. Am J Clin Pathol 58:554, 1972.

706. Zimmerman RA, Miller WT: Pulmonary aspergillosis. Am J Roentgenol 109:505, 1970.

707. Laham MN, Carpenter JL: *Aspergillus terreus*, a pathogen capable of causing infective endocarditis, pulmonary mycetoma, and allergic bronchopulmonary aspergillosis. Am Rev Respir Dis 125:769, 1982.

708. Gerber J, Chomicki J, Brandsberg JW, et al: Pulmonary aspergillosis caused by *Aspergillus fischeri* var. *spinosus*: Report of a case and value of serologic studies. Am J Clin Pathol 60:861, 1973.

709. Novey HS, Wells ID: Allergic bronchopulmonary aspergillosis caused by *Aspergillus ochraceus*. Am J Clin Pathol 70:840, 1978.

710. Weiss LM, Thiemke WA: Disseminated *Aspergillus ustus* infection following cardiac surgery. Am J Clin Pathol 80:408, 1983.

711. Tracy SL, McGinnis MR, Peacock JE Jr: Disseminated infection by *Aspergillus terreus*. Am J Clin Pathol 80:728, 1983.

712. Akiyama K, Takizawa H, Suzuki M, et al: Allergic bronchopulmonary aspergillosis due to *Aspergillus oryzae*. Chest 91:285, 1987.

713. Metzger JB, Garagusi VF, Kerwin DM: Pulmonary oxalosis caused by *Aspergillus niger*. Am Rev Respir Dis 129:501, 1984.

714. Mahgoub ES, El Hassan AM: Pulmonary aspergillosis caused by *Aspergillus flavus*. Thorax 27:33, 1972.

715. Yeghen T, Fenelon L, Campbell CK, et al: Chaetomium pneumonia in patient with acute myeloid leukaemia. J Clin Pathol 49:184, 1996.

716. Aisner J, Murillo J, Schimpff SC, et al: Invasive aspergillosis in acute leukemia: Correlation with nose cultures and antibiotic use. Ann Intern Med 90:4, 1979.

717. Kagen SL: Aspergillus: An inhalable contaminant of marihuana. N Engl J Med 304:483, 1981.

718. Hamadeh R, Ardehali A, Locksley RM, et al: Fatal aspergillosis associated with smoking contaminated marijuana, in a marrow transplant recipient. Chest 94:432, 1988.

719. Marks WH, Florence L, Lieberman J, et al: Successfully treated invasive pulmonary aspergillosis associated with smoking marijuana in a renal transplant recipient. Transplantation 61:1771, 1996.

720. Llamas R, Hart DR, Schneider NS: Allergic bronchopulmonary aspergillosis associated with smoking moldy marihuana. Chest 73:871, 1978.

721. Elstad MR: Aspergillosis and lung defenses. Semin Respir Infect 6:27, 1991.

722. Tang CM, Cohen J, Reese AJ, et al: Molecular epidemiological study of invasive pulmonary aspergillosis in a renal transplantation unit. Eur J Clin Microbiol Infect Dis 13:318, 1994.

723. Mondon P, Thelu J, Lebeau B, et al: Virulence of *Aspergillus fumigatus* strains investigated by random amplified polymorphic DNA analysis. J Med Microbiol 42:299, 1995.

724. Henwick S, Hetherington SV, Patrick CC: Complement binding to aspergillus conidia correlates with pathogenicity. J Lab Clin Med 122:27, 1993.

725. Mondon P, De Champs C, Donadille A, et al: Variation in virulence of *Aspergillus fumigatus* strains in a murine model of invasive pulmonary aspergillosis. J Med Microbiol 45:186, 1996.

726. Dixon DM, Polak A, Walsh TJ: Fungus dose-dependent primary pulmonary aspergillosis in immunosuppressed mice. Infect Immunol 57:1452, 1989.

727. Tilden EB, Hatton EH, Freeman S, et al: Preparation and properties of the endotoxins of *Aspergillus fumigatus* and *Aspergillus flavus*. Mycopathologia 14:325, 1961.

728. De E, De Bracco MM, Budzko DB, et al: Mechanisms of activation of complement by extracts of *Aspergillus fumigatus*. Clin Immunol Immunopathol 5:339, 1976.

729. Markaryan A, Morozova I, Yu H, et al: Purification and characterization of an elastinolytic metalloprotease from *Aspergillus fumigatus* and immunoelectron microscopic evidence of secretion of this enzyme by the fungus invading the murine lung. Infect Immun 62:2149, 1994.

730. Moutaouakil M, Monod M, Prevost MC, et al: Identification of the 33-kDa alkaline protease of *Aspergillus fumigatus* in vitro and in vivo. J Med Microbiol 39:393, 1993.

731. Kolattukudy PE, Lee JD, Rogers LM, et al: Evidence for possible involvement of an elastolytic serine protease in aspergillosis. Infect Immun 61:2357, 1993.

732. Tomee JF, Wierenga AT, Hiemstra PS, et al: Proteases from *Aspergillus fumigatus* induce release of proinflammatory cytokines and cell detachment in airway epithelial cell lines. J Infect Dis 176:300, 1997.

733. Holden DW, Tang CM, Smith JM: Molecular genetics of aspergillus pathogenicity. Antonie van Leeuwenhoek 65:251, 1994.

734. Frosco MB, Chase T Jr, Macmillan JD: The effect of elastase-specific monoclonal and polyclonal antibodies on the virulence of *Aspergillus fumigatus* in immunocompromised mice. Mycopathologia 125:65, 1994.

735. Tang CM, Cohen J, Krausz T, et al: The alkaline protease of *Aspergillus fumigatus* is not a virulence determinant in two murine models of invasive pulmonary aspergillosis. Infect Immun 61:1650, 1993.

736. Waldorf AR, Levitz SM, Diamond RD: In vivo broncho-alveolar macrophage defence against *Rhizopus oryzae* and *Aspergillus fumigatus*. J Infect Dis 150:752, 1984.

737. Schaffner A, Douglas H, Braude A: Selective protection against conidia by mononuclear and against mycelia by polymorphonuclear phagocytes in resistance to aspergillus. J Clin Invest 69:617, 1982.

738. Levitz SM, Selsted ME, Ganz T, et al: In vitro killing of spores and hyphae of *Aspergillus fumigatus* and *Rhizopus oryzae* by rabbit neutrophil cationic peptides and broncho-alveolar macrophages. J Infect Dis 154:483, 1986.

739. Madan T, Eggleton P, Kishore U, et al: Binding of pulmonary surfactant proteins A and D to *Aspergillus fumigatus* conidia enhances phagocytosis and killing by human neutrophils and alveolar macrophages. Infect Immun 65:3171, 1997.

740. Taramelli D, Malabarba MG, Sala G, et al: Production of cytokines by alveolar and peritoneal macrophages stimulated by *Aspergillus fumigatus* conidia or hyphae. J Med Vet Mycol 34:49, 1996.

741. Murayama T, Amitani R, Ikegami Y, et al: Suppressive effects of *Aspergillus fumigatus* culture filtrates on human alveolar macrophages and polymorphonuclear leucocytes. Eur Respir J 9:293, 1996.

742. Robertson MD, Seaton A, Milne LJR, et al: Suppression of host defences by *Aspergillus fumigatus*. Thorax 42:19, 1987.

743. Müllbacher A, Eichner RD: Immunosuppression in vitro by a metabolite of a human pathogenic fungus. Proc Natl Acad Sci U S A 81:3835, 1984.

744. Washburn RG, Hammer CH, Benneth JE: Inhibition of complement by culture supernatants of *Aspergillus fumigatus*. J Infect Dis 154:944, 1986.

745. Nime FA, Hutchins GM: Oxalosis caused by *Aspergillus* infection. Johns Hopkins Med J 133:183, 1973.

746. Kurrein F, Green GH, Rowles SL: Localized deposition of calcium oxalate around a pulmonary *Aspergillus niger* fungus ball. Am J Clin Pathol 64:556, 1975.

747. Muller H-M, Frosch S: Oxalate accumulation from citrate by *Aspergillus niger*: II. Involvement of the tricarboxylic acid cycle. Arch Microbiol 104:159, 1975.

748. Reyes CV, Kahuria S, MacGlashan A: Diagnostic value of calcium oxalate crystals in respiratory and pleural fluid cytology: A case report. Acta Cytol 23:65, 1979.

749. Cho C, Asuncion A, Tatum AH: False-positive antineutrophil cytoplasmic antibody in aspergillosis with oxalosis. Arch Pathol Lab Med 119:558, 1996.

750. Ghio AJ, Peterseim DS, Roggli VL, et al: Pulmonary oxalate deposition associated with aspergillus niger infection: An oxidant hypothesis of toxicity. Am Rev Respir Dis 145:1499, 1992.

751. Lee SH, Barnes WG, Schaetzel WP: Pulmonary aspergillosis and the importance of oxalate crystal recognition in cytology specimens. Arch Pathol Lab Med 110:1176, 1986.

752. Farley ML, Mabry L, Munoz LA, et al: Crystals occurring in pulmonary cytology specimens: Association with Aspergillus infection. Acta Cytol 29:737, 1985.

753. Benoit G, Feuilhade de Chauvin M, Cordonnier C, et al: Oxalic acid level in bronchoalveolar lavage fluid from patients with invasive pulmonary aspergillosis. Am Rev Respir Dis 132:748, 1985.

754. Kahanpää A: Bronchopulmonary occurrence of fungi in adults. Acta Pathol Microbiol Scand B (Suppl)227:1, 1972.

755. Tang CM, Holden DW, Aufauvre-Brown A, et al: The detection of *Aspergillus* spp. by the polymerase chain reaction and its evaluation in bronchoalveolar lavage fluid. Am Rev Respir Dis 148:1313, 1993.

756. Nomoto Y, Kuwano K, Hagimoto N, et al: *Aspergillus fumigatus* Asp f1 DNA is prevalent in sputum from patients with coal workers' pneumoconiosis. Respiration 64:291, 1997.

757. Nelson LA, Callerame ML, Schwartz RH: Aspergillosis and atopy in cystic fibrosis. Am Rev Respir Dis 120:863, 1979.

758. Paradowski LJ: Saprophytic fungal infections and lung transplantation—revisited. J Heart Lung Transplant 16:524, 1997.

759. Milla CE, Wielinski CL, Regelmann WE: Clinical significance of the recovery of *Aspergillus* species from the respiratory secretions of cystic fibrosis patients. Pediatr Pulmonol 21:6, 1996.

760. Bhargava V, Tomashefski JF Jr, Stern RC, et al: The pathology of fungal infection and colonization in patients with cystic fibrosis. Hum Pathol 20:977, 1989.

761. Amitani R, Taylor G, Elezis EN, et al: Purification and characterization of factors produced by *Aspergillus fumigatus* which affect human ciliated respiratory epithelium. Infect Immun 63:3266, 1995.

762. Bardana EJ Jr: The clinical spectrum of aspergillosis: Part 2. Classification and description of saprophytic, allergic, and invasive variants of human disease. CRC Crit Rev Clin Lab Sci 13:85, 1980.

762a. Chatzimichalis A, Massard G, Kessler R, et al: Bronchopulmonary aspergilloma: A reappraisal. Ann Thorac Surg 65:927, 1998.

763. Research Committee of British Thoracic and Tuberculosis Association: *Aspergillus* in persistent lung cavities after tuberculosis. Tubercle (Lond) 49:1, 1968.

764. Research Committee of the British Thoracic and Tuberculosis Association: Aspergilloma and residual tuberculous cavities—the results of a resurvey. Tubercle 51:227, 1970.

765. Battaglini JW, Murray GF, Keagy BA, et al: Surgical management of symptomatic pulmonary aspergilloma. Ann Thorac Surg 39:512, 1985.

766. Wollschlager C, Khan F: Aspergillomas complicating sarcoidosis: A prospective study in 100 patients. Chest 86:585, 1984.

767. Campbell MJ, Clayton YM: Bronchopulmonary aspergillosis: A correlation of the clinical and laboratory findings in 272 patients investigated for bronchopulmonary aspergillosis. Am Rev Respir Dis 89:186, 1964.

768. Maguire CP, Hayes JP, Hayes M, et al: Three cases of pulmonary aspergilloma in adult patients with cystic fibrosis. Thorax 50:805, 1995.

769. Procknow JJ, Loewen DF: Pulmonary aspergillosis with cavitation secondary to histoplasmosis. Am Rev Respir Dis 82:101, 1960.

770. Sarosi GA, Silberfarb PM, Saliba NA, et al: Aspergillomas occurring in blastomycotic cavities. Am Rev Respir Dis 104:581, 1971.

771. Rosenheim SH, Schwarz J: Cavitary pulmonary cryptococcosis complicated by aspergilloma. Am Rev Respir Dis 111:549, 1975.

772. Fahey PJ, Utell MJ, Hyde RW: Spontaneous lysis of mycetomas after acute cavitating lung disease. Am Rev Respir Dis 123:336, 1981.

773. Addrizzo-Harris DJ, Harkin TJ, McGuinness G, et al: Pulmonary aspergilloma and AIDS: A comparison of HIV-infected and HIV-negative individuals. Chest 111:612, 1997.

774. McGregor DH, Papasian CJ, Pierce PD: Aspergilloma within cavitating pulmonary adenocarcinoma. Am J Clin Pathol 91:100, 1989.

775. Ward MJ, Davies D: Pulmonary aspergilloma after radiation therapy. Br J Dis Chest 76:361, 1982.

776. Petrie JP, Caughey DE: Bilateral apical fibrobullous disease complicated by bilateral *Aspergillus* mycetomata in rheumatoid arthritis. N Z Med J 96:7, 1983.

777. Krohn J, Halvorsen JH: Aspergilloma of the lung in ankylosing spondylitis. Scand J Respir Dis 63(Suppl):131, 1968.

778. Aslam PA, Eastridge CE, Hughes FA Jr: Aspergillosis of the lung—an eighteen-year experience. Chest 59:28, 1971.

779. Freixinet J, de Cos J, Rodriguez de Castro F, et al: Colonisation with Aspergillus of an intralobar pulmonary sequestration. Thorax 50:810, 1995.

780. Sawasaki H, Horie K, Yamada M, et al: Bronchial stump aspergillosis: Experimental and clinical study. J Thorac Cardiovasc Surg 58:198, 1969.

781. Parry MF, Coughlin FR, Zambetti FX: Aspergillus empyema. Chest 81:768, 1982.

782. Costello P, Rose RM: CT findings in pleural aspergillosis. J Comput Assist Tomogr 9:760, 1985.

783. Tomee JF, Wierenga AT, Hiemstra PS, et al: Proteases from *Aspergillus fumigatus* induce release of proinflammatory cytokines and cell detachment in airway epithelial cell lines. J Infect Dis 176:300, 1997.

784. McCarthy DS, Pepys J: Pulmonary aspergilloma: Clinical immunology. Clin Allergy 3:57, 1973.

785. Jaques D, Bonzon M, Polla BS: Serological evidence of aspergillus type I hypersensitivity in a subgroup of pulmonary aspergilloma patients. Int Arch Allergy Immunol 106:263, 1995.

786. Ein ME, Wallace RJ Jr, Williams TW Jr: Allergic bronchopulmonary aspergillosis-like syndrome consequent to aspergilloma. Am Rev Respir Dis 119:811, 1979.

787. Davies D, Somner AR: Pulmonary aspergillomas treated with corticosteroids. Thorax 27:156, 1972.

788. McCarthy DS, Pepys J: Pulmonary aspergilloma—clinical immunology. Clin Allergy 3:57, 1973.

789. Henderson AH: Allergic aspergillosis: Review of 32 cases. Thorax 23:501, 1968.

790. Israel RH, Poe RH, Bomba PA, et al: The rapid development of an aspergilloma secondary to allergic bronchopulmonary aspergillosis. Am J Med Sci 280:41, 1980.

791. Anderson CJ, Craig S, Bardana EJ Jr: Allergic bronchopulmonary aspergillosis and bilateral fungal balls terminating in disseminated aspergillosis. J Allerg Clin Immunol 65:140, 1980.

792. Causey WA, Arnell P, Brinker J: Systemic *Nocardia caviae* infection. Chest 65:360, 1974.

793. Meyer RD, Rosen P, Armstrong D: Phycomycosis complicating leukemia and lymphoma. Ann Intern Med 77:871, 1972.

794. Mohr JA, Patterson CD, Eaton BG, et al: Primary pulmonary sporotrichosis (case report). Am Rev Respir Dis 106:260, 1972.

795. Weese WC, Helms CM: *Trichophyton*: A new cause of pulmonary mycetoma. Am Rev Respir Dis 108:643, 1973.

796. Belgrad R: Fungus ball—an unusual manifestation of coccidioidomycosis: A case report. Radiology 101:289, 1971.

797. Hainer JW, Ostrow JH, Mackenzie DWR: Pulmonary monosporosis: Report of a case with precipitating antibody. Chest 66:601, 1974.

798. Kathuria SK, Rippon J: Non-*aspergillus* aspergillosis. Am J Clin Pathol 78:870, 1982.

799. Kirkpatrick MB, Pollock HM, Wimberley NE, et al: An intracavitary fungus ball composed of syncephalastrum. Am Rev Respir Dis 120:943, 1979.

800. Kwon-Chung KJ, Schwartz IS, Rybak BJ: A pulmonary fungus ball produced by *Cladosporium cladosporioides*. Am J Clin Pathol 64:564, 1975.

801. Awe RJ, Greenberg SD, Mattox KL: The source of bleeding in pulmonary aspergillomas. Texas Med 80:58, 1984.

802. Goldberg B: Radiological appearances in pulmonary aspergillosis. Clin Radiol 13:106, 1962.

803. Saliba A, Pacini L, Beatty OA: Intracavitary fungus balls in pulmonary aspergillosis. Br J Dis Chest 55:65, 1961.

804. Levin EJ: Pulmonary intracavitary fungus ball. Radiology 66:9, 1956.

805. Libshitz HI, Atkinson GW, Israel HL: Pleural thickening as a manifestation of *Aspergillus* superinfection. Am J Roentgenol 120:883, 1974.

806. Le Hegarat R, Vie A, Allain YM, et al: L'épaississement des parois, signe précoce et peu connu dans l'aspergillome pulmonaire. [Thickening of the walls, early and little known sign of pulmonary aspergilloma.] J Radiol Electrol Med Nucl 47:535, 1966.

807. Donohoo CM: Bronchopulmonary aspergillosis. Aust Radiol 10:225, 1966.

808. Irwin A: Radiology of the aspergilloma. Clin Radiol 18:432, 1967.

809. Tellesson WG: Pulmonary mycetoma. J Coll Radiol Aust 7:193, 1963.

810. Pimentel JC: Pulmonary calcification in the tumor-like form of pulmonary aspergillosis: Pulmonary aspergillosis. Am Rev Respir Dis 94:208, 1966.

811. Nomori H, Horio H, Hasegawa T, et al: Retained sponge after thoracotomy that mimicked aspergilloma. Ann Thorac Surg 61:1535, 1996.

812. Roberts CM, Citron KM, Strickland B: Intrathoracic aspergilloma: Role of CT in diagnosis and treatment. Radiology 165:123, 1987.

813. Gefter WB: The spectrum of pulmonary aspergillosis. J Thorac Imaging 7:56, 1992.

813a. Fujimoto K, Meno S, Nishimura H, et al: Aspergilloma within cavitary lung cancer: MR imaging findings. Am J Roentgenol 163:565, 1994.

814. Pennington JE: *Aspergillus* lung disease. Med Clin North Am 64:475, 1980.

815. Freundlich IM, Israel HL: Pulmonary aspergillosis. Clin Radiol 24:248, 1973.

816. Faulkner SL, Vernon R, Brown PP, et al: Hemoptysis and pulmonary aspergilloma: Operative versus nonoperative treatment. Ann Thorac Surg 25:389, 1978.

817. Jewkes J, Kay PH, Paneth M, et al: Pulmonary aspergilloma: Analysis of prognosis in relation to haemoptysis and survey of treatment. Thorax 38:572, 1983.

818. Butz RO, Zvetina JR, Leininger BJ: Ten-year experience with mycetomas in patients with pulmonary tuberculosis. Chest 87:356, 1985.

819. Rafferty P, Biggs B-A, Crompton GK, et al: What happens to patients with pulmonary aspergilloma? Analysis of 23 cases. Thorax 38:579, 1983.

820. Hillerdal G: Pulmonary *Aspergillus* infection invading the pleura. Thorax 36:745, 1981.

821. Wagner DK, Varkey B, Sheth NK, et al: Epidural abscess, vertebral destruction, and paraplegia caused by extending infection from an aspergilloma. Am J Med 78:518, 1985.

822. Polatty RC, Cooper KR, Kerkering TM: Spinal cord compression due to an aspergilloma. South Med J 77:645, 1984.

823. Leading article: Pulmonary aspergilloma. BMJ 2:124, 1971.

824. Longbottom JL, Pepys J, Clive FT: Diagnostic precipitin test in *Aspergillus* pulmonary mycetoma. Lancet 1:588, 1964.

825. Tomee JF, van der Werf TS, Latge JP, et al: Serologic monitoring of disease and treatment in a patient with pulmonary aspergilloma. Am J Respir Crit Care Med 151:199, 1995.

826. Hammerman KJ, Christianson CS, Huntington I, et al: Spontaneous lysis of aspergillomata. Chest 64:697, 1973.

827. Fahey PJ, Utell MJ, Hyde RW: Spontaneous lysis of mycetomas after acute cavitating lung disease. Am Rev Respir Dis 123:336, 1981.

828. Rosenberg RS, Creviston SA, Schonfeld AJ: Invasive aspergillosis complicating resection of a pulmonary aspergilloma in a nonimmunocompromised host. Am Rev Respir Dis 126:1113, 1982.

829. Buchanan DR, Lamb D: Saprophytic invasion of infarcted pulmonary tissue by *Aspergillus* species. Thorax 37:693, 1982.

830. Przyjemski C, Mattii R: The formation of pulmonary mycetomata. Cancer 46:1701, 1980.

831. Hinojosa M, Fraj J, De la Hoz B, et al: Hypersensitivity pneumonitis in workers exposed to esparto grass (*Stipa tenacissima*) fibers. J Allergy Clin Immunol 98:985, 1996.

832. Channell S, Blyth W, Lloyd M, et al: Allergic alveolitis in maltworkers: A clinical, mycological, and immunological study. QJM 38:351, 1969.

833. Riddle HFV, Channell S, Blyth W, et al: Allergic alveolitis in a maltworker. Thorax 23:271, 1968.

834. Smyth JT, Adkins GE, Lloyd M, et al: Farmer's lung in Devon. Thorax 30:197, 1975.

835. Matsen D, Klock LE, Wensel FJ, et al: The prevalence of farmer's lung in an agricultural population. Am Rev Respir Dis 113:171, 1976.

836. Rosenberg M, Patterson R, Mintzer R: Clinical and immunologic criteria for the diagnosis of allergic bronchopulmonary aspergillosis. Ann Intern Med 86:405, 1977.

837. Rosenberg M, Mintzer R, Aaronson DW, et al: Allergic bronchopulmonary aspergillosis in three patients with normal chest x-ray films. Chest 72:597, 1977.

838. Mintzer RA, Rogers LF, Kruglik GD, et al: The spectrum of radiologic findings in allergic bronchopulmonary aspergillosis. Radiology 127:301, 1978.

838a. Angus RM, Davies M-L, Cowman MD, et al: Computed tomographic scanning of the lung in patients with allergic bronchopulmonary aspergillosis and in asthmatic patients with a positive skin test to *Aspergillus fumigatus*. Thorax 49:586, 1994.

839. Ricketti AJ, Greenberger PA, Mintzer RA, et al: Allergic bronchopulmonary aspergillosis. Chest 86:773, 1984.

840. Berkin KE, Vernon DRH, Kerr JW: Lung collapse caused by allergic bronchopulmonary aspergillosis in nonasthmatic patients. BMJ 285:552, 1982.

841. Glancy JJ, Elder JL, McAleer R: Allergic bronchopulmonary fungal disease without clinical asthma. Thorax 36:345, 1981.

842. Breslin AB, Jenkins CR: Experience with allergic bronchopulmonary aspergillosis: Some unusual features. Clin Allergy 14:21, 1984.

843. Imbeau SA, Nichols D, Flaherty D, et al: Relationships between prednisone therapy, disease activity, and the total serum IgE in allergic bronchopulmonary aspergillosis. J Allergy Clin Immunol 62:91, 1978.

844. Malo J-L, Longbottom J, Mitchell J, et al: Studies in chronic allergic bronchopulmonary aspergillosis: 3. Immunological findings. Thorax 32:269, 1977.

845. Glimp RA, Bayer AS: Fungal pneumonias: Part 3. Allergic bronchopulmonary aspergillosis. Chest 80:85, 1981.

846. Ricketti AJ, Greenberger PA, Patterson R: Serum IgE as an important aid in management of allergic bronchopulmonary aspergillosis. J Allergy Clin Immunol 74:68, 1984.

846a. Aubry M-C, Fraser R: The role of bronchial biopsy and washing in the diagnosis of allergic bronchopulmonary aspergillosis. Mod Pathol 11:607, 1998.

847. Lee TM, Greenberger PA, Patterson R, et al: Stage V (fibrotic) allergic bronchopulmonary aspergillosis: A review of 17 cases followed from diagnosis. Arch Intern Med 147:319, 1987.

848. Longbottom JJ, Pepys J: Pulmonary aspergillosis: Diagnostic immunological significance of antigens and C-substance in *Aspergillus fumigatus*. J Pathol Bacteriol 88:141, 1964.

849. Kauffman HF, Beaumont F, Sluiter HJ, et al: Immunologic observations in sera of a patient with allergic bronchopulmonary aspergillosis by means of the enzyme-linked immunosorbent assay. J Allergy Clin Immunol 74:741, 1984.

850. Safirstein BH: Aspergilloma consequent to allergic bronchopulmonary aspergillosis. Am Rev Respir Dis 108:940, 1973.

851. Benatar SR, Allan B, Hewitson RP, et al: Allergic bronchopulmonary stemphyliosis. Thorax 35:515, 1980.

852. McAleer R, Kroenert DB, Elder JL, et al: Allergic bronchopulmonary disease caused by *Curvularia lunata* and *Drechslera hawaiiensis*. Thorax 36:338, 1981.

853. Halwig JM, Brueske DA, Greenberger PA, et al: Allergic bronchopulmonary curvulariosis. Am Rev Respir Dis 132:186, 1985.

854. Kamei K, Unno H, Nagao K, et al: Allergic bronchopulmonary mycosis caused by the basidiomycetous fungus *Schizophyllum commune*. Clin Infect Dis 18:305, 1994.

855. Backman KS, Roberts M, Patterson R: Allergic bronchopulmonary mycosis caused by *Fusarium vasinfectum*. Am J Respir Crit Care Med 152:1379, 1995.

856. Bromley IM, Donaldson K: Binding of Aspergillus proteins: Relevance to the asthmatic lung. Thorax 51:1203, 1996.

857. Starke ID: Asthma and allergic aspergillosis in monozygotic twins. Br J Dis Chest 79:295, 1985.

858. Halwig JM, Kurup VP, Greenberger PA, et al: A familial occurrence of allergic bronchopulmonary aspergillosis: A probable environmental source. J Allergy Clin Immunol 76:55, 1985.

859. Graves TS, Fink JN, Patterson R, et al: A familial occurrence of allergic bronchopulmonary aspergillosis. Ann Intern Med 91:378, 1979.

860. Flaherty DK, Surfus JE, Geller M, et al: HLA antigen frequencies in allergic bronchopulmonary aspergillosis. Clin Allergy 8:73, 1978.

861. Vernon DRH, Allan F: Environmental factors in allergic bronchopulmonary aspergillosis. Clin Allergy 10:217, 1980.

862. Beaumont F, Kauffmann HF, Sluiter HJ, et al: Environmental aerobiological studies in allergic bronchopulmonary aspergillosis. Allergy 39:183, 1984.

863. Halwig JM, Kurup VP, Greenberger PA, et al: A familial occurrence of allergic bronchopulmonary aspergillosis: A probable environmental source. J Allergy Clin Immunol 76:55, 1985.

864. Malo J-L, Hawkins R, Pepys J: Studies in chronic allergic bronchopulmonary aspergillosis: 1. Clinical and physiological findings. Thorax 32:254, 1977.

865. Shaw RR: Mucoid impaction of bronchi. Thorac Surg 22:149, 1951.

866. Johnson RS, Sita-Lumsden EG: Plastic bronchitis. Thorax 15:325, 1960.

867. Voss MJ, Bush RK, Mischler EH, et al: Association of allergic bronchopulmonary aspergillosis and cystic fibrosis. J Allergy Clin Immunol 69:539, 1982.

868. Mroueh S, Spock A: Allergic bronchopulmonary aspergillosis in patients with cystic fibrosis. Chest 105:32, 1994.

869. Feanny S, Forsyth S, Corey M, et al: Allergic bronchopulmonary aspergillosis in cystic fibrosis: A secretory immune response to a colonizing organism. Ann Allergy 60:64, 1988.

870. Chung Y, Kraut JR, Stone AM, et al: Disseminated aspergillosis in a patient with cystic fibrosis and allergic bronchopulmonary aspergillosis. Pediatr Pulmonol 17:131, 1994.

871. Laufer P, Fink JN, Bruns WT, et al: Allergic bronchopulmonary aspergillosis in cystic fibrosis. J Allergy Clin Immunol 73:44, 1984.

872. Schonheyder H, Jensen T, Hoiby N, et al: Frequency of Aspergillus fumigatus isolates and antibodies to Aspergillus antigens in cystic fibrosis. Acta Pathol Microbiol Immunol Scand [B] 93:105, 1985.

873. Katzenstein A-L, Liebow AA, Friedman PJ: Bronchocentric granulomatosis, mucoid impaction, and hypersensitivity reactions to fungi. Am Rev Respir Dis 111:497, 1975.

874. Hinson KFW, Moon AJ, Plummer NS: Broncho-pulmonary aspergillosis: A review and a report of eight new cases. Thorax 7:317, 1952.

875. Bosken CH, Myers JL, Greenberger PA, et al: Pathologic features of allergic bronchopulmonary aspergillosis. Am J Surg Pathol 12:216, 1988.

876. Liebow AA: Pulmonary angiitis and granulomatosis. Am Rev Respir Dis 108:1, 1973.

877. Clee MD, Lamb D, Urbaniak SJ, et al: Progressive bronchocentric granulomatosis: Case report. Thorax 37:947, 1982.

878. Jelihovsky T: The structure of bronchial plugs in mucoid impaction, bronchocentric granulomatosis and asthma. Histopathology 7:153, 1983.

879. Chan-Yeung M, Chase WH, Trapp W, et al: Allergic bronchopulmonary aspergillosis: Clinical and pathologic study of three cases. Chest 59:33, 1971.

880. Koss MN, Robinson RG, Hochholzer L: Bronchocentric granulomatosis. Hum Pathol 12:632, 1981.

881. Maguire GP, Lee M, Rosen Y, et al: Pulmonary tuberculosis and bronchocentric granulomatosis. Chest 89:606, 1986.

882. Hertog RWD, Wagenaar SS, Westermar CJJ: Bronchocentric granulomatosis and pulmonary echinococcosis: Case reports. Am Rev Respir Dis 126:344, 1982.

883. Hellems SO, Kanner RE, Renzetti AD Jr: Bronchocentric granulomatosis associated with rheumatoid arthritis. Chest 83:831, 1983.

884. Travis WD, Kwon-Chung KJ, Kleiner DE, et al: Unusual aspects of allergic bronchopulmonary fungal disease: Report of two cases due to Curvularia organisms associated with allergic fungal sinusitis. Hum Pathol 22:1240, 1991.

885. Rohatgi PK, Turrisi BC: Bronchocentric granulomatosis and ankylosing spondylitis. Thorax 39:317, 1984.

886. Warnock ML, Fennessy J, Rippon J: Chronic eosinophilic pneumonia, a manifestation of allergic aspergillosis. Am J Clin Pathol 62:73, 1974.

887. Urschel HC, Paulson DL, Shaw RR: Mucoid impaction of the bronchi. Ann Thorac Surg 2:1, 1966.

888. Ellis RH: Total collapse of the lung in aspergillosis. Thorax 20:118, 1965.

889. Lipinski JK, Weisbrod GL, Sanders DE: Unusual manifestations of pulmonary aspergillosis. J Can Assoc Radiol 29:216, 1978.

890. Pepys J, Riddell RW, Citron KM, et al: Clinical and immunologic significance of Aspergillus fumigatus in the sputum. Am Rev Respir Dis 80:167, 1959.

891. Fisher MR, Mendelson EB, Mintzer RA: Allergic bronchopulmonary aspergillosis: A pictorial essay. Radiographics 4:445, 1984.

892. Murphy D, Lane DJ: Pleural effusion in allergic bronchopulmonary aspergillosis: 2 case reports. Br J Dis Chest 75:91, 1981.

893. Ricketti AJ, Greenberger PA, Glassroth J: Spontaneous pneumothorax in allergic bronchopulmonary aspergillosis. Arch Intern Med 144:151, 1984.

894. Kullnig P, Pongratz M, Kopp W, et al: Computerized tomography in the diagnosis of allergic bronchopulmonary aspergillosis. Radiology 29:228, 1989.

895. Neeld DA, Goodman LR, Gurney JW, et al: Computerized tomography in the evaluation of allergic bronchopulmonary aspergillosis. Am Rev Respir Dis 142:1200, 1990.

896. Angus RM, Davies M-L, Cowman MD, et al: Computed tomographic scanning of the lung in patients with allergic bronchopulmonary aspergillosis and in asthmatic patients with a positive skin test to Aspergillus fumigatus. Thorax 49:586, 1994.

897. Logan PM, Müller NL: High-attenuation mucous plugging in allergic bronchopulmonary aspergillosis. Can Assoc Radiol J 47:374, 1996.

898. Kang EY, Miller RR, Müller NL: Bronchiectasis: Comparison of preoperative thin-section CT and pathologic findings in resected specimens. Radiology 195:649, 1995.

899. Reiff DB, Wells AU, Carr DH, et al: CT findings in bronchiectasis: Limited value in distinguishing between idiopathic and specific types. Am J Roentgenol 165:261, 1995.

900. Ricketti AJ, Greenberger PA, Patterson R: Immediate-type reactions in patients with allergic bronchopulmonary aspergillosis. J Allergy Clin Immunol 71:541, 1983.

901. Glimp RA, Bayer AS: Fungal pneumonias: Part 3. Allergic bronchopulmonary aspergillosis. Chest 80:85, 1981.

902. Wang JLF, Patterson R, Roberts M, et al: The management of allergic bronchopulmonary aspergillosis. Am Rev Respir Dis 120:87, 1979.

903. Patterson R, Greenberger PA, Radin RC, et al: Allergic bronchopulmonary aspergillosis: Staging as an aid to management. Ann Intern Med 96:286, 1982.

904. Dick JD, Rosengard BR, Merz WG, et al: Fatal disseminated candidiasis due to amphotericin-B-resistant Candida quilliermondi. Ann Intern Med 102:67, 1985.

905. Leggat PO, De Kretser DMH: Aspergillus pneumonia in association with an aspergilloma. Br J Dis Chest 62:147, 1968.

906. Riley DJ, MacKenzie JW, Uhlman WE, et al: Allergic bronchopulmonary aspergillosis: Evidence of limited tissue invasion. Am Rev Respir Dis 111:232, 1975.

907. Meyer RD, Young LS, Armstrong D, et al: Aspergillosis complicating neoplastic disease. Am J Med 54:6, 1973.

908. Young RC, Bennett JE, Vogel CL, et al: Aspergillosis: The spectrum of the disease in 98 patients. Medicine 49:147, 1970.

909. Kuhlman JE, Fishman EK, Burch PA, et al: Invasive pulmonary aspergillosis in acute leukemia: The contribution of CT to early diagnosis and aggressive management. Chest 92:95, 1987.

910. Robertson MJ, Larson RA: Recurrent fungal pneumonias in patients with acute nonlymphocytic leukemia undergoing multiple courses of intensive chemotherapy. Am J Med 84:233, 1988.

911. Klimowski LL, Rotstein C, Cummings KM: Incidence of nosocomial aspergillosis in patients with leukemia over a twenty-year period. Infect Control Hosp Epidemiol 10:299, 1989.

912. Gerson SL, Talbot GH, Hurwitz S, et al: Prolonged granulocytopenia: The major risk factor for invasive pulmonary aspergillosis in patients with acute leukemia. Ann Intern Med 100:345, 1984.

913. Weiland D, Ferguson RM, Peterson PK, et al: Aspergillosis in 25 renal transplant patients: Epidemiology, clinical presentation, diagnosis and management. Ann Surg 198:622, 1983.

913a. Salerno CT, Ouyang DW, Pederson TS, et al: Surgical therapy for pulmonary aspergillosis in immunocompromised patients. Ann Thorac Surg 65:1415, 1998.

914. Kramer MR, Denning DW, Marshall SE, et al: Ulcerative tracheobronchitis after lung transplantation: A new form of invasive aspergillosis. Am Rev Respir Dis 144:552, 1991.

915. Yeldandi V, Laghi F, McCabe MA, et al: Aspergillus and lung transplantation. J Heart Lung Transplant 14:883, 1995.

916. Horn CR, Wood NC, Hughes JA: Invasive aspergillosis following post-influenzal pneumonia. Br J Dis Chest 77:407, 1983.

917. Lewis M, Kallenbach J, Ruff P, et al: Invasive pulmonary aspergillosis complicating influenza A pneumonia in a previously healthy patient. Chest 87:691, 1985.

918. Tazelaar HD, Baird AM, Mill M, et al: Bronchocentric mycosis occurring in transplant recipients. Chest 96:92, 1989.

919. Park GR, Drummond GB, Lamb D, et al: Disseminated aspergillosis occurring in patients with respiratory, renal and hepatic failure. Lancet 2:179, 1982.

920. Walsh TJ, Hamilton SR: Disseminated aspergillosis complicating hepatic failure. Arch Intern Med 143:1189, 1983

921. Pizzani JN, Knapp A: Diabetic ketoacidosis and invasive aspergillosis. Lung 159:43, 1981.

922. Zellner SR, Selby JB, Loughrin JJ: Aspergillosis: An unusual presentation. Am Rev Respir Dis 100:217, 1969.

923. Blum J, Reed JC, Pizzo SV, et al: Miliary aspergillosis associated with alcoholism. Am J Roentgenol 131:707, 1978.

924. Denning DW, Follansbee SE, Scolaro M, et al: Pulmonary aspergillosis in the acquired immunodeficiency syndrome. N Engl J Med 324:654, 1991.

925. Keating JJ, Rogers T, Petrou M, et al: Management of pulmonary aspergillosis in AIDS: An emerging clinical problem. J Clin Pathol 47:805, 1994.

926. Lake KB, Browne PM, Van Dyke JJ, et al: Fatal disseminated aspergillosis in an asthmatic patient treated with corticosteroids. Chest 83:138, 1983.

927. Guidotti TL, Luetzeler J, Di Sant'Agnese PA, et al: Fatal disseminated aspergillosis in a previously well young adult with cystic fibrosis. Am J Med Sci 283:157, 1982.

928. Palmer LB, Greenberg HE, Schiff MJ: Corticosteroid treatment as a risk factor for invasive aspergillosis in patients with lung disease. Thorax 46:15, 1991.

929. Karim M, Alam M, Shah AA, et al: Chronic invasive aspergillosis in apparently immunocompetent hosts. Clin Infect Dis 24:723, 1997.

929a. Nagata N, Sueishi K, Tanaka K, et al: Pulmonary aspergillosis with bronchocentric granulomas. Am J Surg Pathol 14:485, 1990.

930. Cooper JAD, Weinbaum DL, Aldrich TK, et al: Invasive aspergillosis of the lung and pericardium in a nonimmunocompromised 33 year old man. Am J Med 71:903, 1981.

931. D'Silva H, Burke JF Jr, Cho SY: Disseminated aspergillosis in a presumably immunocompetent host. JAMA 248:1495, 1982.

932. Karam GH, Griffin FM Jr: Invasive pulmonary aspergillosis in nonimmunocompromised, nonneutropenic hosts. Rev Infect Dis 8:357, 1986.

932a. Clancy CJ, Nguyen MH: Acute community-acquired pneumonia due to Aspergillus in presumably immunocompetent hosts: Clues for recognition of a rare but fatal disease. Chest 114:629, 1998.

933. Walsh TJ, Mendelsohn G: Invasive aspergillosis complicating Cushing's syndrome. Arch Intern Med 141:1227, 1981.

934. Vieira DF, Van Saene HK, Miranda DR: Invasive pulmonary aspergillosis after near-drowning. Intensive Care Med 10:203, 1984.

935. Berner R, Sauter S, Michalski Y, et al: Central venous catheter infection by *Aspergillus fumigatus* in a patient with B-type nonHodgkin lymphoma. Med Pediatr Oncol 27:202, 1996.

936. Gage AA, Dean DC, Schimert G, et al: Aspergillus infection after cardiac surgery. Arch Surg 101:384, 1970.

937. Dewhurst AG, Cooper MJ, Khan SM, et al: Invasive aspergillosis in immunosuppressed patients: Potential hazard of hospital building work. BMJ 301:802, 1990.

938. Perraud M, Piens MA, Nicoloyannis N, et al: Invasive nosocomial pulmonary aspergillosis: Risk factors and hospital building works. Epidemiol Infect 99:1147, 1987.

939. Rose HD, Hirsch SR: Filtering hospital air decreases *Aspergillus* spore counts. Am Rev Respir Dis 114:511, 1979.

940. Sarubbi FA Jr, Kopf HB, Wilson MB, et al: Increased recovery of *Aspergillus flavus* from respiratory specimens during hospital construction. Am Rev Respir Dis 125:33, 1982.

941. Pittet D, Huguenin T, Dharan S, et al: Unusual cause of lethal pulmonary aspergillosis in patients with chronic obstructive pulmonary disease. Am J Respir Crit Care Med 154:541, 1996

942. Sidransky H, Verney E, Beede H: Experimental pulmonary aspergillosis. Arch Pathol 79:299, 1965.

943. Merkow LP, Epstein SM, Sidransky H, et al: The pathogenesis of experimental pulmonary aspergillosis. Am J Pathol 62:57, 1971.

944. Turner KJ, Hackshaw R, Papadimitriou J, et al: The pathogenesis of experimental pulmonary aspergillosis in normal and cortisone-treated rats. J Pathol 118:65, 1975.

945. Albelda SM, Gefter WB, Epstein DM, et al: Bronchopleural fistula complicating invasive pulmonary aspergillosis. Am Rev Respir Dis 126:163, 1982.

946. Walsh TJ, Bulkley BH: *Aspergillus* pericarditis: Clinical and pathologic features in the immunocompromised patient. Cancer 49:48, 1982.

947. Müller NL, Miller RR, Ostrow DN, et al: Tension pneumopericardium: An unusual manifestation of invasive pulmonary aspergillosis. Am J Roentgenol 148:678, 1987.

948. Klein DL, Gamsu G: Review: Thoracic manifestations of aspergillosis. Am J Roentgenol 134:543, 1980.

949. Fraser RS: Pulmonary aspergillosis: Pathologic and Pathogenetic Features. *In* Rosen PP, Fechner RE (eds): Pathology Annual Part 1. Vol 28. Norwalk, CT, Appleton & Lange, 1993, p 231.

950. Young RC, Bennett JE, Vogel CL, et al: Aspergillosis: The spectrum of the disease in 98 patients. Medicine 49:147, 1970.

951. Sieber SC, Cole SR, McNab JM, et al: Bronchiolitis associated with the finding of the fungus aspergillus: Report of two cases. Conn Med 58:13, 1994.

952. Cohen DM, Goggans EA: Sclerosing mediastinitis and terminal valvular endocarditis caused by fungus suggestive of *Aspergillus* species. Am J Clin Pathol 56:91, 1970.

953. Meredith HC, Cogan BM, McLaulin B: Pleural aspergillosis. Am J Roentgenol 130:164, 1978.

954. Macartney JN: Pulmonary aspergillosis: A review and a description of three new cases. Thorax 19:287, 1964.

955. Young RC, Vogel CL, DeVita VT: Aspergillus lobar pneumonia. JAMA 208:1156, 1969.

956. Herbert PA, Bayer AS: Fungal pneumonia (Part 4): Invasive pulmonary aspergillosis. Chest 80:220, 1981.

957. Logan PM, Primack SL, Miller RR, Müller NL: Invasive aspergillosis of the airways: Radiographic, CT, and pathologic findings. Radiology 193:383, 1994.

957a. Brown MJ, Worthy SA, Flint JDA, Müller NL: Invasive aspergillosis in the immunocompromised host: Utility of computed tomography and bronchoalveolar lavage. Clin Radiol 53:255, 1997.

958. Orr DP, Myerowitz RL, Dubois PJ: Pathoradiologic correlation of invasive pulmonary aspergillosis in the compromised host. Cancer 41:2028, 1978.

959. Kibbler CC, Milkins SR, Bhamra A, et al: Apparent pulmonary mycetoma following invasive aspergillosis in neutropenic patients. Thorax 43:108, 1988.

960. Przyjemski C, Mattii R: The formation of pulmonary mycetomata. Cancer 46:1701, 1980.

961. Pai U, Blinkhorn RJ Jr, Tomashefski JF Jr: Invasive cavitary pulmonary aspergillosis in patients with cancer: A clinicopathologic study. Hum Pathol 25:293, 1994.

962. Pagani JJ, Libshitz HI: Opportunistic fungal pneumonias in cancer patients. Am J Roentgenol 137:1033, 1981.

963. Libshitz HI, Pagani JJ: Aspergillosis and mucormycosis: Two types of opportunistic fungal pneumonia. Radiology 140:301, 1981.

964. Kirshenbaum JM, Lorell BH, Schoen FJ, et al: Angioinvasive pulmonary aspergillosis: Presentation as massive pulmonary saddle embolism in an immunocompromised patient. J Am Coll Cardiol 6:486, 1985.

965. Curtis AM, Smith GJW, Ravin CE: Air crescent sign of invasive aspergillosis. Radiology 133:17, 1979.

966. Albeda SM, Talbot GH, Gerson SL, et al: Pulmonary cavitation and massive hemoptysis in invasive pulmonary aspergillosis: Influence of bone marrow recovery in patients with acute leukemia. Am Rev Respir Dis 131:115, 1985.

967. Slevin ML, Knowles GK, Phillips MJ, et al: The air crescent sign of invasive pulmonary aspergillosis in acute leukaemia. Thorax 37:554, 1982.

968. Kuhlman JE, Fishman EK, Siegelman SS: Invasive pulmonary aspergillosis in acute leukemia: Characteristic findings on CT, the CT halo sign, and the role of CT in early diagnosis. Radiology 157:611, 1985.

969. Young RC, Vogel CL, Devita VT: *Aspergillus* lobar pneumonia. JAMA 208:1156, 1969.

970. Albelda SM, Gefter WB, Epstein DM, et al: Bronchopleural fistula complicating invasive pulmonary aspergillosis. Am Rev Respir Dis 126:163, 1982.

971. van Ede AE, Meis JF, Koot RA, et al: Pneumopericardium complicating invasive pulmonary aspergillosis: Case report and review. Infection 22:102, 1994.

972. Hruban RH, Meziane MA, Zerhouni EA, et al: Radiologic-pathologic correlation of the CT halo sign in invasive pulmonary aspergillosis. J Comput Assist Tomogr 11:534, 1987.

973. Blum U, Windfuhr M, Buitrago-Tellez C, et al: Invasive pulmonary aspergillosis: MRI, CT, and plain radiographic findings and their contribution for early diagnosis. Chest 106:1156, 1994.

974. Mori M, Galvin JR, Barloon TJ, et al: Fungal pulmonary infections after bone marrow transplantation: Evaluation with radiography and CT. Radiology 178:721, 1991.

974a. Won HJ, Lee KS, Cheon J-E, et al: Invasive pulmonary aspergillosis: prediction at thin-section CT in patients with neutropenia—a prospective study. Radiology 208:777, 1998.

975. Gerson SL, Talbot GH, Lusk E, et al: Invasive pulmonary aspergillosis in adult acute leukemia: Clinical clues to its diagnosis. J Clin Oncol 3:1109, 1985.

976. Borkin MH, Arena FP, Brown AE, et al: Invasive aspergillosis with massive fatal hemoptysis in patients with neoplastic disease. Chest 781:835, 1980.

977. Pagano L, Ricci P, Nosari A, et al: Fatal haemoptysis in pulmonary filamentous mycosis: An underevaluated cause of death in patients with acute leukaemia in haematological complete remission: A retrospective study and review of the literature. Br J Haematol 89:500, 1995.

978. Kirshenbaum JM, Lorell BH, Schoen FJ, et al: Angioinvasive pulmonary aspergillosis: Presentation as massive pulmonary saddle embolism in an immunocompromised patient. J Am Coll Cardiol 6:486, 1985.

979. Vlasveld LTh, Delemarre JFM, Beynen JH, et al: Invasive aspergillosis complicated by subclavian artery occlusion and costal osteomyelitis after autologous bone marrow transplantation. Thorax 47:136, 1992.

980. Albelda SM, Gefter WB, Epstein DM, et al: Bronchopleural fistula complicating invasive pulmonary aspergillosis. Am Rev Respir Dis 126:163, 1982.

981. Galigiuri P, MacMahon M, Courtney J, et al: Opportunistic pulmonary aspergillosis with chest wall invasion: Plain film and computed tomographic findings. Arch Intern Med 143:2323, 1983.

982. Clarke A, Skelton J, Fraser RS: Fungal tracheobronchitis: Report of 9 cases and review of the literature. Medicine 70:1, 1991.

983. Pervez NK, Kleinerman J, Kattan M, et al: Pseudomembranous necrotizing bronchial aspergillosis: A variant of invasive aspergillosis in a patient with hemophilia and acquired immune deficiency syndrome. Am Rev Respir Dis 131:961, 1985

984. Berlinger NT, Freeman TJ: Acute airway obstruction due to necrotizing tracheobronchial aspergillosis in immunocompromised patients: A new clinical entity. Ann Otol Rhinol Laryngol 98:718, 1989.

985. Hines DW, Haber MH, Yaremko L, et al: Pseudomembranous tracheobronchitis caused by aspergillus. Am Rev Respir Dis 143:1408, 1991.

986. Kessler R, Massard G, Warter A, et al: Bronchial-pulmonary artery fistula after unilateral lung transplantation: A case report. J Heart Lung Transplant 16:674, 1997.

987. Gowing NFC, Hamlin IME: Tissue reactions to *Aspergillus* in cases of Hodgkin's disease and leukaemia. J Clin Pathol 13:396, 1960.

988. Tait RC, O'Driscoll BR, Denning DW: Unilateral wheeze caused by pseudomembranous aspergillus tracheobronchitis in the immunocompromised patient. Thorax 48:1285, 1993.

989. Mineur PH, Ferrant A, Wallon J, et al: Bronchoesophageal fistula caused by pulmonary aspergillosis. Eur J Respir Dis 66:360, 1985.

990. Binder RE, Faling LJ, Pugatch RD, et al: Chronic necrotizing pulmonary aspergillosis: A discrete clinical entity. Medicine 61:109, 1982.

991. Gefter WB, Weingrad TR, Epstein DM, et al: "Semi-invasive" pulmonary aspergillosis: A new look at the spectrum of *Aspergillus* infections of the lung. Radiology 140:313, 1981.

992. Yousem SA: The histologic spectrum of chronic necrotizing forms of pulmonary aspergillosis. Hum Pathol 28:650, 1997

993. Yamaguchi M, Nishiya H, Mano K, et al: Chronic necrotising pulmonary aspergillosis caused by *Aspergillus niger* in a mildly immunocompromised host. Thorax 47:570, 1992.

994. Tron V, Churg A: Chronic necrotizing pulmonary aspergillosis mimicking bronchocentric granulomatosis. Pathol Res Pract 181:621, 1986.

995. Vogeser M, Haas A, Aust D, et al: Postmortem analysis of invasive aspergillosis in a tertiary care hospital. Eur J Clin Microbiol Infect Dis 16:1, 1997.

996. Horvath JA, Dummer S: The use of respiratory-tract cultures in the diagnosis of invasive pulmonary aspergillosis. Am J Med 100:171, 1996.

997. Yu VL, Muder RR, Poorsattar A: Significance of isolation of *Aspergillus* from the respiratory tract in diagnosis of invasive pulmonary aspergillosis: Results from a three-year prospective study. Am J Med 81:249, 1986.

998. Kahn FW, Jones JM, England DM: The role of bronchoalveolar lavage in the diagnosis of invasive pulmonary aspergillosis. Am J Clin Pathol 86:518, 1986.

999. Chung C, Lord PL, Krumpe PE: Diagnosis of invasive pulmonary aspergillosis by fiberoptic transbronchial lung biopsy. JAMA 239:749, 1978.

1000. Aisner J, Murillo J, Schimpff SC, et al: Invasive aspergillosis in acute leukemia: Correlation with nose cultures and antibiotic use. Ann Intern Med 90:4, 1979.

1001. Weiner MH, Talbot GH, Gerson SL, et al: Antigen detection in the diagnosis of invasive aspergillosis: Utility in controlled, blinded trials. Ann Intern Med 99:777, 1983.

1002. Tomee JF, Mannes GP, van der Bij W, et al: Serodiagnosis and monitoring of *Aspergillus* infections after lung transplantation. Ann Intern Med 125:197, 1996.

1002a. Yuasa K, Goto H, Iguchi M, et al: Evaluation of the diagnostic value of the measurement of (1–>3)-beta-D-glucan in patients with pulmonary aspergillosis. Respiration 63:78, 1996.

1003. Verweij PE, Dompeling EC, Donnelly JP, et al: Serial monitoring of *Aspergillus* antigen in the early diagnosis of invasive aspergillosis. Preliminary investigations with two examples. Infection 25:86, 1997.

1004. Verweij PE, Latge JP, Rijs AJ, et al: Comparison of antigen detection and PCR assay using bronchoalveolar lavage fluid for diagnosing invasive pulmonary aspergillosis in patients receiving treatment for hematological malignancies. J Clin Microbiol 33:3150, 1995.

1005. Melchers WJ, Verweij PE, van den Hurk P, et al: General primer-mediated PCR for detection of aspergillus species. J Clin Microbiol 32:1710, 1994.

1006. Einsele H, Hebart H, Roller G, et al: Detection and identification of fungal pathogens in blood by using molecular probes. J Clin Microbiol 35:1353, 1997.

1007. Andrews CP, Weiner MH: Immunodiagnosis of invasive pulmonary aspergillosis in rabbits: Fungal antigen detected by radioimmunoassay in bronchoalveolar lavage fluid. Am Rev Respir Dis 124:60, 1981.

1008. Fisher BD, Armstrong D, Yu B, et al: Invasive aspergillosis: Progress in early diagnosis and treatment. Am J Med 71:571, 1981.

1009. Aisner J, Schimpff SC, Wiernik PH: Treatment of invasive aspergillosis: Relation of early diagnosis and treatment to response. Ann Intern Med 86:539, 1977.

1010. Burch PA, Karp JE, Merz WG, et al: Favorable outcome of invasive aspergillosis in patients with acute leukemia. J Clin Oncol 5:1985, 1987.

1011. Walsh TJ, Renshaw G, Andrews J, et al: Invasive zygomycosis due to *Conidiobolus incongruus*. Clin Infect Dis 19:423, 1994.

1012. El-Ani AS, Dhar V: Disseminated mucormycosis in a case of metastatic carcinoma. Am J Clin Pathol 77:110, 1981.

1013. Torell J, Cooper BH, Helgeson NGP: Disseminated *Saksenaea vasiformis* infection. Am J Clin Pathol 76:116, 1981.

1014. McGinnis MR, Walker DH, Dominy IE, et al: Zygomycosis caused by *Cunninghamella bertholletiae*: Clinical and pathologic aspects. Arch Pathol Lab Med 106:282, 1982.

1015. Kwon-Chung KJ, Young RC, Orlando M: Pulmonary mucormycosis caused by *Cunninghamella elegans* in a patient with chronic myelogenous leukemia. Am J Clin Pathol 64:544, 1975.

1016. Kolbeck PC, Makhoul RG, Bollinger RR, et al: Widely disseminated *Cunninghamella* mucormycosis in an adult renal transplant patient: Case report and review of the literature. Am J Clin Pathol 83:747, 1985.

1017. Ventura GJ, Kantarjian HM, Anaissie E, et al: Pneumonia with *Cunninghamella* species in patients with hematologic malignancies. Cancer 58:1534, 1986.

1018. O'Connell MA, Pluss JL, Schkade P, et al: Rhizopus-induced hypersensitivity pneumonitis in a tractor driver. J Allergy Clin Immunol 95:779, 1995.

1019. Marchevsky AM, Bottone EJ, Geller SA, et al: The changing spectrum of disease, etiology, and diagnosis of mucormycosis. Hum Pathol 11:457, 1980.

1020. Melnick JZ, Latimer J, Lee El, et al: Systemic mucormycosis complicating acute renal failure: Case report and review of the literature. Ren Fail 17:619, 1995.

1021. Tedder M, Spratt JA, Anstadt MP, et al: Pulmonary mucormycosis: Results of medical and surgical therapy. Ann Thorac Surg 57:1044, 1994.

1022. Funada H, Matsuda T: Pulmonary mucormycosis in a hematology ward. Intern Med 35:540, 1996.

1023. Rangel-Guerra RA, Martinez HR, Saenz C, et al: Rhinocerebral and systemic mucormycosis: Clinical experience with 36 cases. J Neurol Sci 143:19, 1996.

1024. Ispinoza CG, Halkias DG: Pulmonary mucormycosis as a complication of chronic salicylate poisoning. Am J Clin Pathol 80:508, 1983.

1025. Matsushima T, Soejima R, Nakashima T: Solitary pulmonary nodule caused by phycomycosis in a patient without obvious predisposing factors. Thorax 35:877, 1980.

1026. Majid AA, Yii NW: Granulomatous pulmonary zygomycosis in a patient without underlying illness: Computed tomographic appearances and treatment by pneumonectomy. Chest 100:560, 1991.

1027. Straatsma BR, Zimmerman LE, Gass JDM: Phycomycosis: A clinicopathologic study of fifty-one cases. Lab Invest 11:963, 1962.

1028. Leong ASY: Granulomatous mediastinitis due to *Rhizopus* species. Am J Clin Pathol 70:103, 1978.

1029. Chandler FW, Watts JC, Kaplan W, et al: Zygomycosis: Report of four cases with formation of chlamydoconidia in tissue. Am J Clin Pathol 84:99, 1985.

1030. McAdams HP, Rosado de Christenson M, Strollo DC, et al: Pulmonary mucormycosis: Radiologic findings in 32 cases. Am J Roentgenol 168:1541, 1997.

1031. McBride RA, Corson JM, Dammin GJ: Mucormycosis: Two cases of disseminated disease with cultural identification of rhizopus: Review of literature. Am J Med 28:832, 1960.

1032. Donner MW, McAfee JG: Roentgenographic manifestations of diabetes mellitus. Am J Med Sci 239:622, 1960.

1033. Gabriele EF: Mucormycosis. Am J Roentgenol 83:227, 1960.

1034. Rubin SA, Chaljub G, Winer-Muram HT, et al: Pulmonary zygomycosis: A radiographic and clinical spectrum. J Thorac Imaging 7:85, 1992.

1035. Gale AM, Kleitsch WP: Solitary pulmonary nodule due to phycomycosis (mucormycosis). Chest 62:752, 1972.

1036. Reich J, Renzetti AD Jr: Pulmonary phycomycosis: Report of a case of broncho-

1037. cutaneous fistula formation and pulmonary arterial mycothrombosis. Am Rev Respir Dis 102:959, 1970.

1037. Funada H, Misawa T, Nakao S, et al: The air crescent sign of invasive pulmonary mucormycosis in acute leukemia. Cancer 53:2721, 1984.

1038. Zagoria RJ, Choplin RH, Karstaedt N: Pulmonary gangrene as a complication of mucormycosis. Am J Roentgenol 144:1195, 1985.

1039. Silver SF, Grymaloski MR, Bosken CH, et al: Clinico-radiologic-pathologic conference: Pulmonary consolidation with an air crescent sign in an immunocompromised woman. J Can Assoc Radiol 40:167, 1989.

1040. Aderka A, Sidi Y, Garfinkel D, et al: Roentgenologically invisible mucormycosis pneumonia. Respiration 44:158, 1983.

1041. Abter EI, Lutwick SM, Chapnick EK, et al: Mucormycosis of a median sternotomy wound. Cardiovasc Surg 2:474, 1994.

1042. Gaziev D, Baronciani D, Galimberti M, et al: Mucormycosis after bone marrow transplantation: report of four cases in thalassemia and review of the literature. Bone Marrow Transplant 17:409, 1996.

1043. Bertocchi M, Thevenet F, Bastien O, et al: Fungal infections in lung transplant recipients. Transplant Proc 27:1695, 1995.

1044. Malnick SD, Eliraz A, Goland S, et al: Fatal pulmonary mucormycosis in a well controlled diabetic patient. Presse Med 24:225, 1995.

1045. Murray HW: Pulmonary mucormycosis with massive fatal hemoptysis. Chest 68:65, 1975.

1046. Dykhuizen RS, Kerr KN, Soutar RL: Air crescent sign and fatal haemoptysis in pulmonary mucormycosis. Scand J Infect Dis 26:498, 1994.

1047. Harada M, Manabe T, Yamashita K, et al: Pulmonary mucormycosis with fatal massive hemoptysis. Acta Pathol Jpn 42:49, 1992.

1048. Yagihashi S, Watanabe K, Nagai K, et al: Pulmonary mucormycosis presenting as massive fatal hemoptysis in a hemodialytic patient with chronic renal failure. Klin Wochenschr 69:224, 1991.

1049. Coffey MJ, Fantone J, Stirling MC, et al: Psudoaneurysm of pulmonary artery in mucormycosis. Radiographic characteristics and management. Am Rev Respir Dis 145:1487, 1992.

1050. Loevner LA, Andrews JC, Francis IR: Multiple mycotic pulmonary artery aneurysms: A complication of invasive mucormycosis. Am J Roentgenol 158:761, 1992.

1051. Muhm M, Zuckermann A, Prokesch R, et al: Early onset of pulmonary mucormycosis with pulmonary vein thrombosis in a heart transplant recipient. Transplantation 62:1185, 1996.

1052. Watts WJ: Bronchopleural fistula followed by massive fatal hemoptysis in a patient with pulmonary mucormycosis: Case report. Arch Intern Med 143:1029, 1983.

1053. Helenglass G, Elliot JA, Lucie NP: An unusual presentation of opportunistic mucormycosis. BMJ 282:108, 1981.

1054. Watts WJ: Bronchopleural fistula followed by massive fatal hemoptysis in a patient with pulmonary mucormycosis: Case report. Arch Intern Med 143:1029, 1983.

1055. von Pohle WR: Disseminated mucormycosis presenting with lower extremity weakness. Eur Respir J 9:1751, 1996.

1056. Andrews DR, Allan A, Larbalestier RI: Tracheal mucormycosis. Ann Thorac Surg 63:230, 1997.

1057. Schwartz JRL, Nagle MG, Elkins RC, et al: Mucormycosis of the trachea. Chest 81:653, 1982.

1058. Husari AW, Jensen WA, Kirsch CM, et al: Pulmonary mucormycosis presenting as an endobronchial lesion. Chest 106:1889, 1994.

1059. al-Majed S, al-Kassimi F, Ashour M, et al: Removal of endobronchial mucormycosis lesion through a rigid bronchoscope. Thorax 47:203, 1992.

1060. Fishbach RS, White ML, Finegold SM: Bronchopulmonary geotrichosis. Am Rev Respir Dis 108:1388, 1973.

1061. Morenz J: Geotrichosis. In Baker RD (ed): Human Infection with Fungi, Actinomycetes and Algae. New York, Springer-Verlag, 1971, p 919.

1062. Bell D, Brodie J, Henderson A: A case of pulmonary geotrichosis. Br J Dis Chest 56:26, 1962.

1063. Ross JD, Reid KDG, Speirs CF: Bronchopulmonary geotrichosis with severe asthma. BMJ 1:1400, 1966.

1064. Chang WWL, Buerger L: Disseminated geotrichosis. Arch Intern Med 113:356, 1964.

1065. Ghamande AR, Landis FB, Snider GL: Bronchial geotrichosis with fungemia complicating bronchogenic carcinoma. Chest 59:98, 1971.

1066. Conant NF, Martin DS, Smith DT, et al: Manual of Clinical Mycology. (Prepared under the auspices of the Division of Medical Sciences of the National Research Council.) 3rd ed. Philadelphia, WB Saunders, 1971.

1067. Evers RH, Whereatt RR: Pulmonary sporotrichosis. Chest 66:91, 1974.

1068. Dahl BA, Stilberfarb PM, Sarosi GA, et al: Sporotrichosis in children: Report of an epidemic. JAMA 215:1980, 1971.

1069. D'Alessio DJ, Leavens LJ, Strumpf GB, et al: An outbreak of sporotrichosis in Vermont associated with sphagnum moss as the source of infection. N Engl J Med 272:1054, 1965.

1070. Lurie HI: Sporotrichosis. In Baker RD (ed): Human Infection with Fungi, Actinomycetes and Algae. New York, Springer-Verlag, 1971, p 614.

1071. Coles FB, Schuchat A, Hibbs JR, et al: A multistate outbreak of sporotrichosis associated with sphagnum moss. Am J Epidemiol 136:475, 1992.

1072. England DM, Hochholzer L: Primary pulmonary sporotrichosis: Report of eight cases with clinicopathologic review. Am J Surg Pathol 9:193, 1985.

1073. Naimark A, Tiu S: Primary pulmonary sporotrichosis. J Can Assoc Radiol 30:129, 1979.

1074. Satterwhite TK, Kageler WV, Conklin RH, et al: Disseminated sporotrichosis. JAMA 240:771, 1978.

1075. Pueringer RJ, Iber C, Deike MA, et al: Spontaneous remission of extensive pulmonary sporotrichosis. Ann Intern Med 104:366, 1986.

1076. England DM, Hochholzer L: *Sporothrix* infection of the lung without cutaneous disease. Arch Pathol Lab Med 111:298, 1987.

1077. Plouffe JF Jr, Silva J Jr, Fekety R, et al: Cell-mediated immune responses in sporotrichosis. J Infect Dis 139:152, 1979.

1078. Heller HM, Fuhrer J: Disseminated sporotrichosis in patients with AIDS: Case report and review of the literature. AIDS 5:1243, 1991.

1079. Smith AG, Morgan WKC, Hornick RB, et al: Chronic pulmonary sporotrichosis: Report of a case, including morphologic and mycologic studies. Am J Clin Pathol 54:401, 1970.

1080. England DM, Hochholzer L: Primary pulmonary sporotrichosis. Am J Surg Pathol 9:193, 1985.

1081. Lei PC, Yoshiike T, Yaguchi H, et al: Histopathological studies of *Sporothrix schenckii*-inoculated mice: Possible functions of polymorphonuclear leukocytes in normal and immunocompromised (congenitally athymic nude) mice. Mycopathologia 122:89, 1993.

1082. Hiruma M, Kawada A, Noda T, et al: Tissue response in sporotrichosis: Light and electron microscopy studies. Mycoses 35:35, 1992.

1083. Jay SJ, Platt MR, Reynolds RC: Primary pulmonary sporotrichosis. Am Rev Respir Dis 115:1051, 1977.

1084. Marques MEA, Coelho KIR, Sotto MN, et al: Comparison between histochemical and immunohistochemical methods for diagnosis of sporotrichosis. J Clin Pathol 45:1089, 1992.

1085. Cruthirds TP, Patterson DO: Primary pulmonary sporotrichosis. Am Rev Respir Dis 95:845, 1967.

1086. Beland JE, Mankiewicz E, MacIntosh DJ: Primary pulmonary sporotrichosis: Case report. Can Med Assoc J 99:813, 1968.

1087. Michelson E: Primary pulmonary sporotrichosis. Ann Thorac Surg 24:83, 1977.

1088. Trevathan RD, Phillips S: Primary pulmonary sporotrichosis: Case report. JAMA 195:965, 1966.

1089. Boehm D, Lynch JM, Hodges GR, et al: Disseminated sporotrichosis presenting as sarcoidosis: Electron microscopic and immunologic studies. Am J Med Sci 283:71, 1982.

1090. Comstock C, Wolson AH: Roentgenology of sporotrichosis. Am J Roentgenol 125:651, 1975.

1091. Friedman SJ, Doyle JA: Extracutaneous sporotrichosis. Int J Dermatol 22:171, 1983.

1092. Farley ML, Fagan MF, Mabry LC, et al: Presentation of *Sporothrix schenckii* in pulmonary cytology specimens. Acta Cytol 35:389, 1991.

1093. Gori S, Lupetti A, Moscato G, et al: Pulmonary sporotrichosis with hyphae in a human immunodeficiency virus-infected patient: A case report. Acta Cytol 41:519, 1997.

1094. Lowenstein M, Markowitz SM, Nottebart HC, et al: Existence of *Sporothrix schenckii* as a pulmonary saprophyte. Chest 73:419, 1978.

1095. Agger WA, Seager GM: Granulomas of the vocal cords caused by *Sporothrix schenckii*. Laryngoscope 95:595, 1985.

1096. Pluss JL, Opal SM: Pulmonary sporotrichosis: Review of treatment and outcome. Medicine 65:143, 1986.

1097. Ingrish FM, Schneidau JD: Cutaneous hypersensitivity to sporotrichin in Maricopa County, Arizona. J Invest Dermatol 49:146, 1967.

1098. Schneidau JD, Lamar LM, Hairston MA: Cutaneous hypersensitivity to sporotrichin in Louisiana. JAMA 188:371, 1964.

1099. Salfelder K, Fingerland A, de Mendelovici M, et al: Two cases of adiaspiromycosis. Beitr Path Bd 148:94, 1973.

1100. Schwarz J: Adiaspiromycosis. *In* Schwarz J (ed): Pathology Annual, Part 1. Vol 13. New York, Appleton-Century-Crofts, 1978, p 41.

1101. Nuorva K, Pitkanen R, Issakainen J, et al: Pulmonary adiaspiromycosis in a two year old girl. J Clin Pathol 50:82, 1997.

1102. Kodousek R, Vortel V, Fingerland A, et al: Pulmonary adiaspiromycosis in man caused by *Emmonsia crescens*: Report of a unique case. Am J Clin Pathol 56:394, 1971.

1103. Watts JC, Callaway CS, Chandler FW, et al: Human pulmonary adiaspiromycosis. Arch Pathol 99:11, 1975.

1104. England DM, Hochholzer L: Adiaspiromycosis: An unusual fungal infection of the lung: Report of 11 cases. Am J Surg Pathol 17:876, 1993.

1105. Cueva JA, Little MD: *Emmonsia crescens* infection (adiaspiromycosis) in man in Honduras: Report of a case. Am J Trop Med Hyg 20:282, 1971.

1106. Rippon JW, Carmichael JW: Petriellidiosis (allescheriosis): Four unusual cases and review of literature. Mycopathologia 58:117, 1976.

1107. McCarthy DS, Longbottom JL, Riddell RW, et al: Pulmonary mycetoma due to *Allescheria boydii*. Am Rev Respir Dis 100:213, 1969.

1108. Travis RE, Ulrich EW, Phillips S: Pulmonary allescheriasis. Ann Intern Med 54:141, 1961.

1109. Rosen P, Adelson HT, Burleig E: Bronchiectasis complicated by the presence of *Monosporium apiospermum* and *Aspergillus fumigatus*. Am J Clin Pathol 52:182, 1969.

1110. Travis LB, Roberts GD, Wilson WR: Clinical significance of *Pseudallescheria boydii*: Review of 10 years' experience. Mayo Clin Proc 60:531, 1985.

1111. Miller MA, Greenberger PA, Amerian R, et al: Allergic bronchopulmonary mycosis caused by *Pseudallescheria boydii*. Am Rev Respir Dis 148:810, 1993.

1112. Lutwick LI, Galgiani JN, Johnson RH, et al: Visceral fungal infections due to *Petriellidium boydii (Allescheria boydii)*: In vitro drug sensitivity studies. Am J Med 61:632, 1976.

1113. Alture-Werber E, Edberg SC, Singer JM: Pulmonary infection with *Allescheria boydii*. Am J Clin Pathol 66:1019, 1976.

1114. Rosen F, Deck JHN, Newcastle NB: *Allescheria boydii*—unique systemic dissemination to thyroid and brain. Can Med Assoc 93:1125, 1965.

1115. Galgiani JN, Stevens DA, Graybill JR, et al: *Pseudallescheria boydii* infections treated with ketoconazole: Clinical evaluations of seven patients and in vitro susceptibility results. Chest 86:219, 1984.

1116. Scherr GR, Evans SG, Kiyabu MT, et al: *Pseudallescheria boydii* infection in the acquired immunodeficiency syndrome. Arch Pathol Lab Med 116:535, 1992.

1117. Saadah HA, Dixon T: *Petriellidum boydii (Allescheria boydii)*: Necrotizing pneumonia in a normal host. JAMA 245:605, 1981.

1118. Hung CC, Chang SC, Yang PC, et al: Invasive pulmonary pseudallescheriasis with direct invasion of the thoracic spine in an immunocompetent patient. Eur J Clin Microbiol Infect Dis 13:749, 1994.

1119. Louria DB, Lieberman PH, Collins HS, et al: Pulmonary mycetoma due to *Allescheria boydii*. Arch Intern Med 117:748, 1966.

1120. Reddy PC, Christianson CS, Gorelick DF, et al: Pulmonary monosporosis: An uncommon pulmonary mycotic infection. Thorax 24:722, 1969.

1121. Shih L, Lee N: Disseminated petriellidiosis (allescheriasis) in a patient with refractory acute lymphoblastic leukemia. J Clin Pathol 37:78, 1984.

1122. Enggano IL, Hughes WT, Kalwinsky DK, et al: *Pseudallescheria boydii* in a patient with acute lymphoblastic leukemia. Arch Pathol Lab Med 108:619, 1984.

1123. Schwartz DA: Organ-specific variation in the morphology of the fungomas (fungus balls) of *Pseudallescheria boydii*. Arch Pathol Lab Med 113:476, 1989.

1124. Bakerspigel A, Wood T, Burke S: Pulmonary allescheriasis: Report of a case from Ontario. Am J Clin Pathol 68:299, 1977.

1125. Tsang DNC, Chan JKC, Lau YT, et al: *Penicillium marneffei* infection: An underdiagnosed disease? Histopathology 13:311, 1988.

1126. Piehl MR, Kaplan RL, Haber MH: Disseminated penicilliosis in a patient with acquired immunodeficiency syndrome. Arch Pathol Lab Med 112:1262, 1988.

1127. Chan JKC, Tsang DNC, Wong DKK: *Penicillium marneffei* in bronchoalveolar lavage fluid. Acta Cytol 33:523, 1989.

1127a. de la Camara R, Pinilla I, Munoz E, et al: *Penicillium brevicompactum* as the cause of a necrotic lung ball in an allogeneic bone marrow transplant recipient. Bone Marrow Transplant 18:1189, 1996.

1128. Deng Z, Connor DH: Progressive disseminated penicilliosis caused by *Penicillium marneffei*. Am J Clin Pathol 84:323, 1985.

1129. Case report: A case of invasive penicilliosis in Hong Kong with immunologic evaluation. Am Rev Respir Dis 131:662, 1985.

1130. Fenech FF, Mallie CP: Pleural effusion caused by *Penicillium lilacinum*. Br J Dis Chest 66:284, 1972.

1131. Duong TA: Infection due to *Penicillium marneffei*, an emerging pathogen: Review of 155 reported cases. Clin Infect Dis 23:125, 1996.

1132. Philips P: *Penicillium marneffei*—part of Southeast Asian AIDS. JAMA 276:86, 1996.

1133. Kudeken N, Kawakami K, Kusano N, et al: Cell-mediated immunity in host resistance against infection caused by *Penicillium marneffei*. J Med Vet Mycol 34:371, 1996.

1134. Cooper CR Jr, McGinnis MR: Pathology of *Penicillium marneffei*: An emerging acquired immunodeficiency syndrome-related pathogen. Arch Pathol Lab Med 121:798, 1997.

1135. Ko KF: Retropharyngeal abscess caused by *Penicillium marneffei*: An unusual cause of upper airway obstruction. Otolaryngol Head Neck Surg 110:445, 1994.

1136. Kaufman L, Standard PG, Jalbert M, et al: Diagnostic antigenemia tests for penicilliosis marneffei. J Clin Microbiol 34:2503, 1996.

1136a. Kaufman L, Standard PG, Anderson SA, et al: Development of specific fluorescent antibody test for tissue form of *Penicillium marneffei*. J Clin Microbiol 33:2136, 1995.

1137. Powell DA, Marcon MJ, Durrell DE, et al: Scanning electron microscopy of *Malassezia furfur* attachment to broviac catheters. Hum Pathol 18:740, 1987.

1138. Redline RW, Redline SS, Boxerbaum B, et al: Systemic *Malassezia furfur* infections in patients receiving intralipid therapy. Hum Pathol 16:815, 1985.

1139. Anaissie E, Kantarjian H, Jones P, et al: *Fusarium:* A newly recognized fungal pathogen in immunosuppressed patients. Cancer 57:2141, 1986.

1140. Leblond V, Saint-Jean O, Datry A, et al: Systemic infections with *Trichosporon beigelii (cutaneum)*. Cancer 58:2399, 1986.

1141. Miro O, Sacanella E, Nadal P, et al: *Trichosporon beigelii* fungemia and metastatic pneumonia in a trauma patient. Eur J Clin Microbiol Infect Dis 13:604, 1994.

1142. Ito T, Ishikawa Y, Fujii R, et al: Disseminated *Trichosporon capitatum* infection in a patient with acute leukemia. Cancer 61:585, 1988.

1143. Lutwick LI, Phaff HJ, Steven DA: *Kluyveromyces fragilis* as an opportunistic fungal pathogen in man. Sabouraudia 18:69, 1980.

1144. McGinnis MR, Walker DH, Folds JD: *Hansenula polymorpha* infection in a child with chronic granulomatous disease. Arch Pathol Lab Med 104:290, 1980.

1145. de la Monte SM, Hutchins GM: Disseminated *Curvularia* infection. Arch Pathol Lab Med 109:872, 1985.

1146. Miyazaki E, Sugisaki K, Shigenaga T, et al: A case of acute eosinophilic pneumonia caused by inhalation of *Trichosporon terrestre*. Am J Respir Crit Care Med 151:541, 1995.

1147. Adam RD, Paquin ML, Petersen EA, et al: Phaeohyphomycosis caused by the fungal genera *Bipolaris* and *Exserohilum*: A report of 9 cases and review of the literature. Medicine 65:203, 1986.

1148. Fink JN, Schlueter DP, Barboriak JJ: Hypersensitivity pneumonitis due to exposure to *Alternaria*. Chest 63(Suppl):4, 1973.

1149. Lobritz RW, Roberts TH, Marraro RV, et al: Granulomatous pulmonary disease secondary to *Alternaria*. JAMA 241:596, 1979.
1150. Schiff MJ, Kaplan MH: *Rothia dentocariosa* pneumonia in an immunocompromised patient. Lung 165:279, 1987.
1151. Bassiri AG, Girgis RE, Theodore J: Actinomyces odontolyticus thoracopulmonary infections: Two cases in lung and heart-lung transplant recipients and a review of the literature. Chest 109:1109, 1996.
1152. Thadepalli H, Rao B: *Actinomyces viscosus* infections of the chest in humans. Am Rev Respir Dis 120:203, 1979.
1153. Suzuki JB, Delisle AL: Pulmonary actinomycosis of periodontal origin. J Periodontol 55:581, 1984.
1154. Karetzky MS, Garvey JW: Empyema due to *Actinomyces naeslundi*. Chest 65:229, 1974.
1155. Eng RHK, Corrado ML, Cleri D, et al: Infections caused by *Actinomyces viscosus*. Am J Clin Pathol 75:113, 1981.
1156. Spiegel CA, Telford G: Isolation of *Wolinella recta* and *Actinomyces viscosus* from an actinomycotic chest wall mass. J Clin Microbiol 20:1187, 1984.
1157. Apotheloz C, Regamey C: Disseminated infection due to *Actinomyces meyeri*: Case report and review. Clin Infect Dis 22:621, 1996.
1158. Funke G, von Graevenitz A: Infections due to *Actinomyces neuii* (former "CDC coryneform group 1" bacteria). Infection 23:73, 1995
1159. Gahrn-Hansen B, Frederiksen W: Human infections with *Actinomyces pyogenes* (*Corynebacterium pyogenes*). Diagn Microbiol Infect Dis 15:349, 1992.
1160. Pine L: Actinomyces and microaerophilic actinomycetes. *In* Braude AI, Davis CE, Fierer J (eds): Medical Microbiology and Infectious Diseases. Philadelphia, WB Saunders, 1981, p 448.
1161. Brock DW, Georg LK, Brown JM, et al: Actinomycosis caused by *Arachnia propionica*: Report of 11 cases. Am J Clin Pathol 59:66, 1973.
1162. Brown JR: Human actinomycosis: A study of 181 subjects. Hum Pathol 4:319, 1973.
1163. Robboy SJ, Vickery AL Jr: Tinctorial and morphologic properties distinguishing actinomycosis and nocardiosis. N Engl J Med 282:593, 1970.
1164. Dicpinigaitis PV, Bleiweiss IJ, Krellenstein DJ, et al: Primary endobronchial actinomycosis in association with foreign body aspiration. Chest 101:283, 1992.
1165. Julia G, Rodriguez de Castro F, Caminero J, et al: Endobronchial actinomycosis associated with a foreign body. Respiration 58:229, 1991.
1166. Kasano Y, Tanimura H, Yamaue H, et al: Hepatic actinomycosis infiltrating the diaphragm and right lung. Am J Gastroenterol 91:2418, 1996.
1167. Parker JS, deBoisblanc BP: Case report: Actinomycosis: Multinodular pulmonary involvement. Am J Med Sci 307:418, 1994.
1168. Snape PS: Thoracic actinomycosis: An unusual childhood infection. South Med J 86:222, 1993.
1169. Cendan I, Klapholz A, Talavera W: Pulmonary actinomycosis: A cause of endobronchial disease in a patient with AIDS. Chest 103:1886, 1993.
1170. Bennhoff DF: Actinomycosis: Diagnostic and therapeutic considerations and a review of 32 cases. Laryngoscope 94:1198, 1984.
1171. Oddó D, González S: Actinomycosis and nocardiosis: A morphologic study of 17 cases. Pathol Res Pract 181:320, 1986.
1172. Bates M, Cruickshank G: Thoracic actinomycosis. Thorax 12:99, 1957.
1173. Slade PR, Slesser BV, Southgate J: Thoracic actinomycosis. Thorax 28:73, 1973.
1174. Epidemiology. BMJ 1:1037, 1977.
1175. Flynn MW, Felson B: The roentgen manifestations of thoracic actinomycosis. Am J Roentgenol 110:707, 1970.
1176. Frank P, Strickland B: Pulmonary actinomycosis. Br J Radiol 47:373, 1974.
1177. Kwong JS, Müller NL, Godwin JD, et al: Thoracic actinomycosis: CT findings in eight patients. Radiology 183:189, 1992.
1178. Balatsouras DG, Kaberos AK, Eliopoulos PN, et al: Cervicofacial actinomycosis presenting as acute upper respiratory tract obstruction. J Laryngol Otol 108:801, 1994.
1179. Luff RD, Gupta PK, Spence MR, et al: Pelvic actinomycosis and the intrauterine contraceptive device: A cytohistomorphologic study. Am J Clin Pathol 69:581, 1978.
1180. McBride WJ, Hill DR, Gordon DL: Chest wall actinomycosis in association with the use of an intra-uterine device. Aust N Z J Surg 65:141, 1995.
1181. Morris JF, Sewell DL: Necrotizing pneumonia caused by mixed infection with *Actinobacillus actinomycetemcomitans* and *Actinomyces israelii*: Case report and review. Clin Infect Dis 18:450, 1994.
1182. Kuijper EJ, Wiggerts HO, Jonker GJ, et al: Disseminated actinomycosis due to *Actinomyces meyeri* and *Actinobacillus actinomycetemcomitans*. Scand J Infect Dis 24:667, 1992.
1183. Tyrrell J, Noone P, Prichard JS: Thoracic actinomycosis complicated by actinobacillus *Actinomycetem comitans*: Case report and review of literature. Respir Med 86:341, 1992.
1184. Behbehani MJ, Heeley JD, Jordan HV: Comparative histopathology of lesions produced by *Actinomyces israelii*, *Actinomyces naeslundii*, and *Actinomyces viscosus* in mice. Am J Pathol 110:267, 1983.
1185. Weed LA, Baggenstoss AH: Actinomycosis: A pathologic and bacteriologic study of twenty-one fatal cases. Am J Clin Pathol 19:201, 1949.
1186. Cendan I, Klapholz A, Talavera W: Pulmonary actinomycosis: A cause of endobronchial disease in a patient with AIDS. Chest 103:1886, 1993.
1187. Lazzari G, Vineis C, Cugini A: Cytologic diagnosis of primary pulmonary actinomycosis. Report of two cases. Acta Cytol 25:299, 1981.
1188. Pollock PG, Meyers DS, Frable WJ, et al: Rapid diagnosis of actinomycosis by thin-needle aspiration biopsy. Am J Clin Pathol 70:27, 1978.

1189. Das DK: Actinomycosis in fine needle aspiration cytology. Cytopathology 5:243, 1994.
1190. Flynn MW, Felson B: The roentgen manifestations of thoracic actinomycosis. Am J Roentgenol 110:707, 1970.
1191. Eiben C, Indihar FJ, Hunter SW: Thoracic actinomycosis mimicking the pancoast syndrome. Minn Med 66:541, 1983.
1192. Balikian JP, Cheng TH, Costello P, et al: Pulmonary actinomycosis: A report of three cases. Radiology 128:613, 1978.
1193. Hsieh MJ, Liu HP, Chang JP, et al: Thoracic actinomycosis. Chest 104:366, 1993.
1194. Multz AS, Cohen R, Azeuta V: Bacterial pseudomycosis: A rare cause of haemoptysis. Eur Respir J 7:1712, 1994.
1195. Schwarz J, Baum GL: Actinomycosis. Semin Roentgenol 5:58, 1970.
1196. Coodley EL, Yoshinaka R: Pleural effusion as the major manifestation of actinomycosis. Chest 106:1615, 1994.
1197. Harrison RN, Thomas DJB: Acute actinomycotic empyema. Thorax 34:406, 1979.
1198. Merdler C, Greif J, Burke M, et al: Primary actinomycotic empyema. South Med J 76:411, 1983.
1199. Dalhoff K, Wallner S, Finck C, et al: Endobronchial actinomycosis. Eur Respir J 7:1189, 1994.
1200. Dontfraid F, Ramphal R: Bilateral pulmonary infiltrates in association with disseminated actinomycosis. Clin Infect Dis 19:143, 1994.
1201. Morgan DE, Nath H, Sanders C, et al: Mediastinal actinomycosis. Am J Roentgenol 155:735, 1990.
1202. Greer AE: Disseminating Fungus Diseases of the Lung. Springfield, IL, Charles C Thomas, 1962.
1203. Harvey JC, Cantrell JR, Fisher AM: Actinomycosis: Its recognition and treatment. Ann Intern Med 46:868, 1957.
1204. Webb WR, Sagel SS: Actinomycosis involving the chest wall: CT findings. Am J Roentgenol 139:1007, 1982.
1205. Dershaw DD: Actinomycosis of the chest wall: Ultrasound findings in empyema necessitans. Chest 86:779, 1984.
1206. Peabody J Jr, Seabury JH: Actinomycosis and nocardiosis: A review of basic differences in therapy. Am J Med 28:99, 1960.
1207. Tolentino A, Ahkee S, Ramirez J: Pancoast's syndrome secondary to thoracic actinomycosis. J Kansas Med Assoc 94:500, 1996.
1208. Datta JS, Raff MJ: Actinomycotic pleuropericarditis. Am Rev Respir Dis 110:338, 1974.
1209. Zijlstra EE, Swart GR, Godfroy FJ, et al: Pericarditis, pneumonia and brain abscess due to a combined actinomyces—*Actinobacillus actinomycetemcomitans* infection. J Infect 25:83, 1992.
1210. Knoepfli HJ, Friedli B: Systemic-to-pulmonary artery fistula following actinomycosis. Chest 67:494, 1975.
1211. Jepson EM, Rose FC, Tonkin RD: Thoracic actinomycosis. BMJ 1:1025, 1958.
1212. Smith DL, Lockwood WR: Disseminated actinomycosis. Chest 67:242, 1975.
1213. Varkey B, Landis FB, Tang TT, et al: Thoracic actinomycosis: Dissemination to skin, subcutaneous tissue, and muscle. Arch Intern Med 134:689, 1974.
1214. Legum LL, Greer KE, Glessner SF: Disseminated actinomycosis. South Med J 71:463, 1978.
1215. Ariel I, Breuer R, Kamal NS, et al: Endobronchial actinomycosis simulating bronchogenic carcinoma: Diagnosis by bronchial biopsy. Chest 99:493, 1991
1216. Hamer DH, Schwab LE, Gray R: Massive hemoptysis from thoracic actinomycosis successfully treated by embolization. Chest 101:1442, 1992.
1217. Georghiou PR, Blacklock ZM: Infection with nocardia species in Queensland: A review of 102 clinical isolates. Med J Aust 156:692, 1992.
1218. Wallace RJ Jr, Brown BA, Blacklock Z, et al: New *Nocardia taxon* among isolates of *Nocardia brasiliensis* associated with invasive disease. J Clin Microbiol 33:1528, 1995.
1219. Miron D, Dennehy PH, Josephson SL, et al: Catheter-associated bacteremia with *Nocardia nova* with secondary pulmonary involvement. Pediatr Infect Dis J 13:416, 1994.
1220. Weinberger M, Eid A, Schreiber L, et al: Disseminated *Nocardia transvalensis* infection resembling pulmonary infarction in a liver transplant recipient. Eur J Clin Microbiol Infect Dis 14:337, 1995.
1221. Marrie TJ: Pneumonia caused by *Nocardia* species. Semin Respir Infect 9:207, 1994.
1222. Curry WA: Human nocardiosis: A clinical review with selected case reports. Arch Intern Med 140:818, 1980.
1223. Coker RJ, Bignardi G, Horner P, et al: Nocardia infection in AIDS: A clinical and microbiological challenge. J Clin Pathol 45:821, 1992.
1224. Roberts GD, Brewer NS, Hermans PE: Diagnosis of nocardiosis by blood culture. Mayo Clin Proc 49:293, 1974.
1225. Avram MM, Nair SR, Lipner HI, et al: Persistent nocardemia following renal transplantation: Association with pulmonary nocardiosis. JAMA 239:2779, 1978.
1226. Lovett IS, Houang ET, Burge S, et al: An outbreak of *Nocardia asteroides* infection in a renal transplant unit. QJM 50:123, 1981.
1227. Stevens DA, Pier AC, Beaman BL, et al: Laboratory evaluation of an outbreak of nocardiosis in immunocompromised hosts. Am J Med 71:928, 1981.
1228. Cox F, Hughes WT: Contagious and other aspects of nocardiosis in the compromised host. Pediatrics 55:135, 1975.
1229. Frazier AR, Rosenow EC III, Roberts GD: Nocardiosis: A review of 25 cases occurring during 24 months. Mayo Clin Proc 50:657, 1975.
1230. Hosty TS, McDurmont C, Ajello L, et al: Prevalence of *Nocardia asteroides*

in sputa examined by a tuberculosis diagnostic laboratory. J Lab Clin Med 58:107, 1961.

1231. Rosett W, Hodges GR: Recent experiences with nocardial infections. Am J Med Sci 276:279, 1978.

1232. Wongthim S, Charoenlap P, Udompanich V, et al: Pulmonary nocardiosis in Chulalongkorn Hospital. J Med Assoc Thai 74:271, 1991.

1233. Menendez R, Cordero PJ, Santos M, et al: Pulmonary infection with *Nocardia* species: A report of 10 cases and review. Eur Respir J 10:1542, 1997.

1234. Murray JF, Finegold SM, Froman S, et al: The changing spectrum of nocardiosis: A review and presentation of nine cases. Am Rev Respir Dis 83:315, 1961.

1235. Young LS, Armstrong D, Blevins A, et al: *Nocardia asteroides* infection complicating neoplastic disease. Am J Med 501:356, 1971.

1236. Pinkhas J, Oliver I, De Vries A, et al: Pulmonary nocardiosis complicating malignant lymphoma successfully treated with chemotherapy. Chest 63:367, 1973.

1237. Krick JA, Stinson EB, Remington JS: *Nocardia* infection in heart transplant patients. Ann Intern Med 82:18, 1975.

1238. Bach MC, Sahyoun A, Adler JL, et al: Influence of rejection therapy on fungal and nocardial infections in renal transplant recipients. Lancet 1:180, 1973.

1239. Taleghani-Far M, Barber JB, Sampson C, et al: Cerebral nocardiosis and alveolar proteinosis. Am Rev Respir Dis 89:561, 1964.

1240. Burbank B, Morrione TG, Cutler SS: Pulmonary alveolar proteinosis and nocardiosis. Am J Med 28:1002, 1960.

1241. Andriole VT, Ballas M, Wilson GL: The association of nocardiosis and pulmonary alveolar proteinosis: A case study. Ann Intern Med 60:266, 1964.

1242. Mok CC, Yuen KY, Lau CS: Nocardiosis in systemic lupus erythematosus. Semin Arthritis Rheum 26:675, 1997.

1243. Presant CA, Wiernik PH, Serpick AA: Factors affecting survival in nocardiosis. Am Rev Respir Dis 108:1444, 1973.

1244. Pesce CM, Quaglia AC: *Nocardia* lung infection with hematogenous spread in a woman with adrenal cortical hyperfunction. Eur J Respir Dis 65:613, 1984.

1245. Pizzolato P: Nocardiosis. *In* Baker RD (ed): Human Infection with Fungi, Actinomycetes and Algae. New York, Springer-Verlag, 1971, p 1059.

1246. Neu HC, Silva M, Hazen E, et al: Necrotizing nocardial pneumonitis. Ann Intern Med 66:274, 1967.

1247. Hathaway BM, Mason KN: Nocardiosis: A study of fourteen cases. Am J Med 32:903, 1962.

1248. Weed LA, Anderson HA, Good CA, et al: Nocardiosis: Clinical, bacteriologic and pathological aspects. N Engl J Med 253:1137, 1955.

1249. Raich RA, Casey F, Hall WH: Pulmonary and cutaneous nocardiosis: The significance of the laboratory isolation of *Nocardia*. Am Rev Respir Dis 83:505, 1961.

1250. Feigin DS: Nocardiosis of the lung: Chest radiographic findings in 21 cases. Radiology 159:9, 1986.

1251. Grossman CB, Bragg DG, Armstrong D: Roentgen manifestations of pulmonary nocardiosis. Radiology 96:325, 1970.

1252. Neu HC, Silva M, Hazen E, et al: Necrotizing nocardial pneumonitis. Ann Intern Med 66:274, 1967.

1253. Weed LA, Anderson HA: Etiology of broncholithiasis. Dis Chest 37:270, 1960.

1254. Balikian JP, Herman PG, Kopit S: Pulmonary nocardiosis. Radiology 126:569, 1978.

1255. Raby N, Forbes G, Williams R. *Nocardia* infection in patients with liver transplants or chronic liver disease: Radiologic findings. Radiology 174:713, 1990.

1256. Yoon HK, Im J-G, Ahn JM, et al: Pulmonary nocardiosis: CT findings. J Comput Assist Tomogr 19:52, 1995

1257. van Kralingen KW, Hekker TA, Bril H, et al: Haemoptysis and an abnormal x-ray after prolonged treatment in the ICU. Eur Respir J 7:419, 1994.

1258. Abdelkafi S, Dubail D, Bosschaerts T, et al: Superior vena cava syndrome associated with *Nocardia farcinica* infection. Thorax 52:492, 1997.

1259. Busmanis I, Harney M, Hellyar A: Nocardiosis diagnosed by lung FNA: A case report. Diagn Cytopathol 12:56, 1995.

1260. Geiseler PJ, Andersen BR: Results of therapy in systemic nocardiosis. Am J Med Sci 278:188, 1980.

1261. Stamm AM, McFall DW, Dismukes WE: Failure of sulfonamides and trimethoprim in the treatment of nocardiosis. Arch Intern Med 143:383, 1983.

1262. Mok CC, Yuen KY, Lau CS: Nocardiosis in systemic lupus erythematosus. Semin Arthritis Rheum 26:675, 1997.

1263. Winslow DJ: Botryomycosis. Am J Pathol 35:153, 1959.

1264. Greenblatt M, Heredia R, Rubenstein L, et al: Bacterial pseudomycosis ("Botryomycosis"). Am J Clin Pathol 41:188, 1964.

1264a. Shih J-Y, Hsueh P-R, Chang Y-L, et al: Tracheal botryomycosis in a patient with tracheopathia osteochondroplastica. Thorax 53:73, 1998.

1265. Katznelsen D, Vawter GF, Foley GE, et al: Botryomycosis, a complication in cystic fibrosis. J Pediatr 65:525, 1964.

1266. Katapadi K, Pujol F, Vuletin JC, et al: Pulmonary botryomycosis in a patient with AIDS. Chest 109:276, 1996.

1267. Winslow DJ, Chamblin SA: Disseminated visceral botryomycosis: Report of a fatal case probably caused by *Pseudomonas aeruginosa*. Am J Clin Pathol 33:43, 1960.

1268. Kimmelstiel P, Easley CA Jr: Experimental botryomycosis. Am J Pathol 16:95, 1940.

1269. Mackinnon JE, Conti-Diaz A, Galiana GJ, et al: Experimental botryomycosis produced by *Pseudomonas aeruginosa*. J Med Microbiol 2:369, 1969.

CHAPTER 29

Viruses, Mycoplasmas, Chlamydiae, and Rickettsiae

    Many respiratory infections caused by viruses begin in the upper respiratory tract. Some of these organisms, including certain enteroviruses and the chickenpox and measles viruses, propagate there and then disseminate throughout the body, usually without producing lower respiratory tract symptoms. Others typically remain confined to the respiratory mucosa, where they cause a spectrum of disease, including rhinitis, pharyngitis, laryngotracheitis (croup), bronchitis, bronchiolitis, and pneumonia (primary atypical pneumonia*). Although specific respiratory viruses tend to produce fairly well-defined clinical syndromes, each can cause several forms of upper or lower respiratory tract disease, depending on the virulence and dose of the organism and the host resistance.[2, 2a]

Viruses are usually transmitted from one individual to another, either by hand contact with contaminated skin or mucosa or by aerosol inhalation. As might be expected, the size of the virus-carrying aerosol particle can play a major role in determining the site of initial infection:[3] large aerosol particles tend to deposit in the nasopharynx, resulting in rhinitis with little or no involvement of the lower respiratory tract, whereas small particles are carried into the lungs, where they tend to cause bronchitis, bronchiolitis, or interstitial pneumonitis.

Once deposited on the mucosa of the respiratory tract, a virus must gain access to the underlying epithelial cells to propagate. It does this by means of molecules that interact with specific receptors on the surface of the host cells; the presence and nature of these molecules and receptors are important in determining the infectivity of the virus and the site at which it causes disease. After penetration of the cell membrane, viral DNA (or newly constituted DNA in the case of RNA viruses) acts as a template for the production of various molecules required for the formation of new viruses. Depending on the virulence and nature of the virus and the adequacy of host defense, a variety of outcomes may ensue: (1) the host cell may die, releasing its newly formed viruses to infect other cells; (2) the host cell may remain viable with continuing production and release of new virions, a process that may be associated with a host-mediated immune reaction to viral antigens expressed on the cell surface; and (3) the virus may remain within the cell in a latent state for extended periods of time (e.g., after incorporation of viral DNA with host DNA), reappearing to cause disease only when the general immunity of the host is impaired.

As with infections caused by other microorganisms, a variety of factors influence the likelihood of infection and the development of clinically evident disease as well as the form such disease takes. Host resistance is clearly one of the most important of these factors. Immunity is conferred to most individuals after infection with a specific virus, in most cases probably by a combination of humoral (locally produced IgA and systemic IgG) and cell-mediated mechanisms. The numerous antigenic subtypes of some species (e.g., rhinovirus) and the ability of others to undergo antigenic change (e.g., influenza A), however, mean that protection from repeated infection is not absolute. Conversely, conditions that affect the host's immune reaction, such as malignancy, hereditary immunodeficiency states, acquired immunodeficiency syndrome (AIDS), and iatrogenic immunosuppression, all increase individual susceptibility to newly acquired viral infection as well as reactivation of previously acquired (dormant) viruses.

The patient's age is also related to the presence, form, and severity of infection;[3a] for example, although rhinovirus usually causes only coryza in adults, it may produce croup, bronchitis, bronchiolitis, and bronchopneumonia in children.[2] In addition to being more common in younger individuals, such complications are generally more severe; in developing countries, it has been estimated that lower respiratory tract viral infections are the leading cause of death in children under 5 years of age.[2] Viruses usually associated with childhood infection, such as respiratory syncytial virus, can also cause serious disease in adults, particularly military recruits, immunocompromised patients, and people in close contact with children (such as in day-care centers or hospital clinics).[4]

Underlying airway disease also appears to play a role in determining the risk and form of viral infection. For example, patients who have chronic obstructive pulmonary disease (COPD) have an increased susceptibility to respiratory tract infections, many of them viral or chlamydial in origin. The pathogenesis of this increased susceptibility is unclear, but may be related to structural changes in airway epithelium (e.g., squamous metaplasia and goblet cell hyperplasia), abnormal mucociliary clearance, or impairment of the local inflammatory reaction. Children who have bronchopulmonary dysplasia also appear to have an increased risk of serious viral infection;[5] whether this risk will persist as these patients age is unclear. Other factors that influence the likelihood of developing viral infection and its severity include crowded living or working conditions, tobacco smoke, occupational dust or gas exposure, and nutritional status.[2, 6]

Although viruses can clearly cause pulmonary disease by themselves, the course of the disease can be affected by superimposed bacterial pneumonia. This complication is particularly common in influenza virus infection, but can also occur with other organisms, such as parainfluenza, measles and adenoviruses.[7] The propensity for the development of such superinfection is probably related to several factors, including:[8, 9] (1) deficiency of mucociliary clearance caused by either the loss of airway and alveolar lining cells[10, 11] or ciliary abnormalities;[12] (2) the presence of intra-alveolar edema fluid containing nutrients that can be used for bacterial growth;[9] (3) impairment of alveolar macrophage phagocytosis[13, 14] and bactericidal efficiency;[9] (4) interference with polymorphonuclear leukocyte chemotaxis;[15] and (5) the enhancement of bacterial adherence to damaged epithelium.[16, 16a] It has also been suggested that viruses may enhance the bacterial colonization of and damage to airways in some chronic pulmonary diseases, such as cystic fibrosis.[17]

In addition to the acute effects of direct viral and secondary bacterial infection, viral disease may have important long-term sequelae for the lungs. For example, experimental evidence suggests that neonatal infection may impair subsequent lung development,[18] and viral-induced childhood bronchiolitis is well recognized as a precursor of adult bronchiectasis. Viral respiratory tract infection can clearly induce acute symptoms of asthma in patients who have this disease; moreover, there is evidence that such infection in childhood is involved in the pathogenesis of asthma in later life.[18a] It has also been hypothesized that measles infection in early childhood[19] or latent adenovirus infection during adulthood[20]

---

*The term *primary atypical pneumonia* was coined to describe a form of pneumonia that differs clinically and radiographically from classic bacterial pneumonia.[1] Onset is insidious, fever mild to moderate, and cough nonproductive (at least initially); the chest radiograph typically shows a localized interstitial or bronchopneumonic pattern, and there is little or no response to antibiotics. Although the term initially served some purpose by describing a respiratory disorder of unknown cause, it is logical that with the discovery of the various responsible organisms that it will eventually be discarded.

may contribute to the pathogenesis of COPD. Finally, several viruses, such as Epstein-Barr virus (EBV), herpesvirus 8, papillomavirus, and simian virus 40, have been implicated in the development of some pleural and pulmonary neoplasms.

The following discussion documents the features of disease that occur with viral infection of the lower respiratory tract. The chlamydiae and rickettsiae, although properly classified as bacteria, are also considered at this point because they are obligate intracellular organisms that cause disease that is similar to that of many viruses. Disease caused by *Mycoplasma pneumoniae*, an organism that possesses characteristics intermediate between bacteria and viruses, is described as well.

VIRUSES

The respiratory viruses can be divided into two large groups according to the type of nucleic acid they contain: (1) the RNA group, which includes the myxoviruses, picornaviruses, reoviruses, arenaviruses, coronaviruses, hantaviruses, togaviruses, and retroviruses; and (2) the DNA group, which contains poxviruses, papovaviruses, adenoviruses, and herpesviruses. Lower respiratory tract disease caused by these organisms, particularly pneumonia, is relatively uncommon; however, in specific populations (e.g., recent military recruits, young children, and some immunocompromised patients[24]), the incidence of such infection as well as clinically significant disease is high.

The diagnosis of viral pneumonia is often one of exclusion and is based on an absence of sputum production, a failure to culture pathogenic bacteria, a relatively benign clinical presentation, a white blood cell count that is normal or only slightly elevated, a chest radiograph that reveals bronchopneumonia or localized interstitial disease, and a lack of response to antibiotic therapy. Confirmation of the diagnosis and identification of its cause may be accomplished by a variety of means, including standard tube culture (which has the disadvantage of taking up to several weeks), shell-vial culture (in which centrifugation and the use of monoclonal antibodies can decrease the identification time to a few days), serology (again limited by the time taken for seroconversion to occur), detection of viral antigens within respiratory tract secretions or blood by monoclonal antibodies (by immunofluorescent or immunohistochemical techniques), detection of virus-associated molecules by in situ hybridization or polymerase chain reaction (PCR), and observation of virus-induced changes cytologically or histologically.[21] With respect to the last-mentioned of these, nuclear or cytoplasmic inclusions diagnostic of infection may be present in the absence of tissue damage (as in some cases of cytomegalovirus [CMV] infection) and may not be evident in other cases in which the organism is presumed to be pathogenic. The use of immunohistochemistry or molecular biologic techniques such as PCR may facilitate identification of the organism in the latter situation.[22, 23] Because of their high degree of sensitivity, however, such identification must be interpreted with caution in the absence of evidence of viral replication or tissue damage. A similar proviso holds for diagnosis using specimens obtained by bronchoalveolar lavage.

RNA VIRUSES

Myxoviruses

Four types of myxovirus cause tracheobronchial and pulmonary parenchymal disease in humans. *Influenza virus* infection usually involves only the upper respiratory passages, including the trachea and major bronchi, and chiefly affects children and young adults; however, in a small percentage of patients, particularly the aged or chronically ill, it may be responsible for fulminating pneumonia. *Parainfluenza viruses* are the cause of croup; in infants and young children, they can also cause severe bronchiolitis and pneumonitis. The *respiratory syncytial virus* also tends to affect infants and small children, in some with bronchiolitis and pneumonitis. Although *measles virus* can cause pneumonia, the majority of affected patients with this complication have secondary bacterial infection.

Influenza Virus

Influenza viruses range from 80 to 120 nm in diameter and are pleomorphic, varying in shape from spherical to elongated and filamentous. They are divided into three groups—A, B, and C—on the basis of internal membrane (M) and nucleoprotein (NP) antigens that are demonstrable by complement-fixation tests. Group A, in turn, can be subdivided into a variety of antigenic subtypes related to the presence of two structurally, functionally, and genetically distinct surface glycoproteins, hemagglutinin (H) and neuraminidase (N).[25] The former is necessary for binding of the virus to the host cell surface and is involved in viral penetration of the host cell membrane;[26] antibody to it is protective against infection. Interactions between host proteases and the hemagglutinin molecule have important implications for the development of infection and disease;[26] in addition, variation in the structure of the molecule has been shown in experimental animal studies to be related to different histologic reactions in the lung.[27] Neuraminidase aids in the release and spread of replicated virus particles; although the antibody against it is not as important in immunity as anti-H antibody, it is capable of limiting the severity of the disease.

The viruses have the important ability to change the structural (and hence antigenic) nature of these glycoproteins spontaneously, the variant forms possessing a virulence different from that of their progenitors. Types A, B, and C can all undergo minor structural changes; however, only type A has been found to produce immunologically distinct forms, designated by numerical subscripts in the H and N loci. Because immunity to infection is conferred by antibodies to the H and N glycoproteins, such antigenic changes are of major importance in explaining the pathogenesis of disease; they may be relatively minor (antigenic drift) or major (antigenic shift) in degree.[28, 29]

Epidemiology

Influenza can occur in pandemics, epidemics, or sporadically in individual or small clusters of patients. Almost all severe epidemics and all pandemics are caused by type A viruses. Although outbreaks of type B disease can occur, they are less frequent, more localized, and more common in schoolchildren than in the general population;[30] in addition, this form usually causes only brief coryzal illness, although it has occasionally been associated with Reye's syndrome and fatal pneumonia.[31, 32] Sporadic cases of clinically recognized influenza are usually mild and are caused largely by type C organisms;[30] rarely, influenza C is the cause of localized outbreaks or is responsible for disease that is just as severe as that caused by influenza A.[33, 34]

Although the influenza A virus is generally transmitted from person to person by droplet infection, antigenically similar viruses also infect a wide range of animals and birds, and it is likely that human disease is occasionally derived from these sources. In fact, it has been hypothesized that birds such as aquatic wildfowl and animals such as pigs may be important natural reservoirs of the organism and a milieu for genetic recombination, leading to new, virulent strains capable of causing human disease.[35, 36] Antibody formation to specific strains by either infection or vaccination confers immunity for 1 to 2 years. In addition to strain-specific hemagglutination inhibition antibody, there appears to be a naturally acquired immunity to influenza type A infection, which may last as long as 20 years.[37]

Influenza outbreaks tend to occur on an annual basis, typically during the winter in temperate climates; a seasonal association is less clear-cut in tropical areas. Attack rates are highest in schoolchildren; complications and hospitalization are also more likely in these individuals and in the elderly (particularly those in nursing homes). The incubation period is 24 to 48 hours, allowing rapid spread of the disease. It is highly contagious, and during epidemics and pandemics, the majority of the population contracts the infection in some degree. Serologic studies have shown a higher frequency of antibodies to both influenza A and B in health care workers than in comparable controls;[38] in addition, transmission of disease can occur to these individuals and subsequently to other patients.[39] Viral shedding (and thus infectivity) can persist for as long as 2 weeks in children,[40] but probably less in adults.

Pneumonia is an uncommon but serious complication of influenza infection, usually caused by type A and occasionally type B organisms.[31, 32] Although it is often localized and of only mild-to-moderate severity, it can be overwhelming and fatal within 24 hours.[41] Most cases are recognized during epidemics or pandemics; when sporadic, they are often misdiagnosed. The risk of developing pneumonia as well as its severity is increased in cigarette smokers.[42] In approximately one third of cases of severe pneumonia, the illness develops abruptly in apparently healthy persons.[43, 44] Many of the remainder have a predisposing condition, such as heart disease (particularly mitral stenosis),[45, 46] pregnancy,[47, 48] chronic bronchitis, cystic fibrosis,[49] diabetes,[50] or nephrosis.[51] Elderly individuals are at particular risk for serious disease.[52] The complication has also been reported in immunocompromised individuals.[53, 54]

Although the virus is the only pathogen recovered from the lungs in some patients at autopsy,[55, 56] implying that it can cause fatal pneumonia, in many cases death is related to bacterial superinfection. In the 1918–1919 influenza pandemic, hemolytic *Streptococcus* was a common cause of this complication. In the pandemic of 1957–1958, *Staphylococcus aureus* replaced *Streptococcus* and undoubtedly was the pathogen that contributed to the fatal outcome in a large proportion of cases. Superinfection with *S. aureus* was also common in the Hong Kong influenza epidemic of 1968.[57] Influenza also predisposes to pneumococcal pneumonia[57] and infection by *Meningococcus*, manifested either as a carrier state[58] or as invasive disease.[59] Although secondary infections are usually caused by bacteria, fungi have been documented in some patients.[60]

Pathogenesis and Pathologic Characteristics

Electron microscopic studies of infected organ cultures have shown adherence of viruses to cilia and microvilli of epithelial cells from which they enter the cell cytoplasm.[61] This adherence is modulated, at least in part, by virus surface hemagglutinin that binds to *N*-acetylneuraminic acid residues present in the cell membrane. In experimental animals, viral replication and release are accompanied by degeneration and sloughing of the lining cells of bronchi, bronchioles, and alveoli.[27, 62] Similar abnormalities have been documented in biopsy specimens of bronchial mucosa from individuals with minimal clinical evidence of lower respiratory tract disease.[39] Host defense against the organism is related to a variety of factors, including interferon-mediated production of Mx proteins that appear to inhibit viral replication,[63] an appropriate immune response,[64] and the presence of surfactant-related lectins capable of mediating viral aggregation.[65, 66]

Experimental data in mice suggest that pneumonitis can persist for a long time after the resolution of the acute infection;[67] although the pathogenesis of this reaction is unclear, it has been associated with persistence of viral antigen within the lung, leading to speculation that an immune reaction may be responsible.[67] The propensity and possible mechanisms for the development of bacterial superinfection have been discussed previously (*see* page 980). It is also possible that such superinfection may enhance the viral disease; staphylococci have an enzyme that appears to facilitate cleavage of viral hemagglutinin and increase infectivity.[68]

The pathologic characteristics of fatal influenza pneumonia have been described in several reports;[46, 53, 55] similar histopathologic changes have been observed in the occasional patient on whom bronchial or open-lung biopsy has been performed.[69–71] Grossly, the lungs are characteristically dusky red to plum colored and are large and heavy. The cut surface exudes frothy, blood-tinged fluid. In the most severe cases, this appearance is more or less diffuse throughout the parenchyma; in others, the distribution is patchy and sometimes lobular in distribution.[46, 72] The lining of the airways is usually markedly congested, and their lumens contain hemorrhagic fluid.

The typical microscopic appearance is diffuse alveolar damage, the parenchyma showing capillary congestion; a variably severe interstitial mononuclear inflammatory infiltrate; consolidation of alveolar air spaces by hemorrhage, edema, and fibrin; type II cell hyperplasia; and hyaline membranes.[53] Airway walls are congested and contain a mononuclear inflammatory infiltrate; although usually not prominent except in association with bacterial superinfection, a polymorphonuclear infiltrate may also be seen in apparently pure viral infection.[69] Invariably, marked epithelial changes are present, consisting in early stages of degeneration and desquamation of the superficial epithelial cells with persistence of the basal layer and in the later stages by regeneration (Fig. 29–1).[69, 70] The latter can occur as early as 5 to 7 days after onset of clinical illness[53, 72] and appears as stratified cuboidal cells or, in later stages, as squamous epithelium.[53] Bronchiolitis obliterans with organizing pneumonia is seen in some patients.[71] Interstitial fibrosis occasionally develops.[73]

In a high proportion of cases, the virus can be isolated from postmortem lung parenchyma or airway epithelium, as in 121 of 148 proven cases in one study;[72] however, it can be detected with a greater degree of accuracy and sensitivity by immunofluoresence than by culture.[74] Intranuclear fibrillary inclusions, possibly representing virus-induced structures, have been identified by electron microscopy in airway and alveolar lining cells and in endothelial cells;[75] inclusions representing viral aggregates cannot be seen with light microscopy.

Radiologic Manifestations

Involvement may be local or general. The former usually is in the form of lower-lobe segmental consolidation that may be either homogeneous or patchy and unilateral or bilateral.[76, 77] Serial radiographs may show poorly defined, patchy areas of consolidation, 1 to 2 cm in diameter, which rapidly become confluent. In one series, disease was unilateral and bilateral in approximately the same number of cases and widely disseminated in roughly a quarter of the latter cases.[77] Radiographically, there was bilateral, patchy airspace disease resembling high permeability pulmonary edema, an appearance that has been noted by others (Fig. 29–2).[46] Pleural effusion is comparatively rare.[77] Resolution averages about 3 weeks.[77]

Clinical Manifestations

The clinical manifestations of influenza depend to some extent on the age and underlying health of the patient.[78] In young children, croup is common. In young adults, a flulike syndrome without significant pulmonary complaints predominates. This syndrome has a rapid onset and consists of dry cough, myalgia, chills, headache, conjunctivitis, and a temperature of 38.5° C or more. Substernal burning pain is sometimes present; signs of otitis media and sinusitis may be apparent. Significant rhinorrhea and pharyngitis are seldom seen, and gastrointestinal symptoms occur in a minority of patients.[79] In older patients, there is a greater tendency for the development of lower respiratory tract disease in addition to flulike symptoms. Infection may also cause exacerbation of underlying disease in patients with asthma,[81, 82] cystic fibrosis,[83] and COPD.[84]

When pneumonia develops, symptoms and signs depend on the nature and extent of the infection. Three distinct lower respiratory tract syndromes were described in the 1957–1958 pandemic.[44] The mildest is believed to represent bronchitis/bronchiolitis and produces no radiographic abnormality; patients may have hemoptysis with or without local or diffuse crackles and rhonchi. A second form of disease develops within 12 to 36 hours after the onset of the initial symptoms and is caused by the spread of the virus to the lung parenchyma. Affected patients may be extremely ill, with the rapid progression of tachypnea, dyspnea, cyanosis, and hypoxemia;[85, 86] as indicated previously, many have mitral stenosis or chronic bronchitis or are pregnant.

The third form of influenza-associated pneumonia occurs when there is superinfection with *S. aureus, Haemophilus influenzae,* streptococci, or other bacteria. This complication develops within 2 weeks (most often within a few days) after the initial viral infection. The patient—who may have been improving—begins to expectorate purulent sputum, which may be rusty or bloody, and may complain of pleural pain. (As in other viral infections involving mucous membranes,[87] however, the production of purulent expectoration does not necessarily signify a superimposed bacterial infection.) Complications of such bacterial superinfection include all those normally associated with these organisms, such as

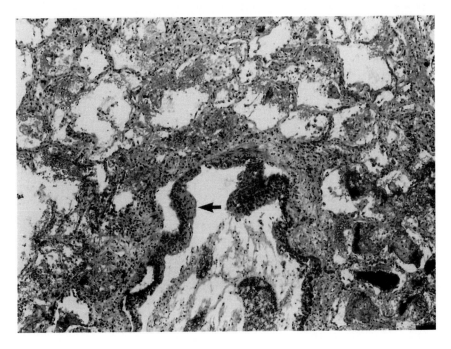

Figure 29–1. Influenza A Pneumonia. The section shows air spaces consolidated by proteinaceous material and mild interstitial thickening. Note the focus of squamous metaplasia in the small bronchiole *(arrow).* The patient was a 34-year-old man with inactive Hodgkin's disease. Influenza A was cultured from tracheal secretions 10 days before death. (×64.)

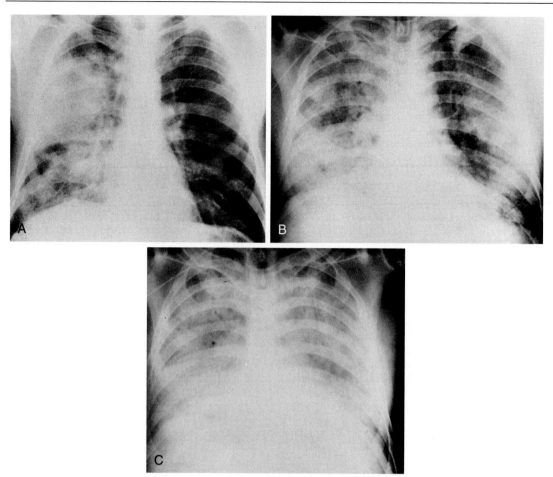

Figure 29–2. Acute Influenza Virus Pneumonia. This 32-year-old man was admitted to the hospital with a 3-day history of progressive dyspnea, cough productive of whitish yellow sputum, right-sided pleuritic chest pain, chills, and fever. His white cell count was 3,500, consisting of 54% lymphocytes and 46% neutrophils. A posteroanterior chest radiograph on the day of admission *(A)* reveals extensive homogeneous air-space consolidation of the right upper lobe, with patchy shadows of air-space consolidation of the right lower lobe; the left lung is clear. Two days later *(B)*, consolidation of the right lower lobe has become almost uniform, and the air-space disease has extended throughout the whole of the left lung. Twenty-four hours later *(C)*, both lungs are almost completely consolidated, the only visible air being present within the bronchial tree (a diffuse air bronchogram). Shortly after admission, the patient became comatose and never regained consciousness; even with assisted ventilation on 100% oxygen, the Po_2 was below 40 and the Pco_2 between 80 and 90. Serologic studies revealed a titer of 1:128 (complement-fixation test [CFT]) for influenza A_2 and of 1:32 CFT for influenza B; a hemagglutination inhibition test was positive to a titer of 1:160 for influenza A_2, Hong Kong variant. Respiratory syncytial virus and influenza virus were cultured from the blood, the sputum, and directly from the lung at autopsy.

abscess formation, sepsis, empyema, and (rarely) toxic shock syndrome.[88]

A variety of complications of influenza virus infection have been reported in addition to bacterial superinfection. Neurologic sequelae (including transverse myelopathy) are thought to be due to autoimmunity or hypersensitivity because influenza virus has not been isolated from the brain.[89, 90] Neurologic manifestations of acute disease, particularly convulsions, appear to be especially common in infants and young children.[91] Guillain-Barré syndrome can develop several weeks after the onset of infection and, rarely, after immunization with some anti-influenza vaccines.[92] Severe myositis associated with elevation of serum creatinine and phosphokinase and the acute onset of bilateral lower limb weakness and tenderness may develop after the acute respiratory symptoms abate (in contrast to the simple myalgia that commonly develops during the acute stage);[93–95] neurologic signs may or may not be present,[96] and myoglobinuria may occur.[97–99] Other rare complications include Reye's

syndrome,[99, 100] thrombocytopenia, renal failure, myocarditis, and disseminated intravascular coagulation.[98, 101]

Laboratory Findings

The white blood cell count is usually normal in uncomplicated influenza; however, leukopenia develops in some cases, and overwhelming infection may result in a neutrophilia of 20,000/mm³ or more. Superinfection with staphylococci or other bacteria is manifested by the production of purulent sputum and similar neutrophilia. The majority of patients with mild, uncomplicated influenza have small airway obstruction, as evidenced by slightly but consistently decreased flow rates at low lung volumes[102, 103] and an increased A-a gradient for oxygen.[104] The virus can be grown by culture of respiratory tract secretions (sputum or nasopharyngeal swabs) in monkey kidney cells or chick embryo, growth occurring in 3 to 21 days. Using these media, it can be readily isolated from specimens obtained during the first few days of illness; however, the success of culture decreases rapidly thereafter and is typically negative at 1 week. The virus can be specifically identified in cell cultures by hemadsorption or hemagglutination methods; infected cells can also be detected by immunofluorescent techniques before the virus is sufficiently concentrated to give a positive result by complement-fixation test. Immunoelectron microscopy has been used to identify the virus in nasopharyngeal washings, but is relatively expensive and time-consuming.[105] A more efficient and rapid method of diagnosis consists of staining nasal secretions directly with monoclonal antibody to influenza viruses.[106] Confirmation of infection can also be done by measurement of acute and convalescent antibody titers to components of a viral strain known to be epidemic at the time a patient is ill.

Prognosis and Natural History

Although there may be substantial morbidity, most cases of uncomplicated influenza are associated with complete clinical recovery. The development of pneumonia portends a more serious course and an increased risk of death, particularly in the very young or very old and in patients with underlying cardiac or pulmonary disease. Severe leukopenia is associated with a poor prognosis. A relationship between influenza epidemics and subsequent increased incidence of congenital neurologic malformations has been postulated.[107, 108] In addition, several investigators have reported an apparent association between influenza in the mother during pregnancy and leukemia in the child.[109, 110] Patients surviving pulmonary infection may have residual, functionally significant fibrosis.[111, 112]

Epidemiologic studies performed during influenza epidemics[47, 113] and in sporadic infections[114] have revealed increased morbidity and mortality from both respiratory and cardiovascular disease. The cause of the excess mortality is age related and is often pneumonia and cerebrovascular disease in patients over 65 years of age and myocardial infarction in patients 40 to 64 years of age.[115, 116] At greatest risk are elderly individuals, particularly those in nursing homes, in whom the mortality rate can be as high as 30%.[117, 118] In fact, it has been estimated that greater than 90% of influenza-related fatalities occur in individuals over 65 years of age.[52] Although underlying chronic disease is a factor in many of these patients, a significant number are judged to be otherwise healthy.[119] Decreased immunity may be important in these individuals.

Parainfluenza Virus

Parainfluenza viruses can be classified into types 1, 2, 3, and 4, of which the first three are responsible for the vast majority of respiratory tract disease. In adults, the organisms are responsible for pharyngitis and a small percentage of cases of coryza; in infants and young children, they cause the majority of cases of severe croup.[120] Symptomatic lower respiratory tract disease also occurs, particularly in the young;[30, 121] in one large prospective study of such infections in children in the first 3 years of life, the virus was found to be the cause in approximately 25% of cases.[122] Immunocompromised individuals also appear to be at increased risk for

this form of disease.[123–125] Recurrent infection in later life is probably not uncommon, usually in a mild form.

Infections caused by parainfluenza virus types 1 and 2 occur predominantly in the autumn and early winter.[1, 120] They can achieve epidemic proportions and can account for a high proportion of cases of pneumonia, croup, and acute bronchiolitis in nursery outbreaks.[126] Lower respiratory tract infection in adults is uncommon. In one study of acute respiratory illness in 200 adult students, 8.5% were found to be caused by type 1 and 1.5% by type 2;[127] the majority of the infections were restricted to the upper respiratory tract, only two being associated with pneumonia. Disease is presumably transmitted by inhalation of microorganisms in droplet form.

Parainfluenza type 3 infection tends to occur in the spring and is an important cause of bronchiolitis or pneumonia in infants and children.[129] The virus may persist for long periods in respiratory tract secretions.[130] Changes in serum antibody titer do not seem to correlate with protection from persistent infection; in fact, prolonged infection with this virus has been reported in patients whose titers of serum hemagglutination-inhibition antibody exceeded those in persons with intact local defense mechanisms who rapidly eliminated the organism.[130] As with influenza virus, parainfluenza virus infection predisposes to bacterial superinfection.[131] Experimental studies have shown that infection of alveolar macrophages *in vitro* induces phagocytic defects that are accentuated by the addition to the macrophage culture of antiparainfluenzal antibody.[132]

Pathologic characteristics of human infections have rarely been described because virtually all are mild and self-limiting. The pattern of giant cell pneumonia has been reported in infants with immunodeficiency syndromes[125, 133] and in children with AIDS and leukemia.[134] Studies of experimentally infected hamsters[135] and of organ cultures of human tracheobronchial tissue[136] have shown a variety of epithelial cytopathologic effects, including multinucleation, nuclear enlargement and pleomorphism, cytoplasmic vacuolization, and the appearance of nuclear and cytoplasmic inclusions. In infected animals, a mononuclear and sometimes polymorphonuclear peribronchial and peribronchiolar inflammatory infiltrate has also been observed in association with epithelial sloughing and regeneration.[135, 137, 138]

Radiographic findings are nonspecific, consisting of diffuse or local accentuation of lung markings in the lower lobes, presumably caused by peribronchial and peribronchiolar inflammation.[128] In one series of 26 children with lower respiratory tract infection, bronchial wall thickening and peribronchial infiltrates were seen in 21, patchy consolidation in 14, and air trapping in 12.[139]

In children, the symptoms are usually those of croup or acute tracheitis; sometimes, crackles indicate the presence of bronchiolitis.[140] The typical manifestation in adults is acute pharyngitis and tonsillitis. In one investigation of five cases of parainfluenza-related pneumonia requiring hospitalization in naval recruits, the clinical presentation was indistinguishable from that of other viral or *Mycoplasma* infection.[128] The white blood cell count usually is normal, but in croup or pneumonia may increase to 15,000/mm³. The organism can be isolated by culture of sputum in monkey tissue; growth requires 3 to 21 days. Immunofluorescent antibody is useful for rapid identification of the virus in nasopharyngeal secretions.[141] Serologic diagnosis can be achieved by agglutinin neutralization and complement-fixation tests and by hemadsorption with guinea pig erythrocytes.

Respiratory Syncytial Virus

Epidemiology

Respiratory syncytial virus (RSV) is particularly important as a cause of disease in infants and small children.[121, 142] In one investigation of such individuals, the organism was found to be responsible for approximately 15% of all cases of mild upper respiratory illness and 45% of lower respiratory tract disease.[143] In another more recent, prospective study of respiratory infections in the first 3 years of life, RSV was identified as the cause of 50% of cases.[122] It has been estimated that the organism is responsible for about 90,000 hospitalizations and 4,500 deaths per year in infants and children in the United States.[144]

The virus can be separated into types A and B on the basis of surface glycoprotein; there is evidence that the former is responsible for more severe disease.[145] Infection occurs predominantly during the winter months and early spring; the incubation period is 3 to 5 days.[146, 147] Disease may occur sporadically, as localized outbreaks in schools or nursing homes, or in epidemics.[146, 148, 149] Transmission is by airborne droplets or hand-to-hand contact. The disease is highly contagious, and infection rates in relatively enclosed places, such as day-care centers, nursing homes, nurseries, and hospital pediatric wards, may be high.[150, 151] As might be expected from these observations, there is evidence that health care workers are at increased risk for infection.[38]

Infants in the first 6 weeks of life appear to be at decreased risk, possibly reflecting the presence of maternal IgG;[152] alternatively, if lower respiratory tract disease caused by this virus is immunologically mediated (*see* farther on), the immaturity of the neonate's immune system might be protective.[153] By contrast, infants and children between 2 months and 2 years are particularly susceptible to respiratory syncytial virus infection,[121, 142, 154] the lower respiratory tract being affected in one third to one half of patients.[146, 155] Individuals with underlying disease, such as bronchopulmonary dysplasia or congenital cardiac anomalies, are especially at risk.[156, 157] Boys have been found to be affected approximately twice as often as girls.[121, 154]

Disease in adults is usually mild and limited to the upper respiratory tract, presumably reflecting immunity as a result of childhood infection; however, significant lower respiratory tract involvement can occur, particularly in elderly or chronically ill patients in nursing homes or hospitals[158–160] and in immunocompromised individuals.[161, 162] Rarely, there is acute onset of pneumonia with rapid progression to the adult respiratory distress syndrome (ARDS).[163] Serologic testing of a group of Dutch military recruits with acute respiratory disease showed pulmonary infection to be caused by RSV in about 5%.[164] A 10-year retrospective study in Sweden uncovered 36 cases of pneumonia in adults in which RSV was recovered, usually accompanied by bacteria; 20% of patients had symptoms of underlying obstructive airway disease.[165]

Pathogenesis

Although the bronchiolar damage in RSV infection is most logically related to direct viral toxicity, it has also been postulated to represent a hypersensitivity reaction. This concept was supported by the findings in the lungs of three infants studied with fluorescent antibodies to determine the distribution of respiratory syncytial virus and human immunoglobulin.[166] In the two cases with bronchiolitis, the lungs contained similarly small amounts of virus and immunoglobulin; the third had pneumonia, and the virus was abundant but immunoglobulin was absent. The authors postulated that the essential process in bronchiolitis is a widespread hypersensitivity reaction, whereas in RSV pneumonia, the mucosal necrosis and alveolar and interstitial inflammation result from direct viral damage to the lung parenchyma. Similar findings have been noted by others, although with the interpretation that the different pattern of inflammation is caused by differences in host immune response and size of viral inoculum rather than by intrinsically different disease processes.[167] It is possible that alveolar macrophages infected by the virus may have a role in the pathogenesis of the inflammatory reaction.[168]

Pathologic Characteristics

Experiments with human tracheal organ cultures have shown that the virus primarily infects ciliated epithelial cells, with the subsequent development of multinucleation and cytoplasmic inclusions.[169] Histologically, fatal human RSV infection may involve the airways or the lung parenchyma predominantly.[167] In the latter instance, disease is manifested mainly as a mononuclear infiltrate in the alveolar interstitium; in more severe cases, there may be a pattern of giant cell pneumonia[171] or diffuse alveolar damage.[161] Multinucleated giant cells containing basophilic cytoplasmic inclusions can sometimes be identified in sputum or BAL specimens, suggesting the diagnosis. When airway involvement predominates, the most severe changes occur in small membranous and respiratory bronchioles;[167] these consist of epithelial degeneration and desquamation accompanied by a variably intense mononuclear inflammatory infiltrate. Round-to-oval, eosinophilic cytoplasmic inclusions adjacent to the nucleus and surrounded by a halo can occasionally be seen in the degenerating epithelial cells.[167]

Radiologic Manifestations

A disparity has been noted between the severity of respiratory symptoms and the relative paucity of radiographic findings.[149] In infants, the chest radiograph shows patchy areas of consolidation interspersed with zones of overinflation.[146] In one study of 65 patients, the dominant findings in 60 cases were bronchial wall thickening, peribronchial infiltrates, and perihilar linearity.[139] Patchy sublobular or lobular consolidation was present in 39 cases, whereas more homogeneous consolidation was present in 10; multiple areas of involvement were common. Air trapping was evident in 41 cases. Although hilar lymphadenopathy was seen in only one patient in this study, an investigation of 35 infants and children with RSV infection in Nigeria found hilar enlargement in 10 (30%; 7 unilateral and 3 bilateral).[172] Other radiologic findings in this study included bilateral pulmonary interstitial and air-space opacities in two cases, atelectasis in one, and severe air trapping in another.

Clinical Manifestations

Symptoms of RSV infection include those of rhinitis, pharyngitis, otitis media, and conjunctivitis.[155] In the presence of bronchiolitis or pneumonia, wheezing, dyspnea, cyanosis, signs of parenchymal consolidation, and retraction of the rib cage may be present. Episodes of apnea are seen in some infants.[173] In contrast to influenza and measles virus, infection by RSV is associated with relatively little risk of bacterial superinfection.[174] Some authors have found an increased incidence of prior atopy in infants with acute RSV infection;[175] however, this has not been the experience of others.[176]

Laboratory Findings

The organism can be propagated in cell culture, in which it forms characteristic syncytia; however, shell-vial culture has been shown to be both more rapid and more sensitive.[177, 178] A variety of serologic tests are available for antibody detection,[179] the most sensitive using enzyme-linked immunosorbent assay (ELISA).[180] In one study of 229 nasopharyngeal aspirates (of which shell-vial culture was positive in 104), the sensitivity of dot-blot enzyme immunoassay was 63% and of direct immunofluorescence 87% (compared with culture).[177] A monoclonal antibody has been described that can detect the virus in formalin-fixed, paraffin-embedded tissue specimens.[181] PCR has also been shown by one group of investigators to be more sensitve than culture in detecting the presence of the virus.[182]

Prognosis and Natural History

Infection is mild and self-limited in the vast majority of patients. In the immunocompromised and in infants and young children with underlying cardiac or pulmonary disease, it may be severe and rapidly fatal.[156, 157]

The results of studies of the long-term sequelae of RSV bronchiolitis vary. In one investigation of 10 adults exposed to the virus in an infants' ward during a community outbreak, elevation of airway resistance persisted for at least 8 weeks.[165] Moreover, in some follow-up studies of infants and children, many patients have been found to have episodes of wheezing, persistent reduction in maximal expiratory flow, and greater bronchial lability than control subjects.[184] Acute infection in experimental animals has also been followed by evidence for bronchial hyperresponsiveness.[185] IgE has been reported to be bound to exfoliated nasopharyngeal epithelial cells in most patients during the acute phase of infection, and it tends to persist in those who suffer from recurrent wheezing.[186] Despite these observations, some investigators have found pulmonary function to be normal after the acute infection.[187] It is possible that in some children, bronchiolitis accompanying RSV infection may be the first manifestation of an asthmatic state (i.e., the viral infection acts as an environmental factor that unmasks a genetic predisposition to airway hyperresponsiveness); alternatively, the viral infection itself may alter the host immune response and initiate IgE-mediated airway disease.[188]

Measles Virus

Epidemiology

Measles (rubeola) is a highly contagious systemic viral disease that occurs predominantly in the late winter and early spring. It is most frequent in highly populated areas, where sporadic cases and small epidemics occur. Before measles vaccine was available, serologic evidence of infection could be seen in the vast majority of individuals before adolescence. Since the introduction of active immunization programs in the 1960s, however, there has been a remarkable reduction in the number of reported cases. Despite this, miniepidemics are still reported in developed countries,[189] and the disease remains a significant problem worldwide, particularly in regions lacking effective immunization programs.[190]

In its natural form, measles is found principally in small children. In societies with active immunization programs, however, a significant number of older individuals contract the illness,[191, 192] presumably because of a combination of nonimmunization, vaccine failure (which occurs in about 5% of individuals), and decreased likelihood of childhood exposure to the organism. The infection is highly contagious and is probably spread largely be airborne droplets. The incubation period is about 10 days to 2 weeks.

Pulmonary disease is the most common complication (3% to 4% of cases) and takes one of three distinct forms: (1) primary measles virus pneumonia; (2) secondary bacterial pneumonia; and (3) atypical measles pneumonia.[193] The majority of cases are caused by bacterial superinfection. In one large series of 3,220 Air Force recruits with measles, 106 (3.3%) developed pneumonia. Although there were no deaths, the disease was clinically severe;[194] transtracheal aspiration revealed pathogenic bacteria in one third of the cases—*H. influenzae* in half of these and *Neisseria meningitidis* in a quarter. An association between risk of superinfection and vitamin A deficiency has been reported.[195] It is possible that pulmonary involvement is more common than generally appreciated; in one study of 75 adult patients with a clinical diagnosis of measles seen at an emergency department, 43 were considered to have pneumonitis on the basis of an abnormal radiograph and/or an A-a gradient of more than 30 mm Hg;[196] in fact, 27 of the 43 had normal radiographs.

The risk of complications, especially primary measles pneumonia, appears to be higher in pregnant women[197] and individuals who are immunocompromised as a result of congenital immunodeficiency syndromes,[198, 199] malignancy (usually lymphoma or leukemia),[202] AIDS, or immunosuppressive therapy.[200, 200a] Immunocompromised patients frequently have a clinical course different from patients with typical measles, characterized chiefly by the absence of rash (as a result of the lack of a delayed hypersensitivity reaction) and, in some cases, by prolonged illness;[198, 201, 202] most are children with readily identified immunodeficiency, although occasionally the risk factor is unrecognized.

In the 1970s, an entirely different form of disease was

noted in individuals in whom measles developed or who received live measles virus vaccine[203, 204] after being immunized with killed or live attenuated[205] measles vaccine. In this *altered measles syndrome (atypical measles)*, a maculopapular rash appeared first on the extremities and spread centrifugally, with limb edema and pneumonia in many cases and moderate eosinophilia in some. Although the precise mechanisms by which these pathologic changes occurred are unknown, their radiographic appearance (interstitial edema and pleural effusion) and rapid clearing suggest an immune response.[206, 207] Since the use of the killed vaccine has been abandoned, this form of disease has virtually disappeared.

Pathologic Characteristics

Pathologic characteristics of fatal cases of typical measles pneumonia without bacterial superinfection are those of giant cell pneumonia. Histologically, epithelial hyperplasia can be seen in bronchioles and in the adjacent parenchyma, which contains many foci of metaplastic squamous cells.[188, 202] Epithelial hyperplasia has also been described in the tracheobronchial epithelium, associated with cystic dilation of underlying mucous glands.[199] Alveolar air spaces are filled with edema fluid, fibrin, and a variable cellular infiltrate; hyaline membranes may be present (Fig. 29–3). The interstitium is thickened by edema and a mononuclear inflammatory infiltrate.

Characteristically, multinucleated giant cells containing up to 50 nuclei are present in variable numbers lining the alveolar air spaces and, to a lesser extent, within the bronchiolar and tracheobronchial epithelium (*see* Fig. 29–3). These contain eosinophilic nuclear and cytoplasmic viral inclusions, the latter surrounded by indistinct halos. The giant cells may be seen in expectorated sputum or bronchoalveolar lavage specimens on cytologic examination before and dur-

ing the presence of the skin rash.[208] Although the pattern of giant cell pneumonia is caused most often by measles, a similar pattern has been reported in respiratory syncytial virus and parainfluenza virus infections.

Radiologic Manifestations

Primary pneumonia caused by the measles virus produces a reticular pattern and patchy consolidation throughout the lungs, indicating the location of the disease in the interstitium and air spaces (Fig. 29–4).[139, 194] In children, the most common findings are patchy air-space consolidation, bronchial wall thickening, peribronchial infiltrates, perihilar linearity, and small nodules.[139, 210] Other abnormalities include evidence of lymph node enlargement and (rarely) mediastinal emphysema.[211, 213] In contrast to its frequency in children, radiologic evidence of lymph node enlargement in adults is uncommon.[194, 214] In one review of the radiologic findings in 11 adults with measles pneumonia, 4 patients had abnormalities on the chest radiograph and all 11 on CT;[212] the latter abnormalities consisted of areas of ground-glass attenuation in eight patients, small nodular opacities in seven, and consolidation in three.

Clinical Manifestations

In the typical case, prodromal symptoms of fever, malaise, myalgia, headaches, conjunctivitis, sneezing, coughing, and nasal discharge are present for 2 to 6 days before the characteristic maculopapular erythematous rash appears. The latter begins on the head and spreads to the trunk and limbs over the next few days. Koplik's spots (erythematous macules with central pallor) develop on the buccal mucosa toward the end of the prodromal period.

Although it has been estimated that only 1 of 15 pa-

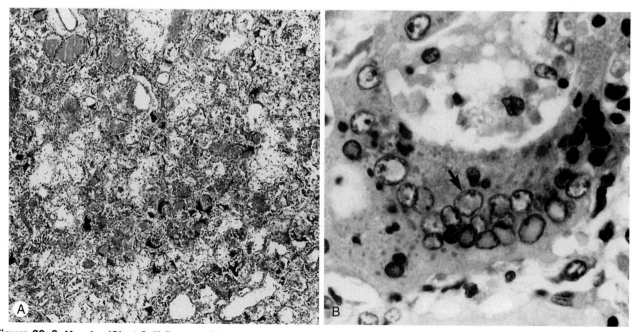

Figure 29–3. Measles (Giant Cell) Pneumonia. Low-power view *(A)* showing extensive air-space consolidation by proteinaceous fluid, macrophages, and red blood cells. Irregular or sickle cell–shaped giant cells are clearly visible. A magnified view *(B)* of giant cell shows numerous nuclei, some of which contain lightly stained but well-defined viral inclusions *(arrow)*. (A, ×40; B, ×800.)

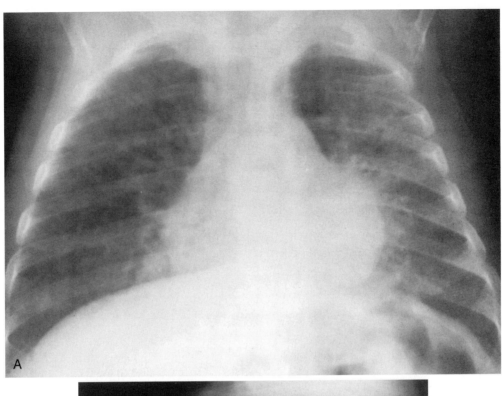

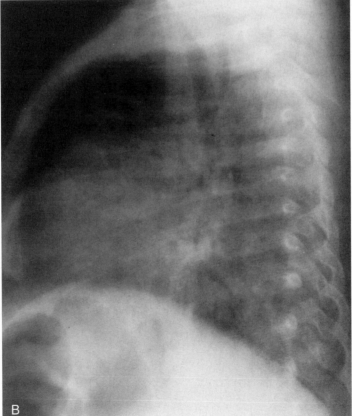

Figure 29–4. Acute Measles Pneumonia. Anteroposterior *(A)* and lateral *(B)* chest radiographs show patchy areas of air-space consolidation throughout the left lung and right lower lobe. The upper lobes are moderately overinflated. The findings are consistent with bronchiolitis and air-space pneumonia. At autopsy, the findings were those of giant cell pneumonia.

tients suffers an additional complication,[212a] some workers have reported a rate of almost 45%.[212b] Primary measles pneumonia characteristically develops before or coincident with the peak of the measles exanthem and is manifested by cough and, in severe cases, hemoptysis, dyspnea, and features of ARDS.[213] Bacterial superinfection usually occurs several days after the rash, when the patient's condition has begun to improve. It should be suspected when cough, purulent expectoration, tachycardia, rise in temperature, and (sometimes) pleural pain develop during early convalescence. Evidence of infection in the paranasal sinuses and middle ear is a common accompaniment of measles pneumonia in adults.[196] Other complications include encephalitis, enteritis with diarrhea, hepatitis, and myositis.[170]

The diagnosis of atypical measles syndrome should be considered in an individual who has previously received killed or live attenuated measles virus vaccine and who has a hemorrhagic vesicular rash on peripheral limb areas.[214] Because use of the inactivated form of the vaccine has been discontinued, however, patients with this form of disease are unlikely to be encountered.

Laboratory Findings

The white blood cell count in primary measles pneumonia may be normal but is often low, particularly in the early stage; in the presence of secondary bacterial infection, polymorphonuclear leukocytosis commonly develops. Thrombocytopenia and hypocalcemia occur rarely.[170] The diagnosis is usually evident from the clinical picture, including the characteristic rash. In atypical cases, the virus can be isolated on tissue cultures of throat washings or blood or identified by immunohistochemical means in biopsy or cytology specimens.[215] A variety of serologic tests are also available to detect the antibody reaction to the organism.[216] Characteristic giant cells may be seen in respiratory tract secretions.

Prognosis

Pulmonary sequelae of primary pneumonia are typically absent or mild. The overall fatality rate in developed countries is probably less than 0.1%; however, it is significantly greater in developing countries, in which hundreds of thousands of infants and children succumb. Most deaths are caused by pneumonia.

Picornaviruses

The picornaviruses are a group of small, icosahedral, RNA-containing organisms that include two subgroups pathogenic for humans: the enteroviruses and the rhinoviruses. The latter subgroup contains many serotypes and is responsible for greater than 50% of cases of coryza.[217] Lower respiratory tract infection is rare but can occur in both children and adults.[218, 219]

The enteroviruses include coxsackie, ECHO, and poliovirus; these organisms are transmitted predominantly by the fecal-oral route and because of acid resistance are able to pass through the stomach and replicate in the lower intestinal tract. Children and young adults are most commonly af-

fected. The incubation period ranges from 7 to 12 days. In temperate climates, illnesses caused by the enteroviruses occur chiefly in the late summer and autumn months, but in the tropics they occur at any time.[220, 221] Respiratory infection caused by the coxsackie and ECHO viruses is usually limited to the upper tract and tends to be mild; pneumonia is rare.[222]

The effects of the polioviruses on the thorax are usually indirect, paralysis of the muscles of respiration sometimes resulting in respiratory failure in the acute disease and often in pulmonary function abnormalities in the postpolio syndrome.[223] Iatrogenic disease of the upper airways as a result of intubation, including tracheal stenosis, tracheomalacia, and vocal cord paralysis, also leads to respiratory symptoms in some patients.[224] Because chest radiographs are usually normal, this subject is dealt with in Chapter 79 (*see* page 3061). It has also been hypothesized that infection by simian virus 40 contained in polio vaccines given between 1959 and 1961 may be involved in the pathogenesis of some cases of mesothelioma.[225]

Coxsackievirus

Coxsackieviruses can be divided into two major groups: *group A*, which is distinguished by its ability to induce flaccid paralysis in mice, and *group B*, which causes spastic paralysis. Group A coxsackieviruses (particularly type A10) typically produce vesicular and ulcerative lesions on the soft palate and (occasionally) aseptic meningitis; strains A21 and A24 account for a small proportion of upper respiratory tract infections resembling the common cold. Group B coxsackieviruses cause a great variety of clinical diseases, including aseptic meningitis, myocarditis, pericarditis, acute meningoencephalitis, and orchitis.[226] Infections occur in local or widespread epidemics, usually during the summer months and early autumn. In one study of 311 patients whose throat or rectal swabs grew group B coxsackieviruses, 227 had upper respiratory tract disease, many with streptococcal-like pharyngitis.[227] Pneumonia rarely develops in association with coxsackievirus A infection[228] or with pleurodynia caused by coxsackievirus B.[222, 229] The B5 strain has been associated with linear atelectasis and pleural effusion.[230]

The pulmonary pathology of coxsackievirus infection has been described only rarely because the disease is seldom fatal. In one case in which coxsackievirus A was isolated from lung tissue at autopsy,[228] multifocal hemorrhagic areas measuring 0.5 to 1 cm were observed in the parenchyma. Histologic examination revealed a pattern of diffuse alveolar damage. The radiographic pattern is said to consist of "fine perihilar infiltrates."[228] Parenchymal consolidation in the lung bases may develop when pleurodynia is present.[229]

Symptoms may be limited to the upper respiratory tract, with rhinitis, pharyngitis, and a dry cough, or may consist of severe aching and gripping pain in the lower thoracic and upper abdominal regions (epidemic pleurodynia). The latter usually is accompanied by difficulty in breathing and by fever. We have also seen several cases of pleurodynia with persistent widespread bilateral pleural friction rub. The disease is characterized by remissions and exacerbations that may last several weeks. It may be associated with meningitis (evidenced by headache), myocarditis, pericarditis, and orchitis. The white blood cell count ranges from slight leukopenia to mild leukocytosis.[228]

ECHO Virus

The enteric cytopathic human orphan (ECHO) viruses include approximately 30 strains that cause a variety of clinical manifestations,[30, 231] including fever, diarrhea, maculopapular and petechial rashes, and aseptic meningitis. Pneumonia, which occurs predominantly in infants, is caused primarily by the type 19 strain.[232, 233] In adults, infection usually simulates the common cold; however, a few cases of pleurodynia have been reported.[234]

Involvement of the lung by this organism produces a radiographic pattern of increased bronchovascular markings and bilateral hilar lymph node enlargement.[232] In one report of eight premature infants affected during an epidemic involving a hospital nursery, chest radiographs of the seven survivors showed cystic changes in the lungs.[233]

The white blood cell count usually is within normal limits, with relative lymphocytosis; leukocytosis develops in some cases. Diagnosis depends on demonstration of the organism in tissue culture, by immunochemical tests, or by a fourfold increase in titer of neutralization or complement-fixation antibodies.

Rhinovirus

Rhinoviruses are most closely associated with the common cold, of which they are the cause in approximately 40% to 50% of cases. Clinically significant lower respiratory tract infection is uncommon but includes croup, acute bronchitis, bronchiolitis, and bronchopneumonia, in both children and adults.[218, 235] There is evidence that children with bronchopulmonary dysplasia[5] and elderly adults with COPD[236] are at increased risk of clinically significant disease.

In one series of 20 cases diagnosed in military trainees on the basis of virus recovery and antibody production without similar support for other viral or mycoplasmal origin, the radiographic and clinical presentations were identical to those of other viral pneumonias;[218] in most cases, the disease was localized to one or more segments of a lower lobe. Leukocyte counts exceeded 10,000/mm^3 in 13 of the 20 patients, and the duration of illness—which was not influenced by treatment with antibiotics—was approximately 1 week. Some investigators have shown a correlation between severity of infection and both lymphopenia, particularly of T4 cells, and polymorphonuclear leukocytosis.[237] Impairment in diffusing capacity has been observed in some patients with rhinovirus coryza, possibly reflecting diffuse bronchiolitis.[239] The virus has been isolated from the lower respiratory tract at autopsy[238] and by fiberoptic bronchoscopy[240] of patients with symptomatic infection.

Perhaps more important than direct infection is the indirect effect that rhinovirus may have on patients with asthma. Although some studies of experimentally infected asthmatic volunteers have shown a minority to develop clinical exacerbation associated with only a mild decrease in flow rates,[241] there is little doubt that the virus can cause clinically significant airway narrowing in some patients (*see* page 2111).[242–244] Rhinovirus infection has also been associated with exacerbation of clinical symptoms and with worsening pulmonary function in some patients with COPD.[245, 246]

Retroviruses

Retroviruses are RNA viruses that are characterized by a unique mode of replication in which viral RNA is converted to DNA by the process of reverse transcription; the latter is then incorporated into the host cell DNA and acts as a template for the formation of new virions. Human retroviruses can be categorized in two groups: human T-cell leukemia viruses (HTLV) and human immunodeficiency viruses (HIV). Although each is more closely associated with extrathoracic or systemic disease—leukemia and degenerative neurologic disease in the former and AIDS in the latter—there is also evidence that they may have a direct pathogenic effect in the lungs in some patients. Viruses in both groups share a pronounced tropism for cells expressing CD4 receptors (particularly lymphocytes) and the ability to persist for prolonged periods of time as clinically latent infection.

Human T-Cell Leukemia Virus

Two variants of HTLV have been identified: HTLV-I, the cause of T-cell leukemia/lymphoma and tropical spastic paraparesis (HTLV-1-associated myelopathy), and HTLV-II, a possible cause of some cases of T-cell leukemia. In one study of six patients with spastic paraparesis who underwent bronchoalveolar lavage, five had an increased cell count associated with an increased proportion of lymphocytes.[247] In another investigation of 23 seropositive patients, including 6 who had neurologic disease, PCR analysis of bronchoalveolar lavage fluid revealed the presence of an HTLV-1-associated gene in all those who had disease and in 8 of the 17 carriers.[248] Histologic examination of the lungs of some patients has shown a parenchymal interstitial lymphocytic infiltrate[247, 249] or bronchiolitis.[250]

Human Immunodeficiency Virus

HIV-I is by far the best known of the two types of HIV. As the cause of AIDS, it has become one of the most important viruses of the late twentieth century. The vast majority of the pulmonary manifestations of infection are secondary to viral-induced immunodeficiency and are discussed elsewhere (*see* page 1643). There is also evidence, however, that the virus directly affects the lungs, most likely via circulating monocytes or lymphocytes emigrating from the blood into the alveolar interstitium and air spaces (*see* page 1685).[251] Such infection likely occurs early in the course of the disease, because the virus can be detected in bronchoalveolar lavage fluid from HIV-positive individuals without clinical disease.

The infection is manifested in bronchoalveolar lavage fluid by an increased number of lymphocytes, mostly CD8 +; this is associated with a decreased number of CD4 + lymphocytes, the ratio of the two increasing with the development of clinical disease and with increasing severity of such disease.[252] A variety of other abnormalities of bronchoalveolar lavage cell type and function have also been documented.[253–255] It has been hypothesized that the presence of infected cells in the lung parenchyma may increase the likelihood of opportunistic infections by interfering with normal cellular defense mechanisms.[251] It has also been suggested that HIV may be directly involved in the pathogenesis of lymphocytic interstitial pneumonitis (*see* page 1685)[256] and pulmonary emphysema[257] in patients who have AIDS.

Hantaviruses

Hantaviruses are lipid-enveloped, single-stranded RNA viruses that typically cause a symptom complex referred to as *hemorrhagic fever with renal syndrome*. Five antigenically different viruses from various parts of the world—Hantaan, Seoul, Puumala, Dobrava, and Prospect Hill—have been found to cause the syndrome, which is variable in severity and is characterized clinically by fever, hypotension, and renal failure. In the early 1990s, a sixth organism—Sin Nombre virus—was identified as the agent responsible for a frequently more fulminant and clinically severe disease with prominent pulmonary involvement—the hantavirus pulmonary syndrome.[258-260] Additional varieties of the virus (e.g., the Bayou and Black Creek canal viruses[261, 262]) have been recognized to cause similar disease since the documentation of this syndrome.[263] Although recognized relatively recently, it is clear that the syndrome is not as new as initially believed; in a retrospective review of 82 autopsies in which there was unexplained noncardiogenic pulmonary edema, immunohistochemical evidence of hantavirus was detected in 12, the earliest case dating from 1978.[264] Other reviewers have found cases dating from 1959.[260]

The natural reservoir of all hantaviruses is wild rodents, the deer mouse being the most important animal harboring the Sin Nombre variant in the United States.[258] Climatic or other environmentally driven changes in the local rodent population are believed to be at least partly responsible for variations in the incidence of disease and the development of local outbreaks. The organism is thought to be transmitted by inhalation of dried rodent excreta, and activities associated with an increased risk of such exposure, such as cleaning barns, trapping, and plowing with hand tools, have been associated with development of infection.[258] Presumably because of this association, most cases have been identified in rural areas. A small number of cases of community-acquired pneumonia in large urban centers have been found to be caused by the virus.[265] Although the possibility of person-to-person transmission has been raised,[268] this is thought to be rare if it occurs at all.[266]

With the exception of the Seoul virus, whose reservoir is *Rattus norvegicus* and is thus found worldwide, specific hantaviruses are found in relatively localized regions. Most cases of Sin Nombre virus infection have been identified in the southwestern United States; however, outbreaks have also been reported in South America (Paraguay and Argentina)[267, 268] and western Canada.[269] Infections with the Black Creek and Bayou viruses have occurred in Texas and southeastern states such as Florida.[261] The majority of affected patients have been between the ages of 20 and 40 years; there is no sex predominance.[260]

Pathologic examination of the lungs of patients dying from hantavirus pulmonary syndrome show interstitial and air-space edema with a mild-to-moderate interstitial infiltrate of cytologically mature and activated lymphocytes.[270] Evidence of viral-induced tissue damage, such as epithelial necrosis, vascular thrombosis, or hyaline membranes, is typically sparse or absent; however, diffuse alveolar damage can be seen.[270] Virus-like particles can be identified in endothelial cells and alveolar macrophages by electron microscopic examination. The pathogenesis of the edema is not well understood; however, the histologic findings suggest that it is not related to a direct cytopathic effect. Viral antigens can be detected by immunohistochemistry in endothelial cells of the alveolar capillaries, arterioles, and venules.

The radiographic findings were described in 16 patients seen during an epidemic in the southwestern United States in 1993.[271] In 13 of the 16, the initial chest radiographs revealed changes indicative of interstitial pulmonary edema, including septal (Kerley B) lines, hilar indistinctness, and peribronchial cuffing (Fig. 29–5). In the three patients with normal radiographs at presentation, findings consistent with interstitial pulmonary edema developed within 48 hours. Four of the 16 patients had radiographic findings consisting

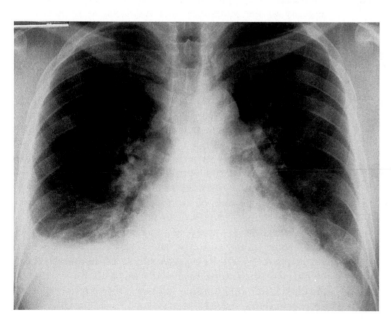

Figure 29–5. Hantavirus Pneumonia. A chest radiograph in a patient with hantavirus pulmonary syndrome demonstrates mild cardiomegaly with prominence of the pulmonary vascular markings and small bilateral pleural effusions. These findings resolved rapidly after renal dialysis. (Case courtesy of Dr. Eun-Young Kang, Department of Radiology, Korea University Medical Center, Guro Hospital, Seoul, Korea.)

predominantly or exclusively of interstitial edema at 48 hours; all 4 survived, and their radiographs returned to normal within 5 days after admission. Six of the 16 patients had air-space consolidation on the initial chest radiograph; this was perihilar in 3 and involved the basal segments in 2 and the central upper lobe in 1 (Fig. 29–6). Within 48 hours after admission, 11 patients developed extensive air-space consolidation. The distribution was bibasilar or perihilar in 10 and predominantly peripheral in 1. The time to resolution of the radiographic findings in the nine patients who survived ranged from 5 days to more than 3 weeks. Pleural effusions were present on the initial chest radiographs in two patients and developed within 48 hours in nine other patients. The effusions were small in five and large in six.

The hemorrhagic fever with renal syndrome typically begins abruptly with fever, headache, abdominal pain, and petechiae. This preliminary phase is followed by hypotension and oliguric renal failure; respiratory symptoms as a result of pulmonary edema occur occasionally, but are believed to be related to fluid overload rather than primary viral disease.[258] The hantavirus pulmonary syndrome typically begins with a 2- to 3-day prodrome of fever, myalgia, and (sometimes) abdominal pain and headache; skin rash and features of coryza and pharyngitis are usually absent.[258, 272] The prodrome is followed after 3 to 6 days by progressive cough and dyspnea, tachypnea, tachycardia, and hypotension. Respiratory failure with worsening hypoxemia may ensue and, in combination with intractable hypotension, often results in death. Disseminated intravascular coagulation develops in some cases. Patients who survive these acute events enter a convalescent phase, which may be

remarkably rapid, presumably reflecting the lack of significant pulmonary tissue damage.

Laboratory findings include leukocytosis (sometimes to 25,000 cells/mm^3 and often with a shift to the left), thrombocytopenia, increased lactate dehydrogenase and aspartate aminotransferase, and hemoconcentration. Mild-to-moderate proteinuria and a slight elevation of serum creatinine may be present, but clear-cut renal failure as seen in the hemorrhagic fever with renal syndrome is unusual. The diagnosis can be confirmed by the demonstration of virus-specific IgM antibodies or a fourfold rise in IgG antibodies.[273] A strip immunoblot assay using four antigens has been found by one group of investigators to be a reliable and rapid means of diagnosis.[274] The virus can also be detected in tissue samples by immunohistochemical examination or PCR.[264, 270, 275]

Hemorrhagic fever with renal syndrome is fatal in a minority of patients, the incidence depending on the specific virus. By contrast, hantavirus pulmonary syndrome is a serious disease, the case fatality rate being about 50%.[258, 260] Long-term sequelae in patients who survive appear to be minimal.[258]

Reoviruses

There have been sporadic reports of pneumonia caused by reoviruses.[276, 277] One patient was a 5-year-old child who had a maculopapular rash and diffuse bilateral bronchopneumonia;[276] at autopsy, the trachea and proximal bronchi were obstructed by a large mucous plug, which on culture grew reovirus type 3. Histologically the lungs showed interstitial pneumonitis with a mononuclear infiltrate.

Togaviruses

Togaviruses are spherical, single-stranded RNA viruses of which only the rubella virus is important in respiratory disease. Postnatal infection with this organism is characterized by fever, a maculopapular rash, and lymph node enlargement; to our knowledge, lower respiratory tract involvement has not been reported. Approximately 10% to 15% of infants born to mothers infected during the first trimester of pregnancy have congenital teratogenic anomalies that not uncommonly include the respiratory system. The most frequent abnormalities are pulmonary artery stenosis[278–280] and interstitial pneumonitis.[280–282] The former may affect the main pulmonary artery, its major branches, or, less commonly, the muscular arteries in either isolated or multiple locations. Histopathologic studies have shown fibromuscular thickening of the intima with concomitant luminal narrowing;[278] the underlying media is usually normal. These changes may be mild and unassociated with clinical evidence of stenosis[278] or may be severe enough to result in pulmonary hypertension. Survival into adulthood can occur, sometimes with the development of cor pulmonale.[283] Other congenital cardiovascular defects are found in many symptomatic patients.[279]

Interstitial pneumonitis presents during infancy and varies from an acute necrotizing process with edema, hyaline membrane formation, and a prominent inflammatory cellular infiltrate to less active disease manifested by an intersti-

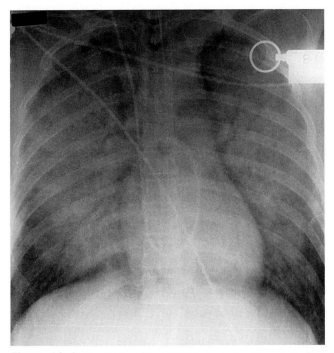

Figure 29–6. Hantavirus Pneumonia. A chest radiograph in a 31-year-old woman demonstrates extensive, predominantly perihilar parenchymal consolidation. The patient presented with respiratory failure and rapidly progressed to adult respiratory distress syndrome. Despite this, a follow-up chest radiograph 1 month after admission was entirely normal. The patient had no recent travel history outside of British Columbia, and the infection was presumably related to contact with deer mice.

tial mononuclear infiltrate and a variable degree of fibrosis.[281, 282] The virus can be cultured from the lungs in some cases.[281]

Arenaviruses

The virus of lymphocytic choriomeningitis has rarely been identified as the cause of pulmonary disease. In one epidemic of this condition, 34 patients had a flulike syndrome, with cough in 6; the authors of the report did not mention the presence of abnormal chest radiographs.[284] Fatal hemorrhagic bronchopneumonia has also been documented in some cases.[285]

Coronaviruses

Coronavirus typically causes coryza and pharyngitis, usually during the winter and spring.[286] Studies on volunteers inoculated intranasally with the organism suggest that disease is limited to the upper respiratory tract in the vast majority of cases.[287, 288] In fact, there are few well-documented reports of pneumonia caused by the virus;[289] in one epidemic of lower respiratory tract infection in military recruits, most of the 39 patients also had evidence of adenovirus or *Mycoplasma* infection.[290] Despite this, the virus has been associated with exacerbations of asthma[291] and COPD.[292] In addition, in one study of 443 individuals (some healthy and some with acute or chronic respiratory disease), an indirect enzyme immunoassay was used to detect an antibody to the coronaviral protein OC43;[293] investigators found approximately 4% of acute respiratory infections to be caused by the virus.

DNA VIRUSES

Adenovirus

Adenoviruses are nonenveloped, DNA-containing organisms of which approximately 50 human serotypes have been identified. All types have a common complement-fixing antibody and can be differentiated by serum neutralization tests. They grow readily in tissue culture of human and simian cells, producing a distinctive cytopathologic appearance.

Epidemiology

Adenovirus infection forms a small but significant proportion of viral-induced respiratory disease. In one investigation of more than 18,000 infants and children followed for 10 years, at least 7% of respiratory infections were estimated to be caused by the virus,[294] although other groups have reported a much lower incidence.[121] Disease may occur as pharyngitis, pharyngoconjunctivitis, laryngotracheobronchitis, bronchiolitis, pneumonia, or a nonspecific acute respiratory syndrome; there is also evidence that the organism may be involved in the pathogenesis of some cases of bronchiectasis.[294a]

Infections may occur sporadically or in epidemic form,

the latter especially in association with military populations recently removed from civilian life;[164, 295] if the period of basic combat training is during the colder months, infection rates of susceptible recruits have been reported to approach 100% in some studies.[296] The majority of sporadic respiratory infections are caused by types 1, 2, and 5;[121, 294] epidemics are more frequently associated with types 3, 4, 7, and 21. Most severe cases are associated with types 3 and 7.[297-300] Epidemics have also been reported in children in association with swimming pools and summer camps.[301, 302] Localized outbreaks of nosocomial infection have been reported.[303]

Pathologic Characteristics

Grossly, the lungs of patients who have died of acute adenovirus pneumonia are large and heavy and show patchy areas of hemorrhagic consolidation alternating with areas of overinflation or atelectasis. Airways frequently contain mucopurulent or hemorrhagic material, and their walls are usually markedly congested. Microscopically, there is necrotizing bronchitis and bronchiolitis most prominent in the smaller airways and frequently associated with epithelial desquamation and occlusion of the lumens by necrotic material and inflammatory exudate.[297-299] Bronchial mucous glands often show similar changes.[299, 304] Airway walls contain a largely mononuclear infiltrate, although in areas of ulceration, polymorphonuclear leukocytes may be prominent.

The lung parenchyma may show similar necrotic changes, with intra-alveolar hemorrhage, edema, and hyaline membrane formation associated with interstitial mononuclear inflammatory cells. Some cases, presumably representing a milder form of infection, show predominantly interstitial inflammation with little evidence of tissue necrosis (Fig. 29–7).[305] Depending on the time between the onset of the infection and the examination of the tissue, airways may show only chronic inflammation and evidence of epithelial regeneration (Fig. 29–8).

Two forms of nuclear inclusion may be identified in infected cells: the first and less common consists of small, eosinophilic globules surrounded by indistinct halos that gradually coalesce to form a single, relatively well-defined, central inclusion.[306] Within a relatively short time, this inclusion enlarges to become a homogeneous, basophilic mass without a peripheral halo, occupying the whole of the cell nucleus (*see* Fig. 29–7);[306] this second inclusion is the basis of the *smudge cell* and is characteristic of adenovirus infection. The inclusions are most prominent in alveolar lining cells but may be seen in airway epithelium; their presence in expectorated sputum may provide a clue to the diagnosis.

Radiologic Manifestations

One of the most extensive reviews of adenoviral pneumonia and its complications in infancy and childhood consisted of a study of 69 patients conducted over a 5-year period.[307] Forty-six (67%) of the patients were North American Indian, Métis, or Inuit, and the majority were younger than 1 year of age. The most common radiographic findings consisted of diffuse bilateral bronchopneumonia and severe overinflation. Lobar collapse was a frequent complication, in the right upper lobe in 20 instances and the left lower

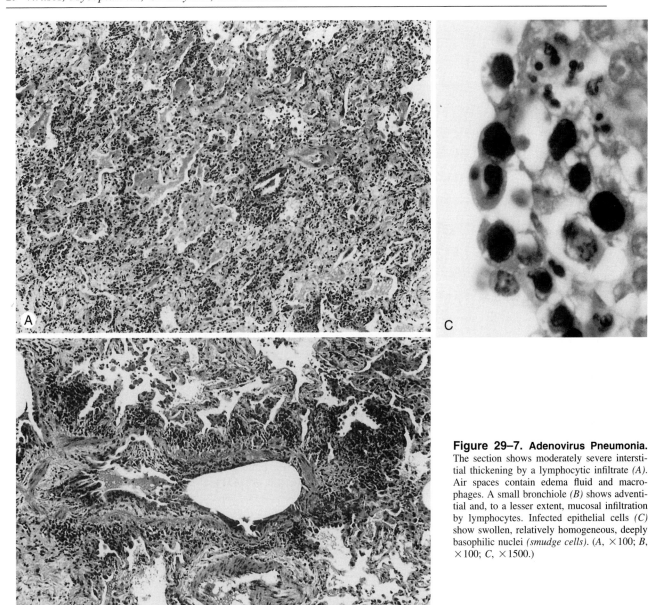

Figure 29–7. Adenovirus Pneumonia. The section shows moderately severe interstitial thickening by a lymphocytic infiltrate *(A)*. Air spaces contain edema fluid and macrophages. A small bronchiole *(B)* shows adventitial and, to a lesser extent, mucosal infiltration by lymphocytes. Infected epithelial cells *(C)* show swollen, relatively homogeneous, deeply basophilic nuclei *(smudge cells)*. (A, ×100; B, ×100; C, ×1500.)

lobe in 6; re-expansion did not occur in 10. For unknown reasons, collapse of the right upper lobe occurred mainly in infants younger than 18 months of age and of the left lower lobe in older children. In uncomplicated cases, the radiographic abnormalities resolved within 2 weeks; however, of the 58 children adequately followed up, 21 (53%) had some form of chronic pulmonary disease. The likelihood of chronic disease was considerably greater in children under 2 years of age at the time of the acute illness than in the older patients. Similar findings to those of this investigation were documented by the same investigators in a subsequent study.[308]

Clinical Manifestations

In another investigation of the radiographic findings in 21 children who had lower respiratory tract adenovirus infection, the main abnormalities consisted of segmental or nonsegmental consolidation (in 19 patients), overinflation (in 12), atelectasis (in 7), and pleural effusion (in 13).[308a] The air-space consolidation was bilateral in 12 patients.

The adenoviruses are perhaps the most common cause of the *acute respiratory disease syndrome*, a somewhat ill-defined condition consisting of fever, pharyngitis, cough, hoarseness, chest pain, and conjunctivitis. Chills and myalgia may be present, simulating influenza infection. Tracheobronchitis is prominent in some cases. Infection occasionally presents clinically as whooping cough indistinguishable from the classic disease caused by *Bordetella pertussis*.[309]

Pneumonia usually is mild and associated with typical upper respiratory symptoms in addition to those of the pneumonia.[310] Occasionally, it is severe, with productive cough, dyspnea, and hypoxemia; pleural pain occurs rarely. Physical findings include those of pharyngitis, which frequently is

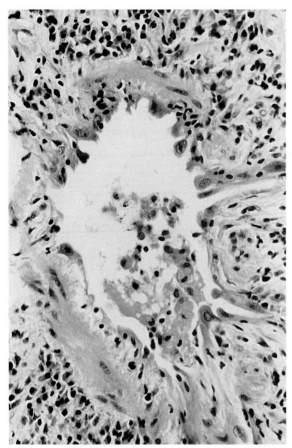

Figure 29–8. Adenovirus Bronchiolitis—Healing. The section shows a small membranous bronchiole with enlarged, cytologically atypical epithelial cells, representing a reparative process after virus-induced epithelial necrosis. The airway wall contains a mononuclear (predominantly lymphocyte) infiltrate.

exudative and resembles that produced by streptococcal infection, and diffuse crackles and rhonchi indicative of bronchiolitis; in some cases, there are signs of consolidation.[301, 310]

Complications of the primary infection are relatively uncommon. Bacterial superinfection occurs in some cases, in one series with a preponderance of group Y *N. meningitidis.*[311] Disseminated infection is most frequent in immunocompromised patients and may result in death.[312–314] Pneumonia is only rarely fatal in otherwise healthy adult patients.[315] Rare complications include rhabdomyolysis and myoglobinuria[316] and Reye's syndrome.[317] Long-term sequelae include bronchiectasis, bronchiolitis obliterans,[318–321] and hyperlucent lung syndrome.[322, 323] It has also been proposed that chronic (subclinical) airway infection may be involved in the pathogenesis COPD.[20] Using *in situ* hybridization and PCR, some investigators have demonstrated the presence of adenoviral genome in the lung tissue of a high percentage of smokers;[324] a disproportionate amount of such viral DNA has been found in the lungs of smokers who have significant air-flow obstruction compared with individuals who have smoked a similar amount but do not have significant obstruction, suggesting a role for the virus in the pathogenesis of the airway disease.

Laboratory Findings

The white blood cell count usually is normal, but may be slightly increased and in very ill patients may exceed 30,000/mm³.[325] Although the cold agglutination test is usually negative,[301, 325] titers of 1:32 or higher were recorded in 17% of patients in one series;[310] however, none had a four-fold rise in titer.

Herpesviruses

Herpesviruses are double-stranded DNA viruses that range in diameter from 150 to 200 nm. The viral particle is surrounded by a lipid envelope derived from the host nuclear membrane, within which are located viral glycoproteins that mediate cell surface attachment. Once within the cell, the organisms or their genomes are able to remain dormant without causing recognizable disease, apparently for the lifetime of the individual. In certain circumstances, often of an immunocompromising nature but sometimes without obvious clinical correlate, reactivation occurs and clinical disease ensues. Such disease is usually localized and well tolerated in otherwise healthy individuals; however, in the immunocompromised, disease is frequently disseminated and severe.

The organisms can be subdivided antigenically into more than 70 subtypes, of which only a small number have been implicated in human pleuropulmonary disease: herpes simplex *(Herpesvirus hominis)* types 1 and 2, herpesvirus 6, herpesvirus 8, *Varicellavirus* (varicella-zoster virus), CMV, and EBV. Humans are also rarely infected with *Herpesvirus simiae,* an organism naturally pathogenic for monkeys; the disease can be transmitted by direct inoculation via bites or scratches from infected animals or by contact with laboratory media, such as tissue cultures of monkey cells. The most prominent clinical features are those of encephalomyelitis (usually fatal); however, upper respiratory tract symptoms and pneumonia may occur.[326]

Latent herpesviruses reside within specific cells.[327] Herpes simplex virus (HSV) is found in sensory ganglia of nerves that innervate the site of recurrent mucocutaneous infection[328] and in cervical and vagal ganglia.[329] Sensory ganglia are also the likely source of latent infection with varicella-zoster virus. CMV persistently infects epithelial cells of the salivary gland, the kidney, and potentially other organs of the genitourinary system; the virus can also persist in B lymphocytes and neutrophils in peripheral blood. Herpesvirus 6 infects T and B lymphocytes and neural cells and is possibly persistent in salivary gland tissue.[330] EBV appears to infect predominantly B lymphocytes and pharyngeal epithelial cells.[331]

Herpes Simplex Type I

HSV-I is transmitted in situations of close personal contact through saliva or vesicle fluid and is most commonly associated with oral disease. This may be either primary, as in acute gingivostomatitis in children, or as recurrent coldsores (herpes labialis) in older individuals, representing reactivation of latent virus. Such recurrent disease can develop as a result of such simple stimuli as fever and sunlight. Urogenital infection, keratitis, dermatitis, pharyngitis, esophagitis, and meningoencephalitis occur with lesser frequency. Infection is common and is usually acquired in childhood or adolescence.

Infection of the lower respiratory tract may be much more common than is generally appreciated: in one investigation of 308 consecutive patients with severe respiratory tract infection, it was the most frequent microorganism identified.[332] Such infection almost always represents reactivation of latent virus, most often affects the tracheobronchial mucosa alone, and may occur by several mechanisms. Extension from a focus of active disease in the oropharynx or esophagus is supported by the finding in some series of concomitant mucocutaneous disease in many affected patients.[333] Although some of these cases may result from aspiration or direct mucosal spread of the organism, many such patients have undergone tracheal intubation,[334, 335] suggesting that iatrogenic introduction, trauma, or both may also be pathogenetic factors. Despite these observations, several investigators have found no evidence of oral herpetic infection and no history of intubation,[336] indicating that other mechanisms of respiratory tract infection must occur in some patients. Some of these may involve hematogenous transmission from a site of extrapulmonary disease. It has also been hypothe-

sized that there may be direct tracheobronchial spread of reactivated virus originally present within vagal ganglia.[329]

Some investigators have found an association between herpetic tracheobronchitis and cigarette smoking;[334] because the virus typically infects squamous epithelium, it has been hypothesized that this association may be related to tobacco-induced squamous metaplasia. Most patients with HSV-I pulmonary or tracheobronchial disease have an underlying predisposing condition, such as severe burns,[337] AIDS, malignancy, or organ transplants.[332–334, 338] Tracheobronchitis has also been reported occasionally in nonimmunocompromised patients with recent myocardial infarcts or COPD[334] and in elderly but otherwise healthy individuals.[336, 339]

Pathologically, disease caused by HSV-I is manifested by focal or diffuse ulcers in the tracheobronchial epithelium (Fig. 29–9) with or without necrotizing bronchopneumonia.[338, 340, 343] The former is characterized histologically by epithelial necrosis and ulceration, frequently with bacterial or fungal superinfection in cases of longer duration. Cells at the margins of the ulcers show cytologic features characteristic of HSV infection—small eosinophilic intranuclear inclusions surrounded by a clear halo and single or multinucleated cells with ground-glass, basophilic, molded nuclei (Fig. 29–

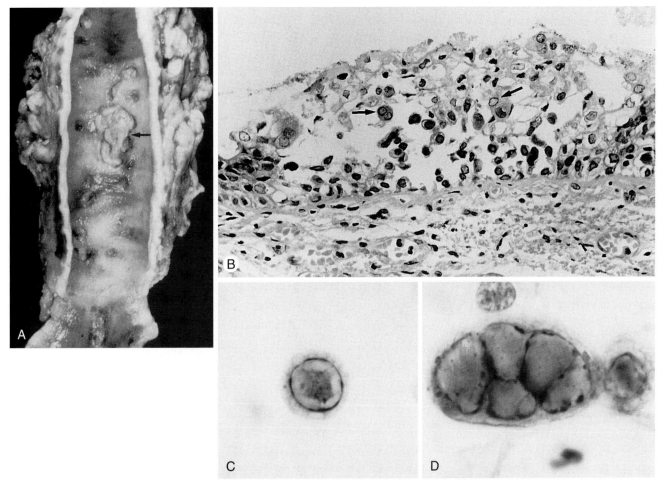

Figure 29–9. Herpes Simplex Tracheitis. The trachea *(A)* of this 40-year-old burn patient has been opened posteriorly and reveals multiple foci of ulceration, some covered with a pyogenic membrane *(arrow)*. A section of tissue at the edge of an ulcer *(B)* shows dissolution of the epithelium and scattered cells showing nuclear changes *(arrows)* suggestive of herpetic viral infection. Magnified views of cells from a cytology brush preparation show a well-defined, angulated viral inclusion *(C)* and a multinucleated giant cell with typical herpes-related nuclear smudging *(D)*. (*B*, ×250; *C* and *D*, ×1500.)

9).[306] Such cells may be detected in expectorated sputum or in bronchial washings or brushings[341] and constitute strong evidence of lower respiratory tract HSV infection in the absence of oropharyngeal herpetic disease (which can cause specimen contamination). Pneumonia is usually characterized by alveolar necrosis and a proteinaceous exudate with a variable polymorphonuclear inflammatory response (Fig. 29–10).[337] Radiologic manifestations of herpes simplex pneu-

monia have been described in a small number of patients and most commonly consist of bilateral areas of air-space consolidation.[338] Occasionally, there are poorly defined nodular opacities, corresponding on HRCT to small (3- to 20-mm diameter) soft tissue nodules associated with areas of ground-glass attenuation (Fig. 29–11).[342]

Tracheobronchial involvement is manifested by fever, productive cough, and, in some patients, signs of broncho-

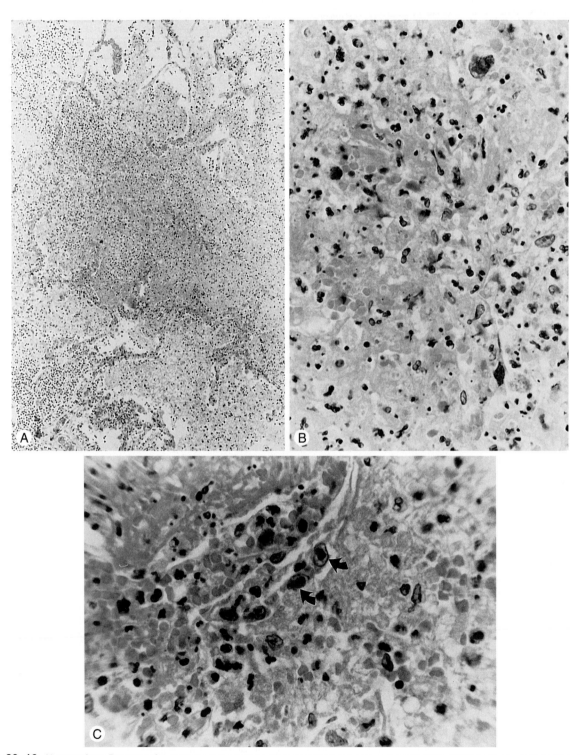

Figure 29–10. Herpesvirus Pneumonia. Sections show a focus of parenchymal necrosis and neutrophilic infiltrate (many cells having undergone leukocytoclasis). Occasional intranuclear viral inclusions are evident *(arrows in C).*

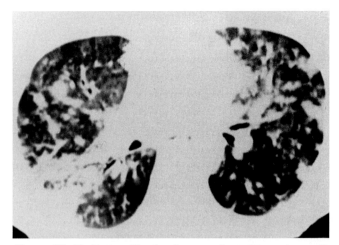

Figure 29–11. Herpes Simplex Pneumonia. A CT scan from a 42-year-old immunocompromised woman after bone marrow transplantation demonstrates bilateral nodules ranging from 3 to 15 mm in diameter. Focal areas of consolidation in the right lower lobe and lingula are also present.

spasm;[332, 336] hemoptysis occurs occasionally. Pseudomembranes related to tracheal ulcers may be large enough to cause upper airway obstruction.[332] Symptoms of pneumonia are nonspecific and depend on the extent of disease. The presence of mucocutaneous coldsores should raise suspicion of the disease; however, these are often absent and may be seen in association with other diseases.

The virus has also been associated with the development of ARDS. In one investigation of 54 patients who died as a result of burns, the immunohistochemical reaction to HSV was positive in alveolar epithelial cells and macrophages in 27 (50%);[343] 13 (81%) of the 16 patients with ARDS showed a positive reaction compared with 14 (37%) of 38 without, leading the authors to speculate that the two were pathogenetically linked. In fact, it is likely that the presence of the virus has different significance in different patients. In some, the ARDS is probably a manifestation of fulminant viral-induced pulmonary injury;[344] in others, it likely represents a secondary reaction similar to that sometimes seen with other pulmonary infections;[345] in still others, the virus may be simply a nonpathogenic "bystander," similar to CMV.[345]

The diagnosis of HSV tracheobronchitis or pneumonia is usually based on cytologic and histologic findings in specimens obtained by tracheobronchial brushing or biopsy;[337, 339] confirmation can be obtained by viral cultures or by immunofluorescent or immunohistochemical studies. Bronchoscopy is valuable for identifying ulceration in the trachea and proximal bronchi and for improving the sensitivity and specificity of the cytologic diagnosis.[338] Antibody levels tend to be low in patients who develop active disease with dissemination after transplantation;[346] however, a rise during the infection is a good prognostic sign because a lack of humoral response is associated with a bad prognosis.[338, 345] The virus can be distinguished from HSV-II by detecting appropriate antibodies in serum or antigens in formalin-fixed, paraffin-embedded tissue.[347]

Herpes Simplex Type II

HSV-II is best known as the cause of herpes genitalis, a sexually transmitted disease characterized by ulcers of the vagina, vulva, and perineum in women and glans penis, prepuce, and penile shaft in men. Recurrent disease results from reactivation of latent virus in sensory neurons of the sacral ganglia. Neonatal infection, which may be severe and disseminated, is usually acquired during passage of the infant through an infected birth canal.[348] Pulmonary infection may occur as part of the systemic disease, typically via hematogenous dissemination. Such infection tends to show less prominent airway involvement than HSV-I. The histologic pattern is usually diffuse alveolar damage or interstitial pneumonitis.[348] Clinical manifestations include cutaneous or conjunctival vesicles, fever, jaundice, seizures, and signs of pneumonia. Pleural effusion has been reported rarely.[347a]

Herpesvirus 6

Herpesvirus 6 is closely related to CMV. It is best known as the cause of childhood roseola (exanthem subitum), but has also been tentatively associated with a variety of other conditions.[348a] There is evidence that the viral carrier state can be reactivated by other organisms, such as CMV and EBV.[348a] Pulmonary disease caused by the virus appears to be rare. It has been reported, however, to cause interstitial pneumonitis in bone marrow transplant recipients.[349] A possible synergistic role with *Legionella* in a case of fatal pneumonia has also been postulated.[350]

Herpesvirus 8

Herpesvirus 8 (also known as *Kaposi's sarcoma-associated herpesvirus*), as the name suggests, has been implicated in the pathogenesis of Kaposi's sarcoma (*see* page 1677).[351] In fact, measurement of sequences of the organism in bronchoalveolar lavage fluid specimens by nested PCR has been found by some investigators to be a sensitive and specific technique for diagnosis of pulmonary Kaposi's sarcoma.[352] A strong association of the virus with primary lymphoma of serosal surfaces (including the pleura) (*see* page 2759) and with multicentric Castleman's disease has also been documented.[351]

Varicellavirus

Varicellavirus (varicella-zoster virus) is seen in two clinical forms: (1) chickenpox (varicella), representing primary and usually disseminated disease in previously uninfected individuals; and (2) zoster (shingles), representing reactivation of latent virus, typically as a unilateral dermatomal skin eruption. Although either form may be associated with pneumonia, the majority of cases with this complication occur after chickenpox.[353] In addition, zoster may be complicated by unilateral diaphragmatic paralysis, presumably as a result of extension of infection from the dorsal root to the adjacent posterior and lateral spinal cord and anterior horn cells.[354, 355]

Epidemiology

Chickenpox is a highly contagious, predominantly mucocutaneous disease that tends to occur during the colder months in temperate climates.[356] It is thought to be transmitted by droplet infection. Humans are the only known reservoir, and the incubation period averages 14 days.[357] Infection rates are high, seropositivity in urban centers in the United States approaching 100% in populations of older individuals.[356] In developed countries, most cases are recognized in childhood, with fewer than 20% occurring in adults;[358] in developing countries, disease is more common in adolescents and young adults.[356]

The overall incidence of pneumonia is about 15%,[357, 359] although in adults admitted to the hospital it may be as high as 50%.[360] Most cases occur in young children or adults.[356] In both groups, pre-existing neoplastic disease—particularly leukemia and lymphoma—and immunodeficiency are predisposing factors.[361, 362] Both the incidence and the severity of such pneumonia are also significantly greater in pregnant women.[357, 363]

In contrast to chickenpox, zoster is usually a localized cutaneous eruption that occurs most frequently in the elderly.

The precise mechanisms responsible for viral reactivation are not known, but in many cases there appears to be a relationship with acquired immunodeficiency;[364] thus, the disease is seen most frequently and is most severe in patients with lymphoreticular neoplasms (particularly Hodgkin's disease) or in those who received recent irradiation or immunosuppressive therapy. Dissemination of the infection outside the initially affected dermatome occurs in a minority of patients; an increased incidence of such disseminated infection has been described in patients with small cell carcinoma of the lung.[365, 366]

Pathogenesis and Pathologic Characteristics

In chickenpox, viremia develops promptly after deposition of the virus in the upper respiratory tract. Replication of disseminated virus occurs within the reticuloendothelial

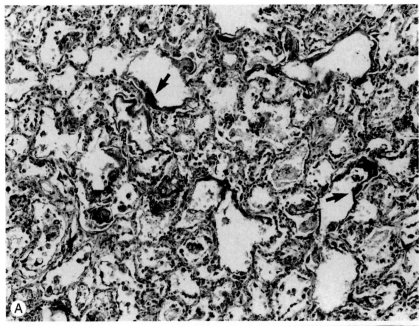

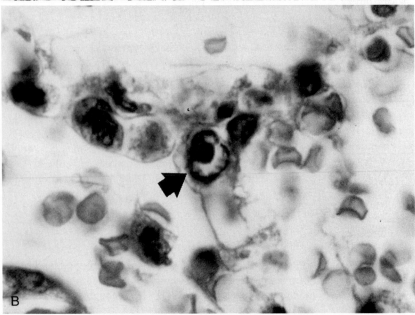

Figure 29–12. Pneumonia Caused by Herpes Zoster. Section *(A)* shows mild interstitial thickening, extensive type II cell hyperplasia, and proteinaceous material within air spaces. Well-defined hyaline membranes are present *(arrows)*. A type II pneumocyte *(B)* shows a well-defined intranuclear viral inclusion surrounded by a clear halo *(arrow)*. The sections are from an 8-year-old boy with leukemia who developed disseminated chickenpox and rapidly progressive pneumonia. (*A*, ×100; *B*, ×1500.)

system, and when host defenses are overwhelmed, a second viremia occurs with dissemination to mucocutaneous sites and the appearance of the characteristic rash.

Histologic features of pneumonitis in chickenpox and zoster are similar and consist of an interstitial mononuclear inflammatory infiltrate, associated with intra-alveolar proteinaceous exudate, edema, hemorrhage, hyaline membranes, and type 2 cell hyperplasia (diffuse alveolar damage) (Fig. 29–12). A pattern of giant cell pneumonia has also been described.[367] Somewhat angular, eosinophilic intranuclear inclusions surrounded by a halo and indistinguishable from those of herpes simplex may be seen in type 2 cells, in airway epithelial cells, and (occasionally) in desquamated cells in pleural fluid.[368] Vesicles similar to those on the skin and mucous membranes may be seen in the trachea and larger bronchi and on the pleural and peritoneal surfaces.[357, 369]

Pathologic features of remote chickenpox infection consist of spherical nodules with an average diameter of 2 mm scattered randomly and without confluence throughout the lung parenchyma.[370] Histologically, they are composed of a fibrous capsule surrounding a focus of hyalinized collagen or necrotic tissue; calcification is variable.

Radiologic Manifestations

The characteristic radiographic pattern of acute pneumonia consists of multiple 5- to 10-mm diameter nodular opacities (Fig. 29–13). Smaller nodular opacities and miliary-like nodules also may be seen but are uncommon.[371, 372] The opacities usually are fairly discrete in the lung periphery but tend to coalesce near the hila and in the lung bases.[357,

[369, 373] Progression to extensive air-space consolidation can occur rapidly (Fig. 29–14). In a minority of cases, the changes have been described as transitory, some areas of air-space consolidation clearing while new areas appear.[369, 372] Occasionally, the nodular opacities mimic pulmonary metastases.[372a, 374] Hilar lymph node enlargement occurs, but may be difficult to appreciate because of contiguity of the consolidation in the parahilar parenchyma.[357, 369, 372, 373] Central rarefaction in a zone of confluent consolidation was reported in one case.[374] Pleural effusion is uncommon and never large.[375]

Radiographic clearing usually takes from 10 days to several months;[372, 376] however, in one series of 20 patients, chest radiographs of 6 showed widespread nodulation considered to represent scarring 6 years after the infection.[369] In one case, fibrosis appeared to increase in extent over a period of 3 to 4 years after the initial infection.[377]

An apparently unique manifestation of chickenpox pneumonia, first described in 1960,[378] consists of tiny widespread foci of calcification throughout both lungs in persons who had chickenpox many years before (typically in adulthood) (Fig. 29–15).[379, 380] The foci of calcification vary in size and number but seldom exceed 2 to 3 mm in diameter; they predominate in the lower half of the lungs. Hilar lymph nodes do not calcify. The complication is relatively uncommon: in one survey of almost 17,000 individuals, 463 (2.7%) had a history of chickenpox as adults;[381] only 8 (1.7%) of these had multifocal calcification.

Clinical Manifestations

Although the initial site of varicella infection is thought to be the respiratory tract, clinical signs related to this are

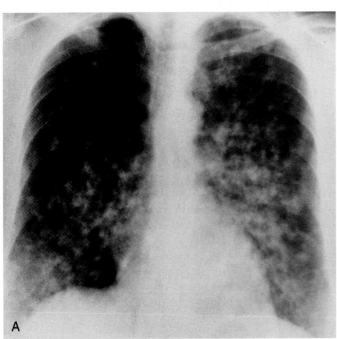

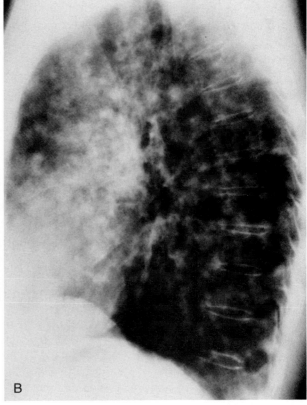

Figure 29–13. Acute Varicella Zoster Pneumonia. Posteroanterior *(A)* and lateral *(B)* radiographs reveal widespread pulmonary disease possessing a pattern characteristic of patchy air-space consolidation. Also seen are multiple, poorly defined nodular opacities. The patient was a 42-year-old woman who had non-Hodgkin's lymphoma.

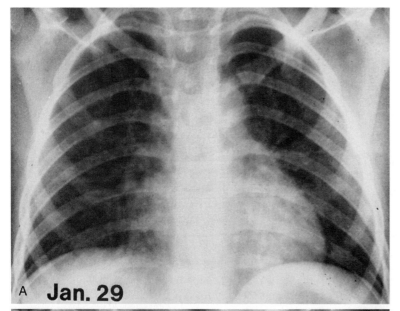

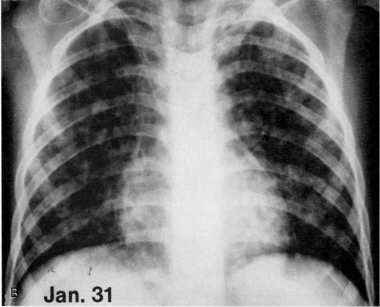

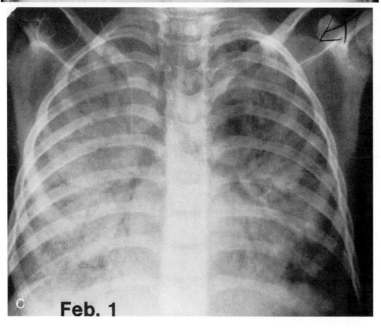

Figure 29–14. Acute Varicella Zoster Pneumonia.
Shortly after the onset of an acute respiratory illness, a
radiograph *(A)* of this 6-year-old boy with acute leukemia
revealed poorly defined opacities scattered widely throughout
both lungs; the film was exposed at a poor inspiratory position. A rash characteristic of chickenpox had appeared 2
days previously. Two days later *(B)*, the rounded opacities
had become more pronounced. Twenty-four hours later *(C)*,
both lungs had become uniformly opacified by extensive air-
space consolidation; an air bronchogram is clearly visible
bilaterally. The child died shortly thereafter.

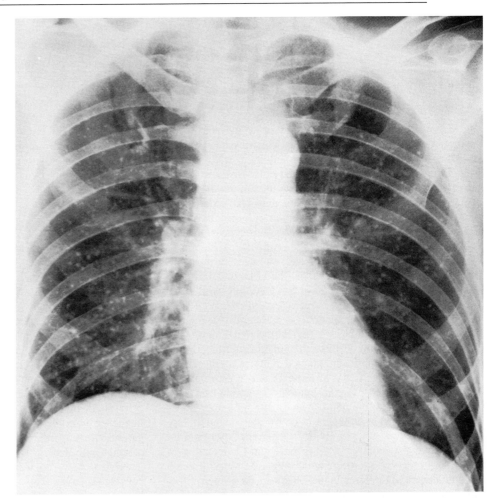

Figure 29–15. Healed Varicella Zoster (Chickenpox) Pneumonia. A posteroanterior radiograph demonstrates a multitude of tiny calcific shadows measuring 1 to 2 mm in diameter scattered widely and uniformly throughout both lungs. This 42-year-old asymptomatic man had had florid chickenpox 15 years previously; the presence of acute pneumonia was recognized at the time. (Courtesy of Dr. Romeo Ethier, Montreal Neurological Hospital.)

almost invariably absent. In most cases, there is a history of contact with an affected child 3 to 21 days before onset of the acute illness. The onset often is marked by high fever, which may precede the rash by 2 to 3 days. The rash itself may be scarlatiniform in its early stages but rapidly becomes maculopapular, vesicular, and pustular. It is often preceded by pain and, at least initially, has a distinct dermatomal distribution. Thoracic dermatomes are affected in approximately one half of cases.

Acute chickenpox pneumonia is most common in adults with severe cutaneous disease. Symptoms and signs usually develop 2 to 3 days after the appearance of the skin eruption and consist of cough, dyspnea, tachypnea, pleuritic chest pain, and, in severe cases, hemoptysis and cyanosis. The temperature may be high. Expectoration is not purulent, unless there is secondary bacterial infection (a relatively uncommon complication compared to influenza virus infection). The rash often extends onto the mucosa of the mouth and pharynx.[369] Abdominal pain may be suggestive of acute abdomen,[382] and back pain may simulate that caused by a herniated intervertebral disc.[357] Complications include hepatitis, nephritis, myocarditis, meningoencephalitis, thrombocytopenia, thromboembolism, and adrenal hemorrhage.[357, 383, 384] Clinical improvement usually antedates radiographic clearing by several weeks.

Laboratory Findings

In approximately one third of cases, the white blood cell count exceeds 10,000/mm³ and is associated with polymorphonuclear leukocytosis.[357, 369] The virus can be cultured from fluid derived from early vesicles.[385] Cytologic examination of vesicle scrapings for the presence of viral inclusions is a more rapid and frequently diagnostic procedure. Immunofluorescent studies may be used if routine microscopy is equivocal. Characteristic intranuclear inclusion bodies can also be found in the sputum specimens of patients with pneumonia.[386] Antibodies can be detected in both varicella and zoster, from about the fifth day of illness, and paired titers (in the acute and convalescent stages) can be used to confirm the diagnosis.[357]

Prognosis and Natural History

Although it is probable that many cases of varicella pneumonia are mild and are overlooked, a mortality as high as 10% has been reported,[369] and patients with acute pneumonia may die suddenly.[373] Pulmonary function studies of adult patients with acute varicella, with and without pneumonia, have shown normal values in the latter and decreased diffusing capacity (sometimes persisting for many years after the acute illness) but normal ventilatory function in the former.[387]

Cytomegalovirus

Epidemiology

CMV is a common human pathogen that has been associated with a wide variety of illnesses, the manifestations of which depend largely on the immunologic status of the host. Congenital infection occurs most often by transplacental spread of organisms from an asymptomatic mother. Subsequent disease is usually benign but may lead to death in utero or to clinically evident congenital cytomegalic inclusion disease. In neonates and infants, disease is usually acquired during passage through an infected birth canal, from maternal milk, or from infected neonates in the newborn nursery.[388] In older individuals, the virus is believed to be transmitted predominantly by direct contact with body secretions (e.g., saliva, tears, urine, semen) of an infected individual.[389] As such, populations at increased risk include children in day-care centers[390] and homosexual men. The virus can also be acquired through contaminated blood during transfusion[391] and from infected cells in organ transplants.[392] Excretion of CMV in urine or saliva, especially in immunocompromised patients, can last for months and even years after the initial infection.[393]

Acquired CMV infection is common, seropositivity rates varying from 40% to 100% in different adult populations around the world.[388] Higher rates tend to be seen in groups with lower socioeconomic status.[388] Most affected individuals are asymptomatic, the only sequela of their infection being the presence of latent virus as a potential source of reinfection. As a corollary, CMV is an uncommon cause of community-acquired pneumonia; for example, in one study of 443 patients with this condition, the virus was etiologically related in only 4 (0.9%).[394] By contrast, pneumonia as well as other clinical manifestations of active infection is much more frequent in patients with underlying disease, particularly immunodeficiency related to organ transplantation (*see* page 1716)[395, 396, 401] or AIDS (*see* page 1674).

Both humoral and cell-mediated defense mechanisms appear to be important in the control of human CMV infection. Patients who have CMV-specific antibodies before institution of immunosuppressive therapy and who respond to CMV infection with an increase in antibody production usually shed virus asymptomatically rather than develop clinically significant disease.[458] By contrast, patients with clinically severe CMV infection typically fail to mount a significant complement-fixing antibody response.[397] Moreover, intravenous immunoglobulin has been shown to modify the severity of CMV infection.[398, 399] Despite these observations, patients at risk for clinical disease are most often particularly deficient in cell-mediated immunity. In addition to intrinsic immunodeficiency associated with the primary disease, corticosteroids and immunosuppressive drugs undoubtedly contribute significantly to the impaired host response.[388]

Serologic studies indicate that many patients who develop clinical disease have had prior exposure to CMV[393, 400] (i.e., the infection represents reactivation of latent [endogenous] virus). As with primary disease, this *secondary* form of infection can elicit an antibody response and patients remain asymptomatic, the principal manifestation of the infection being asymptomatic shedding of virus in various body secretions.[397, 400, 401] It is also clear that seropositive patients can be reinfected from an exogenous source and that infection with two strains can occur at the same time.[402] From a practical point of view, clinically evident disease tends to be more common and more severe in immunosuppressed patients with primary disease (e.g., seronegative recipients of an organ transplant from a seropositve donor).[388]

Pathogenesis and Pathologic Characteristics

Pathologic characteristics of pulmonary CMV infection are variable and reflect the complex interaction between viral reproduction and host immunologic control. The organism is sometimes cultured from the lung at autopsy of individuals who have manifested no clinical symptoms and who show neither histologic evidence of disease nor the typical cytologic inclusions associated with the presence of the virus. In other cases, such inclusions can be identified focally in occasional cells[403] or diffusely throughout the parenchyma,[404] without evidence of pulmonary injury or inflammation. The frequency of these findings in unselected autopsies ranges from 0 to 10%, with an average of about 1%;[405, 406] the incidence is higher in immunosuppressed hosts than in apparently healthy subjects and is particularly common in patients with AIDS. The cell in which CMV resides in an inactive state is unclear;[407] however, blood leukocytes are considered to be likely candidates.[388]

The pathogenesis of CMV-induced pulmonary disease is complex and not completely understood. It is clear from a variety of experimental and pathologic observations that the virus causes direct tissue damage in many cases.[408] In addition, clinical studies of patients who have had bone marrow transplants and experimental animal studies[409] have provided evidence that an immunologically mediated mechanism may be involved in the pathogenesis of disease in some cases (*see* page 1716).[408, 410] The not infrequent presence of other pathogens when CMV is isolated from tissue, the failure of therapy to alter the course of established CMV pneumonia in some investigations, the frequent identification of inclusion-bearing cells lining the alveolar air spaces without underlying inflammatory reaction in patients who have AIDS, and the observation that the presence of CMV in the lung does not appear to affect mortality[411] strongly suggest that CMV is not pathogenic in every case in which it is detected.

Two morphologic patterns have been described in CMV pneumonia, the first and most common consisting of multiple, relatively well-defined, hemorrhagic nodules 0.1 to 1.5 cm in diameter scattered randomly throughout the parenchyma and separated by more or less normal lung.[403, 412–414] Histologically the nodules consist of foci of intra-alveolar hemorrhage, edema, and fibrin deposition accompanied by necrotic debris and acute and chronic inflammatory cells. Hyaline membranes can be seen, and a mononuclear cell interstitial infiltrate of variable severity is usually present. Infected cells are easily identified in the abnormal areas, both singly and in small clusters. The second pattern affects most of the parenchyma, with histologic features of either diffuse alveolar damage[403, 412] or interstitial pneumonitis (Fig. 29–16). It has been speculated that the nodular form of disease results from hematogenous seeding of the lungs from an extrapulmonary source and that the diffuse type may represent either endogenous pulmonary infection or an extension of the nodular form to involve more of the lung.[412]

CMV-infected cells are characteristic, and their presence in tissue or in cytologic specimens is diagnostic of infection (although, as is evident from the previous discussion, not necessarily of disease). In the lung, inclusions are usually seen in alveolar lining cells, but may be present in alveolar macrophages and endothelial cells and airway epithelial cells. Infected cells are significantly enlarged (30 to 50 μm in diameter) and, in fully developed infection, contain round-to-oval, homogeneous, basophilic intranuclear inclusions that fill most of the nucleus and are separated

from the nuclear membrane by a distinct halo *(owl-eye nucleus)* (Fig. 29–17).[306] Intracytoplasmic inclusions, which appear after the nuclear inclusions are well developed, are small, usually multiple, and basophilic. Although both inclusions may be identified with hematoxylin and eosin stain, Wright-Giemsa staining of touch imprints of open-lung biopsy specimens has been reported to be a relatively quick and easy, although less sensitive, method of identification.[415] They may also be identified with the Papanicolaou's stain.[416, 417] Histochemical staining and ultrastructural characteristics of the inclusions have been described.[418–420] Care must be taken not to confuse nucleoli of reactive type II cells with viral inclusions (Fig. 29–18); although the distinction is usually possible on standard hematoxylin and eosin–stained sections, immunohistochemical analysis can usually settle the matter in doubtful cases.

CMV pulmonary infection not infrequently coexists

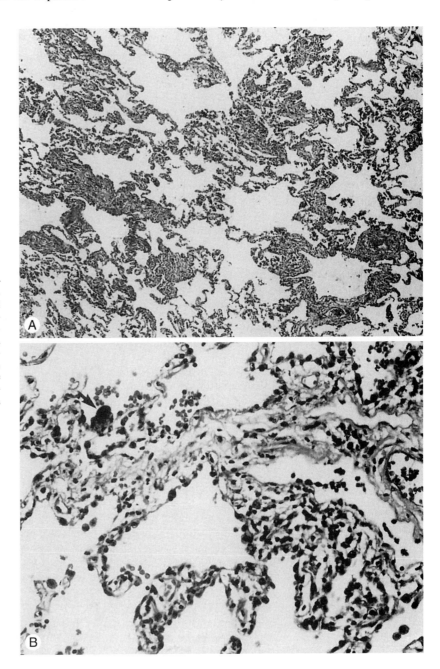

Figure 29–16. Interstitial Pneumonia— Cytomegalovirus. A 68-year-old man had a thymoma and red cell aplasia, for which he was treated with transfusions and prednisone. He subsequently developed cough and increasing dyspnea. A posteroanterior chest radiograph showed a fine reticular pattern. Open-lung biopsy *(A)* shows more or less diffuse interstitial pneumonitis; the air spaces are unaffected. Higher magnification *(B)* shows a lymphocytic infiltrate and a single large cell *(arrow)*, representing a cytomegalovirus-infected type II pneumocyte. (*A*, ×48; *B*, ×250.)

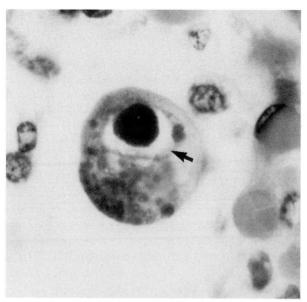

Figure 29–17. Cytomegalovirus. Infected pulmonary epithelial cell, showing a deeply basophilic round nuclear inclusion that is surrounded by a clear halo (the nuclear membrane is indicated by an *arrow*). Numerous discrete intracytoplasmic inclusions are also present. (×1500.)

with pneumonia caused by other organisms.[421] *Toxoplasma gondii,*[422] *Aspergillus* species, *Nocardia asteroides,*[423] herpes simplex,[424] and *Pneumocystis carinii* have all been reported, the last being the most frequent.[425–427] It is possible that the association with *Pneumocystis* is more than just a chance dual infection in an immunocompromised host; in two cases, small, round bodies resembling viral particles have been found within *P. carinii* trophozoites on electron microscopic examination,[426, 427] suggesting that the organism might act as an intermediate host for the virus. Alveolar proteinosis has occasionally been reported in association with CMV infection.[428]

Radiologic Manifestations

The most common radiographic findings in CMV pneumonia are bilateral linear opacities (reticular pattern), ground-glass opacities, and parenchymal consolidation (Fig. 29–19).[429–431] Less common manifestations include small nodular opacities, a reticulonodular pattern, and lobar consolidation.[432–434]

In one investigation of 31 patients who had CMV pneumonia after bone marrow transplantation, radiographic abnormalities consisted of air-space consolidation in 12 (39%), linear opacities (reticular pattern) in 7 (23%), and ground-glass opacities in 4 (13%);[431] a combination of the three patterns was seen in 8 (26%). These abnormalities were first seen 26 to 270 days (median, 96 days) after transplantation, were bilateral in 22 patients and unilateral in 9, and most commonly involved the lower lung zones. Although pleural effusions were present in six patients, they could usually be attributed to other causes, most commonly renal failure. In another study of six patients with cardiac transplants, the radiographic findings included diffuse bilateral haze (ground-glass opacities), lobar consolidation with small pleural effusion, and focal subsegmental consolidation.[430]

Findings of CMV pneumonia on CT include areas of ground-glass attenuation, parenchymal consolidation, and nodular or reticulonodular opacities.[435–437] In one investigation of eight patients, seven had a combination of linear opacities and parenchymal consolidation, and one had only consolidation.[435] All abnormalities were bilateral. The consolidation most commonly consisted of poorly marginated opacities that were predominantly peripheral in distribution. Pleural effusion was present in four cases and was bilateral in three. No enlarged hilar or mediastinal nodes were identified.

In a second study of 10 patients, the CT findings included small nodules in 6, consolidation in 4, ground-glass attenuation in 4, and irregular lines in 1 (Figs. 29–20 and 29–21).[436] The nodules had a bilateral and symmetric distribution and involved all lung zones. The areas of consolidation were nonsegmental and involved the lower lung zones. Neither nodules nor consolidation showed a tendency toward a peribronchial or subpleural distribution. Pathologic correlation showed the nodules to correspond to foci of hemorrhage, necrosis and inflammation, or organizing pneumonia; the areas of ground-glass attenuation corresponded to early changes of diffuse alveolar damage. All four patients with parenchymal consolidation on CT had interstitial pneumonia with associated edema and fibrinous exudate demonstrated histologically in specimens obtained from open-lung biopsy. Pleural effusion was present in 4 of 10 cases (bilateral in 3

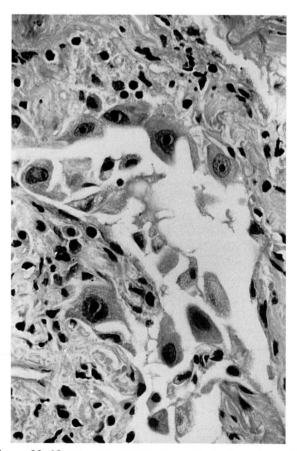

Figure 29–18. Nucleoli Resembling Viral Inclusions. A magnified view of an alveolus from a patient with idiopathic pulmonary fibrosis shows several hyperplastic type II cells with prominent nucleoli, resembling cytomegalovirus-infected cells.

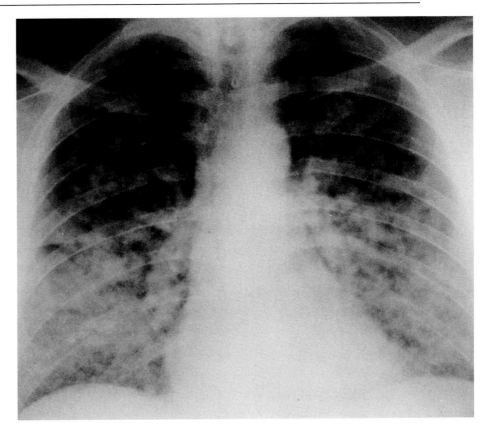

Figure 29–19. Acute Cytomegalovirus Pneumonia in a Renal Transplant Patient. A posteroanterior chest radiograph shows widespread patchy airspace consolidation, more marked in the lower lobes. There is mild left ventricular enlargement. At autopsy several days later, severe cytomegalovirus pneumonia was found.

and unilateral in 1). Mediastinal lymphadenopathy was present in one patient.

Clinical Manifestations

The clinical features of congenital CMV infection include jaundice, hepatosplenomegaly, thrombocytopenic purpura, chorioretinitis, and (sometimes) diffuse interstitial pneumonia.[438] Most of those who survive the acute illness are severely mentally retarded, with microcephaly, seizures, deafness, and other signs of cerebral damage. Acquired postnatal infection in neonates and children is usually subclinical, although symptomatic infection is more frequent than in adults; however, these infants appear to develop normally.[389]

In older children and adults without immunodeficiency, the only symptom of CMV infection may be prolonged fever.[439] Some patients also have malaise, nonexudative pharyngitis, hepatosplenomegaly, lymph node enlargement, jaundice, and atypical lymphocytosis suggestive of infectious mononucleosis.[391, 439, 440] This clinical picture appears in previously healthy individuals or in patients 2 to 4 weeks after surgery or transfusion and is associated with a rise in titer of CMV antibody (with or without positive culture of the organism). Pneumonia is an uncommon manifestation.[441, 442] CMV is also a rare cause of community-acquired pneumonia without associated mononucleosis symptoms.[394] Clinical evidence of pneumonia is much more common in immunocompromised individuals. Signs and symptoms of pulmonary involvement are nonspecific and include nonproductive cough, progressive dyspnea, and cyanosis; paroxysms of coughing and hemoptysis have been reported.[443, 444] Features of disease in patients who have received transplants or who have AIDS are discussed elsewhere (*see* pages 1674 and 1716).

Laboratory Findings

As with other organisms, several techniques are available to detect CMV, each with its own advantages and limitations.[445] The virus can be isolated from various body secretions, blood, or tissue; it appears to be particularly plentiful in leukocytes, and buffy coat culture may be useful.[446] The organism can be grown on human fibroblasts, in which it produces characteristic cell rounding and enlargement.[389] The major problem with culture is time; 2 to 3 weeks are required with standard methods before the virus can be definitvely identified. Use of the shell-vial technique—which combines inoculation of centrifuged specimens and staining of infected cells with monoclonal antibodies—is a distinct improvement, results being available within 24 to 36 hours.[447] Additional, even more sensitive techniques, such as immunoglobulin-labelled immunomagnetic beads,[447a] fluorescent antibody staining,[448] *in situ* hybridization,[449] and PCR,[449a] have also been used to identify CMV antigen in bronchoalveolar lavage fluid and tissue specimens.

A major limitation of these diagnostic studies is the fact that the identification of CMV, particularly in specimens such as urine and bronchoalveolar lavage fluid, does not necessarily indicate concomitant disease.[450, 451] As a result, it is necessary in some cases to identify CMV in association with tissue damage in biopsy specimens to be certain that the virus is truly pathogenic. In this situation, the organism is most easily identified by the characteristic light microscopic

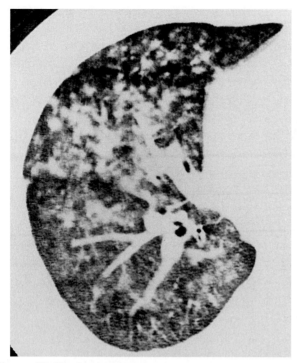

Figure 29–20. Cytomegalovirus Pneumonia. An HRCT scan targeted to the right lung demonstrates small nodular opacities ranging from 3 to 10 mm in diameter and areas of ground-glass attenuation. Similar abnormalities were evident in the left lung. The patient was a 24-year-old man who had undergone renal transplantation.

appearance of infected cells. As in the examination of bronchoalveolar lavage fluid, however, additional techniques, including immunofluorescent or immunohistochemical analysis,[452, 453] *in situ* hybridization,[454] and PCR,[455–457] have been employed to increase sensitivity.

Complement-fixation, agglutination, ELISA, and radioimmunoassay methods have also been used to diagnose CMV infection serologically and may be useful even in immunosuppressed patients.[458] As with other viral infections, a fourfold rise in titer is considered to be a positive test result; however, similar to standard culture, the time delay is such that the tests have limited practical value. The detection of IgM is of some value, particularly in infants, because it is specific for CMV infection and cannot be the result of passive transfer of maternal antibodies across the placenta.

Epstein-Barr Virus

EBV has been associated with a wide variety of human disease, including that involving the lungs. The virus infects B lymphocytes, pharyngeal epithelial cells, and (possibly) epithelial cells of the lower respiratory tract,[459] in all of which it can remain dormant for prolonged periods of time; clinical manifestations of disease are largely related to organs and tissues containing these cells. Infection can be transmitted by blood transfusion or extracorporeal circulation;[460] however, it occurs much more often by direct person-to-person spread.[461]

Infectious Mononucleosis

EBV is perhaps best known as the cause of infectious mononucleosis, a syndrome that affects predominantly

young adults and consists of pharyngitis; fever; more or less diffuse lymph node enlargement; splenomegaly; and an increase in lymphocytes, often cytologically atypical, in peripheral blood. Intrathoracic disease is uncommon and is manifested most often by lymph node enlargement (Fig. 29–22), interstitial pneumonitis, or both.[462] In one series of 556 patients, 30 had abnormal physical findings in the chest, and 14 of these had radiographic evidence of interstitial pneumonitis.[463] In another series of 59 patients, the radiographic findings were as follows:[464] hilar lymph node enlargement in 8 (13%); a diffuse reticular pattern in 3 (5%), one of these also showing an air-space pattern; and pleural effusions in 3 (small and bilateral in 2 and moderate and unilateral in the other). More sophisticated imaging techniques, such as CT[465] and magnetic resonance imaging,[466] are capable of documenting mediastinal and hilar adenopathy in patients whose chest radiographs are normal.

The most common radiologic finding in infectious mononucleosis is splenomegaly: in the study of 59 patients cited previously, it was observed in 28 (47%);[464] in an ultrasonographic investigation of 29 patients, it was identified in all (hepatomegaly was also found in 50%).[467] It has been suggested that this finding, in association with hilar lymph node enlargement, pleural effusion, or a diffuse reticular pattern, should alert the radiologist to the possibility of the disease.[464]

Pathologic features of the pulmonary abnormalities consist of a predominantly peribronchovascular interstitial infiltrate of mature-appearing lymphocytes, plasmacytoid lymphocytes, and immunoblasts.[468, 469] A similar lymphoid population can be seen in enlarged lymph nodes and, sometimes, in distended alveolar capillaries.[469]

Patients typically complain of the insidious onset of weakness, malaise, fever, and sore throat. Examination of the throat may reveal signs of pharyngitis, a palatal rash consisting of well-circumscribed red spots, and tonsillar enlargement. The last-mentioned may be severe enough to cause dysphagia and dyspnea, particularly in children;[471, 472] rarely, upper airway obstruction is fatal.[468, 473] Spasmodic

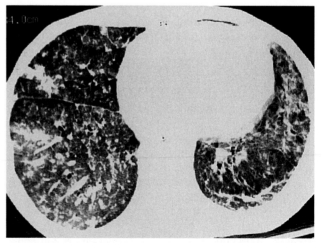

Figure 29–21. Cytomegalovirus Pneumonia. An HRCT scan demonstrates bilateral nodular opacities with irregular margins and areas of ground-glass attenuation. Irregular linear opacities are present in the left lower lobe. The patient was a 38-year-old man who had undergone bilateral lung transplantation.

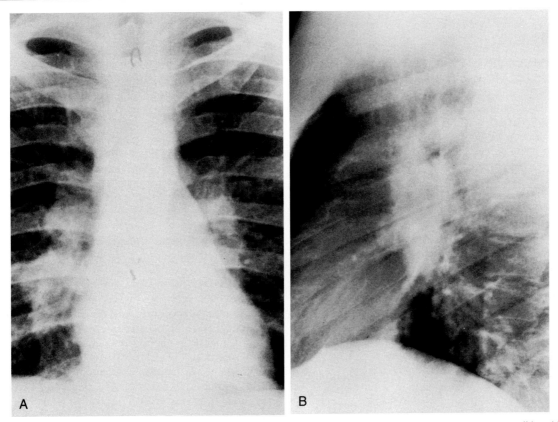

Figure 29–22. Infectious Mononucleosis. This 17-year-old boy presented with a history and physical findings compatible with infectious mononucleosis; he had a leukocytosis of 18,000, 50% of which were atypical lymphocytes; serial studies revealed a rising heterophil antibody titer. Views from posteroanterior *(A)* and lateral *(B)* radiographs demonstrate marked enlargement of both hila, the lobulated contour being typical of lymph node enlargement. There is no evidence of mediastinal lymphadenopathy or of pulmonary or pleural disease. One month later, a chest radiograph was normal.

cough productive of small amounts of tenacious sputum has been a frequently reported symptom in some series.[463] Significant infiltration of the pulmonary interstitium by lymphoid cells can also result in dyspnea and, rarely, respiratory failure.

In one study of nine patients, pulmonary function tests performed at the onset and termination of the illness and 5 months later were normal except for the maximal inspiratory pressures, which were reduced during and at the end of the illness but had returned to normal at the 5-month follow-up.[474] This finding presumably reflects a transient weakening of the respiratory muscles.

The diagnosis can be confirmed in most cases by a positive heterophil antibody test. This test is negative in up to 20% of patients, however, and a negative test is of little diagnostic value. In the latter circumstance, measurement of virus-specific antibodies in the serum or of viral DNA in blood or tissue cells by PCR may be helpful.

Other Epstein-Barr Virus–Related Diseases

EBV has been strongly implicated in the development of several lymphoproliferative disorders. This association has been best documented in Burkitt's lymphoma and in lymphomas complicating systemic immunodeficiency, particularly AIDS, congenital immunodeficiency states, and post-transplant lymphoproliferative disorders (including those of the lung) *(see* page 1711).[475] Infectious mononucleosis itself is rarely complicated by lymphoma.[476] There is also

evidence that the virus may play a role in Hodgkin's disease,[470, 477] angioimmunoblastic lymphadenopathy,[478] some primary pleural lymphomas associated with chronic pyothorax,[479, 480] and pulmonary angiocentric immunoproliferative lesions (lymphomatoid granulomatosis).[481] EBV has also been implicated in the pathogenesis of lymphocytic interstitial pneumonitis (in association with either Sjögren's syndrome or AIDS),[482] idiopathic pulmonary fibrosis *(see* page 1079),[483] and the lymphoepithelioma variant of pulmonary carcinoma.[484]

Poxviruses

Poxviruses include the variola virus (responsible for smallpox) and the vaccinia virus, which was used in an attenuated form as a smallpox vaccine. Now that the former virus has been eradicated as a cause of human infection, acute manifestations of disease are no longer seen; however, long-term radiologic sequelae—manifested as punctate calcifications throughout the lungs—may still be encountered.[485]

Papovaviruses

Papillomaviruses are a subgroup of papovaviruses that are responsible for a variety of hyperplastic lesions of the skin and mucous membrane, variously described as papillomas, condylomas, and warts. They have been shown to be present in laryngeal papillomas[486] and are undoubtedly responsible for similar lesions in the lower respiratory tract (*see* page 1262).[487] There is also evidence that the viruses are pathogenetically related to the occasional development of pulmonary carcinoma in patients with tracheobronchial papillomatosis[487] and, possibly, in some individuals with *de novo* bronchial squamous cell carcinoma (see page 1079).[488] As mentioned previously, there is also some evidence that iatrogenic infection by simian virus 40 (a papovavirus that does not normally infect humans) may be responsible for some cases of mesothelioma.[225]

Parvoviruses

Parvoviruses form a group of extremely small, ether-resistant organisms that cause a variety of forms of disease whose severity depends on the immunocompetence of the affected individual.[488a] Pulmonary disease may occur as part of systemic infection.[488b] An association of the organism with the development of the acute chest syndrome in patients who have sickle cell disease has also been reported.[488c]

MYCOPLASMAS

The mycoplasmas (pleuropneumonia-like organisms) are the smallest free-living organisms that can be cultured on artificial media. They share a number of bacterial attributes, including the presence of replicative DNA and RNA, susceptibility to antibiotics, and reproduction by binary fission. Their small size (about 0.2×0.8 μm), absence of a cell wall, and genetic features set them apart from most bacteria, and they are usually considered as a separate group. Of the several species that have been recognized, *Mycoplasma pneumoniae* is associated with the vast majority of cases of human respiratory disease. Although other species cultured from the respiratory tract are usually considered to be commensals,[489] there is evidence that *M. hominis* is the occasional cause of penumonia or pleural effusion[490] or diffuse alveolar hemorrhage.[490a] In addition, *M. fermentans* has been associated with ARDS and fulminant, fatal infection in previously healthy individuals.[491] *M. genitalium* has also been detected rarely in bronchoalveolar lavage fluid by PCR analysis;[492] however, the clinical significance of this finding is unclear.

Although the organisms are pleomorphic, they tend to be filamentous or rod shaped in tissue. At one end is a specialized terminal structure that is believed to be necessary for attachment of the organism to epithelial surfaces.[493] *M. pneumoniae* grows readily on sterol-enriched media[494] and has been cultured in tissue and in the chorioallantoic membrane of chick embryos.[495]

Epidemiology

M. pneumoniae is one of the more common causes of community-acquired pneumonia, having been estimated to account for 10% to 15% of cases in the population as a whole[496–500] and up to 50% of cases in specific groups, such as military recruits.[494, 501] Infections occur throughout the year, with a peak during the autumn and early winter. Dis-ease is most common in individuals between 5 and 20 years of age, and the incubation period is 1 to 3 weeks.[502]

Transmission of the organism usually occurs from person to person by droplet inhalation secondary to coughing. One exceptional outbreak was associated with a fine-particle aerosol generated from abrasive drilling of contaminated false teeth.[503] Another unusual mechanism of transmission is via a donor lung during transplantation.[504] Shedding of *Mycoplasma* organisms may persist for several months after the patient has recovered from the acute infection.[505, 506] These carriers have been found in both military populations[507] and civilian communities.[508] Presumably because of the cessation of cough with the resolution of active disease, transmission of organisms by these individuals appears to be minimal.[509]

Despite the high incidence of pneumonia in the general population, the organism does not appear to be particularly contagious, disease usually being transmitted after prolonged contact in families or close communities. In these settings, however, the infection rate is high; careful inquiry into family groups usually reveals symptoms of upper or lower respiratory tract involvement in most individuals.[505, 508, 510, 511] Schoolchildren are probably a major source of dispersal. Local outbreaks of relatively severe infection can occur, again usually in families or community groups.[503, 510, 512, 513] More widespread epidemics affecting cities or entire countries and occurring over an extended period of time have also been reported.[511, 514]

Pathogenesis

The pathogenesis of *M. pneumoniae* infection has been related to several mechanisms, including: (1) a direct cytotoxic effect of the organism; (2) tissue damage as a result of a host immune reaction; and (3) cytotoxic and inflammatory changes resulting from contact of macrophages with the organism. In experimental and natural human infection, the organism is initially localized along the tracheobronchial epithelium, where it is in intimate contact with the surface of ciliated cells,[493, 515] apparently by attachment to its terminal unit. Both scanning and transmission electron microscopy have revealed cytopathologic changes and exfoliation of these cells in infected tracheal organ cultures, suggesting a direct toxic action by the organism.[515, 516] The possibility that tissue damage is related to the local effects of toxic enzymes and oxygen free radical released from macrophages has also been proposed.[517]

Immune mechanisms not only play a protective role in *M. pneumoniae* infection, but also are almost certainly implicated in the pathogenesis of disease itself.[518, 519] Infection is associated with an IgM followed by IgG response, but these serum antibodies do not confer long-lasting immunity;[494, 518] in addition, some IgG antibodies are nonspecific and react with measles, rubella, and HSV.[520] Despite these findings, rechallenge of previously infected animals with organisms has been shown to result in less severe pneumonia, implying some degree of immunity.[521] IgA produced locally in the nasopharynx appears to be effective in inhibiting the initial binding of *M. pneumoniae* to the respiratory epithelium and may be responsible for the protective effect.[518]

The concept that immune mechanisms play a role in

the pathogenesis of the disease is supported by the fact that immunodeficient animals and patients appear to be relatively resistant to the development of mycoplasmal pneumonia. Additional evidence is provided by the protection against disease afforded by antithymocyte serum and corticosteroid therapy[518, 519] and by the observation that the neurologic deficit associated with some cases of mycoplasmal pneumonia can be reversed by plasma exchange.[522] The pathogenesis of these effects is not known but may lie in the production of a variety of autoantibodies and in the formation of immune complexes.[522, 523]

Pathologic Characteristics

Because the disease is rarely fatal and because bacterial superinfection or other complications are common in patients who do die, pathologic changes in pure human *Mycoplasma* infection have been described infrequently. In animal experiments, histopathologic findings consist principally of a peribronchial and peribronchiolar mononuclear inflammatory infiltrate; epithelial ulceration and a neutrophilic infiltrate occur in some cases.[524] Chronic inflammation and type II cell hyperplasia occur to a variable degree in adjacent parenchyma, probably corresponding to the severity of infection. Similar changes have been found in the rare instances of human *Mycoplasma* infection studied at autopsy[525, 526] and in open-lung biopsy specimens (Fig. 29–23).[527] Other histologic patterns occasionally reported include diffuse alveolar damage, organizing pneumonia, alveolar hemorrhage, and an alveolar proteinosis–like picture.[524, 527, 528] To what extent these represent a direct effect of the *Mycoplasma* organism or are secondary to other mechanisms is not clear. Interstitial fibrosis may develop as a long-term complication.[529]

Radiologic Manifestations

The radiographic pattern of acute mycoplasmal pneumonia is indistinguishable from that of many viral pneumonias,[530] the manifestations consisting of interstitial or airspace opacities or a combination of both.[531] In the early stages, the interstitial inflammation is associated with a fine reticular pattern, followed by signs of air-space consolidation of patchy distribution (Fig. 29–24).[530, 532, 533] With resolution, the process is reversed, the air-space consolidation disappearing first. In one series of 60 adults with mycoplasmal pneumonia proven serologically, 40% showed clearing of chest radiographs by 4 weeks and 96% by 8 weeks.[534] However, in another study of 116 cases, resolution averaged only 11 days, and was complete in all cases within 25 days.[310]

In contrast to the nonsegmental distribution of acute bacterial air-space pneumonia (e.g., caused by *Streptococcus pneumoniae*), mycoplasmal pneumonia tends to be segmental (Fig. 29–25). In one series of 79 cases, only 2 had a radiographic picture that could be confused with bacterial pneumonia; both of these were readily identified clinically and from the leukocyte count as of mycoplasmal or viral origin.[535] Disease is manifested predominantly in the lower lobes: only 5 of 39 cases in one series had upper-lobe involvement.[536] Hilar lymph node enlargement is rare in adults,[530, 537] but occurs in approximately 30% of children.[538, 539]

In one investigation of 100 patients with serologically proven pneumonia, two distinct clinical and radiologic presentations were recognized.[540] The largest group (48 patients) presented with symptoms of short duration characteristic of acute pneumonia, including nonpleuritic chest pain, cough, myalgias, and fever. The chest radiographs demonstrated segmental or lobar consolidation associated with an air bronchogram and sometimes with atelectasis; pleural effusion was evident on erect posteroanterior and lateral radiographs of nine patients (19%). Hypoxemia (PO_2 75 mm Hg) was found in 4 (28%) of 14 patients. Ten of the 48 patients (20%) had associated disease (systemic lupus erythematosus in 4, sickle cell disease in 3, and Hodgkin's disease in 3).

The second group (28 patients) presented with symptoms of malaise, lethargy, and dyspnea ranging in duration from 1 to 4 weeks. In contrast to the first group, most of these patients were afebrile and were free from cough, myalgia, and chest pain. The chest radiographs demonstrated a diffuse, bilateral reticulonodular pattern (Fig. 29–26), sometimes associated with septal (Kerley B) lines; none showed lobar or segmental consolidation. Pleural effusion was observed in only one patient. Hypoxemia was evident in 13 (68%) of 19 patients. Nine patients in this group had associated disease (sarcoidosis in eight and Hodgkin's disease in one). The remaining 24 patients (group 3) had clinical and radiologic manifestations that overlapped with the other two groups. The authors surmised that three factors may be involved in these apparently different responses to the same infecting agent:[540] pre-existing pulmonary disease, previous infection by *Mycoplasma*, and differing immune reactions.

Pleural effusions occur in approximately 20% of patients, but are usually small and unilateral;[540–542] radiographs obtained in lateral decubitus position may be necessary to demonstrate their presence.[543] In children with underlying disease, however, the pneumonia is often more severe and usually accompanied by effusion.[544, 545] Unusual findings include Kerley B lines and pneumatoceles.[310] ARDS has been reported occasionally.[546] Similar to the radiograph, the CT scan demonstrates interstitial thickening and areas of segmental, subsegmental, or lobular consolidation (Fig. 29–27).[547, 547a] Nodular and branching areas of attenuation may also be apparent in the centrilobular region. Correlation between the HRCT and histopathologic findings has demonstrated that these areas correspond to the presence of bronchiolitis and exudate within the bronchiolar lumen (Fig. 29–28).[547]

Clinical Manifestations

The typical case of *Mycoplasma* infection begins insidiously with fever, nonproductive cough, headache, malaise, and (rarely) chills.[518, 548, 549] Myalgia, arthralgia, and gastrointestinal symptoms are usually mild or absent. Upper respiratory tract involvement, characterized predominantly by sore throat and symptoms of rhinitis, is present in about 50% of cases;[310, 502] bullous myringitis occurs occasionally.[508, 510, 512]

The major symptom of lower respiratory tract involvement is cough, which may be hacking and paroxysmal in nature. Although initially nonproductive, it may become associated with mucoid or frankly purulent sputum if infection is prolonged. Hemoptysis and pleuritic chest pain are uncommon; however, pneumonia occasionally mimics pulmonary thromboembolism with infarction[550] or diffuse alveo-

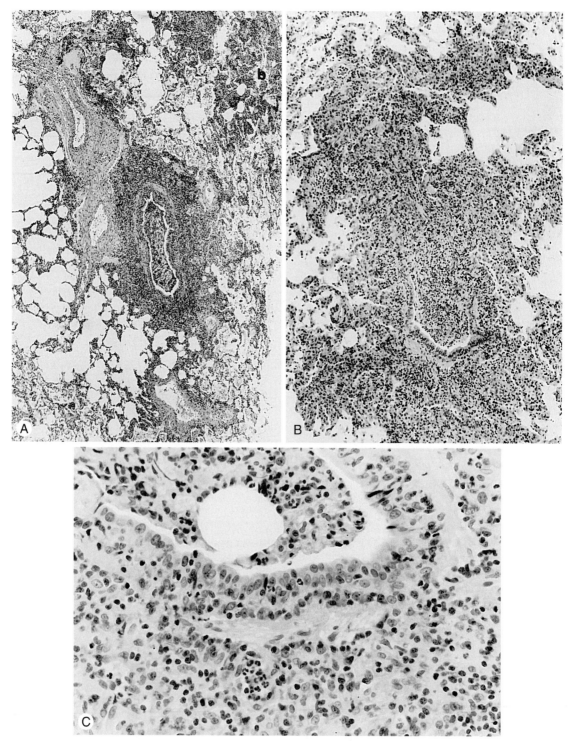

Figure 29–23. *Mycoplasma pneumoniae*—**Bronchiolitis and Pneumonitis**. A section of an open-lung biopsy specimen from a 23-year-old man with rapidly progressive respiratory failure *(A)* shows patchy, overall mild-to-moderate interstitial pneumonitis and severe inflammation centered about a membranous bronchiole and a respiratory bronchiole (b). A mild degree of alveolar interstitial inflammation is also evident. Another view from the same biopsy specimen *(B)* shows the same reaction in a proximal respiratory bronchiole. High magnification *(C)* shows a mixed lymphocytic and neutrophilic infiltrate in the bronchiolar wall. (*A*, ×70; *B*, ×120; *C*, ×220.)

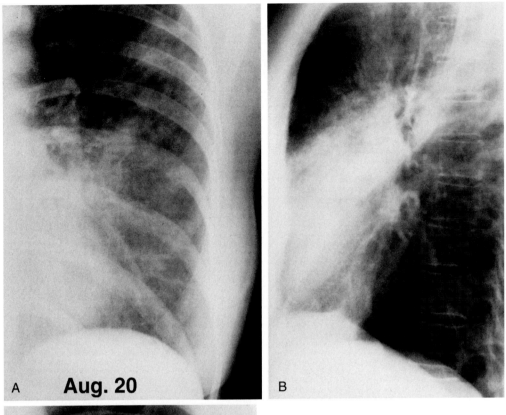

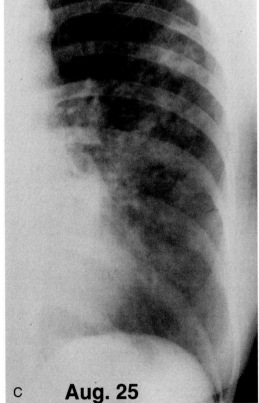

Figure 29–24. Acute Pneumonia Caused by *Mycoplasma pneumoniae*. Views of the left lung from posteroanterior *(A)* and lateral *(B)* radiographs demonstrate patchy air-space consolidation in the distribution of the lingular and posterior segments of the left upper lobe. The consolidation is not homogeneous, as would be anticipated in acute bacterial pneumonia caused by, for example, *Streptococcus pneumoniae*. Immunofluorescence microscopy of sputum revealed the presence of *M. pneumoniae*. Five days later *(C)*, considerable improvement had occurred, particularly in the lingula.

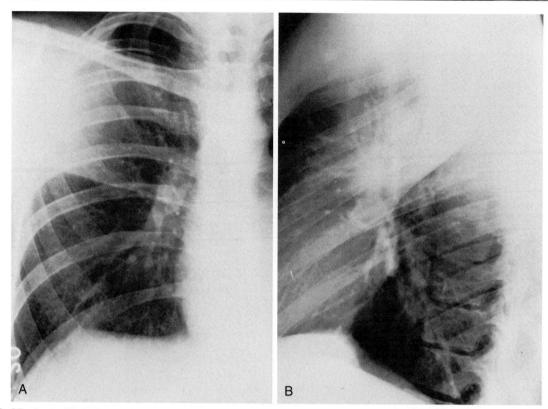

Figure 29–25. Acute *Mycoplasma* Pneumonia. Views of the right hemithorax from posteroanterior *(A)* and lateral *(B)* radiographs demonstrate homogeneous consolidation of the posterior segment of the right upper lobe. The consolidation abuts the posterior portion of the minor fissure, in keeping with the anatomic distribution of this segment. The patient was a 28-year-old man. Tests showed moderate leukopenia and positive complement fixation to *Mycoplasma pneumoniae*. Although this pattern of homogeneous consolidation occurs in some cases of acute viral or *Mycoplasma* pneumonia, in our experience it is not as common (or as characteristic) as a mixed interstitial and air-space pattern.

lar hemorrhage.[551] Patients have been described in whom the infection appeared to be followed by the development of asthma.[552] ARDS develops occasionally.[546] Rare cases present with profound hypoxemia and symptoms and signs of obstructive airway disease with carbon dioxide retention, presumably as a result of widespread bronchiolitis.[553, 554] A particularly severe form of pneumonia, with multiple lobe involvement, prolonged fever, respiratory distress, and pleural effusion, has been described in some patients with sickle cell disease.[544, 555]

Complications and extrapulmonary manifestations of *M. pneumoniae* infection are not uncommon and often more serious than respiratory tract disease.[548, 556] Manifestations of *central nervous system* involvement include meningoencephalitis, aseptic meningitis, brainstem encephalitis, ascending paralysis, transverse myelitis, acute psychosis, cerebellar ataxia, and Miller-Fisher syndrome; polyradiculitis and cranial nerve palsies can also be encountered.[522, 557–560] *Hematologic* complications include hemagglutination; hemolysis (related to the presence of cold agglutinins); thrombocytopenic purpura; acquired Pelger-Huët anomaly;[561] and peripheral venous thrombosis, sometimes associated with pulmonary thromboembolism. These complications usually occur in patients who have high titers of cold agglutinins.[562, 563]

Arthritis and *arthralgia* are relatively uncommon but may accompany a significant increase in complement-fixing antibodies;[564, 565] multiple joints are usually affected, and pain can persist for up to 18 months.[566] *Pericarditis* and *myopericarditis* sometimes cause serious morbidity or mor-

tality.[567–569] Similar to other complications, pericarditis typically becomes evident 2 to 3 weeks after the initial infection, suggesting an immunologic mechanism in its pathogenesis. *Cutaneous* disease includes maculopapular rash (sometimes simulating varicella[566]), urticaria, erythema nodosum, and erythema multiforme.[570, 571] The last-named is sometimes accompanied by a systemic reaction that includes high fever, stomatitis, and ophthalmia (Stevens-Johnson syndrome).[549, 572] *Glomerulonephritis* has been reported rarely.[573]

Laboratory Findings

The white blood cell count in mycoplasmal pneumonia is usually normal; however, levels above 10,000/mm³ have been recorded in one quarter to one third of patients.[494, 518] Eosinophilia occurs in some patients.[574] Cold agglutinins are present in a titer of greater than 1:32 in most patients. In fact, *M. pneumoniae* infection is the most common respiratory cause of cold agglutinin production.[502, 549, 575] Despite this, their presence is of little diagnostic value because approximately one quarter of cold agglutinin–positive pneumonias are caused by organisms other than *M. pneumoniae* (usually viruses).[502]

M. pneumoniae can be cultured on artificial media,[576] the organism being presumptively identified by the ability of colonies to hemolyze guinea pig erythrocytes. When positive specimens are obtained, they are almost invariably from the throat or sputum; the organism has occasionally been recovered from middle ear or skin vesicle fluid and rarely

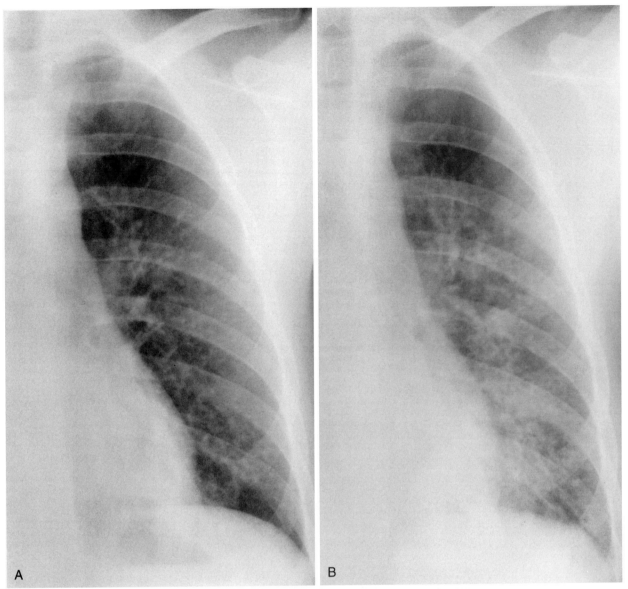

Figure 29–26. Acute *Mycoplasma* Pneumonia Demonstrating Sequential Interstitial and Air-Space Features. A detail view *(A)* of the left lung from a posteroanterior chest radiograph reveals a loss of definition and thickening of the bronchovascular bundles in the left lower lobe. A faint reticulation is suggested in some areas. Several days later *(B)*, after unsuccessful therapy with penicillin, considerable progression of the disease had occurred; patchy air-space opacities now obscure the previous interstitial abnormality. A subsequent chest radiograph showed complete resolution after tetracycline therapy. The patient was a young college student who complained of the acute onset of cough, fever, myalgia, and headache.

from blood or other body fluids.[518] Because isolation takes 1 week or longer, at which time clinical recovery is well underway in most patients, culture usually is useful only to confirm the diagnosis. Similarly a fourfold rise in specific IgG antibody titer or in cold agglutinins, by complement-fixation test, radioimmunoassay, or ELISA,[577] usually takes several weeks and is therefore of little diagnostic value during the acute phase of the disease.[578] Demonstration of the presence of *Mycoplasma*-specific IgA or IgM antibodies has been advocated as a more rapid and reliable test for early diagnosis.[549, 579]

As with other pulmonary infections, molecular diagnostic techniques can be particularly useful. Using a probe to mycoplasmal RNA, sensitivities and specificities of 75% to 100% and 85% to 95% have been reported.[580–582] PCR also yields rapid results and is highly sensitive.[583–585]

Prognosis and Natural History

Although nearly all infections caused by *M. pneumoniae* are mild,[586] pneumonia is usually more prolonged and severe than that caused by the viruses.[587] Rarely, disease is fulminant and fatal.[546, 588, 589] In a few patients, diffuse pulmonary disease results in residual dysfunction, either restrictive[590, 591] or obstructive.[592, 593] Fatal bronchiectasis has also been reported.[594]

CHLAMYDIAE

Chlamydiae are small, obligate intracellular organisms that at various times have been considered to be both viruses and protozoans. However, the presence of a cell wall and

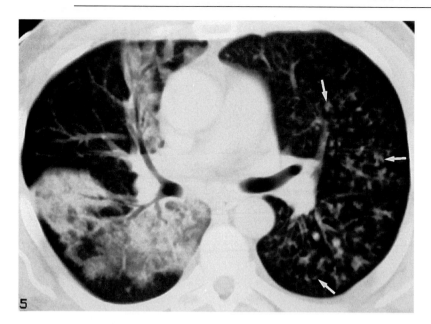

Figure 29–27. *Mycoplasma* Pneumonia. A conventional 10-mm collimation CT scan demonstrates areas of lobular and segmental consolidation in the right lung and branching linear and nodular areas of attenuation in the left lung *(arrows)*.

of DNA and RNA, the susceptibility of the organisms to antibiotics, and their capacity to synthesize limited amounts of protein and nucleic acid all indicate that they are properly classified as bacteria. They differ from the latter (including intracellular forms such as rickettsiae) chiefly by their unique mode of reproduction and by their inability to synthesize

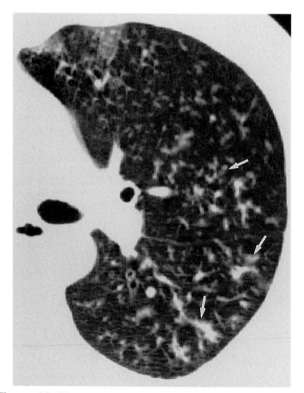

Figure 29–28. *Mycoplasma pneumoniae* Bronchiolitis. HRCT targeted to the left lung demonstrates small nodular and branching areas of increased attenuation in a centrilobular distribution *(arrows)*, consistent with bronchiolitis. Also noted are localized areas of ground-glass attenuation anteriorly, consistent with lobular pneumonia. Serologic tests were positive for *Mycoplasma pneumoniae*; open-lung biopsy demonstrated severe bronchiolitis. (From Müller NL, Miller RR: Radiology 196:3,1995.)

high-energy compounds such as adenosine triphosphate (ATP) and guanosine triphosphate (GTP).[595] The organisms are grouped in the family Chlamydiaceae; three species—*Chlamydia trachomatis, Chlamydia pneumoniae* and *Chlamydia psittaci*—can cause pulmonary disease in humans.

The organisms exist in an extracellular form as *elementary bodies* measuring 0.2 to 0.3 μm in diameter.[595] These attach to and enter susceptible cells,[595a] within which they convert to large *reticulate bodies* measuring 0.5 to 1.0 μm that undergo division to form intracellular colonies. This process occurs within the host phagosome, which remains intact as the colonies develop. The reticulate bodies themselves are noninfectious and eventually undergo conversion into numerous elementary bodies, at which point the phagosome membrane disrupts, the cell dies, and the elementary bodies are released. On disruption of the membrane, the release of phagolysosomal enzymes is believed to be responsible for cell lysis; whether this is the cause of cell death or only a reflection of it is not known.[595]

Chlamydia pneumoniae

In the mid-1980s, a new strain of *Chlamydia* was isolated from patients with pneumonia and labeled *TWAR* because of its similarity to isolates previously designated *TW-183* and *AR-39*. Subsequent genetic analysis showed the organism to be distinct from *C. trachomatis* and *C. psittaci*, and it was renamed *C. pneumoniae*. Clinical and epidemiologic studies since have found it to be one of the more common causes of community-acquired pneumonia. Possible associations between infection and the development of pulmonary carcinoma[598] and asthma[599, 599a] have also been suggested.

Seroepidemiologic studies have detected antibodies to the organism in a substantial number of individuals in several countries.[600–602] The prevalence of antibodies is relatively low in children but increases progressively thereafter to reach a level of about 50%. The incidence of clinically evident disease appears to be about 5% to 10% of cases of nonbacterial lower respiratory tract infection.[122, 602, 603] Although it usually occurs sporadically, outbreaks of disease in families and in local communities have been described.[604–606, 614] There is some evidence for an increased prevalence of antibodies and, possibly, risk of pneumonia in patients with AIDS.[606] Patients who have COPD[607, 608] or cystic fibrosis[610] also appear to have an increased risk of infection; there is evidence that disease in the former group may be chronic.[612] The mode of transmission and natural reservoir of the organism are uncertain. Pathologic features of the infection are poorly documented because the disease is rarely fatal.

Radiographic manifestations have been described in one series of 55 adults hospitalized for community-acquired pneumonia.[609] Based on serologic criteria, the patients were categorized as having either acute primary (17 patients, 31%) or recurrent (38 patients, 69%) infection. Radiographic findings in the first group included air-space consolidation in 11 patients, interstitial opacities in 2, combined interstitial and air-space opacities in 3, and a normal chest radiograph in 1. The consolidation was unilateral in 12, lobar in 9, and multifocal in 3. Pleural effusions were present in only three patients. Of the 38 patients with recurrent infection, 11 had air-space consolidation; 14 had interstitial opacities; 6 had a combination of air-space and interstitial opacities; and 7 had other findings, including areas of atelectasis, small nodules, and biapical cavitation. Fourteen of the 38 had unilateral abnormalities, and 24 had bilateral disease. Eleven had pleural effusion, typically of small-to-medium size. In both groups, the radiographic abnormalities tended to progress to bilateral, mixed, interstitial, and air-space opacities during the course of infection.

The most common clinical manifestations are sore throat, nonproductive cough, and fever; hoarseness occurs in some patients. In one study of 65 patients presenting to the emergency department with a principal symptom of cough lasting longer than 2 weeks and less than 3 months, 13 (20%) were found to have serologic evidence of recent *C. pneumoniae* infection.[611] There is some evidence that the organism can cause systemic vasculitis.[613] Disease is usually mild, self-limited, and without sequela. However, fatalities have been reported in some patients with underlying disease; moreover, in one epidemiologic study of 61 patients who had severe community-acquired pneumonia, 10% were found to be infected by *C. pneumoniae*.[615]

The virus can be isolated on tissue culture and identified with specific antibodies.[596] A direct immunofluorescence test using *C. pneumoniae* antigen is both sensitive and specific and is widely used for diagnosis; it has been performed successfully on both throat swabs and on specimens derived from the lower respiratory tract.[615a] IgM-capture ELISA[616] and ELISPOT[617] tests have also been reported to be reliable. The use of PCR as a diagnostic tool is likely to become even more important in the future.[597]

Chlamydia trachomatis

Strains of *C. trachomatis* can be divided into two major groups: (1) those that cause genitourinary infections in adults and conjunctivitis and pneumonia in infants born to infected mothers; and (2) those that show tropism for lymph nodes (lymphogranuloma venereum strains) and that occasionally cause interstitial pneumonitis or a granulomatous proctitis that resembles Crohn's disease.[618]

It has been estimated that 2% to 13% of women in city hospitals in the United States are infected with *C. trachomatis* and that infants born to such mothers have a 50% chance of acquiring conjunctivitis and a 10% to 20% risk of developing pneumonia.[618, 619] The latter invariably occurs before the age of 6 months (usually from 2 to 14 weeks). Affected infants typically have paroxysmal "staccato" cough and tachypnea, sometimes associated with otitis media. Fever is usually mild or absent. The organism can be grown from the upper respiratory passages; blood eosinophilia and markedly elevated IgM antibody titers to *C. trachomatis* are usually present.[619–621] *C. trachomatis* has also been recovered from the lower respiratory tract of adults[622] and has been shown to cause pneumonia in both immunocompromised[623–625] and immunocompetent individuals.[626, 627]

There are few reports of the pathologic findings in cases of *C. trachomatis* pneumonia. Peribronchiolar foci of chronic interstitial and air-space inflammation have been described in one patient who had undergone bone marrow transplantation.[623] Similar findings as well as lymphocytic, plasmacytic, and eosinophilic infiltration of tracheobronchial epithelium have been reported in experimental infection in baboons.[628]

In infants with *C. trachomatis* pneumonia, the chest radiograph has been described as showing bilateral diffuse interstitial and air-space disease associated with areas of overinflation and atelectasis.[620, 629] In one study of six adults, streaky, multilobar interstitial disease with areas of plate-like atelectasis were documented.[630] Pleural effusion[631, 632] and mediastinal lymph node enlargement[631] have also been described in some cases.

Clinically, lower respiratory tract infection in adults ranges from acute bronchitis to severe diffuse interstitial pneumonia.[622] Symptoms and signs are nonspecific. Limited experience with infection in adults indicates that specific antibodies to *C. trachomatis* do not reach levels as high as in children.[622, 626] A simple, sensitive enzyme-linked fluorescence immunoassay has been described in which reticulate and elementary bodies from *C. trachomatis* are employed as antigens to detect IgM antibody.[633] The complement-fixation test is genus specific, and positive results may lead to an erroneous diagnosis of ornithosis;[627] microimmunofluorescence is required to reveal species-specific antibodies.

Chlamydia psittaci

C. psittaci is a common pathogen of many birds and mammals that only occasionally infects humans. Because human illness was initially associated with parrots, parakeets, and other members of the order Psittaciformis, it has been widely known as *psittacosis*, although the presence of disease in many other birds suggests that the term *ornithosis* is more appropriate. Even this term, however, is not strictly correct because the disease is acquired occasionally from mammals (usually ewes) stricken with enzootic abortion.[634, 635]

Epidemiology

Although *C. psittaci* has been reported to infect more than 100 species of birds,[636] most human cases in which a history of exposure can be obtained are acquired from parakeets,[637] pigeons, or poultry.[638, 639] Pathologic changes in infected birds occur much more often in the abdominal organs than in the respiratory tract, and the organisms are excreted in the feces and urine, especially at breeding time or in crowded and unsanitary conditions. Organisms are resistant to drying and remain viable for at least a month at ambient temperature; thus, in most cases, human infection results from the inhalation of dried, contaminated bird excreta. The disease can be acquired at any time of the year, although the incidence has been found to be slightly greater during the cold months and early spring by some investigators.[640] The incubation period ranges from 6 to 20 days.[638]

When considering the potential risk of avian exposure in the clinical history, several features must be remembered. Although the bird or birds responsible may have been obviously ill or may have died from the disease, this is not invariable.[641, 642] In addition, infection may be acquired from a recently purchased bird that, having acquired immunity, remains healthy. Finally, a history of avian exposure is not always obtained;[643] for example, only 17% of the patients in sporadic cases in England in 1980 had known contact with birds.[636] The mode of infection in such cases is often unclear. Person-to-person transmission has been documented[644] or suspected[642] in some cases. Rare examples of human pneumonia have also been associated with chlamydial animal infection, usually abortion in domestic animals, such as cattle, sheep, or goats.[634, 635]

Although the incidence of disease is probably low, it is likely that it is underdiagnosed and that some cases labeled as primary atypical or viral pneumonia could be proved to be ornithosis with careful history taking and appropriate serologic testing. Asymptomatic or mild infection is also likely more frequent than might be considered from the number of reported cases; for example, after an unusually large outbreak of infection that originated from sick parakeets in a department store in Hamilton, Ontario, a survey of 83 persons who might have been exposed revealed specific serum agglutinins in 38 (45%).[645]

Disease can occur sporadically or in epidemics, the latter usually among poultry workers.[637–639] An occasional rather abrupt increase in incidence of the disease—in the United Kingdom in 1964, 61 cases were recorded compared with an average of 2 or 3 in previous years[644]—suggests that epidemics may originate from an infected wild bird population when climatic conditions allow desiccation of excreta and subsequent dissemination of contaminated dust.

Pathologic Characteristics

The pathologic characteristics of mild disease have been studied in experimentally infected monkeys.[646] The earliest findings consist of small aggregates of mononuclear and polymorphonuclear inflammatory cells in the vicinity of the respiratory bronchioles, followed by extension of the infiltrate into contiguous alveoli. Older lesions show intra-alveolar fibrin and abundant mononuclear cells without evidence of necrosis. Alveolar epithelial cells are hyperplastic, especially at the periphery of individual inflammatory foci. Histologic resolution begins 2 to 3 weeks after exposure, and by the end of the fifth week the only evidence of prior disease is mild pleural fibrosis.

Pathologic features of fatal human disease consist of intra-alveolar edema, hemorrhage, fibrin, and a mononuclear inflammatory infiltrate.[647–649] The interstitium is mildly to moderately thickened by mononuclear cells and edema; type II cells are usually hyperplastic, and hyaline membranes may be present (diffuse alveolar damage).[635] Focal areas of airway ulceration and epithelial hyperplasia have also been documented in some cases.[648] Intracytoplasmic inclusions can be identified, but usually with difficulty. With Macchiavellos' stain, the fully developed intracytoplasmic bodies may be identified as small, somewhat rod-shaped inclusions.

Radiologic Manifestations

The chest radiograph is usually abnormal; in one outbreak, evidence of pneumonia was present in 21 (72%) of 29 patients.[650] The pattern has been described as a homogeneous ground-glass opacity, sometimes containing small areas of radiolucency,[644] a patchy reticular pattern radiating from the hilar areas or involving the lung bases,[651–653] and segmental or nonsegmental consolidation with or without atelectasis (Fig. 29–29). Enlargement of hilar lymph nodes was a common feature in one series of 29 patients,[651] and a miliary pattern has been described in one patient.[654]

Radiographic resolution often is delayed for many weeks after clinical cure has occurred. The interval between the first abnormal radiograph and complete resolution averages about 6 weeks, with a range of 1 to 20 weeks;[636, 644, 654] in one series of 29 cases, radiologic abnormalities were still apparent at 6 weeks in 48% and for more than 9 weeks in 17%.[651]

Clinical Manifestations

Ornithosis varies in intensity from a mild febrile episode to severe pneumonia indistinguishable from an acute bacterial infection;[652] it can also be manifested as chronic, recurrent disease. Onset may be insidious or abrupt. In more severe cases, the presentation tends to simulate typhoid, including bradycardia and even "rose spots."[654, 655] Headaches, fever, and chills are almost invariable.[650, 656] The most prominent respiratory symptom is cough, which is usually dry but may be productive of nonpurulent mucoid material;[652] hemoptysis occurs occasionally. Pleuritic pain and dyspnea may develop in cases of overwhelming infection. Systemic symptoms and signs include malaise, anorexia, nausea and vomiting, pharyngitis, polyarthritis, myalgia, and abdominal pain.[644, 652]

Physical signs may consist only of basal crackles;[644] however, signs of frank parenchymal consolidation have been described, and a friction rub may be heard.[652] Hepatosplenomegaly and superficial lymph node enlargement may be present.[653] An association between *C. psittaci* bacteremia and a clinical picture of sarcoidosis has been reported in a single patient.[657] Fulminant, often fatal disease with respiratory insufficiency and disseminated intravascular coagulation can occur.[642, 658, 659]

Laboratory Findings

The white blood cell count ranges from normal to moderately increased, with or without eosinophilia.[652] Hemo-

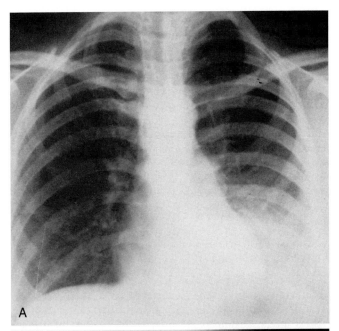

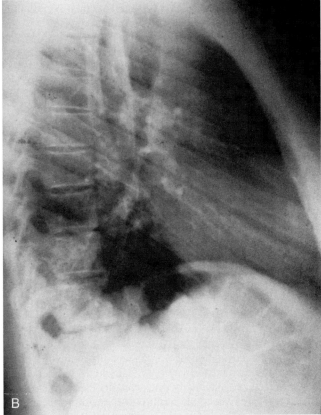

Figure 29–29. Acute Psittacosis (Ornithosis). Posteroanterior *(A)* and lateral *(B)* radiographs reveal homogeneous consolidation of the basal segments of the left lower lobe associated with slight loss of volume; an air bronchogram is not visualized, and there is no evidence of left hilar lymph node enlargement. This 34-year-old woman had recently acquired a parakeet; *Chlamydia psittaci* was recovered from the sputum.

lytic anemia was present in one patient in the absence of cold agglutinins.[660] Proteinuria may occur, and liver function may be disturbed.[652]

The organism can be recovered from the blood during the first 4 days and from the sputum during the first 2 weeks of illness. It can be isolated by culture of spleen or liver tissue in the intraperitoneal cavity of mice, in chicken embryos, and on tissue; growth occurs in 5 to 30 days. Complement-fixation antibodies appear in the second to fourth week of the disease, and the diagnosis can be confirmed by a fourfold rise in paired samples.

RICKETTSIAE

Rickettsiae are small (0.3 to 0.7 μm × 1.0 to 2.0 μm), obligate, intracellular organisms that are properly classified as bacteria. They are found naturally in a variety of arthropods and are transmitted to humans and animals by their bites. Four groups cause disease in humans, of which the major organism responsible for respiratory disease is *Coxiella burnetii*. Pneumonia may also occur occasionally in endemic (scrub) typhus. Although usually not clinically prominent, pulmonary involvement in Rocky Mountain spotted fever is commonly present at autopsy. Similar disease is seen occasionally in fulminant Mediterranean spotted fever.

Coxiella burnetii

Q fever is caused by *C. burnetii,* an organism distinguished from other rickettsiae by its gram positivity with alcoholic iodine, lack of pathogenicity for mice, and a variety of antigenic and metabolic characteristics.[661] It is exceptionally resistant to drying and to chemical agents and can survive for many months in a hostile extracellular environment. The organism can be isolated by inoculation of infected material into the peritoneal cavity of guinea pigs and can be cultured in chick embryos, growth occurring in 4 to 14 days.

Epidemiology

C. burnetii has been isolated from insects; arachnids; birds; and a variety of wild and domestic animals, particularly sheep, cattle, and goats.[662] Its natural reservoir appears to be ticks, from which it is transmitted to other hosts by bites. The resistance of the organism to drying favors transmission by inhalation, and most infections emanate from laboratory cultures[663] or from infected animals used in research[664–667] or slaughtered in abattoirs.[668–670] Animals are especially contagious after parturition (the organism grows well in the reproductive tract of cows and can be recovered from the placenta);[671] an outbreak has even been described after exposure to a parturient cat.[672] Although most miniepidemics can be traced to domestic animals, there has been a report of an outbreak associated with exposure to wild rabbits[673] and one in an urban area in which the source was never discovered.[674] The organism can be recovered from milk, although pasteurization destroys it, and ingestion is a relatively unimportant mechanism of spread in developed countries. The possibility that the organism may primarily infect tissue adjacent to ventriculoperitoneal drains or artificial cardiac valves has been postulated.[675] Person-to-person transmission is rare.[676]

Q fever is worldwide in distribution, having been described originally in Australia (Queensland fever) and subsequently in the United States, Europe, and elsewhere. Pneumonia has been estimated to occur in about 5% of cases in Australia, in contrast to an incidence of approximately 50% in patients in the United States and the United Kingdom,[670] a finding that may reflect a difference in the virulence of strains of the organism. As might be expected from the discussion of transmission, there is a strong occupational association; farmers, abattoir and stock-yard workers, and veterinary and medical laboratory personnel are at particular risk. The incubation period ranges from 1 to 6 weeks, averaging about 14 days.[663, 670]

Pathologic Characteristics

Pathologic characteristics of Q fever pneumonia have seldom been documented, usually in single case reports.[677–680] According to these, histologic findings are nonspecific and consist predominantly of mild interstitial inflammation and alveolar air-space filling by a combination of blood, edema fluid, fibrin, and mononuclear inflammatory cells (both lymphocytes and macrophages); necrosis may be present.[677] Airways contain a similar exudate, and their walls may show focal areas of epithelial ulceration and a mononuclear inflammatory infiltrate. Organisms may be identified in some cases both intracellularly and extracellularly by Macchiavellos' stain and by Wolbach's modifications of the Giemsa stain.

Several cases have presented as inflammatory pseudotumors.[681] In one that appeared grossly as a nonencapsulated mass in the left upper lobe, histologic examination showed an infiltrate of lymphocytes, plasma cells, macrophages, and fibroblasts that surrounded and obliterated bronchioles and alveolar air spaces;[682] organisms consistent with *C. burnetii* were identified within the mass by both electron microscopy and immunofluorescence.

Radiologic Manifestations

In a review of 35 patients with serologically confirmed Q fever, the most common radiographic findings consisted of multiple areas of rounded consolidation that measured 5 to 20 cm in diameter and were usually situated in the lower lobes.[683] Some patients had lobar or sublobar consolidation associated with loss of volume (Fig. 29–30). A small pleural effusion was present in three patients. Basal linear opacities interpreted by the author as "linear atelectasis" were frequent. Resolution tended to be slow, ranging from 10 to 70 days and averaging 30 days. The high frequency of rounded pneumonias with *C. burnetii* infection has also been documented by other investigators.[684, 685] However, in another review of 21 cases, the most common radiographic finding consisted of segmental consolidation (in 17 of 21 patients); lobar consolidation was found in 5 patients and rounded areas of consolidation in only 4.[686]

Clinical Manifestations

Onset of the disease is usually insidious, with malaise for several days followed by headache (sometimes severe), chills, myalgia, and arthralgia; nausea, vomiting, and diarrhea occur in a minority of cases.[667] Pulmonary involvement is characterized by dry cough and, in severe cases, dyspnea

and chest pain. Fever is frequently remittent and may last for several weeks.[687] Extrapulmonary disease is common and includes hepatitis, endocarditis,[688] myocarditis,[689] meningoencephalitis,[690] and phlebitis; complications from the latter can be more prolonged and disabling than the original infection.[687] The illness may have a chronic progressive course or relapse and recur;[663, 681] in most such cases, the heart is the principal site of disease.

The organism can be isolated from the urine, blood, sputum, or pleural fluid. Complement-fixing and agglutinating antibodies appear within 2 to 3 weeks, and the titer is maximal approximately 30 days after onset of clinical symptoms.[663, 670] The disease is usually self-limited, and few patients develop long-term sequelae. The mortality is probably less than 1%.[687]

Rickettsia tsutsugamushi

R. tsutsugamushi is the cause of scrub typhus, a disease occurring primarily in the southwest Pacific, southeast Asia, Australia, and Japan. Its incidence is highest during the hottest months. Humans are infected by the bite of a mite, causing a local lesion followed by enlargement of draining lymph nodes; pneumonia occurs occasionally.

Histologic findings of pulmonary infection are nonspecific, consisting of an interstitial mononuclear infiltrate and alveolar consolidation by edema, fibrin, and mononuclear cells. Radiographically the pneumonia may be interstitial or, less often, in the form of homogeneous consolidation. Affected patients have a maculopapular rash, fever, splenomegaly, cough (often with hemoptysis), myocarditis, and encephalitis. The white blood cell count may be normal, or there may be leukopenia. The organism is recoverable from the peritoneal cavity of mice injected with blood from patients with the disease. Agglutinins to *Proteus* OX-K antigen appear during the second or third week, and specific complement-fixing antibodies also may be demonstrable.

Rickettsia rickettsii

Rocky Mountain spotted fever is an acute and often fulminant disease caused by *Rickettsia rickettsii*. It is found exclusively in North and South America and, despite its name, is most prevalent in the eastern United States. Humans are infected by the bite of several species of tick, so that the majority of cases occur during the warm months. From the initial site of inoculation, the organisms disseminate via the bloodstream and invade capillary endothelial cells, where they multiply and eventually cause endothelial necrosis, vasculitis, and thrombosis; the result is widespread tissue necrosis and hemorrhage. The skin, subcutaneous tissues, and central nervous system are most severely affected. Although respiratory involvement is usually not a prominent clinical feature of the disease, findings indicating lower respiratory tract involvement (crackles, abnormal chest radiograph, impaired gas exchange) were observed in about 40% of patients in one series at some time in the course of the illness.[691]

Pathologic changes in the lungs have been found in a high proportion of patients who have undergone autopsy.[692–694] Gross examination reveals edema, congestion, focal hemorrhage, and (occasionally) bronchopneumonia. Microscopically, there is a diffuse interstitial mononuclear

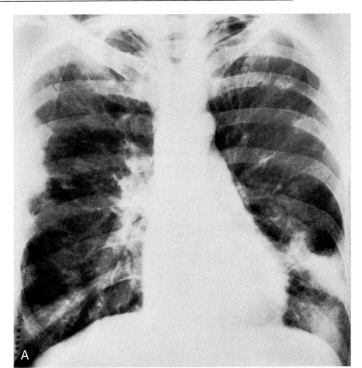

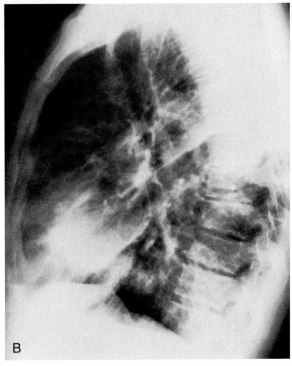

Figure 29–30. Q Fever Pneumonia. This 37-year-old man had had mild symptoms described as a "chest cold" for 3 weeks before admission; on the morning of admission, he was awakened with a severe pain in the left side of the chest, made worse by deep breathing. Posteroanterior *(A)* and lateral *(B)* radiographs show local areas of homogeneous consolidation in the right upper and lower lobes, the lingula, and the left lower lobe. In no area is the consolidation truly segmental, although the pattern is typically one of air-space consolidation. Four serum samples showed a rising titer of complement-fixing antibodies to *Coxiella burnetii* during the 4 weeks following these radiographs, maximum being 1:256. Radiologic resolution was slow and was not complete at the time of the last available radiograph 5 weeks later. (Courtesy of Sherbrooke Hospital, Sherbrooke, Quebec.)

inflammatory infiltrate, intra-alveolar edema and hemorrhage, and vasculitis and thrombosis of pulmonary capillaries and small venules and arterioles. The organisms can be demonstrated along vascular walls by immunofluorescence, presumably within endothelial cells as in other tissues.

Radiologic manifestations in the chest are quite variable. In one study, six patients were described in whom diffuse pulmonary opacities were associated with cardiac enlargement and presumably represented pulmonary edema resulting from cardiac decompensation;[695] it was suggested that the latter was secondary to myocardial vasculitis. Of 13

patients with abnormal chest radiographs in another investigation, the predominant abnormalities were focal air-space consolidation (in 3 patients), diffuse air-space consolidation (in 4), diffuse interstitial disease (in 6), and pleural effusion (in 4);[696] cardiac enlargement was observed in only 1 patient. Diffuse parenchymal consolidation has also been thought to be caused by noncardiogenic pulmonary edema.[691]

Clinically, patients present with fever, rash, headaches, and myalgia. Involvement of the respiratory tract is typically manifested by cough.[691] An association of particularly severe disease with glucose-6-phosphate dehydrogenase deficiency has been noted.[692] Patients with radiologic evidence of diffuse interstitial and air-space disease have been found to have a mortality rate of about 50%, whereas patients with focal disease tend to recover.[696]

Rickettsia conorii

Mediterranean spotted fever (South African tick bite fever, African or Indian tick typhus, boutonneuse fever) is an acute febrile illness, usually of mild-to-moderate severity, caused by *Rickettsia conorii*. Disease is transmitted by ticks[697] and is found principally in Southern Europe, Africa, the Middle East, and India. Travelers to these regions who subsequently develop the disease in their own country are being recognized with increased frequency.[698]

The majority of infections caused by *R. conorii* are mild and self-limited, the usual manifestations being a primary skin ulcer that develops a black eschar (the *tache noire*, corresponding to the site of the initial tick bite), regional lymphadenitis, and a disseminated maculopapular skin rash. Headache, fever, and myalgia are frequent. Symptoms and signs of visceral disease, including pneumonia, occur in a minority of patients. Pathologic findings in the lungs in the few reported patients who have had autopsies have been similar to those of Rocky Mountain spotted fever.[697, 699] Organisms can be identified within alveolar vessels by immunofluorescent techniques.

REFERENCES

1. Denny FW: Atypical pneumonia and the Armed Forces Epidemiological Board. J Infect Dis 143:305, 1981.
2. Denny FW Jr: The clinical impact of human respiratory virus infections. Am J Respir Crit Care Med 152:S4, 1995.
2a. Andersen P: Pathogenesis of lower respiratory tract infections due to Chlamydia, Mycoplasma, Legionella and viruses. Thorax 53:302, 1998.
3. Spickard A: The common cold: Past, present and future research. Survey of the literature. Dis Chest 48:545, 1965.
3a. Falsey AR, McCann RM, Hall WJ, et al: Acute respiratory tract infection in daycare centers for older persons. J Am Geriatr Soc 43:30, 1995.
4. Yang E, Rubin BK: "Childhood" viruses as a cause of pneumonia in adults. Semin Respir Infect 10:232, 1995.
5. Chidekel AS, Rosen CL, Bazzy AR: Rhinovirus infection associated with serious lower respiratory illness in patients with bronchopulmonary dysplasia. Pediatr Infect Dis J 16:43, 1997.
6. Omenaas E, Bakke P, Haukenes G, et al: Respiratory virus antibodies in adults of a Norwegian community: Prevalences and risk factors. Int J Epidemiol 24:223, 1995.
7. Ellenbogen C, Graybill JR, Silva J, et al: Bacterial pneumonia complicating adenoviral pneumonia. Am J Med 56:169, 1974.
8. How does influenza virus pave the way for bacteria [editorial]? Lancet 1:485, 1982.
9. Jakab GJ: Pulmonary defense mechanisms and the interaction between viruses and bacteria in acute respiratory infections. Bull Eur Physiopathol 13:119, 1977.
10. Gerrard CS, Levandowski RA, Gerrity TR, et al: The effects of acute respiratory virus infection upon tracheal mucous transport. Arch Environ Health 40:322, 1985.
11. Levandowski RA, Gerrity TR, Garrard CS, et al: Modifications of lung clearance mechanisms by acute influenza A infection. J Lab Clin Med 106:428, 1985.
12. Carson JL, Collier AM, Hu S-CS: Acquired ciliary defects in nasal epithelium of children with acute viral upper respiratory infections. N Engl J Med 312:463, 1985.
13. Jakab GJ: Immune impairment of alveolar macrophage phagocytosis during influenza virus pneumonia. Am Rev Respir Dis 126:778, 1982.
14. Jakab GJ, Warr GA: Immune-enhanced phagocytic dysfunction in pulmonary macrophages infected with parainfluenza 1 (Sendai) virus. Am Rev Respir Dis 124:575, 1981.
15. Larson HE, Parry RP, Tyrrell DAJ: Impaired polymorphonuclear leucocyte chemotaxis after influenza virus infection. Br J Dis Chest 74:56, 1980.
16. Plotkowski M-C, Puchelle E, Beck G, et al: Adherence of Type I Streptococcus pneumoniae to tracheal epithelium of mice infected with influenza A/PR8 virus. Am Rev Respir Dis 134:1040, 1986.
16a. Wadowsky RM, Mietzner SM, Skoner DP, et al: Effect of experimental influenza A virus infection on isolation of Streptococcus pneumoniae and other aerobic bacteria from the oropharynges of allergic and nonallergic adult subjects. Infect Immun 63:1153, 1995.
17. Shale DJ: Viral infections: A role in the lung disease of cystic fibrosis? Thorax 47:69, 1992.
18. Castleman WL, Sorkness RL, Lemanske RF, et al: Neonatal viral bronchiolitis and pneumonia induces bronchiolar hypoplasia and alveolar dysplasia in rats. Lab Invest 59:387, 1988.
18a. Folkerts G, Busse WW, Nijkamp FP, et al: Virus-induced airway hyperresponsiveness and asthma. Am J Respir Crit Care Med 157:1708, 1998.
19. Shaheen SO, Barker DJ, Shiell AW, et al: The relationship between pneumonia in early childhood and impaired lung function in late adult life. Am J Respir Crit Care Med 149:616, 1994.
20. Matsuse T, Hayashi S, Kuwano K, et al: Latent adenoviral infection in the pathogenesis of chronic airways obstruction. Am Rev Respir Dis 148:177, 1992.
21. Shelhamer JH, Gill VJ, Quinn TC, et al: The laboratory evaluation of opportunistic pulmonary infections. Ann Intern Med 124:585, 1996.
22. Akhtar N, Ni J, Langston C, et al: PCR diagnosis of viral pneumonitis from fixed-lung tissue in children. Biochem Mol Med 58:66, 1996.
23. Oda Y, Katsuda S, Okada Y, et al: Detection of human CMV, Epstein-Barr virus, and herpes simplex virus in diffuse interstitial pneumonia by polymerase chain reaction and immunohistochemistry. Am J Clin Pathol 102:495, 1994.
24. Connolly MG Jr, Baughman RP, Dohn MN, et al: Recovery of viruses other than CMV from bronchoalveolar lavage fluid. Chest 105:1775, 1994.
25. Skehel JJ, Wiley DC: Influenza viruses and cell membranes. Am J Respir Crit Care Med 152:S13, 1995.
26. Rott RR, Klenk HD, Nagai Y, et al: Influenza viruses, cell enzymes, and pathogenicity. Am J Respir Crit Care Med 152:S16, 1995.
27. Smeenk CA, Wright KE, Burns BF, et al: Mutations in the hemagglutinin and matrix genes of a virulent influenza virus variant, A/FM/1/47-MA, control different stages in pathogenesis. Virus Res 44:79, 1996.
28. Nolan TF Jr: Influenza vaccine efficacy. JAMA 245:1762, 1981.
29. Piedra PA: Influenza virus pneumonia: Pathogenesis, treatment, and prevention. Semin Respir Infect 10:216, 1995.
30. Hobson D: Acute respiratory virus infections. BMJ 2:229, 1973.
31. Nolan TF Jr, Goodman RA, Hinman AR, et al: Morbidity and mortality associated with influenza B in the United States, 1979–1980: A report from the Centers for Disease Control. J Infect Dis 142:360, 1980.
32. Glezen WP: Viral pneumonia as a cause and result of hospitalization. J Infect Dis 147:765, 1983.
33. Glezen WP: Influenza C virus infection. Arch Intern Med 140:1278, 1980.
34. Dykes AC, Cherry JD, Nolan CE: A clinical, epidemiologic, serologic, and virologic study of influenza C virus infection. Arch Intern Med 140:1295, 1980.
35. Wentworth DE, Thompson BL, Xu X, et al: An influenza A (H_1N_1) virus, closely related to swine influenza virus, responsible for a fatal case of human influenza. J Virol 68:2051, 1994.
36. Webster RG, Sharp GB, Claas EC: Interspecies transmission of influenza viruses. Am J Respir Crit Care Med 152:S16, 1995.
37. Gill PW, Murphy AM: Naturally acquired immunity to influenza type A: Lessons from two coexisting subtypes. Med J Aust 142:94, 1985.
38. Davies KJ, Herbert AM, Westmoreland D, et al: Seroepidemiological study of respiratory virus infections among dental surgeons. Br Dent J 176:262, 1994.
39. Van Voris LP, Belshe RB, Shaffer JL: Nosocomial influenza B virus infection in the elderly. Ann Intern Med 96:153, 1982.
40. Frank AL, Taber LH, Wells CR, et al: Patterns of shedding of myxoviruses and paramyxoviruses in children. J Infect Dis 144:433, 1981.
41. Harford CG: Influenza viral pneumonia of human beings. Am J Med 29:907, 1960.
42. Kark JD, Lebiush M, Rannon L: Cigarette smoking as a risk factor for epidemic A(H_1N_1) influenza in young men. N Engl J Med 307:1042, 1982.
43. Neilson DB: Sudden death due to fulminating influenza. BMJ 1:420, 1958.
44. Louria DB, Blumenfeld HL, Ellis JT, et al: Studies on influenza in the pandemic of 1957–1958: II. Pulmonary complications of influenza. J Clin Invest 38:213, 1959.
45. Kaye D, Rosenbluth M, Hood EW, et al: Endemic influenza: II. The nature of the disease in the post-pandemic period. Am Rev Respir Dis 85:9, 1962.
46. Soto PJ, Broun GO, Wyatt JP: Asian influenzal pneumonitis: A structural and virologic analysis. Am J Med 27:18, 1959.
47. Tillett HE, Smith JWG, Clifford RE: Excess morbidity and mortality associated with influenza in England and Wales. Lancet 1:793, 1980.
48. Mullooly JP, Barker WH, Nolan TF Jr: Risk of acute respiratory disease among pregnant women during influenza A epidemics. Public Health Rep 101:205, 1986.
49. Conway SP, Simmonds EJ, Littlewood JM: Acute severe deterioration in cystic fibrosis associated with influenza A virus infection. Thorax 47:112, 1992.
50. Leading article: Epidemic influenza and general hospitals. BMJ 4:655, 1968.
51. Monto AS, Kendal AP: Effect of neuraminidase antibody on Hong Kong influenza. Lancet 1:623, 1973.
52. Bradley SF: Influenza in the elderly: Prevention is the best strategy in high-risk populations. Postgrad Med 99:138, 1996.
53. Feldman PS, Cohan MA, Hierholzer WJ Jr: Fatal Hong Kong influenza: A clinical microbiological and pathological analysis of nine cases. Yale J Biol Med 45:49, 1972.
54. Patriarca PA, Kendal AP, Zakowski PC, et al: Lack of significant person-to-person spread of swine influenza-like virus following fatal infection in an immunocompromised child. Am J Epidemiol 119:152, 1984.
55. Oseasohn R, Adelson L, Kaji M: Clinicopathologic study of thirty-three fatal cases of Asian influenza. N Engl J Med 260:509, 1959.
56. Kilbourne ED: Studies on influenza in the pandemic of 1957–1958: III. Isolation of influenza A (Asian strain) viruses from influenza patients with pulmonary complications: Details of virus isolation and characterization of isolates, with quantitative comparison of isolation methods. J Clin Invest 38:266, 1959.
57. Schwarzmann SW, Adler JL, Sullivan RJ Jr, et al: Bacterial pneumonia during the Hong Kong influenza epidemic of 1968–1969: Experience in a city-county hospital. Arch Intern Med 127:1037, 1971.
58. Young LS, LaForce FM, Head JJ, et al: A simultaneous outbreak of meningococcal and influenza infections. N Engl J Med 287:5, 1972.
59. Cartwright KAV, Jones DM, Smith AM, et al: Influenza A and meningococcal disease. Lancet 338:554, 1991.
60. Fischer JJ, Walker DH: Invasive pulmonary aspergillosis associated with influenza. JAMA 241:1493, 1979.
61. Dourmashkin RR, Tyrrell DAJ: Attachment of two myxoviruses to ciliated epithelial cells. J Gen Virol 9:77, 1970.
62. Stinson SF, Ryan DP, Hertweek MS, et al: Epithelial and surfactant changes in influenzal pulmonary lesions. Arch Pathol Lab Med 100:147, 1976.
63. Horisberger MA: Interferons, Mx genes, and resistance to influenza virus. Am J Respir Crit Care Med 152:S67, 1995.
64. McMichael A: Cytotoxic T lymphocytes specific for influenza virus. Curr Top Microbiol Immunol 189:75, 1994.
65. Hartshorn KL, Reid KB, White MR, et al: Neutrophil deactivation by influenza A viruses: Mechanisms of protection after viral opsonization with collectins and hemagglutination-inhibiting antibodies. Blood 87:3450, 1996.
66. Benne CA, Kraaijeveld CA, van Strijp JA, et al: Interactions of surfactant protein A with influenza A viruses: Binding and neutralization. J Infect Dis 171:335, 1995.
67. Jakab GJ, Astry CL, Warr GA: Alveolitis induced by influenza virus. Am Rev Resp Dis 128:730, 1983.
68. Tashiro M, Ciborwski P, Klenk H-D, et al: The role of Staphylococcus protease in the development of influenza pneumonia. Nature 325:536, 1987.

69. Noble RL, Lillington GA, Kempson RL: Fatal diffuse influenzal pneumonia: Premortem diagnosis by lung biopsy. Chest 63:644, 1973.
70. Walsh JJ, Dietlein LF, Low FN, et al: Bronchotracheal response in human influenza type A, Asian strain, as studied by light and electron microscopic examination of bronchoscopic biopsies. Arch Intern Med 108:376, 1961.
71. Yeldandi AV, Colby TV: Pathologic features of lung biopsy specimens from influenza pneumonia cases. Hum Pathol 25:47, 1994.
72. Hers JFPh, Masurel N, Mulder J: Bacteriology and histopathology of the respiratory tract and lungs in fatal Asian influenza. Lancet 2:1141, 1958.
73. Pinsker KL, Schneyer B, Becker N, et al: Usual interstitial pneumonia following Texas A2 influenza infection. Chest 80:1123, 1981.
74. McQuillin J, Gardner PS, McGuckin R: Rapid diagnosis of influenza by immunofluorescent techniques. Lancet 2:690, 1970.
75. Tamura H, Aronson BE: Intranuclear fibrillary inclusions in influenza pneumonia. Arch Pathol Lab Med 102:252, 1978.
76. Fry J: Influenza A (Asian) 1957: Clinical and epidemiological features in a general practice. BMJ 1:259, 1959.
77. Galloway RW, Miller RS: Lung changes in the recent influenza epidemic. Br J Radiol 32:28, 1959.
78. Monto AS, Koopman JS, Longini IM Jr: Tecumseh study of illness: XIII. Influenza infection and disease, 1976–1981. Am J Epidemiol 121:811, 1985.
79. Taylor R, Nemaia H, Tukuitonga C, et al: An epidemic of influenza in the population of Niue. J Med Virol 16:127, 1985.
80. Spelman DW, McHardy CJ: Concurrent outbreaks of influenza A and influenza. Br J Hyg 94:331, 1905.
81. Little JW, Hall WJ, Douglas RG, et al: Airway hyperreactivity and peripheral airway dysfunction in influenza A infection. Am Rev Respir Dis 118:295, 1978.
82. Roldaan AC, Masural N: Viral respiratory infections in asthmatic children staying in a mountain resort. Eur J Respir Dis 63:140, 1982.
83. Wang EEL, Probers CG, Manson B, et al: Association of respiratory viral infections with pulmonary deterioration in patients with cystic fibrosis. N Engl J Med 311:1653, 1984.
84. Smith CB, Golden CA, Kanner RE, et al: Association of viral and *Mycoplasma pneumoniae* infections with acute respiratory illness in patients with chronic obstructive pulmonary diseases. Am Rev Respir Dis 121:225, 1980.
85. O'Brien TG, Sweeney DF: Interstitial viral pneumonitis complicated by severe respiratory failure: Successful management using intensive dehydration and steroids. Chest 63:314, 1973.
86. Roberts GBS: Fulminating influenza. Lancet 2:944, 1957.
87. Winther B, Brofeldt S, Gronborg H, et al: Study of bacteria in the nasal cavity and nasopharynx during naturally acquired common cold. Acta Otolaryngol 98:315, 1984.
88. MacDonald KL, Osterholm MT, Hedberg CW, et al: Toxic shock syndrome: A newly recognized complication of influenza and influenza-like illness. JAMA 257:1053, 1987.
89. Editorial: Influenza and the nervous system. BMJ 1:357, 1971.
90. Wells CEC: Neurological complications of so-called "influenza": A winter study in southeast Wales. BMJ 1:369, 1971.
91. Brocklebank JT, Court SDM, McQuillin J, et al: Influenza-A infection in children. Lancet 2:497, 1972.
92. Marks JS, Halpin TJ: Guillain-Barré syndrome in recipients of A/New Jersey influenza vaccine. JAMA 243:2490, 1980.
93. Middleton PJ, Alexander RM, Szymanski MT: Severe myositis during recovery from influenza. Lancet 2:533, 1970.
94. Stevens S, Burman D, Clarke SKR, et al: Temporary paralysis in childhood after influenza B. Lancet 2:1354, 1974.
95. Leebeek FW, Baggen MG, Mulder LJ, et al: Rhabdomyolysis associated with influenza A virus infection. Neth J Med 46:189, 1995.
96. Kessler HA, Trenholme GM, Harris AA, et al: Acute myopathy associated with influenza A/Texas/1/77 infection. JAMA 243:461, 1980.
97. Minow RA, Gorbach S, Johnson BL Jr, et al: Myoglobinuria associated with influenza A infection. Ann Intern Med 80:359, 1974.
98. Morgensen JL: Myoglobinuria and renal failure associated with influenza. Ann Intern Med 80:362, 1974.
99. Baine WB, Luby JP, Martin SM: Severe illness with Influenza B. Am J Med 68:181, 1980.
100. Reye syndrome—United States, 1985. MMWR 35:66, 73, 1986.
101. Luksza AR, Jones DK: Influenza B virus infection complicated by pneumonia, acute renal failure and disseminated intravascular coagulation. J Infect 9:174, 1984.
102. Horner GJ, Gray FD Jr: Effect of uncomplicated, presumptive influenza on the diffusing capacity of the lung. Am Rev Respir Dis 108:866, 1973.
103. Rosenzweig DY, Dwyer DJ, Ferstenfeld JE, et al: Changes in small airway function after live attenuated influenza vaccination. Am Rev Respir Dis 111:399, 1975.
104. Johanson WG Jr, Pierce AK, Sanford JP: Pulmonary function in uncomplicated influenza. Am Rev Respir Dis 100:141, 1969.
105. Ptakova M, Tumova B: Detection of type A and B influenza viruses in clinical materials by immunoelectronmicroscopy. Acta Virol 29:19, 1985.
106. Doller G, Schuy W, Tjhen KY, et al: Direct detection of influenza virus antigen in nasopharyngeal specimens by direct enzyme immunoassay in comparison with quantitating virus shedding. J Clin Microbiol 30:866, 1992.
107. Hakosalo J, Saxén L: Influenza epidemic and congenital defects. Lancet 2:1346, 1971.
108. Janerich DT: Relationship between the influenza pandemic and the epidemic of neurological malformations. Lancet 1:1165, 1971.
109. Fedrick J, Alberman ED: Reported influenza in pregnancy and subsequent cancer in the child. BMJ 2:485, 1972.
110. Bithell JF, Draper GJ, Gorbach PD: Association between malignant disease in children and maternal virus infections. BMJ 1:706, 1973.
111. Laraya-Cuasay LR, Deforest A, et al: Chronic pulmonary complications of early influenza virus infection in children. Am Rev Respir Dis 116:617, 1977.
112. Winterbauer RH, Ludwig WR, Hammar SP: Clinical course, management, and long-term sequelae of respiratory failure due to influenza viral pneumonia. Johns Hopkins Med J 141:148, 1977.
113. Cameron AS, Roder DM, Esterman AJ, et al: Mortality from influenza and allied infections in South Australia during 1968–1981. Med J Aust 142:14, 1985.
114. Sprenger MJ, Mulder PG, Beyer WE, et al: Impact of influenza on mortality in relation to age and underlying disease, 1967–1989. Int J Epidemiol 22:334, 1993.
115. Tillett HE, Smith JW, Gooch CD: Excess deaths attributable to influenza in England and Wales: Age at death and certified cause. Int J Epidemiol 12:344, 1983.
116. Scragg R: Effect of influenza epidemics on Australian mortality. Med J Aust 142:98, 1985.
117. Prevention and control of influenza. Recommendation of the Immunization Practices Advisory Committee. Centers for Disease Control, Department of Health and Human Services. Ann Intern Med 103:560, 1985.
118. Horman JT, Stetler MC, Israel E, et al: An outbreak of influenza A in a nursing home. Am J Public Health 76:501, 1986.
119. Glezen WP, Payne AA, Snyder DN, et al: Mortality and influenza. J Infect Dis 146:313, 1982.
120. Herrmann EC Jr, Hable KA: Experiences in laboratory diagnosis of parainfluenza viruses in routine medical practice. Mayo Clin Proc 45:177, 1970.
121. Glezen WP, Denny FW: Epidemiology of acute lower respiratory disease in children. N Engl J Med 288:498, 1973.
122. Taussig LM, Wright AL, Morgan WJ, et al: The Tucson Children's Respiratory Study: I. Design and implementation of a prospective study of acute and chronic respiratory illness in children. Am J Epidemiol 129:1219, 1989.
123. Wendt CH, Weisdorf DJ, Jordan MC, et al: Parainfluenza virus respiratory infection after bone marrow transplantation. N Engl J Med 326:921, 1992.
124. Jarvis WR, Middleton PJ, Gelfand EW: Parainfluenza pneumonia in severe combined immunodeficiency disease. J Pediatr 94:423, 1979.
125. Lauzon D, Delage G, Brochu P, et al: Pathogens in children with severe combined immune deficiency disease or AIDS. Can Med Assoc J 135:33, 1986.
126. Chanock R, Chambon L, Chang W, et al: WHO respiratory disease survey in children: A serological study. Bull WHO 37:363, 1967.
127. Evans AS: Infections with hemadsorption virus in University of Wisconsin students. N Engl J Med 263:233, 1960.
128. Wenzel RP, McCormick DP, Beam WE Jr: Parainfluenza pneumonia in adults. JAMA 221:294, 1972.
129. Glezen WP, Frank AL, Taber LH, et al: Parainfluenza virus type 3: Seasonality and risk of infection and re-infection in young children. Infect Dis 150:851, 1984.
130. Gross PA, Green RH, Curmen MGM: Persistent infection with parainfluenza type 3 virus in man. Am Rev Respir Dis 108:894, 1973.
131. Fekety FR Jr, Caldwell J, Gump D, et al: Bacteria, viruses, and mycoplasmas in acute pneumonia in adults. Am Rev Respir Dis 104:499, 1971.
132. Jakab GJ, Warr GA: Immune-enhanced phagocytic dysfunction in pulmonary macrophages infected with parainfluenza 1 (Sendai) virus. Am Rev Respir Dis 124:575, 1981.
133. Delage G, Brochu P, Pelletier M, et al: Giant-cell pneumonia caused by parainfluenza virus. J Pediatr 94:426, 1979.
134. Weintrub PS, Sullender WM, Lombard C, et al: Giant cell pneumonia caused by parainfluenza type 3 in a patient with acute myelomonocytic leukemia. Arch Pathol Lab Med 111:569, 1987.
135. Buthala DA, Soret MG: Parainfluenza type 3 virus infection in hamsters: Virologic, serologic, and pathologic studies. J Infect Dis 114:226, 1964.
136. Craighead JE, Brennan BJ: Cytopathic effects of parainfluenza virus type 3 in organ cultures of human respiratory tract tissue. Am J Pathol 52:287, 1968.
137. Wagener JS, Minnich L, Sobonya R, et al: Parainfluenza type II infection in dogs. Am Rev Respir Dis 127:771, 1983.
138. Castleman WL, Brundage-Anguish LJ, Kreitzer L, et al: Pathogenesis of bronchiolitis and pneumonia induced in neonatal and weanling rats by parainfluenza (sendai) virus. Am J Pathol 129:277, 1987.
139. Osborne D: Radiologic appearance of viral disease of the lower respiratory tract in infants and children. Am J Roentgenol 130:29, 1978.
140. Horstmann DM, Hsiung GD: Myxovirus infections and respiratory illness in children. Clin Pediatr 2:378, 1963.
141. Gardner PS, McQuillin J, McGuckin R, et al: Observations on clinical and immunofluorescent diagnosis of parainfluenza virus infections. BMJ 2:7, 1971.
142. Downham MAPS, Gardner PS, McQuillin J, et al: Role of respiratory viruses in childhood mortality. BMJ 1:235, 1975.
143. Reilly CM, Stokes J Jr, McClelland L, et al: Studies of acute respiratory illnesses caused by respiratory syncytial virus. Am J Dis Child 102:763, 1961.
144. Anonymous: From the Centers for Disease Control and Prevention. Update: Respiratory syncytial virus activity—United States, 1994–95 season. JAMA 273:282, 1995.
145. Hall CB, Walsh EE, Schnabel KC, et al: Occurrence of groups A and B of respiratory syncytial virus over 15 years: Associated epidemiologic and clinical characteristics in hospitalized and ambulatory children. J Infect Dis 162:1283, 1990.
146. Sterner G, Wolontis S, Bloth B, et al: Respiratory syncytial virus—an outbreak

of acute respiratory illnesses in a home for infants. Acta Paediatr Scand 55:273, 1966.

147. Knight V, Kapikian AZ, Kravetz HM, et al: Ecology of a newly recognized common respiratory agent RS-virus. Combined clinical staff conference at the National Institutes of Health. Ann Intern Med 55:507, 1961.

148. Crone PB, Heycock JB, Noble TC, et al: Serological evidence of infection by respiratory syncytial virus in outbreak of acute bronchiolitis. BMJ 1:1539, 1964.

149. Forbes JA, Bennett NMcK, Gray NJ: Epidemic bronchiolitis caused by a respiratory syncytial virus: Clinical aspects. Med J Aust 2:933, 1961.

150. Mathur U, Bentley DW, Hall CB: Concurrent respiratory syncytial virus and influenza A infections in the institutionalized elderly and chronically ill. Ann Intern Med 93:49, 1980.

151. Hall CB: The nosocomial spread of respiratory syncytial virus infections. Ann Rev Med 34:311, 1983.

152. Glezen WP, Paredes A, Allison JE, et al: Risk of respiratory syncytial virus infection for infants from low-income families in relationship to age, sex, ethnic group and maternal antibody level. J Pediatr 98:708, 1981.

153. Hall CB, Kopelman AE, Douglas RG Jr, et al: Neonatal respiratory syncytial virus infection. N Engl J Med 300:393, 1979.

154. Brodie HR, Spence LP: Respiratory syncytial virus infections in children in Montreal: A retrospective study. Can Med Assoc J 109:1199, 1973.

155. McLelland L, Hilleman MR, Hamparian VV, et al: Studies of acute respiratory illnesses caused by respiratory syncytial virus: 2. Epidemiology and assessment of importance. N Engl J Med 264:1169, 1961.

156. Groothuis JR, Gutierrez KM, Lauer BA: Respiratory syncytial virus infection in children with bronchopulmonary dysplasia. Pediatrics 82:199, 1988.

157. MacDonald NE, Hall CB, Suffin SC, et al: Respiratory syncytial viral infection in infants with congenital heart disease. N Engl J Med 307:397, 1982.

158. Garvie DG, Gray J: Outbreak of respiratory syncytial virus infection in the elderly. BMJ 281:1253, 1980.

159. Sorvillo FJ, Huie SF, Strassburg MA, et al: An outbreak of respiratory syncytial virus pneumonia in a nursing home for the elderly. J Infect 9:252, 1984.

160. Morales F, Calder MA, Inglis JM, et al: A study of respiratory infections in the elderly to assess the role of respiratory syncytial virus. J Infect 7:236, 1983.

161. Parham DM, Bozeman P, Killian C, et al: Cytologic diagnosis of respiratory syncytial virus infection in a bronchoalveolar lavage specimen from a bone marrow transplant recipient. Am J Clin Pathol 99:588, 1993.

162. van Dissel JT, Zijlmans JM, Kroes AC, et al: Respiratory syncytial virus, a rare cause of severe pneumonia following bone marrow transplantation. Ann Hematol 71:253, 1995.

163. Zaroukian MH, Kashyap GH, Wentworth BB: Case report: Respiratory syncytial virus infection: A cause of respiratory distress syndrome and pneumonia in adults. Am J Med Sci 295:218, 1988.

164. Hers JF, Masurel N, Gans JC: Acute respiratory disease associated with pulmonary involvement in military servicemen in the Netherlands: A serologic and bacteriologic survey. January, 1967–1968. Am Rev Respir Dis 100:499, 1969.

165. Vikerfors T, Gradien M, Olcen P: Respiratory syncytial virus infections in adults. Am Rev Respir Dis 136:561, 1987.

166. Gardner PS, McQuillin J, Court SDM: Speculation on pathogenesis of death from respiratory syncytial virus infection. BMJ 1:327, 1970.

167. Aherne W, Bird T, Court SDM, et al: Pathological changes in virus infections of the lower respiratory tract in children. J Clin Pathol 23:7, 1970.

168. Midulla F, Villani A, Panuska JR, et al: Respiratory syncytial virus lung infection in infants: Immunoregulatory role of infected alveolar macrophages. J Infect Dis 168:1515, 1993.

169. Henderson FW, Hu S-C, Collier AM: Pathogenesis of respiratory syncytial virus infection in ferret and fetal human tracheas in organ culture. Am Rev Respir Dis 118:29, 1978.

170. Forni AL, Schluger NW, Roberts RB: Severe measles pneumonitis in adults: Evaluation of clinical characteristics and therapy with intravenous ribavirin. Clin Infect Dis 19:454, 1994.

171. Delage G, Brochu P, Robillard L, et al: Giant cell pneumonia due to respiratory syncytial virus. Arch Pathol Lab Med 108:623, 1984.

172. Odita JC, Nwankwo M, Aghahowa JE: Hilar enlargement in respiratory syncytial virus pneumonia. Eur J Radiol 9:155, 1989.

173. Anas N, Boettrich C, Hall CB, et al: The association of apnea and respiratory syncytial virus infection in infants. J Pediatr 101:65, 1982.

174. Hall CB, Powell KR, Schnabel KC, et al: Risk of secondary bacterial infection in infants hospitalized with respiratory syncytial viral infection. J Pediatr 113:266, 1988.

175. Laing I, Riedel F, Yap PL, et al: Atopy predisposing to acute bronchiolitis during an epidemic of respiratory syncytial virus. BMJ 284:1070, 1982.

176. Sims DG, Gardner PS, Weightman D, et al: Atopy does not predispose to respiratory syncytial virus bronchiolitis or postbronchiolitic wheezing. BMJ 282:2086, 1981.

177. Reina J, Ros MJ, Del Valle JM, et al: Evaluation of direct immunofluorescence, dot-blot enzyme immunoassay, and shell-vial culture for detection of respiratory syncytial virus in patients with bronchiolitis. Eur J Clin Microbiol Infect Dis 14:1018, 1995.

178. Johnston SLG, Siegel CS: Evaluation of direct immunofluorescence, enzyme immunoassay, centrifugation culture, and conventional culture for the detection of respiratory syncytial virus. J Clin Microbiol 28:2394, 1990.

179. Gardner PS, McQuillin J: Application of immunofluorescent antibody technique in rapid diagnosis of respiratory syncytial virus infection. BMJ 3:340, 1968.

180. Meurman O, Ruuskanen O, Sarkkinen H, et al: Immunoglobulin class-specific

antibody response in respiratory syncytial virus infection measured by enzyme immunoassay. J Med Virol 14:67, 1984.

181. Wright C, Oliver KC, Fenwick FI, et al: A monoclonal antibody pool for routine immunohistochemical detection of human respiratory syncytial virus antigens in formalin-fixed, paraffin-embedded tissue. J Pathol 182:238, 1997.

182. Gilbert LL, Dakhama A, Bone BM, et al: Diagnosis of viral respiratory tract infections in children using a reverse transcription-PCR panel. J Clin Microbiol 34:140, 1996.

183. Hall WJ, Hall CB, Speers DM: Respiratory syncytial virus infection in adults: Clinical, virologic, and serial pulmonary function studies. Ann Intern Med 88:203, 1978.

184. Pullan CR, Hey EN: Wheezing, asthma, and pulmonary dysfunction 10 years after infection with respiratory syncytial virus in infancy. BMJ 284:1665, 1982.

185. Schwarze J, Hamelmann E, Bradley KL, et al: Respiratory syncytial virus infection results in airway hyperresponsiveness and enhanced airway sensitization to allergen. J Clin Invest 100:226, 1997.

186. Welliver RC, Kaul TN, Ogra PL: The appearance of cell-bound IgE in respiratory-tract epithelium after respiratory-syncytial-virus infection. N Engl J Med 303:1198, 1980.

187. McConnochie KM, Mark JD, McBride JT, et al: Normal pulmonary function measurements and airway reactivity in childhood after mild bronchiolitis. J Pediatr 107:54, 1985.

188. Hegele RG, Hayashi S, Hogg JC, et al: Mechanisms of airway narrowing and hyperresponsiveness in viral respiratory tract infections. Am J Respir Crit Care Med 151:1659, 1995.

189. Mason WH, Ross LA, Lanson J, et al: Epidemic measles in the postvaccine era: Evaluation of epidemiology, clinical presentation and complications during an urban outbreak. Pediatr Infect Dis J 12:42, 1993.

190. Markowitz LE, Nieburg P: The burden of acute respiratory infection due to measles in developing countries and the potential impact of measles vaccine. Rev Infect Dis 13:S555, 1991.

191. Hinman AR, Orenstein WA, Bloch AB, et al: Impact of measles in the United States. Rev Infect Dis 5:439, 1983.

192. Weiner LB, Corwin RM, Nieburg PI, et al: A measles outbreak among adolescents. J Pediatr 90:17, 1977.

193. Barkin RM: Measles mortality: Analysis of the primary cause of death. Am J Dis Child 129:307, 1975.

194. Gremillion DH, Crawford GE: Measles pneumonia in young adults: An analysis of 106 cases. Am J Med 71:539, 1981.

195. Hussey GD, Klein M: A randomized, controlled trial of vitamin A in children with severe measles. N Engl J Med 323:160, 1990.

196. Henneman PL, Birnbaumer DM, Cairns CB: Measles pneumonitis. Ann Emerg Med 26:278, 1995.

197. Atmar RI, Englund JA, Hammill H: Complications of measles during pregnancy. Clin Infect Dis 14:217, 1992.

198. Lipsey AI, Kahn MJ, Bolande RP: Pathologic variants of congenital hypogammaglobulinemia: An analysis of 3 patients dying of measles. Pediatrics 39:659, 1967.

199. Becroft DMO, Osborne DRS: The lungs in fatal measles infection in childhood: Pathological, radiological and immunological correlations. Histopathology 4:401, 1980.

200. Kaplan LJ, Daum RS, Smaron M, et al: Severe measles in immunocompromised patients. JAMA 267:1237, 1992.

200a. Sobonya RE, Hiller FC, Pingleton W, et al: Fatal measles (rubeola) pneumonia in adults. Arch Pathol Lab Med 102:366, 1978.

201. Enders JF, McCarthy K, Mitus A, et al: Isolation of measles virus at autopsy in cases of giant-cell pneumonia without rash. N Engl J Med 261:875, 1959.

202. Joliat G, Abetel G, Schindler A-M, et al: Measles giant cell pneumonia without rash in a case of lymphocytic lymphosarcoma: An electron microscopic study. Virchows Arch 358:215, 1973.

203. Editorial: Pneumonia in atypical measles. BMJ 2:235, 1971.

204. McLean DM, Kettyls GDM, Hingston J, et al: Atypical measles following immunization with killed measles vaccine. Can Med Assoc J 103:743, 1970.

205. Henderson JAM, Hammond DI: Delayed diagnosis in atypical measles syndrome. Can Med Assoc J 133:211, 1985.

206. Gokiert JG, Beamish WE: Altered reactivity to measles virus in previously vaccinated children. Can Med Assoc J 103:724, 1970.

207. Fulginiti VA, Arthur JH: Altered reactivity to measles virus: Skin test reactivity and antibody response to measles virus antigens in recipients of killed measles virus vaccine. J Pediatr 75:609, 1969.

208. Harboldt SL, Dugan JM, Tronic BS: Cytologic diagnosis of measles pneumonia in a bronchoalveolar lavage specimen: A case report. Acta Cytol 38:403, 1994.

209. Quinn JL III: Measles pneumonia in an adult. Am J Roentgenol 91:560, 1964.

210. Fawcitt J, Parry HE: Lung changes in pertussis and measles in childhood: A review of 1894 cases with a follow-up study of the pulmonary complications. Br J Radiol 30:76, 1957.

211. Gilmartin D: Mediastinal emphysema in Melbourne children: With particular reference to measles and giant-cell pneumonia. Australas Radiol 15:27, 1971.

212. Tanaka H, Honma S, Yamagishi M, et al: Clinical features of measles pneumonia in adults: Usefulness of computed tomography. Jpn J Thorac Dis 31:1129, 1993.

212a. Barkin RM: Measles mortality: Analysis of the primary cause of death. Am J Dis Child 129:307, 1975.

212b. Mason WH, Ross LA, Lanson J, et al: Epidemic measles in the postvaccine era: Evaluation of epidemiology, clinical presentation, and complications during an urban outbreak. Pediatr Infect Dis J 12:42, 1993.

213. Abramson O, Dagan R, Tal A, et al: Severe complications of measles requiring intensive care in infants and young children. Arch Pediatr Adolesc Med 149:1237, 1995.

214. Martin DB, Weiner LB, Nieburg PI, et al: Atypical measles in adolescents and young adults. Ann Intern Med 90:877, 1979.

215. Minnich LL, Goodenough F, Ray CG: Use of immunofluorescence to identify measles virus infections. J Clin Microbiol 29:1148, 1991.

216. Kleiman MB, Blackburn CKL, Zimmerman SE, et al: Comparison of enzyme-linked immunosorbent assay for acute measles with hemagglutination inhibition, complement fixation, and fluorescent-antibody methods. J Clin Microbiol 14:147, 1981.

217. Editorial: Upper respiratory tract infections. BMJ 3:101, 1971.

218. Hilleman MR, Reilly CM, Stokes J Jr, et al: Clinical-epidemiologic findings in coryzavirus infections. Am Rev Respir Dis 88(Suppl):274, 1963.

219. George RB, Mogabgab WJ: Atypical pneumonia in young men with rhinovirus infections. Ann Intern Med 71:1073, 1969.

220. Brown EH: Enterovirus infections. BMJ 2:169, 1973.

221. Herrmann EC Jr, Person DA, Smith TF: Experience in laboratory diagnosis of enterovirus infections in routine medical practice. Mayo Clin Proc 47:577, 1972.

222. Altman R: Clinical aspects of enterovirus infection. Postgrad Med 35:451, 1964.

223. Stanghelle JK, Festvag LV: Postpolio syndrome: A 5 year follow-up. Spinal Cord 35:503, 1997.

224. Knobil K, Becker FS, Harper P, et al: Dyspnea in a patient years after severe poliomyelitis: The role of cardiopulmonary exercise testing. Chest 105:777, 1994.

225. Pepper C, Jasani B, Navabi H, et al: Simian virus 40 large T antigen (SV40LTAg) primer specific DNA amplification in human pleural mesothelioma tissue. Thorax 51:1074, 1996.

226. Leading article: Coxsackie virus infections. BMJ 3:70, 1968.

227. Hable KA, O'Connell EJ, Hermann EC Jr: Group B Coxsackieviruses as respiratory viruses. Mayo Clin Proc 45:170, 1970.

228. Lerner AM, Klein JO, Levin HS, et al: Infections due to Coxsackie virus group A, type 9, in Boston, 1959, with special reference to exanthems and pneumonia. N Engl J Med 263:1265, 1960.

229. Disney ME, Howard EM, Wood BSB, et al: Bornholm disease in children. BMJ 1:1351, 1953.

230. Helin M, Savola J, Lapinleimu K: Cardiac manifestations during a Coxsackie B5 epidemic. BMJ 3:97, 1968.

231. Brown EH: Enterovirus infections. Br Med J 2:169, 1973.

232. Cramblett HG, Rosen L, Parrott RH, et al: Respiratory illness in six infants infected with a newly recognized ECHO virus. Pediatrics 21:168, 1958.

233. Butterfield J, Moscovici C, Berry C, et al: Cystic emphysema in premature infants: A report of an outbreak with the isolation of type 19 ECHO virus in one case. N Engl J Med 268:18, 1963.

234. Bell EJ, Grist NR: Echoviruses, carditis, and acute pleurodynia. Lancet 1:326, 1970.

235. Cherry JD, Diddams JA, Dick EC: Rhinovirus infections in hospitalized children: Provocative bacterial interrelationships. Arch Environ Health 14:390, 1967.

236. Wald TG, Shult P, Krause P, et al: A rhinovirus outbreak among residents of a long-term care facility. Ann Intern Med 123:588, 1995.

237. Levandowski RA, Ou DW, Jackson GG: Acute-phase decrease of T lymphocyte subsets in rhinovirus infection. J Infect Dis 153:743, 1986.

238. Craighead JE, Meier M, Cooley MH: Brief recordings: Pulmonary infection due to rhinovirus type 13. N Engl J Med 281:1403, 1969.

239. Cate TR, Roberts JS, Russ MA, et al: Effects of common colds on pulmonary function. Am Rev Respir Dis 108:858, 1975.

240. Halperin SA, Eggleston PA, Hendley JO, et al: Pathogenesis of lower respiratory tract symptoms in experimental rhinovirus infection. Am Rev Respir Dis 128:806, 1983.

241. Halperin SA, Eggleston PA, Beasley P, et al: Exacerbations of asthma in adults during rhinovirus infection. Am Rev Respir Dis 132:976, 1985.

242. Minor TE, Dick EC, Baker JW, et al: Rhinovirus and influenza type A infections as precipitants of asthma. Am Rev Respir Dis 113:149, 1976.

243. Johnston SL: Natural and experimental rhinovirus infections of the lower respiratory tract. Am J Respir Crit Care Med 152:S46, 1995.

244. Gern JE, Calhoun W, Swenson C, et al: Rhinovirus infection preferentially increases lower airway responsiveness in allergic subjects. Am J Respir Crit Care Med 155:1872, 1997.

245. Smith CB, Kanner RE, Golden CA, et al: Effect of viral infections on pulmonary function in patients with chronic obstructive pulmonary diseases. J Infect Dis 141:271, 1985.

246. Stenhouse AC: Rhinovirus infection in acute exacerbations of chronic bronchitis: A controlled prospective study. BMJ 3:461, 1967.

247. Sugimoto M, Nakashima H, Watanabe S, et al: T-lymphocyte alveolitis in HTLV-I-associated myelopathy. Lancet 2:1220, 1987.

248. Higashiyama Y, Katamine S, Kohno S, et al: Expression of human T lymphotropic virus type 1 (HTLV-1) tax/rex gene in fresh bronchoalveolar lavage cells of HTLV-1-infected individuals. Clin Exp Immunol 96:193, 1994.

249. Kuwabara H, Katanaka J, Nagai M, et al: Human T lymphotropic virus type I associated myelopathy with pulmonary and cutaneous lesions. J Clin Pathol 46:273, 1993.

250. Kikuchi T, Saijo Y, Sakai T, et al: Human T-cell lymphotropic virus type I (HTLV-I) carrier with clinical manifestations characteristic of diffuse panbronchiolitis. Intern Med 35:305, 1996.

251. Chayt KJ, Harper ME, Marselle L, et al: Detection of HTLV-III RNA in lungs of patients with AIDS and pulmonary involvement. JAMA 256:2356, 1986.

252. Agostini C, Zambello R, Trentin L, et al: Prognostic significance of the evaluation of bronchoalveolar lavage populations in patients with HIV-1 infection and pulmonary involvement. Chest 100:1601, 1991.

253. Agostini C, Zambello R, Trentin L, et al: Gamma delta T-cell receptor subsets in the lung of patients with HIV-1 infection. Cell Immunol 153:194, 1994.

254. Twigg HL 3rd, Soliman DM, Spain BA: Impaired alveolar macrophage accessory cell function and reduced incidence of lymphocytic alveolitis in HIV-infected patients who smoke. AIDS 8:611, 1994.

255. Sadat-Sowti B, Parrot A, Quint L, et al: Alveolar CD8 + CD57 + lymphocytes in human immunodeficiency virus infection produce an inhibitor of cytotoxic functions. Am J Respir Crit Care Med 149:972, 1994.

256. Travis WD, Fox CH, Devaney KO, et al: Lymphoid pneumonitis in 50 adult patients infected with human immunodeficiency virus: Lymphocytic interstitial pneumonitis versus nonspecific interstitial pneumonitis. Hum Pathol 23:529, 1992.

257. Diaz PT, Clanton TL, Pacht ER: Emphysema-like pulmonary disease associated with human immunodeficiency virus infection. Ann Intern Med 116:124, 1992.

258. Butler JC, Peters CJ: Hantaviruses and hantavirus pulmonary syndrome. Clin Infect Dis 19:387, 1994.

259. Moolenaar RL, Breiman RF, Peters CJ: Hantavirus pulmonary syndrome. Semin Respir Infect 12:31, 1997.

260. Khan AS, Khabbaz RF, Armstrong LR, et al: Hantavirus pulmonary syndrome: The first 100 US cases. J Infect Dis 173:1297, 1996.

261. Hjelle B, Goade D, Torrez-Martinez N, et al: Hantavirus pulmonary syndrome, renal insufficiency, and myositis associated with infection by Bayou hantavirus. Clin Infect Dis 23:495, 1996.

262. Khan AS, Gaviria M, Rollin PE, et al: Hantavirus pulmonary syndrome in Florida: Association with the newly identified Black Creek Canal virus. Am J Med 100:46, 1996.

263. Schmaljohn C, Hjelle B: Hantaviruses: A global disease problem. Emerg Infect Dis 3:95, 1997.

264. Zaki SR, Khan AS, Goodman RA, et al: Retrospective diagnosis of hantavirus pulmonary syndrome, 1978–1993: Implications for emerging infectious diseases. Arch Pathol Lab Med 120:134, 1996.

265. Auwaerter PG, Oldach D, Mundy LM, et al: Hantavirus serologies in patients hospitalized with community-acquired pneumonia. J Infect Dis 173:237, 1996.

266. Wells RM, Young J, Williams RJ, et al: Hantavirus transmission in the United States. Emerg Infect Dis 3:361, 1997.

267. Williams RJ, Bryan RT, Mills JN, et al: An outbreak of hantavirus pulmonary syndrome in western Paraguay. Am J Trop Med Hyg 57:274, 1997.

268. Wells RM, Sosa Estani S, Yadon ZE, et al: An unusual hantavirus outbreak in southern Argentina: Person-to-person transmission? Hantavirus Pulmonary Syndrome Study Group for Patagonia. Emerg Infect Dis 3:171, 1997.

269. Anonymous: Hantavirus pulmonary syndrome in Canada: Update. Can Med Assoc J 153:1303, 1995.

270. Zaki SR, Greer PW, Coffield LM, et al: Hantavirus pulmonary syndrome: Pathogenesis of an emerging infectious disease. Am J Pathol 146:552, 1995.

271. Ketai LH, Williamson MR, Telepak RJ, et al: Hantavirus pulmonary syndrome: Radiographic findings in 16 patients. Radiology 191:665, 1994.

272. Duchin JS, Koster FT, Peters CJ, et al: Hantavirus pulmonary syndrome: A clinical description of 17 patients with a newly recognized disease. The Hantavirus Study Group. N Engl J Med 330:949, 1994.

273. Jenison S, Yamada T, Morris C, et al: Characterization of human antibody responses to four corners hantavirus infections among patients with hantavirus pulmonary syndrome. J Virol 68:3000, 1994.

274. Hjelle B, Jenison S, Torrez-Martinez N, et al: Rapid and specific detection of Sin Nombre virus antibodies in patients with hantavirus pulmonary syndrome by a strip immunoblot assay suitable for field diagnosis. J Clin Microbiol 35:600, 1997.

275. Schwarz TF, Zaki SR, Morzunov S, et al: Detection and sequence confirmation of Sin Nombre virus RNA in paraffin-embedded human tissues using one-step RT-PCR. J Virol Methods 51:349, 1995.

276. Tillotson JR, Lerner AM: Reovirus type 3 associated with fatal pneumonia. N Engl J Med 276:1060, 1967.

277. El-Rai FM, Evans AS: Reovirus infections in children and young adults. Arch Environ Health 7:700, 1963.

278. Esterly JR, Oppenheimer EH: Vascular lesions in infants with congenital rubella. Circulation 36:544, 1967.

279. Rowe RD: Maternal rubella and pulmonary artery stenoses: Report of eleven cases. Pediatrics 32:180, 1963.

280. Williams HJ, Carey LS: Rubella embryopathy: Roentgenologic features. Am J Roentgenol 97:92, 1966.

281. Phelan P, Campbell P: Pulmonary complications of rubella embryopathy. J Pediatr 75:202, 1969.

282. Esterly JR, Oppenheimer EH: Pathological lesions due to congenital rubella. Arch Pathol 87:380, 1969.

283. Waller BF, Smith FA, Kerwin DM, et al: Structure-function correlations in cardiovascular and pulmonary diseases. Chest 81:735, 1982.

284. Deibel R, Woodall JP, Decher WJ, et al: Lymphocytic choriomeningitis virus in man: Serologic evidence of association with pet hamsters. JAMA 232:501, 1975.

285. Smadel JE, Green RH, Paltauf RM, et al: Lymphocytic choriomeningitis: Two human fatalities following an unusual febrile illness. Soc Exp Biol Med Proc 49:683, 1942.

286. Hendley JO, Fishburne HB, Gwaltney JM Jr: Coronavirus infections in working adults: Eight-year study with 229 E and OC 43. Am Rev Respir Dis 105:805, 1972.

287. Reed SE: The behaviour of recent isolates of human respiratory coronavirus in vitro and in volunteers: Evidence of heterogeneity among 229 E-related strains. J Med Virol 13:179, 1984.

288. Callow KA: Effect of specific humoral immunity and some non-specific factors on resistance of volunteers to respiratory coronavirus infection. J Hyg 95:173, 1985.

289. McIntosh K, Chao RK, Krause HE, et al: Coronavirus infection in acute lower tract disease of infants. J Infect Dis 130:502, 1974.

290. Wenzel RP, Hendley JO, Davies JA, et al: Coronavirus infections in military recruits: Three-year study with coronavirus strains OC 43 and 229 E. Am Rev Respir Dis 109:621, 1974.

291. McIntosh K, Ellis EF, Hoffman LS, et al: The association of viral and bacterial respiratory infections with exacerbations of wheezing in young children. J Pediatr 82:578, 1973.

292. Smith CB, Golden CA, Kanner RE, et al: Association of viral and *Mycoplasma pneumoniae* infections with acute respiratory illness in patients with chronic obstructive pulmonary diseases. Am Rev Respir Dis 121:225, 1980.

293. Gill EP, Dominguez EA, Greenberg SB, et al: Development and application of an enzyme immunoassay for coronavirus OC43 antibody in acute respiratory illness. J Clin Microbiol 32:2372, 1994.

294. Brandt CD, Kim HW, Vargosko AJ, et al: Infections in 18,000 infants and children in a controlled study of respiratory tract disease: I. Adenovirus pathogenicity in relation to serologic type and illness syndrome. Am J Epidemiol 90:484, 1969.

294a. Bateman ED, Hayashi S, Kuwano K, et al: Latent adenoviral infection in follicular bronchiectasis. Am J Respir Crit Care Med 151:170, 1995.

295. Miller LF, Rytel M, Pierce WE, et al: Epidemiology of non-bacterial pneumonia among naval recruits. JAMA 185:92, 1963.

296. Buescher EL: Respiratory disease and adenoviruses. Med Clin North Am 51:769, 1967.

297. Chih-Ch'uan H: Adenovirus pneumonia in infants and children: Pathologic studies of 40 cases. Chin Med J 82:390, 1963.

298. Wright HT Jr, Beckwith JB, Gwinn JL: A fatal case of inclusion body pneumonia in an infant infected with adenovirus type 3. J Pediatr 64:528, 1964.

299. Becroft DMO: Histopathology of fatal adenovirus infection of the respiratory tract in young children. J Clin Pathol 20:561, 1967.

300. Murtagh P, Cerqueiro C, Halac A, et al: Adenovirus type 7h respiratory infections: A report of 29 cases of acute lower respiratory disease. Acta Paediatr 82:557, 1993.

301. Adams JM, Loosli CG: Viral pharyngitis, laryngitis and pneumonitis: The myxoviruses, adenoviruses and enteroviruses in respiratory disease. Med Clin North Am 43:1335, 1959.

302. Martone WJ, Hierholzer JC, Keenlyside RA, et al: An outbreak of adenovirus type 3 disease at a private recreation center swimming pool. Am J Epidemiol 111:229, 1980.

303. Brummitt CF, Cherrington JM, Katzenstein DA, et al: Nosocomial adenovirus infections: Molecular epidemiology of an outbreak due to adenovirus 3a. J Infect Dis 158:423, 1988.

304. Brown RS, Nogrady MB, Spence L, et al: An outbreak of adenovirus type 7 infection in children in Montreal. Can Med Assoc J 108:434, 1973.

305. Kawai T, Fujiwara T, Aoyama Y, et al: Diffuse interstitial fibrosing pneumonitis and adenovirus infection. Chest 69:692, 1976.

306. Strano AJ: Light microscopy of selected viral disease (morphology of inclusion bodies). *In* Sommers SC (ed): Pathology Annual. Vol 11. New York, Appleton-Century-Crofts, 1976, p 53.

307. Gold R, Wilt JC, Adhikari PK, et al: Adenoviral pneumonia and its complications in infancy and childhood. J Can Assoc Radiol 20:218, 1969.

308. Wenman WM, Pagtakhan RD, Reed MH, et al: Adenovirus bronchiolitis in Manitoba: Epidemiologic, clinical, and radiologic features. Chest 81:605, 1982.

308a. Han BK, Son JA, Yoon H-K, Lee S-I: Epidemic adenoviral lower respiratory tract infection in pediatric patients: Radiographic and clinical characteristics. Am J Roentgenol 170:1077, 1998.

309. Connor JD: Evidence for an etiologic role of adenoviral infection in pertussis syndrome. N Engl J Med 283:390, 1970.

310. George RB, Ziskind MM, Rasch Jr, et al: *Mycoplasma* and adenovirus pneumonias: Comparison with other atypical pneumonias in a military population. Ann Intern Med 65:931, 1966.

311. Ellenbogen C, Graybill JR, Silva J Jr, et al: Bacterial pneumonia complicating adenoviral pneumonia: A comparison of respiratory tract bacterial culture sources and effectiveness of chemoprophylaxis against bacterial pneumonia. Am J Med 56:169, 1974.

312. Hierholzer JC, Wigand R, Anderson LJ, et al: Adenoviruses from patients with AIDS: A plethora of serotypes and a description of five new serotypes of subgenus D (types 43-37). J Infect Dis 158:804, 1988.

313. Zahradnik JM, Spencer MJ, Porter DD: Adenovirus infection in the immunocompromised patient. Am J Med 68:725, 1980.

314. Shields AF, Hackman RC, Fife KH, et al: Adenovirus infections in patients undergoing bone-marrow transplantation. N Engl J Med 312:529, 1985.

315. Field PR, Patwardhan J, McKenzie JA, et al: Fatal adenovirus type 7 pneumonia in an adult. Med J Aust 2:445, 1978.

316. Wright J, Couchonnal G, Hodges GR: Adenovirus type 21 infection: Occurrence with pneumonia, rhabdomyolysis, and myoglobinuria in an adult. JAMA 241:2420, 1979.

317. Morgan PN, Moses EB, Fody EP, et al: Association of adenovirus type 16 with Reye's syndrome-like illness and pneumonia. South Med J 77:827, 1984.

318. Lang WR, Howden CW, Laws J, et al: Bronchopneumonia with serious sequelae in children with evidence of adenovirus type 21 infection. BMJ 1:73, 1969.

319. Osborne D, White P: Radiology of epidemic adenovirus 21 infection of the lower respiratory tract in infants and young children. Am J Roentgenol 133:379, 1979.

320. Becroft DMO: Bronchiolitis obliterans, bronchiectasis, and other sequelae of adenovirus type 21 infection in young children. J Clin Pathol 24:72, 1971.

321. Castleman WL: Bronchiolitis obliterans and pneumonia induced in young dogs by experimental adenovirus infection. Am J Pathol 119:495, 1985.

322. Spigelblatt L, Rosenfeld R: Hyperlucent lung: Long-term complication of adenovirus type 7 pneumonia. Can Med Assoc J 128:47, 1983.

323. MacPherson RI, Cumming GR, Chernick V: Unilateral hyperlucent lung: A complication of viral pneumonia. J Can Assoc Radiol 20:225, 1969.

324. Elliot WM, Hayashi S, Hogg JC: Immunodetection of adenoviral e1a protein in human lung tissue. Am J Respir Crit Care Med 12:642, 1995.

325. Dascomb HE, Hilleman MR: Clinical and laboratory studies in patients with respiratory disease caused by adenoviruses (RI-APC-ARD agents). Am J Med 21:161, 1956.

326. Hull RN: The Simian herpesviruses. *In* Kaplan AS (ed): The Herpesviruses. New York, Academic Press, 1973, p 389.

327. Overall JC Jr: Persistent problems with persistent herpesviruses. N Engl J Med 305:95, 1981.

328. Croen KD, Ostrove JM, Dragovic LJ, et al: Latent herpes simplex virus in human trigeminal ganglia: Detection of an immediate early gene "anti-sense" transcript by in situ hybridization. N Engl J Med 317:1427, 1987.

329. Warren KG, Brown SM, Wroblewska A: Isolation of latent herpes simplex from the superior cervical ganglion and vagus ganglions of human beings. N Engl J Med 298:1068, 1978.

330. Horwitz CA, Beneke J: Human herpesvirus-6 revisited. Am J Clin Pathol 99:533, 1993.

331. Sixbey JW, Nedrud JG, Raab-Traub N, et al: Epstein-Barr virus replication in oropharyngeal epithelial cells. N Engl J Med 310:1225, 1984.

332. Prellner T, Flamholc L, Haidl S, et al: Herpes simplex virus—the most frequently isolated pathogen in the lungs of patients with severe respiratory distress. Scand J Infect Dis 24:283, 1992.

333. Ramsey PG, Fife KH, Hackman RC, et al: Herpes simplex virus pneumonia: Clinical, virologic, and pathologic features in 20 patients. Ann Intern Med 97:813, 1982.

334. Schullere D, Spessert C, Fraser VJ, et al: Herpes simplex virus from respiratory tract secretions: Epidemiology, clinical characteristics, and outcome in immunocompromised and nonimmunocompromised hosts. Am J Med 94:29, 1993.

335. Nash G: Necrotizing tracheobronchitis and bronchopneumonia consistent with herpetic infection. Hum Pathol 3:283, 1972.

336. Sherry MK, Klainer AS, Wolff M, et al: Herpetic tracheobronchitis. Ann Intern Med 109:229, 1988.

337. Nash G, Foley FD: Herpetic infection of the middle and lower respiratory tract. Am J Clin Pathol 54:857, 1970.

338. Graham BS, Snell JD Jr: Herpes simplex virus infection of the adult lower respiratory tract. Medicine 62:384, 1983.

339. Vernon SE: Herpetic tracheobronchitis: Immunohistologic demonstration of herpes simplex virus antigen. Hum Pathol 13:683, 1982.

340. Herout V, Vortel V, Vondrackova A: Herpes simplex involvement of the lower respiratory tract. Am J Clin Pathol 46:411, 1966.

341. Vernon SE: Cytologic features of nonfatal herpesvirus tracheobronchitis. Acta Cytol 26:237, 1982.

342. Brown MJ, Miller RR, Müller NL: Acute lung disease in the immunocompromised host: CT and pathologic examination findings. Radiology 190:247, 1994.

343. Byers RJ, Hasleton PS, Quigley A, et al: Pulmonary herpes simplex in burn patients. Eur Respir J 9:2313, 1996.

344. L'Heureux P, Verhest A, Vincent JL, et al: Herpes virus infection, an unusual source of adult respiratory distress syndrome. Eur J Respir Dis 67:72, 1985.

345. Tuxen DV, Cade JF, McDonald MI, et al: Herpes simplex virus from the lower respiratory tract in adult respiratory distress syndrome. Am Rev Respir Dis 126:416, 1982.

346. Mazur MH, Whitley RJ, Dolin R: Serum antibody levels as risk factors in the dissemination of herpes zoster. Arch Intern Med 139:1341, 1979.

347. Martin JR, Holt RK, Langston C, et al: Type-specific identification of herpes simplex and varicella-Zoster virus antigen in autopsy tissues. Hum Pathol 22:75, 1991.

374a. Trudo FJ, Gopez EV, Gupta PK, et al: Pleural effusion due to herpes simplex type II infection in an immunocompromised host. Am J Respir Crit Care Med 155:371, 1997.

348. Singer DB: Pathology of neonatal herpes simplex virus infection. Perspect Pediatr Pathol 6:243, 1981.

348a. Horwitz CA, Beneke J: Human herpesvirus-6 revisited. Am J Clin Pathol 99:533, 1993.

349. Carrigan DR, Drobyski WR, Russler SK, et al: Interstitial pneumonitis associated with human herpesvirus-6 infection after marrow transplantation. Lancet 338:147, 1991.

350. Russler SK, Tapper MA, Knox KK, et al: Pneumonitis associated with coinfection by human herpes virus 6 and legionella in an immunocompetent adult. Am J Pathol 138:1405, 1991.

351. Cesarman E, Knowles DM: Kaposi's sarcoma-associated herpesvirus: A lymphotropic human herpesvirus associated with Kaposi's sarcoma, primary effusion lymphoma, and multicentric Castleman's disease. Semin Diagn Pathol 14:54, 1997.

352. Benfield TL, Dodt KK, Lundgren JD: Human herpes virus-8 DNA in bronchoalveolar lavage samples from patients with AIDS-associated pulmonary Kaposi's sarcoma. Scand J Infect Dis 29:13, 1997.
353. Pek S, Gikas PW: Pneumonia due to herpes zoster: Report of a case and review of the literature. Ann Intern Med 62:350, 1965.
354. Dutt AK: Diaphragmatic paralysis caused by herpes zoster (case report). Am Rev Respir Dis 101:755, 1970.
355. Soler JJ, Perpina M, Alfaro A: Hemidiaphragmatic paralysis caused by cervical herpes zoster. Respiration 63:403, 1996.
356. Weller TH: Varicella and herpes zoster: Changing concepts of the natural history, control, and importance of a not-so-benign virus (first of two parts). N Engl J Med 309:1434, 1983.
357. Triebwasser JH, Harris RE, Bryant RE, et al: Varicella pneumonia in adults: A report of seven cases and a review of literature. Medicine 46:409, 1967.
358. Guess HA, Broughton DD, Melton LJ III: Chickenpox hospitalizations among residents of Olmsted County, Minnesota, 1962 through 1981: A population-based study. Am J Dis Child 138:1055, 1984.
359. Weber DM, Pellecchia JA: Varicella pneumonia: Study of prevalence in adult men. JAMA 192:572, 1965.
360. Mermelstein RH, Freireich AW: Varicella pneumonia. Ann Intern Med 55:456, 1961.
361. Jura E, Chadwick EG, Josephs SH, et al: Varicella-Zoster virus infections in children infected with human immunodeficiency virus. Pediatr Infect J 8:586, 1989.
362. Locksley RM, Flournoy N, Sullivan KM, et al: Infection with varicella-zoster virus after marrow transplantation. J Infect Dis 152:1172, 1985.
363. Esmonde TF, Herdman G, Anderson G: Chickenpox pneumonia: An association with pregnancy. Thorax 44:812, 1989.
364. Dolin R, Reichman RC, Mazur MH, et al: Herpes zoster-varicella infections in immunosuppressed patients. Ann Intern Med 89:375, 1978.
365. Huberman M, Fossieck BE Jr, Bunn PA Jr, et al: Herpes zoster and small cell bronchogenic carcinoma. Am J Med 68:214, 1980.
366. Feld R, Evans WK, DeBoer G: Herpes zoster in patients with carcinoma of the lung. Am J Med 73:795, 1982.
367. Saito F, Yutani C, Imakita M, et al: Giant cell pneumonia caused by Varicella Zoster virus in a neonate. Arch Pathol Lab Med 113:201, 1989.
368. Charles RE, Katz RL, Ordóñez NG, et al: Varicella-zoster infection with pleural involvement. Am J Clin Pathol 85:522, 1986.
369. Sargent EN, Carson MJ, Reilly ED: Roentgenographic manifestations of varicella pneumonia with postmortem correlation. Am J Roentgenol 98:305, 1966.
370. Knyvett AF: The pulmonary lesions of chicken pox. QJM 39:313, 1966.
371. Southard ME: Roentgen findings in chickenpox pneumonia: Review of the literature and report of five cases. Am J Roentgenol 76:533, 1956.
372. Tan DYM, Kaufman SA, Levene G: Primary chickenpox pneumonia. Am J Roentgenol 76:527, 1956.
373. Burton GC, Sayer WJ, Lillington GA: Varicella pneumonitis in adults: Frequency of sudden death. Dis Chest 50:179, 1966.
373a. Picken G, Booth AJ, Williams MV. Case report: the pulmonary lesions of chickenpox pneumonia-revisited. Br J Radiol 67:659, 1994.
374. Levin HG: A case of chicken-pox pneumonia with x-ray findings suggesting metastatic carcinoma. N Engl J Med 257:461, 1957.
375. Charles RE, Katz RL, Ordonez NG, et al: Varicella-zoster infection with pleural involvement: A cytologic and ultrastructural study of a case. Am J Clin Pathol 85:522, 1986.
376. Kriss N: Chickenpox pneumonia: A case report. Radiology 66:727, 1956.
377. Raider L: Calcification in chickenpox pneumonia. Chest 60:504, 1971.
378. MacKay JB, Cairney P: Pulmonary calcification following varicella. N Z Med J 59:453, 1960.
379. Abrahams EW, Evans C, Knyvett AF, et al: Varicella pneumonia: A possible cause of subsequent pulmonary calcification. Med J Aust 2:781, 1964.
380. Knyvett AF, Stringer RE, Abrahams EW: The radiology of chickenpox lung. J Coll Radiol Australas 9:134, 1965.
381. Brunton FJ, Moore ME: A survey of pulmonary calcification following adult chicken-pox. Br J Radiol 42:256, 1969.
382. Morgan ER, Smalley LA: Varicella in immunocompromised children: Incidence of abdominal pain and organ involvement. Am J Dis Child 137:883, 1983.
383. Krugman S, Goodrich CH, Ward R: Primary varicella pneumonia. N Engl J Med 257:843, 1957.
384. Glick N, Levin S, Nelson K: Recurrent pulmonary infarction in adult chickenpox pneumonia. JAMA 222:173, 1972.
385. Levin MJ, Leventhal S, Masters HA: Factors influencing quantitative isolation of varicella-zoster virus. J Clin Microbiol 19:880, 1984.
386. Williams B, Caper TH: The demonstration of intranuclear inclusion bodies in sputum from a patient with varicella pneumonia. Am J Med 27:836, 1959.
387. Bocles JS, Ehrenkranz NJ, Marks A: Abnormalities of respiratory function in varicella pneumonia. Ann Intern Med 60:183, 1964.
388. Ho M: Epidemiology of CMV infections. Rev Infect Dis 12:S701, 1990.
389. Nankervis GA, Kumar ML: Diseases produced by cytomegaloviruses. Med Clin North Am 62:1021, 1978.
390. Adler SP: Cytomegalovirus and child daycare: Evidence for an increased infection rate among daycare workers. N Engl J Med 321:1290, 1989.
391. Drew WL, Miner RC: Transfusion-related CMV infection following noncardiac surgery. JAMA 247:2389, 1982.
392. Craighead JE, Hanshaw JB, Carpenter CB: Cytomegalovirus infection after renal allotransplantation. JAMA 201:725, 1967.
393. Friedman HM: Cytomegalovirus: Subclinical infection or disease? Am J Med 70:215, 1981.
394. Marrie TJ, Janigan DT, Haldane EV, et al: Does CMV play a role in community-acquired pneumonia? Clin Invest Med 8:286, 1985.
395. Ettinger NA, Bailey TC, Trulock EP, et al: Cytomegalovirus infection and pneumonitis: Impact after isolated lung transplantation. Am Rev Respir Dis 147:1017, 1993.
396. Meyers JD, Flournoy N, Thomas ED: Nonbacterial pneumonia after allogeneic marrow transplantation: A review of ten years' experience. Rev Infect Dis 4:1119, 1982.
397. Skinhoj P, Andersen HK, Moller J, et al: Cytomegalovirus infection after bone marrow transplantation: Relation of pneumonia to postgrafting immunosuppressive treatment. J Med Virol 14:91, 1984.
398. Winston DJ, Ho WG, Lin C-H, et al: Intravenous immunoglobulin for modification of CMV infections associated with bone marrow transplantation. Am J Med 76:128, 1984.
399. Condie RM, O'Reilly RJ: Prevention of CMV infection by prophylaxis with an intravenous, hyperimmune, native, unmodified CMV globulin: Randomized trial in bone marrow transplant recipients. Am J Med 76:134, 1984.
400. Meyers JD, Flournoy N, Thomas ED: Risk factors for CMV infection after human marrow transplantation. J Infect Dis 153:478, 1986.
401. Dummer JS, White LT, Ho M, et al: Morbidity of CMV infection in recipients of heart or heart-lung transplants who received cyclosporine. J Infect Dis 152:1182, 1985.
402. Chou S: Reactivation and recombination of multiple CMV strains from individual organ donors. J Infect Dis 160:11, 1989.
403. Craighead JE: Pulmonary CMV infection in the adult. Am J Pathol 63:487, 1971.
404. Heard BE, Hassan AM, Wilson SM: Pulmonary cytomegalic inclusion-body disease in a diabetic. J Clin Pathol 15:17, 1962.
405. Smith TF, Holley KE, Keys TF, et al: Cytomegalovirus studies of autopsy tissue: I. Virus isolation. Am J Clin Pathol 63:854, 1975.
406. Macasaet FF, Holley KE, Smith TF, et al: Cytomegalovirus studies of autopsy tissue: II. Incidence of inclusion bodies and related pathologic data. Am J Clin Pathol 63:859, 1975.
407. Fajac A, Vidaud M, Lebargy F, et al: Evaluation of human CMV latency in alveolar macrophages. Am J Respir Crit Care Med 149:495, 1994.
408. Grundy JE: Virologic and pathogenetic aspects of CMV infection. Rev Infect Dis 12:S711, 1990.
409. Shanley JD, Pesanti EL, Nugent KM: The pathogenesis of pneumonitis due to murine CMV. J Infect Dis 146:388, 1982.
410. Shepp DH, Dandliker PS, de Miranda P, et al: Activity of 9-[2-hydroxy-1-(hydroxymethyl)ethoxymethyl]-guanine in the treatment of CMV pneumonia. Ann Intern Med 103:368, 1985.
411. Millar AB, Patou G, Miller RF, et al: Cytomegalovirus in the lungs of patients with AIDS: Respiratory pathogen or passenger? Am Rev Respir Dis 141:1474, 1990.
412. Beschorner WE, Hutchins GM, Burns WH, et al: Cytomegalovirus pneumonia in bone marrow transplant recipients: Miliary and diffuse patterns. Am Rev Respir Dis 122:107, 1980.
413. Millard PR, Herbertson BM, Nagington J, et al: The morphological consequences and the significance of CMV infection in renal transplant patients. QJM 42:585, 1973.
414. Peace RJ: Cytomegalic inclusion disease in adults: A complication of neoplastic disease of the hemopoietic and reticulohistiocytic systems. Am J Med 24:48, 1958.
415. Shulman HM, Hackman RC, Sale GE, et al: Rapid cytologic diagnosis of CMV interstitial pneumonia on touch imprints from open-lung biopsy. Am J Clin Pathol 77:90, 1982.
416. Jain U, Mani K, Frable WJ: Cytomegalic inclusion disease: Cytologic diagnosis from bronchial brushing material. Acta Cytol 17:467, 1973.
417. Delfs-Jegge S, Dalquen P, Hurwitz N: Cytomegalovirus-infected cells in a pleural effusion from an acquired immunodeficiency syndrome patient: A case report. Acta Cytol 38:70, 1994.
418. Gorelkin L, Chandler FW, Ewing EP: Staining qualities of CMV inclusions in the lungs of patients with the acquired immunodeficiency syndrome: A potential source of diagnostic misinterpretation. Hum Pathol 17:926, 1986.
419. Martin AM, Kurtz SM: Cytomegalic inclusion disease: An electron microscopic histochemical study of the virus at necropsy. Arch Pathol 82:27, 1966.
420. Browning JD, More IAR, Boyd JF: Adult pulmonary cytomegalic inclusion disease: Report of a case. J Clin Pathol 331:11, 1980.
421. Peterson PK, Balfour HH Jr, Marker SC, et al: Cytomegalovirus disease in renal allograft recipients: A prospective study of the clinical features, risk factors and impact on renal transplantation. Medicine 59:283, 1980.
422. Luna MA, Lichtiger B: Disseminated toxoplasmosis and CMV infection complicating Hodgkin's disease. Am J Clin Pathol 55:499, 1971.
423. Wong T-W, Warner NE: Cytomegalic inclusion disease in adults. Arch Pathol 74:17, 1961.
424. Weiss RL, Colby TV, Spruance S, et al: Simultaneous CMV and herpes simplex virus pneumonia. Arch Pathol Lab Med 111:242, 1987.
425. Rosen P, Hajdu S: Cytomegalovirus inclusion disease at autopsy of patients with cancer. Am J Clin Pathol 55:749, 1971.
426. Ernst P, Chen M-F, Wang N-S, et al: Symbiosis of *Pneumocystis carinii* and CMV in a fatal pneumonia. Can Med Assoc J 128:1089, 1983.
427. Wang N-S, Huang S-N, Thurlbeck WM: Combined *Pneumocystis carinii* and CMV infection. Arch Pathol 90:529, 1970.

428. Ranchod M, Bissell M: Pulmonary alveolar proteinosis and CMV infection. Arch Pathol Lab Med 103:139, 1979.

429. Webb W, Gamsu G, Rohlfing B, et al: Pulmonary complications of renal transplantation: A survey of patients treated by low-dose immunosuppression. Radiology 126:1, 1978.

430. Austin JHM, Schulman LL, Mastrobattista JD: Pulmonary infection after cardiac transplantation: Clinical and radiologic correlations. Radiology 172:259, 1989.

431. Olliff JFC, Williams MP: Radiological appearances of CMV infections. Clin Radiol 40:463, 1989.

432. Schulman LL: Cytomegalovirus pneumonitis and lobar consolidation. Chest 91:558, 1987.

433. Moore EH, Webb WR, Amend WJC: Pulmonary infections in renal transplantation patients treated with cyclosporine. Radiology 167:97, 1988.

434. Janzen DL, Padley SPG, Adler BD, et al: Acute pulmonary complications in immunocompromised non-AIDS patients: Comparison of diagnostic accuracy of CT and chest radiography. Clin Radiol 47:159, 1993.

435. Aafedt BC, Halvorsen RA, Tylen U, et al: Cytomegalovirus pneumonia: Computed tomography findings. J Can Assoc Radiol 41:276, 1990.

436. Kang E-Y, Patz EF, Müller NL: Cytomegalovirus pneumonia in transplant patients: CT findings. J Comput Assist Tomogr 20:295, 1996.

437. McGuinness G, Scholes JV, Garay SM, et al: Cytomegalovirus pneumonitis: Spectrum of parenchymal CT findings with pathologic correlation in 21 AIDS patients. Radiology 192:451, 1994.

438. Hanshaw JB: Clinical significance of CMV infection. Postgrad Med 35:472, 1964.

439. Cohen JI, Corey GR: Cytomegalovirus infection in the normal host. Medicine 64:100, 1985.

440. Pannuti CS, Vilas Boas LS, Angelo MJ, et al: Cytomegalovirus mononucleosis in children and adults: Differences in clinical presentation. Scand J Infect Dis 17:153, 1985.

441. Idell S, Johnson M, Beauregard L, et al: Pneumonia associated with rising CMV antibody titres in a healthy adult. Thorax 38:957, 1983.

442. Klemola E, Stenström R, von Essen R: Pneumonia as a clinical manifestation of CMV infection in previously healthy adults. Scand J Infect Dis 4:7, 1972.

443. Medearis DN Jr: Observations concerning human CMV infection and disease. Bull Johns Hopkins Hosp 114:181, 1964.

444. Jeffery JR, Guttmann RD, Becklake MR, et al: Recovery from severe CMV pneumonia in a renal transplant patient. Am Rev Respir Dis 109:129, 1974.

445. Chou S: Newer methods for diagnosis of CMV infection. Rev Infect Dis 12:S727, 1990.

446. Smith TF: Cytomegalovirus infections: Current diagnostic methods. Mayo Clin Proc 56:767, 1981.

447. Shuster EA, Beneke JS, Tegtmeier GE, et al: Monoclonal antibody for rapid laboratory detection of CMV infections: Characterization and diagnostic application. Mayo Clin Proc 60:577, 1985.

447a. Heurlin N, Markling L, Barkholt L, et al: Rapid detection of cytomegalovirus antigen on alveolar cells in bronchoalveolar fluid from transplant patients with cytomegalovirus pneumonia. Clin Transplant 8:466, 1994.

448. Emanuel D, Peppard J, Stover D, et al: Rapid immunodiagnosis of CMV pneumonia by bronchoalveolar lavage using human and murine monoclonal antibodies. Ann Intern Med 104:476, 1986.

449. Hilborne LH, Nieberg RK, Cheng L, et al: Direct in situ hybridization for rapid detection of cytomegalovirus in bronchoalveolar lavage. Am J Clin Pathol 87:766, 1987.

449a. Aspin MM, Gallez-Hawkins GM, Giugni TD, et al: Comparison of plasma PCR and bronchoalveolar lavage fluid culture for detection of cytomegalovirus infection in adult bone marrow transplant recipients. J Clin Microbiol 32:2266, 1994.

450. Ruutu P, Ruutu T, Volin L, et al: Cytomegalovirus is frequently isolated in bronchoalveolar lavage fluid of bone marrow transplant recipients without pneumonia. Ann Intern Med 112:913, 1990.

451. Zaia JA, Forman SJ, Gallagher MT, et al: Prolonged human CMV viremia following bone marrow transplantation. Transplantation 37:315, 1984.

452. Hackman RC, Myerson D, Meyers JD: Rapid diagnosis of CMV pneumonia by tissue immunofluorescence with a murine monoclonal antibody. J Infect Dis 151:325, 1985.

453. Solans EP, Yong S, Husain AN, et al: Bronchioloalveolar lavage in the diagnosis of CMV pneumonitis in lung transplant recipients: An immunocytochemical study. Diagn Cytopathol 16:350, 1997.

454. Myerson D, Hackman RC, Meyers JD: Diagnosis of cytomegaloviral pneumonia by in situ hybridization. J Infect Dis 150:272, 1984.

455. Jiwa M, Steenbergen RDM, Zwaan FE, et al: Three sensitive methods for the detection of CMV in lung tissue of patients with interstitial pneumonitis. Am J Clin Pathol 93:491, 1990.

456. Shibata M, Terashima M, Kimura H, et al: Quantitation of CMV DNA in lung tissue of bone marrow transplant recipients. Hum Pathol 23:911, 1992.

457. Burgart LJ, Heller MJ, Reznicek MJ, et al: Cytomegalovirus detection in bone marrow transplant patients with idiopathic pneumonitis: A clinicopathologic study of the clinical utility of the polymerase chain reaction on open lung biopsy specimen tissue. Am J Clin Pathol 96:572, 1991.

458. Rasmussen L, Kelsall D, Nelson R, et al: Virus-specific IgG and IgM antibodies in normal and immunocompromised subjects infected with CMV. J Infect Dis 145:191, 1982.

459. Lung ML, Lam WK, So SL, et al: Evidence that respiratory tract is major reservoir for Epstein-Barr virus. Lancet 1:889, 1985.

460. Henle W, Henle G, Scriba M, et al: Antibody responses to the Epstein-Barr virus and cytomegaloviruses after open-heart and other surgery. N Engl J Med 282:1068, 1970.

461. Pereira MS, Field AM, Blake JM, et al: Evidence for oral excretion of E.B. virus in infectious mononucleosis. Lancet 1:710, 1972.

462. Hoagland RJ: The clinical manifestations of infectious mononucleosis: A report of two hundred cases. Am J Med Sci 240:21, 1960.

463. Wechsler HF, Rosenblum AH, Sills CT: Infectious mononucleosis: Report of an epidemic in an army post. Ann Intern Med 25:113, 1946.

464. Lander P, Palayew MJ: Infectious mononucleosis—a review of chest roentgenographic manifestations. J Can Assoc Radiol 25:303, 1974.

465. Garten AJ, Mendelson DS, Halton KP: CT manifestations of infectious mononucleosis. Clin Imaging 16:114, 1992.

466. Goddard P, Kinsella D, Duncan AW, et al: Magnetic resonance imaging of the chest in infectious mononucleosis. Br J Radiol 63:138, 1990.

467. Dommerby H, Stangerup S-E, Stangerup M, et al: Hepatosplenomegaly in infectious mononucleosis, assessed by ultrasonic scanning. J Laryngol Otol 100:573, 1986.

468. Britton S, Andersson-Anvret M, Gergely P, et al: Epstein-Barr-virus immunity and tissue distribution in a fatal case of infectious mononucleosis. N Engl J Med 298:89, 1978.

469. Ziegler EE: Infectious mononucleosis: Report of a fatal case with autopsy. Arch Pathol 37:196, 1944.

470. Weiss LM, Chang KL: Molecular biologic studies of Hodgkin's disease. Semin Diagn Pathol 9:272, 1992.

471. Sato Y, Dunbar JS: Abnormalities of the pharynx and prevertebral soft tissues in infectious mononucleosis. Am J Roentgenol 134:149, 1980.

472. Johnsen T, Katholm M, Stangerup S-E: Otolaryngological complications in infectious mononucleosis. J Laryngol Otol 98:999, 1984.

473. Carrington P, Hall JI: Fatal airway obstruction in infectious mononucleosis. BMJ 292:195, 1986.

474. Morgan EJ, Altmeyer R, Khakoo R, et al: Pulmonary function in infectious mononucleosis. Chest 81:699, 1982.

475. Cohen JI: Epstein-Barr virus lymphoproliferative disease associated with acquired immunodeficiency. Medicine 70:137, 1991.

476. Jones JF, Shurin S, Abramowsky C, et al: T-cell lymphomas containing Epstein-Barr viral DNA in patients with chronic Epstein-Barr virus infections. N Engl J Med 318:733, 1988.

477. Evans AS, Comstock GW: Presence of elevated antibody titres to Epstein-Barr virus before Hodgkin's disease. Lancet 1:1183, 1981.

478. Seigneurin JM, Mingat J, Lenoir SM, et al: Angioimmunoblastic lymphadenopathy after infectious mononucleosis. BMJ 282:1574, 1981.

479. Martin A, Capron F, Liguory-Brunaud MD, et al: Epstein-Barr virus-associated primary malignant lymphomas of the pleural cavity occurring in longstanding pleural chronic inflammation. Hum Pathol 25:1314, 1994.

480. Aozasa K: Pyothorax-associated lymphoma. Int J Hematol 65:9, 1996.

481. Katzenstein A-LA, Peiper SC: Detection of Epstein-Barr virus genomes in lymphomatoid granulomatosis: Analysis of 29 cases by the polymerase chain reaction technique. Mod Pathol 3:435, 1990.

482. Barbera JA, Hayashi S, Hegele RG, et al: Detection of Epstein-Barr virus in lymphocytic interstitial pneumonia in situ hybridization. Am Rev Respir Dis 145:940, 1992.

483. Vergnon JM, Vincent M, De Thé G, et al: Cryptogenic fibrosing alveolitis and Epstein-Barr virus: An association? Lancet 2:768, 1984.

484. Butler AE, Colby TV, Weiss L, et al: Lymphoepithelioma-like carcinoma of the lung. Am J Surg Pathol 13:632, 1989.

485. Ross PJ, Seaton A, Foreman HM, et al: Pulmonary calcification following smallpox handler's lung. Thorax 29:659, 1974.

486. Steinberg BM, Topp WC, Schneider PS, et al: Laryngeal papillomavirus infection during clinical remission. N Engl J Med 308:1261, 1983.

487. Byrne JC, Tsao MS, Fraser RS, et al: Human papillomavirus-11 DNA in a patient with chronic laryngotracheobronchial papillomatosis and metastatic squamous-cell carcinoma of the lung. N Engl J Med 317:873, 1987.

488. Béjui-Thivolet F, Liagre N, Chignol MC, et al: Detection of human papillomavirus DNA in squamous bronchial metaplasia and squamous cell carcinoma of the lung by in situ hybridization using biotinylated probes in paraffin-embedded specimens. Hum Pathol 21:111, 1990.

488a. Balkhy HH, Sabella C, Goldfarb J: Parvovirus: A review. Bull Rheum Dis 47:4, 1998.

488b. Kolquist KA, Vnencak-Jones CL, Swift L, et al: Fatal fat embolism syndrome in a child with undiagnosed hemoglobin s/beta + thalassemia: A complication of acute parvovirus B19 infection. Pediatr Pathol Lab Med 16:71, 1996.

488c. Lowenthal EA, Wells A, Emanuel PD, et al: Sickle cell acute chest syndrome associated with parvovirus B19 infection: Case series and review. Am J Hematol 51:207, 1996.

489. Embree JE, Embil JA: Mycoplasmas in diseases of humans. Can Med Assoc J 123:105, 1980.

490. Norton R, Mollison L: *Mycoplasma hominis* pneumonia in aboriginal adults. Pathology 27:58, 1995.

490a. Kane JR, Shenep JL, Krance RA, et al: Diffuse alveolar hemorrhage associated with *Mycoplasma hominis* respiratory tract infection in a bone marrow transplant recipient. Chest 105:1891, 1994.

491. Lo SC, Wear DJ, Green SL, et al: Adult respiratory distress syndrome with or without systemic disease associated with infections due to *Mycoplasma fermentans*. Clin Infect Dis 17:S259, 1993.

492. de Barbeyrac B, Bernet-Poggi C, Febrer F, et al: Detection of *Mycoplasma pneumoniae* and *Mycoplasma genitalium* in clinical samples by polymerase chain reaction. Clin Infect Dis 17(Suppl 1):S83, 1993.

493. Collier AM, Clyde WA Jr: Appearance of *Mycoplasma pneumoniae* in lungs of experimentally infected hamsters and sputum from patients with natural disease. Am Rev Respir Dis 110:765, 1974.

494. Levine DP, Lerner AM: The clinical spectrum of *Mycoplasma pneumoniae* infections. Med Clin North Am 62:961, 1978.

495. Taylor-Robinson D: The biology of mycoplasmas. J Clin Pathol 21(Suppl 2):38, 1968.

496. Ortqvist A, Jedlund A, Grillner I, et al: Etiology, outcome and prognostic factors in community-acquired pneumonia requiring hospitalization. Eur Respir J 3:1105, 1990.

497. Karalus NC, Cursons RT, Leng RA, et al: Community acquired pneumonia: Etiology and prognostic index evaluation. Thorax 46:413, 1991.

498. Almirall J, Morato I, Riera F, et al: Incidence of community-acquired pneumonia and *Chlamydia pneumoniae* infection: A prospective multicentre study. Eur Respir J 6:14, 1993.

499. Berntsson E, Blomberg J, Lagergard T, et al: Etiology of community-acquired pneumonia in patients requiring hospitalization. Eur J Clin Microbiol 4:268, 1985.

500. Foy HM, Kenny GE, Cooney MK, et al: Long-term epidemiology of infections with *Mycoplasma pneumoniae*. J Infect Dis 139:681, 1979.

501. Amundson DE, Weiss PJ: Pneumonia in military recruits. Milit Med 159:629, 1994.

502. Purcell RH, Chanock RM: Role of mycoplasmas in human respiratory disease. Med Clin North Am 51:791, 1967.

503. Sande MA, Gadot F, Wenzel RP: Point source epidemic of *Mycoplasma pneumoniae* infection in a prosthodontics laboratory. Am Rev Respir Dis 112:213, 1975.

504. Gass R, Fisher J, Badesch D, et al: Donor-to-host transmission of *Mycoplasma hominis* in lung allograft recipients. Clin Infect Dis 22:567, 1996.

505. Balassanian N, Robbins FC: *Mycoplasma pneumoniae* infection in families. N Engl J Med 27:719, 1967.

506. Smith CB, Friedewald WT, Chanock RM: Shedding of *Mycoplasma pneumoniae* after tetracycline and erythromycin therapy. N Engl J Med 276:1172, 1967.

507. Forsyth BR, Bloom HH, Johnson KM, et al: Etiology of primary atypical pneumonia in a military population. JAMA 191:364, 1965.

508. Foy HM, Grayston JT, Kenny GE, et al: Epidemiology of *Mycoplasma pneumoniae* infection in families. JAMA 197:859, 1966.

509. Foy HM, Kenny GE, McMahan R, et al: *Mycoplasma pneumoniae* in the community. Am J Epidemiol 93:55, 1971.

510. Copps SC, Allen VD, Sueltmann S, et al: A community outbreak of *Mycoplasma* pneumonia. JAMA 204:123, 1968.

511. Noah ND: *Mycoplasma pneumoniae* infection in the United Kingdom—1967–73. BMJ 2:544, 1974.

512. Evatt BL, Dowdle WR, Johnson M Jr, et al: Epidemic *Mycoplasma* pneumonia. N Engl J Med 285:374, 1971.

513. Khatib R, Schnarr D: Point-source outbreak of *Mycoplasma pneumoniae* infection in a family unit. J Infect Dis 151:186, 1985.

514. Foy HM, Kenny GE, McMahan R, et al: *Mycoplasma pneumoniae* pneumonia in an urban area: Five years of surveillance. JAMA 214:1666, 1970.

515. Murphy GF, Brody AR, Craighead JE: Exfoliation of respiratory epithelium in hamster tracheal organ cultures infected with *Mycoplasma pneumoniae*. Virchows Arch 389:93, 1980.

516. Woodruff KH: Scanning electron microscopy of *Mycoplasma*-infected tracheal rings. Arch Pathol Lab Med 100:360, 1976.

517. Kist M, Koester H, Bredt W: *Mycoplasma pneumoniae* induces cytotoxic activity in guinea pig bronchoalveolar cells. Am Rev Respir Dis 131:669, 1985.

518. Murray HW, Tuazon C: Atypical pneumonias. Med Clin North Am 64:507, 1980.

519. Cassell GH, Cole BC: Mycoplasmas as agents of human disease. N Engl J Med 304:80, 1981.

520. Biberfeld G, Arneborn P, Forsgren M, et al: Nonspecific polyclonal antibody response induced by *Mycoplasma pneumoniae*. Yale J Biol Med 56:639, 1983.

521. Taylor G: Immunity to *Mycoplasma* infections of the respiratory tract: A review. J R Soc Med 72:520, 1979.

522. Cotter FE, Bainbridge D, Newland AC: Neurological deficit associated with *Mycoplasma pneumoniae* reversed by plasma exchange. BMJ 286:22, 1983.

523. Mizutani H, Mizutani H: Circulating immune complexes in patients with mycoplasmal pneumonia. Am Rev Respir Dis 130:627, 1984.

524. Dajani AS, Clyde WA, Denny FW: Experimental infection with *Mycoplasma pneumoniae* (Eaton's agent). J Exp Med 121:1071, 1965.

525. Koletsky RJ, Weinstein AJ: Fulminant *Mycoplasma pneumoniae* infection: Report of a fatal case and a review of the literature. Am Rev Respir Dis 122:491, 1980.

526. Maisel JC, Babbitt LH, John TJ: Fatal *Mycoplasma pneumoniae* infection with isolation of organisms from lung. JAMA 202:287, 1967.

527. Rollins S, Colby T, Clayton F: Open lung biopsy in *Mycoplasma pneumoniae* pneumonia. Arch Pathol Lab Med 110:34, 1986.

528. Benisch BM, Fayemi A, Gerber MA, et al: Mycoplasmal pneumonia in a patient with rheumatic heart disease. Am J Clin Pathol 58:343, 1972.

529. Kaufman JM, Cuvelier CA, Van der Straeten M: *Mycoplasma* pneumonia with fulminant evolution into diffuse interstitial fibrosis. Thorax 35:140, 1980.

530. Rosmus HH, Paré JAP, Masson AM, et al: Roentgenographic patterns of acute *Mycoplasma* and viral pneumonitis. J Can Assoc Radiol 19:74, 1968.

531. Brolin I, Wernstedt L: Radiographic appearance of mycoplasmal pneumonia. Scand J Respir Dis 59:179, 1978.

532. Borthwick RC, Cameron DC, Philp T: Radiographic patterns of pulmonary involvement in acute mycoplasmal infections. Scand J Respir Dis 59:190, 1978.

533. Cameron DC, Borthwick RN, Philp T: The radiographic patterns of acute myco-plasma pneumonitis. Clin Radiol 28:173, 1977.

534. Finnegan OC, Fowles SJ, White RJ: Radiographic appearances of *Mycoplasma* pneumonia. Thorax 36:469, 1981.

535. Alexander ER, Foy JM, Kenny GE, et al: Pneumonia due to *Mycoplasma pneumoniae*: Its incidence in the membership of a cooperative medical group. N Engl J Med 275:131, 1966.

536. Grayston JT, Alexander ER, Kenny GE, et al: *Mycoplasma pneumoniae* infections: Clinical and epidemiologic studies. JAMA 191:369, 1965.

537. Izumikawa K, Hara K: Clinical features of mycoplasmal pneumonia in adults. Yale J Biol Med 56:505, 1983.

538. Thombs DD: Cold agglutinin-positive pneumonia: A review of thirty cases in children. Ohio State Med J 63:1171, 1967.

539. Nitu Y: *M. pneumoniae* respiratory diseases: Clinical features—children. Yale J Biol Med 56:493, 1983.

540. Putman CE, Curtis AM, Simeone JF, et al: *Mycoplasma* pneumonia: Clinical and roentgenographic patterns. Am J Roentgenol 124:417, 1975.

541. Lambert HP: *Mycoplasma pneumoniae* infections. J Clin Pathol 21(Suppl 2):52, 1968.

542. Dean NL: Mycoplasma pneumonias in the community hospital: The "unusual" manifestations become common. Clin Chest Med 2:121, 1981.

543. Fine NL, Smith LR, Sheedy PF: Frequency of pleural effusions in *Mycoplasma* and viral pneumonias. N Engl J Med 283:790, 1970.

544. Shulman ST, Bartlett J, Clyde WA Jr, et al: The unusual severity of mycoplasmal pneumonia in children with sickle-cell disease. N Engl J Med 287:164, 1972.

545. Grix A, Giammona ST: Pneumonitis with pleural effusion in children due to *Mycoplasma pneumoniae*. Am Rev Respir Dis 109:665, 1974.

546. Fischman RA, Marschall KE, Kislak JW, et al: Adult respiratory distress syndrome caused by *Mycoplasma* pneumonia. Chest 74:471, 1974.

547. Müller NL, Miller RR. State-of-the-art diseases of the bronchioles: CT and histopathologic findings. Radiology 196:3, 1995.

547a. Tanaka N, Matsumoto T, Kuramitsu T, et al: High-resolution CT findings in community-acquired pneumonia. J Comput Assist Tomogr 20:600, 1996.

548. Lind K: Manifestations and complications of *Mycoplasma pneumoniae* disease: A review. Yale J Biol Med 56:461, 1983.

549. Ali NJ, Sillis M, Andrews BE, et al: The clinical spectrum and diagnosis of *Mycoplasma pneumoniae* infection. QJM 58:241, 1986.

550. Simmons BP, Aber RC: *Mycoplasma pneumoniae* pneumonia: Symptoms mimicking pulmonary embolism with infarction. JAMA 241:1268, 1979.

551. Kane JR, Shenep JL, Krance RA, et al: Diffuse alveolar hemorrhage associated with *Mycoplasma hominis* respiratory tract infection in a bone marrow transplant recipient. Chest 105:1891, 1994.

552. Yano T, Ichikawa Y, Komatu S, et al: Association of *Mycoplasma pneumoniae* antigen with initial onset of bronchial asthma. Am J Respir Crit Care Med 149:1348, 1994.

553. Nastro JA, Littner MR, Tashkin DP, et al: Diffuse, pulmonary, interstitial infiltrate and mycoplasmal pneumonia: Case report. Am Rev Respir Dis 110:659, 1974.

554. Zack MB, Kazemi H: Carbon dioxide retention in *Mycoplasma* pneumonia. Am Rev Respir Dis 107:1052, 1973.

555. Solanki DL, Berdoff RL: Severe mycoplasma pneumonia with pleural effusions in patient with sickle cell-hemoglobin C(SC) disease: Case report and review of the literature. Am J Med 66:707, 1979.

556. Foy HM, Nolan CM, Allan ID: Epidemiologic aspects of *M. pneumoniae* disease complications: A review. Yale J Biol Med 56:469, 1983.

557. Merkx H, De Keyser J, Ebinger G: Miller Fisher syndrome associated with *Mycoplasma pneumoniae* infection: Report of a case. Clin Neurol Neurosurg 96:96, 1994.

558. Hely MA, Williamson PM, Terenty TR: Neurological complications of *Mycoplasma pneumoniae* infection. Clin Exp Neurol 20:153, 1984.

559. Ponka A, von Bonsdorff M, Farkkila M: Polyradiculitis associated with *Mycoplasma pneumoniae* reversed by plasma exchange [letter]. BMJ 286:475, 1983.

560. MacFarlane PI, Miller V: Transverse myelitis associated with *Mycoplasma pneumoniae* infection. Arch Dis Child 59:80, 1984.

561. van Hook L, Spivack C, Duncanson FP: Acquired Pelger-Huet anomaly associated with *Mycoplasma pneumoniae* pneumonia. Am J Clin Pathol 84:248, 1985.

562. Mickley H, Sorensen PG: Immune haemolytic anaemia associated with ampicillin-dependent warm antibodies and high titre cold agglutinins in a patient with *Mycoplasma* pneumonia. Scand J Haematol 32:323, 1984.

563. Schulman P, Piemonte TC, Singh B: Acute renal failure, hemolytic anemia, and *Mycoplasma* pneumonia. JAMA 244:1823, 1980.

564. Lambert HP: Syndrome with joint manifestations in association with *Mycoplasma pneumoniae* infection. BMJ 3:156, 1968.

565. Jones MC: Arthritis and arthralgia in infection with *Mycoplasma pneumoniae*. Thorax 25:748, 1970.

566. Sequeira W, Jones E, Bronson DM: *Mycoplasma* pneumonia infection with arthritis and varicella-like eruption. JAMA 246:1936, 1981.

567. El Khatib MR, Lerner AM: Myocarditis in *Mycoplasma pneumoniae* pneumonia: Occurrence with hemolytic anemia and extraordinary titers of cold isohemagglutinins. JAMA 231:493, 1975.

568. Sands MJ Jr, Satz JE, Turner WE Jr, et al: Pericarditis and perimyocarditis associated with active *Mycoplasma pneumoniae* infection. Ann Intern Med 86:544, 1977.

569. Sands MJ, Rosenthal R: Progressive heart failure and death associated with *Mycoplasma pneumoniae* pneumonia. Chest 81:763, 1982.

570. Cherry JD, Hurwitz ES, Welliver RC: *Mycoplasma pneumoniae* infections and exanthems. J Pediatr 87:369, 1975.

571. Turner JAP, Burchak EC, Bannatyne RM, et al: The protean manifestations of *Mycoplasma* infections in childhood. Can Med Assoc J 99:633, 1968.

572. Teisch JA, Shapiro L, Walzer RA: Vesiculopustular eruption with *Mycoplasma* infection. JAMA 211:1694, 1970.

573. Von Bonsdorff M, Ponka A, Tornroth T: Mycoplasmal pneumonia associated with mesangiocapillary glomerulonephritis type II (dense deposit disease). Acta Med Scand 216:427, 1984.

574. Yamashitga R, Kitahara H, Kanemitsu T, et al: Eosinophil cationic protein in the sera of patients with *Mycoplasma pneumonia*. Pediatr Infect Dis J 13:379, 1994.

575. Sterner G, Svedmyr A, Tunevall G, et al: Infections with Eaton agent in pneumonia. Acta Med Scand 178:751, 1965.

576. Tully JG, Rose DL, Whitcomb RF, et al: Enhanced isolation of *Mycoplasma pneumoniae* from throat washings with a newly modified culture medium. J Infect Dis 139:478, 1979.

577. Dussaix E, Slim A, Tournier P: Comparison of enzyme-linked immunosorbent assay (ELISA) and complement fixation test for detection of *Mycoplasma pneumoniae* antibodies. J Clin Pathol 36:228, 1983.

578. Clyde WA Jr: *Mycoplasma pneumoniae* respiratory disease symposium: Summation and significance. Yale J Biol Med 56:523, 1983.

579. Granstrom M, Holme T, Sjogren AM, et al: The role of IgA determination by ELISA in the early serodiagnosis of *Mycoplasma pneumoniae* infection, in relation to IgG and mu-capture IgM methods. J Med Microbiol 40:288, 1994.

580. Dular R, Kajioka R, Kasatiya S: Comparison of Gen-Probe commercial kit and culture technique for the diagnosis of *Mycoplasma pneumoniae* infection. J Clin Microbiol 26:1068, 1988.

581. Tilton RC, Dias F, Kidd H, et al: DNA probe versus culture for detection of *Mycoplasma pneumoniae* in clinical specimens. Diagn Microbiol Infect Dis 10:109, 1988.

582. Kleemola SRM, Karjalainen JE, Raty RKH: Rapid diagnosis of *Mycoplasma pneumoniae* infection: Clinical evaluation of a commercial probe test. J Infect Dis 162:70, 1990.

583. Bernet C, Garret M, DeBarbeyrac B, et al: Detection of *Mycoplasma pneumoniae* by using the polymerase chain reaction. J Clin Microbiol 27:2492, 1989.

584. Luneberg E, Jensen JS, Frosch M: Detection of *Mycoplasma pneumoniae* by polymerase chain reaction and nonradioactive hybridization in microtiter plates. J Clin Microbiol 31:1088, 1993.

585. Falguera M, Nogues A, Ruiz-Gonzalez A, et al: Detection of *Mycoplasma pneumoniae* by polymerase chain reaction in lung aspirates from patients with community-acquired pneumonia. Chest 110:972, 1996.

586. Chanock RM: *Mycoplasma* infections of man (concluded). N Engl J Med 273:1257, 1965.

587. Mufson MA, Manko MA, Kingston JR, et al: Eaton agent pneumonia—clinical features. JAMA 178:369, 1961.

588. Harris LF, Swann P: Mycoplasmal pneumonia: Three severe cases of a common infection. Postgrad Med 76:71, 1984.

589. Koletsky RJ, Weinstein AJ: Fulminant *Mycoplasma pneumoniae* infection: Report of a fatal case and a review of the literature. Am Rev Respir Dis 122:491, 1980.

590. McFarlane JT, Morris MJ: Abnormalities in lung function following clinical recovery from *Mycoplasma pneumoniae* pneumonia. Eur J Respir Dis 63:337, 1982.

591. Tablan OC, Reyes MP: Chronic interstitial pulmonary fibrosis following *Mycoplasma pneumoniae* pneumonia. Am J Med 79:268, 1985.

592. Reyes de la Rocha S, Leonard JC, Demetriou E: Potential permanent respiratory sequela of Stevens-Johnson syndrome in an adolescent. J Adolesc Health Care 6:220, 1985.

593. Sabato AR, Martin AJ, Marmion BP, et al: *Mycoplasma pneumoniae:* Acute illness, antibiotics, and subsequent pulmonary function. Arch Dis Child 59:1034, 1984.

594. Halal F, Brochu P, Delage G, et al: Severe disseminated lung disease and bronchiectasis probably due to *Mycoplasma pneumoniae.* Can Med Assoc J 117:1055, 1977.

595. Ward ME: Chlamydial classification, development and structure. Br Med Bull 39:109, 1983.

595a. Campbell S, Larsen J, Knight ST, et al: Chlamydial elementary bodies are translocated on the surface of epithelial cells. Am J Pathol 152:1167, 1998.

596. Montalban GS, Roblin PM, Hammerschlag MR: Performance of three commercially available monoclonal reagents for confirmation of *Chlamydia pneumoniae* in cell culture. J Clin Microbiol 32:1406, 1994.

597. Gaydos CA, Roblin PM, Hammerschlag MR, et al: Diagnostic utility of PCR-enzyme immunoassay, culture, and serology for the detection of *Chlamydia pneumoniae* in symptomatic and asymptomatic patients. J Clin Microbiol 32:903, 1994.

598. Laurila AL, Anttila T, Laara E, et al: Serological evidence of an association between *Chlamydia pneumoniae* infection and lung cancer. Int J Cancer 74:31, 1997.

599. Hahn DL, Anttila T, Saikku P: Association of *Chlamydia pneumoniae* IgA antibodies with recently symptomatic asthma. Epidemiol Infect 117:513, 1996.

599a. Cook PJ, Davies P, Tunnicliffe W, et al: *Chlamydia pneumoniae* and asthma. Thorax 53:254, 1998.

600. Ben-Yaakov M, Lazarovich Z, Beer S, et al: Prevalence of *Chlamydia pneumoniae* antibodies in patients with acute respiratory infections in Israel. J Clin Pathol 47:232, 1994.

601. Einarsson S, Sigurdsson HK, Magnusdottir SD, et al: Age specific prevalence of antibodies against *Chlamydia pneumoniae* in Iceland. Scand J Infect Dis 26:393, 1994.

602. Herrmann B, Salih MA, Yousif BE, et al: *Chlamydia* etiology of acute lower respiratory tract infections in children in the Sudan. Acta Paediatr 83:169, 1994.

603. Thorn DH, Grayston JT, Campbell LA, et al: Respiratory infection with *Chlamydia pneumoniae* in middle-aged and older adult outpatients. Eur J Clin Microbiol Infect Dis 13:785, 1994.

604. Pether JVS, Wang S-P, Grayston JT: *Chlamydia pneumoniae*, strain TWAR, as the cause of an outbreak in a boy's school previously called psittacosis. Epidemiol Infect 103:395, 1989.

605. Blasi F, Cosentini R, Denti F, et al: Two family outbreaks of *Chlamydia pneumoniae* infection. Eur Respir J 7:102, 1994.

606. Blasi F, Boschini A, Cosentini R, et al: Outbreak of *Chlamydia pneumoniae* infection in former injection-drug users. Chest 105:812, 1994.

607. Von Hertzen L, Alakarppa H, Koskinen R, et al: *Chlamydia pneumoniae* infection in patients with chronic obstructive pulmonary disease. Epidemiol Infect 118:155, 1997.

608. von Hertzen L, Isoaho R, Leinonen M, et al: *Chlamydia pneumoniae* antibodies in chronic obstructive pulmonary disease. Int J Epidemiol 25:658, 1996.

609. McConnell CT, Plouffe JF, File TM, et al, CBPIS Study Group: Radiographic appearance of *Chlamydia pneumoniae* (TWAR Strain) respiratory infections. Radiology 192:819, 1994.

610. Emre U, Bernius M, Roblin PM, et al: *Chlamydia pneumoniae* infection in patients with cystic fibrosis. Clin Infect Dis 22:819, 1996.

611. Wright SW, Edwards KM, Decker MD, et al: Prevalence of positive serology for acute *Chlamydia pneumoniae* infection in emergency department patients with persistent cough. Acad Emerg Med 4:179, 1997.

612. von Hertzen L, Leinonen M, Surcel HM, et al: Measurement of sputum antibodies in the diagnosis of acute and chronic respiratory infections associated with *Chlamydia pneumoniae.* Clin Diagn Lab Immunol 2:454, 1995.

613. Ljungstrom L, Franzen C, Schlaug M, et al: Reinfection with *Chlamydia pneumoniae* may induce isolated and systemic vasculitis in small and large vessels. Scand J Infect Dis 104(Suppl):37, 1997.

614. Kleemola M, Saikku P, Visakorpi R, et al: Epidemics of pneumonia caused by TWAR, a new chlamydia organism, in military trainees in Finland. J Infect Dis 157:230, 1988.

615. Cosentini R, Blasi F, Raccanelli R, et al: Severe community-acquired pneumonia: a possible role for *Chlamydia pneumoniae.* Respiration 63:61, 1996.

615a. Garnett P, Brogan O, Lafong C, et al: Comparison of throat swabs with sputum specimens for the detection of *Chlamydia pneumoniae* antigen by direct immunofluorescence. J Clin Pathol 51:309, 1998.

616. Poussin M, Fuentes V, Corbel C, et al: Capture-ELISA: A new assay for the detection of immunoglobulin M isotype antibodies using Chlamydia trachomatis antigen. J Immunol Methods 204:1, 1997.

617. Daugharty H, Messmer TO, Fields BS: ELISPOT assay for Chlamydia-specific, antibody-producing cells correlated with conventional complement fixation and microimmunofluorescence. J Clin Lab Anal 11:45, 1997.

618. Schachter J: Chlamydial infections (three parts). N Engl J Med 298:428, 490, 540, 1978.

619. Hieber JP: Infections due to *Chlamydia.* J Pediatr 91:864, 1977.

620. Radkowski MA, Kranzler JK, Beem MO, et al: *Chlamydia* pneumonia in infants: Radiography in 125 cases. Am J Roentgenol 137:703, 1981.

621. Hammerschlag MR: Chlamydial pneumonia: Not for babies only? JAMA 245:1346, 1981.

622. Tack KJ, Peterson PK, Rasp PL, et al: Isolation of *Chlamydia trachomatis* from the lower respiratory tract of adults. Lancet 1:116, 1980.

623. Ito JE Jr, Comess KA, Alexander ER, et al: Pneumonia due to *Chlamydia trachomatis* in an immunocompromised adult. N Engl J Med 307:95, 1982.

624. Moncada JV, Schachter J, Wofsy C: Prevalence of *Chlamydia trachomatis* lung infection in patients with acquired immune deficiency syndrome. J Clin Microbiol 23:986, 1986.

625. Meyers JD, Hackman RC, Stamm WE: *Chlamydia trachomatis* infection as a cause of pneumonia after human marrow transplantation. Transplantation 36:130, 1983.

626. Komaroff AL, Aronson MD, Schachter J: *Chlamydia trachomatis* infection in adults with community-acquired pneumonia. JAMA 245:1319, 1981.

627. Sundkvist R, Mardh PA: Serological evidence of *Chlamydia trachomatis* infection in non-immunocompromised adults with pneumonia. J Infect 9:143, 1984.

628. Harrison HR, Alexander ER, Chiang W-T, et al: Experimental nasopharyngitis and pneumonia caused by *Chlamydia trachomatis* in infant baboons: Histopathologic comparison with a case in a human infant. J Infect Dis 139:141, 1979.

629. Goldbloom RB: Chlamydial pneumonia and human sexuality [editorial]. Can Med Assoc J 119:1153, 1978.

630. Edelman RR, Hann LE, Simon M: *Chlamydia trachomatis* pneumonia in adults: Radiographic appearance. Radiology 152:279, 1984.

631. Bernstein DI, Hubbard T, Wenman WM, et al: Mediastinal and supraclavicular lymphadenitis and pneumonitis due to *Chlamydia trachomatis* serovars L1 and L2. N Engl J Med 311:1543, 1984.

632. Stutman HR, Rettig PJ, Reyes S: *Chlamydia trachomatis* as a cause of pneumonitis and pleural effusion. J Pediatr 104:588, 1984.

633. Numazaki K, Chiba S, Yamanaka T, et al: Detection of IgM antibodies against *Chlamydia trachomatis* by enzyme linked fluorescence immunoassay. J Clin Pathol 38:733, 1985.

634. Beer RJS, Bradford WP, Hart RJC: Pregnancy complicated by psittacosis acquired from sheep. BMJ 284:1156, 1982.

635. Barnes MG, Brainerd H: Pneumonitis with alveolar-capillary block in a cattle rancher exposed to epizootic bovine abortion. N Engl J Med 271:981, 1964.

636. MacFarlane JT, MacRae AD: Psittacosis. Br Med Bull 39:163, 1983.

637. McKendrick GDW, Davies J, Dutta T: A small outbreak of psittacosis. Lancet 2:1255, 1973.

638. Palmer SR, Andrews BE, Major R: A common-source outbreak of ornithosis in veterinary surgeons. Lancet 2:798, 1981.

639. Andrews BE, Major R, Palmer SR: Ornithosis in poultry workers. Lancet 1:632, 1981.

640. Grist NR, McLean C: Infections by organisms of psittacosis/lymphogranuloma venereum group in the west of Scotland. BMJ 2:21, 1964.

641. Editorial: Psittacosis. BMJ 1:1, 1972.

642. Byrom NP, Walls J, Mair HJ: Fulminant psittacosis. Lancet 1:353, 1979.

643. Saikku P, Wang SP, Kleemola M, et al: An epidemic of mild pneumonia due to an unusual strain of *Chlamydia psittaci.* J Infect Dis 151:832, 1985.

644. Barrett PKM, Greenberg MJ: Outbreak of ornithosis. BMJ 2:206, 1966.

645. Cunningham AI, Walker WJ: Psittacosis in Hamilton: A case report and epidemiological study. Can Med Assoc J 102:69, 1970.

646. McGavran MH, Beard CW, Berendt RF, et al: The pathogenesis of psittacosis: Serial studies on rhesus monkeys exposed to a small-particle aerosol of the Borg strain. Am J Pathol 40:653, 1962.

647. Walton KW: The pathology of a fatal case of psittacosis showing intracytoplasmic inclusions in the meninges. J Pathol Bacteriol 68:565, 1954.

648. Yow EM, Brennan JC, Preston J, et al: The pathology of psittacosis: A report of two cases with hepatitis. Am J Med 27:739, 1959.

649. Lillie RD: I. The pathology of psittacosis in man. II. The pathology of psittacosis in animals and the distribution of *Rickettsia psittachi* in the tissues of man and animals. National Institutes of Health Bulletin No. 161, pp 1–66, May, 1933.

650. Kuritsky JN, Schmid GP, Potter ME, et al: Psittacosis: A diagnostic challenge. J Occup Med 26:731, 1984.

651. Stenström R, Jansson E, Wager O: Ornithosis pneumonia with special reference to roentgenological lung findings. Acta Med Scand 171:349, 1962.

652. Schaffner W, Brutz DJ, Duncan GW, et al: The clinical spectrum of endemic psittacosis. Arch Intern Med 119:433, 1967.

653. Kroening PM: Ornithosis: Report of a case. Am J Roentgenol 92:1370, 1964.

654. Cornog JL Jr, Hanson CW: Psittacosis as a cause of miliary infiltrates of the lung and hepatic granulomas. Am Rev Respir Dis 98:1033, 1968.

655. Editorial: Psittacosis. Lancet 2:1246, 1973.

656. Psittacosis associated with turkey processing. MMWR 30:638, 1982.

657. Harris AA, Pottage JC Jr, Kessler HA, et al: Psittacosis bacteremia in a patient with sarcoidosis. Ann Intern Med 101:502, 1984.

658. Hamilton DV: Psittacosis and disseminated intravascular coagulation. BMJ 2:370, 1975.

659. van Berkel M, Dik H, van der Meer JWM, et al: Acute respiratory insufficiency from psittacosis. BMJ 290:1503, 1985.

660. Geddes DM, Skeates SJ: Ornithosis pneumonia associated with haemolysis. Br J Dis Chest 71:135, 1977.

661. Antony SJ, Schaffner W: Q fever pneumonia. Semin Respir Infect 12:2, 1997.

662. Brown GL: Q fever. BMJ 2:43, 1973.

663. Johnson JE, Kadull PJ: Laboratory-acquired Q fever: A report of 50 cases. Am J Med 41:391, 1966.

664. Simor AE, Brunton JL, Salit IE, et al: Q-fever: Hazard from sheep used in research. Can Med Assoc J 130:1013, 1984.

665. Meiklejohn G, Reimer LG, Graves PS, et al: Cryptic epidemic of Q fever in a medical school. J Infect Dis 144:107, 1981.

666. Ruppanner R, Brooks D, Morrish D, et al: Q-fever hazards from sheep and goats used in research. Arch Environ Health 37:103, 1982.

667. Rauch AM, Tanner M, Pacer RE, et al: Sheep-associated outbreak of Q fever, Idaho. Arch Intern Med 147:341, 1987.

668. McKelvie P: Q fever in a Queensland meatworks. Med J Aust 1:590, 1980.

669. Buckley B: Q fever epidemic in Victorian general practice. Med J Aust 1:593, 1980.

670. Spelman DW: Q fever: A study of 111 consecutive cases. Med J Aust 1:547, 1982.

671. Occasional survey: World-wide Q fever. Lancet 265:616, 1953.

672. Kosatsky T: Household outbreak of Q-fever pneumonia related to a parturient cat. Lancet 2:1447, 1984.

673. Marrie TJ, Schlech WF III, Williams JC, et al: Q fever pneumonia associated with exposure to wild rabbits. Lancet 1:427, 1986.

674. Salmon MM, Howells B, Glencross EJG, et al: Q fever in an urban area. Lancet 1:1002, 1982.

675. Lohuis PJ, Ligtenberg PC, Diepersloot RJ, et al: Q-fever in a patient with a ventriculo-peritoneal drain: Case report and short review of the literature. Neth J Med 44:60, 1994.

676. Pavilanis V, Duval L, Foley AR, et al: An epidemic of Q fever at Princeville, Quebec. Can J Public Health 49:520, 1958.

677. Urso FP: The pathologic findings in rickettsial pneumonia. Am J Clin Pathol 64:335, 1975.

678. Perrin TL: Histopathologic observations in a fatal case of Q fever. Arch Pathol 47:361, 1949.

679. Whittick JW: Necropsy findings in a case of Q fever in Britain. BMJ 1:979, 1950.

680. Lillie RD, Perrin TL, Armstrong C: An institutional outbreak of pneumonitis: III. Histopathology in man and rhesus monkeys in the pneumonitis due to the virus of "Q" fever. Public Health Rep 56:149, 1941.

681. Brouqui P, Dupont HT, Drancourt M, et al: Chronic Q fever: Ninety-two cases from France, including 27 cases without endocarditis. Arch Intern Med 153:642, 1993.

682. Janigan DT, Marrie TJ: An inflammatory pseudotumor of the lung in Q fever pneumonia. N Engl J Med 308:86, 1983.

683. Millar JK: The chest film findings in "Q" fever—a series of 35 cases. Clin Radiol 29:371, 1978.

684. Gordon JD, MacKeen AD, Marrie TJ, et al: The radiographic features of epidemic and sporadic Q fever pneumonia. J Can Assoc Radiol 35:293, 1984.

685. Lipton JH, Fong TC, Gill MJ, et al: Q fever inflammatory pseudotumor of the lung. Chest 92:756, 1987.

686. Pickworth FE, El-Soussi M, Wells IP, et al: The radiological appearances of Q fever pneumonia. Clin Radiol 44:150, 1991.

687. Ramos HS, Hodges RE, Meroney WH: Q fever: Report of a case simulating lymphoma. Ann Intern Med 47:1030, 1957.

688. Editorial: Epidemiology Q fever. BMJ 2:780, 1971.

689. Sheridan P, MacCaig JN, Hart RJC: Myocarditis complicating Q fever. BMJ 2:155, 1974.

690. Marrie TJ: Pneumonia and meningo-encephalitis due to *Coxiella burnetii.* J Infect 11:59, 1985.

691. Donohue JF: Lower respiratory tract involvement in Rocky Mountain spotted fever. Arch Intern Med 140:223, 1980.

692. Walker DH, Hawkins HK, Hudson P: Fulminant Rocky Mountain spotted fever. Arch Pathol Lab Med 107:121, 1983.

693. Walker DH, Crawford CG, Cain BG: Rickettsial infection of the pulmonary microcirculation: The basis for interstitial pneumonitis in Rocky Mountain spotted fever. Hum Pathol 2:263, 1980.

694. Roggli VL, Keener S, Bradford WD, et al: Pulmonary pathology of Rocky Mountain spotted fever (RMSF) in children. Pediatr Pathol 4:47, 1985.

695. Lees RF, Harrison RB, Williamson BRJ, et al: Radiographic findings in Rocky Mountain spotted fever. Radiology 129:17, 1978.

696. Martin W III, Choplin RH, Shertzer ME: The chest radiograph in Rocky Mountain spotted fever. Am J Roentgenol 139:889, 1982.

697. Walker DH, Gear JHS: Correlation of the distribution of *Rickettsia conorii,* microscopic lesions and clinical features in South African tick bite fever. Am J Trop Med Hyg 34:361, 1985.

698. Harris RL: Concise communications: Boutonneuse fever in American travelers. J Infect Dis 153:126, 1986.

699. Walker DH, Herrero-Herrero JI, Ruiz-Beltrán R, et al: The pathology of fatal Mediterranean spotted fever. Am J Clin Pathol 87:669, 1987.

700. Picken G, Booth AJ, Williams MV: Case report: The pulmonary lesions of chickenpox pneumonia—revisited. Br J Radiol 67:659, 1994.

701. Luby JP, Ware AJ, Hull AR, et al: Disease due to CMV and its long-term consequences in renal transplant recipients: Correlation of allograft survival with disease due to CMV and rubella antibody level. Arch Intern Med 143:1126, 1983.

CHAPTER 30

Protozoa, Helminths, Arthropods, and Leeches

Pulmonary disease caused by parasites (including protozoa; worms of the nematode, trematode and cestode groups; arthropods; and leeches) is most prevalent and serious in tropical and subtropical, relatively unindustrialized countries and rare in those that are "developed." However, an ever-increasing amount of travel to countries in which parasitic infestations are endemic, the migration of people from such countries, and the increasing prevalence of immunodeficient individuals (as a result of such conditions as acquired immunodeficiency syndrome [AIDS] and organ transplantation) require that every physician be knowledgeable about parasitic diseases and their diagnostic features.

In many cases, a suspicion of parasitic disease is aroused by the discovery of peripheral blood eosinophilia in a patient who resides or has traveled in an endemic area; unfortunately, this clue is often absent in immunosuppressed patients, particularly those receiving corticosteroids. Strong circumstantial evidence of pleuropulmonary involvement is the finding of ova or larvae in stool, although confirmation requires their demonstration in the sputum, bronchial or bronchoalveolar washings, pleural fluid, or lung tissue. Even though recovery of the organism may be readily accomplished in the presence of overwhelming infestation, such is the exception rather than the rule; as a result, considerable emphasis has been placed on the development of serologic methods of detection. Unfortunately, there have been major problems in the purification and standardization of antigen and in the specificity of serologic tests because of cross-reactivity between antigens of a number of parasites. Despite these obstacles, major advances have been made in diagnostic parasite serology, particularly in enzyme-linked immunosorbent assay (ELISA) methods and the use of monoclonal antibodies.[1, 2, 2a]

PROTOZOA

Amebiasis

Although human infestation is sometimes caused by other entamoebae, the term *amebiasis* is usually reserved for that caused by *Entamoeba histolytica,* an organism most often associated with colonic disease (amebic dysentery). Species of the *Hartmanella-Acanthamoeba* group typically cause encephalitis, but can (rarely) cause pneumonia.[3] It has also been hypothesized that some amoeba species may be involved in the pathogenesis of asthma.[3a]

E. histolytica exists in humans as both cysts and trophozoites. The former are spherical structures measuring 5 to 20 μm and are found only in the feces; the latter are motile organisms that are somewhat larger in size (15 to 25 μm in diameter) and possess a characteristic circular nucleus containing finely clumped peripheral chromatin and a prominent central karyosome; ingested red blood cells can be seen within the cytoplasm.

Epidemiology

Although amebic dysentery is found throughout the world, the highest rates of infection are seen in regions where hygiene and therapeutic measures are relatively inadequate. The disease has been estimated to affect approximately 10% of the world's population and is the third most important parasitic cause of death (after malaria and schistosomiasis).[4] Epidemics can occur, although they are uncommon in "developed" societies.[5] In most cases, cysts are passed in the feces of affected individuals (who are frequently asymptomatic) and are ingested by the new host in contaminated water or food. Person-to-person venereal and nonvenereal transmission has been said to be a more common mode of spread in the United States.[5] Despite this, most cases in the United States develop in immigrants from endemic regions who have been in the country for less than 2 years.[4]

Whereas amebic dysentery shows no age or sex predominance, pleuropulmonary disease develops most frequently between the ages of 20 and 40 years and is 10 to 15 times more common in men.[6] Such disease has been estimated to occur in only 1 in 1,000 patients;[6] however, when the liver is involved, it may develop in as many as 15% to 35%.[4, 7, 8]

Pathogenesis

The cysts of *E. histolytica* are acid resistant and able to travel through the stomach to the small intestine, where the trophozoites excyst. The latter migrate to the colon where they multiply and, in some cases, pass through the epithelium into the submucosa. The factors that determine this invasive property are not well understood, but may relate to the production of enzymes or toxins such as proteases and epithelial binding proteins.[9] Several bacteria have been shown to enhance the pathogenicity of the organism,[9] and it is possible that their presence is necessary for invasive disease.[5] It has also been speculated that antineutrophil cytoplasmic antibodies (ANCAs) may have a role in pathogenesis.[10] Penetration of the mucosa is associated with necrosis, ulceration, and the characteristic symptoms of amebic dysentery. The organism may subsequently enter the colonic venous circulation and pass via the portal veins to the liver, where microabscesses and eventually macroabscesses may develop.

Pleuropulmonary manifestations of amebiasis can occur by several mechanisms, the most frequent of which is direct extension of disease from a hepatic abscess, usually located in the right lobe.[11, 12] Such abscesses may extend into the subphrenic space and form a separate subdiaphragmatic abscess, in which circumstance intrathoracic complications such as pleural effusion and basal pulmonary disease result from the subphrenic inflammation rather than from direct invasion by the parasite. In other instances, empyema or basal pulmonary disease results from direct transdiaphragmatic extension of infection, either in association with a hepatic abscess alone or with combined hepatic and subphrenic abscesses. A hepatobronchial fistula sometimes develops without associated radiographic changes in the lungs or pleura.[13]

Occasionally, pulmonary amebiasis is seen without evidence of hepatic involvement; in such cases it has been hypothesized that the organism reaches the lungs or pleura by one of three routes: (1) via the hemorrhoidal veins in association with lower rectal disease; (2) via transdiaphragmatic lymphatics or hepatic veins in association with inapparent hepatic disease; or (3) via the thoracic duct.[9] Infection occasionally develops in sites other than the lungs and pleura, principally the brain (representing hematogenous dissemination with abscess formation) and pericardium (almost invariably by direct extension through the tendinous portion of the diaphragm from the left hepatic lobe).[14, 15]

Pathologic Characteristics

Over 95% of amebic lung abscesses develop in parenchyma contiguous to the diaphragm (in the lower lobes, middle lobe, or lingula); in about 75% of such cases, extension is demonstrable from the liver through the diaphragm into the lungs.[16] Fibrous pleural adhesions are frequently present. Gross sections of the lung show poorly defined areas of necrosis that are frequently soft or semifluid in consistency and possess a characteristic mucinous appearance;[9] the necrotic tissue has been likened to anchovy paste or chocolate sauce. Histologically, the necrotic tissue is associated with a variable degree of peripheral fibrosis and mononuclear inflammatory infiltrate; despite the frequent use of the term *abscess* to describe this lesion, polymorphonuclear leukocytes are rarely found. Trophozoites may be identified at the margins of the necrotic areas contiguous to normal lung.

Radiologic Manifestations

Elevation of the right hemidiaphragm and right-sided pleural effusion, with or without basal pulmonary disease, constitute the usual picture (Fig. 30–1). The effusion may

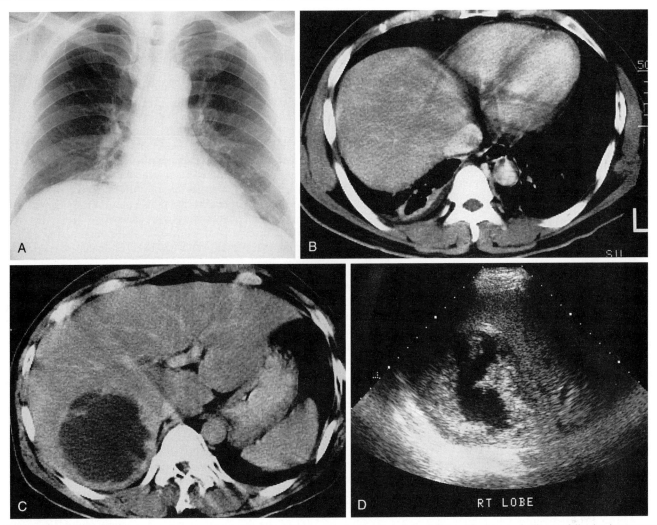

Figure 30–1. Amebiasis. A posteroanterior chest radiograph *(A)* demonstrates elevation of the right hemidiaphragm. A CT scan following intravenous administration of contrast *(B)* demonstrates a small right pleural effusion and areas of atelectasis in the right lower lobe. A scan through the liver *(C)* demonstrates a large cystic lesion in the right lobe of the liver. Ultrasonographic examination *(D)* demonstrates echogenic material within the lesion consistent with an abscess. The diagnosis of amebiasis was proved by fine-needle aspiration under ultrasound guidance. The patient was a 42-year-old South Korean man with a 1-week history of fever and chills; physical examination demonstrated tenderness in the right upper quadrant. (Case courtesy of Dr. Soon Ju Cha, Inje University Hospital, Seoul, Korea.)

be sufficient to result in total or nearly total opacification of the right hemithorax and a marked mediastinal shift to the left.[17] The parenchymal abnormality may be no more than horizontal line shadows just above an elevated hemidiaphragm;[13, 18] more commonly, however, the abnormality consists of ill-defined homogeneous consolidation of the right lower or middle lobe without a clear-cut segmental distribution. Some of these areas of consolidation progress to abscess formation and cavitation.[18, 19] In a small number of patients, parenchymal consolidation, with or without cavitation, develops at a site remote from the diaphragm such as the upper lobes, presumably by direct spread to the lungs from the colon without an intermediate liver abscess. In cases of hepatobronchial fistula, a band-like shadow may be seen extending from the pulmonary hilum to the diaphragm, unassociated with parenchymal consolidation.[13, 18] Rarely, the cardiac silhouette is enlarged as a result of extension of an abscess into the pericardial sac.[17]

Ultrasonography can be useful in evaluating suspected liver abscesses.[20, 21] Ultrasonically guided percutaneous fine-needle aspiration can be used not only in the diagnosis of abscesses but also for definitive therapy by instillation of metronidazole[22] or percutaneous drainage.[21] The diagnosis can also be made with CT[23] or magnetic resonance imaging.[24]

Clinical Manifestations

The possibility of pleuropulmonary amebiasis should be considered in any patient who is or has been a resident of an endemic area and who complains of right upper quadrant abdominal pain and a dry cough. The latter is characteristic of the early stages of pleuropulmonary involvement; in more advanced disease, cough may become productive of sputum resembling "chocolate sauce" or "anchovy paste," which is indicative of hepatobronchial communication. Expectoration of bile (biloptysis) may also occur as a result of a bronchohepatic or, less often, bronchobiliary fistula.[25] Wheezing and hemoptysis are present in a small number of patients.[4] Occasionally, pulmonary symptoms are accompanied by severe cachexia, suggesting the possibility of tuberculosis or cancer. Physical examination may reveal a palpable, tender liver, lower intercostal tenderness, or both.[26] Signs of consolidation may be evident. Clubbing is said not to be a feature.[4]

Patients are usually febrile. Gastrointestinal symptoms, including diarrhea, constipation, flatulence, and bloody or mucoid stool, may or may not be present.[4] In one series, the clinical course before the onset of pleural complications averaged 71 days (range, 3 days to 8 months);[17] rupture into the pleural cavity was heralded by the acute onset of sharp, tearing lower thoracic pain that frequently radiated to the ipsilateral shoulder, as well as progressive dyspnea and evidence of sepsis.

Laboratory Findings

Leukocytosis is usually moderate and may be associated with anemia. Eosinophilia is typically absent.[4] The results of liver function tests may be completely normal. A positive diagnosis can be made by the demonstration of trophozoites in the sputum, pleural exudate, or material obtained by needle aspiration;[22, 27] however, recovery of the organism from these sources is difficult in most patients.[7, 17] Care must be taken in the cytologic analysis of sputum to distinguish *E. histolytica* from *Entamoeba gingivalis*, a relatively common saprophyte of the oral cavity.[28] A presumptive diagnosis can be made in cases of pleuropulmonary disease if stool contains trophozoites or cysts; however, it is often not possible to isolate the organism from this source.[29]

Results of serologic tests for amebiasis are positive in almost all cases.[7] A gel diffusion test has a sensitivity of about 95%, and indirect hemagglutinin and ELISA tests are almost 100% sensitive.[4] However, most such tests cannot distinguish between active and remote disease. A possible exception is an ELISA test directed to a recombinant serine-rich protein, which has been reported to have a sensitivity of almost 80% and a specificity of 87% for the presence of acute disease.[30] C-ANCAs were found in a large proportion of patients in one investigation.[10]

The overall mortality rate associated with thoracic amebiasis has been estimated to range from 10%[31] to 15%.[17] Pericardial involvement, although rare, is particularly ominous.[14]

Toxoplasmosis

Toxoplasmosis is caused by *Toxoplasma gondii*, an obligate intracellular protozoan causing widespread infestation that is rarely manifested clinically. In humans, the organisms appear as rounded or crescent-shaped trophozoites that measure 6 to 7 by 2 to 4 μm; they multiply quickly in acute infestation (tachyzoites) and slowly in chronic infestation (bradyzoites). In the latter form, large (200 to 1,000 μm) intracellular cysts develop that contain numerous bradyzoites and are enclosed by a *Toxoplasma*-produced membrane. The organism can be seen with hematoxylin and eosin (H&E) and Giemsa stains; its nucleus stains red and its cytoplasm blue with Romanovsky's stain.

Epidemiology

Toxoplasmosis occurs in many wild and domestic warm-blooded animals throughout the world. Its definitive hosts are members of the cat family, in which the sexual phase of reproduction (accompanied by oocyst formation) takes place in the intestine. Humans usually acquire the infestation by contact with material contaminated by oocyst-infected stool (such as "kitty litter") or by eating poorly cooked, cyst-containing meat,[32] particularly lamb.[33] Mice, rats, and sparrows serve as intermediate hosts.[34] The disease can also be transmitted in the laboratory,[35] in organ transplants,[36] and by transfusion of infected blood products.[37] Transplacental spread to the fetus can occur in women who acquire the infestation during pregnancy.

The disease is of worldwide distribution and is a common human infestation. It has been estimated that approximately 50% of the world's population is affected.[38] According to serologic studies, evidence of prior infection has been identified in 5% to 70% of the population of the United States.[38, 39] In the United Kingdom, approximately half the population over 60 years of age has been found to have antibodies to the parasite;[33] in France, it has been estimated that approximately two thirds of adults and almost 95% of pregnant women over the age of 35 have been infected.[38]

Although usually innocuous in both the chronic stage and following the initial infestation, disease can be categorized into four clinicopathologic forms—congenital, ocular, lymphatic, and generalized. The congenital form is perhaps the most important because of its effects on the central nervous system, including hydrocephalus and microcephalus;[40] pulmonary involvement, however, is rare even following widespread dissemination of the organism. Lymph node enlargement, with or without symptoms similar to infectious mononucleosis, is the most common clinically recognized form of the disease in immunocompetent adults;[39] a variety of lymph node groups, including those in the mediastinum, may be affected. Disease in adults usually occurs in immunocompromised hosts, mostly in patients with AIDS (*see* page 1675), organ transplants, leukemia, or lymphoma[41-43] and (occasionally) in association with other malignancies or autoimmune disease.[41] The most common clinical features are related to the central nervous system, but pneumonitis, carditis, and hepatitis are also seen frequently.[41, 44] Occasionally, patients who have these manifestations have no evidence of underlying immunosuppression.[45]

Pathogenesis and Pathologic Characteristics

Upon ingestion, the oocysts are disrupted by digestive enzymes and release trophozoites that enter the intestinal mucosa and disseminate via the bloodstream. In immunologically competent individuals, the disease is usually limited, intracellular infestation and occasional cell death occurring predominantly in cardiac and skeletal muscle and in the brain. The organisms encyst in these and (occasionally) other sites, where they remain viable and are presumably the source of disease in individuals who subsequently lose their immunologic competence.

Pathologic changes in lymph nodes in acquired toxoplasmosis are so characteristic that the diagnosis can be suggested on the basis of histologic examination.[46] Findings include follicular hyperplasia associated with cortical and paracortical clusters of epithelioid cells that typically encroach upon and blur the margins of the germinal centers. Sinus histiocytosis caused by a proliferation of monocytoid cells is also observed. *Toxoplasma* cysts are identified rarely.

Cases of disseminated disease involving the lungs are manifested by interstitial pneumonitis, with or without necrosis, and a largely mononuclear inflammatory infiltrate (Fig. 30–2).[41, 47] A pattern of diffuse alveolar damage is seen in some cases.[47] Trophozoites can be identified free in tissue, and cysts are found in macrophages and in alveolar epithelial and capillary endothelial cells.[48] The trophozoites may be difficult to see and can be confused with a variety of other organisms, including *Histoplasma capsulatum* and *Pneumocystis carinii*; although electron microscopic features permit differentiation,[49] immunohistochemical testing is more rapid, easier to perform, and more sensitive.[47]

Radiologic Manifestations

In apparently immunocompetent individuals, pulmonary toxoplasmosis usually results in a focal reticular pattern resembling acute viral pneumonia; air-space consolidation occurs in some cases.[50, 51] The findings may also consist of poorly defined areas of ground-glass opacity that are easier to appreciate on HRCT scans than on radiographs (Fig. 30–3). Hilar lymph node enlargement is common.[52, 53]

The findings tend to be different in immunocompromised individuals.[54] In one study of nine patients with AIDS, six demonstrated a bilateral, predominantly coarse nodular pattern and three had a diffuse reticulonodular pattern;[54a] the nodular opacities had poorly defined margins. Two patients had pleural effusion and none had hilar or mediastinal lymphadenopathy. Manifestation as a solitary lung nodule has also been reported in one patient with AIDS.[55]

Clinical Manifestations

The clinical features of toxoplasmosis in immunocompetent adults commonly resemble those of infectious mononucleosis.[56] Patients may be asymptomatic or may manifest low-grade fever and lymph node enlargement (usually cervical), with or without a rash, over a period of several weeks or months. Anemia and lymphocytosis (frequently with some atypia) are common. Epstein-Barr virus and heterophil antibodies are absent. Evidence of pleuropulmonary disease is rare.

The disseminated form of disease is characterized by fever, disorientation, confusion, headache, and manifestations of myocarditis.[42] Pneumonia is commonly associated with nonproductive cough and dyspnea;[38] physical examination reveals crackles in a minority of patients. Some individuals have a syndrome resembling Rocky Mountain spotted fever, with pneumonia[51] or polymyositis;[57] the latter manifes-

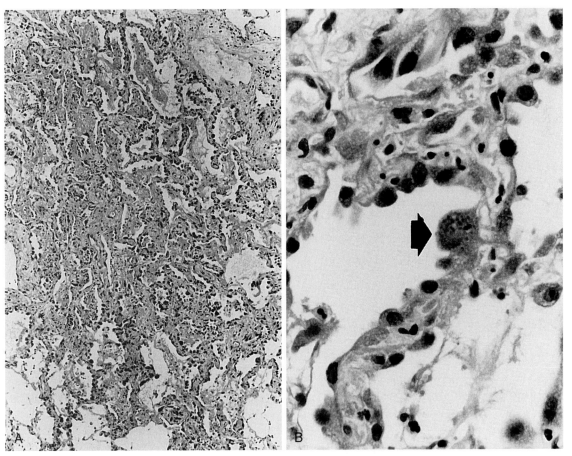

Figure 30–2. Toxoplasmosis. A section from an open lung biopsy *(A)* of a heart transplant patient shows moderately severe alveolar interstitial thickening by fibrous tissue and a mild lymphocytic infiltrate. A magnified view of an alveolus *(B)* shows hyperplastic Type II cells, one of which *(arrow)* contains numerous intracytoplasmic dots representing *Toxoplasma* organisms. *(A,* ×80; *B,* ×500.)

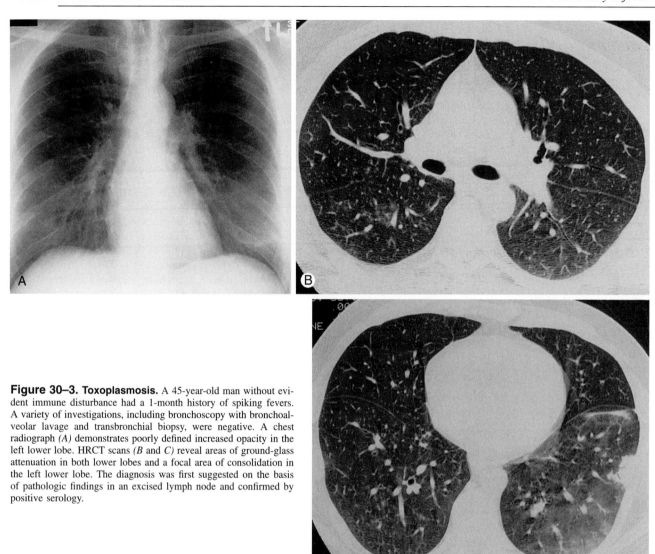

Figure 30–3. Toxoplasmosis. A 45-year-old man without evident immune disturbance had a 1-month history of spiking fevers. A variety of investigations, including bronchoscopy with bronchoalveolar lavage and transbronchial biopsy, were negative. A chest radiograph *(A)* demonstrates poorly defined increased opacity in the left lower lobe. HRCT scans *(B and C)* reveal areas of ground-glass attenuation in both lower lobes and a focal area of consolidation in the left lower lobe. The diagnosis was first suggested on the basis of pathologic findings in an excised lymph node and confirmed by positive serology.

tation may represent activation of latent *Toxoplasma* infestation in patients with immune-related myositis or dermatomyositis who are receiving corticosteroid therapy.

Laboratory Findings

High levels of serum lactate dehydrogenase (LDH) have been detected in some patients with pneumonia;[58] however, the finding can also be seen in other etiologies. Several serologic tests have been used in the diagnosis of toxoplasmosis, including the Sabin-Feldman dye test and a variety of indirect antibody tests that detect antitoxoplasmal IgG or IgM antibodies. For the dye test, *Toxoplasma* organisms are incubated in serum from patients with suspected disease; methylene blue stains the *Toxoplasma* organisms injured by the patient's antibodies.[59] A positive test result (1:8) indicates that the patient has or has had the disease; a fourfold rise in titer is required for the diagnosis of active disease. An IgM titer of 1:160 or greater or a fourfold rise in IgG titer is the best indicator of recent infestation.[60] However, such results are distinctly uncommon in immunocompromised patients,

particularly those with AIDS,[61] and the use of these tests is equivocal at best in these individuals. Because of these limitations, demonstration of the organism in tissue or in bronchoalveolar lavage (BAL) fluid is usually necessary to confirm the diagnosis;[61, 62] identification has also been achieved by polymerase chain reaction analysis of BAL fluid.[63]

Miscellaneous Protozoa

Babesiosis. Babesiosis is an acute febrile illness caused by protozoa of the genus *Babesia*. The organisms infect primarily wild and domestic animals, between whom they are transmitted by ticks; about 200 human cases were reported in the United States in the 1980s.[64] Individuals who have undergone splenectomy appear to be particularly at risk.[65] Human disease is characterized by fever, myalgia, hemolytic anemia, hemoglobinuria, and jaundice. Pulmonary complications, including cough[66] and adult respiratory distress syndrome (ARDS),[67, 68] are rare.

Malaria. Malaria is caused by species of the *Plasmodium* genus, of which the most virulent is *Plasmodium falciparum*. Clinically significant pulmonary disease ("malarial lung") is seen in 2% to 5% of patients infested with this organism;[69, 70] it is likely that the incidence of subclinical or mild symptomatic disease is much greater in patients with less severe systemic infection.[71] The clinical picture ranges from mild cough to fulminant respiratory failure and death, the latter usually being the result of ARDS.[72, 73] Patients with severe disease typically have a large number of parasites and signs of cerebral dysfunction; expectoration of blood-tinged fluid may occur. Radiologically, the findings are those of interstitial and air-space edema associated with small pleural effusions.[74, 75] Disseminated intravascular coagulation may occur.[76]

Trichomoniasis. Three species of trichomonads—*Trichomonas tenax*, *Trichomonas vaginalis*, and *Trichomonas hominis*—are known to infest humans; all have been identified in sputum, pleural fluid, and pulmonary tissue.[77] Although these organisms may be contaminants or saprophytes in some cases, in others there is evidence of tissue damage. *T. tenax* is frequently found in the mouth and bronchial washings of patients with poor oral hygiene.[78–80] Its presence in pleural effusion, empyema, BAL fluid, and necrotic lung tissue,[79, 81, 82, 82a] as well as the clinical response to drainage and metronidazole in some cases, suggests that it is pathogenic. The organisms are best demonstrated by culture[80] or by wet mounts and direct microscopic examination without fixation or staining;[79] they have also been identified on Wright-Giemsa– and Papanicolaou-stained smears.[80, 82]

Cryptosporidiosis. Cryptosporidia are well recognized as a cause of chronic diarrhea in patients with AIDS. They have also been identified in tracheobronchial secretions (sputum and BAL fluid[83, 84]), on the surface of the airway epithelium (*see* page 1676), and in the bronchial glands of these same patients.[84, 85] Occasional instances of infection in individuals with other immunosuppressive diseases have also been reported.[86] The organisms most likely gain access to the lungs by aspiration from the small intestine; however, it has also been suggested that pulmonary disease may occur by inhalation or by hematogenous spread via infected blood monocytes.[84] The predominant clinical finding is cough.

Microsporidiosis. Microsporidia are obligate intracellular protozoa that have been increasingly recognized as a cause of disease in patients with AIDS. Several genera, including *Enterocytozoon* and *Encephalitozoon*, have been identified. Although most commonly associated with intestinal or ocular disease (causing chronic diarrhea or keratoconjunctivitis, respectively), involvement of the lungs has been reported in several patients.[87–89] Clinical findings include nonproductive cough and chest pain. Histologic examination has shown tracheobronchitis and/or bronchiolitis and the presence of organisms in the supranuclear cytoplasm of airway epithelial cells.[90] The organism can also be detected in macrophages obtained from specimens of sputum or BAL.[87]

Leishmaniasis. *Leishmania donovani*, the protozoan that causes visceral leishmaniasis (kala-azar), is found predominantly within macrophages in the bone marrow, liver, spleen, lymph nodes, gastrointestinal tract, and skin. Clinical signs and symptoms are caused by infestation of these sites and include hepatosplenomegaly, lymph node enlargement, pan-

cytopenia, fever, and cachexia. Although pulmonary disease that causes symptoms and radiographic abnormalities is rare, histologic involvement of the lungs has been identified in a number of cases; in one autopsy study of five untreated children, four showed a mild, diffuse interstitial mononuclear infiltrate with occasional macrophages that contained characteristic Leishman-Donovan bodies.[91] The organism has also been identified in macrophages obtained by BAL.[92]

Giardiasis. *Giardia lamblia* has been suspected as the cause of pneumonitis in a patient with cancer from whom it was isolated from BAL fluid.[93]

NEMATODES (ROUNDWORMS)

Ascariasis

In the great majority of cases, human ascariasis is caused by *Ascaris lumbricoides*, a cylindrical nematode measuring up to 35 cm in length and 0.5 cm in width. *Ascaris suum*, normally a parasite of pigs, has also been reported to cause disease in humans following the ingestion of food maliciously seasoned with ova.[94]

The adult female worm lives in the small intestine, where it may live for up to 2 years and produce as many as 250,000 eggs per day. The fertilized eggs, which are passed in the feces, are about 40 by 60 μm in diameter and possess a smooth or roughly mamillated surface. They are resistant to drying and freezing and can remain viable for many years.[95] In moist, warm, and shady soil, the first two larval stages develop within the shell of the ovum. When ingested, the ovum hatches in the small intestine, and the larvae enter the portal veins or intestinal lymphatics. From there they pass to the lungs, where they are trapped by the alveolar capillaries and exit into the air spaces. At this point they molt and develop into third-stage larvae that measure up to 2 mm in length and 75 μm in width; these larvae possess a characteristic morphology that can be recognized on histologic examination.[95] The third-stage larvae migrate up the airways to the larynx, where they are swallowed to complete their odyssey by developing into mature worms in the small intestine.

Human infestation is common, approximately 25% of the world's population having been estimated to be infected.[96] About 75% of affected individuals live in Southeast Asia; most of the remainder reside in Africa or Central and South America. It has been estimated that approximately 4 million individuals in the United States are infested, mostly in the southeast.[96] Since larval development in the soil is inhibited by direct sunlight and excessive heat, a peak incidence of disease is usually reported during seasons when the soil is moist and cool. The disease is more common in children than in adults and is acquired by the ingestion of eggs in water or food or from contaminated soil under the fingernails.

Pulmonary disease is most often caused by passage of the third-stage larvae through the lungs. Occasionally, clinically unimportant granulomas can be seen histologically at autopsy in relation to *Ascaris* ova within lung parenchyma;[95] adult worms have been identified within the biliary tract in these cases, and it has been hypothesized that the eggs reach the lungs by way of the hepatic circulation. Adult

Ascaris worms have rarely been found within the bronchi in association with foci of bronchopneumonia;[95] it has been assumed that they are aspirated during vomiting and that the pneumonia is related to the aspiration rather than the organism itself. Rare complications include migration of adult worms across the diaphragm (sometimes associated with a pattern of chronic eosinophilic pneumonia)[97] and upper airway obstruction.[98]

Pathologic descriptions of pulmonary ascariasis during larval migration are rare since the disease is seldom fatal. In one case, the gross and histologic descriptions were essentially those of asthma, although patchy alveolar interstitial thickening and intra-alveolar fibroblastic tissue were also noted;[99] occasional larvae were identified within bronchial lumens. In a second case, the lungs showed a combination of bronchopneumonia (in which the inflammatory exudate was composed largely of eosinophils and fibrin) and patchy interstitial pneumonia with alveolar hemorrhage and edema;[95] tissue necrosis was absent, and numerous larvae were seen within alveolar walls and air spaces and in the airways. As indicated previously, granulomatous inflammation (sometimes associated with eosinophils) is seen occasionally in relation to embolized ova.[95]

Radiographic findings consist of patchy areas of homogeneous consolidation. In many cases, the consolidation is transient and without clear-cut segmental distribution in the characteristic pattern originally described by Löffler (Fig. 30–4). The shadows may be several centimeters in diameter and, in cases of mild to moderate disease, tend to be rather discrete and concentrated in the perihilar regions; with more severe involvement, they tend to coalesce and assume a lobular pattern.[100]

The vast majority of patients are asymptomatic. When symptoms are present, they are usually related to the gastrointestinal tract, the most serious being associated with obstruction of the intestine or the biliary or pancreatic ducts (caused by the migration of organisms through the ampulla of Vater). Pulmonary symptoms consist of cough (usually nonproductive), retrosternal ("burning") chest pain, and in more severe cases, hemoptysis and dyspnea. Of 108 patients in one series, 16 (15%) complained of a transient, intensely pruritic skin eruption that appeared within 4 or 5 days after the onset of respiratory symptoms.[100] One group has found evidence that the infestation may be more severe in patients who have experienced smoke inhalation.[101] Low-grade fever may be present, and scattered rhonchi and crackles may be heard over the lungs. Leukocytosis of 20,000 to 25,000/mm^3 is common, with an eosinophilia of 30% to 70%. Pulmonary disease is usually self-limited.

The diagnosis of pulmonary ascariasis can be confirmed by the discovery of larvae in the sputum or a gastric aspirate,[102] although this finding is uncommon. The identification of adult worms or ova in the stool strongly supports the diagnosis; however, in patients with recently acquired infection, worms or ova may not be present. The presence of specific IgE antibodies to *Ascaris* has been shown to correlate with positive skin prick reactions to *Ascaris* antigen;[103] however, serologic tests are not useful in differentiating ascariasis from other roundworm infestations.[7]

Strongyloidiasis

The great majority of cases of strongyloidiasis are caused by the nematode *Strongyloides stercoralis*, a parasite prevalent in tropical and temperate climates throughout the world.[104] In addition, *Strongyloides fülleborni,* a parasite of monkeys and apes, often infests humans in Africa and has been shown to produce clinical disease similar to that caused by *S. stercoralis*.[105] Infestation by a related organism, *Angiostrongyloides costaricensis,* has been reported in Central and South America; it has been accompanied by extensive thrombosis of vessels of the greater omentum and by pulmonary manifestations of a Löffler-like syndrome.[106]

Life Cycle

The adult female of *S. stercoralis* lives in the human small intestine and measures 2 to 3 mm in length by 30 to 60 μm in width; the existence of a parasitic male is not certain, and it is believed that parthenogenesis is the rule. The life cycle of the organism is complex. Free-living filariform larvae penetrate the undamaged skin and pass via the blood to the lung, where they migrate from the capillaries into the alveoli and thence up the airways to the larynx and down the esophagus to the gut. Within the small intestine they develop into adult females that take up residence and lay eggs in the mucosal crypts. In their subsequent passage through the gut, the eggs develop into noninfectious rhabditiform larvae that may take three courses: (1) they may be passed in the stool and develop directly into filariform larvae

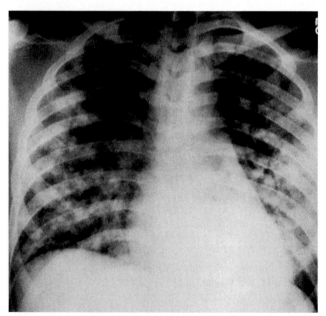

Figure 30–4. *Ascaris suum* Infestation. A radiograph exposed in the supine position reveals widespread, patchy air-space consolidation reminiscent of acute pulmonary edema. Two weeks previously, this 25-year-old man had ingested a meal maliciously seasoned with large quantities of embryonated *Ascaris suum* ova. At the time of this radiograph, he was cyanotic and in acute respiratory failure. Arterial Po$_2$ was 37 mm Hg and Pco$_2$ was 25 mm Hg. The white cell count was 21,000 with 14% eosinophils. *A. suum* larvae were recovered from both sputum and gastric washings but not from stools. The patient had an uneventful recovery. The pulmonary reaction represents severe edema occasioned by an allergic response to the passage of larvae through the pulmonary circulation. (From Phills JA, Harrold AJ, Whiteman GV, et al: N Engl J Med 286:965, 1972.)

in the soil; (2) they may be passed in the stool and develop into free-living adults, which in turn produce filariform larvae; or (3) they may transform directly into the filariform larvae within the gut and lead to autoinfection through direct penetration of the intestinal mucosa or perianal skin. The ability of the organism to migrate through the lungs without a soil cycle permits chronic infestation, in some cases as long as 65 years.[107]

Epidemiology

The disease is endemic in tropical and subtropical areas where the climate is warm and the soil moist; depending on the particular geographic region, infestation has been estimated to affect approximately 10% to 50% of the population.[108] One comprehensive analysis of epidemiology reports revealed the following groups to have an increased risk of disease in the United States: residents and immigrants from "developing" countries and from southern, eastern, and central Europe; travelers and soldiers from the same areas; residents of the Appalachian region; and individuals residing in institutions.[108] Individuals with achlorhydria also appear to be at increased risk.[109]

In many cases the infestation is accompanied by mild or no clinical symptoms. However, severe disease can occur with accelerated larval differentiation and mucosal penetration ("hyperinfection syndrome"), in which case both the load of pathogenic organisms is increased and involvement of organs outside the typical migration route is not uncommon. This complication is rarely seen in otherwise healthy individuals,[110, 111] and generally develops in individuals whose defenses are compromised by malignancy, malnutrition, alcoholism, or therapy with cytotoxic or immunosuppressive drugs or corticosteroids.[112–115] Respiratory physicians should be particularly aware that the latter therapy also increases the risk in patients with asthma[117] or chronic obstructive pulmonary disease;[118] interestingly, infestation has also been first manifested as new onset of asthma or worsening of asthmatic symptoms concurrent with the use

of systemic corticosteroids.[119] The infestation is relatively uncommon in patients with AIDS.[120, 121]

Pathogenesis and Pathologic Characteristics

Pulmonary disease is caused principally by the migration of larvae through alveolar capillaries into air spaces. Experimentally, infestation of rats with *Strongyloides ratti* results in only mild intra-alveolar hemorrhage and occasional microabscesses without residual damage,[122] minimal findings that correspond to the paucity of pulmonary symptoms in chronic human infestation. However, the greater number of organisms seen in hyperinfection is often associated with significant alveolar injury. In addition to the damage caused by the organisms and the inflammatory reaction to them, it has been suggested that enteric bacteria carried by migrating worms may cause sepsis and secondary ARDS.[104]

Morphologic changes at autopsy of immunocompromised patients with severe disease have not been extensively documented;[117, 123] larvae can be found in capillaries or free within alveolar air spaces, often in association with intra-alveolar hemorrhage and edema.[117, 123] There may be minimal or no associated inflammatory reaction, or a prominent cellular infiltrate of polymorphonuclear leukocytes, lymphocytes, and macrophages. Isolated multinucleated giant cells may be seen, and granulomas occasionally develop in relation to larvae.[124] A pattern of interlobular septal fibrosis has also been reported.[125] Although filaria are the most common form of the organism to be identified, fully developed adult females and ova are seen occasionally, implying maturation *in situ*.[117, 126] The organism (in both filarial and mature forms) can be identified by H&E and Gram stains of expectorated sputum and in BAL specimens stained by the Papanicolaou method (Fig. 30–5).[126]

Radiologic Manifestations

Radiographic manifestations are similar to those seen in ascariasis or hookworm infestation—nonsegmental, patchy areas of consolidation (Fig. 30–6), presumably caused by an

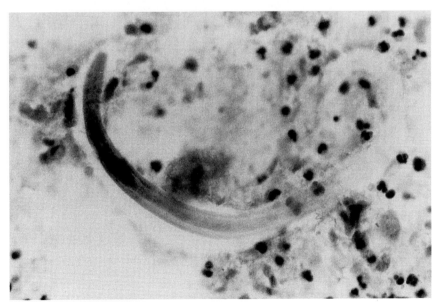

Figure 30–5. Strongyloidiasis. A bronchial wash specimen shows a background of polymorphonuclear leukocytes and an elongated larva consistent with *Strongyloides stercoralis.* (× 650.)

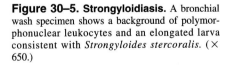

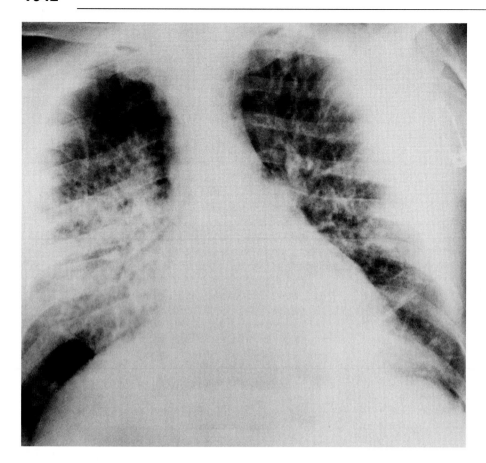

Figure 30–6. Pulmonary Strongyloidiasis. An anteroposterior radiograph exposed in the supine position reveals widespread disease of both lungs in a pattern suggesting involvement of both the interstitium and air spaces. Confluent air-space consolidation is particularly evident in the right lung. The larvae of *Strongyloides stercoralis* were identified in both the sputum and stool. This diffuse disease is thought to represent alveolar hemorrhage and edema. (Courtesy of the General Hospital, Wayne County, Michigan.)

allergic reaction to migration of the filariform larvae through the lungs. Hyperinfection may be associated with air-space consolidation,[7, 127] focal opacities,[128, 129] or diffuse reticulonodular[112, 130] or nodular patterns.[131] The nodules may have poorly defined or well-defined margins and generally measure 2 to 5 mm in diameter (Fig. 30–7), an appearance that may simulate miliary tuberculosis.[132, 133] Diffuse pulmonary opacities may lead to a clinical and radiographic picture of ARDS.[132, 134] Pleural effusions may be seen, usually in association with parenchymal abnormalities but occasionally as the only radiographic manifestation.[134] Cavitary disease has been described in an asthmatic patient receiving predni-

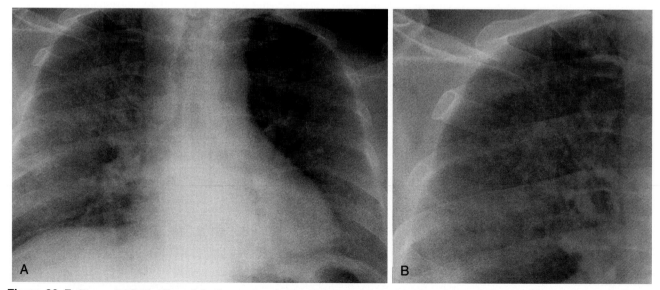

Figure 30–7. Strongyloidiasis: Hyperinfection. A 53-year-old man undergoing chemotherapy for pancreatic lymphoma was evaluated for periumbilical abdominal pain, fever, and diarrhea. The admission chest radiograph was normal. Two days after admission, rapidly progressive shortness of breath developed. An anteroposterior chest radiograph *(A)* demonstrates a miliary pattern, better visualized on the magnified image of the right upper lobe *(B)*. Fiberoptic bronchoscopy and bronchoalveolar lavage demonstrated pulmonary hemorrhage and numerous filariform larvae of *Strongyloides stercoralis*.

sone;[135] however, since this patient also had copious foul-smelling sputum, it is likely that there was associated anaerobic infection.

Clinical Manifestations

Larval penetration of the skin may be associated with an erythematous papular eruption. In one study of 40 former Allied prisoners of war, 27 (68%) had a history of nonspecific urticaria and 13 (33%) had transient urticarial eruptions that migrated in a serpiginous fashion (larva currens), a pathognomonic feature.[136] Abdominal pain and diarrhea—or diarrhea alternating with constipation—are common features of chronic infestation.[136] Pulmonary symptoms are usually mild or absent, the most common being productive cough; hemoptysis and dyspnea occur occasionally. As indicated previously, signs and symptoms of asthma develop or worsen in some patients. Patients with hyperinfection have nausea, vomiting, and colicky abdominal pain;[137] life-threatening gastrointestinal hemorrhage may occur.[116]

Laboratory Findings

Although affected patients are usually immunosuppressed, they can still manifest significant peripheral eosinophilia unless they are receiving large doses of corticosteroids.[123, 127] Some patients are anemic.

A definitive diagnosis of pulmonary strongyloidiasis can be made by finding larvae in the sputum or BAL fluid.[120, 138, 139] A presumptive diagnosis can be based on their detection in stool; however, although this is usually not difficult in immunocompromised patients with hyperinfection, large amounts of stool might need to be examined in otherwise healthy individuals, and the overall sensitivity of the test varies between 30% and 75%.[104] Organisms have also been detected in specimens derived by BAL[120] and duodenal aspiration.[140] An ELISA test using antigen extracted from filariform larvae has been found to have a sensitivity of about 85% to 90% and a specificity of 97% to 99%;[104] in immunocompromised patients, however, this test is of limited value.[141]

The disease is self-limited or chronic with minimal clinical significance in many individuals. Some patients have chronic or recurrent gastrointestinal or skin involvement resulting in malabsorption and weight loss. By contrast, disseminated disease and hyperinfection syndrome may be fulminant with multiorgan failure and death.

Ancylostomiasis (Hookworm Disease)

Hookworm disease is caused by the nematodes *Ancylostoma duodenale* and *Necator americanus*. The organisms exist as filariform larvae in soil and infest humans by penetrating the skin; as a result, a combination of warm climate, moist contaminated soil, poor hygiene, and bare feet is required for completion of the life cycle. Having penetrated the skin, the larvae migrate to the pulmonary capillaries by way of the systemic veins, cross into the alveolar air spaces, and migrate up the bronchi and trachea and into the esophagus and small intestine. In the last site they mature into adult hookworms that produce eggs, which are passed in the feces.

The major complication of hookworm disease is anemia, which is caused by the worms' tendency to feed mainly on blood. Pulmonary manifestations are similar to those of *Strongyloides* and *Ascaris* infestation and are the result of larval migration through the alveolus;[96] they include wheezing, cough, and hemoptysis. Nonsegmental homogeneous consolidation may be apparent on radiographs. Patients are typically pale, weak, and emaciated, with anemia and blood eosinophilia. The diagnosis is made by finding ova or mature worms in the stool.

Trichinosis

Trichinosis results from ingestion of the larvae of *Trichinella spiralis*. The disease is worldwide in distribution and is found where contaminated meat, particularly pork, is eaten raw or undercooked. Encysted larvae in the meat reach the small intestine, where they mature into adult worms that mate and produce eggs. When the latter hatch, the larvae penetrate the duodenal wall and are carried to the lungs, thence through the pulmonary circulation into the systemic circulation, and finally to striated muscle throughout the body. Although any muscle may be affected, the diaphragm is perhaps the most frequently involved, followed by the tongue and the masseter, intercostal, ocular, laryngeal, and paravertebral muscles.[142] Within muscle, the coiled *Trichinella* larvae encyst and become surrounded by a layer of connective tissue that frequently calcifies 6 to 18 months after infestation. Adjacent muscle fibers are usually atrophic and surrounded by a chronic inflammatory infiltrate that is sometimes granulomatous.[142]

Radiographically, there are no abnormalities related to the lungs, since the larvae produce minimal reaction in their passage through the pulmonary circulation. Pleural effusion is seen rarely. Calcified walls of larval cysts within the respiratory muscles may be visible as oval opacities 0.8 to 1.0 mm in their longest diameter.

Diarrhea develops 2 to 4 days after the ingestion of contaminated meat; fever, muscular pains, facial edema, and in some cases, central nervous system symptoms may develop by the seventh day. Pulmonary symptoms are usually absent during passage of the parasite through the lungs; blood-tinged sputum or frank hemoptysis has been reported in some cases.[143] If the respiratory muscles are affected, the patient may complain of dyspnea; severe disease may result in respiratory failure requiring assisted ventilation.[144]

Leukocytosis with some degree of eosinophilia is common. Skin and serologic test results become positive 3 weeks after infestation; by that time, however, the diagnosis has generally been made on the basis of the clinical picture, particularly if a clear history of ingesting uncooked pork has been obtained.

Tropical Eosinophilia

As the name suggests, tropical eosinophilia is a disease largely confined to the tropics and characterized clinically by asthma associated with moderate to severe leukocytosis and eosinophilia. The etiologic agents are believed to be the parasitic microfilariae *Wuchereria bancrofti* and *Brugia malayi*, best known as the causes of Bancroft's and Malayan filariasis;[145, 146] infestation with animal microfilariae has also been implicated rarely.[145]

In classic filarial disease such as Bancroft's filariasis, humans are infected by the bite of a mosquito, which introduces filariform larvae into the skin. The latter mature into adult worms in draining lymphatics and there produce microfilariae that eventually reach the bloodstream; these are ingested by an uninfected mosquito, thus completing the cycle. Although the precise pathogenesis of tropical eosinophilia is unclear, it is probably related to a hypersensitivity reaction to filariae trapped within pulmonary capillaries,[145] in the case of *B. malayi* possibly a reaction to the cuticular antigen Bm 23-25.[146] This hypothesis is supported by the observations that the antigen can induce T-cell proliferation[146] and that levels of antifilarial antibodies are typically elevated in both blood and BAL fluid of affected patients.[147]

Disease is usually seen in regions in which the appropriate mosquito vectors live—the Indian subcontinent, Sri Lanka, Southeast Asia, the West Indies, and certain areas of northwest and central Africa.[145] Patients with tropical eosinophilia whose disease is recognized in other geographic locations invariably give a history of travel to or immigration from one of the endemic regions. Although unusual, the latter may have occurred many months or even years before the diagnosis is established.[148] Most patients are adult men between the ages of 20 and 40 years.[149]

Pathologic characteristics have been described in several series of patients who have undergone open-lung biopsy.[111, 150, 151] In the majority of those in whom biopsy is performed early in the course of the disease, a prominent eosinophilic leukocytic infiltrate is located within the alveolar interstitium and air spaces and the bronchovascular interstitium; the severity of the response ranges from focal collections of inflammatory cells to an extensive infiltrate accompanied by eosinophil microabscess formation. Multinucleated giant cells and well-formed granulomas may be present. Tissue necrosis is seldom evident. Older lesions are characterized by interstitial, peribronchial, and perivascular fibrosis. Fragmented or degenerated microfilariae can be identified within the areas of eosinophilic and granulomatous inflammation, but with great difficulty; they were seen in four of five patients in one series, but only after examination of 2,000 serial sections of lung tissue![151]

Radiographically, lung involvement is diffuse and symmetric and characterized by a reticulonodular pattern, sometimes accompanied by nodules 2 to 5 mm in diameter; the mid and lower lung zones are predominantly affected (Fig. 30–8). Hilar lymph node enlargement occurs in some cases,[149, 152, 153] and pleural effusion is rare.[154] HRCT is superior to the radiograph in the depiction of the reticulonodular opacities and the lymphadenopathy.[154a]

The main symptom is cough, usually paroxysmal and productive of small amounts of mucoid or mucopurulent material. It tends to be particularly bothersome at night, sometimes with the production of blood-streaked sputum. Attacks of coughing and dyspnea may be so severe as to suggest status asthmaticus. Weight loss, fatigue, low-grade fever, and slight enlargement of the liver and spleen are frequent.[153, 155] Superficial lymph node enlargement is rare.

Leukocytosis is usually present and may be as high as

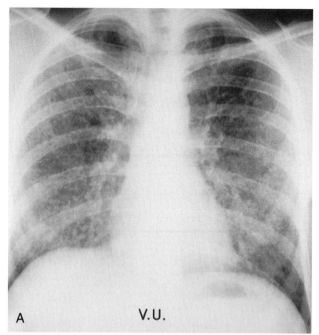

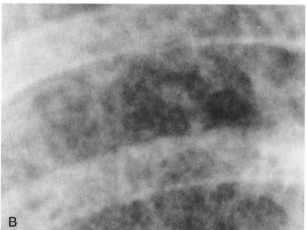

Figure 30–8. Tropical Eosinophilia. A posteroanterior chest radiograph *(A)* and a magnified view of the right upper lobe *(B)* reveal multiple discrete and confluent nodular opacities throughout both lungs ranging in diameter from 3 to 5 mm. There is no evidence of hilar or mediastinal lymph node enlargement. The patient was a young man from East India with gradual onset of nocturnal cough, fever, and high blood eosinophilia. Recovery was complete following appropriate chemotherapy.

100,000/mm³ with eosinophilia up to 80%. An absolute eosinophil count greater than 3,000 to 3,500 is seen in most patients.[145] Eosinophils as well as total and filarial-specific IgE are also prominent in sputum and BAL specimens.[147, 156] Serum IgE levels are raised (often greater than 5,000 ng/ml[157]) and may be higher during relapses than during the initial evaluation.[158] The serum level of α_1-antitrypsin is often low.[159] Hypergammaglobulinemia is common.[146]

Pulmonary function tests show either a restrictive pattern or a combined restrictive and obstructive pattern.[160] In the latter, flow rates, residual volume, and vital capacity are diminished; the decrease in flow rate is disproportionately greater than the decrease in vital capacity. Evidence of airway hyper-responsiveness is common in acute disease.[161] In one epidemiologic study in the Philippines in which village populations with and without a high incidence of parasitemia were compared,[162] a relationship between the presence of microfilariae and the degree of air-flow obstruction was demonstrated.

The diagnosis should be suspected from the clinical picture combined with a diffuse reticulonodular pattern on the radiograph in a patient who resides or has traveled in an endemic zone. Confirmation can be provided by a complement fixation or a skin test using *Dirofilaria immitis* antigen. Microfilariae have been identified in lung biopsy tissue, in transthoracic needle aspiration specimens,[163] in specimens of pulmonary secretions submitted for cytologic examination,[164, 165] in pleural fluid,[166] and (rarely) in specimens of blood obtained at night.

The chest radiograph usually shows complete clearing with appropriate therapy; however, the changes may be permanent[167] and may be associated with irreversible pulmonary function abnormalities,[168, 169] presumably reflecting the fibrosis observed pathologically. The relapse rate in patients treated with diethylcarbamazine is about 10% to 20%.[146]

Dirofilariasis

Dirofilariasis is caused by nematodes of the genus *Dirofilaria*, several species of which cause human infestation. Pulmonary disease caused by *D. immitis* has been recognized with increasing frequency since its original description in 1961,[170] and about 150 cases had been reported by 1992.[171–173] (Although usually residing outside the thorax and causing pulmonary disease via microfilariae [tropical eosinophilia], adult worms resembling *W. bancrofti* and *B. malayi* have rarely been identified in pulmonary arteries, where they have been associated with focal necrosis similar to that of dirofilariasis.[174–176])

D. immitis is found worldwide as a natural parasite of dogs, less commonly of cats and a variety of wild carnivores. In these animals the organisms are initially present in the subcutaneous tissue, from which they migrate to the right heart chambers where one or several worms take up residence and release microfilariae into the blood. Several species of mosquito are known to be intermediaries in the disease and are believed to transmit filariae to both the definitive host and humans.[177] Since humans are not a natural host, the organism does not complete its life cycle and dies before reaching sexual maturity; it is subsequently carried into the pulmonary circulation where it lodges in a peripheral vessel and causes necrosis and inflammation of surrounding tissue. Microfilariae have not been demonstrated in human peripheral blood.

Serologic studies in areas of endemic heartworm infestation suggest that the incidence of human infection is much greater than the number of reported cases of dirofilariasis would suggest.[173] It seems likely that a large proportion of these clinically undetected cases are the result of death of microfilariae at the site of their initial inoculation. However, since the worm can be difficult to detect in pathologic specimens and since it appears that transitory, asymptomatic nodules develop in some patients,[173] it is likely that some cases of pulmonary disease are not recognized.

Although the increase in the number of reported cases may be due partly to improved recognition of the condition, an actual increase in the frequency of canine heartworm disease in the United States suggests a real increase in incidence in this region.[178] The endemic zone of *D. immitis* in dogs was originally confined to the eastern seaboard but has moved inland, and cases of canine disease have been documented in virtually all states.[180] Most reports of human disease come from the eastern and southern coastal United States,[180] but cases have also been seen in Canada, Japan,[179] Brazil,[181] Europe,[182] and New Zealand.[183] All patients have been adults, an age group in which there is a greater likelihood that chest radiography will be performed and in which a malignancy will be suspected when a solitary nodule is found.

As indicated, pulmonary disease occurs when one or more worms embolize into a peripheral pulmonary artery. Since the organisms are dead at this time, active infection is not involved in the pathogenesis of the pulmonary lesion. Although ischemia (i.e., infarction) is probably a factor in some cases, the typical spherical rather than wedge shape of the resulting nodule and the paucity of hemorrhage suggest that tissue necrosis is more likely the result of toxins or enzymes released by the dead worms or host inflammatory cells than of vascular compromise.

Pathologically, the lesions are usually located in the periphery of the lung and appear as well-circumscribed, spherical, or slightly lobulated nodules.[184–186] Histologically there is a central area of coagulative or occasionally caseation-like[186] necrosis surrounded by a variable amount of fibrous tissue and inflammatory infiltrate. The latter is frequently granulomatous; eosinophils are prominent in some cases.[185] One or occasionally several worms may be identified within a pulmonary artery in the central portion of the nodule; they usually measure 100 to 300 μm in diameter and show, in varying stages of preservation, a characteristic thick multilayered cuticle, abundant somatic muscle, internal longitudinal ridges, and broad lateral cords (Fig. 30–9).[186] Silver stains and nonspecific fluorescent whitener stains such as Calcofluor white can facilitate identification of the worm.[188]

Radiologically, the typical manifestation is a solitary spherical or somewhat wedge-shaped, well-circumscribed nodule 1 to 2 cm in diameter.[187] Multiple nodules are seen occasionally,[178, 190] in one report associated with repeated episodes of pulmonary "infarction."[189] A pneumonic pattern has also been described, with eventual evolution to a solitary nodule.

Most patients are asymptomatic, the diagnosis being made after pulmonary resection or (rarely) transthoracic needle aspiration performed because of a suspicion of pulmonary carcinoma;[190] occasionally there is cough, chest pain, and hemoptysis.[177, 191] Laboratory tests are not usually helpful in diagnosis. Systemic eosinophilia is not uncommon, but usually mild (about 5% in most cases).[191] Immunologic tests, including indirect hemagglutination and ELISA,[192, 193] may prove to be helpful but have not yet been shown to permit confident distinction of dirofilariasis from carcinoma.

Visceral Larva Migrans

Visceral larva migrans (toxocariasis) results from infestation by larvae of the dog and cat roundworms *Toxocara*

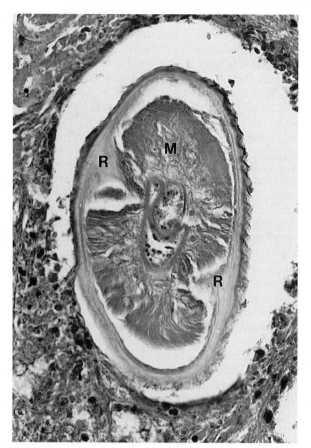

Figure 30–9. *Dirofilaria immitis.* Partly degenerated organism within a pulmonary artery. Muscle (M) and cuticle with longitudinal ridges (R) are shown. (×375.) (Reprinted from Thurlbeck WM, Churg AM: Pathology of the Lung. 2nd ed. New York, Thieme Medical Publishers, 1995, with permission.)

canis and *Toxocara cati.*[146] Animal disease is found throughout the world but is particularly common in temperate and tropical regions. Symptomatic human disease appears to be relatively rare, at least in temperate climates; for example, only 18 cases were recognized at Toronto's Hospital for Sick Children over a period of 27 years.[194] As a result of the mode of transmission (*see* farther on), toxocariasis occurs predominantly in children; however, disease also occurs occasionally in adults.[195]

Human infestation typically begins when an individual swallows soil containing eggs passed in the feces of dogs or cats. The eggs develop into larvae in the intestine, pass into the bloodstream, and are carried to various organs, including the liver, brain, eyes, heart, and lungs. Since humans are not the definitive host, the larvae cannot complete their life cycle; they become trapped within small blood vessels, penetrate their walls, and migrate into contiguous tissue. Here they may either remain dormant or die and provoke an inflammatory reaction that is largely responsible for clinical disease.

Histologically, granulomas may be found in many organs and consist of a central zone of necrotic tissue surrounded by epithelioid and multinucleated giant cells, lymphocytes, and eosinophils.[196, 197] Larvae can often be identified within the necrotic material. Long-standing granulomas may be completely organized into fibrous tissue.[196]

Approximately 50% of patients with pulmonary symptoms have transient, local, or diffuse patchy areas of ill-defined air-space opacification on radiographs.[7] Patients are often asymptomatic but may complain of cough, wheezing, dyspnea, abdominal pain, and neurologic symptoms; rapidly progressive and/or fatal disease is seen rarely.[198] Hepatosplenomegaly and a pruritic skin rash are common. Systemic symptoms such as fever, weight loss, and malaise are also frequent. Leukocytosis of 40,000/mm³ or more is common, usually with eosinophilia of at least 30%. Marked eosinophilia may also be seen in BAL fluid.[199] Hypergammaglobulinemia and anemia may develop.

The diagnosis can be made by the identification of granulomas containing larvae on liver biopsy. Since the larvae do not mature in humans, eggs are not passed in the stool. An immunofluorescent antibody test has been considered practical and reliable;[200] an ELISA has been reported to have a sensitivity of 78% and a specificity of 92% and may be a more efficient diagnostic test.[194]

Syngamosis

The parasite *Mammomanogamus (Syngamus) laryngeus* is found in wild and domestic birds and mammals in the tropics and subtropics. Virtually all instances of human infestation have been reported in natives or travelers to the Caribbean or Brazil.[201, 202] Approximately 100 cases had been reported by 1995.[202] Humans are only accidental hosts and probably become infested from eating vegetables contaminated by respiratory secretions from affected animals (probably cattle) or an undetermined intermediate host.

The worms first attach themselves to the pharyngeal mucosa and then migrate into the larynx, trachea, or proximal bronchi, where they produce severe paroxysmal cough, particularly at night and sometimes accompanied by hemoptysis. A characteristic feature is a tantalizing "crawling" sensation that may become extremely unpleasant and annoying to the patient, sometimes to the point of desperation. The clinical picture in some patients mimics that of asthma.[203]

Males (measuring 3 mm in length) and females (10 mm) are found *in copula* when expectorated or when removed from the trachea through a bronchoscope. Endoscopically they appear as red Y-shaped "filaments" moving over the mucosa. The couple is usually solitary but may be multiple. The eggs have a characteristic morphology and may be seen in the sputum or feces.[203, 204]

Gnathostomiasis

Human gnathostomiasis is caused principally by *Gnathostoma spinigerum*; occasional cases associated with *Gnathostoma hispidum, Gnathostoma nipponicum,* and *Gnathostoma doloresi* have also been reported.[205] The disease is endemic in Southeast Asia, Australia, Mexico, and parts of South America.[205] It is usually acquired by the ingestion of raw or undercooked fish, poultry, or pork. Larvae present within the food penetrate the gastric wall and migrate through the liver to skeletal muscle and connective tissue. In the definitive hosts (domestic dogs and cats and a variety of wild animals), the larvae then travel back to the stomach where they form a tumor-like mass within the mucosa from which eggs are laid. In humans, this last migratory phase does not occur, and the larvae continue to wander, largely in subcutaneous tissue, for as long as 10 years. At this site they are manifested clinically by intermittent episodes of localized swelling lasting 1 to 2 weeks and associated with pruritus, edema, erythema, and/or pain. Migration of a worm into a visceral organ occurs occasionally.

Pulmonary disease is uncommon and is usually preceded by several years of migratory subcutaneous swelling. Reported manifestations include cough, chest pain, dyspnea, and hemoptysis.[205, 206] Occasionally, the worm is expectorated, with resolution of symptomatology.[205] Pneumothorax, hydropneumothorax, and pleural effusion have also been documented; marked eosinophilia may be present in the aspirated fluid. Peripheral blood eosinophilia is common and ranges from 30% to 70%.

Miscellaneous Nematodes

Cutaneous Larva Migrans. This variety of larva migrans (creeping eruption) is characterized by the migration under the skin of the larvae of *Ancylostoma braziliense* and *Ancylostoma caninum* (cat and dog hookworms). Pulmonary disease is manifested as a Löffler-like syndrome; the combination of typical serpiginous cutaneous tracts, cough, blood eosinophilia, and radiographic evidence of transitory nonsegmental patchy air-space consolidation is virtually diagnostic.[207, 208]

Onchocerciasis. *Onchocerca volvulus* characteristically affects the eyes, skin, and lymph nodes. Treatment of the disease with diethylcarbamazine has been associated with "mobilization" of microfilariae into the systemic and, ultimately, the pulmonary circulation, in some instances with respiratory distress.[209] In one severe case that resulted in death, microfilariae were seen in the pulmonary parenchyma in association with microabscesses.[210] Filariae can also be identified in sputum in these cases.[209]

Capillariasis. This abnormality is caused by several species of *Capillaria*, most often *Capillaria philippinensis* and *Capillaria hepatica*. Pulmonary disease caused by *Capillaria aerophila,* is rare, most cases having been reported from the former Soviet Union.[211] Adult worms live in the conducting airways of the definite hosts (dogs, cats, and various wild carnivores) and produce eggs that are swallowed and shed in the feces. Human infestation probably occurs following contact with contaminated soil. Examination of a lung biopsy specimen in one case showed worms within bronchioles surrounded by a granulomatous inflammatory infiltrate.[211] Chest radiographs of some patients have shown a reticulonodular pattern. Symptoms consist of cough and dyspnea, sometimes described as "asthma-like." Eggs can be identified in sputum samples.

Enterobiasis. The pinworm *Enterobius vermicularis* usually causes disease in the lower intestine or female genital tract. A case of a solitary pulmonary nodule composed of necrotic lung containing numerous eosinophils and scattered adult worms has been reported.[212]

Anisakiasis. Anisakiasis is usually a disease of the gastrointestinal tract that in humans is acquired by eating raw or undercooked fish containing *Anisakis marina*. A single report of pleural effusion probably caused by the organism has been documented.[213]

Metastrongylodiasis. Metastrongylids (lung worms) are nematodes that inhabit the pulmonary arteries, bronchi, and lung parenchyma of a number of animals throughout the world. A single case has been reported of overwhelming infestation leading to death in an apparently immunocompetent man;[214] pathologic examination showed necrotizing granulomatous vasculitis simulating Wegener's granulomatosis.

TREMATODES (FLATWORMS)

Paragonimiasis

Paragonimiasis is caused by flukes of the genus *Paragonimus*. Although the most frequent etiologic agent is *Paragonimus westermani*,[215] several other species also cause pulmonary disease. For example, *Paragonimus uterobilateralis* and *Paragonimus africanus* are known to infest humans in parts of Africa,[216] *Paragonimus mexicanus* is the most commonly implicated organism in Mexico and Central America, and *Paragonimus kellicotti* infestation has been identified in North America.[217, 218] The adult fluke measures about 7.5 to 20 mm in length by 4 to 6 mm in width and possesses oral and ventral suckers for attachment to the lung parenchyma. The eggs measure 80 to 120 by 45 to 65 μm and have a somewhat flattened operculum at one end; their outer wall is birefringent.

Epidemiology

Paragonimiasis is seen most frequently in Southeast Asia, especially in Korea, Japan, the Philippines, Taiwan, and parts of China; it occurs with lesser frequency in Nepal and in parts of South America (especially Brazil, Peru, Ecuador, and Venezuela), Central America (Costa Rica, Honduras, and Mexico), and western Africa. The prevalence of the disease in the Philippines has been estimated to be between 1% and 10% and in Korea about 4%.[215] Migration of Southeast Asian refugees has resulted in an increased recognition of the disease in North America.[219–221]

Humans typically acquire the disease by ingesting raw or undercooked crabs or crayfish or by drinking water contaminated by them; as a result the disease tends to occur in families because of common dietary exposure. It has also been suggested that person-to-person transmission via intermediate hosts may occur in areas of high disease prevalence.[215]

Life Cycle

The life cycle of *P. westermani* is one of the most fascinating of all parasites. Within the lungs of humans or animals, the larval forms (metacercariae) develop into adult flukes that deposit eggs in burrows in the lung parenchyma. The eggs are coughed up or swallowed and excreted in the feces. Under suitable conditions, the eggs develop into ciliated miracidia, which infest freshwater snails. Within the snail, further larval forms develop that are liberated as cercariae after about 2 months; these actively motile parasites penetrate the soft periarticular tissues of certain species of crayfish and crabs.

When ingested by the definitive host, metacercariae are liberated in the jejunum, from which they migrate through the wall of the small bowel into the peritoneal cavity, burrow through the diaphragm into the pleural space, and finally invade the lung. Within the lung—usually a lower lobe—the metacercariae mature into adult flukes, which produce ova to repeat the cycle. Migration of flukes to extrapulmonary sites such as the brain or skin occurs rarely. The mature parasite can live for many years in the lung and produce ova continuously.

Pathogenesis and Pathologic Characteristics

In the typical case of paragonimiasis examined at autopsy, there are single or multiple 1- to 3-cm cystic spaces containing reddish brown mucinous fluid and usually a single adult parasite.[222] The cysts are frequently located near larger bronchioles or bronchi; although predominantly subpleural, they can occur anywhere within the lung parenchyma.

Microscopically, the parasites are initially surrounded by polymorphonuclear leukocytes and eosinophils. Fibrosis and a mononuclear inflammatory infiltrate, sometimes granulomatous (Fig. 30–10), eventually develop at the periphery of the cystic cavities; the contents of the cyst at this stage consist of the adult worm, numerous ova, and necrotic debris. When erosion occurs into a draining airway, the contents of the cyst may be coughed up or may spread to other portions of the lung parenchyma and result in bronchopneumonia; granulomas may develop in relation to ova disseminated by this mechanism. Bronchial arteries in the vicinity of the cysts undergo hypertrophy and are probably the source of hemoptysis.[222]

Radiologic Manifestations

The chest radiograph is normal in approximately 20% of patients in whom *Paragonimus* eggs are identified in the sputum.[7, 223] The most common abnormalities consist of parenchymal opacities and cystic lesions, each seen in approximately 50% of patients (Fig. 30–11).[224, 225] The parenchymal opacities may be poorly defined or homogeneous, single or multiple, nodular, subsegmental, or segmental[223, 225] (Fig. 30–12). The cystic lesions may be single or multiple, measure 0.5 to 5 cm in diameter, and are usually thin walled (Fig. 30–13).[224, 225] They may be seen in areas of consolidation or as isolated thin-walled ring shadows.[223, 225] They often have a crescent-shaped or oval opacity along one aspect of the inner lining;[224] this opacity has soft tissue attenuation on CT and presumably represents the worm.[225]

Communication between the cysts and a bronchus has been demonstrated by bronchography[224] and by CT[225] and may mimic bronchiectasis. Irregular tracks or burrows measuring up to 5 mm in diameter and connecting adjacent cysts have been identified on both radiographs[224] and on CT[225] in a small number of patients. In one case of disseminated paragonimiasis from Thailand,[226] CT demonstrated multiple irregularly marginated nodules in the left lung, a large suprahilar cystic mass extending into the mediastinum, and cysts in the thoracic wall. Abdominal CT revealed cystic masses and liver abscesses. Head CT demonstrated a mixed-density mass with a cystic component in the frontotemporal region of the brain.

Pleural abnormalities were identified in approximately 60% of 71 patients in one study and included unilateral or bilateral effusion (37%), hydropneumothorax (17%), and pleural thickening (7%).[225] Massive effusion occurs in some patients.[220, 227, 228]

Studies of immigrants to the United States who have resided in various endemic areas have shown a somewhat different chest radiographic pattern. The opacities tend to

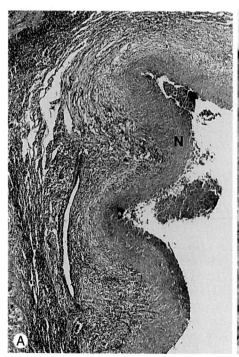
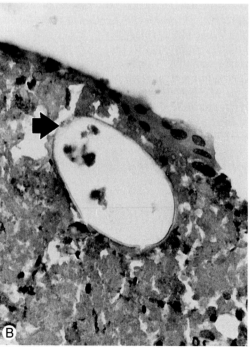

Figure 30–10. Paragonimiasis. A low-magnification view *(A)* shows a focus of necrotic tissue (N) adjacent to a cavity and bordered by granulomatous inflammatory tissue. An egg with a flattened operculum *(B, arrow)* is present within the necrotic tissue *(A, ×40; B, ×500.)* (Reprinted from Thurlbeck WM, Churg AM: Pathology of the Lung. 2nd ed. New York, Thieme Medical Publishers, 1995, with permission.)

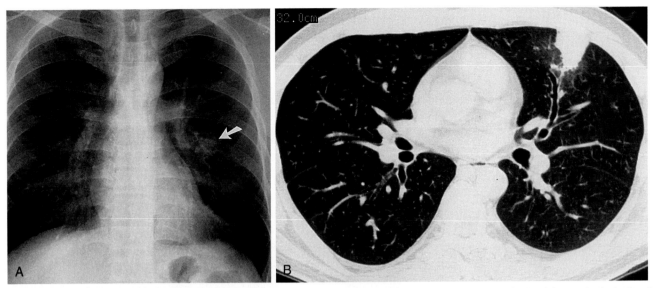

Figure 30–11. Paragonimiasis: Single Opacity. A posteroanterior chest radiograph *(A)* demonstrates a poorly defined nodular opacity in the lingula *(arrow)*. An HRCT scan *(B)* demonstrates this opacity to represent a subsegmental pleural-based area of consolidation. The appearance is consistent with a pulmonary infarct. The diagnosis of paragonimiasis was confirmed by open-lung biopsy in this 39-year-old South Korean man seen for left chest pain. (Case courtesy of Dr. Kyung Soo Lee, Samsung Medical Center, Seoul, Korea.)

mimic postprimary tuberculosis, particularly in the upper lobes, and it is probable that some patients have been treated erroneously for this disease.[220] This error in diagnosis perhaps applies mostly to patients who have pleural effusion in addition to parenchymal disease. In the late stages, some lesions calcify.[226]

Clinical Manifestations

Symptoms of acute pleuropulmonary disease occur during the migration of metacercariae and include cough, dyspnea, and chest pain; signs of pneumothorax or pleural effusion may be evident.[229] Symptoms of chronic disease may not develop for 1 year or more after the presumed time of the infestation. Tuberculosis is initially diagnosed in a significant number of patients.[215] Although hemoptysis has been considered to be an almost invariable symptom of this phase, it was noted in only 64% of cases in one series of 25 patients;[220] it tends to occur sporadically for months or even years in the absence of other signs of illness.[229, 230] Episodic pleural pain is common.[215] Low-grade fever, anorexia, clubbing, and/or weight loss may be present. Both flukes and ova can be carried to the brain from the lungs and cause epileptic seizures, hemiplegia, and fatal encephalitis. Diarrhea occurs occasionally.

Laboratory Findings

Eosinophilia (absolute level greater than 500 cells/mm³) is seen in about two thirds of cases;[215] very high levels are uncommon.[231] Some patients are anemic. Pleural fluid has been reported to show eosinophilia, a low sugar level and low pH, and high protein and LDH levels.[227]

The diagnosis can be made readily in most patients by identifying the typical operculated eggs in sputum, stool, or pleural fluid.[220, 228, 232] The sensitivity of a single sputum examination is about 30% to 40%;[215] sensitivity increases to 50% to 90% with repeated examinations. When considered in association with the clinical and radiographic findings, the complement fixation test is also a useful method of diagnosis.[220] An indirect ELISA has been found by one group of investigators to be highly sensitive and specific for the detection of circulating antibody to the organism.[233] Another group has documented similar results with an ELISA using fluke cysteine proteinases as antigens.[234]

Schistosomiasis

Schistosoma mansoni, Schistosoma japonicum, and *Schistosoma haematobium* are the most important agents of human schistosomiasis. *Schistosoma mekongi* has been identified as an important etiologic agent in parts of Southeast Asia;[235] occasional examples of infestation by other species such as *Schistosoma intercalatum* and *Schistosoma malayensis* have also been reported.[236]

Adult worms are flat and elongated and possess oral and ventral suckers for attachment to the luminal surface of veins. Size varies with the sex and species,[237] but the worm is generally 0.6 to 20 mm in length by 0.3 to 1.0 mm in width. The eggs of the various species differ morphologically, thus permitting their distinction in well-preserved specimens. The eggs of *S. mansoni* and *S. haematobium* measure about 110 to 175 μm by 40 to 70 μm; the former possess a prominent lateral spine, and the latter a terminal spine. The eggs of *S. japonicum* are smaller (70 to 100 μm by 50 to 65 μm) and possess only a minute lateral spine. When stained by a modified Ziehl-Neelsen technique, the outer portion of the eggs of both *S. mansoni* and *S. japonicum* is acid fast; that of *S. haematobium* is not.[237]

Epidemiology

Schistosomiasis is one of the most important parasitic infestations of humans and has been estimated to affect more

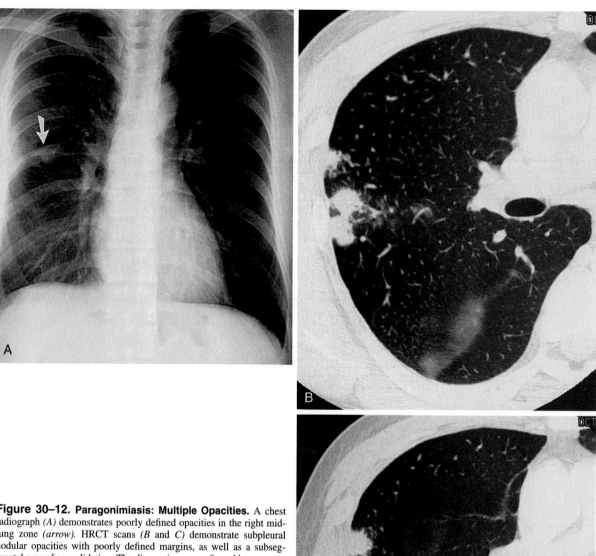

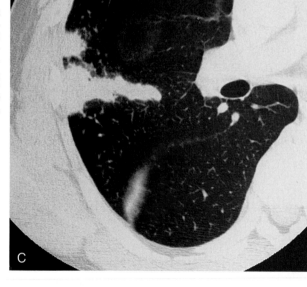

Figure 30–12. Paragonimiasis: Multiple Opacities. A chest radiograph *(A)* demonstrates poorly defined opacities in the right mid-lung zone *(arrow)*. HRCT scans *(B* and *C)* demonstrate subpleural nodular opacities with poorly defined margins, as well as a subsegmental area of consolidation. The diagnosis was confirmed by enzyme-linked immunosorbent assay and transthoracic needle aspiration, which demonstrated characteristic ova. The patient was a 38-year-old South Korean man evaluated for vague chest pain and cough. (Case courtesy of Dr. Kyung Soo Lee, Samsung Medical Center, Seoul, Korea.)

than 200 million people worldwide.[238] Acquisition of disease is limited to areas inhabited by the intermediate host, the snail. With increasing development of agriculture and associated irrigation projects, proliferation of these hosts may result in an increased prevalence of disease.[239] Humans are the only important definitive hosts of *S. mansoni* and *S. haematobium*; wild and domestic animals are additional important reservoirs of *S. japonicum*.[237]

The geographic distribution of schistosomiasis varies with the specific etiologic agent. Both *S. mansoni* and *S. haematobium* are endemic in the Middle East (especially Egypt and parts of Saudi Arabia) and in large areas of central and southern Africa; *S. mansoni* is also found in the Caribbean Islands and in South America, particularly Brazil. *S. japonicum* is predominantly seen in China, Japan, and the Philippines and *S. mekongi* in Laos, Kampuchea, and

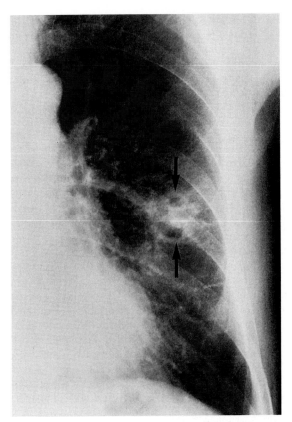

Figure 30–13. Paragonimiasis: Cystic Lesion. A view of the left lung from a posteroanterior chest radiograph shows aggregated, uniform-sized, thin-walled cysts *(arrows)* in the left upper lobe. The diagnosis was proved by a positive serologic test for *Paragonimus*-specific antibody. The patient was a 51-year-old South Korean man with a history of blood-tinged sputum for several months. (From Im JG, Whang NY, Kim WS, et al: Am J Roentgenol 159:39, 1992.)

Thailand.[235] Although disease is most commonly identified in endemic regions, increased emigration from these regions in the recent past means that it is likely to be more frequently encountered elsewhere; for example, it has been estimated that approximately 400,000 infected immigrants reside in the United States.[236]

Life Cycle

The life cycle of *Schistosoma* is complex. Humans acquire the infestation by drinking, swimming, working, or washing in fresh water containing infective cercariae. The latter penetrate the skin or, less commonly, the mucosa of the mouth or pharynx and pass as schistosomules via the venous circulation to the pulmonary capillaries. They pass through these vessels to the systemic circulation and traverse the mesenteric vessels into the intrahepatic portion of the portal system. There they develop into adolescent worms that migrate to the superior mesenteric (*S. japonicum* and *S. mekongi*), inferior mesenteric (*S. mansoni*), or vesical (*S. haematobium*) veins. The adult male and female worms copulate in these venules, and the females then lodge in smaller venous channels in the submucosa and mucosa of the bowel or bladder, where they lay eggs. Many eggs are extruded into the lumen of the bowel or urinary bladder and are passed in the feces or urine; those that reach fresh water develop into miracidia, which enter snails. Several transformations take place within the snail, infective cercariae eventually emerging; penetration of the skin of a person in contact with the contaminated water completes the odyssey.

Pathogenesis and Pathologic Characteristics

Tissue damage in schistosomiasis almost always results from the release of eggs into host tissues with subsequent immunologic reaction, inflammation, and fibrosis.[238] These effects may be related to entrapment of eggs during their extrusion into the lumen of the bowel or bladder, damage thus remaining localized to the gastrointestinal or vesical mucosa. Some eggs may also be released directly into venous blood: in the case of *S. mansoni, S. japonicum,* and *S. mekongi,* release usually occurs into the portal system with deposition in the liver; with *S. haematobium,* release is into the inferior vena cava with direct embolization to the lungs. Eggs of the former three species can also reach the lungs once the liver has become cirrhotic as a result of schistosoma-related fibrosis, the development of anastomotic channels permitting passage of the ova between the portal and systemic venous systems.[240]

Once they reach the lungs, most embolized eggs become impacted in pulmonary arterioles measuring 50 to 100 μm in diameter, following which they are extruded into the perivascular tissue. The host reaction to the eggs may be associated with an obliterative arteriolitis that, when widespread, can result in pulmonary hypertension. Less often, pulmonary disease occurs by other pathogenetic mechanisms. The passage of cercariae through the pulmonary capillaries can cause a transitory process that simulates Löffler's syndrome; although well documented radiographically, the pathologic features of this form have been incompletely described. Rarely, focal accumulation of extruded eggs with surrounding inflammation and fibrosis is manifested as a nodule or mass ("bilharzioma").[241]

Schistosoma ova are commonly identified at autopsy in the lungs of individuals with schistosomiasis.[242, 243] In the majority of the cases, they are present in small numbers and are unassociated with significant vascular changes or with a clinical history of cardiopulmonary disease. Histologically they are usually located adjacent to small pulmonary arteries or arterioles or in contiguous alveolar interstitial tissue and are surrounded by an inflammatory infiltrate composed of lymphocytes, histiocytes, eosinophils, and scattered multinucleated giant cells; granulomas may also be apparent. Fibrosis eventually ensues, and in some instances scars may be the only residua. The eggs themselves often show degenerative changes, occasionally with calcification; sometimes they are sufficiently well preserved to permit histologic identification of a particular species.

Occasionally, focal or diffuse vasculopathy is present in association with the ova. This has several histologic patterns, including intimal fibroelastosis and medial hypertrophy of small arteries and arterioles, angiomatoid and plexiform lesions virtually identical to those of plexogenic pulmonary arteriopathy, necrotizing arteritis with or without thrombosis, and obliterative endarteritis.[244–246] When severe enough, the latter is associated with arterial hypertension and cor pulmonale.

Adult worms, either histologically viable or showing degenerative changes, may also be found within medium-sized pulmonary arteries,[242] usually at branch points. Live worms appear to cause no tissue necrosis or vascular thrombosis; by contrast, dead parasites are generally associated with surrounding tissue necrosis and inflammation, the extent of which may be sufficient to cause radiographically visible nodules.[247]

Radiologic Manifestations

The appearance of the chest radiograph varies considerably, depending on the number of eggs that reach the lung and the time interval since the formation of perivascular granulomas following extrusion of the eggs. Some cases—perhaps the majority—show a diffuse miliary or reticulonodular pattern presumably caused by the migration of ova through vessel walls and subsequent reaction to these foreign bodies.[249–251] Areas of pneumonic consolidation can develop around dead adult worms and occluded arteries.[247, 251] Pleural effusion does not occur, although focal pleural thickening may develop. Pulmonary arterial hypertension caused by schistosomiasis is indistinguishable from that resulting from any other cause, there being a marked degree of dilatation of the main pulmonary artery and its branches with rapid tapering toward the periphery.[248]

Clinical Manifestations

Clinical manifestations occur in several distinct time intervals following parasitization. During the early stage of infestation, migration of the schistosomules from the skin through the pulmonary circulation may be associated with an acute syndrome consisting of fever, cough, diarrhea, arthralgia, anorexia, malaise, and hives; leukocytosis and eosinophilia are almost invariable. It is at this stage that transitory opacities may be seen on the chest radiograph.[240]

Somewhat later (following the deposition of eggs in the intestinal and bladder venules), cough, dyspnea, hypoxemia, palpitation, and pulmonary edema can develop acutely, findings that are believed to constitute an allergic reaction to the sudden mobilization of many eggs to the lungs.[252] A similar syndrome may be observed when therapy is instituted in patients with known schistosomiasis; in such circumstances, BAL and transbronchial biopsy specimens have revealed interstitial and alveolar eosinophilia.[253] These acute forms of disease are seldom seen in inhabitants of endemic areas and are instead usually seen in visitors.[254] Such disease is usually mild and self-limited; however, fatalities can occur.[236]

The most important pulmonary manifestation of schistosomiasis—hypertension—develops after years of persistent infestation and continuous exposure,[253] usually in a relatively small percentage of the affected population.[248] With the development of this complication, an ejection systolic murmur (with or without an early diastolic murmur), a loud second pulmonic sound, and a left parasternal heave may appear; signs of cardiac decompensation may develop. Diffuse scattered crackles or rhonchi may be the only audible sounds on auscultation of the lungs. Hemoptysis is rare; when present, it is apparently caused by larval erosion of a pulmonary artery.[255]

Signs of extrathoracic disease are almost invariably present in chronic disease. The eggs of *S. mansoni* and *S. japonicum* are deposited mainly in the liver, so symptoms and signs of cirrhosis and hepatosplenomegaly predominate; diarrhea can occur and be accompanied by blood, pus, and mucus in the stool. *S. haematobium* infestation is associated with dysuria and terminal hematuria.

Laboratory Findings

In patients with suspected schistosomiasis, concentrated specimens of stool and urine should be examined repeatedly for ova. Infestation is demonstrable in many cases by the presence of eggs in biopsy specimens of the rectal and bladder mucosa; however, examination of the sputum seldom reveals ova, and lung biopsy may be necessary to unequivocally establish the presence of pulmonary involvement.[256, 257] Specific IgE against soluble egg antigen is found in high titer during the acute but not the chronic stage of disease. Levels of IgM and IgG antibody to cercarial antigen are increased in acute disease, and levels of IgG to the adult worm are increased in the chronic form.[258] Specific skin tests and precipitin tests are available for individual species.[249] Moderate leukocytosis and eosinophilia are usual, the latter reaching as high as 33%.[251]

Pulmonary function tests in pulmonary schistosomiasis associated with cor pulmonale may yield normal results even in the presence of high pulmonary artery pressures. A slight reduction in vital capacity and flow rates has been recorded in some studies.[251, 259] Patients tend to hyperventilate and have raised ventilatory equivalents and increased dead space. Compliance is reduced, presumably as a result of interstitial fibrosis.[260] One group of investigators found arterial oxygen saturations of 89% to 94% in fewer than 10% of their patients and only in those with pulmonary hypertension at rest or during exercise.[261] The hypoxemia is probably caused by shunting between portal and pulmonary veins.

Miscellaneous Trematodes

Hepatic Flukes. As their name implies, hepatic flukes (including *Clonorchis sinensis*, *Opisthorchis felineus*, *Opisthorchis viverrini*, and *Fasciola hepatica*) typically affect the liver. Complicating pleuropulmonary disease can be manifested in two ways:[262, 263] (1) Löffler-like syndrome can develop some months after the ingestion of undercooked freshwater fish or watercress contaminated with encysted metacercariae, during the period when larvae are migrating from the duodenum to the biliary tree and liver; and (2) somewhat later, a liver abscess caused by the presence of the adult worm can extend into the right hemithorax (a complication with a much lower incidence than seen with amebic infestation).

Alariasis. This disease is caused by metacercariae of *Alaria americana*. The organism has a complicated life cycle that at one point involves the accumulation of larvae in the hind legs of frogs. A single fatal case of human disease presumed to be acquired from eating such legs has been reported;[264] cough, increasing dyspnea, and hemoptysis were prominent features.

CESTODES (TAPEWORMS)

Echinococcosis (Hydatid Disease)

Echinococcosis is caused by small (3 to 6 mm) larvae of the subclass Cestoda, two species of which, *Echinococcus granulosus* and *Echinococcus multilocularis,* are responsible for the vast majority of human infestations;[265] *Echinococcus vogeli* and *Echinococcus oligarthrus* have been implicated rarely (causing a form of disease similar to that of *E. multilocularis*).[266] The adult worms are morphologically similar (although *E. multilocularis* is somewhat smaller[267]) and consist of four segments, a head (scolex, composed of four suckers and a rostellum that contains a double row of hooklets for attachment to the intestinal mucosa) and three proglottids, the last of which is the egg-laying organ.

Echinococcus granulosus (Cystic Hydatid Disease)

Epidemiology

E. granulosus is the cause of most cases of human hydatid disease and occurs in two varieties, pastoral and sylvatic, that differ in their definitive and intermediate hosts, their geographic distributions, and to a limited extent their clinical and radiologic features. The *pastoral* variety is the more common of the two and, as the name implies, occurs in rural settings in which sheep, cows, horses, or pigs are the intermediate hosts and dogs the usual definitive hosts. Different strains of the organism occur in association with different host pairs; such strains appear to have different pathogenicity, that of the sheep/dog being the most pathogenetic for humans whereas that of horse/dog rarely causes human disease.[265]

Humans typically acquire the disease by direct contact with infested dogs or by ingestion of contaminated water, food, or soil, thus becoming accidental intermediate hosts. The disease is particularly common in the sheep-raising regions of southeastern Europe, the Middle East, North Africa, parts of the former Soviet Union, South America (particularly Argentina, Chile, and Uruguay), Australia, and New Zealand. Cases that are seen outside these regions most often occur in immigrants from them.

The *sylvatic* variety of echinococcosis has as its definitive hosts several species of the Canidae family, including the dog, wolf, arctic fox, and coyote. A variety of herbivores, including the moose, white-tailed and coast deer, reindeer, elk, caribou, and bison, serve as intermediate hosts. This variety is seen primarily in Alaska and northern Canada, where it affects mostly native Indians and Inuits.[268] A similar form of disease has been described in Australia in association with the dingo dog and the wallaby.[265]

The infestation is usually first noted in young adults,[265] about one third of affected patients being under the age of 20 years.[269, 270] Pulmonary disease in particular appears to be relatively more common in younger individuals.[271] Ethnic and cultural differences in the handling of potentially infected material and in farming have profound effects on the prevalence of disease in certain groups;[265] for example, it has been estimated that the risk of disease is 1,340 times greater in Californians of Basque origin than other California residents as a result of their use of sheep dogs.[265] The theory that most infestations are acquired in childhood only to become manifested in adulthood has been questioned by the relatively rapid reduction in incidence of the disease in adults following the institution of control programs.[272]

Life Cycle

The mature adult worms, of which there may be thousands, live in the small intestine of the definitive host. Millions of eggs are passed in the feces to grazing land, ground vegetation, or water and are ingested by the intermediate hosts. In these, larvae develop in the duodenum, penetrate its wall, and pass via the portal system to the liver, where the majority are trapped in hepatic sinusoids; most of those that escape are trapped in the alveolar capillaries. The majority of entrapped larvae are killed by the host; the few that survive develop into solitary or multiple cysts that produce brood capsules containing immature worms (protoscoleces). The life cycle of the parasite is completed when the definitive host feeds on the remains of an intermediate host that harbors cysts, with the subsequent intraintestinal development of adult worms.

Pathogenesis and Pathologic Characteristics

The effect of the hepatic and pulmonary capillary sieves in containing the larvae is largely responsible for the distribution of disease—approximately 65% to 70% of *E. granulosus* cysts occur in the liver and 15% to 30% in the lungs. The remaining 3% to 5% can be found virtually anywhere in the body, but most commonly in the spleen, kidney, brain, and bones. The anatomic bias for the liver or lung varies in different series; for example, in pastoral echinococcosis, lung cysts have been reported to be more common than,[273] less common than,[274] and equally as common as liver cysts.[275, 276] In sylvatic hydatid disease, however, lung cysts show a clear preponderance over those in the liver.[277] Review of the literature suggests that the prevalence of lung cysts is higher today than formerly, possibly a result of the more common use of screening chest radiography in endemic areas.

As indicated previously, larvae that survive the host defenses develop into unilocular cysts that gradually enlarge, sometimes taking many years before giving rise to symptoms.[278] Although a growth rate of 1 cm/yr is considered typical, rates up to 5 cm/yr have been recorded.[265] (The growth rate of cysts in the sylvatic variety is thought to be less, averaging about 0.5 cm/yr.[265]) It has been speculated that the organism may be able to produce a substance homologous to human cyclophilin (a molecule that interacts with cyclosporin A to induce T-cell suppression) and thereby induce local depression of host defense.[265]

Within the lung, the cyst is typically spherical or oval (Fig. 30–14) and surrounded by a pericyst consisting of fibrous tissue containing a nonspecific chronic inflammatory infiltrate; the surrounding lung is usually atelectatic owing to compression. The hydatid cyst itself is composed of two layers: a laminated outer membrane (the exocyst) that serves to protect the developing organisms from the host and a thin inner layer formed by a syncytium of cells (the endocyst) that constitutes the germinal layer (Fig. 30–15).[267] The latter produces intracystic fluid and gives origin to numerous

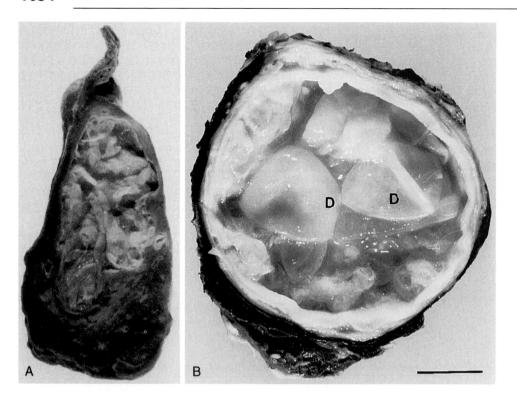

Figure 30–14. Hydatid Cysts.
Lesions from two patients are illustrated, one irregular in shape *(A)* and the other spherical *(B)*. Daughter cysts (D) are better appreciated in the latter. (*Bar,* 1 cm.)

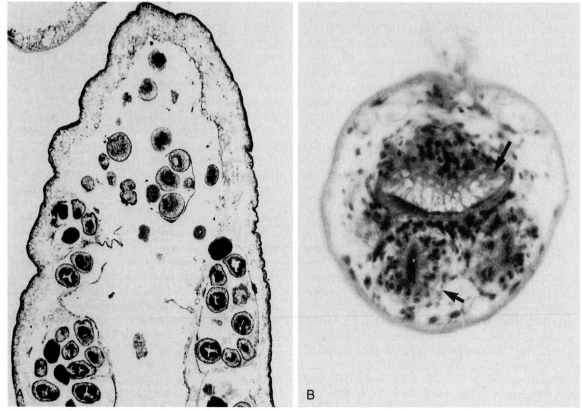

Figure 30–15. *Echinoccocus granulosus.* A section of a daughter cyst *(A)* shows the endocyst and multiple larval scolices. A magnified view of a scolex *(B)* shows the sucker *(short arrow)* and hooklets *(long arrow)*. (*A,* ×56; *B,* ×720.)

brood capsules within which develop larval protoscoleces. Daughter cysts with poorly formed endocysts may also develop directly from the exocyst or free protoscoleces; these cysts can be numerous and can give rise to "granddaughter" cysts and the subsequent creation of a "multicystic" structure.

Although intrathoracic hydatid cysts can cause symptoms by direct compression of surrounding structures, disease most often becomes clinically evident as a result of rupture. Within the lungs, rupture usually occurs into adjacent bronchi in one of two ways: (1) rupture through the pericyst, exocyst, and endocyst, the contents being expelled into the airway and replaced by air, commonly followed by secondary bacterial infection, which tends to kill the organism; and (2) rupture through the pericyst only, with communication established between the bronchi and the potential space between the exocyst and pericyst; when such communication occurs, air accumulates around the exocyst and the endocyst tends to collapse. A cyst can also rupture directly into lung parenchyma and induce an intense inflammatory reaction that may contain well-formed granulomas in relation to fragments of exocyst. A histologic pattern of bronchocentric granulomatosis can also occur.[279] Rarely, a cyst ruptures into the pleural cavity and produces a pyopneumothorax. Rupture is said to occur far more frequently in the pastoral than in the sylvatic type.[277]

In addition to the development of cysts from entrapped larvae, *Echinococcus* can also affect the lung secondary to hepatic disease, usually by direct extension of disease across the diaphragm.[280, 281] Once an enlarging hepatic cyst communicates with the biliary system, it often becomes secondarily infected; the resulting inflammatory mass expands superiorly, traverses the diaphragm, and ruptures into the lung, most commonly into the right lower lobe.[280] The result is the formation of either a hepatobronchial fistula or a parenchymal "abscess" with cavitation. Such fistulas are a complication of hydatid cysts in approximately 2% of cases.[283, 284] Occasional instances of spread into the left lower lobe, pericardium, or pleural space have also been recorded.[280, 281] Rarely, hepatic cysts rupture into the hepatic veins or inferior vena cava with subsequent embolization of the cyst contents to the lungs.[285, 286]

Radiologic Manifestations

Pulmonary echinococcal cysts are characteristically seen as solitary, sharply circumscribed, spherical or oval masses surrounded by normal lung (Fig. 30–16).[270, 277, 287, 288] They are multiple in 20% to 30% of patients (Fig. 30–17).[270, 287] Their size ranges from 1 cm to over 20 cm in diameter;[289] the larger cysts are usually seen in the pastoral type of disease, those in the sylvatic variety rarely exceeding 10 cm.[265, 277] The majority of cysts are located in the lower lobes, more often posteriorly than anteriorly and somewhat more commonly on the right;[270, 290, 291] however, in one study of 75 cases of sylvatic disease upper lobe predominance was found in the right lung and lower lobe in the left.[292] In a study of cyst growth rates in 10 patients, the doubling time was found to be 16 to 20 weeks.[287] In contrast to liver cysts—in which calcification occurs in 20% to 30%—calcification of pulmonary hydatid cysts is rare.[270, 287, 291, 293, 294]

Although often spherical or oval, cysts sometimes have a "bizarre," irregular shape attributed by some to the fact that they impinge on relatively rigid structures such as bronchovascular bundles as they grow and then become indented and lobulated.[270, 275] A cyst that is near the diaphragm, chest wall, or mediastinum also tends to flatten against it, although compression of mediastinal structures may occur and rib erosion has been observed occasionally.[295] The fluid content of a cyst may be demonstrated by a change in shape on radiographs exposed after maximal inspiration and expiration or with the patient in erect and recumbent positions.[292, 294]

As discussed previously, when communication develops between the cyst and the bronchial tree, air may enter the space between the pericyst and exocyst and produce a thin

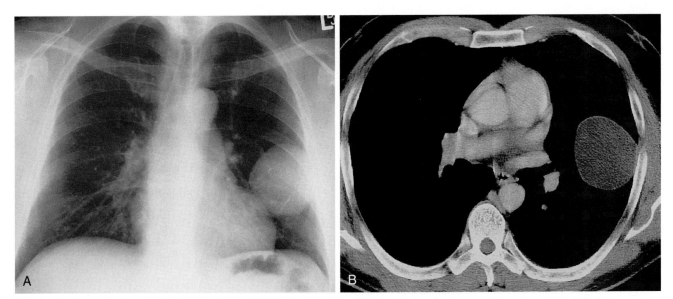

Figure 30–16. Hydatid Cyst: Radiographic and CT Findings. A posteroanterior chest radiograph *(A)* demonstrates a smoothly marginated 6-cm-diameter mass in the left lung. A CT scan *(B)* demonstrates a cystic lesion containing fluid with attenuation values similar to water (0 HU). The patient was a 51-year-old asymptomatic man who hunted for several years in northern Canada.

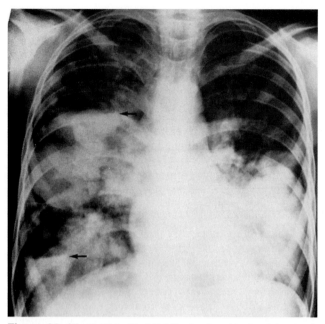

Figure 30–17. Multiple Hydatid Cysts. A multitude of sharply circumscribed masses ranging from 1 to 7 cm in diameter are widely scattered throughout both lungs. The majority of the cysts are intact; however, at least four have ruptured into the tracheobronchial tree and show prominent fluid levels (two of these are indicated by *arrows*). Note the irregular configuration of the air-fluid interface caused by floating membranes (the water-lily sign or sign of the camalote). The patient, a 14-year-old Iranian girl, died of the disease. (Courtesy of Dr. Hassan Fateh, Teheran, Iran.)

crescent of air around the periphery of the cyst—the "meniscus" or "crescent" sign.[270, 278, 287] Despite the emphasis that has been placed on this sign in published reports, it was observed in only 5% of 49 patients with the pastoral type of infestation in one study.[270] The sign appears to be even more rare in the sylvatic form; for example, it was observed in none of the 101 patients in a study from Alaska.[277] When bronchial communication occurs directly with the endocyst (Fig. 30–18), expulsion of the cyst contents produces an air-fluid level on the radiograph; cyst fluid that spreads into surrounding parenchyma may result in consolidation.[270] Occasionally, both forms of communication are manifested—a fluid level within the cyst and a crescent sign around its periphery.[278, 296]

After the cyst has ruptured into the bronchial tree, its membrane may float on the fluid within the cyst and give rise to the classic "water-lily sign" or "sign of the camalote" (*see* Fig. 30–18).[287, 297, 298] This sign may also be seen in pleural fluid when rupture of the cyst into the pleural space has resulted in hydropneumothorax or pyopneumothorax;[299] in such circumstances, the pneumothorax may be under "tension."[300] The water-lily sign is rare in the sylvatic form of the disease; in the series cited previously it was observed in only 1 of 101 patients.[277]

CT allows ready distinction of hydatid cysts from soft tissue nodules by demonstrating a thin-walled fluid-filled cyst. The fluid has attenuation values close to 0 Hounsfield units (*see* Fig. 30–16).[301, 302] CT can also be helpful in identifying pathognomonic features in ruptured or complicated hydatid cysts such as detached or collapsed endocyst membranes, collapsed daughter cyst membranes, and intact

daughter cysts.[301, 302, 304] However, rupture of the cysts may occur without such characteristic signs being evident (Fig. 30–19). MR imaging also allows reliable differentiation of fluid-filled hydatid cysts from solid tumors.[305, 306] The cysts have low signal intensity on T1-weighted images and high signal intensity on T2-weighted MR images (Fig. 30–20).

Clinical Manifestations

The majority of intact pulmonary hydatid cysts cause no symptoms. Occasionally, an unruptured cyst is associated with nonproductive cough and minimal hemoptysis.[275] When a cyst ruptures, either spontaneously or as a result of secondary infection, there is an abrupt onset of cough, expectoration, and fever; an acute hypersensitivity reaction may develop, with urticaria, pruritus, and in some cases hypotension.[290] The patient may complain of chest pain, and the sputum may become purulent. A few cases have been described of a cyst developing at the thoracic inlet and causing symptoms and signs resembling those of an apical pulmonary carcinoma.[307, 308]

Laboratory Findings

Laboratory aids in diagnosis include a variety of serologic tests (indirect hemagglutination, latex agglutination, complement fixation, and ELISA).[265, 273, 292, 309] They are superior to the Casoni and other skin tests and have been shown to have a sensitivity ranging from 80% to 100% and specificity of 88% to 98% for hepatic cysts;[265] however, the sensitivity for the detection of pulmonary cysts is only 50% to 55%. In addition, the specificity of serologic tests is limited by cross-reactions with antigens of other parasites[310] and some pulmonary carcinomas.[311, 312] Blood eosinophilia, usually mild, occurs in 25% to 50% of cases;[269, 288, 293] it may be severe when associated with anaphylaxis following cyst rupture.

Papanicolaou-stained specimens of pleural fluid[313] or sputum[314] may reveal scoleces or hooklets to confirm the diagnosis. In addition, paraffin-embedded cell blocks derived from centrifuged sputum specimens may show fragments of exocyst;[315] although these can be seen with H&E stain, they are reportedly more easily identified after staining with silver methenamine or Best's carmine.[315] Although percutaneous aspiration of pulmonary echinococcal cysts has not been considered a safe procedure because of the possibility of allergic reaction or spread of the disease, in our experience and that of others, such a response is certainly not invariable.[316]

Sylvatic hydatid disease appears to be a relatively benign disease.[268, 277] By contrast, cysts caused by the pastoral variety have been considered to need surgical resection;[290, 317] it has even been recommended that accessible liver cysts be excised at the same time as thoracotomy.[318]

Echinococcus multilocularis (Alveolar Hydatid Disease)

As with *E. granulosus*, the principal definitive hosts of *E. multilocularis* are members of the Canidae family, particularly dogs, foxes, and wolves; cats can also harbor

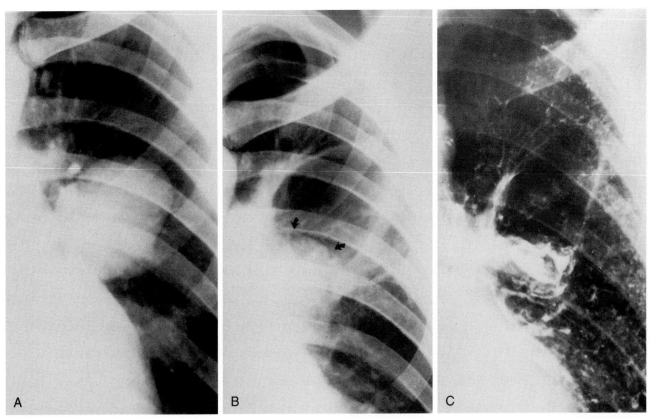

Figure 30–18. Hydatid Cyst with Rupture. A sharply circumscribed homogeneous mass *(A)* visible in the left midlung has a smooth but somewhat lobulated contour. Four years later *(B)*, the cyst has expelled all its liquid contents into the tracheobronchial tree and now contains air; an irregular mass present at the bottom of the cyst *(arrows)* represents collapsed membranes. A bronchogram *(C)* shows contrast material within the cyst outlining the membranes. (Courtesy of Alfred Hospital, Melbourne, Australia.)

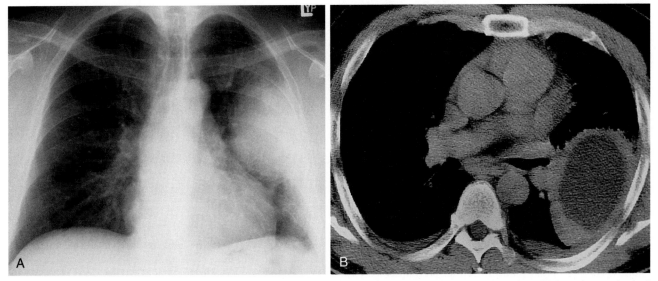

Figure 30–19. Ruptured Hydatid Cyst. A posteroanterior chest radiograph *(A)* demonstrates a large mass-like lesion with irregular margins in the left lung. A CT scan following intravenous administration of contrast *(B)* demonstrates a cystic lesion with a thick wall and small bilateral pleural effusions. At surgery, there was evidence of extravasation of fluid from the cyst into the left pleural space. The cause of the small right pleural effusion is unclear. The patient was evaluated for sudden onset of left pleuritic chest pain. He is the same patient illustrated in Figure 30–16. He had initially refused surgery.

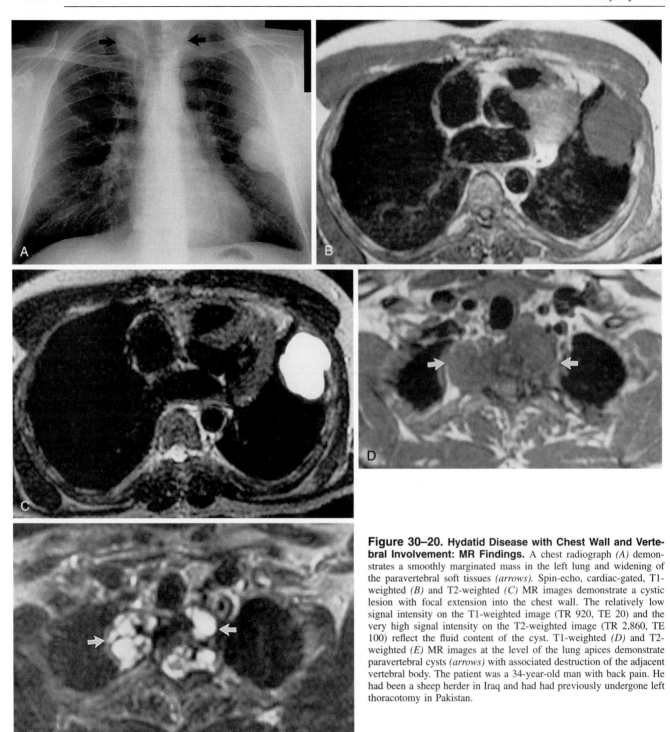

Figure 30–20. Hydatid Disease with Chest Wall and Vertebral Involvement: MR Findings. A chest radiograph *(A)* demonstrates a smoothly marginated mass in the left lung and widening of the paravertebral soft tissues *(arrows)*. Spin-echo, cardiac-gated, T1-weighted *(B)* and T2-weighted *(C)* MR images demonstrate a cystic lesion with focal extension into the chest wall. The relatively low signal intensity on the T1-weighted image (TR 920, TE 20) and the very high signal intensity on the T2-weighted image (TR 2,860, TE 100) reflect the fluid content of the cyst. T1-weighted *(D)* and T2-weighted *(E)* MR images at the level of the lung apices demonstrate paravertebral cysts *(arrows)* with associated destruction of the adjacent vertebral body. The patient was a 34-year-old man with back pain. He had been a sheep herder in Iraq and had had previously undergone left thoracotomy in Pakistan.

the organism.[267] The intermediate hosts are a variety of rodents, including voles, muskrats, and house mice. The disease is seen principally in central Europe (particularly in southern Germany and Switzerland), Alaska, islands in the Bering Sea, and parts of the former Soviet Union and Canadian arctic.[319] For unknown reasons, the frequency of HLA-DR13 is greatly increased in patients infested by the organism.[265]

Humans acquire the infestation in the same manner as in pastoral echinococcosis. Although the life cycle of the organism is essentially the same as that of *E. granulosus,* development of hydatid disease within the intermediate host, including humans, is quite different. Typically, only a poorly developed exocyst is formed, and the host-derived pericyst characteristic of *E. granulosus* infestation does not develop. Foci of disease thus appear grossly as poorly defined masses of gelatinous, somewhat spongy tissue. Histologically, these masses are composed of a series of interconnected spaces containing thin strands of hyaline material and only occasional scoleces. The inflammatory reaction is typically intense. Endarteritis obliterans in surrounding parenchyma is common and may be responsible for the central necrosis in the larger masses. The infestation is locally invasive, expanding and infiltrating in the fashion of a malignant neoplasm, with which it may be confused grossly.[319]

In the vast majority of cases, alveolar hydatid disease is confined to the liver,[282] in which it may resemble primary hepatic or gallbladder carcinoma both clinically and pathologically. Direct extension into the diaphragm[320] and "metastases" to the lungs[321, 322] have occasionally been described. Clinical symptoms are usually related to hepatic dysfunction and include anorexia, weight loss, epigastric and right upper quadrant pain, and jaundice; dyspnea can occur in patients with pulmonary involvement.[323] An ELISA test using an antigen specific for *E. multilocularis* has been found to be useful in distinguishing alveolar and cystic forms of hydatid disease and in follow-up after therapy.[324] The disease is particularly serious, with a mortality rate of about 70% in untreated individuals.[323]

Echinococcus vogeli (Polycystic Hydatid Disease)

This variety of hydatid disease has been reported rarely in individuals in northwestern South America and parts of Central America.[266] The infestation is somewhat similar to that of alveolar hydatid disease, except that the cysts are much larger. The intermediate host is the paca and the definitive host is most probably the wild or domestic dog.

Cysticercosis

Cysticercosis is caused by larvae of the pork tapeworm *Taenia solium*. Humans are the definitive hosts of mature worms, whose presence in the intestinal tract usually produces no symptoms or causes only mild, nonspecific gastrointestinal complaints. Although the pig is the most common intermediate host, a variety of other vertebrates that are rarely ingested by humans can also serve in that capacity. The disease is most common in eastern Europe, Spain, Portugal, Mexico, Central America, and parts of Africa and Asia.[324]

Humans acquire the disease by ingesting meat contaminated with viable cysticerci, most often incompletely cooked pork. Mature larvae (known as *Cysticercus cellulosae*) are liberated in the gut and grow into adult worms that attach to the mucosa and generate numerous proglottids. The latter release eggs that are found in soil contaminated by feces; following ingestion by the intermediate host (usually pigs), the eggs hatch into oncospheres (immature larvae). These penetrate the mucosa, enter the mesenteric veins, and are carried to various organs and tissues where they mature into cysticerci. In addition to functioning as a definitive host for the adult worm, humans can act as intermediate hosts—and thus acquire cysticercosis—in three ways: (1) by ingesting eggs in contaminated soil or water; (2) by autoinfection from anus to mouth in patients infested with adult worms; and (3)

rarely, by autoinfection through regurgitation of eggs from the lower intestine to the stomach. Following the ingestion or regurgitation of eggs, the course of events in humans is identical to that in other intermediate hosts.

Morphologically, cysticerci are composed of round or oval cysts containing a yellowish fluid and an invaginated larval scolex. While they remain viable (usually 3 to 6 years), there is little associated tissue reaction;[324] their death is followed by an inflammatory reaction and, eventually, pericystic fibrosis and calcification. Multinucleated foreign body giant cells may be seen in relation to fragments of the cyst wall.[324]

Although cysticerci can be found in any organ or tissue, they are seen most commonly in the brain, skeletal muscles, and eyes. Thoracic involvement usually results from the deposition of cysticerci in the respiratory muscles, where their presence may occasion pain. Radiographically, they appear as oval, calcified shadows ranging from 3 to 10 mm in diameter; they are usually multiple but are occasionally solitary.[325] Uncommonly, cysticerci are present in visceral organs, including the lungs and pleura (Fig. 30–21); associated clinical signs and symptoms are usually absent.[326–328]

Miscellaneous Cestodes

Sparganosis. Sparganosis is a rare infestation caused by immature forms of various cestodes that fail to mature in their host and migrate aimlessly, usually in subcutaneous tissue. Involvement of the pleural space and lung has been reported rarely.[329]

ARTHROPODS

Pentastomiasis

Pentastomiasis is caused by several species of blood-sucking invertebrate parasites whose larval stage occasionally infests humans. The vast majority of reported cases have been caused by *Armillifer armillatus,* a parasite that normally inhabits the nasopharynx of carnivorous mammals, and *Linguatula serrata,* which is found principally in the lungs of reptiles. Occasional instances of infestation by *Armillifer moniliformis, Armillifer grandis*, and *Leiperia cincinnalais* have also been documented.[330]

L. serrata is said to be present on every continent,[331] although most reports of human infestation have originated in southern Germany, Switzerland, Brazil, and Chile.[332, 333] The adults of this arachnid live in the upper respiratory passages of pigs, foxes, and wolves; the females lay eggs that are discharged in sputum and mucus from the respiratory tract of these animals. The larval hosts include rabbits and hares, domestic animals, and occasionally humans. The eggs hatch when swallowed by the larval host; four- to six-legged larvae emerge in the intestine and migrate to the liver, spleen, lymph nodes, and lungs, where they are transformed into nymphs, which become encapsulated and eventually calcified. *A. armillatus* has a similar life cycle. It has been described chiefly in blacks in central Africa, but cases have also been reported from Indonesia, Malaysia, the Philippines,

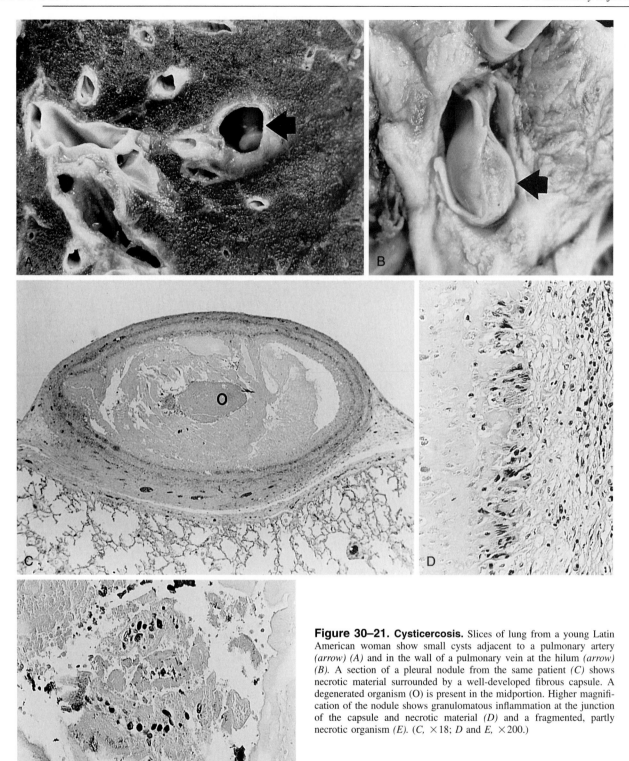

Figure 30–21. Cysticercosis. Slices of lung from a young Latin American woman show small cysts adjacent to a pulmonary artery *(arrow) (A)* and in the wall of a pulmonary vein at the hilum *(arrow) (B)*. A section of a pleural nodule from the same patient *(C)* shows necrotic material surrounded by a well-developed fibrous capsule. A degenerated organism (O) is present in the midportion. Higher magnification of the nodule shows granulomatous inflammation at the junction of the capsule and necrotic material *(D)* and a fragmented, partly necrotic organism *(E)*. *(C, ×18; D and E, ×200.)*

and China. The adult arachnid lives in the respiratory passages and body cavities of reptiles, birds, and mammals.

Humans can acquire disease by ingesting eggs in contaminated food or water or by direct contact with the definitive host. The eggs are sticky and adhere readily to hands or clothing; in some parts of the world they are ingested directly during the preparation or eating of snakes and liz-

ards.[330] In some regions, the incidence of infestation is high; for example, the parasite has been found at autopsy in 25% of individuals in some areas of Africa and in up to 45% of aborigines in Malaysia.[16]

In humans, the larvae are found most frequently in the abdominal cavity, particularly the liver, intestinal wall, and mesentery;[330] the lungs are involved less often. Morphologically, the migrating and encysted larvae appear to cause little tissue reaction while alive; however, when dead, they are associated with a marked inflammatory response, fibrosis, and eventually calcification.[330] Chest radiographs may reflect the latter changes with numerous discrete foci of calcification 4 to 6 mm in diameter, usually in the form of incomplete ring shadows.[331, 334] In the great majority of cases, infestation does not produce symptoms and is discovered only at autopsy or on a screening chest radiograph. However, in one instance an enlarging "cyst" was reported to cause compression of a contiguous bronchus with distal obstructive effects.[330]

Myiasis

The term *myiasis* refers to parasitic infestation of vertebrate tissue by dipteran larvae. Structures that are usually affected in humans are the skin, nasal or ocular mucous membranes, and genitourinary tract. A single case has been reported of a solitary pulmonary nodule discovered in an asymptomatic man.[335] On microscopic examination the excised nodule showed vascular thrombosis and necrosis, in the center of which was a degenerated and calcified parasite presumptively identified as a second-stage larva of the horse bot (*Gasterophilus* species). A second instance was documented in a 19-year-old Japanese man with chronic productive cough and ill-defined nodules on the chest radiograph; larvae of the genus *Megaselia* were identified at thoracotomy.[336]

Acariasis

Acariasis is caused by ticks and mites of the class Arachnida. Human infestation is almost always limited to the skin; however, the organisms are allergenic and inhalation has been shown to result in a decrease in FEV_1 in some individuals.[337] In addition, there is a remarkable case report of a 53-year-old woman who was evaluated for hemoptysis and chest pain and whose expectorated sputum contained mites identified as *Tyroglyphus* species.[338] A resected upper lobe showed multiple small structures within respiratory bronchioles that were presumed to be ova; the surrounding parenchyma showed nonspecific chronic inflammation.

LEECHES

Although infestation by leeches (hirudiniasis) is best known to affect the skin, involvement of the mucous membranes (so-called internal hirudiniasis) also occurs and may result in respiratory disease. Species of the genus *Limnatis*, particularly *Limnatis nilotica*, have been most frequently implicated.[339] The organism normally lives in quiet streams and pools. Human infestation is probably acquired in most instances by drinking water containing the leech.[340] Although the pharynx and nose are most commonly affected, the larynx and upper part of the trachea may also be involved. After attaching itself to the mucosa, the organism sucks blood, increases in size, and produces hemoptysis and, occasionally, upper airway obstruction.

REFERENCES

1. Leading article: Immunodiagnosis in parasitic disease. BMJ 283:1349, 1981.
2. Bruckner DA: Serologic and intradermal tests for parasitic infections. Pediatr Clin North Am 32:1063, 1985.
2a. Singh B: Molecular methods for diagnosis and epidemiologic studies of parasitic infections. Int J Parasitol 27:1135, 1997.
3. Visvesvara GS, Mirra SS, Brandt FH, et al: Isolation of two strains of *Acanthamoeba castellani* from human tissue and their pathogenicity and isoenzyme profiles. J Clin Microbiol 18:1405, 1983.
3a. Ribas A, Mosquera J-A: Ameboflagellates in bronchial asthma. Acta Cytol 42:685, 1998.
4. Lyche KD, Jensen WA: Pleuropulmonary amebiasis. Semin Respir Infect 12:106, 1997.
5. Krogstad DJ, Spencer HC Jr, Healy GR: Current concepts in parasitology. N Engl J Med 298:262, 1978.
6. Takaro T, Bond WM: Pleuropulmonary, pericardial, and cerebral complications of amebiasis: A twenty-year survey. Int Abstr Surg 107:209, 1958.
7. Barrett-Connor E: Parasitic pulmonary disease. Am Rev Respir Dis 126:558, 1982.
8. Webster BH: Pleuropulmonary amebiasis: A review with an analysis of ten cases. Am Rev Respir Dis 81:683, 1960.
9. Brandt H, Tamayo RP: Pathology of human amebiasis. Hum Pathol 1:351, 1970.
10. Pudifin DJ, Duursma J, Gathiram V, et al: Invasive amoebiasis is associated with the development of anti-neutrophil cytoplasmic antibody. Clin Exp Immunol 97:48, 1994.
11. Ochsner A, DeBakey M: Pleuropulmonary complications of amebiasis: An analysis of 153 collected and 15 personal cases. J Thorac Surg 5:225, 1936.
12. Ibarra-Perez C: Thoracic complications of amebic abscesses of the liver: Report of 501 cases. Chest 79:672, 1981.
13. Herrera-Llerandi R: Thoracic repercussions of amebiasis. J Thorac Cardiovasc Surg 52:361, 1966.
14. Adayemo AO, Aderounmu A: Intrathoracic complications of amoebic liver abscess. J R Soc Med 77:17, 1984.
15. Ibarra-Perez C, Green L, Calvillo-Juarez M, et al: Diagnosis and treatment of rupture of amebic abscess of the liver into the pericardium. J Thorac Cardiovasc Surg 64:11, 1972.
16. Spencer H: Pathology of the Lung. 2nd ed. Oxford, Pergamon, 1968.
17. Ibarra-Perez C, Selman-Lama M: Diagnosis and treatment of amebic "empyema." Report of 88 cases. Am J Surg 134:283, 1977.
18. Ducloux JM, Ducloux M, Calvez F, et al: Les pleuropneumopathies amibiennes: Étude radiologique. (Amebic pleuropneumopathies. A radiologic study.) Ann Radiol (Paris) 10:341, 1967.
19. Bohrer SP: Right lower lobe abscess in a Nigerian. Chest 61:379, 1972.
20. Wilson SR, Arenson AM: Sonographic evaluation of hepatic abscesses. J Can Assoc Radiol 35:174, 1984.
21. Shamsi K, DeSchepper A, Deckers F, et al: Role of ultrasound in the diagnosis and treatment follow-up of amoebic liver abscess. Eur Radiol 3:434, 1993.
22. Walsh TJ, Berkman W, Brown NL, et al: Cytopathologic diagnosis of extracolonic amebiasis. Acta Cytol 27:671, 1983.
23. Radin DR, Ralls PW, Colletti PM, et al: CT of amebic liver abscess. Am J Roentgenol 150:1297, 1988.
24. Elizander G, Weissleder R, Stark DD, et al: Amebic liver abscess: Diagnosis and treatment evaluation with MR. Radiology 165:795, 1987.
25. Roy DC, Ravindran P, Padmanabhan R: Bronchobiliary fistula secondary to amebic liver abscess. Chest 62:523, 1972.
26. Vickers PJ, Bohra RC, Sharma GC: Hepatopulmonary amebiasis: A review of 40 cases. Int Surg 67(Suppl):427, 1982.
27. Walsh TJ, Berkman W, Brown NL, et al: Cytopathologic diagnosis of extracolonic amebiasis. Acta Cytol 27:671, 1983.
28. Dao AH: *Entamoeba gingivalis* in sputum smears. Acta Cytol 29:632, 1984.
29. Wilson ES: Pleuropulmonary amebiasis. Am J Roentgenol 111:518, 1971.
30. Myung K, Burch D, Jackson TF, et al: Serodiagnosis of invasive amebiasis using a recombinant *Entamoeba histolytica* antigen-based ELISA. Arch Med Res 23:285, 1992.
31. Ibarra-Perez C: Thoracic complications of amebic abscesses of the liver: Report of 501 cases. Chest 79:672, 1981.
32. Kean BH, Kimball AC, Christenson WN: An epidemic of acute toxoplasmosis. JAMA 208:1002, 1969.
33. Leading article: Toxoplasmosis. BMJ 282:249, 1981.
34. Editorial: The epidemiology of toxoplasmosis. Lancet 2:1148, 1981.
35. Feldman HA: Toxoplasmosis. N Engl J Med 279:1370, 1431, 1968.
36. Ryning FW, McLeod R, Maddox JC, et al: Probable transmission of *Toxoplasma gondii* by organ transplantation. Ann Intern Med 90:47, 1979.
37. Siegel SE, Lunde MN, Gelderman AH: Transmission of toxoplasmosis by leukocyte transfusion. Blood 37:388, 1971.
38. Campagna AC: Pulmonary toxoplasmosis. Semin Respir Infect 12:98, 1997.
39. Krick JA, Remington JS: Current concepts in parasitology: Toxoplasmosis in the adult—an overview. N Engl J Med 298:550, 1978.
40. Carter AO, Frank JW: Congenital toxoplasmosis: Epidemiologic features and control. Can Med Assoc J 135:618, 1986.
41. Gleason TH, Hamlin WB: Disseminated toxoplasmosis in the compromised host: A report of five cases. Arch Intern Med 134:1059, 1974.
42. Luft BJ, Naot Y, Araujo FG, et al: Primary and reactivated toxoplasma infection in patients with cardiac transplantation. Ann Intern Med 99:27, 1983.
43. Saad R, Vincent JF, Cimon B, et al: Pulmonary toxoplasmosis after allogeneic bone marrow transplantation: Case report and review. Bone Marrow Transplant 18:211, 1996.
44. Carey RM, Kimball AC, Armstrong D, et al: Toxoplasmosis: Clinical experiences in a cancer hospital. Am J Med 54:30, 1973.
45. Candolfi E, de Blay F, Rey D, et al: A parasitologically proven case of *Toxoplasma* pneumonia in an immunocompetent pregnant woman. J Infect 26:79, 1993.
46. Dorfman RF, Remington JS: Value of lymph node biopsy in the diagnosis of acute acquired toxoplasmosis. N Engl J Med 289:878, 1973.
47. Nash G, Kerschmann RL, Herndier B, et al: The pathological manifestations of pulmonary toxoplasmosis in the acquired immunodeficiency syndrome. Hum Pathol 25:652, 1994.
48. Luna MA, Lichtiger B: Disseminated toxoplasmosis and cytomegalovirus infection complicating Hodgkin's disease. Am J Clin Pathol 55:499, 1971.
49. Callaway CS, Walls KW, Hicklin MD: Electron-microscopic studies of toxoplasmosis. Arch Pathol 86:484, 1968.
50. Sante LR: Roentgen manifestations of adult toxoplasmosis. Am J Roentgenol 47:825, 1942.
51. Pinkerton H, Henderson RG: Adult toxoplasmosis: A previously unrecognized disease entity simulating typhus–spotted fever group. JAMA 116:807, 1941.
52. Theologides A, Kennedy BJ: Clinical manifestations of toxoplasmosis in the adult. Arch Intern Med 117:536, 1966.
53. Thalhammer O: Die Diagnose der Toxoplasmose. [The diagnosis of toxoplasmosis.] Wien Med Wochenschr 108:499, 1958.
54. Prosmanne O, Chalaoui J, Sylvestre J, et al: Small nodular pattern in the lungs due to opportunistic toxoplasmosis. J Can Assoc Radiol 35:186, 1984.
54a. Goodman PC, Schnapp LM: Pulmonary toxoplasmosis in AIDS. Radiology 184:791, 1992.
55. Tawney S, Masci J, Berger HW, et al: Pulmonary toxoplasmosis: An unusual nodular radiographic pattern in a patient with AIDS. Mt Sinai J Med 53:683, 1986.
56. Quinn EL, Fisher EJ, Cox F Jr, et al: The clinical spectrum of toxoplasmosis in the adult. Cleve Clin Q 42:71, 1975.
57. Kagen LJ, Kimball AC, Christian CL: Serologic evidence of toxoplasmosis among patients with polymyositis. Am J Med 56:186, 1974.
58. Pugin J, Vanhems P, Hirschel B, et al: Extreme elevations of serum lactate dehydrogenase differentiating pulmonary toxoplasmosis from *Pneumocystis* pneumonia. N Engl J Med 326:1226, 1992.
59. Sabin AB, Feldman HA: Dyes as microchemical indicators of a new immunity phenomenon affecting a protozoon parasite *(Toxoplasma)*. Science 108:660, 1948.
60. Welch PC, Masur H, Jones TC, et al: Serologic diagnosis of acute lymphadenopathic toxoplasmosis. J Infect Dis 142:256, 1980.
61. Pomeroy C, Filice GA: Pulmonary toxoplasmosis: A review. Clin Infect Dis 14:863, 1992.
62. Gordon SM, Gal AA, Hertzler GL, et al: Diagnosis of pulmonary toxoplasmosis by bronchoalveolar lavage in cardiac transplant recipients. Diagn Cytopathol 9:650, 1993.
63. Bretagne S, Costa JM, Vidaud M, et al: Detection of *Toxoplasma gondii* by competitive DNA amplification of bronchoalveolar lavage samples. J Infect Dis 168:1585, 1993.
64. Alward W, Javaid M, Garner J: Babesiosis in a Connecticut resident. Conn Med 54:425, 1990.
65. Rosner F, Zarrabi MH, Benach JL, et al: Babesiosis in splenectomized adults—review of 22 reported cases. Am J Med 76:696, 1981.
66. Fransioli PB, Keithly JS, Jones TC, et al: Response of babesiosis to pentamidine therapy. Ann Intern Med 94:326, 1981.
67. Gordon S, Cordon RA, Mazdzer EJ, et al: Adult respiratory distress syndrome in babesiosis. Chest 86:633, 1984.
68. Horowitz ML, Coletta F, Fein AM: Delayed-onset adult respiratory distress syndrome in babesiosis. Chest 106:1299, 1994.
69. Duarte MIS, Corbett CEP, Boulos M, et al: Ultrastructure of the lung in *falciparum* malaria. Am J Trop Med Hyg 34:31, 1985.
70. Lichtman AR, Mohrcken S, Engelbrecht M, et al: Pathophysiology of severe forms of *falciparum* malaria. Crit Care Med 18:666, 1990.
71. Gozal D: The incidence of pulmonary manifestations during *Plasmodium falciparum* malaria in non-immune subjects. Trop Med Parsitol 43:6, 1992.
72. Charoenpan P, Indraprasit S, Kiaboonsri S, et al: Pulmonary edema in severe *falciparum* malaria—hemodynamic study and clinicophysiologic correlation. Chest 97:1190, 1990.
73. James MF: Pulmonary damage associated with *falciparum* malaria: A report of ten cases. Ann Trop Med Parasitol 79:123, 1985.
74. Godard JE, Hansen RA: Interstitial pulmonary edema in acute malaria. Radiology 101:523, 1971.
75. Cayea PD, Rubin E, Teixidor HS: Atypical pulmonary malaria. Am J Roentgenol 137:51, 1981.
76. Punyagupta S, Scichaikul T, Nitiyanant P, et al: Acute pulmonary insufficiency in *falciparum* malaria: Summary of 12 cases with evidence of disseminated intravascular coagulation. Am J Trop Med 23:551, 1974.

77. Osborne PT, Giltman LI, Uthman EO: Trichomonads in the respiratory tract. Acta Cytol 28:136, 1984.
78. Walton BC, Bacharach T: Occurrence of trichomonads in the respiratory tract: Report of three cases. J Parasitol 49:35, 1963.
79. Osborne PT, Giltman CI, Uthman EO: Trichomonads in the respiratory tract: A case report and literature review. Acta Cytol 28:136, 1984.
80. Hersh SM: Pulmonary trichomoniasis and *Trichomonas tenax*. J Med Microbiol 20:1, 1985.
81. Ohkura T, Suzuki N, Hashiguchi Y: Invasion of the human respiratory tracts by trichomonads. Am J Trop Med Hyg 34:823, 1985.
82. Walzer PD, Rutherford I, East R: Empyema with *Trichomonas* species. Am Rev Respir Dis 118:415, 1978.
82a. El Kamel A, Rouetbi N, Chakroun M, et al: Pulmonary eosinophilia due to *Trichomonas tenax*. Thorax 51:554, 1996.
83. Stemmermann GN, Hayashi T, Glober GA, et al: Cryptosporidiosis: Report of a fatal case complicated by disseminated toxoplasmosis. Am J Med 69:637, 1980.
84. Kemper CA: Pulmonary disease in selected protozoal infections. Semin Respir Infect 12:113, 1997.
85. Brady EM, Margolis ML, Korzeniowski OM: Pulmonary cryptosporidiosis in acquired immunodeficiency syndrome. JAMA 252:89, 1984.
86. Immunodeficiency and cryptosporidiosis (Clinicopathologic Conference). BMJ 281:1123, 1980.
87. Schwartz DA, Visvesvara GS, Leitch GJ, et al: Pathology of symptomatic microsporidial *(Encephalitozoon hellem)* bronchiolitis in the acquired immunodeficiency syndrome: A new respiratory pathogen diagnosed from lung biopsy, bronchoalveolar lavage, sputum, and tissue culture. Hum Pathol 24:937, 1993.
88. Weber R, Kuster H, Keller R, et al: Pulmonary and intestinal microsporidiosis in a patient with the acquired immunodeficiency syndrome. Am Rev Respir Dis 146:1603, 1992.
89. Schwartz DA, Bryan RT, Hewan-Lowe KO, et al: Disseminated microsporidiosis *(Encephalitozoon hellem)* and acquired immunodeficiency syndrome: Autopsy evidence for respiratory acquisition. Arch Pathol Lab Med 116:660, 1992.
90. Mertens RB, Didier ES, Fishbein MC, et al: *Encephalitozoon cuniculi* microsporidiosis: Infection of the brain, heart, kidneys, trachea, adrenal glands, and urinary bladder in a patient with AIDS. Mod Pathol 10:68, 1997.
91. Daneshbod K: Visceral leishmaniasis (kala-azar) in Iran: A pathologic and electron-microscopic study. Am J Clin Pathol 57:156, 1972.
92. Rosenthal E, Marty P, Pesce A: *Leishmania* in bronchoalveolar lavage. Ann Intern Med 114:1064, 1991.
93. Stevens WJ, Vermeire PA: *Giardia lamblia* in bronchoalveolar lavage fluid. Thorax 36:875, 1981.
94. Phills JA, Harrold AJ, Whiteman GV, et al: Pulmonary infiltrates, asthma, and eosinophilia due to *Ascaris suum* infestation in man. N Engl J Med 286:965, 1972.
95. Piggott J, Hansbarger EA Jr, Neafie RC: Human ascariasis. Am J Clin Pathol 53:223, 1970.
96. Sarinas PS, Chitkaraa RK: Ascariasis and hookworm. Semin Respir Infect 12:130, 1997.
97. Rexroth G, Keller C: Chronic course of eosinophilic pneumonia in infection with *Ascaris lumbricoides*. Pneumologie 49:77, 1995.
98. Faraj JH: Upper airway obstruction by *Ascaris* worm. Can J Anaesth 40:471, 1993.
99. Beaver PC, Danaraj TJ: Pulmonary ascariasis resembling eosinophilic lung. Am J Trop Med Hyg 7:100, 1958.
100. Gelpi AP, Mustafa A: *Ascaris* pneumonia. Am J Med 44:377, 1968.
101. Heggers JP, Muller MJ, Elwood E, et al: Ascariasis pneumonitis: A potentially fatal complication in smoke inhalation injury. Burns 21:149, 1995.
102. Proffitt RD, Walton BC: *Ascaris* pneumonia in a two-year-old girl: Diagnosis by gastric aspirate. N Engl J Med 266:931, 1962.
103. Joubert JR, van Schalkwyk DJ, Turner KJ: *Ascaris lumbricoides* and the human immunogenic response: Enhanced IgE-mediated reactivity to common inhaled allergens. S Afr Med J 57:409, 1980.
104. Wehner JH, Kirsch CM: Pulmonary manifestations of strongyloidiasis. Semin Respir Infect 12:122, 1997.
105. Pampiglione S, Ricciardi ML: Experimental infestation with human strain *Strongyloides fülleborni* in man. Lancet 1:663, 1972.
106. Fisher E: Personal communication.
107. Leighton PM, MacSween HM: *Strongyloides stercoralis:* The cause of an urticarial-like eruption of 65 years' duration. Arch Intern Med 150:1747, 1990.
108. Genta RM: Global prevalence of *Strongyloides:* Critical review with epidemiologic insights into the prevention of disseminated disease. Rev Infect Dis 11:755, 1989.
109. Davidson RA, Fletcher RH, Chapman LE: Risk factors for *Strongyloides:* A case control study. Arch Intern Med 144:321, 1984.
110. Wilson S, Thompson AE: A fatal case of strongyloidiasis. J Pathol Bacteriol 87:169, 1964.
111. Udwadia FE, Joshi VV: A study of tropical eosinophilia. Thorax 19:548, 1964.
112. Berger R, Kraman S, Paciotti M: Pulmonary strongyloidiasis complicating therapy with corticosteroids. Am J Trop Med Hyg 29:31, 1980.
113. Fowler CG, Lindsay I, Lewin J, et al: Recurrent hyperinfestation with *Strongyloides stercoralis* in a renal allograft recipient. BMJ 285:1394, 1982.
114. Gocek LA, Siekkinen PJ, Lankerani MR: Unsuspected *Strongyloides* coexisting with adenocarcinoma of the lung. Acta Cytol 29:628, 1985.
115. Cruz T, Reboucas G, Tocha H: Fatal strongyloidiasis in patients receiving corticosteroids. N Engl J Med 275:1093, 1966.

116. Powell RW, Moss JP, Nagar D, et al: Strongyloidiasis in immunosuppressed hosts: Presentation as massive lower gastrointestinal bleeding. Arch Intern Med 140:1061, 1980.
117. Higenbottam TW, Heard BE: Opportunistic pulmonary strongyloidiasis complicating asthma treated with steroids. Thorax 31:226, 1976.
118. Reddy KR, Laurain AR, Thomas E: Strongyloidiasis: When to suspect the wily nematode. Postgrad Med 74:273, 279, 1983.
119. Sen P, Gil C, Estrellas B, et al: Corticosteroid-induced asthma: A manifestation of limited hyperinfection syndrome due to *Strongyloides stercoralis*. South Med J 88:923, 1995.
120. Schainberg L, Schainberg MA: Recovery of *Strongyloides stercoralis* by bronchoalveolar lavage in a patient with acquired immunodeficiency syndrome. Am J Med 87:486, 1989.
121. Netto VA, Pasternak J, Moreira AA, et al: *Strongyloides stercoralis* hyperinfection in the acquired immunodeficiency syndrome. Am J Med 87:602, 1989.
122. Genta RM, Ward PA: The histopathology of experimental strongyloidiasis. Am J Pathol 99:207, 1980.
123. Purtilo DT, Meyers WM, Connor DH: Fatal strongyloidiasis in immunosuppressed patients. Am J Med 56:488, 1974.
124. Marcial-Rojas RA: Strongyloidiasis. *In* Marcial-Rojas RA (ed): Pathology of Protozoal and Helminthic Diseases with Clinical Correlation. Baltimore, Williams & Wilkins, 1971, p 711.
125. Lin AL, Kessimian N, Benditt JO: Restrictive pulmonary disease due to interlobular septal fibrosis associated with disseminated infection by *Strongyloides stercoralis*. Am J Respir Crit Care Med 151:205, 1995.
126. Humpherys K, Hieger LR: *Strongyloides stercoralis* in routine Papanicolaou-stained sputum smears. Acta Cytol 23:471, 1979.
127. Weller IVD, Copland P, Gabriel R: *Strongyloides stercoralis* infection in renal transplant recipients. BMJ 282:524, 1981.
128. Maayan S, Wormser GP, Widerhorn J, et al: *Strongyloides stercoralis* hyperinfection in a patient with the acquired immune deficiency syndrome. Am J Med 83:945, 1987.
129. Gompels MM, Todd J, Peters BS, et al: Disseminated strongyloidiasis in AIDS: Uncommon but important. AIDS 5:329, 1991.
130. Kramer MR, Gregg PA, Goldstein M, et al: Disseminated strongyloidiasis in AIDS and non-AIDS immunocompromised hosts: Diagnosis by sputum and bronchoalveolar lavage. South Med J 83:1226, 1990.
131. Venizelos PC, Lopata M, Bardawil WA, et al: Respiratory failure due to *Strongyloides stercoralis* in a patient with a renal transplant. Chest 78:104, 1980.
132. Krysl J, Müller NL, Miller RR, et al: Clinico-radiologic-pathologic conference: Patient with miliary nodules and diarrhea. Can Assoc Radiol J 42:363, 1991.
133. Makris AN, Sher S, Bertoli C, et al: Pulmonary strongyloidiasis: An unusual opportunistic pneumonia in a patient with AIDS. Am J Roentgenol 161:545, 1993.
134. Woodring JH, Halfhill H II, Reed JC: Pulmonary strongyloidiasis: Clinical and imaging features. Am J Roentgenol 162:537, 1994.
135. Ford J, Reiss-Levy E, Clark E, et al: Pulmonary strongyloidiasis and lung abscess. Chest 79:239, 1981.
136. Grove DI: Strongyloidiasis in Allied ex-prisoners of war in southeast Asia. BMJ 280:598, 1980.
137. Rivera E, Maldonado N, Vélez-García E, et al: Hyperinfection syndrome with *Strongyloides stercoralis*. Ann Intern Med 72:199, 1970.
138. Harris RA Jr, Musher DM, Fainstein V, et al: Disseminated strongyloidiasis: Diagnosis made by sputum examination. JAMA 244:65, 1980.
139. Williams J, Nunley D, Dralle W, et al: Diagnosis of pulmonary strongyloidiasis by bronchoalveolar lavage. Chest 94:643, 1988.
140. Grove DI, Warren KS, Mahmoud AAF: Algorithms in the management of exotic diseases: Strongyloidiasis. J Infect Dis 131:755, 1975.
141. Neva FA, Gam AA, Burke J: Comparison of larval antigens in an enzyme-linked immunosorbent assay for strongyloidiasis in humans. J Infect Dis 144:427, 1981.
142. Ribas-Mujal D: Trichinosis. *In* Marcial-Rojas RA (ed): Pathology of Protozoal and Helminthic Diseases with Clinical Correlation. Baltimore, Williams & Wilkins, 1971, p 677.
143. Goldwater LJ, Steinberg I, Most H, et al: Hemoptysis in trichiniasis. N Engl J Med 213:849, 1935.
144. Robin ED, Crump CH, Wagman RJ: Low sedimentation rate, hypofibrinogenemia, and restrictive pseudo-obstructive pulmonary disease associated with trichinosis. N Engl J Med 262:758, 1960.
145. Udwadia FE: Tropical eosinophilia: A review. Respir Med 87:17, 1993.
146. Chitkara RK, Sarinas PS: Dirofilaria, visceral larva migrans, and tropical pulmonary eosinophilia. Semin Respir Infect 12:138, 1997.
147. Nutman TB, Vijayan VK, Pinkston P, et al: Tropical pulmonary eosinophilia: Analysis of antifilarial antibody localized to the lung. J Infect Dis 160:1042, 1989.
148. Jones DA, Pillai DK, Rathbone BJ, et al: Persisting "asthma" in tropical pulmonary eosinophilia. Thorax 38:692, 1983.
149. Udwadia FE: Tropical eosinophilia—a correlation of clinical, histopathologic, and lung function studies. Dis Chest 52:531, 1967.
150. Udwadia FE: Pulmonary eosinophilia. *In* Herzog H (ed): Tropical Eosinophilia. Vol. 7. Progress in Respiration Research. New York, 1975.
151. Danaraj TJ, Pacheco G, Shanmugaratnam K, et al: The etiology and pathology of eosinophilic lung (tropical eosinophilia). Am J Trop Med Hyg 15:183, 1966.
152. Khoo FY, Danaraj TJ: The roentgenographic appearance of eosinophilic lung (tropical eosinophilia). Am J Roentgenol 83:251, 1960.
153. Herlinger H: Pulmonary changes in tropical eosinophilia. Br J Radiol 36:889, 1963.

154. Boornazian JS, Fagan MJ: Tropical pulmonary eosinophilia associated with pleural effusions. Am J Trop Med Hyg 34:473, 1985.

154a. Sandhu M, Muchopadhyay S, Sharma SK: Tropical pulmonary eosinophilia: A comparative evaluation of plain chest radiography and computed tomography. Australas Radiol 40:32, 1996.

155. Kariks J: Tropical pulmonary eosinophilia. Med J Aust 2:773, 1958.

156. Pinkston P, Vijayan VK, Nutman TB, et al: Acute tropical pulmonary eosinophilia: Characterization of the lower respiratory tract inflammation and its response to therapy. J Clin Invest 80:216, 1987.

157. Hussain R, Hamilton RG, Kumaraswami V, et al: IgE responses in human filariasis: Quantitation of filaria-specific IgE. J Immunol 127:1623, 1981.

158. Ray D, Saha K: Serum immunoglobulin and complement levels in tropical pulmonary eosinophilia and their correlation with primary and relapsing stages of the illness. Am J Trop Med Hyg 27:503, 1978.

159. Ray D, Sri Krishna K: Alpha$_1$-antitrypsin in tropical pulmonary eosinophilia. Chest 104:487, 1993.

160. Peter RH, Campbell MF: Tropical pulmonary eosinophilia, cause unknown, treatment dramatically effective. Ann Intern Med 59:231, 1963.

161. Vijayan VK, Kuppu Rao KV, Sankaran K, et al: Tropical eosinophilia: Clinical and physiological response to diethylcarbamazine. Respir Med 85:17, 1991.

162. Enarson DA: Microfilaremia and peak expiratory flow rate, Philippines. Trop Geogr Med 36:17, 1984.

163. Avasthi R, Jain AP, Swaroop, et al: *Bancrofti* microfiliariasis in association with pulmonary tuberculosis. Report of a case with diagnosis by fine needle aspiration. Acta Cytol 35:717, 1991.

164. Walter A, Krishnaswami H, Cariappa A: Microfilariae of *Wuchereria bancrofti* in cytologic smears. Acta Cytol 27:432, 1983.

165. Anupindi L, Sahoo R, Rao RV, et al: Microfiariae in bronchial brushing cytology of symptomatic pulmonary lesions. A report of two cases. Acta Cytol 37:398, 1993.

166. Aggarwal J, Kapila K, Gaur A, et al: Bancroftian filarial pleural effusion. Postgrad Med J 69:869, 1993.

167. Danaraj TJ: The treatment of eosinophilic lung (tropical eosinophilia) with diethylcarbamazine. Q J Med 27:243, 1958.

168. Nesarajah MS: Pulmonary function in tropical eosinophilia. Thorax 27:185, 1972.

169. Poh SC: The course of lung function in treated tropical pulmonary eosinophilia. Thorax 29:710, 1974.

170. Dashiell GF: A case of dirofilariasis involving the lung. Am J Trop Med Hyg 10:37, 1961.

171. Kochar AS: Human pulmonary dirofilariasis. Am J Clin Pathol 84:19, 1985.

172. Tsung SH, Lin JI, Han D: Pulmonary dirofilariasis in man. Am J Med Sci 283:106, 1982.

173. Cordero M, Muro A, Simon F, et al: Are transient pulmonary solitary nodules a common event in human dirofilariosis? Clin Invest 70:437, 1992.

174. Beaver PC, Fallon M, Smith GH: Pulmonary nodule caused by a living *Brugia malayi*–like filaria in an artery. Am J Trop Med Hyg 20:661, 1971.

175. Scully RE, McNeely BU: Case records of the Massachusetts General Hospital. N Engl J Med 291:35, 1974.

176. Beaver PC, Cran IR: *Wuchereria*-like filaria in an artery, associated with pulmonary infarction. Am J Trop Med Hyg 23:869, 1974.

177. Dayal Y, Neafie RC: Human pulmonary dirofilariasis: A case report and review of the literature. Am Rev Respir Dis 112:437, 1975.

178. Awe RJ, Mattox KL, Alvarez BA, et al: Solitary and bilateral pulmonary nodules due to *Dirofilaria immitis*. Am Rev Respir Dis 112:445, 1975.

179. Makiya K, Tsukamoto M, Kagei N: Fifty-six cases of human dirofilariasis reported from Japan—a compiled table. J UOEH 9:233, 1987.

180. Asimacopoulos PJ, Katras A, Christie B: Pulmonary dirofilariasis—the largest single-hospital experience. Chest 102:851, 1992.

181. Milanez de Campos JR, Barbas CS, Filomeno LT, et al: Human pulmonary dirofilariasis: Analysis of 24 cases from Sao Paulo, Brazil. Chest 112:729, 1997.

182. Pampiglione S, Del Maschio O, Pagan V, et al: Pulmonary dirofilariasis in man: A new Italian case. Review of the European literature. Parasite 1:379, 1994.

183. Jagusch MF, Roberts RM, Rea HH, et al: Human pulmonary dirofilariasis. N Z Med J 97:556, 1984.

184. Navarrete-Reyna A, Noon G: Pulmonary dirofilariasis manifested as a coin lesion. Arch Pathol 85:266, 1968.

185. Harrison EG, Thompson JH: Dirofilariasis of human lung. Am J Clin Pathol 43:224, 1965.

186. Neafie RC, Piggott J: Human pulmonary dirofilariasis. Arch Pathol 92:342, 1971.

187. Levinson ED, Ziter FMH Jr, Westcott JL: Pulmonary lesions due to *Dirofilaria immitis* (dog heartworm): Report of four cases with radiologic findings. Radiology 131:305, 1979.

188. Green LK, Ansari MQ, Schwartz MR, et al: Nonspecific fluorescent whitener stains in the rapid recognition of pulmonary dirofilariasis: A report of 20 cases. Thorax 49:590, 1994.

189. Kochar AS: Human pulmonary dirofilariasis: Report of three cases and brief review of the literature. Am J Clin Pathol 84:19, 1985.

190. Hawkins AG, Hsiu J-G, Smith RM, et al: Pulmonary dirofilariasis diagnosed by fine needle aspiration biopsy. Acta Cytol 29:19, 1985.

191. Ciferri F: Human pulmonary dirofilariasis in the United States: A critical review. Am J Trop Med Hyg 31:302, 1982.

192. Glickman LT, Grieve RB, Schantz PM: Serologic diagnosis of zoonotic pulmonary dirofilariasis. Am J Med 80:161, 1986.

193. Perera L, Muro A, Cordero M, et al: Evaluation of a 22-kDa *Dirofilaria immitis* antigen for the immunodiagnosis of human pulmonary dirofilariosis. Trop Med Parasitol 45:249, 1994.

194. Fanning M, Hill A, Langer HM, et al: Visceral larva migrans (toxocariasis) in Toronto. Can Med Assoc J 124:21, 1981.

195. Glickman LT, Magnaval JF, Domanski LM, et al: Visceral larva migrans in French adults: A new disease syndrome. Am J Epidemiol 125:1019, 1987.

196. Dent JH, Nichols RL, Beaver PC, et al: Visceral larva migrans: With a case report. Am J Pathol 32:777, 1956.

197. Brill R, Churg M, Beaver PC: Allergic granulomatosis associated with visceral larva migrans: Case report with autopsy findings of *Toxocara* infection in a child. Am J Pathol 23:1208, 1953.

198. Sarda AK, Kannan R, Sharma DK, et al: Visceral larva migrans. J Postgrad Med 39:155, 1993.

199. Roig J, Romeu J, Riera C, et al: Acute eosinophilic pneumonia due to toxocariasis with bronchoalveolar lavage findings. Chest 102:294, 1992.

200. Woodruff AW: Toxocariasis. BMJ 3:663, 1970.

201. Timmons RF, Bowers RE, Price DL: Infection of the respiratory tract with *Mammomanogamus (Syngamus) laryngeus:* A new case in Largo, Florida, and a summary of previously reported cases. Am Rev Respir Dis 128:566, 1983.

202. Nosanchuk JS, Wade SE, Landolf M: Case report of and description of parasite in *Mammomonogamus laryngeus* (human syngamosis) infection. J Clin Microbiol 33:998, 1995.

203. Lears WD, Sarin MK, Arthurs K: Syngamosis, an unusual cause of asthma: The first reported case in Canada. Can Med Assoc J 132:269, 1985.

204. Weinstein L, Molavi A: *Syngamus laryngeus* infection (syngamosis) with chronic cough. Ann Intern Med 74:577, 1971.

205. Rusnak JM, Lucey DR: Clinical gnathostomiasis: Case report and review of the English-language literature. Clin Infect Dis 16:33, 1993.

206. Houston S: Gnathostomiasis: Report of a case and brief review. Can J Infect Dis 5:125, 1994.

207. Guill MA, Odom RB: Larva migrans complicated by Loeffler's syndrome. Arch Dermatol 114:1525, 1978.

208. Butland RJA, Coulson IH: Pulmonary eosinophilia associated with cutaneous larva migrans. Thorax 40:76, 1985.

209. Fuglsang H, Anderson J: Effect of diethylcarbamazine and suramin on *Onchocerca volvulus* microfilariae in urine. Lancet 2:321, 1973.

210. Meyers WM, Neafie RC, Connor DH: Onchocerciasis: Invasion of deep organs by *Onchocerca volvulus:* Autopsy findings. Am J Trop Med Hyg 26:650, 1977.

211. Aftandelians R, Raafat F, Taffazoli M, et al: Pulmonary capillariasis in a child in Iran. Am J Trop Med Hyg 26:64, 1977.

212. Beaver PC, Kriz JJ, Lau TJ: Pulmonary nodule caused by *Enterobius vermicularis*. Am J Trop Med Hyg 22:711, 1973.

213. Kobayashi A, Tsuji M, Wilbur DL: Probable pulmonary anisakiasis accompanying pleural effusion. Am J Trop Med Hyg 34:310, 1985.

214. Pirisi M, Gutierrez Y, Minini C, et al: Fatal human pulmonary infection caused by an *Angiostrongylus*-like nematode. Clin Infect Dis 20:59, 1995.

215. Kagawa FT: Pulmonary paragonimiasis. Semin Respir Infect 12:149, 1997.

216. Monson MH, Koenig JW, Sachs R: Successful treatment with praziquantel of six patients infected with the African lung fluke, *Paragonimus uterobilateralis*. Am J Trop Med Hyg 32:371, 1983.

217. Béland JE, Boone J, Donevan RE, et al: Paragonimiasis (the lung fluke): Report of four cases. Am Rev Respir Dis 99:261, 1969.

218. Mariano EG, Borja SR, Vruno MJ: A human infection with *Paragonimus kellicotti* (lung fluke) in the United States. Am J Clin Pathol 86:685, 1986.

219. Taylor CR, Swett HA: Pulmonary paragonimiasis in Laotian refugees. Radiology 143:411, 1982.

220. Johnson RJ, Johnson JR: Paragonimiasis in Indochinese refugees: Roentgenographic findings with clinical correlations. Am Rev Respir Dis 128:534, 1983.

221. Johnson JR, Falk A, Iber C, et al: Paragonimiasis in the United States: A report of 9 cases in Hmong immigrants. Chest 82:168, 1982.

222. Chung CH: Human paragonimiasis (pulmonary distomiasis, endemic hemoptysis). *In* Marcial-Rojas RA (ed): Pathology of Protozoal and Helminthic Diseases with Clinical Correlation. Baltimore, Williams & Wilkins, 1971, p 504.

223. Ogakwu M, Nwokolo C: Radiological findings in pulmonary paragonimiasis as seen in Nigeria: A review based on one hundred cases. Br J Radiol 46:699, 1973.

224. Suwanik R, Harinsuta C: Pulmonary paragonimiasis: An evaluation of roentgen findings in 38 positive sputum patients in an endemic area in Thailand. Am J Roentgenol 81:236, 1959.

225. Im JG, Whang HY, Kim WS, et al: Pleuropulmonary paragonimiasis: Radiologic findings in 71 patients. Am J Roentgenol 159:39, 1992.

226. Singcharoen T, Silprasert W: CT findings in pulmonary paragonimiasis. J Comput Assist Tomogr 11:1101, 1987.

227. Romeo DP, Pollock JJ: Pulmonary paragonimiasis: Diagnostic value of pleural fluid analysis. South Med J 79:241, 1986.

228. Minh V-D, Engle P, Greenwood JR, et al: Pleural paragonimiasis in a Southeast Asian refugee. Am Rev Respir Dis 124:186, 1981.

229. Béland JE, Boone J, Donevan RE, et al: Paragonimiasis (the lung fluke): Report of four cases. Am Rev Respir Dis 99:261, 1969.

230. Eikas J, Kim PK: Clinical investigation of paragonimiasis. Acta Tuberc Scand 39:140, 1960.

231. Kan H, Ogata T, Taniyama A, et al: Extraordinarily high eosinophilia and elevated serum interleukin-5 level observed in a patient infected with *Paragonimus westermani*. Pediatrics 96:351, 1995.

232. Johnson RJ, Jong EC, Dunning SB, et al: Paragonimiasis: Diagnosis and the use of praziquantel in treatment. Rev Infect Dis 7:200, 1985.

233. Maleewong W, Intapan PM, Priammuenwai M, et al: Monoclonal antibodies to *Paragonimus heterotremus* and their potential for diagnosis of paragonimiasis. Am J Trop Med Hyg 56:413, 1997.

234. Ikeda T, Oikawa Y, Nishiyama T: Enzyme-linked immunosorbent assay using cysteine proteinase antigens for immunodiagnosis of human paragonimiasis. Am J Trop Med Hyg 55:435, 1996.

235. Hofstetter M, Nash TE, Cheever AW, et al: Infection with *Schistosoma mekongi* in Southeast Asian refugees. J Infect Dis 144:420, 1981.

236. Morris W, Knauer CM: Cardiopulmonary manifestations of schistosomiasis. Semin Respir Infect 12:159, 1997.

237. McCully RM, Barron CN, Cheever AW: Diseases caused by trematodes: Schistosomiasis. *In* Binford CH, Connor DH (eds): Pathology of Tropical and Extraordinary Diseases. Vol 2. Washington, DC, Armed Forces Institute of Pathology, 1976, p 482.

238. Cheever AW: Schistosomiasis. Infection versus disease and hypersensitivity versus immunity. Am J Pathol 142:699, 1993.

239. Mahmoud AA: Medical intelligence: Current concepts in schistosomiasis. N Engl J Med 297:1329, 1977.

240. Macieira-Coelho E, Duarte CS: The syndrome of portopulmonary schistosomiasis. Am J Med 43:944, 1967.

241. Thompson HT, Pettigrew R, Johnson EA: Short reports: Solitary pulmonary bilharzioma. Thorax 34:401, 1979.

242. Shaw AFB, Ghareeb AA: The pathogenesis of pulmonary schistosomiasis in Egypt with special reference to Ayerza's disease. J Pathol Bacteriol 146:401, 1938.

243. Andrade ZA, Andrade SG: Pathogenesis of schistosomal pulmonary arteritis. Am J Trop Med Hyg 19:305, 1970.

244. Marcial-Rojas RA: Schistosomiasis mansoni. *In* Marcial-Rojas RA (ed): Pathology of Protozoal and Helminthic Diseases with Clinical Correlation. Baltimore, Williams & Wilkins, 1971, p 373.

245. El-Gazayreli M: Pulmonary bilharziasis. *In* Liebow AA (ed): The Lung. Baltimore, Williams & Wilkins, 1968, p 245.

246. Sadigursky M, Andrade ZA: Pulmonary changes in schistosomal cor pulmonale. Am J Trop Med Hyg 31:779, 1982.

247. El Mallah SH, Hashem M: Localized bilharzial granuloma of the lung simulating a tumour. Thorax 8:148, 1953.

248. Faird Z, Greer JW, Ishak KG, et al: Chronic pulmonary schistosomiasis. Am Rev Respir Dis 79:119, 1959.

249. Kagan IG, Rairigh DW, Kaiser RL: A clinical, parasitologic, and immunologic study of schistosomiasis in 103 Puerto Rican males residing in the United States. Ann Intern Med 56:457, 1962.

250. Marchand E, Marcial-Rojas R, Rodriguez R, et al: The pulmonary obstruction syndrome in *Schistosoma mansoni* pulmonary endarteritis: Report of five cases. Arch Intern Med 100:965, 1957.

251. Faird Z, Greer JW, Ishak KG, et al: Chronic pulmonary schistosomiasis. Am Rev Respir Dis 79:119, 1959.

252. Wessell HU, Sommers HM, Cugell DW, et al: Variants of cardiopulmonary manifestations of Manson's schistosomiasis: Report of two cases. Ann Intern Med 62:757, 1965.

253. Davidson BL, el-Kassimi F, Uz-Zaman A, et al: The "lung shift" in treated schistosomiasis: Bronchoalveolar lavage evidence of eosinophilic pneumonia. Chest 89:455, 1986.

254. Nash TE, Cheever AW, Ottesen EA, et al: Schistosome infections in humans: Perspectives and recent findings. Ann Intern Med 97:740, 1982.

255. Rodríguez HF, Rivera E: Pulmonary schistosomiasis. N Engl J Med 258:1196, 1958.

256. Cortes FM, Winters WL: Schistosomiasis cor pulmonale. Am J Med 31:808, 1961.

257. Rickert JH, Krakaur RB: Diffuse pulmonary schistosomiasis: Report of two cases proved by lung biopsy. JAMA 169:1302, 1959.

258. Lunde MN, Ottesen EA: Enzyme-linked immunosorbent assay (ELISA) for detecting IgM and IgE antibodies in human schistosomiasis. Am J Trop Med Hyg 29:82, 1980.

259. Frayser R, de Alonso AE: Studies of pulmonary function in patients with schistosomiasis mansoni. Am Rev Respir Dis 95:1036, 1967.

260. Zaky HA, El-Heneidy AR, El-Maksoud Tarabeih AA: Hyperventilation and effort dyspnea in porto-pulmonary bilharziasis. Dis Chest 53:163, 1968.

261. Zaky HA, El-Heneidy AR, Khalil M: Use of krypton 85 in the study of hypoxia in porto-pulmonary bilharziasis (schistosomiasis). BMJ 1:1021, 1964.

262. Prijyanonda B, Tandhanand S: Opisthorchiasis with pulmonary involvement. Ann Intern Med 54:795, 1961.

263. Flores M, Merino-Angulo J, Aguirre Errasti C: Pulmonary infiltrates as first sign of infection by *Fasciola hepatica*. Eur J Respir Dis 63:231, 1982.

264. Freeman RS, Stuart PF, Cullen JB, et al: Fatal human infection with mesocercariae of the trematode *Alaria americana*. Am J Trop Med Hyg 25:803, 1976.

265. Bhatia G: Echinococcus. Semin Respir Infect 12:171, 1997.

266. D'Alessandro A: Polycystic echinococcosis in tropical America: *Echinococcus vogeli* and *E. oligarthrus*. Acta Trop 67:43, 1997.

267. Poole JB, Marcial-Rojas RA: Echinococcosis. *In* Marcial-Rojas RA (ed): Pathology of Protozoal and Helminthic Diseases with Clinical Correlation. Baltimore, Williams & Wilkins, 1971, p 635.

268. Moore RD, Urschel JD, Fraser RE, et al: Cystic hydatid lung disease in northwest Canada. Can J Surg 37:20, 1994.

269. Jerray M, Benzarti M, Garrouche A, et al: Hydatid disease of the lungs: Study of 386 cases. Am Rev Respir Dis 146:185, 1992.

270. McPhail JL, Arora TS: Intrathoracic hydatid disease. Dis Chest 52:772, 1967.

271. Ozcelik C, Inci I, Toprak M, et al: Surgical treatment of pulmonary hydatidosis in children: Experience in 92 patients. J Pediatr Surg 29:392, 1994.

272. Beard TC: Evidence that a hydatid cyst is seldom "as old as the patient." Lancet 2:30, 1978.

273. Parija SC, Rao RS, Badrinath S, et al: Hydatid disease in Pondicherry. J Trop Med Hyg 86:113, 1983.

274. Karpathios T, Fretzayas A, Nicolaidou P, et al: Statistical aspects of hydatid disease in Greek adults. Am J Trop Med Hyg 34:124, 1985.

275. Sadrieh M, Dutz W, Navabpoor MS: Review of 150 cases of hydatid cyst of the lung. Dis Chest 52:662, 1967.

276. Nicks R: Thoracic hydatid cysts. Med J Aust 1:999, 1967.

277. Wilson JF, Diddams AC, Rausch RL: Cystic hydatid disease in Alaska: A review of 101 autochthonous cases of *Echinococcus granulosus* infection. Am Rev Respir Dis 98:1, 1968.

278. Kegel RFC, Fatemi A: The ruptured pulmonary hydatid cyst. Radiology 76:60, 1961.

279. Hertog RWD, Wagenaar SS, Westermann CJJ: Bronchocentric granulomatosis and pulmonary echinococcosis. Am Rev Respir Dis 126:344, 1982.

280. Xanthankis DS, Katsaras E, Efthimiadis M, et al: Hydatid cyst of the liver with intrathoracic rupture. Thorax 36:497, 1981.

281. Toole J, Propatoridis J, Pangalos N: Intrapulmonary rupture of hydatid cysts of the liver. Thorax 8:274, 1953.

282. Sailer M, Soelder B, Allerberger F, et al: Alevolar echinococcosis of the liver in a six-year-old girl with acquired immunodeficiency syndrome. J Pediatr 130:320, 1997.

283. Borrie J, Shaw JHF: Hepatobronchial fistula caused by hydatid disease: The Dunedin experience 1952–79. Thorax 36:25, 1981.

284. Matar K, Gardner MAH, Courtice BH, et al: Bronchobiliary fistula due to hydatid disease: A case report. Aust N Z J Surg 48:559, 1978.

285. Richmond DR, Bernstein L: Hydatid pulmonary embolism: Case report. Aust Ann Med 17:270, 1968.

286. Hirzalla MO, Samara N, Ateyat B, et al: Recurrent hydatid pulmonary emboli. Am Rev Respir Dis 140:1082, 1989.

287. Bloomfield JA: Protean radiological manifestations of hydatid infestation. Aust Radiol 10:330, 1966.

288. Perianayagam WJ, Freitas E, Sharma SS, et al: Pulmonary hydatid cyst: A 25-year experience. Aust N Z J Surg 49:450, 1979.

289. Halezeroglu S, Celik M, Uysal A, et al: Giant hydatid cysts of the lung. J Thorac Cardiovasc Surg 113:712, 1997.

290. Ozdemir IA, Kalaycioglu E: Surgical treatment and complications of thoracic hydatid disease: Report of 61 cases. Eur J Respir Dis 64:217, 1983.

291. Borrie J: Fifty thoracic hydatid cysts. Br J Surg 50:268, 1962.

292. Cuthbert R: Sylvatic pulmonary hydatid disease: A radiologic survey. J Can Assoc Radiol 26:132, 1975.

293. Beggs I: The radiology of hydatid disease. Am J Roentgenol 145:639, 1985.

294. Taiana JA: Thoracic hydatid echinococcosis: Diagnosis and treatment. Dis Chest 49:8, 1966.

295. Jonathan OM: Hydatid disease in North Wales. BMJ 1:1246, 1960.

296. Aggarwal ML: Hydatid disease of the lung. Indian J Radiol 10:10, 1956.

297. Fainsinger MH: Pulmonary hydatid disease: The sign of the camalote. S Afr Med J 23:723, 1949.

298. Ozer Z, Cetin M, Kahraman C: Pleural involvement by hydatid cysts of the lung. Thorac Cardiovasc Surg 33:103, 1985.

299. Rakower J, Milwidsky H: Hydatid pleural disease. Am Rev Respir Dis 90:623, 1964.

300. Bakir F, Al-Omeri MM: Echinococcal tension pneumothorax. Thorax 24:547, 1969.

301. Saksouk FA, Fahl MH, Rizk GK: Computed tomography of pulmonary hydatid disease. J Comput Assist Tomogr 10:226, 1986.

302. Von Sinner WN: Radiographic, CT, and MRI spectrum of hydatid disease of the chest: Pictorial essay. Eur Radiol 3:62, 1993.

303. Müller NL: A northern hunter with a cavitating nodule. J Respir Dis 11:933, 1990.

304. von Sinner WN: New diagnostic signs in hydatid disease: Radiography, ultrasound, CT and MRI correlated to pathology. Eur J Radiol 12:150, 1991.

305. von Sinner WN, Rifai A, teStrake L, et al: Magnetic resonance imaging of thoracic hydatid disease: Correlation with clinical findings, radiography, ultrasonography, CT, and pathology. Acta Radiol 31:59, 1990.

306. von Sinner WN, Linjawi T, Al Watban J: Mediastinal hydatid disease: Report of three cases. J Can Assoc Radiol 41:79, 1990.

307. Massenti S, Racugno V: The Ciuffini-Pancoast syndrome due to extrapleural apical *Echinococcus* cysts. Radiol Med Milan 43:63, 1957.

308. Purriel P, Armand U: Bernard-Horner syndrome in thoracic hydatid cyst. Tórax 2:131, 1962.

309. Xu MQ: Hydatid disease of the lung. Am J Surg 150:568, 1985.

310. Iacona A, Pini C, Vicari G: Enzyme-linked immunosorbent assay (ELISA) in the serodiagnosis of hydatid disease. Am J Trop Med Hyg 29:95, 1980.

311. van Knapen F: Echinococcus granulosus infection and malignancy. BMJ 281:195, 1980.

312. Yong W, Heath DD, Savage T: Possible antigenic similarity between pulmonary carcinoma and cysts of *Echinococcus granulosus*. BMJ 1:1463, 1979.

313. Jacobson ES: A case of secondary echinococcosis diagnosed by cytologic examination of pleural fluid and needle biopsy of pleura. Acta Cytol 17:76, 1973.

314. Allen AR, Fullmer CD: Primary diagnosis of pulmonary echinococcosis by the cytologic technique. Acta Cytol 16:212, 1972.

315. Vercelli-Retta J, Manana G, Reissenweber NJ: The cytologic diagnosis of hydatid disease. Acta Cytol 26:159, 1982.

316. McCorkell SJ: Unintended percutaneous aspiration of pulmonary echinococcal cysts. Am J Roentgenol 143:123, 1984.

317. Ayuso LA, de Peralta GT, Lazaro RB, et al: Surgical treatment of pulmonary hydatidosis. J Thorac Cardiovasc Surg 82:569, 1981.

318. Peleg H, Best LA, Gaitini D: Simultaneous operation for hydatid cysts of right lung and liver. J Thorac Cardiovasc Surg 90:783, 1985.

319. Saidi F: Alveolar echinococcosis. *In* Saidi F (ed): Surgery of Hydatid Disease. Philadelphia, WB Saunders, 1976, p 377.

320. Samuels S, Fosmoe R: Alveolar hydatid disease with involvement of the inferior vena cava. Am Surg 36:698, 1970.

321. Sereda MM, Sherman L, Smith EMG: Case reports: Alveolar echinococcosis. Can Med Assoc J 84:1138, 1961.

322. West JT, Hillman FJ, Bausch RL: Alveolar hydatid disease of the liver. Rationale and technics of surgical treatment. Ann Surg 157:548, 1963.

323. Wilson JF, Rausch RL: Alveolar hydatid disease. A review of clinical features of 33 indigenous cases of *Echinococcus multilocularis* infection in Alaskan Eskimos. Am J Trop Med Hyg 29:1340, 1980.

324. Gottsein B: Molecular and immunological diagnosis of echinococcosis. Clin Microbiol Rev 5:248, 1992.

325. Lennon E, Longo G: The recognition of cysticercosis on chest radiographs. Aust Radiol 10:14, 1966.

326. Mayo F, Baier H: Cysticercotic cyst involving the pleura: An unusual case of an abnormal chest roentgenogram. Arch Intern Med 139:115, 1979.

327. Kaplan JO, Weinfeld A: Cysticercosis: A report of thoracic disease. Br J Radiol 52:841, 1979.

328. Walts AE, Nivatpumin T, Epstein A: Pulmonary cysticercus. Mod Pathol 8:299, 1995.

329. Beaver PC, Rolon FA: Proliferating larval cestode in a man in Paraguay. Am J Trop Med Hyg 30:625, 1981.

330. Hopps HC, Keegan HL, Price DL, et al: Pentastomiasis. *In* Marcial-Rojas RA (ed): Pathology of Protozoal and Helminthic Diseases with Clinical Correlation. Baltimore, Williams & Wilkins, 1971, p 970.

331. González de Vega N, Gómez-Moreno C, Aguilar MR: Probable pulmonary linguatulosis cases. Enferm Torax 4:381, 1962.

332. Faust EC, Russell PF: Craig and Faust's Clinical Parasitology. 7th ed. Philadelphia, Lea & Febiger, 1964.

333. Manson-Bahr PH (ed): Manson's Tropical Diseases: A Manual of the Diseases of Warm Climates. 15th ed. London, Cassell, 1960.

334. Bretland PM: *Armillifer armillatus* infestation. Radiological diagnosis in two Ghanaian soldiers. Br J Radiol 35:603, 1962.

335. Ahmed MJ, Miller A: Pulmonary coin lesion containing a horse bot, *Gasterophilus:* Report of a case of myiasis. Am J Clin Pathol 52:414, 1969.

336. Komori K, Hara K, Smith KGV, et al: A case of lung myiasis caused by larvae of *Megaselia spiracularis* Schmitz. Trans R Soc Trop Med Hyg 72:467, 1978.

337. Ingram CG, Jeffrey IG, Symington IS, et al: Bronchial provocation studies in farmers allergic to storage mites. Lancet 2:1330, 1979.

338. Kijima S: Medical memoranda. A case of pulmonary acariasis—histopathological findings of resected lungs. BMJ 1:451, 1963.

339. Almallah Z: Internal hirudiniasis as an unusual cause of haemoptysis. Br J Dis Chest 62:215, 1968.

340. Boye ES, Joshi DC: Occurrence of the leech *Limnatis paluda* as a respiratory parasite in man: Case report from Saudi Arabia. J Trop Med Hyg 97:18, 1994.

Pulmonary Carcinoma

Pulmonary neoplasms are among the most common conditions encountered in respiratory medicine and enter into the differential diagnosis of many lesions seen on chest radiographs. Partly because of the many cell types that exist in the normal lung and the associated range of histogenetic possibilities, there are numerous histologically defined types of neoplasm. A variety of classification schemes have been proposed to categorize these tumors. That proposed by the World Health Organization (WHO) (Table 31–1) is one of the best known and most widely used and, with minor modifications, is followed in this and subsequent chapters.[1]

This chapter deals with carcinoma that arises from the surface epithelium of the airways and alveoli and, for practi-cal purposes, is concerned with six histologic types of neoplasm: (1) squamous cell carcinoma, (2) small cell carcinoma, (3) adenocarcinoma, (4) large cell carcinoma, (5) adenosquamous carcinoma, and (6) sarcomatoid (pleomorphic) carcinoma. Although these tumors are commonly referred to collectively as *bronchogenic carcinoma*, we prefer to use the designation *pulmonary carcinoma* in recognition of the fact that most adenocarcinomas probably arise from bronchiolar or alveolar epithelial cells. Although also derived from the airway epithelium, tracheobronchial gland tumors and pulmonary tumors other than small cell carcinoma that show neuroendocrine differentiation are discussed separately because of somewhat different etiologic, prognostic, and clinical characteristics. Subsequent chapters deal with the numerous other neoplasms derived from pulmonary mesenchymal or lymphoid cells.

Although the number of types of neoplasm other than pulmonary carcinoma is large and the space dedicated to a discussion of their characteristics is out of proportion to that allocated to pulmonary carcinoma, the latter is by far the most important group. For example, in one review of 150,854 histologically confirmed invasive lung cancers seen at the U.S. National Cancer Institute between 1973 and 1987, 147,637 (98%) were carcinomas: 31.1% were categorized as squamous cell carcinoma; 29% adenocarcinoma (including 0.1% bronchial gland carcinomas, 1.2% adenosquamous carcinomas, and 3.0% bronchioloalveolar carcinomas); 16.8%, small cell carcinoma; and 10.7%, large cell or undifferentiated carcinoma; other (unspecified) carcinomas constituted 8.6% of cases.

EPIDEMIOLOGY

Pulmonary carcinoma is the most frequently diagnosed "major" cancer in the world[2] and the most common cause of cancer-related death in both men and women in North America and worldwide.[3–8] In 1997, there were an estimated 170,000 deaths from pulmonary carcinoma in the United States,[9] accounting for more than one third of all cancer deaths in men and close to one quarter in women.[3, 10] Because many of these individuals are between 50 and 70 years of age at the time of death, the neoplasm is responsible for the most years of life lost of any cancer.[11]

The incidence of the tumor has increased progressively during the twentieth century. In the United States, the overall incidence rose from 38.5 per 100,000 person-years in 1969–1971 to 60.2 in 1989–1991. A variety of factors, such as ethnicity, age, gender, geographic location, and socioeconomic status, influence the rate in specific groups. Rates in men exceed those in women, and rates in African American men exceed those in white men.[3, 12, 13] In the United States, rates in men peaked in the 1980s and are currently in decline,[8, 14] both in elderly and in younger populations.[3] However, rates in white and African American women are similar and have continued to rise.[3, 15] The increasing incidence in women has also been seen in other countries: between 1969 and 1989, deaths from pulmonary carcinoma in women more than doubled in Japan, Norway, Poland, Sweden, and the United Kingdom; increased by more than 200% in Australia, Denmark, and New Zealand; and increased by more than 300% in Canada and the United

Table 31–1. 1999 WHO HISTOLOGICAL CLASSIFICATION OF LUNG AND PLEURAL TUMORS

EPITHELIAL TUMOURS

Benign

Papillomas
Squamous cell papilloma
Exophytic
Inverted
Glandular papilloma
Mixed squamous cell and glandular papilloma
Adenomas
Alveolar adenoma
Papillary adenoma
Adenomas of salivary gland type
Mucous gland adenoma
Pleomorphic adenoma
Others
Mucinous cystadenoma
Others

Preinvasive lesions

Squamous dysplasia/carcinoma *in situ*
Atypical adenomatous hyperplasia
Diffuse idiopathic pulmonary neuroendocrine cell hyperplasia

Malignant

Squamous cell carcinoma
Variants
Papillary
Clear cell
Small cell
Basaloid
Small cell carcinoma
Variant
Combined small cell carcinoma
Adenocarcinoma
Acinar
Papillary
Bronchioloalveolar carcinoma
Nonmucinous
Mucinous
Mixed mucinous and nonmucinous or indeterminate
Solid adenocarcinoma with mucin
Adenocarcinoma with mixed subtypes
Variants
Well-differentiated fetal adenocarcinoma
Mucinous ("colloid") adenocarcinoma
Mucinous cystadenocarcinoma
Signet ring adenocarcinoma
Clear cell adenocarcinoma
Large cell carcinoma
Variants
Large cell neuroendocrine carcinoma
Combined large cell neuroendocrine carcinoma
Basaloid carcinoma
Lymphoepithelioma-like carcinoma
Clear cell carcinoma
Large cell carcinoma with rhabdoid phenotype
Adenosquamous carcinoma
Carcinomas with pleomorphic, sarcomatoid, or sarcomatous elements
Carcinomas with spindle and/or giant cells
Pleomorphic carcinoma
Spindle cell carcinoma
Giant cell carcinoma
Carcinosarcoma
Pulmonary blastoma
Other

Carcinoid tumour
Typical carcinoid
Atypical carcinoid
Carcinomas of salivary gland type
Mucoepidermoid carcinoma
Adenoid cystic carcinoma
Others
Unclassified carcinoma

SOFT TISSUE TUMOURS

Localized fibrous tumour
Epithelioid hemangioendothelioma
Pleuropulmonary blastoma
Chondroma
Calcifying fibrous pseudotumour of the pleura
Congenital peribronchial myofibroblastic tumour
Diffuse pulmonary lymphangiomatosis
Desmoplastic round cell tumour
Others

MESOTHELIAL TUMOURS

Benign

Adenomatoid tumour

Malignant mesothelioma

Epithelioid mesothelioma
Sarcomatoid mesothelioma
Desmoplastic mesothelioma
Biphasic mesothelioma
Other

MISCELLANEOUS TUMOURS

Hamartoma
Sclerosing hemangioma
Clear cell tumour
Germ cell tumours
Teratoma, mature or immature
Other germ cell tumours
Thymoma
Malignant melanoma
Others

LYMPHOPROLIFERATIVE DISEASES

Lymphoid interstitial pneumonia
Nodular lymphoid hyperplasia
Low-grade marginal zone B-cell lymphoma of the Mucosa-Associated Lymphoid Tissue (MALT)
Lymphomatoid granulomatosis

SECONDARY TUMOURS

UNCLASSIFIED TUMOURS

TUMOUR-LIKE LESIONS

Tumourlet
Minute meningothelioid nodule
Langerhans cell histiocytosis
Inflammatory pseudotumour (inflammatory myofibroblastic tumour)
Localized organizing pneumonia
Amyloid tumour
Hyalinizing granuloma
Lymphangioleiomyomatosis
Micronodular pneumocyte hyperplasia
Endometriosis
Bronchial inflammatory polyp
Others

From Travis WD, Colby TV, Corrin B, et al, and Collaborators from 14 Countries: World Health Organization Pathology Panel: World Health Organization. Histological Typing of Lung and Pleural Tumours: International Histological Classification of Tumours, 3rd ed. Berlin, Springer-Verlag, In press.

States.[16, 17] Such increases are reflected in the proportion of cases seen in the two sexes: the ratio of men to women was reported to be 15:1 in the United Kingdom in 1955–1959[18] and 6.8:1 in a series reported from the Lahey Clinic in 1957–1960,[19] whereas it is currently less than 1.5:1.[3] As discussed farther on, the declining incidence rates for men and the increasing rates in women are related largely to parallel trends in smoking prevalence before the development of carcinoma.[20] There is some evidence, however, that women are more susceptible to the development of pulmonary carcinoma than men after controlling for amount smoked and body size.[5, 13, 21–24]

Despite a plateau in the overall incidence of pulmonary carcinoma and a decline in incidence in countries such as the United States, it has been estimated that 3 million deaths a year (many owing to cancer) occur worldwide as a result of cigarette smoking.[25] It is possible that this figure will increase to 10 million per year in 30 to 40 years' time. This suggests that with current smoking patterns, somewhat more than 20% of deaths in individuals living in "developed" countries will be related to tobacco smoke.[26]

Certain variations in the epidemiologic features of the different histologic subtypes of pulmonary carcinoma warrant specific comment. Compared to the 1970s, an increased proportion of adenocarcinoma has been documented by several groups of investigators.[15, 27–29] Although partly explained by changes in histologic criteria, the increase may also be the result of changes in cigarette composition, pattern of cigarette smoke inhalation,[30] and (possibly) exposure to various substances in food and the atmosphere (e.g., environmental tobacco smoke and occupational carcinogens).[27, 31] In the United States, the overall rate for adenocarcinoma has not declined in men (although a peak for African American men was noted in 1987).[3] By contrast, squamous cell carcinoma is decreasing in both African American and white men less than 75 years old.[3] The proportion of cases of small cell carcinoma is higher in white than African American men, a difference that is particularly marked in younger individuals.[12] This difference does not seem to be related to smoking habits or diet.[3] Among women, there may be a plateau in the incidence rate for large cell carcinoma;[3] there is also evidence that the rate of squamous cell carcinoma is decreasing in white women, especially those less than 65 years of age.

The incidence of pulmonary carcinoma increases with age among both smokers and nonsmokers, a finding more likely related to cumulative exposure to carcinogens than to aging itself.[32] Even so, nearly 3% of pulmonary carcinomas occur in patients less than 40 years of age.[33] The relative risk for carcinoma of smokers compared with nonsmokers is not constant across age groups: an increased relative risk is first seen in the mid to late forties, peaks rapidly, and declines with increasing age.[3] The higher relative risk at younger ages is a reflection of the low incidence of pulmonary carcinoma among young nonsmokers, rather than a large mortality effect from smoking at a younger age.

There is an inverse relationship between the risk for pulmonary carcinoma and increasing socioeconomic status.[34, 35] Although variations in smoking behavior likely account for a significant part of this difference, some investigators have shown that it persists after smoking is taken into account;[36, 37] differences in occupational exposure to potential carcinogens also do not appear to be involved.[38]

ETIOLOGY

The most important etiologic agent of pulmonary carcinoma is tobacco smoke. Although the attributable proportion of carcinomas caused by this agent varies with smoking prevalence and intensity in any given population,[11] it has been estimated that approximately 85% of all cases in North America and Europe are the result of cigarette consumption.[11, 39–42] This estimate does not take into account the impact of environmental tobacco smoke in nonsmokers (*see* farther on). Moreover, it is clear that tobacco also has a significant role in the pathogenesis of other neoplasms and a variety of nonneoplastic diseases. Mortality rates from all causes in smokers aged 35 to 54 years have been shown to be more than double those of nonsmokers of similar age.[43] It has been estimated that 38% of all cancer deaths in men and 23% in women are caused by cigarette smoking.[10]

A variety of particulate and chemical substances inhaled in occupational and other settings have also been implicated in the etiology of lung cancer. Although many of these appear to have an intrinsic carcinogenic potential of their own, in most cases, this is augmented substantially by concomitant exposure to tobacco smoke. Pulmonary fibrosis, either focal or diffuse and related to a variety of causes, has been hypothesized to be important in the development of some tumors.[44] Other factors, such as radiation and viral infection, play an important role in occasional neoplasms. Finally, although the mechanisms are not yet fully understood, it is likely that genetic susceptibility, immunologic status, and diet also have some effects.

Tobacco Smoke

The suspicion that tobacco could cause cancer was first suggested in 1761, when Hill reported the occurrence of polyps in snuff takers;[45] two of his patients had all the features of malignancy, an association well documented since that time.[45] Although Ochsner has been given credit for recognizing the parallel between smoking and the increased incidence of pulmonary carcinoma,[46] it appears that Ochsner and DeBakey's first reference to this association was in 1939.[47] In 1941, these authors reviewed the subject of carcinoma of the lung in some detail and recognized a German author, Fahr, who suspected tobacco as a major cause of pulmonary carcinoma in 1923.[48] In 1927, in a letter to the editor commenting on an article describing what appeared to be a rising incidence of cancer of the lung, a British physician, Tylecote, stated, "I have no statistics with regard to tobacco but I think that in almost every case I have seen and known of, the patient has been a regular smoker, generally of cigarettes."[49] This observation is still relevant today.[50]

The relationship between smoking and pulmonary carcinoma meets virtually all the criteria for causality as outlined by Hill in 1965.[51] These include the strength of the association (a relative risk of > 2 after standardization for age usually being considered to indicate clear causality), consistent data, and a specific causative agent. The relationship must be both biologically plausible (i.e., supported by known biologic mechanisms and animal studies) and temporally plausible (i.e., associated with an exposure that precedes the disease and, in the case of malignancy, precedes it with an appropriate latency). The demonstration of an increase in disease with increasing exposure—a dose-response phenomenon—strengthens the argument for causality.

As indicated previously, cigarette smoke is not the only cause of pulmonary carcinoma, and the precise substance it contains that is responsible for the development of cancer is unclear. Nevertheless, the evidence for causality is so overwhelming that the relationship is universally accepted. Short of an impractical and unethical prospective, randomized, control trial of the health effects of cigarette smoking, the best information on the adverse effects of cigarette smoking is derived from prospective cohort studies of rigorous design.[52] Only a fraction of the published reports that document these effects is presented here for illustrative purposes.

The epidemiologic features of pulmonary carcinoma largely parallel those of tobacco use. For example, in one study in which the prevalence of cigarette smoking from 1920 to 1990 was plotted against age-adjusted mortality rates from pulmonary carcinoma from 1930 to 1992, a strong temporal relationship was found for both men and women with an approximately 30-year latency period between smoking and the development of carcinoma.[20]

The mortality from pulmonary carcinoma in nonsmoking population groups, such as the Seventh Day Adventists in the United States[53, 54] and the Parsi in Bombay, India,[55] is much lower than that in smoking populations; in the few cases in which pulmonary carcinoma is found in the former groups, the patient has almost invariably been a heavy cigarette smoker in the past.[54] Similarly, the results of a variety of retrospective and prospective studies have shown that pulmonary carcinoma occurs infrequently in nonsmokers in the general population;[56] for example, in a follow-up investigation of 6,071 men aged 45 or older, pulmonary carcinoma developed in 4% of those who had smoked for 40 years or more but in none of 805 nonsmokers.[57] In another study of 2,668 patients who had pulmonary carcinoma diagnosed between 1971 and 1980, only 134 (5%) were found to be nonsmokers.[58] None of the 1,859 never-smokers in the Multiple Risk Factor Intervention Trial (MRFIT) died from pulmonary carcinoma during 10.5 years of surveillance.[59]

The relative risk for developing pulmonary carcinoma in male smokers compared with male nonsmokers was about 10 in the eight prospective cohort studies reviewed for the 1982 Report of the Surgeon General on the Health Consequences of Smoking;[52] in heavy smokers, carcinoma was 15 to 35 times more common than in nonsmokers.[41, 60] An analysis of a population-based registry of cancers in Orange County in which smoking habits were abstracted from the medical records revealed an odds ratio of 19.2 for ever-smoking men and 15.0 for ever-smoking women for the development of pulmonary carcinoma compared with never-smokers.[61] In two large prospective investigations performed by the American Cancer Society in the United States (Cancer Prevention Studies I and II), each of which enrolled more than 1 million subjects, as much as a 22-fold increase in risk of dying from pulmonary carcinoma was found in current smokers compared with nonsmokers.[62, 63] In MRFIT,[59] virtu-

ally every death from pulmonary carcinoma occurred in current and former smokers.

A clear-cut, dose-response relationship between amount of tobacco smoked and the risk of developing pulmonary carcinoma has been shown by many investigators.[22, 43, 64–67] The duration of smoking also appears to be important (i.e., there is evidence that smoking one pack per day for 40 years is associated with a greater risk than smoking two packs per day for 20 years).[68] It has also been well established that stopping the habit or appreciably reducing the number of cigarettes smoked results in a decreased risk of developing pulmonary carcinoma; however, although the relative risk declines exponentially after the first year,[43, 69, 70] a complete return to the incidence rates of never-smokers has not been documented.[71] Such persistent risk may be related to prolonged tobacco-induced changes in pulmonary epithelial cell function, such as the expression of receptors for mitogenic growth factors.[72] Despite the maintenance of increased risk, smoking cessation may postpone the age at which carcinoma develops.[73]

A number of factors other than number of cigarettes smoked likely determine the "dose" of carcinogens delivered to the lung. These include the pattern and intensity of smoking as well as the composition of the cigarette. High-tar cigarettes are associated with an increased risk for the development of carcinoma,[74] whereas the use of a filter likely reduces exposure to carcinogens as well as the risk.[74] Lowering of the nicotine content of cigarettes leads individuals to inhale more deeply and smoke more intently (larger puff volumes at higher frequency) in an attempt to maintain blood nicotine level;[30, 75] although the net effect of such changes on pulmonary carcinoma rate is modest, it may be related to an increase in the proportion of adenocarcinomas.[30]

Analysis of the dose-response relationship between cigarette smoking and pulmonary carcinoma has revealed a consistent and important increase in risk in men and women who smoke only one to nine cigarettes a day compared with nonsmokers.[76–78] (In fact, even this increase in risk may be an underestimate because of inclusion of ex-smokers in the nonsmoking groups).[78] This observation strongly supports the biologic plausibility of the carcinogenic effect of environmental tobacco smoke. The results of a number of other studies corroborate this association. On the basis of a review of 30 epidemiologic studies conducted worldwide, members of the U.S. Environmental Protection Agency concluded that environmental tobacco smoke is responsible for approximately 3,000 pulmonary carcinoma deaths per year in lifelong nonsmoking Americans.[79] This conclusion is consistent with those of previous reviews of epidemiologic studies by the U.S. National Research Council, the Surgeon General of the U.S. Public Health Service, and the International Agency for Research on Cancer (IARC).[77, 80] All these reviews have demonstrated a small but consistent increase in risk of pulmonary carcinoma in nonsmokers exposed to environmental tobacco smoke (usually nonsmokers whose spouses smoked) compared with those who are not;[77, 81–89] many also show a dose-response relationship. Since the publication of these reviews, data that strengthen the initial conclusions continue to accumulate.[90–94b] Even childhood exposure has been associated with an increased risk[95, 96] (although the assessment of such risk is confounded by possible inheritable risk factors).[97]

More than 4,000 constituents of cigarette smoke have been identified; tobacco itself accounts for 2,550 of these with additives, with pesticides and other organic and metallic compounds accounting for the rest.[98] Radioactive elements in tobacco smoke include radon, lead, bismuth, and polonium. Which of these numerous constituents or elements is responsible for the development of neoplasia has not been identified; however, it is clear from experiments in several animal species that both epithelial atypia and invasive cancer can develop either from inhalation of tobacco smoke or from direct intrapulmonary inoculation of tobacco condensates.[99–101]

Pathologic studies have shown that squamous metaplasia and basal cell hyperplasia of bronchial epithelium, sometimes accompanied by cytologic atypia, are common in cigarette smokers.[102, 103] Furthermore, the degree of atypia as well as its extent throughout the bronchial tree is greater in heavier smokers[102] and decreases in individuals who have stopped smoking.[103] Epithelial atypia has also been found to be greater in individuals who smoked during the years 1955 to 1960 compared with 1970 to 1977,[104] an observation attributed to the increased use of low-tar, low-nicotine cigarettes. Studies of cytologic atypia in sputum specimens have shown a similar association with cigarette smoking;[105] however, some variation has been observed in the degree of atypia with repeated cytologic testing.[106]

The plausibility of the association between environmental tobacco smoke and pulmonary carcinoma in nonsmokers is reinforced by the recognition that such smoke contains carcinogens[81] and that tobacco metabolites can be found in the urine and saliva of individuals exposed to environmental tobacco smoke.[85, 107, 108] Exposure to environmental tobacco smoke has also been shown to cause lung tumors in a murine model.[109] Dysplastic changes in airway epithelium have also been shown in autopsy studies of nonsmokers who have been exposed to environmental tobacco smoke and who have died of nonrespiratory disease.[110, 111]

Other Inhaled Particulate and Chemical Substances

Exposure to a variety of inorganic particulate materials and organic chemicals results in an increased risk for the development of pulmonary carcinoma.[112–114] Because of their mutagenicity in *in vitro* tests and their association with neoplasms in epidemiologic studies, some of these substances are classified as carcinogens. These include asbestos, crystalline silica, polycyclic aromatic hydrocarbons, arsenic, nickel, cadmium, chromium compounds, bis(chloromethyl)ether, chloromethyl methyl ether, mustard gas, beryllium, and vinyl chloride. The greatest risk lies in specific work environments where exposure can occur over long periods of time and the concentration of noxious materials can reach dangerous levels.

Epidemiologic evidence for a causative role of these substances is based largely on the finding of a higher incidence of pulmonary carcinoma in populations engaged in certain occupations than in control populations. Despite the undoubted association between cancer and some occupations, however, it is not always clear in a particular instance which, if any, of the substances previously mentioned is the sole or primary carcinogen; in fact, it is possible that multi-ple agents are involved in some situations. In addition, it is clear that there is a significant synergistic effect of cigarette smoke in many patients.[115]

Estimates of the number of cases of pulmonary carcinoma attributable to occupational carcinogen exposure have varied widely. In one review of five American case-control studies in which there was an attempt to control for cigarette smoking, 3% to 17% of pulmonary carcinomas were considered to be the result of occupational exposures, depending on the study area.[116] This is similar to the 15% estimate of Doll and Peto[117] for occupational lung cancer in the United States. Investigators in Italy and Norway have, in turn, provided estimates of 33%[118] and 13% to 27%.[119] The authors of a more recent and more conservative estimate of work-related lung cancer in the United States concluded that 10,000 to 12,000 cases of pulmonary carcinoma per year can be attributed to exposure to occupational carcinogens;[113] of these, more than half are related to asbestos. Although these figures illustrate the importance of occupational carcinogens in the development of pulmonary carcinoma, there is little doubt that most of the implicated tumors could be prevented by the elimination of cigarette smoking.

Asbestos

Although there has been a debate about when the cancer risk of asbestos was first recognized,[120] since the mid-1950s the relationship has been documented in many pathologic and epidemiologic studies.[121, 122] The mineral is undoubtedly one of the most important causes of pleuropulmonary cancer: of all nonneoplastic pulmonary diseases, those related to asbestos have the highest incidence of associated neoplasia, especially pulmonary carcinoma and pleural mesothelioma (*see* page 2807).[123, 124]

The association between asbestos exposure and pulmonary carcinoma has been demonstrated in workers who have been involved in mining and milling of the mineral as well as in those who have had secondary contact with it in a variety of industries.[125–140] For example, an excess mortality from pulmonary carcinoma has been documented in crocidolite miners in South Africa[141] and Australia,[142] in workers engaged in the manufacture of asbestos friction products and textiles,[143, 144] in workers in asbestos-cement factories,[145, 146] in sheet metal workers,[147] in manufacturers of insulation board in the construction industry,[148] in insulation workers,[148, 149] in shipyard workers,[150–152] and in maintenance shop workers exposed to asbestos in railroad workshops.[153] Although a history of such occupational exposure is usually easily identified, detailed questioning may be required in some patients.[154]

Although some investigators have found an excess of squamous cell carcinoma[140, 155] or adenocarcinoma[156] in patients who have asbestos-related disease, most have found the proportion of histologic types of carcinoma to be similar to that in patients who do not have a history of asbestos exposure.[145, 157, 158]

The risk of pulmonary carcinoma in asbestos-exposed individuals is modified by several factors, including the duration of asbestos exposure, the type of fiber to which the individual is exposed, and the presence or absence of asbestosis or exposure to tobacco smoke; the possibility that pleural plaques may also confer an increased risk has also been investigated.

Fiber Type and Exposure History

The excess risk for pulmonary carcinoma varies in different industries. Although such differences are partly attributable to methods used in calculating risk, there are important real differences related to fiber type and degree of worker exposure.[159, 160] Fiber type is clearly important; exposure to amphibole fibers (crocidolite, amosite, and anthophyllite) is associated with a significantly greater risk of carcinoma compared to chrysotile exposure.[153, 161] The degree of exposure, as indicated by the number of asbestos bodies or fibers in lung tissue, is usually high in individuals who develop carcinoma.[162–168] Despite this, the results of most studies indicate that the relationship between malignancy risk and asbestos exposure is linear.[169–171] There may or may not be a threshold below which there is no risk;[169] however, in practical terms, it may be impossible to prove any measurable increase in risk of carcinoma for low-level exposure to asbestos.[172]

The intensity and duration of asbestos exposure are both important determinants of carcinoma risk.[113, 143, 145, 153, 155, 173–178] In most series in which an increased incidence of carcinoma has been demonstrated, workers have been exposed for at least 20 years.[143, 145, 146, 153, 179] The degree of asbestos exposure is also clearly related to the concentration of fibers in the atmosphere. The latter, in turn, depends in part on the state of the asbestos fibers during the period of contact. For example, once they are incorporated into manufactured products, fibers are relatively well bound and unlikely to cause harm; by contrast, situations in which the mineral is present in the atmosphere, such as building demolition or spraying of insulation material, are potentially hazardous.

Association with Tobacco Smoke

As indicated previously, the increased risk of asbestos-associated pulmonary carcinoma is strongly associated with cigarette smoking,[180] a relationship that is likely to be synergistic.[159, 181] Asbestos exposure is associated with a risk of 20:1 in heavy smokers compared with exposed nonsmokers and a risk as high as 100:1 for heavy smokers compared with unexposed nonsmokers.[182] Although the relatively small number of nonsmoking asbestos workers has created difficulties in identifying large cohorts for investigation, the results of some epidemiologic studies indicate an increased risk of pulmonary carcinoma in these individuals as well.[177, 183, 184] For example, one group of investigators conducted a 10-year follow-up study of 8,220 asbestos insulation workers who had volunteered their histories of smoking at the outset of the study in 1967; 6,841 had a history of cigarette smoking, and 1,379 did not.[180] They were compared to a control group of 73,763 men in the American Cancer Society's prospective cancer prevention study; these men had the same distribution of smoking habits and were alike in most other respects except that they had not been exposed to asbestos. Death rates for pulmonary carcinoma (per 100,000 man-years, standardized for age) were as follows: 11 for men who neither worked with asbestos nor smoked cigarettes, 58 for men who worked with asbestos but did not smoke, 123 for cigarette smokers who had not worked with asbestos, and 602 for men who had been exposed to both cigarettes and asbestos.

Asbestosis

The risk of developing pulmonary carcinoma in asbestos-exposed individuals has also been associated with the presence of asbestosis. In fact, pleuropulmonary malignancy develops in approximately 50% of patients who have the disease;[152, 157, 185] this figure is particularly remarkable in the light of the fact that some patients die of respiratory failure or cor pulmonale before they have the opportunity to develop a neoplastic complication. Whether there is an increased risk of pulmonary carcinoma in asbestos-exposed individuals in the absence of *pathologic* evidence of asbestosis has been a matter of considerable debate.[154, 186–190] The resolution of this debate has important implications for regulation of the industry, workers' compensation, and litigation.[188]

A strong argument has been made that the excess risk of pulmonary carcinoma in asbestos-exposed workers is confined to individuals who have asbestosis.[191–195] There is little doubt that the vast majority of tumors occur in individuals who have this abnormality; for example, in one study of 138 insulation workers who had pulmonary carcinoma, all had pulmonary fibrosis on histologic examination.[193] Many patients also have radiographic evidence of asbestosis. For example, in one group of 839 asbestos cement workers followed prospectively, an excess risk of pulmonary carcinoma (9 observed deaths versus 2.1 expected) was restricted to those who had small irregular opacities on the chest radiograph consistent with asbestosis;[189] similarly exposed workers who did not have radiographic evidence of asbestosis showed no increase in pulmonary carcinoma after controlling for age and smoking history (although the ability of this study to detect a smaller increase in risk in these workers was limited by sample size). Despite the results of this and other studies, it is clear that an excess risk for pulmonary carcinoma exists in asbestos-exposed workers in the absence of *radiographic* evidence for asbestosis.[189, 193, 196–198] For example, in 25 workers (18%) described in the study of insulation workers cited earlier, there was no evidence for fibrosis radiographically.[193] Additional support for an association between asbestosis and the development of carcinoma is provided by animal models of malignancy and fibrotic lung disease and the observation that patients who have diffuse interstitial fibrosis of other causes are at risk for the development of pulmonary carcinoma (*see* page 1080).[188, 199]

Despite these arguments, several observations suggest that the association between asbestosis and pulmonary carcinoma may be neither absolute nor causal, and it is possible that this abnormality is no more than a marker of more intense exposure to asbestos.[201] For example, the results of some experimental studies suggest that fibrogenic growth factors released by asbestos-activated macrophages facilitate the growth of tobacco smoke–damaged cells,[202] that is, that asbestos acts as a promoter of carcinogenesis rather than as an inducer. (Despite this, asbestos fibers have been shown to induce the expression of proto-oncogenes in *in vitro* experiments and can contribute to cell division via induction of growth regulatory polyamine molecules.[203, 204]) The cytotoxic effect of asbestos, which is linked to oxidant production, also leads to a compensatory hyperplasia of surviving cells, facilitating accumulation of genetic error—"mitogenesis increases mutagenesis."[171] Asbestos can facilitate the transfection of exogenous DNA into cells and enhances DNA strand breakage, particularly when combined with cigarette smoke.[204] Some investigators have shown a reduction in peripheral natural killer (NK) lymphocytes, responsible for immune surveillance of tumors, in asbestos-exposed workers;[205, 206] a reduction in NK lymphocyte activity has also been found after exposure of these cells to asbestos *in vitro*.[207] All these effects argue against the necessity for asbestosis in the pathogenesis of asbestos-related pulmonary carcinoma.

Accurate information on dose, radiographic abnormalities, and smoking history is required to give a definitive answer to the asbestosis-carcinoma question; in addition, large populations are required to confirm the negative hypothesis—that those who do not have fibrosis are not at excess risk for lung cancer.[113] However, it seems reasonable to conclude that if there is an increased risk of pulmonary carcinoma in asbestos-exposed workers who do not have asbestosis histologically, it is small. The results of experimental studies, however, suggest that the fiber may have a carcinogenic effect independent of a fibrogenic one, and the hypothesis that asbestosis is a necessary prerequisite for the development of carcinoma cannot be considered to have been definitively proved. Also, asbestosis can be present histologically in the absence of radiographic abnormalities.

Pleural Plaques

The relationship between the presence of pleural plaques and pulmonary carcinoma has also been somewhat controversial. Although plaques are seen in most patients who have pulmonary carcinoma and a history of asbestos exposure,[152] this is not a uniform observation. In addition, on the basis of a review of the English language literature, one group of investigators concluded that in the absence of asbestosis, there was no evidence for an increased risk for pulmonary carcinoma in patients who had plaques.[208]

Arsenic

Occupational exposure to arsenic occurs principally in the mining and smelting of copper, lead, zinc, and other metals and in the production and use of arsenic-containing pesticides. In smelters, it is emitted as an airborne byproduct during processing. Several groups of investigators have shown an increased risk of pulmonary carcinoma in association with high levels of arsenic exposure;[113, 209, 210] the combined relative risk of the largest studies has been about 3.7.[209, 210] This increase in risk seems to be confined to workers who have been exposed to high levels of arsenic in the past; when exposure has been to levels meeting current industry standards, an excess incidence of carcinoma has not been noted.[211]

In addition to arsenic exposure associated with smelting, an increased risk of pulmonary carcinoma has been identified in workers involved in the production of insecticides,[212, 213] in vineyard workers who use such substances,[214] in Italian felt hat makers,[215] and in Swedish glass-

workers.[216] Arsenic was also used intramuscularly in the treatment of syphilis and orally (Fowler's solution) as a treatment for a variety of diseases; as such, it has been associated with the development of visceral, including pulmonary, neoplasms.[217]

Nickel

The principal uses of nickel and nickel salts are in the production of stainless steel and other metal alloys, electroplating, and the manufacture of batteries.[113] Workers engaged in refining nickel ore have been found to have an increased incidence of malignancy affecting both the lungs and the nasal mucosa.[218–222] For example, in one series of 495 workers employed in a nickel sinter plant between 1948 and 1962, 54 (11%) developed pulmonary carcinoma.[223] The standardized mortality rates for lung and nasal carcinoma increased linearly with increasing duration of exposure, and there was no evidence of a threshold.[224] Risk seems confined to exposure to nickel sulfate and to the combination of nickel sulfides and oxides to which workers are exposed in nickel refining industries.[113] By contrast, workers involved in the manufacture of nickel alloys do not seem to be at excess risk for the development of pulmonary carcinoma.[113] The combined effect of smoking is multiplicative.[225] The overall relative risk of 13 studies has been estimated to be about 1.6.[113]

Chromium

The industrial uses of chromium include tanning, pigment production, plating, and alloy formation with other metals, such as nickel and cobalt. Masons who spray wet concrete are also exposed to hexavalent chromium.[226] Historical exposures in chromate production and plating were approximately 10 times higher than current permissible standards.[113] With such exposure, an incidence of pulmonary carcinoma as high as 27 times that expected has been found in workers involved in the use of chromium and its processing into dichromates.[227–229] In one study of three English chromate pigment factories, moderate-to-heavy exposure to zinc chromate but not to lead chromate was found to be associated with a markedly increased risk of pulmonary carcinoma;[230] however, exposure that is relatively mild or that lasts for less than a year may not constitute a significant risk. The requirement for a long period of exposure was borne out by two studies in Japan in which the average duration of exposure was 24 years[231, 232] and in a third study from New Jersey, in which risk was clearly apparent only 30 years after initial exposure.[233] Although many workers in electroplating industries are also exposed to nickel, a significant risk related to chromium exposure can be found after this is taken into account.[234]

The carcinogenic effect of chromium appears to be particularly related to its hexavalent form,[235–237a] a variant also incriminated in the increased incidence of pulmonary carcinoma in arc welders who use coated electrodes.[238] Zinc chromate is also a highly potent carcinogen.[235] The development of carcinoma and the specific histologic subtypes that occur have been associated with different stages of the manufacturing process.[239] Most investigators have found high concentrations of chromium in lung tissue at autopsy, even decades after the most recent exposure.[227, 230, 240, 241]

Silica

There has been considerable controversy concerning the association between silica exposure and the development of pulmonary carcinoma.[113, 242–247] In a 1997 publication, members of IARC concluded that crystalline silica inhaled in the form of quartz or cristobalite from occupational sources is carcinogenic to humans.[248] Although species specific, a number of experimental animal studies have provided evidence for this carcinogenic effect.[244, 249] The time course of exposure to silica and development of cancer is also consistent with causality, because the latency between exposure and cancer is a realistic and biologically plausible one.[244]

The strength of the association is much greater for workers who have silicosis[250–259] than workers who have been exposed to silica but have no evidence of the disease.[260–265] The relative risk for pulmonary carcinoma among the former workers often exceeds 3.0 and is as high as 6.0;[256] by contrast, the relative risk of carcinoma in the absence of silicosis is modest, being estimated at 1.3.[113] The results of many studies, especially those of ore mining and foundry workers, have been confounded by exposure to other carcinogens, such as asbestos,[261, 266, 267] radon,[255, 268–272] polycyclic aromatic hydrocarbons,[271, 273–276] arsenic,[271, 277, 278] chromium, and nickel.[273, 275] However, excess risk has been reported in workers in industries unassociated with exposure to other occupational carcinogens, such as stone cutters.[263, 279–281] The excess risk of carcinoma has been shown to be independent of cigarette smoking,[256, 259, 262, 264, 282, 283] because it is increased in both nonsmoking and never-smoking workers.[256, 284–286]

It is likely that the risk of pulmonary carcinoma in silica-exposed workers can be significantly decreased by decreasing contact with environmental dust. For example, in one investigation of a large hematite mining population in which dust exposure was carefully controlled and exposure to cocarcinogens minimized, no increase in risk of pulmonary carcinoma was identified.[287]

Chloromethyl Methyl Ether and Bis(Chloromethyl)Ether

Chloromethyl methyl ether and bis(chloromethyl)ether are widely used as intermediates in organic synthesis and in the preparation of ion-exchange resins. A survey of 111 workers who had been exposed to fumes of chloromethyl methyl ether in a chemical manufacturing plant for periods ranging from 3 to 14 years revealed pulmonary carcinoma in 14.[288] Their age range (33 to 55 years) was considerably lower than that of patients in the general population; moreover, three had never smoked. All but two of the carcinomas were small cell in type. In a more recent investigation, the risk of developing pulmonary carcinoma was found to be five times greater in exposed than nonexposed workers from the same plant.[289] The average age was about 11 years younger than that reported in nonexposed workers, and the mean time from first exposure to diagnosis was only 13 years. Cancers were again of the small cell type. A dose-response relationship has been established, the degree of exposure being found to be more important than its duration.[289–291]

Mustard Gas

The production of toxic gases for military use during World War II has been associated with an increased incidence of carcinoma involving the upper and lower respiratory tract, chiefly the larynx, trachea, and main bronchi.[292–295] A predominance of squamous cell carcinoma has been found in some studies.[296] In one investigation of a cohort of 2,498 men and 1,032 women employed in the manufacture of mustard gas during World War II, 200 developed pulmonary carcinoma (compared to approximately 138 expected).[295] Former workers who have died from other causes also have been found at autopsy to have a considerably higher incidence of bronchial carcinoma *in situ* than control individuals.[297]

Beryllium

In 1980, workers at IARC concluded that beryllium metal and several beryllium compounds are animal carcinogens.[298] Based on two cohort studies published in the early 1990s, workers at the same organization recognized beryllium as a human carcinogen as well.[299, 300] In a retrospective cohort review of 9,225 male workers employed at seven beryllium processing plants between 1940 and 1969, a higher standardized mortality rate for pulmonary carcinoma (3.33, confidence interval, 1.66 to 5.95) was identified.[299] Tumors were seen primarily in workers who had acute berylliosis, which is associated with especially high exposure levels; however, a smaller but significant risk was also seen in workers from other plants in which exposure was not as high. In both situations, the risk remained after controlling for smoking. In another analysis of 689 patients who had berylliosis, the standardized mortality rate for pulmonary carcinoma was 2.0 compared to the U.S. population as a whole.[300] The risk also remained after taking smoking history into account; other than death from berylliosis itself, no other cause of death was found to be more prevalent in these workers. The excess of carcinoma in this study was also greater in workers who had acute berylliosis than in those who had chronic disease.

Polycyclic Aromatic Hydrocarbons

Polycyclic aromatic hydrocarbons (PAHs) are a group of carcinogenic chemicals formed during the incomplete combustion of organic matter. Depending on the specific occupation, workers may be exposed to a variety of PAHs, including coke oven and coal gasification fumes[301, 302] and soot.[302, 303] A relationship between carcinoma and occupational carbon black exposure was demonstrated in a study of 857 cases of pulmonary carcinoma;[304] the risk was particularly striking for small cell carcinoma. Diesel exhaust is also considered a probable but not proven pulmonary carcinogen by IARC.[305]

Studies of coke oven workers have shown a threefold to sevenfold increase in the risk of pulmonary carcinoma, the highest being seen in those exposed to the highest levels of PAHs on the tops of the ovens.[301, 306–311] Rates of pulmonary carcinoma are currently declining in factories in which there has been effective implementation of environmental protective measures.[306] An excess risk of pulmonary carcinoma has also been documented in workers in other industries in which there is potential exposure to significant amounts of PAHs, such as aluminum production workers,[312, 313] steel foundry workers,[307, 314] and rubber workers.[315, 316]

The carcinogenic potential of soot has been recognized since the eighteenth century when chimney sweeps were observed to develop scrotal cancer. An increased risk for pulmonary carcinoma has also been found in a more recent analysis of 5,542 Swedish chimney sweeps, the risk increasing with increasing duration of employment and remaining significant after controlling for cigarette smoking;[317] in this study, the standardized incidence ratio for pulmonary carcinoma as a whole was 178 and for small cell carcinoma was 240. The indoor soot and combustion emissions from smoky coal have also been blamed for the high rate of pulmonary carcinoma in nonsmoking Chinese women.[318] Resected lung tissue from these patients has been shown to contain significantly higher levels of PAHs than control tissue from Japanese patients who had pulmonary carcinoma.

Concerns regarding possible carcinogenicity of exposure to the low level of PAHs found in the atmosphere[319] are magnified in workers exposed to diesel fumes, such as railroad workers, taxi drivers, and dock workers. Although there is some evidence that prolonged exposure to such fumes can cause pulmonary carcinoma,[320–323a] studies have been criticized for their failure to account properly for smoking intensity[324] and for inconsistency of their data.[325] On the basis of a review of 14 case-control and cohort studies, one group of investigators concluded that exposure of less than 20 years does not result in an increased risk of pulmonary carcinoma;[325] however, a statistically significant association existed between pulmonary carcinoma and long-term exposure to diesel fumes among railroad workers and diesel mechanics. In a meta-analysis of 29 case-control and cohort studies in which the relationship between occupational exposure to diesel exhaust and pulmonary carcinoma had been examined, evidence for an association was found even in studies in which there was adequate control for the effect of cigarette smoking;[325a] a duration-response effect was also evident.

Cadmium

The evidence that cadmium is a pulmonary carcinogen has not been consistent. Several groups of investigators have failed to confirm it in any convincing fashion.[326, 327] However, an increased risk for pulmonary carcinoma was identified in a retrospective cohort study of workers from a cadmium smelter;[328] this risk was greatest among those most heavily exposed (standardized mortality ratio, 272) and among workers who had 20 or more years from first exposure (standardized mortality ratio, 161). Although it has been suggested that the design of this study resulted in inadequate consideration of smoking and arsenic exposure,[329] the results of this and other investigations[330] led workers at IARC to conclude that cadmium is carcinogenic.[331]

Miscellaneous Substances

Other inhaled substances that have been implicated in the etiology of pulmonary carcinoma but for which definitive evidence of causality is lacking include isopropyl oil, chloroprene,[332] aflatoxin,[333] chlorinated toluenes,[334] vinyl and polyvinyl chlorides,[335] and synthetic mineral fibers.[336] Surveys of phosphate workers to identify a possible increase in the incidence of pulmonary carcinoma have produced both positive[337] and negative results.[338] Formaldehyde was not found to be associated with an increased incidence of pulmonary carcinoma in one study;[339] however, reanalysis of the data has led to the suggestion that a risk might be associated with high exposure.[340]

Radiation

Exposure to radiation may be from an external source (such as a therapeutic x-ray apparatus or a nuclear bomb) or by inhalation of radioactive gases. The latter is more important in terms of the number of individuals potentially exposed and is related primarily to radon, a substance formed during the decay of uranium to stable lead. The radioactive decay of radon gas itself releases a number of radioactive isotopes known as *radon daughters*.[113] These progeny are metal ions that adhere to particles suspended in air. When inhaled, they are deposited in the respiratory tract, where they are able to irradiate the surrounding tissue with alpha particles.

Radioactivity related to radon can be measured in several ways. Investigators in occupational studies have reported exposure in working level months. (A working level [WL] represents a release of 1.3×10^5 MeV of alpha energy from any combination of radon progeny in 1 liter of air; exposure to 1 WL for 170 hours represents 1 WL month.) Exposure may also be expressed in becquerels (Bq), which are a measure of the number of radioactive transformations of a radionuclide over time. (A becquerel is equivalent to 1 disintegration per second, activity being reported as Bq/m^3; 1 WL is equivalent to 3.7×10^3 Bq/m^3.) Radon concentration can also be expressed in picocuries per liter (pCi/L), 1 pCi/L being equivalent to 0.005 WL or 37 Bq/m^3.[341]

Occupational exposure to radon and its progeny occurs in workers involved in mining uranium,[342–346] fluorspar,[347, 347a] niobium,[348] and other substances (during which naturally occurring radon leeches from the rock face)[349–352] or in the processing of radioactive materials.[353, 354] In 1988, members of IARC concluded that radon should be classified as a human carcinogen.[355]

Studies of the risk of pulmonary carcinoma in exposed miners have shown a consistent increase compared with nonexposed individuals, the risk being greater in association with younger age at first exposure as well as with longer duration and intensity of exposure.[344, 345, 347, 356–359] The plausibility of these observations is reinforced by animal models in which carcinomas have been produced by exposure to radon and other radioactive products.[360, 361] The risk for developing pulmonary carcinoma in nonsmokers exposed to radon is similar to that of nonexposed active smokers.[359] The risk is greatly increased by concomitant cigarette smoking,[362–364] reported death rates being intermediate to those predicted by additive and multiplicative models of carcinogenesis.[365] Although the incidence of all histologic types is increased, the predominant one is small cell.[366–368] Tumors tend to be more frequently located centrally than those in nonexposed smokers, an observation that could be explained by central deposition of radioactive particles.[367]

Radon is also frequently found in the indoor environment of human habitations. It can be derived from water or natural gas, in which case it may enter buildings through cracks in the foundation, or from building materials themselves.[369] The observation that levels of radon found in some homes—especially those that have poorly ventilated basements—approach those in mines in which an association with carcinoma has been documented[345, 356, 358] has led to concern that radon also may be carcinogenic in the nonoccupational setting. This concern is supported by the results of an analysis of 11 cohort studies of radon-exposed miners, in which a linear relative risk for pulmonary carcinoma was consistently found across the range of exposures, suggesting that even low exposures are dangerous.[370] In fact, according to some investigators, residential radon exposure may account for as many as 10% to 15% of all deaths from pulmonary carcinoma in the United States;[371, 372] however, the assumptions on which these conclusions rest have been challenged.[373]

Studies of the association of domestic radon exposure and pulmonary carcinoma risk have not yielded consistent results, some investigators finding a positive association[374, 375] and others not.[376–379] Study designs describing ecologic associations and case-control studies each have had significant methodologic problems, especially with respect to measurement error, failure to evaluate carefully all potential confounding factors, inadequate statistical power, and mis-specification of the risk model.[380–384] Nevertheless, the authors of a meta-analysis of eight case-control studies concluded that the risk from domestic radon exposure was real, albeit small (relative risk, 1.14, with a 95% confidence interval of 1.0 to 1.3) and that the magnitude of the risk was consistent with that predicted by extrapolation of data available from radon-exposed miners.[385]

The relative contribution of external radiation to the development of pulmonary carcinoma is variable and undoubtedly depends to a great extent on the dose received. The incidence of pulmonary carcinoma in individuals who survived the atomic bombings of Nagasaki and Hiroshima is slightly increased;[386, 387] in one study, the relative risk was 3.9.[387] Such radiation appears to be associated with the development of small cell carcinoma.[388] Patients who have Hodgkin's disease or breast carcinoma and who have been treated with supradiaphragmatic radiation or combined modality therapy also may have a slightly increased risk for the development of pulmonary carcinoma.[389, 390] For example, in one study of 3,537 patients who had breast carcinoma, 19 were identified who had received adjuvant radiation therapy and had developed pulmonary carcinoma a median of 17 years after the irradiation;[391] 15 of these tumors were on the side of the radiation, and only 4 were contralateral, suggesting an etiologic role for the radiation. In a second analysis of 8,976 patients who had breast carcinoma and who survived for at least 10 years, the overall relative risk for pulmonary carcinoma in those initially treated with radiotherapy was 1.8;[392] this relative risk increased to 2.8 for periods greater than 15 years after initial therapy. These results are concordant with those of an analysis of patients from the National Cancer Institute[393] and suggest an excess of nine cases of pulmonary carcinoma among 10,000 treated

women surviving for at least 10 years. Fortunately, current radiation regimens expose the lung to substantially less irradiation than previously, and concern for secondary pulmonary carcinoma should not influence decisions regarding therapy in this respect.

Viral Infection

Although there is abundant evidence linking viral infection with human cancer, there is little to suggest that it is an important factor in most carcinomas of the lung. Jaagsiekte, a disease of sheep morphologically similar to human bronchioloalveolar carcinoma, shows many features consistent with a viral etiology.[394] Epidemiologic studies have shown that this disease can be transmitted from animal to animal, and electron microscopic and virologic investigations, including sophisticated molecular biology techniques, have shown evidence for infection by what is now known as the *jaagsiekte sheep retrovirus*.[395–398] Animal-to-human transmission of the disease has been suggested in some cases,[399] but must be exceedingly rare if it occurs at all. Viral-like inclusions have also been noted in cases of human bronchioloalveolar carcinoma,[400] although their significance is disputed. Thus, although it is theoretically possible that the human tumor is also caused by a virus, evidence for this is tenuous.

Laryngotracheobronchial papillomas are known to be caused by human papillomavirus (HPV);[401] it is likely that the rare cases of pulmonary squamous cell carcinoma that develop in association with these lesions are pathogenetically related to the virus, particularly types 16 and 18 (*see* page 1262).[402, 403] These observations have led to investigation of the possible role of these viruses in the pathogenesis of pulmonary carcinoma unassociated with papillomatosis. Using *in situ* hybridization and polymerase chain reaction techniques, HPV DNA has been identified in 6% to 79% of human pulmonary carcinomas by some investigators;[404–406, 449] however, others have not been able to identify it in any tumors.[407–409] Although there is evidence that the virus can inactivate the tumor-suppressor gene product P53,[404] the precise role and importance of this virus in pulmonary carcinoma have not been clearly defined.

Epstein-Barr viral genome was identified in 9 of 167 (5%) consecutive non–small cell pulmonary carcinomas in one study;[410] all had the morphologic appearance of lymphoepithelioma-like carcinoma, a pattern similar to that of nasopharyngeal tumors of the same name that are also believed to be related to Epstein-Barr virus infection. Eight of the nine patients were men, and smoking was not a risk factor. Other investigators have confirmed the association between this uncommon histologic type of tumor and Epstein-Barr virus expression.[411, 412] The virus is uncommonly associated with other forms of pulmonary carcinoma. In one investigation of 80 adenocarcinomas, it was not identified in any tumor;[413] in another review of 127 cases of non–small cell carcinoma, it was documented by *in situ* hybridization in 5 of 5 lymphoepithelioma-like carcinomas, 6 of 43 squamous cell carcinomas, 0 of 67 adenocarcinomas, and 0 of 12 large cell carcinomas.[450]

Pulmonary Fibrosis

The term *scar carcinoma* refers to a pulmonary carcinoma that is intimately related to a localized area of parenchymal fibrosis. Early investigators who studied this association postulated that the scars preceded the carcinoma and were pathogenetically related to its development,[414, 415] and the term has since come to encompass this concept. The hypothesized cause of the cancer-associated fibrosis has been reported to include tuberculosis,[415, 416] infarction,[415–418] chronic abscess,[415] organized pneumonia,[419] and foreign bodies.[420, 421] In addition to the parenchymal scarring itself, other factors have been implicated in carcinogenesis, the most important being the epithelial metaplasia and hyperplasia that are frequently present at the junction of the fibrotic and unscarred lung.[414, 422, 423] These hyperplastic areas can exhibit cytologic atypia;[415, 419] occasionally, there is apparent transition between such regions and clear-cut carcinoma.

Despite the fact that focal pulmonary fibrosis and carcinoma are frequently associated, especially in peripheral tumors (Fig. 31–1), the idea that the fibrosis antedates and in some way causes the carcinoma is difficult to prove in most cases. The validity of a causal relationship has thus been questioned, and most observers now believe that the cancer induces the fibrosis rather than the other way around.[424–429] Several observations support this viewpoint. It is well known that carcinomas originating in other tissues can induce prominent fibrosis that sometimes resembles that seen in peripheral pulmonary scars; there is no reason why a similar process should not occur in the lung. In support of this interpretation are immunohistochemical and biochemical investigations of peripheral "scar carcinomas" in which evidence has been found for the active production of collagen.[424, 428, 429] It is also possible that other cancer-associated processes can cause focal fibrosis; for example, recent infarcts are occasionally identified between a peripheral carcinoma and the pleura, presumably related to vascular occlusion by the carcinoma. If these organize and are engulfed by

the carcinoma before surgical excision, they could give the appearance of a long-standing scar. Chronic atelectasis secondary to small airway obstruction by tumor may lead to a similar histologic picture.[426] Thus, although focal areas of fibrosis are probably pathogenetically important in the development of carcinoma in some cases,[430, 431] the incidence of true scar carcinomas has undoubtedly been overestimated in the past.[44]

An association between diffuse interstitial pulmonary fibrosis and carcinoma has also been documented. The risk, at times markedly elevated,[432] has been noted in patients who have progressive systemic sclerosis,[433, 434] rheumatoid disease,[435, 436] neurofibromatosis,[437, 438] sarcoidosis,[439, 440] dermatomyositis,[441] and idiopathic pulmonary fibrosis.[441–445] In contrast to carcinoma associated with focal scars, it is often possible to be certain on clinical and radiologic grounds that the fibrosis preceded the development of carcinoma in all these diseases, suggesting that the fibrosis is truly pathogenic. The observation that the carcinomas tend to be peripheral in origin and located in the most advanced areas of fibrosis also supports this interpretation.[445, 446]

The pathogenetic basis for the diffuse fibrosis–carcinoma association is unclear. As with focal scars, epithelial metaplasia and hyperplasia are frequently present in association with the areas of fibrosis; such lesions have been shown to have a high proliferative activity.[447] It is also possible that growth factors, such as transforming growth factor-β_1, elaborated by epithelial cells and macrophages enhance tumor development.[448]

Other Lung Disease

The association of tuberculosis and carcinoma in the same area of the lung has been reported with sufficient frequency to suggest that the combination may be more than coincidental.[451, 452] In occasional cases, the malignancy appears to originate in tuberculous scars, suggesting that the

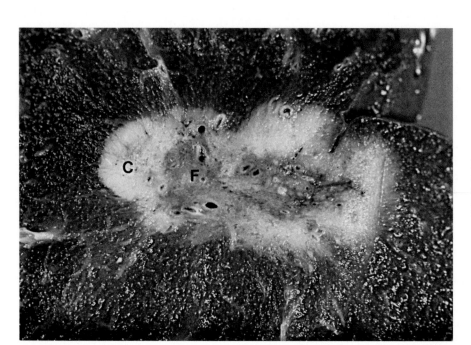

Figure 31–1. Pulmonary "Scar" Carcinoma. A magnified view of a peripheral pulmonary adenocarcinoma shows a central area of gray fibrous tissue (F) surrounded by a variably thick rim of lighter-shaded carcinoma (C).

tumors represent true scar carcinomas. However, the incidence of such a causal relationship must be very small; in two large series of patients who had both tuberculosis and pulmonary carcinoma, the association appeared to be purely coincidental.[454, 455] Whether or not there is a pathogenetic relationship between tuberculosis and pulmonary carcinoma, appreciation of the second lesion may come late.[457] In a cytologic screening study of 800 men aged 40 years or older who had been admitted to an urban sanatorium, malignant cells were found in 57 (10%) of those who provided satisfactory sputum specimens;[458] in 50 of these, follow-up examinations confirmed the diagnosis of carcinoma. Retrospective review of their chest radiographs revealed no evidence of malignancy in 25.

The importance of a previous history of lung disease as a risk factor for the development of pulmonary carcinoma has been the focus of several studies. In a population-based, case-control study of nonsmoking women from five urban areas in the United States, a history of previous lung disease was associated with a significantly increased risk for pulmonary carcinoma (adjusted odds ratio, 1.56);[459] the risk was still evident after consideration of potential confounders, such as lifelong environmental tobacco smoke exposure and diet. (The investigators included the reporting of a history of asthma or tuberculosis before the age of 21, so that there was unlikely to be confusion with early symptoms of lung cancer.) In another study of similar design, an excess risk of pulmonary carcinoma was found in never-smoking women who had a history of pneumonia or asthma;[460] among former smokers, both emphysema and tuberculosis also conferred an increased risk. A study in which the database of the Finnish Social Insurance Institution was linked with that of the Finnish Cancer Registry revealed an excess risk of pulmonary carcinoma in both men and women with asthma.[460] The risk for carcinoma of the larynx, another smoking-related malignancy, was reduced in this asthmatic population.

A significantly higher incidence of pulmonary carcinoma has been documented in cigarette smoking patients who have chronic bronchitis than in those who do not.[462–465] The relationship appears to be independent of age and amount smoked. Abnormalities of lung function also seem to increase the risk for pulmonary carcinoma after correction for amount smoked.[464–467] In a community-based cohort of about 4,000 adults first examined between 1962 and 1965, the risk for pulmonary carcinoma was greatly increased in smokers, as expected;[465] however, after stratifying the population for amount smoked, subjects in the lowest quartile for percent predicted forced expiratory volume in 1 second (FEV_1) had 2.7 times the risk for developing carcinoma than subjects in the highest quartile. Similar results were reported in a cohort of 13,946 Danish subjects[464] and in a group of 6,317 Japanese-American men followed prospectively for a 10-year period.[466] In another study of cigarette smokers, the presence of airway obstruction was a better indicator for the subsequent development of pulmonary carcinoma than age or the intensity of smoking;[467] moreover, the risk of carcinoma increased in proportion to the severity of airway obstruction. Obstructive airway disease may also be an independent risk factor in patients who have asbestos-associated malignancy.[468] Based on a review of the literature and their own experience with six patients,

one group has suggested that there may be an increased risk in patients who have bullous disease;[469] such patients tend to be younger than the average patient with pulmonary carcinoma.

The associations of impaired lung function and chronic bronchitis with pulmonary carcinoma risk seem to be robust. However, whether these risk factors are more accurate representations of amount smoked (intensity, cigarette type, breath-hold) than pack-years, whether chronic obstructive pulmonary disease and carcinoma are related to common susceptibility, and whether chronic mucus hypersecretion or emphysema (or both) play a pathogenic role in pulmonary carcinoma have not been determined.

Dietary Factors

There has been a great deal of interest in the potential benefit of antioxidant vitamins, such as beta-carotene (provitamin A) and alpha-tocopherol (vitamin E), in the prophylaxis of pulmonary carcinoma in both smokers and nonsmokers.[472] Epidemiologic studies of the relationship between dietary intake of these vitamins and pulmonary carcinoma risk have been criticized for their failure to adjust adequately for confounders of cancer risk, such as smoking intensity and indoor air pollutants.[473, 474] Many investigators, however, have shown a small but important inverse relationship between consumption of fruits and vegetables high in vitamin content and pulmonary carcinoma.[453, 475–484] This observation is supported by the results of experimental studies in animals and cell cultures.[485, 486]

On the basis of this finding, several large clinical studies were instituted to investigate the value of vitamins in the prevention of pulmonary carcinoma. In one randomized, double-blind, placebo-controlled, primary prevention trial of daily alpha-tocopherol, beta-carotene, or both, 29,133 male Finnish smokers were followed for 5 to 8 years (the ATBC Cancer Prevention Trial).[487] Investigators found an unexpected 18% higher incidence of pulmonary carcinoma among the subjects who received beta-carotene than among those who did not. The use of alpha-tocopherol had no effect. In a second multicenter, randomized, double-blind, placebo-controlled primary prevention trial (the CARET trial), the effects of a combination of beta-carotene and retinol (vitamin A) were compared to placebo in 18,314 smokers, former smokers, and asbestos-exposed workers followed for a 4-year period.[488] The trial was ended prematurely when a relative risk of pulmonary carcinoma of 1.28 was found in the active treatment group after 73,135 person-years of follow-up.

Whether vitamin supplementation of the type administered in these studies is harmful has not been conclusively proven; however, it must be concluded that it is unlikely to be of benefit. Many foods contain a variety of substances in addition to beta-carotene and vitamin E that are anticarcinogens.[479, 481, 486, 489, 490] It is conceivable that these underlie the discrepancy in the results of these preventive trials as well as in the results of retrospective-cohort studies and case-control studies of vitamin-rich diets, which have been shown to be associated with a decreased risk of carcinoma. If this interpretation is correct, a high blood carotene level is best considered to be a marker for a healthy intake of fruits and vegetables rather than a suppressor of carcinoma.[491]

Other dietary factors have been less thoroughly investigated. A high intake of cholesterol has been found to be a risk factor for pulmonary carcinoma in a multiethnic population in Hawaii,[492] although Japanese men in this state have been shown to have no increased risk no matter how much cholesterol they consume.[493] Increased fatty food intake has been associated with a higher risk of pulmonary carcinoma in many (albeit not all[494, 495]) studies.[478, 491, 496–499] Further work is required to clarify the importance and validity of these observations.

Genetic Factors

Although tobacco smoke and the various occupational carcinogens discussed previously are responsible for most cases of pulmonary carcinoma, it is clear that only a minority of individuals exposed to these agents develop cancer. Such individual susceptibility may be explained, at least in part, by host-specific factors that confer sensitivity or resistance to disease.[500] The results of a number of epidemiologic studies suggest that at least some such factors are inherited. Family clusters of pulmonary carcinoma have been well documented.[501–503] In young individuals who smoke, the risk of developing carcinoma is significantly greater for those who have first-degree relatives with a history of pulmonary carcinoma or other tobacco smoke–related cancer.[456] Retrospective studies in which the morbidity and mortality among first-degree relatives of patients who have the more common malignancies (such as lung, breast, colon, and rectum) have been compared with those of a control group of relatives of the probands' spouses or with the expected population rates have shown a twofold to fourfold increased incidence of cancers of the same[504] or other[505] types. In some studies, the excess for pulmonary carcinoma is evident even after the confounding effects of age, gender, cigarette smoking, and occupational and industrial carcinogen exposure have been controlled.[506–509] Individuals who smoke and who have a family history of pulmonary carcinoma have a 30-fold to 35-fold increased risk of developing pulmonary carcinoma compared with nonsmokers who have no family history.[510, 511] In fact, on the basis of an analysis of 337 families with pulmonary carcinoma, one group of investigators speculated that there is virtually no chance of developing carcinoma in the absence of a genetic susceptibility to the carcinogenic effects of tobacco smoke.[509]

Individual variations in response to environmental carcinogens might be explained by differences in their metabolism that confer sensitivity or resistance to their effects.[500] The carcinogenic effect of PAHs found in cigarette smoke, as measured by their ability to modify cellular DNA, has been positively correlated with the level of aryl hydrocarbon hydroxylase activity in the lung.[512, 513] The latter is genetically determined and is largely dependent on the activity of the cytochrome P450 enzyme complex. Cigarette smoking induces aryl hydrocarbon hydroxylase activity in the lung,[514] an effect that is enhanced in patients who have the CYP1A1 genotype, leading to a significantly higher risk for pulmonary carcinoma.[515–518] Other cytochrome P450 enzyme genotypes have also been associated with an increased risk of pulmo-

nary carcinoma.[519–524] Glutathione-S-transferases are a family of enzymes involved in the inactivation of a variety of toxins; deficiency of a particular isoenzyme has been associated with a significantly increased risk for lung cancer.[525–527]

PATHOGENESIS

The pathogenesis of pulmonary carcinoma—as with other cancers—is a complex and incompletely understood process that is only briefly discussed at this point. Two features that are of particular importance are genetic and molecular abnormalities that result in an alteration of the control of cell growth and the body's immune reaction to the presence of neoplastic cells.

Genetic and Molecular Factors

Pulmonary carcinoma occurs by a multistep process in which progressive accumulation of mutations leads to a loss of normal mechanisms of control of cellular growth.[528–530, 590] It has been estimated that 10 to 20 such mutations may have occurred by the time a carcinoma becomes clinically evident.[529] It is possible that these varied mutations are reflected in the development of different tumor clones and in the histologic heterogeneity of many pulmonary carcinomas (*see* farther on). Genes involved with DNA repair, cell growth, signal transduction, and cell-cycle control may all be damaged during the course of carcinoma progression.[532] Exposure to carcinogens causes both initiating events (mutations) and tumor promotion, which results in the growth of cells containing such mutations.[529] DNA damage can result in the activation of growth-stimulating genes or the inactivation of growth-suppressing genes.[532]

A genetic element that contributes to the neoplastic transformation of cells is called an *oncogene*.[533] Under the influence of carcinogens, oncogenes develop from nuclear proto-oncogenes, which are components of the normal cellular genome with important functions in nonneoplastic cellular processes.[533] Proto-oncogenes are homologous cellular counterparts of a variety of retroviral oncogenes found in nature. They can be activated to oncogenes through gene mutations, deletions, insertions, abnormal regulation, or rearrangement.[534] Oncogenes can be either recessive or dominant.[529] For dominant oncogenes, activation of only one of the two copies of the gene results in oncogenesis; in the case of recessive oncogenes (also known as *tumor-suppressor genes*), two different lesions involving both copies of the gene are required.[529]

Dominant oncogenes may cause cancer by the production of functional but abnormal proteins or by the overexpression of an otherwise normal gene;[535] in both circumstances, the gene product drives cell growth in an unrestrained fashion.[529] Examples of this type of gene include members of the *myc* family, *ras* family, and the HER2/*neu* gene. *Myc* gene amplification is seen in most small cell carcinomas and some non–small cell carcinomas;[536] its presence is associated with aggressive disease, previous exposure to chemotherapy, and poor prognosis.[529] Mutations in *myc* genes lead to overexpression of an otherwise normal protein, which drives cell growth. *Ras* genes are most often identified in non–small cell carcinoma, especially adenocarcinoma and large cell carcinoma;[532] point mutation or overexpression of the plasma membrane guanosine triphosphate–binding protein they encode correlates with poorer survival for any given stage.[529, 535, 537, 538] The HER2/*neu* gene (or c-*erb*B-2) encodes a protein that has structural similarity to epidermal growth factor receptor; overexpression correlates with decreased survival in non–small cell carcinoma.[539] *Bcl*-2 is a novel oncogene that regulates cell death by protecting the cell against apoptosis.[540] It is present in a minority of non–small cell carcinomas[540, 541] and may indicate a favorable prognosis.[540] Many other oncogenes have been described in pulmonary carcinomas, including *Erb*B-1, *fos, jun, raf, met, fes, kit, fms,* and *myb*.[534, 535, 542–545]

Alteration of the activity of the protein products of tumor-suppressor genes, which normally modulate cellular proliferation, may permit the accelerated growth of neoplastic tissue.[546] Two well-described cancer-suppressor genes are the retinoblastoma gene (*Rb*) and P53.[534] *Rb* normally maintains a controlled progression through the cell cycle by repressing the promoter activity of several growth-promoting genes; inactivation of *Rb* disrupts constraints on cell growth.[546] Most small cell carcinomas do not express the *Rb* protein; its inactivation is generally the result of mutation or deletion of the *Rb* gene.[528] Although *Rb* is expressed by most non–small cell carcinomas, it may be inactive in some tumors as a result of hyperphosphorylation.[528, 546] Loss of *Rb* protein function in Stage I and II non–small cell carcinomas is a marker of poor prognosis.[547]

The tumor-suppressor gene P53 probably acts in the nucleus with other proteins as a transcription factor to activate a number of genes responsible for genetic stability, growth arrest, and cell death.[529, 532] Mutation of this gene and abnormal expression of its protein occur in almost all small cell carcinomas and in the majority of non–small cell carcinomas,[470, 529, 548] making this the most commonly identified genetic abnormality in pulmonary carcinoma. The absence of P53 expression in normal and metaplastic bronchial epithelium without atypia, the increasing frequency of its detection in metaplastic epithelium with increasing severity of dysplasia,[549] and its presence in virtually all cases of carcinoma *in situ* suggest that it plays a role in carcinogenesis and that its detection might prove useful in early diagnosis.[532, 535] Its presence in areas of squamous metaplasia has also been shown to be a marker of increased risk for the presence of synchronous or metachronous carcinoma.[550] The identification of a P53 protein in resected tumors by immunohistochemistry correlates with poor prognosis in patients who have non–small cell carcinoma.[470, 529, 551, 552]

Growth factors are a group of signaling molecules that take part in the control of cell proliferation.[553] When secreted by tumor cells or adjacent stromal cells, they augment cell growth in an autocrine or paracrine fashion and thereby assume a promoter function for neoplastic cells.[529] They require specific receptors and intracellular signal transduction pathways to stimulate cell division.[553] The best known of these are the autocrine polypeptide bombesin (which is active in small cell carcinoma) and transforming growth factor alpha, epidermal growth factor, and heregulin (all of which are found in non–small cell carcinoma).[528, 554] Cell surface peptidases can degrade and thereby regulate the

effects of growth factors; they seem to be absent or present at low levels in pulmonary carcinoma cell lines and tumors.[531]

Genetic deletions and translocations are common in pulmonary carcinoma.[531, 555] Such alterations may cause the loss of tumor-suppressor genes or activate oncogenes through the abnormal control of oncogene expression.[555] A loss of the short arm of chromosome 3 is particularly frequent; however, the large region deleted has made it difficult to identify specific tumor-suppressor genes.[529] Changes to chromosome 3 have also been observed in premalignant lesions of the bronchial epithelium, suggesting that damage to this chromosome is an early event in carcinogenesis.[556] Deletions have also been reported in a number of other chromosomes.[471, 531, 534, 555, 557–559]

Immunologic Factors

Cell-mediated immunity has an important role in the host response to neoplastic cells. Convincing evidence for this is provided by observing the consequence of deficiencies in cell-mediated immunity, such as the development of Kaposi's sarcoma and lymphoma in patients who have acquired immunodeficiency syndrome and of lymphoproliferative disorders in patients who have undergone organ transplantation. It is thus possible that abnormalities in immune function might be involved in the pathogenesis of pulmonary carcinoma. Evidence of such abnormalities has been found by a number of investigators.[560–562] For example, in one study of 219 patients who had pulmonary carcinoma, a correlation was found between delayed cutaneous hypersensitivity and the degree of differentiation of the tumor, stage of the disease, response to chemotherapy, and prognosis and survival.[563] However, it is not clear which, if any, of these immunologic abnormalities are related to the development of the carcinoma and which are simply a reaction to its presence. The four major cell types implicated in cell-mediated immunity are NK cells, lymphokine-activated killer cells, cytotoxic T cells, and monocytes-macrophages;[564] each of these may have a role to play in the pathogenesis of pulmonary carcinoma.

NK cells are believed to be the first line of defense in the immune surveillance of tumors.[564, 565] Their activity is decreased in the peripheral blood of patients who have pulmonary carcinoma,[566] particularly those who have advanced disease. In fact, in patients undergoing resection for non–small cell carcinoma, the conservation of NK cell activity in peripheral blood lymphocytes in the immediate postoperative period has been shown to be a favorable prognostic marker independent of tumor stage.[567] Lymphocytes obtained from lung specimens resected from patients who have pulmonary carcinoma show a significant reduction in NK cell activity;[568] however, the significance of this is unclear because quantitative NK cell deficits have also been described in smokers who do not have carcinoma.[569]

Lymphocytes that depend on cytokines to have a cytotoxic effect on tumor cells are known as *lymphokine-activated killer cells*.[564] Their importance in tumor control is suggested by the observation of a significant antitumor effect when they are activated by interleukin-2 in clinical trials.[570] Analysis of bronchoalveolar lavage fluid has shown lymphokine-activated killer cell lytic activity directed against tumor cells in some patients.[571] *In vitro* studies suggest that this effect is dependent on adhesion molecule expression by the tumor cells.[572, 573]

Cytotoxic T cells are likely responsible for *in vitro* cytotoxicity directed against autologous tumor. Their ability to recognize autologous tumor cells *in vivo* also may be among the more important of host responses to cancer.[564] Direct examination of activation-related molecules on regional lymph node lymphocytes in patients who have pulmonary carcinoma has revealed that they are more activated than peripheral blood lymphocytes, especially in patients who have Stage I and II tumors.[574] Whether these lymphocytes are active against and help control carcinoma has not been determined; however, their presence has significant prognostic value in patients who have resected non–small cell carcinoma,[575] and preliminary work using expanded clones of these cells for adoptive immunotherapy suggests that they might be therapeutically useful.[576] Some investigators have shown that patients who have autologous lymphocyte cytotoxicity in peripheral lymphocytes against single cell suspensions of their tumor live longer than do those lacking this response.[564] Lymphocyte cytotoxicity has also been reported to be deficient in patients who have asbestosis, perhaps explaining, in part, their susceptibility to pulmonary carcinoma.[577]

Pulmonary alveolar macrophage activation and phagocytotic abilities are conserved in patients who have pulmonary carcinoma.[564] However, their cytotoxic function may be reduced; normalization of this function with γ-interferon administration has been demonstrated.[564] The precise role of macrophages in the host reaction to pulmonary carcinoma is uncertain; however, they are found in many tumors, and some have suggested that the effectiveness of their cytostatic function correlates positively with resectability.[578]

The presence of tumor-associated antigens allows for a mechanism by which a humoral immune response to the cancer might be initiated.[564] B lymphocytes, however, are functionally abnormal in untreated patients who have advanced pulmonary carcinoma; some of this impairment is caused by suppressor T-cell activity.[579] Using the T cell–dependent primary immunogen *Helix pomatia*, it has been shown that antibody response and *in vitro* lymphocyte reactivity are impaired in patients who have pulmonary carcinoma compared with matched controls.[580] In addition, cutaneous atopy has been found by some (albeit not all[581]) workers to be less prevalent in patients who have newly diagnosed pulmonary carcinoma compared with those in a control group.[582] Overall, evidence that humoral response to tumor might be important in pathogenesis is weak;[564] however, the presence of antibodies against a variety of tumor antigens has been associated with a favorable prognosis in small cell carcinoma.[583]

PATHOLOGIC CHARACTERISTICS

One of the earliest classifications of pulmonary carcinoma was proposed in 1924 by Marchesani,[584] who enumerated four subtypes corresponding to the current widely used categories of squamous cell carcinoma, small cell carcinoma, large cell carcinoma, and adenocarcinoma. Although there have been several refinements proposed since that time,[417, 585]

this fundamental subdivision is still the basis of most current classifications. Modifications of the original format were introduced by WHO in 1967,[586] by the Veterans' Administration Lung Cancer Therapy Study Group (VALG) in 1965,[587] by the Working Party for the Therapy of Lung Cancer (WPL) in 1973,[588] by a WHO review committee in 1981,[589] and most recently by another WHO group in 1999 (*see* Table 31–1, page 1071).[1] With minor modifications, the last-named schema is the one followed in this chapter.

Despite its widespread use, the WHO classification has not been accepted without criticism. As in many other schemata, its categories are defined by light microscopic criteria; although information is used from standard histochemical reactions such as mucin and silver stains, there is little provision for the use of ancillary techniques to define tumor categories more precisely (exceptions include the immunohistochemical confirmation of neuroendocrine differentiation in large cell neuroendocrine carcinoma and epithelial differentiation in spindle cell carcinoma). Because ultrastructural,[591–594] immunohistochemical,[595] and molecular studies clearly reveal more varied differentiation in many pulmonary carcinomas than is evident from the light microscopic appearance alone, the exclusion of these techniques in classification can be questioned.[592, 593] However, although the use of such techniques can be helpful and is occasionally essential for accurate diagnosis, for practical purposes we describe most carcinomas according to the standard histologic features defined by the WHO classification.

The usefulness of any tumor classification can be evaluated by assessing three attributes: (1) *comprehensiveness*—the proportion of tumors that can be placed within the defined categories; (2) *validity*—the ability to describe categories with well-defined clinicopathologic features; and (3) *reliability*—the presence of a reasonable degree of interobserver and intraobserver agreement in the use of the classification scheme. The comprehensiveness of the original WHO classification was good, the number of tumors in an unclassified category identified in a 1974 study being less than 5%.[596] The validity is also reasonable; although there is some overlap, considerable evidence has accumulated that the major categories of squamous cell carcinoma, small cell carcinoma, adenocarcinoma, carcinoid tumor, and tumors of tracheobronchial glands show fairly characteristic clinical and pathologic features. The existence of large cell carcinoma as a true entity can be debated, however, and it is probably more accurate to view it as a form that overlaps histologically with the other subtypes but possesses none of the specific defining properties of any one of them. There is also some debate whether some of the minor subdivisions within the WHO classification represent distinct entities. These issues are discussed more fully in the following sections on pathologic characteristics.

The issue of reliability is also open to some question, particularly with respect to poorly differentiated tumors and some of the subdivisions of the major categories. Most studies of interobserver agreement in the diagnosis of small cell carcinoma have shown it to be good.[597–600] For example, in one investigation of 93 cases that had this diagnosis, unanimity among three observers was found in 94% of cases categorized according to the 1981 WHO classification.[597] In another investigation of 149 cases of small cell and undifferentiated carcinoma (including 114 of the former), consensus diagnosis (agreement between at least three of five pathologists) was found in 144 (97%).[601] Although the numbers were small, interobserver agreement for diagnoses of mixed and combined subtypes of small cell carcinoma were considerably poorer. Nevertheless, from a practical point of view, the distinction between small cell carcinoma and non–small cell tumors can be made with confidence in the vast majority of cases.

Although intraobserver and interobserver agreement for well-differentiated forms of squamous cell carcinoma and adenocarcinoma is generally good,[587, 602–604] that for poorly differentiated forms and for large cell carcinoma is considerably worse.[602] In one study of 3,600 lung cancer biopsy specimens classified according to the Veterans' Administration schema, unanimity in diagnosis among three observers was found in only 47% of cases designated poorly differentiated squamous cell carcinoma and in 43% of those diagnosed as poorly differentiated adenocarcinoma.[587] In another investigation of 50 specimens, disagreement between first and second readings of the same slides by the same pathologist ranged from 2% for the most consistent reader to 20% for the least consistent;[603] interobserver disagreement was 2% to 5% for well-differentiated squamous cell carcinoma and adenocarcinoma but averaged 25% for large and small cell carcinomas and 40% for poorly differentiated squamous cell carcinomas and adenocarcinomas.

The figures cited previously generally refer to variation among pathologists who have extensive experience and interest in pulmonary carcinoma. If the diagnoses of pathologists who do not have a specific interest in pulmonary disease are examined, variation is probably even greater.[605] For example, in one study in which the classification of pulmonary carcinoma according to the 1967 WHO schema was investigated, wide disagreement was found in the diagnosis of "epidermoid" and large cell carcinoma between a reference pathologist and local pathologists;[606] the authors concluded that the disagreement was caused primarily by a lack of adherence to the structural criteria of keratinization, intercellular bridges, or both in the diagnosis of squamous cell carcinoma.

Although the WHO classification recognizes the possibility of different degrees and types of differentiation in any particular tumor, the portion that is most "highly differentiated" is the one that defines the specific diagnosis. Although this guideline is certainly practical, it is clear that such a "final" diagnosis depends, in part, on the amount of tissue examined. This proviso is particularly relevant when only small tissue fragments, such as those obtained by endoscopy, are available for examination;[607] for example, in one study of 107 pulmonary carcinomas diagnosed initially by fiberoptic bronchoscopy, 41 (38%) were given a different diagnosis on subsequent examination of tissue in lymph nodes or excised lung.[608]

A definitive histologic diagnosis also depends to some extent on the number of sections examined in excised tumors. In one investigation, 100 consecutive cases of pulmonary carcinoma were examined by five pathologists.[598] Either the entire tumor or 10 blocks of tissue were available for each case; all pathologists examined each slide and gave a diagnosis on the basis of the 1981 WHO classification, according to the predominant histologic pattern and any other patterns present. There was unanimity in typing of

major categories (i.e., squamous cell carcinoma, small cell carcinoma, large cell carcinoma, and adenocarcinoma) in 53% of slides; a majority concurrence (i.e., ≥ 3 observers agreeing) was present in 94%. Unanimity was achieved in the distinction between small cell and non–small cell carcinoma in 93% of the slides. Although these figures indicate good diagnostic agreement between observers, in only 34 cases was the tumor considered to have a single histologic pattern; in 45% of tumors, more than one major histologic pattern was found, and in a further 21%, there were minor variations in subtype within a major category. These findings emphasize the importance of adequate sampling before histologic diagnosis is considered definitive and indicate the difficulty that may occur in precisely classifying individual neoplasms. Such histologic heterogeneity is accompanied in some cases by differences in the gross appearance of the tumor and in its immunohistochemical and molecular characteristics (Fig. 31–2).[593, 609]

It is clear that there are valid and important criticisms of the WHO classification of lung carcinoma from both conceptual and practical viewpoints. Nevertheless, the schema is fairly easy to use, shows reasonable correlation with clinical and radiologic findings, can be applied without the use of relatively expensive and time-consuming procedures such as electron microscopy, and is recognized throughout the world. Therefore, the following discussion is based on this classification.

Squamous Cell Carcinoma

Although formerly the most common subtype of pulmonary carcinoma, squamous cell carcinoma has decreased in incidence in many areas since the 1960s and now is generally believed to be second to adenocarcinoma in overall frequency, constituting approximately 30% of all pulmonary carcinomas.

Gross and Histologic Features

Squamous cell carcinoma originates most frequently in a segmental or lobar bronchus.[611, 612] Early lesions, consisting of squamous cell carcinoma *in situ* or minimally invasive carcinoma, may be grossly undetectable or may be recognized as a white, plaquelike swelling or a fine granularity of the bronchial mucosa;[613] such findings appear to be more easily detected at bronchial carinae. These lesions may extend for a considerable distance within the mucosa without significant growth into the airway lumen or invasion of peribronchial tissue;[614] eventually, however, most grow into the bronchial lumen as polypoid or papillary tumors (Fig. 31–3). Rarely, a carcinoma is identified in which there is partial or complete luminal obstruction but little or no invasion of the bronchial wall (Fig. 31–4);[615] much more commonly, tumor has invaded the submucosal and peribronchial connective tissue at the time it becomes evident clinically.

Because of the intraluminal growth, airway obstruction is an almost invariable feature of squamous cell carcinoma; consequently, distal atelectasis, bronchiectasis, and obstructive pneumonitis are present to some degree in most patients at presentation (Fig. 31–5). Proximal extension of tumor from a segmental bronchus or growth of a carcinoma that

Text continued on page 1090

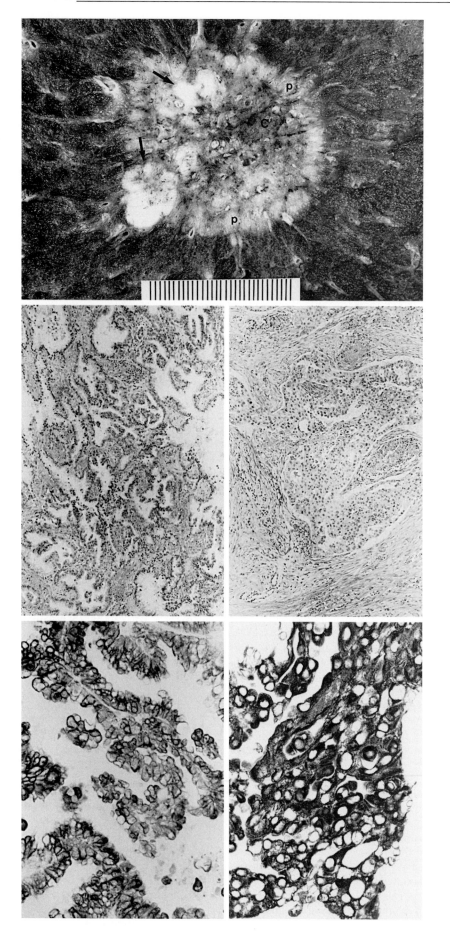

Figure 31–2. Adenocarcinoma—Variable Morphologic Appearance. A magnified view of a peripheral pulmonary adenocarcinoma *(A)* shows three different patterns: a relatively dark central area (c), a peripheral rim of gray tissue (p), and two somewhat lobulated white nodules *(arrows)*. Histologic examination showed the area in p to be composed of well-differentiated carcinoma with a bronchioloalveolar pattern *(B)*. Tumor in c consisted of nests of moderately differentiated carcinoma in a fibroblastic stroma *(C)*. The white nodules showed poorly differentiated carcinoma with focal necrosis (not illustrated). Immunoperoxidase reactions for cytokeratin were positive in the apical cytoplasm of the p tumor *(D)* and throughout the cytoplasm in the *p* variant *(E)*.

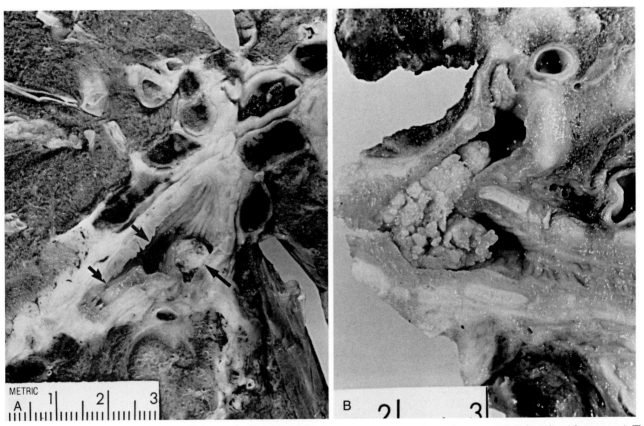

Figure 31–3. Squamous Cell Carcinoma. An oblique section of lower lobe segmental bronchi *(A)* shows two patent branches *(short arrows)*. The origin of a third *(long arrow)* is completely occluded by a polypoid squamous cell carcinoma. A longitudinal section of lower lobe segmental bronchi from another case *(B)* shows a finely papillary tumor occluding two branches.

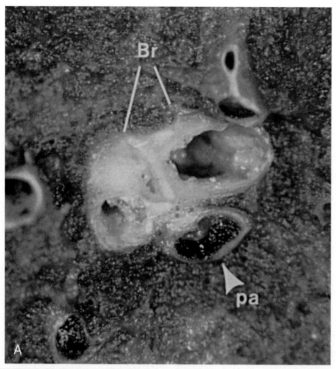

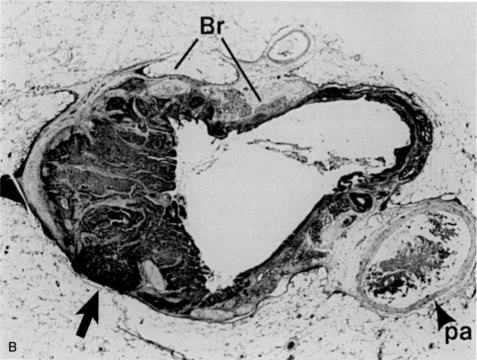

Figure 31–4. Early Squamous Cell Carcinoma. A highly magnified view of two subsegmental bronchi (Br) and their accompanying pulmonary arteries (pa) *(A)* shows partial occlusion of one branch by a solid, white tumor. A section through the tumor *(B)* shows it to extend into the submucosa *(arrow);* however, it has not spread beyond the confines of the bronchial wall. (From Foster WL, Roberts L, McLendon RF, Hill RC: Am J Roentgenol 144:906, 1985.)

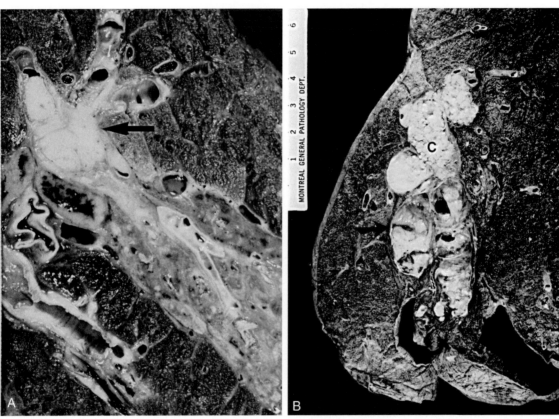

Figure 31–5. Squamous Cell Carcinoma—Obstructive Pneumonitis and Bronchiectasis. A magnified view of a slice of an upper lobe *(A)* shows segmental bronchi to be occluded by tumor that is largely confined to the airway lumen (focal extension into peribronchial tissue is evident *[arrow]*). The anterior segment shows obstructive pneumonitis. A slice of lower lobe from another patient *(B)* also shows carcinoma (C) confined to and distending segmental bronchi. Distal bronchi are markedly ectatic and partly filled with mucus, and the parenchyma is atelectatic.

originates in a lobar or main bronchus can result in collapse of a lobe or even a whole lung (Fig. 31–6). As the carcinoma increases further in size and invades the adjacent lung parenchyma, the original bronchial origin may or may not be apparent (Fig. 31–7). In larger tumors, central necrosis is frequent and may be extensive; drainage of necrotic material leads to cavitation in some cases (Fig. 31–8).

Histologically, carcinoma *in situ* is usually manifested as a thickened epithelium of squamous cells in which nuclear atypia is present from the most basal to the most apical cells (Fig. 31–9).[616, 617] Extension of the neoplasm into bronchial glands without actual tissue invasion is not uncommon (Fig. 31–9); on small endobronchial biopsy specimens, this can be confused with invasive carcinoma. Larger, clearly invasive neoplasms are recognized histologically as squamous cell carcinoma by the presence of intercellular bridges or keratinization (or both) (Fig. 31–10).[1] Such tumors vary from well-differentiated forms that show obvious and abundant keratinization to poorly differentiated forms that may be difficult to distinguish from small or large cell carcinoma with confidence. Although a cobblestone-like arrangement

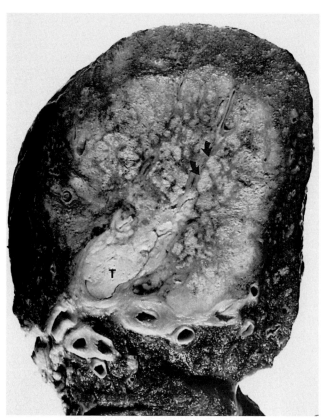

Figure 31–7. Squamous Cell Carcinoma. A slice of right upper lobe shows a fairly well-demarcated tumor that occupies a considerable portion of the parenchyma. Numerous foci of necrosis are evident *(arrows)*. A portion of the carcinoma can be seen within the lobar bronchus (T).

of polygonal cells is designated squamous cell carcinoma by some pathologists ("epidermoid" carcinoma), the presence of this pattern alone is not sufficient evidence of squamous cell differentiation according to the WHO classification.

Several histologic variants of squamous cell carcinoma can be identified. By definition, all show some areas of keratinization, intercellular bridge formation, or both; although the extent of such differentiation necessary to consider a tumor a squamous cell variant is arbitrary, a figure of at least 10% seems reasonable.[1] Depending on the particular histologic pattern, these variants have been termed *papillary*, *clear cell*, *basaloid*, and *small cell*.[1] The last-named is the most important from a diagnostic point of view because of its resemblance to small cell carcinoma. Distinction between the two can be difficult, particularly on small biopsy specimens, and rests predominantly on the presence of a slightly larger cell size, more clumped nuclear chromatin, more prominent nucleoli, and more distinct cell borders in squamous cell carcinoma. Tumors that have a spindle cell (sarcomatoid) component as well as squamous cell carcinoma are now classified as pleomorphic carcinoma (*see* page 1114).

Squamous cell carcinoma is usually an invasive, destructive neoplasm that obliterates the underlying lung parenchyma as it grows. Rarely, a tumor extends along the parenchymal framework without destroying it, as in bronchioloalveolar carcinoma. In contrast to the latter tumor, however, it usually expands to fill the air spaces completely rather than simply lining them. Although such growth is

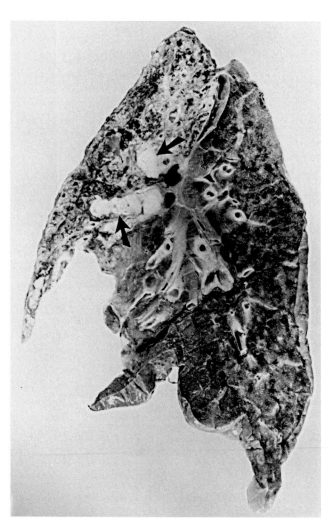

Figure 31–6. Squamous Cell Carcinoma—Lobar Collapse. A slice of the left lung near the hilum shows marked collapse and consolidation of the upper lobe (chronic obstructive pneumonitis). Squamous cell carcinoma appears as a solid white tumor within segmental airways *(arrows)*.

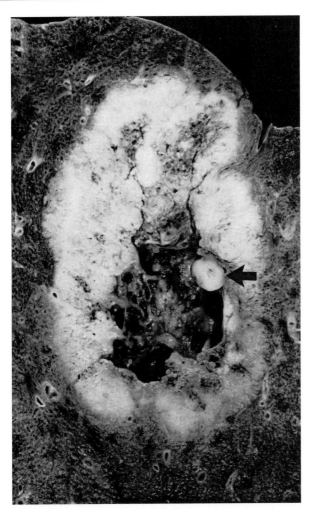

Figure 31–8. Squamous Cell Carcinoma—Cavitation. A large neoplasm arising in an upper lobe possesses a prominent central cavity. The shaggy appearance of the cavity wall is caused by the patchy nature of the necrosis and by nodules of residual viable neoplasm growing into the cavity itself *(arrow).*

usually minimal in extent, exceptionally it may involve entire bronchopulmonary segments.[618]

Ultrastructural Features

The ultrastructure of squamous cell carcinoma has been described by several authors.[619–621] Well-differentiated forms have ample cytoplasm, usually with relatively sparse endoplasmic reticulum, mitochondria, and Golgi complexes but with abundant polyribosomes and intermediate filaments (Fig. 31–11). The latter are typically aggregated into dense, often curved, bundles, many of which attach to well-developed desmosomes. Less well-differentiated tumors show fewer desmosomes and intermediate filaments and an increased proportion of other cytoplasmic organelles. Occasional cells have glandular features, especially in poorly differentiated tumors.[620–623] Unusual granules, some projecting from the cell surface and others associated with mitochondria, have been noted in some cases.[620, 624] Membrane-bound neurosecretory-like granules have also been identified in some tumors;[620, 625] it has been hypothesized that they relate to parathormone production.[625]

Immunohistochemical Features

Virtually all tumors show positive reactions to antikeratin antibodies. The reaction to high-molecular-weight keratin tends to be strong in well-differentiated tumors (i.e., in areas of keratinization), but weak and focal in more poorly differentiated ones.[622, 626, 627] The reaction to carcinoembryonic antigen (CEA) and epithelial membrane antigen is also positive in many cases.[615, 628] Immunoreactive parathormone-like substances have been identified in some tumors.[625]

Small Cell Carcinoma

Small cell carcinoma is an aggressive pulmonary neoplasm that comprises about 15% to 20% of all pulmonary carcinomas. A number of observations indicate that it is a neuroendocrine tumor, including the ultrastructural demonstration of neurosecretory granules,[629] the presence of action potentials in cultured tumor cells similar to those of nerve and muscle,[630] immunohistochemical evidence of cytoplasmic neurofilaments[631] and other neural antigens,[632] and clinical and experimental evidence of the presence and secretion of a variety of polypeptide hormones.[633, 634] Despite these observations, there is little evidence to indicate a direct derivation of the tumor from the normal bronchial neuroendocrine cell; instead, it is widely believed that it is derived from an undifferentiated airway epithelial cell that has the capacity for a variety of forms of differentiation, including neuroendocrine. The identification of squamous and glandular differentiation by both light and electron microscopy in some small cell carcinomas[635, 636] and the electron microscopic and immunohistochemical demonstration of neurosecretory granules and neuroendocrine-associated polypeptides in some non–small cell carcinomas[593, 637, 638] strongly support this hypothesis.

Gross and Histologic Features

Small cell carcinoma is typically located in relation to proximal airways, particularly lobar and main bronchi (Fig. 31–12);[639, 640] occasional tumors (<5%) arise in the lung periphery without an obvious airway association.[641, 642] In the early stage, centrally located tumors tend to be poorly delimited and spread in the submucosa and peribronchovascular connective tissue. As they grow, they extend into the adjacent lung parenchyma and become a more circumscribed mass that obliterates underlying airways and vessels. Endobronchial growth is seen much less frequently than in squamous cell carcinoma; in fact, when airway obstruction occurs, it is usually as a result of compression by the expanding tumor rather than intraluminal growth (Fig. 31–13). Invasion of small blood vessels and lymphatics is evident in most tumors at an early stage, and local lymphangitic spread is not uncommon in the adjacent lung. In addition, regional bronchopulmonary and hilar lymph nodes are almost invariably enlarged as a result of metastatic or invasive carcinoma.

Histologically, three subtypes have been defined by the International Association for the Study of Lung Cancer (IASLC) in 1988—small, mixed, and combined.[643] The first of these encompasses the former WHO oat cell and interme-

Text continued on page 1096

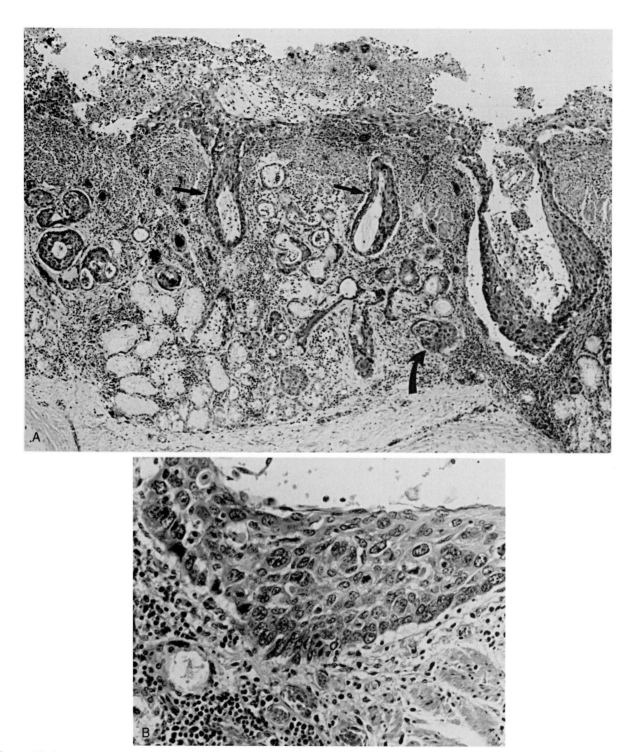

Figure 31–9. Squamous Cell Carcinoma *in Situ*. The surface epithelium of this segmental bronchus *(A)* is partly ulcerated and covered by an acute inflammatory exudate (related to infectious bronchitis). What remains consists of cytologically atypical squamous cells situated entirely above the basement membrane (seen at higher magnification in *B*). Tumor that is present in the mucosa represents extension into bronchial gland ducts *(short arrows)* and acini *(long arrow)* rather than true tissue invasion. *(A,* ×40; *B,* ×250.)

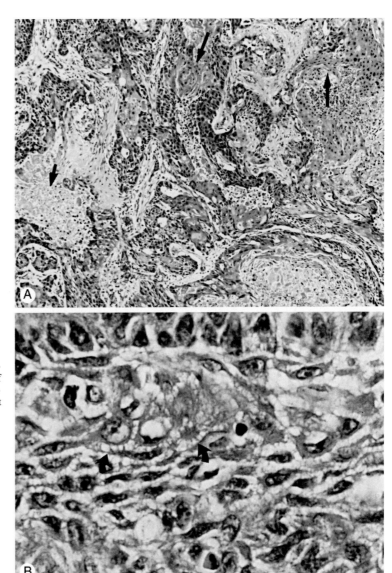

Figure 31–10. Squamous Cell Carcinoma. This moderately differentiated tumor *(A)* shows interconnecting sheets of cells with necrosis *(short arrow)* and multiple foci of keratinization *(long arrows)*. A magnified view *(B)* reveals prominent intercellular bridges *(arrows)*. (A, ×52; B, ×800.)

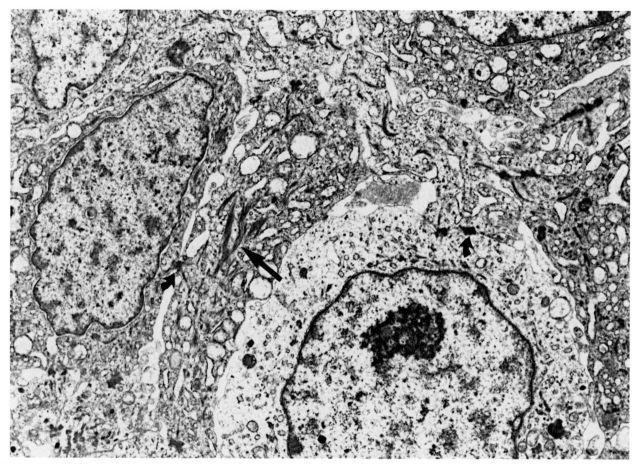

Figure 31–11. Squamous Cell Carcinoma—Ultrastructure. A cluster of several malignant cells shows well-developed intercellular junctions *(short arrows)* and prominent cytoplasmic filaments grouped focally into small aggregates *(long arrow).* (×21,000.)

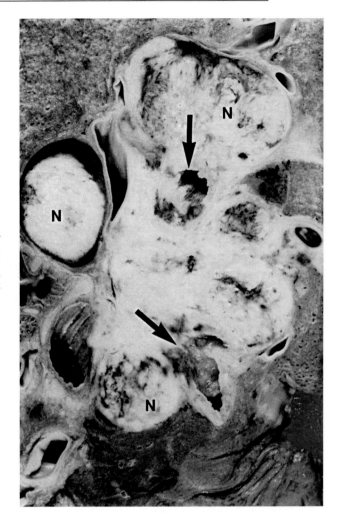

Figure 31–12. Small Cell Carcinoma. A magnified view of the perihilar region of a slice of right lung shows a centrally located tumor that involves lymph nodes (N) and adjacent interstitial tissue; airways *(arrows)* are surrounded and compressed by the tumor but lack the intraluminal growth typical of squamous cell carcinoma. The lung was removed at autopsy from a patient who had had no treatment.

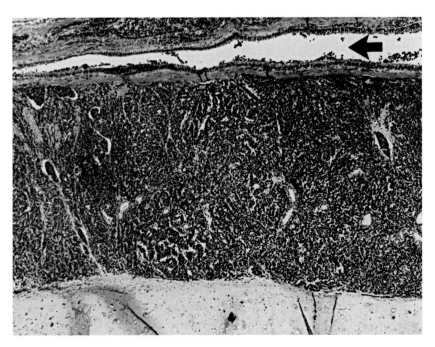

Figure 31–13. Small Cell Carcinoma. A section of a lobar bronchus reveals extensive infiltration of the submucosa by a uniform population of small cells with hyperchromatic nuclei. The surface epithelium is intact, and the bronchial lumen is compressed to a minute slit *(arrow).* (×40.)

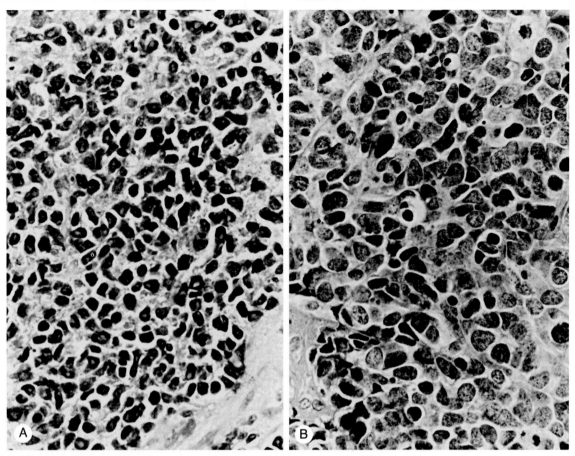

Figure 31–14. Small Cell Carcinoma. Photomicrographs are from different areas in the same carcinoma. Tumor cells in *A* have densely hyperchromatic nuclei and are about one half to one third the size of the cells in *B*. Nuclei in *B* have dispersed, finely granular chromatin and inconspicuous nucleoli. Nuclear molding is evident focally in both, indicative of scanty cytoplasm. The appearance corresponds to the patterns previously designated *oat cell* and *intermediate cell.* (*A, B,* ×500.)

diate types* and consists of cells approximately two to three times the size of a mature lymphocyte. Cytoplasm is scanty, a feature that is often reflected in molding of adjacent cell nuclei (particularly in cytologic specimens). The nuclei themselves may be small and hyperchromatic (corresponding to the oat cell pattern of previous histologic classifications) or may be somewhat vesicular with finely stippled and dispersed chromatin (Fig. 31–14); nucleoli are usually inconspicuous. Tumor cells may be round or fusiform in shape and may be arranged in small clusters, sheets, or anastomosing cords; rosettes are seen occasionally. Stroma is typically scanty, and a desmoplastic reaction and inflammatory cellular infiltrate usually are absent or minimal in extent.

---

*In the 1981 WHO classification of small cell carcinoma, oat cell carcinoma was distinguished from a variant composed of larger cells that had more vesicular, less hyperchromatic nuclei (the intermediate subtype). The observations, however, that cells with hyperchromatic and vesicular nuclei are both seen in some tumors, that interconversion between the two "subtypes" can be seen in tissue culture,[644] that morphometric measurements show a continuum of nuclear and cell size rather than two distinct cell populations,[645, 646] that most investigators have found few or no differences in clinical features or prognosis between the subtypes,[647] and that there is considerable interobserver variation in distinguishing the two patterns[597, 598] all indicate that the distinction between oat cell and intermediate cell types serves little practical purpose and is probably incorrect. As a result, members of IASLC recommended that the two subtypes be considered under the single term *small cell carcinoma*.[643]

Necrosis is common and may be associated with pronounced basophilic staining of blood vessels in the necrotic regions; this finding is caused by incorporation of DNA from necrotic tumor cells in vascular connective tissue and is itself highly suggestive of small cell carcinoma (Fig. 31–15). Artefactual tumor crushing is also common, especially in tissue obtained by endoscopic biopsy; although diagnosis can be difficult in this circumstance, the presence of areas of crushed, hyperchromatic cells is in itself suggestive of small cell carcinoma,[648] and examination of multiple levels almost invariably reveals one or more clusters that are sufficiently preserved to provide a definitive diagnosis. The presence of crush artefact is probably related to a combination of the biopsy procedure, the minimal stroma of the tumor, and the relatively scanty cytoplasm of the tumor cells.

Minute foci of glandular or squamous differentiation may be identified in some tumors, a finding that does not alter the diagnosis of typical small cell carcinoma. In rare instances, however, such foci comprise a significant proportion of the tumor (Fig. 31–16), in which case it is classified as *combined small cell carcinoma*.[643] (A single case in which the combined component had a spindle cell pattern has also been reported.[649]) The precise figure corresponding to *significant* is not well defined, but should probably be at least 10%. This variant is uncommon, constituting no more than about 1% to 3% of all small cell carcinomas.[601, 650]

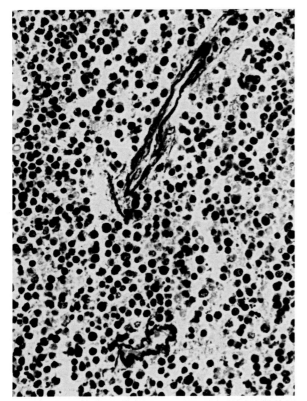

Figure 31–15. Small Cell Carcinoma—Necrosis and DNA Staining. A focus of necrotic tumor cells surrounds two small blood vessels whose walls are outlined by strongly basophilic DNA. (×400.)

Clinical features are similar to those of typical small cell carcinoma;[650] however, there is evidence that they may be more common in the lung periphery than typical tumors and, after resection, may have a better prognosis.[650] Care must be taken in making this diagnosis on small tissue samples, particularly bronchial biopsy specimens. Squamous metaplasia, sometimes with atypia, is frequent in the bronchial epithelium overlying small cell carcinoma; occasionally, the tumor and epithelium are admixed, giving the impression of a combined tumor. Although it is possible that this bronchial epithelial abnormality is related to an effect of tobacco smoke, there is evidence that it may be the result of production of epidermal growth factor by the tumor cells.[610]

A small cell carcinoma may also contain cells, either singly or in clusters, that resemble those of large cell carcinoma (Fig. 31–17); such tumors have been classified as mixed small cell/large cell carcinoma in the classification proposed by IASLC.[643] (In the 1999 WHO schema, these tumors are considered in the same category as combined small cell carcinoma.[1]) As with combined small cell tumors, the precise amount of the large cell component necessary for the diagnosis is uncertain; however, some investigators have stated that as little as 1% is all that is required.[601] This variant is also uncommon, constituting only 5% of small cell tumors in one review.[601] There is evidence from tissue culture studies that the presence of two morphologically different cell types is reflected in different functional characteristics.[652] Although a number of investigators have also found these tumors to have a different natural history from that of other small cell tumors, some have found the prognosis to be better[601] and others worse.[653–655] Large, often irregularly shaped, multinucleated tumor giant cells have also been identified in some small cell carcinomas. In some cases, these may be secondary to irradiation, but in a small proportion they appear to be an inherent feature of the tumor itself.[656]

There is evidence that chemotherapy may affect the morphologic appearance of small cell carcinoma.[657, 658] For example, in one review of 50 consecutive cases of biopsy-proven tumors, evidence of squamous differentiation was found in 5 of 21 patients who underwent autopsy.[659] In another study of 40 autopsied patients, 5 showed features of non–small cell carcinoma—3 squamous cell, 1 adenocarcinoma, and 1 large cell;[660] changes were also demonstrated in the biochemical characteristics of the tumors. Although these observations suggest an effect of chemotherapy on tumor morphology, a similar incidence of histologic changes at autopsy has been documented in patients who have received no intensive chemotherapy.[640]

Ultrastructural Features

Electron microscopic examination of small cell carcinomas shows nuclei to occupy most of the cell volume and to

Figure 31–16. Small Cell Carcinoma—Combined Subtype. A section of a grossly typical, central small cell carcinoma shows a combination of small cells with hyperchromatic nuclei and larger cells that focally show clear-cut squamous differentiation *(arrow).* (×300.)

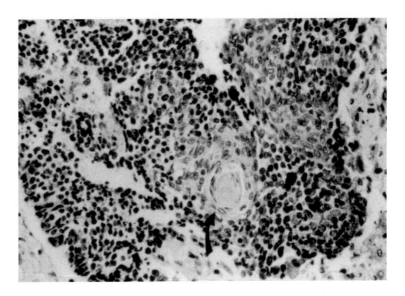

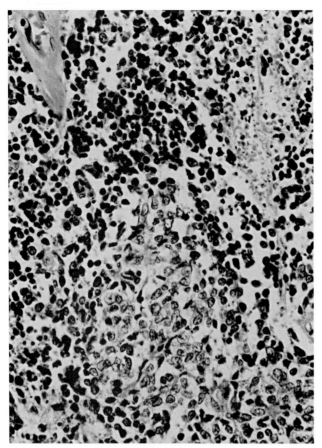

Figure 31–17. Small Cell Carcinoma—Combined Subtype. A magnified view of a bronchial biopsy specimen shows a combination of small cells with hyperchromatic nuclei typical of small cell carcinoma and larger cells without evidence of specific differentiation. This pattern is variably designated *small cell/large cell carcinoma* or *combined small cell carcinoma.*

have dispersed chromatin (Fig. 31–18).[629, 646] Intercellular junctions are generally few and poorly developed; in one study, the presence of well-formed junctions correlated with lower stage and longer survival.[662] Cytoplasm is scanty and usually contains few organelles, although polyribosomes and smooth endoplasmic reticulum are occasionally abundant.[629]

Neurosecretory granules resembling those found in normal neuroendocrine cells of the airway epithelium are found in many cases. They are generally fewer in number and smaller in size than those in carcinoid tumors[663] and are frequently identified in only a small proportion of cells in any particular tumor.[629] Although such granules have been found in almost all cases examined by some authors,[629, 637, 664–666] they have been identified in as few as 30% of those studied by others.[640] Some investigators have suggested that there may be different subtypes of small cell carcinoma based on the morphology of their neurosecretory granules.[667, 668]

Although the previous description is characteristic of the ultrastructural appearance of small cell carcinoma, a small number of cases that are otherwise typical of the tumor at the light microscopic level show ultrastructural features indicative of another form of cytologic differentiation. In addition to the presence of neurosecretory granules, some of these tumors show well-developed intercellular junctions,

cytoplasmic filaments, and intracytoplasmic lumen formation indicative of squamous or glandular differentiation;[622, 635, 646, 669] others show evidence of only squamous or glandular differentiation without neurosecretory granules.[622, 636, 646, 666] Many of these tumors arise in the periphery of the lung; because of the small number of well-documented cases, it is not certain that they represent entities different from pure small cell carcinoma in terms of either response to therapy or natural history.

Immunohistochemical Features

Many small cell carcinomas express markers of neuroendocrine differentiation, such as chromogranin, synaptophysin, and Leu-7.[670, 671] For example, in two investigations of 96 tumors, Leu-7 was detected in 24 of 36 and 31 of 60.[646, 672] In another study of bronchial and open-lung biopsy specimens, positive reactions for chromogranin were detected in 47% and 60%, for Leu-7 in 24% and 40%, and for synaptophysin in 19% and 5%.[670] Most tumors are also positive for CEA and keratin.[670] Many tumors can be shown to have abnormal P53 expression.[673]

A variety of specific neuropeptides have also been identified immunohistochemically in small cell carcinomas. In one study of 33 cases, a positive reaction for one or more of these substances was found in 16, the most common being gastrin-releasing peptide (bombesin), vasoactive intestinal polypeptide, serotonin, and adrenocorticotropic hormone (ACTH);[634] somatostatin and calcitonin were found less frequently. In many cases, several peptides can be identified sometimes, different ones are found in primary and metastatic tumors. The alpha subunit of human chorionic gonadotropin was identified in 9 of 13 tumors in one study.[674] Corticotropin-releasing hormone has been found infrequently—for example, in only 1 of 30 neoplasms in another investigation.[675]

Adenocarcinoma

Pulmonary adenocarcinoma is a neoplasm of varied appearance and histogenesis that is divided into four principal histologic subtypes in the WHO classification—acinar carcinoma, papillary carcinoma, solid carcinoma with mucin formation, and bronchioloalveolar carcinoma.[1] The last-named can be further divided into mucinous and nonmucinous variants.[676] Although the histologic patterns corresponding to all these subgroups are usually easily identifiable, the distinctiveness of the subgroups themselves is open to question. In fact, many investigators consider a more realistic division to be into two types—bronchioloalveolar carcinoma and nonbronchioloalveolar carcinoma. As a group, adenocarcinomas are generally the most common histologic form of pulmonary carcinoma, constituting about 30% to 35% of all cases.

There are several reasons for considering the WHO subgroups as indistinct. First, a mixture of two or more histologic patterns is common in many tumors.[598, 677, 678] That this is the case with the bronchioloalveolar cell pattern as well as the others should not be surprising; because metastatic carcinoma can mimic the pattern of bronchioloalveolar carcinoma,[679, 680] it seems logical that some primary acinar

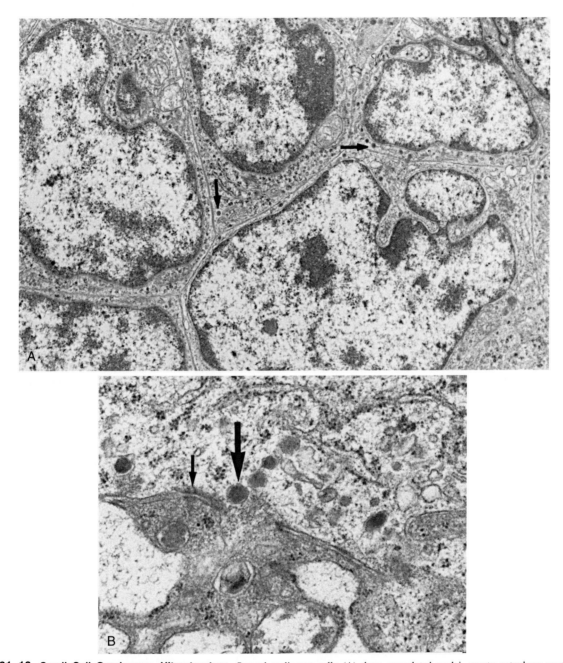

Figure 31–18. Small Cell Carcinoma—Ultrastructure. Several malignant cells *(A)* show convoluted nuclei, scanty cytoplasm containing few organelles, and poorly developed intercellular junctions. Occasional neurosecretory granules are present within the cytoplasm. A magnified view *(B)* depicts an intercellular junction *(short arrow)* and neurosecretory granules *(long arrow)* to better advantage. (A, ×22,800; B, ×69,000.)

or solid adenocarcinomas of the lung should also at times be able to assume a bronchioloalveolar carcinoma pattern. Second, apart from the diffuse form of bronchioloalveolar carcinoma, there is little difference in radiologic or clinical features of the histologic types. Finally, there is little correlation between the histochemical and ultrastructural features of the tumor cells and the light microscopic pattern.[623, 681–684] At the present time, it is thus uncertain whether the principal histologic subtypes of the WHO classification have any substantial clinical or pathologic significance,[685] the exceptions being the solitary nodule that shows a pure bronchioloalveolar growth pattern, the more diffuse form of bronchioloalveolar carcinoma, and (possibly) tumors having a predominantly papillary appearance.[685a]

Other classification schemes of adenocarcinoma based on presumed histogenesis[686] and on cellular morphology and tumor location[678] have also been proposed. Several rare histologic variants or patterns are also classified as adenocarcinoma in the WHO schema, including clear cell carcinoma, colloid carcinoma, mucinous cystadenocarcinoma (*see* page 1265), signet-ring cell carcinoma, and well-differentiated fetal adenocarcinoma (*see* page 1368).[1]

Histogenesis

The histogenesis of pulmonary adenocarcinoma is varied. Its typical peripheral location and lack of obvious association with major airways suggest that it arises from bronchiolar or alveolar epithelium, a hypothesis supported by the results of a variety of ultrastructural,[623, 681, 682] histochemical,[682] immunohistochemical,[687] and autoradiographic[688] studies. The most common feature of cellular differentiation identifiable by light microscopy is mucin secretion. Because

bronchiolar epithelium has the ability to undergo goblet cell metaplasia in response to a variety of noxious stimuli, it is perhaps not surprising that this inherent ability is expressed in neoplasms arising in this region.[623, 689] Clara cell differentiation, manifested by the presence of electron-dense, membrane-bound secretory granules, is present in many tumors,[681, 690] constituting additional evidence for an origin from bronchiolar epithelium. Occasional tumor cells show evidence of cilia formation (usually incomplete).[683, 689, 690] Ultrastructural[691, 692] or immunohistochemical[687, 693] features of type II cell differentiation can also be seen in some tumors.

The origin of more central adenocarcinomas, especially those clearly related to a major bronchus, is less well defined. Presumably, many originate in the surface epithelium, which normally shows glandular differentiation in the form of goblet cells.[694] On the basis of ultrastructural findings, it has also been hypothesized that some proximal adenocarcinomas may be derived from mucous cells of the bronchial glands.[682] In addition, some investigators have found evidence of both Clara and goblet cell differentiation in tumors in this location.[695] Rare bronchioloalveolar carcinomas develop in association with congenital cysts.[696, 697]

Gross and Histologic Features

Nonbronchioloalveolar Adenocarcinoma

The majority of pulmonary adenocarcinomas are located in the periphery of the lung, frequently in a subpleural location.[678] They are often well circumscribed, although an irregular spiculated appearance or clear-cut invasive foci are grossly apparent in some tumors (Fig. 31–19). Focal fibrosis

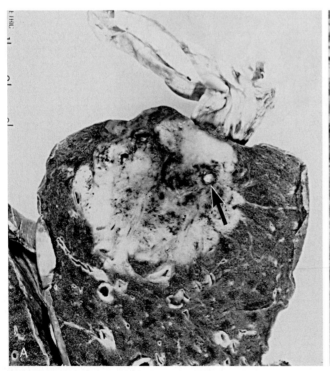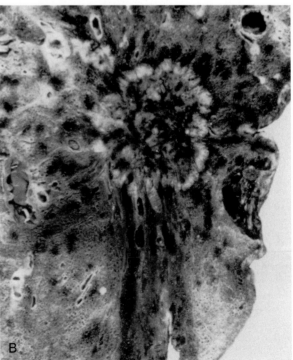

Figure 31–19. Adenocarcinoma. A well-circumscribed tumor *(A)* is present in the apex of the upper lobe immediately adjacent to the pleura. Although it has not extended through the pleura, an inflammatory reaction has caused adhesions. A small focus of remote granulomatous inflammation is incorporated into the tumor mass *(arrow)*. A tumor from another patient *(B)* shows a spiculated appearance caused by irregular outgrowths of tumor into the parenchyma.

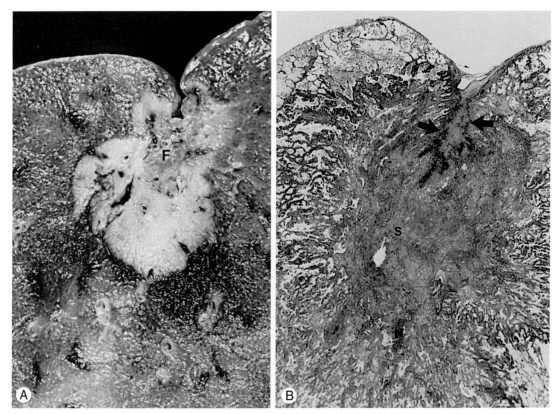

Figure 31–20. Adenocarcinoma with Central Scar and Pleural Puckering. A magnified view *(A)* of a small peripheral carcinoma shows prominent pleural puckering adjacent to a region of fibrosis (F); the latter is surrounded by the carcinoma. A similar appearance can be seen histologically *(B)* in which a focus of fibrous tissue (S) is surrounded by a tumor that lines the alveolar septa (bronchioloalveolar carcinoma). The adjacent pleura *(arrows)* is also fibrotic and has been drawn into the central portion of the scar. (×10.)

is often present in the central portion of the tumor adjacent to the pleura, resulting in a puckered appearance both grossly and microscopically (Fig. 31–20).[698] Although foci of necrosis are fairly common, especially in the larger tumors, only rarely do these become confluent and result in cavitation. Pure adenocarcinoma arising in relation to a major airway is uncommon;[678, 695] when it does occur in this location, it is indistinguishable grossly from squamous cell carcinoma. Spread of individual tumor cells within the bronchial epithelium in a fashion analogous to Paget's disease of the nipple has been reported.[699] Rare mucin-secreting pulmonary tumors have a prominent cystic component; because many of these behave in an indolent fashion, they have been termed *mucinous cystic tumors* rather than *mucinous adenocarcinoma (see* page 1265).[700]

The histologic pattern of nonbronchioloalveolar carcinoma is as indicated in the WHO classification—acini or tubules (with or without intraluminal mucin formation), papillae, or sheets of cells without structural evidence of glandular differentiation (Fig. 31–21). The last-named can be distinguished from large cell carcinoma only by the presence of intracellular mucin in a significant proportion of tumor cells. According to one group of investigators, about 50% to 60% of tumors are acinar in type, 10% are papillary, and 10% to 15% are solid (the remaining cases being bronchioloalveolar or unclassifiable).[701, 702]

Globular eosinophilic, intracytoplasmic inclusions can be seen in some tumors (although they are not specific for adenocarcinoma); in one review of 100 consecutive cases,

these were identified in 6.[703] They may be periodic acid–Schiff (PAS) positive, and some react with antibodies to alpha$_1$-antitrypsin.[703] Histologic findings seen occasionally in association with otherwise typical adenocarcinoma include signet-ring cells,[704] clear cells,[705, 706] choriocarcinoma,[707] and spindle or giant cells (pleomorphic carcinoma, *see* page 1114).[708]

Bronchioloalveolar Carcinoma

Tumors that have a pure bronchioloalveolar pattern histologically may present as a solitary nodule (often in a subpleural location and associated with pleural retraction and a central scar) or as a poorly defined area of parenchymal consolidation (often in association with the mucinous subtype).[708a] The nature of such tumors can often be suspected grossly by the characteristic nondestructive growth. This is somewhat more difficult to appreciate when the lesion is a small nodule; however, when tumor involves more than one or two secondary lobules, underlying anatomic structures such as airways, vessels, and interlobular septa can be readily identified despite being surrounded by tumor (Fig. 31–22). When extensive, this appearance can simulate airspace pneumonia (Fig. 31–23).

Histologically a bronchioloalveolar growth pattern is characterized by tumor cells that spread along the framework of the lung parenchyma without its destruction (Fig. 31–24). Although tumor cells often form a single layer, proliferation may result in crowding into the air space, leading to a

Text continued on page 1106

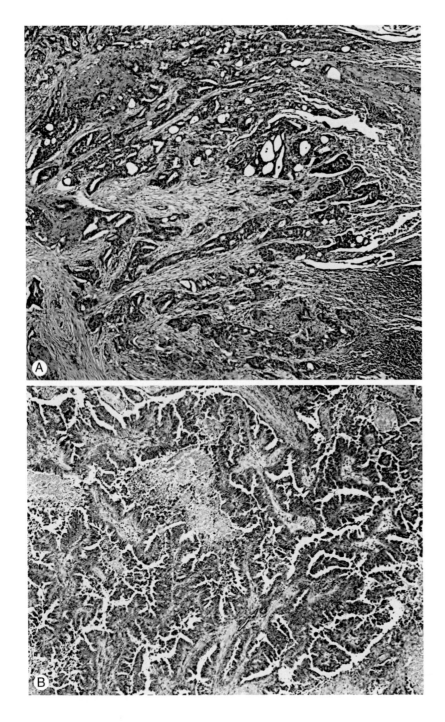

Figure 31–21. Adenocarcinoma. Histologic
sections show two different patterns of adenocarcinoma. In the acinar pattern *(A)*, round or elongated
spaces are almost completely surrounded by one or
two layers of tumor cells. A desmoplastic stromal
reaction is evident near the central portion of the
tumor. In the papillary pattern *(B)*, fibrovascular stalks
are lined by a single, somewhat irregular layer of
tumor cells. *(A, ×40; B, ×60.)*

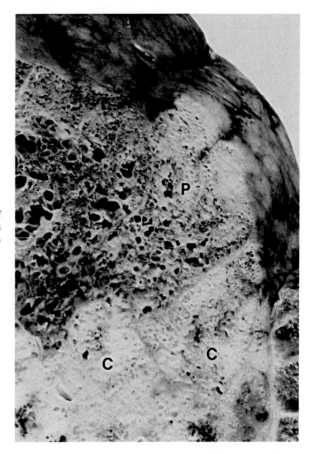

Figure 31–22. Bronchioloalveolar Carcinoma. A highly magnified view of an upper lobe shows complete (C) and partial (P) "consolidation" of several lobules by carcinoma. In both sites, vessels and small airways are patent, and the carcinoma appears to be spreading within the lung without destroying it.

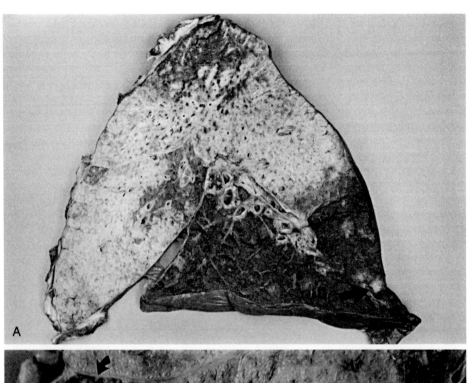

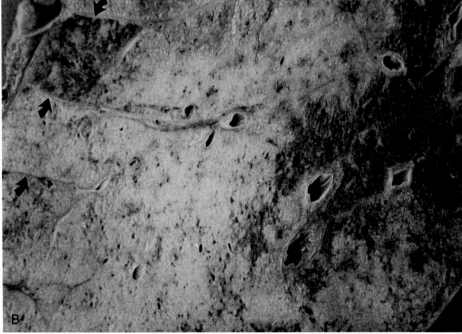

Figure 31–23. Bronchioloalveolar Carcinoma. A sagittal section of the right lung *(A)* shows almost complete "consolidation" of the upper and middle lobes and the superior segment of the lower lobe; several small nodular foci of disease are present in the base of the lower lobe *(arrow)*. On a magnified view *(B)*, the airways, vessels, and interlobular septa *(arrows)* are clearly visible within the tumor mass, indicating spread of carcinoma without destruction of the underlying lung.

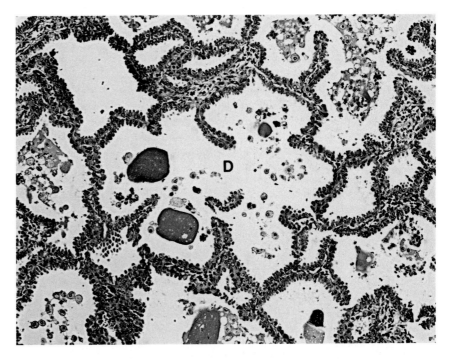

Figure 31–24. Bronchioloalveolar Carcinoma. The section shows an alveolar duct (D) and adjacent alveoli whose epithelium has been completely replaced by a population of cuboidal cells with mild nuclear atypia. Only a mild inflammatory reaction is evident in the interstitial tissue.

papillary appearance. The alveolar interstitium adjacent to the tumor may be virtually normal, but is commonly mildly to moderately thickened by a combination of fibrous tissue and a chronic inflammatory infiltrate (Fig. 31–25); when this fibrotic reaction is prominent, the tumors have been termed *sclerosing carcinoma* (Fig. 31–26).[709] One group of investigators found increased type IV collagenase activity and disruption or absence of basement membrane components adjacent to the neoplastic glands in the central (sclerotic) portion of such tumors;[710] they speculated that these abnormalities might be related to the increased incidence of lymph node metastases seen in this variant.

Individual tumor cells vary from cuboidal to columnar in appearance (*see* Fig. 31–25); cytoplasm may be abundant or sparse and may or may not contain mucin. Rarely, tumors contain abundant glycogen, creating the appearance of a clear cell carcinoma.[690] Variably sized PAS-positive granules in the apical cytoplasm have been found ultrastructurally to correspond to Clara cell differentiation.[709, 711] Similar granules can also be found occasionally in other forms of adenocarcinoma as well as in squamous cell and large cell tumors.[711]

Intra-alveolar secretions derived from the tumor cells may be absent or may be so abundant that they form the major proportion of the tumor volume and fill air spaces a considerable distance from the tumor cells (Fig. 31–27). Such secretions may consist of eosinophilic (proteinaceous) material or (more commonly) mucus. Not uncommonly, the latter substance contains small clusters of tumor cells that have detached from the alveolar walls; it is possible that spread of such "contaminated" material is at least partly responsible for the multifocality seen in some cases. Some investigators have found mucinous tumors to have lower levels of α_2 integrin receptors than other forms of bronchioloalveolar carcinoma, suggesting an explanation of the tendency for the detachment and spread of cells in this variant.[710]

Psammoma bodies can be seen in a small number of tumors, usually in association with a papillary component.[685a, 712] Rarely, they are sufficient in number to result in radiologically evident calcification;[713] their presence in specimens submitted for cytologic analysis occasionally aids in diagnosis.[714, 715] Intranuclear inclusions (sometimes PAS positive) are present in many cases (34% of 38 tumors in one series);[400] in some, they have been found to be associated with ultrastructural or immunohistochemical evidence of type II cell differentiation.[716] Ultrastructurally, the inclusions have been found to consist of cytoplasmic invaginations, membrane-bound granules, collections of 15-nm tubules,[400] or aggregates of dense bodies,[717] either alone or in various combinations. Rare tumors show evidence of neuroendocrine[718] or enteric[719] differentiation in addition to the typical glandular features. Cytologic features of bronchioloalveolar carcinoma have been described by several groups of investigators.[720–723]

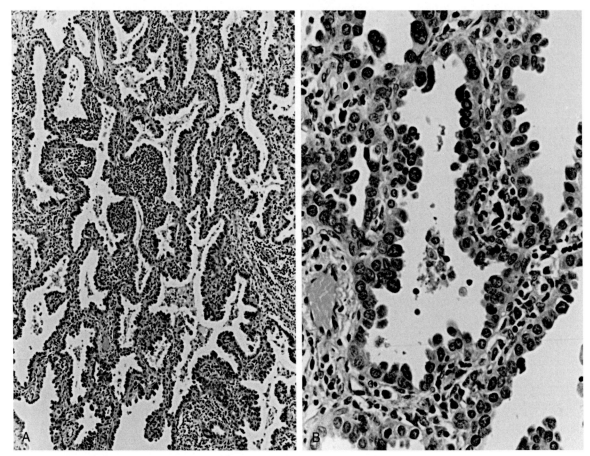

Figure 31–25. Bronchioloalveolar Carcinoma—Inflammatory Reaction. A section of a subpleural tumor *(A)* shows a moderate degree of interstitial thickening, predominantly by lymphocytes and to a lesser extent by fibrous tissue. The normal epithelium is replaced by a population of cuboidal cells with mild nuclear atypia *(B).* The air spaces show no evidence of tumor secretion.

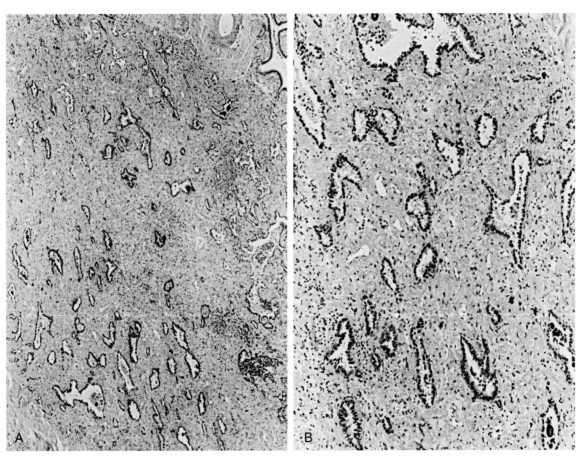

Figure 31–26. Bronchioloalveolar Carcinoma—Sclerosing Subtype. Views of a subpleural tumor *(A and B)* show a marked degree of interstitial thickening, predominantly by mature fibrous tissue. The fairly regular spacing of the glandlike structures indicates that they represent residual air spaces lined by neoplastic cells rather than neoplastic glands in a desmoplastic stroma. The air spaces show no evidence of tumor secretion.

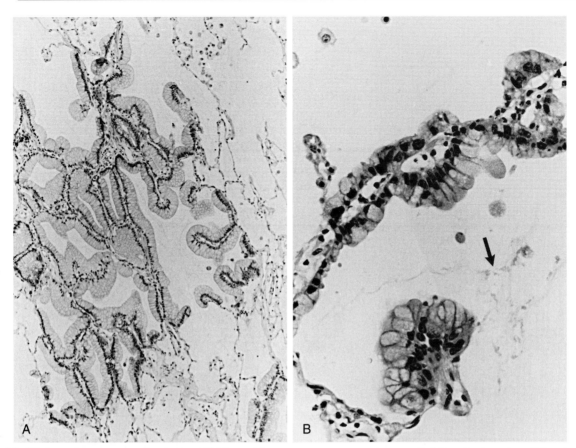

Figure 31–27. Bronchioloalveolar Carcinoma—Mucinous Type. Sections *(A* and *B)* show a well-differentiated neoplasm lining alveolar septa and composed of tall columnar cells with basal nuclei and abundant, mucin-containing cytoplasm. Although it is difficult to appreciate on these H&E-stained sections, the air spaces are filled with mucus (some of which is evident as thin strands in *B [arrow]*).

Focal Alveolar Epithelial Hyperplasia

Careful examination of the lung parenchyma at a distance from a resected adenocarcinoma (either bronchioloalveolar or nonbronchioloalveolar in type) may show small (1 to 5 mm), variably shaped, gray nodules.[724] Histologically, these correspond to foci of alveolar epithelial proliferation, usually associated with a mild degree of interstitial fibrosis (Fig. 31–28).[724–726] The epithelial cells resemble alveolar type II cells and may have uniform nuclei or show varying degrees of atypia; in some cases, the latter may be so marked that distinction from bronchioloalveolar carcinoma is not possible. This observation as well as the results of DNA ploidy analyses and molecular biologic studies[727–729a] strongly suggests that these foci are the result of hyperplasia and dysplasia and are analogous to the squamous metaplasia and dysplasia that occur in bronchi in association with squamous cell carcinoma.

These foci of atypical adenomatous hyperplasia are not uncommon; in two series of 247 carcinomas[724] and 175 adenocarcinomas,[725] they were documented in 23 (9%) and 10 (6%), respectively. In another review of 100 consecutive autopsies (none of which had evidence of pulmonary carcinoma), six cases of alveolar epithelial hyperplasia, two atypical, were identified.[730]

Ultrastructural Features

Ultrastructural features of adenocarcinoma vary with the degree and type of differentiation. In general, the tumors consist of columnar or cuboidal cells that have a variable number of short surface microvilli, relatively abundant endoplasmic reticulum and Golgi complexes, apical tight junctions, and more or less numerous cytoplasmic secretory granules (Fig. 31–29). As indicated previously, several types of granules have been identified—electron-lucent or flocculent inclusions (believed to be mucin and to represent goblet cell or bronchial gland mucous cell differentiation), electron-dense inclusions similar to those of Clara cells, lamellated inclusions similar to those of alveolar type II cells, and (rarely) lysosome-like granules that have been presumed to contain amylase.[686, 709, 731, 732] Some investigators have identified a combination of cell types in individual tumors,[709, 731, 731a] whereas others have found little mixture.[682, 686] In one study, no association was found between ultrastructural type and radiologic pattern or mortality.[731a] The scanning electron microscopic appearance has also been described.[733]

Immunohistochemical Features

Many pulmonary adenocarcinomas express CEA and keratins.[693, 720, 734–737] Approximately 40% to 60% of tumors express surfactant or Clara cell proteins, suggesting type II cell or Clara cell differentiation;[693, 738–741] although some of these proteins can also be found in large cell and squamous cell carcinoma (as in approximately 25% and 15% of cases in one investigation[740]), others appear to have a high degree of specificity for adenocarcinoma.[741] Additional substances that have been identified in a significant proportion of tu-

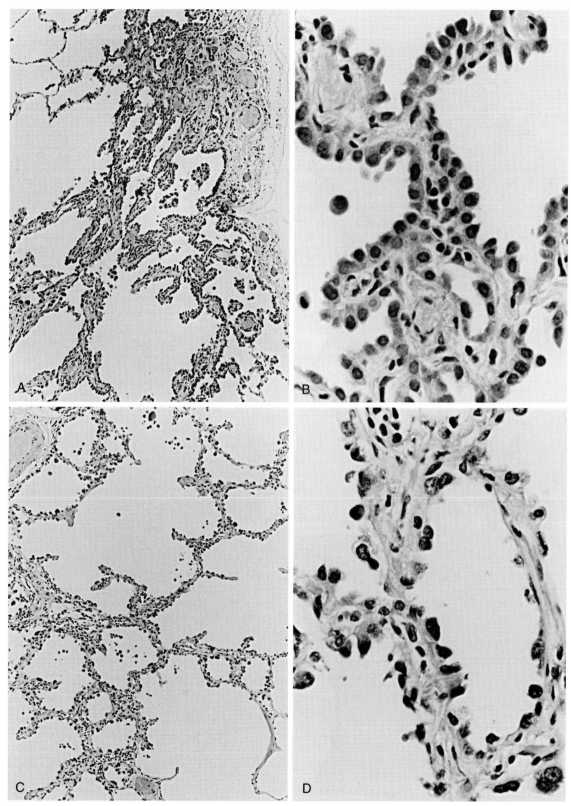

Figure 31–28. Alveolar Epithelial Hyperplasia. A small focus of subpleural lung parenchyma *(A)* shows a moderate degree of interstitial fibrosis associated with extensive type II cell hyperplasia. A magnified view *(B)* shows the cells to have small, fairly uniform nuclei. Photomicrographs taken of another lesion from the same specimen *(C, D)* show more pronounced nuclear atypia (atypical hyperplasia). The patient had a 2.5-cm nonmucinous bronchioloalveolar carcinoma in the resected lobe.

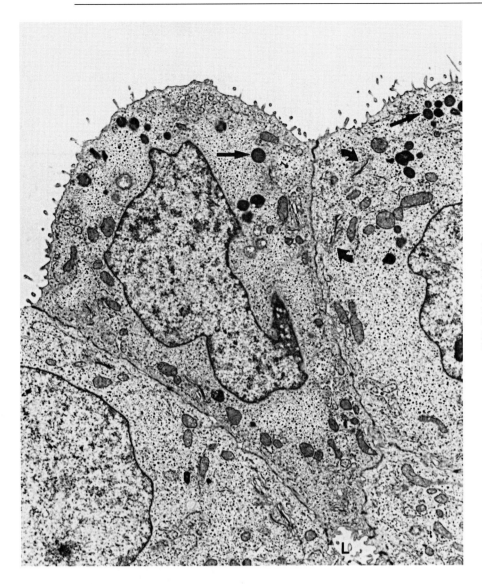

Figure 31–29. Bronchioloalveolar Carcinoma—Ultrastructure. Tumor cells have abundant cytoplasm containing occasional Golgi bodies *(curved arrows)* and electron-dense granules *(straight arrows)* suggestive of Clara cell differentiation. A small intercellular lumen is present at the basal aspect (L). The surface of the cells shows scattered, short microvilli.

mors (30% to 40%) include vimentin,[742] secretory component,[743, 744] and neuroendocrine markers such as chromogranin and synaptophysin;[745, 746] rarely identified substances include estrogen receptors[747] and protein S-100.[745] There is evidence that different histologic subtypes of bronchioloalveolar carcinoma have different immunohistochemical profiles[754] and that different immunohistochemical reactions are seen between bronchioloalveolar and nonbronchioloalveolar tumors.[723a]

Large Cell Carcinoma

According to the WHO classification, the diagnosis of large cell carcinoma is applied to tumors that do not possess the typical appearance of small cell carcinoma and have no evidence at the light microscopic level of either squamous or glandular differentiation. If these criteria are adhered to, the tumor constitutes about 10% to 15% of all pulmonary carcinomas. The incidence varies substantially, however, with the amount of tissue available for examination and the techniques used to study it. Although ultrastructural features

of glandular, neuroendocrine, and squamous cell differentiation are absent in some cases (Fig. 31–30), they are identified frequently, provided that enough tissue is examined, even when they cannot be appreciated by light microscopy.[593, 623, 748–752] Thus, if electron microscopic evidence of cytologic differentiation is used in tumor classification, the incidence of large cell carcinoma is substantially decreased;[593, 753] for example, in one series of 100 consecutive surgically excised carcinomas classified on this basis, no examples of large cell carcinoma were found.[623]

The incidence of large cell carcinoma also tends to diminish as the amount of tissue available for examination increases. Many cases of squamous cell or adenocarcinoma, particularly those that are more poorly differentiated, contain areas that do not exhibit specific cellular differentiation.[598, 753] If a diagnosis is made on small fragments of tissue, such as obtained by endoscopic biopsy or transthoracic needle aspiration, it may be impossible to identify the glandular or squamous features with confidence, and a "false" diagnosis of large cell carcinoma may result.

Grossly, large cell carcinomas tend to be bulky peripheral tumors (Fig. 31–31).[748, 753] Although multiple foci of

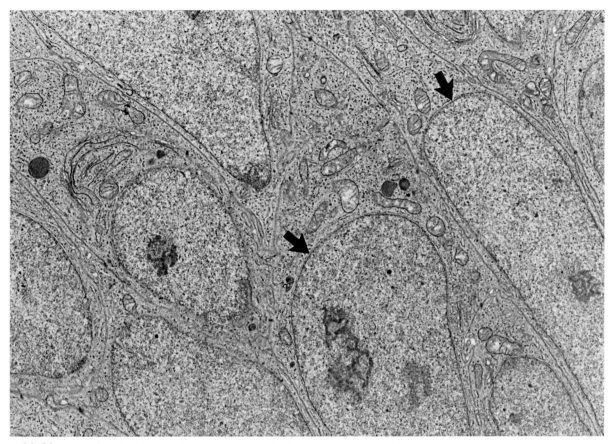

Figure 31–30. Large Cell Carcinoma—Ultrastructure. The section shows a cluster of malignant cells with large vesicular nuclei *(arrows)* and abundant cytoplasm that lacks features of glandular, squamous, or neuroendocrine differentiation. (×14,300.)

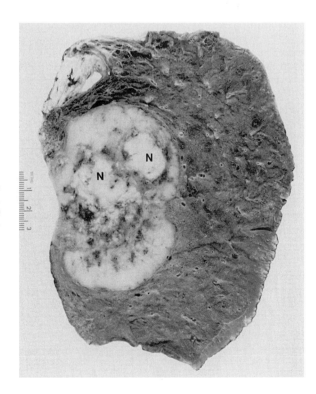

Figure 31–31. Large Cell Carcinoma. A resected upper lobe contains a large, well-circumscribed subpleural tumor with multiple foci of necrosis (N). Although characteristic of a large cell carcinoma, a lesion with this appearance cannot be reliably distinguished from adenocarcinoma or squamous cell carcinoma.

necrosis are characteristic, cavitation is uncommon. Histologically, the tumors consist of sheets of cells that usually contain abundant eosinophilic cytoplasm (Fig. 31–32). Nuclei are large and often vesicular with prominent nucleoli. By definition, intercellular bridges, keratinization, and acinar or papillary structures are absent or are extremely uncommon. Mucin stains show no evidence of intracellular or extracellular secretion. Immunohistochemical studies show positivity of many tumors for keratin, epithelial membrane antigen, B72.3, and CEA.[755, 756]

The WHO classification of large cell carcinoma includes a number of histologic subtypes, including large cell neuroendocrine carcinoma (*see* page 1245), basaloid carcinoma, lymphoepithelioma-like carcinoma, clear cell carcinoma, and large cell carcinoma with rhabdoid phenotype.[1] Several rare tumors, such as pseudoangiomatous carci-

noma[757] and hepatoid carcinoma, may also be appropriately considered in this category.

Clear cell carcinoma is composed of nests or sheets of large cells that have ample, somewhat foamy or clear cytoplasm (Fig. 31–33); mucin stains are negative, and the cleared appearance is believed to be caused by abundant intracytoplasmic glycogen.[705, 706] Immunohistochemical study of one tumor showed the presence of an embryonic carbohydrate antigen.[758] The tumor is rare; in one study of 348 consecutive cases of carcinoma of the lung, only 1 was identified.[705] Despite its separate designation, it is unlikely that clear cell carcinoma represents a distinct entity; because focal clear cell areas can be found in many adenocarcinomas and squamous cell carcinomas,[705, 706] it seems more reasonable to regard tumors with extensive clear cell predominance as simply representing one end of a spectrum. The tumor

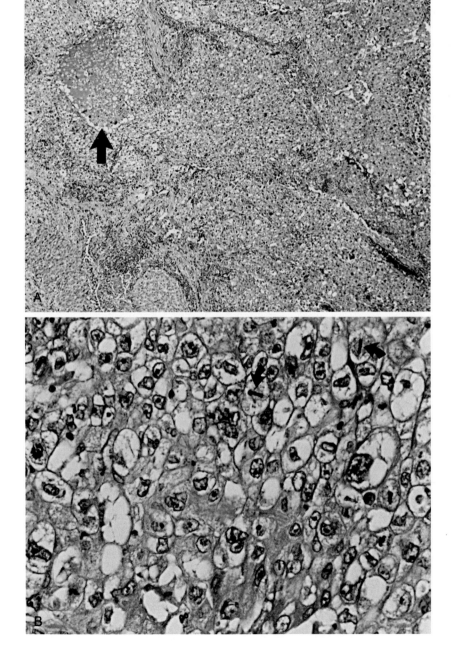

Figure 31–32. Large Cell Carcinoma. Sheets of malignant cells *(A)* contain foci of necrosis *(arrow)* and lack features of glandular or squamous differentiation. A magnified view *(B)* shows abundant cytoplasm, vesicular nuclei with prominent nucleoli, and occasional mitotic figures *(arrows)*. *(A,* ×40; *B,* ×350.)

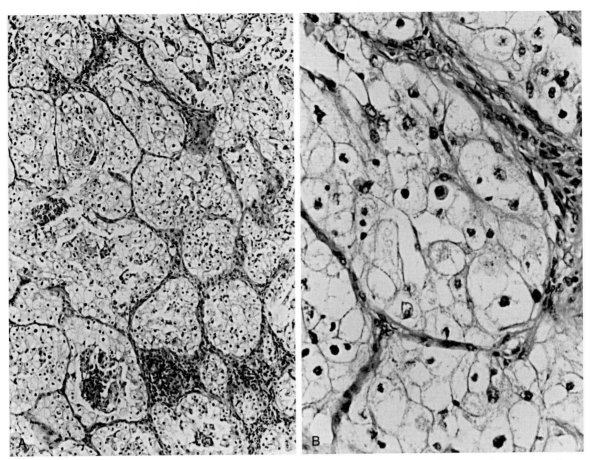

Figure 31–33. Pulmonary Clear Cell Carcinoma. A section of a peripheral lung tumor shows filling of alveolar air spaces by malignant cells *(A)* with abundant finely granular or clear cytoplasm and small, centrally located hyperchromatic nuclei *(B)*. The appearance resembles clear cell carcinoma of the kidney; however, elsewhere the tumor had a pattern typical of bronchioloalveolar carcinoma, and radiologic examination of the kidneys showed no evidence of a primary tumor.

must be differentiated from metastatic renal cell carcinoma, whose histologic appearance may be similar.

As the name suggests, *basaloid carcinoma* resembles basal cell carcinoma of the skin and is composed of lobules of small cells that have scanty cytoplasm and hyperchromatic nuclei;[759, 760] a palisaded arrangement of tumor cells is characteristically present at the periphery of the lobules (Fig. 31–34). In one study of 115 carcinomas initially classified as poorly differentiated or undifferentiated, tumors with a basaloid morphology were identified in pure form in 19 cases and were mixed with other histologic patterns (e.g., squamous cell or adenocarcinoma) in an additional 19 cases.[760] The authors found a significantly worse prognosis for Stage I and II basaloid tumors compared with other poorly differentiated carcinomas.

The term *hepatoid carcinoma* has been used to refer to a rare form of pulmonary carcinoma that consists of tubular, papillary, or solid sheets of cells with abundant eosinophilic cytoplasm and central nuclei.[761, 762] As the name suggests, the tumors resemble hepatocellular carcinoma both histologically and immunohistochemically (α-fetoprotein can be detected in both tumor cells and serum). One tumor has also been associated with the production of an abnormal prothrombin.[763]

Lymphoepithelioma-like carcinoma is histologically similar to its counterpart in the nasopharynx, consisting of

single cells or small nests of cells that have fairly uniform vesicular nuclei and small-to-moderate-sized nucleoli (Fig. 31–35).[764] Numerous lymphocytes characteristically surround and infiltrate the cell nests, in some cases simulating an inflammatory lesion. As discussed previously (*see* page 1079), there is a strong association with the Epstein-Barr virus.[410–412] One tumor has been reported to have arisen in the trachea.[765]

Adenosquamous Carcinoma

The incidence of adenosquamous carcinoma varies greatly, depending on the histologic criteria used for diagnosis and whether or not electron microscopy is employed for classification. If ultrastructural findings are used in typing,[620–622] the incidence in some series is as high as 46% of all pulmonary carcinomas.[623] If only light microscopy is used, however, the number of cases is substantially less, ranging from 0.4% to 4.0%.[766] In two reviews of 626[767] and 2,160[768] pulmonary carcinomas from Japan, the tumor was diagnosed in only 11 (1.8%) and 56 (2.6%) instances, respectively.

As might be expected, lower incidence figures are associated with more rigid criteria for determining cellular differentiation. Thus, based on the identification of clear-cut intra-

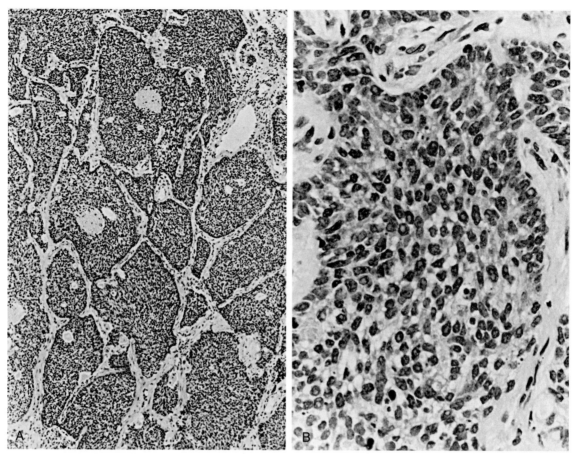

Figure 31–34. Basaloid Carcinoma. Sections *(A* and *B)* show multiple, somewhat irregularly shaped clusters of cells with a moderate amount of cytoplasm and fairly uniform nuclei. Focally *(B),* there is prominent nuclear palisading at the periphery of the cell clusters. *(A,* ×50; *B,* ×380.)

cellular keratinization, squamous pearl formation, or intercellular bridges, one group diagnosed only 7 cases out of a total of 1,125 tumors.[766] In addition to identifying squamous differentiation clearly, it is important not to overestimate glandular features. Glandlike structures can be seen fairly frequently in pulmonary carcinomas as a result of either entrapment of alveolar epithelium within the tumor or apoptosis (single cell necrosis); for example, in one study of 60 tumors, entrapped alveoli were found in 12 (20%).[769] The presence of these "pseudoglands" should be carefully excluded before glandular differentiation is considered to be present. The diagnosis also depends on the amount of squamous and glandular components within a tumor; a figure of 5% for each has been proposed as being necessary by one group of investigators,[767] whereas 10% is required in the WHO classification.[1]

Many adenosquamous carcinomas arise in the periphery of the lung and are grossly indistinguishable from large cell carcinoma or adenocarcinoma.[766] In addition to areas of glandular and squamous differentiation, many show foci of undifferentiated (large cell) carcinoma (Fig. 31–36).

Carcinomas with Pleomorphic, Sarcomatoid, or Sarcomatous Elements

The category of carcinomas with pleomorphic, sarcomatoid, or sarcomatous elements includes a variety of tumors

characterized pathologically by a combination of epithelial and mesenchymal (or mesenchymal-like) elements. A number of terms have been used to describe these tumors, resulting in some confusion in published reports as to their exact nature and making comparisons between such reports difficult. The term *pleomorphic carcinoma* has been used to describe tumors that contain malignant spindle cells, giant cells, or both in association with squamous cell carcinoma, adenocarcinoma, or large cell carcinoma (Fig. 31–37A).[1, 708] Ultrastructural or immunohistochemical features of epithelial differentiation can often be found in the spindle cells in some areas,[771–774] indicating that many, if not all, of these tumors represent poorly differentiated epithelial neoplasms that have a variable histologic pattern. The exceptional tumor that is composed only of spindle cells but that has evidence of epithelial differentiation on immunohistochemical or ultrastructural examination has been termed *spindle cell carcinoma.*[1]

A *carcinosarcoma* can be defined as a neoplasm composed of an admixture of histologically malignant epithelial and mesenchymal tissues, in which the latter have features of specific differentiation (such as bone, cartilage, or muscle) (Fig. 31–37B);[1, 775] some workers also include tumors composed of spindle cells that lack evidence of epithelial differentiation on immunohistochemical analysis in this category.[777] Other investigators believe that pleomorphic carcinoma and carcinosarcoma as defined here represent a spectrum of mesenchymal differentiation in pulmonary

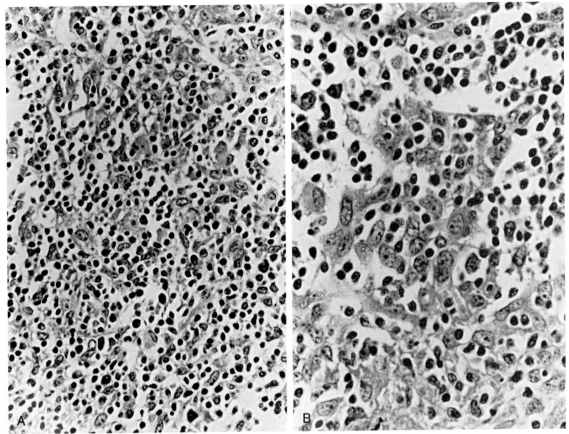

Figure 31–35. Lymphoepithelioma-Like Carcinoma. A section of a peripheral pulmonary nodule *(A)* shows a polymorphous cellular population composed of numerous lymphocytes and lesser numbers of larger histiocyte-like cells. At first glance, the appearance is that of an inflammatory abnormality. Higher magnification *(B)* shows the histiocyte-like cells to have significant nuclear atypia, indicating that they are in fact neoplastic.

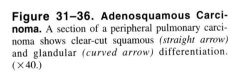

Figure 31–36. Adenosquamous Carcinoma. A section of a peripheral pulmonary carcinoma shows clear-cut squamous *(straight arrow)* and glandular *(curved arrow)* differentiation. (×40.)

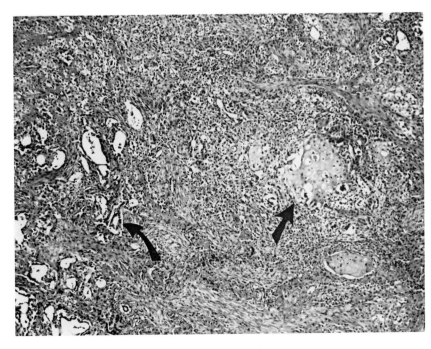

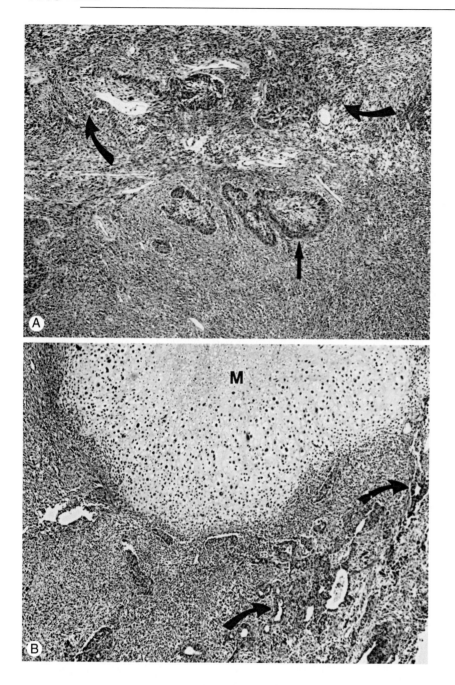

Figure 31–37. Pleomorphic Carcinoma and Carcinosarcoma. Nests of moderately differentiated squamous cell carcinoma *(A, short arrow)* are separated by a poorly differentiated neoplasm, which has a sarcomatous appearance; there is no evidence of specific differentiation in the latter tumor. The two patterns blend imperceptibly into one another in several areas *(long arrows).* The appearance has been designated *pleomorphic carcinoma.* In *B,* there is a mixture of adenocarcinoma *(arrows),* anaplastic neoplasm, and malignant cartilage (M), a histologic appearance designated *carcinosarcoma. (A,* ×44; *B,* ×40.)

carcinoma rather than two separate entities and have advocated the use of terms such as *pulmonary carcinoma with sarcoma-like lesion* or *sarcomatoid carcinoma, monophasic and biphasic types,* to refer to both abnormalities.[778–781] To confuse matters even further, some authors also believe that *pulmonary blastoma* is a variant of carcinosarcoma (or sarcomatoid carcinoma);[781–785] however, because of its distinctive morphology and possible difference in behavior from other forms of carcinosarcoma, we prefer to discuss it separately *(see* page 1367).

Whatever their designation, it is clear that all these tumors are rare. One group of investigators found only 50 cases of "carcinosarcoma" reported in the French and English literature by 1985,[786] and the neoplasm represented only 0.2% of all cases of lung cancer treated at the Mayo Clinic between 1971 and 1982.[787] In one review of 44 patients, the

mean age at the time of diagnosis was 64 (range, 35 to 81 years), and there was a male-to-female predominance of 4:1.[785] Rare cases have been reported of patients who have metachronous carcinosarcoma and carcinoma.[786]

Pathologically, pleomorphic carcinoma and carcinosarcoma can present as a predominantly polypoid intrabronchial tumor (Fig. 31–38), with or without extension into contiguous parenchyma, or as a bulky peripheral mass without an obvious airway association.[783, 788] Only rarely do they occur within the trachea.[789] Histologically, the epithelial component is usually squamous cell carcinoma; adenocarcinoma, small cell carcinoma, and large cell carcinoma have been identified less commonly,[781] and a neuroendocrine component other than small cell carcinoma has been documented rarely.[790] In carcinosarcomas, the mesenchymal component is usually composed of a combination of spindle cells without obvious

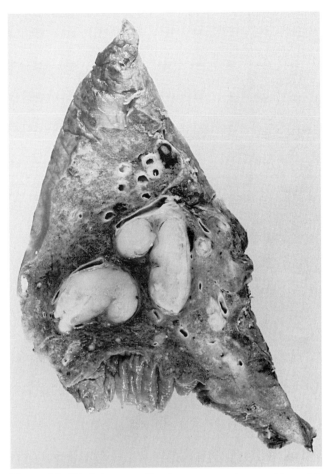

Figure 31–38. Pulmonary Carcinosarcoma. A resected lower lobe shows a fleshy, partly necrotic tumor almost entirely within the lumen of segmental airways. Histologic examination showed adenocarcinoma and chondrosarcoma admixed with anaplastic neoplasm.

differentiation and of malignant cartilaginous, muscular, or osteoid tissue.[791–793] The presence of osteoclast-like giant cells resembling giant cell tumor of bone has been reported in some cases.[779] Ultrastructural and immunohistochemical examination reveals evidence of both mesenchymal and epithelial differentiation in carcinosarcoma[773, 794] and epithelial differentiation only in pleomorphic carcinoma. Metastases may be sarcomatous, epithelial, or a combination of both.[783, 789, 795]

Giant cell carcinoma is also considered to be part of this conglomeration of poorly differentiated neoplasms.[1] As with some other tumors, its separation into a specific histologic category is somewhat arbitrary, and it likely represents one end of a continuum of tumor morphology.[776] Several observations support the latter interpretation, including (1) tumor giant cells are found occasionally in a number of pulmonary carcinomas (e.g., 63 [10%] of 592 cases in one series);[796] (2) histologic features of specific epithelial differentiation, most often glandular, can be identified in many giant cell tumors if enough sections are examined;[598] and (3) a spindle cell component has been noted in many tumors, leading some workers to consider the tumor to be part of a spectrum of pleomorphic carcinoma.[708] Despite these observations, because of the almost uniformly dismal prognosis and the rather distinctive histologic appearance, it may be of

some value to preserve the term. If classification into this subtype is restricted to those cases in which there is no evidence of glandular or squamous differentiation and in which the giant cells form a preponderance of the tumor, the incidence is considerably less than 1%.

Giant cell tumors are usually peripherally located and large; hemorrhage and necrosis are common.[797, 798] Histologically, they are composed of loosely cohesive cells similar to those of large cell carcinoma and numerous intermingled multinucleated giant cells; the cytoplasm of the latter cells characteristically contains polymorphonuclear leukocytes (Fig. 31–39). In an ultrastructural study, one group of investigators found multiple pairs of cytoplasmic centrioles, suggesting that the multinucleation developed as a result of failure of individual tumor cells to divide.[798] Intracytoplasmic inclusions resembling Mallory's (alcoholic) hyaline have been found in some cases.[799] A propensity to metastasize to the gastrointestinal tract was noted in one review.[800] Immunohistochemical studies have shown positive reactions for cytokeratin, epithelial membrane antigen, and vimentin;[801] investigation of one tumor showed reactivity for α-fetoprotein, CEA, and human chorionic gonadotropin (substances that were also detected in serum).[802]

Miscellaneous Pathologic Characteristics

Local Spread

The peripheral portion of many pulmonary carcinomas appears to invade the alveolar air spaces without destroying the adjacent alveolar septa (Fig. 31–40); although this pattern of spread is best recognized in bronchioloalveolar carcinoma, in fact, it is also common in other histologic types of non–small cell carcinoma. Ultrastructural examination of the advancing edge of tumors that infiltrate in this fashion may show malignant cells growing on residual alveolar septal basement membrane.[803] In the vast majority of cases, this intra-alveolar component accounts for only a small amount of the tumor, the remainder being associated with destruction of lung parenchyma and a variably intense inflammatory and fibroblastic reaction; rarely a large proportion of a non-bronchioloalveolar carcinoma is located entirely within air spaces.[618]

Because of their peripheral location, many adenocarcinomas invade the visceral pleura. In the early stage of such invasion, this is best appreciated on sections processed with elastic tissue stains that show disruption of the pleural external elastic lamina.[804] In more advanced disease, thickening of the pleura by an inflammatory infiltrate or fibrous tissue is common.

Vascular Supply

Although there is considerable variation among tumors in the type and origin of vascularization, some tendency toward specific patterns has been found in relation to the location, size, and cell type of the neoplasm.[805–809] Most authors agree that the principal blood supply is derived from the bronchial system, although a component can come from the pulmonary arteries, especially in more peripheral tumors.[809] In addition, as noted earlier, the peripheral portion

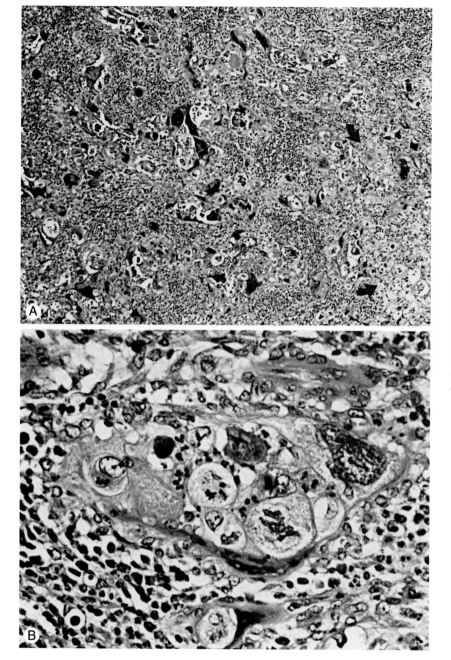

Figure 31–39. Giant Cell Carcinoma. A section *(A)* of a peripheral parenchymal tumor shows sheets of malignant cells that contain numerous giant cells that have bizarre, irregularly shaped, and hyperchromatic nuclei. A prominent inflammatory infiltrate consisting predominantly of lymphocytes and polymorphonuclear leukocytes is evident. A Magnified view *(B)* of one malignant cluster shows highly abnormal nuclei and, characteristically, numerous intracytoplasmic leukocytes. *(A, ×60; B, ×350.)*

of many carcinomas appears to infiltrate the alveolar air spaces; it is likely that such portions derive their nutrition from the pulmonary alveolar capillaries. The size of the tumor can also be related to vascular anatomy: small tumors tend to be associated with straight vessels, whereas larger carcinomas tend to be supplied by vessels whose pattern is much more complex.[808]

Variation in the pattern of vascularization with different cell types has also been noted by several investigators;[805, 808, 809] for example, some have found a denser vascular network in adenocarcinoma than in squamous cell carcinoma.[805] Another group showed a more orderly and well-delineated vascular network in better-differentiated squamous cell carcinomas and adenocarcinomas than in small cell or large cell tumors.[808] Morphometrically derived dimen-

sions and three-dimensional morphology of the microvasculature have been described in detail by some workers;[806, 807] as with the findings in studies of larger vessels, a tendency toward specific patterns with different cell types has been documented.

Vascular Invasion and Proliferation

Pulmonary vascular invasion is common in pulmonary carcinoma. In one study of 109 tumors, arterial infiltration was identified in 63 (58%) and venous invasion in 20 (19%).[810] In another investigation of 87 tumors, vascular invasion was documented in 67 (77%) and lymphatic invasion in 38 (44%);[811] of some interest was the observation that the presence or absence as well as the extent of vascular

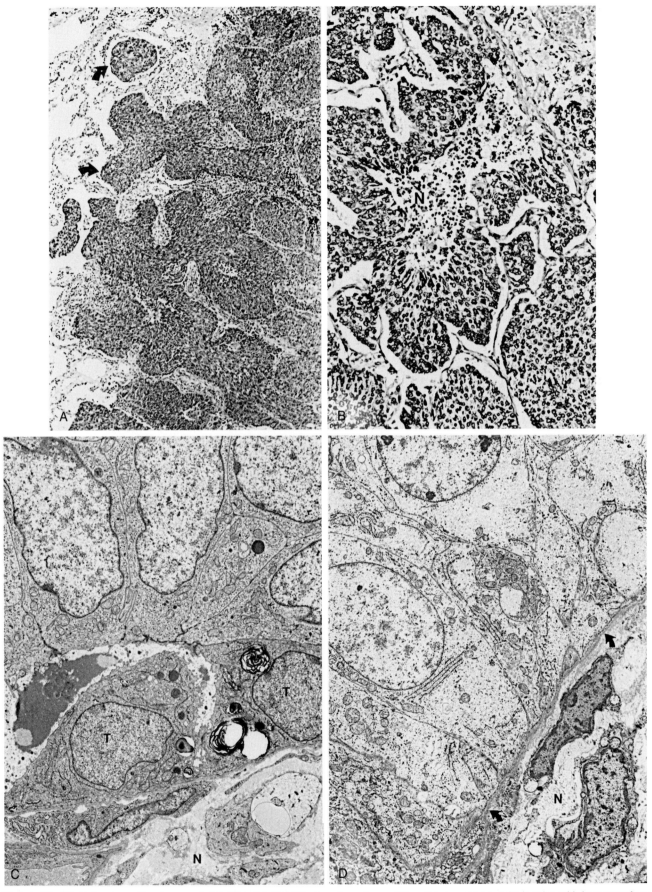

Figure 31–40. Pulmonary Carcinoma—Intra-Alveolar Spread. A section of an undifferentiated carcinoma at its junction with lung parenchyma *(A)* shows several clusters of tumor cells within alveolar air spaces *(arrows)*. A magnified view of another carcinoma *(B)* shows tumor within an alveolar duct and several adjacent alveoli; alveolar septa are essentially normal. (The space between the tumor cells and the septa represents artefactual retraction.) The central portion of the tumor within the alveolar duct is necrotic (N), an effect possibly related to distance from alveolar capillaries. Electron micrographs of the tumor in *B* show malignant cells adjacent to alveolar type II cells *(C)* and directly opposed to the residual alveolar septal basement membrane *(arrows in D)*. T, type II cell; N, alveolar septal interstitium.

infiltration were unrelated to survival, whereas the presence of lymphatic invasion indicated a poor prognosis. As with other malignant neoplasms, pulmonary carcinomas are associated with a proliferation of new vessels (angiogenesis); some investigators have found a greater degree of such proliferation to be associated with an increased risk of metastases.[812]

Inflammatory Reaction

The inflammatory reaction to pulmonary carcinoma is variable, typically being minimal or absent altogether in small cell carcinoma but often present in the other cell types (Fig. 31–41). In one study of 19 surgically excised tumors (including 12 squamous cell carcinomas, 2 adenocarcinomas, 1 bronchioloalveolar carcinoma, and 4 poorly differentiated carcinomas), all were found to be surrounded and, to a lesser extent, infiltrated by T and B lymphocytes, plasma cells, macrophages, and a small number of mast cells.[813] Another group of investigators showed a considerable number of eosinophils and macrophages in many tumors.[814] There is some evidence that the presence of such inflammatory reactions is associated with a better prognosis.[814–816] An accumulation of neutrophils in alveolar air spaces is seen in some bronchioloalveolar carcinomas;[661] it has been speculated that it may be the result of elaboration of IL-8 by the tumor cells and has been associated with a relatively poor prognosis.[661]

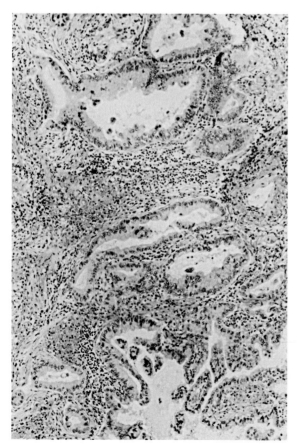

Figure 31–41. Adenocarcinoma—Inflammatory Reaction. The glands of this well-differentiated adenocarcinoma are separated by a moderate amount of fibrous tissue containing a mononuclear inflammatory infiltrate (predominantly lymphocytes).

Langerhans' cells can be found interspersed between tumor cells in a high proportion of pulmonary adenocarcinomas, particularly of the bronchioloalveolar subtype;[817–819] although their function, if any, is not clear, it has been suggested that their presence may be associated with a relatively favorable prognosis.[817] A granulomatous inflammatory reaction is seen rarely;[820] in some cases, it represents a reaction to keratinaceous debris from a squamous cell carcinoma, whereas in others no obvious inciting foreign material is evident.

Three-Dimensional Morphology

One group of investigators divided the three-dimensional macroscopic growth pattern of pulmonary carcinoma into four categories:[821] (1) bizarre with numerous finger-like projections (found most often in squamous cell carcinoma) (Fig. 31–42); (2) spheroid (typically associated with adenocarcinoma); (3) ellipsoid (most frequent in small cell carcinoma); and (4) mixed (found especially in large cell carcinoma but also to some extent in each of the other subtypes). The investigators pointed out that because of the irregular shape of many tumors, estimation of their volume based on measurements of largest diameter can be inaccurate, especially for the larger ones.

RADIOLOGIC MANIFESTATIONS

The radiographic manifestations of pulmonary carcinoma are related to size and anatomic location, particularly with respect to relationship of the carcinoma to an airway. Thus, the earliest finding is often not the lesion itself but the obstructive pneumonitis or atelectasis that the tumor engenders. The ease with which a carcinoma is detected on the radiograph is influenced by the location within the lung, the radiographic density, and the presence or absence of parenchymal disease.[822] For a lesion to be detectable, there needs to be a contrast difference between it and the adjacent parenchyma; both the complexity of adjacent structures and the presence of superimposed structures, such as vessels and ribs, adversely affect early detection.[823] Although the human eye can detect a nodule as small as 3 mm in diameter,[824] a pulmonary carcinoma is seldom evident radiographically until it is 1 cm or greater in diameter.[825]

Anatomic Location

Pulmonary carcinoma occurs with a relative frequency of 3:2 in both the right versus the left lung[826–831] and the upper versus the lower lobe.[611, 827, 830, 832, 833] In one review of almost 25,000 primary pulmonary neoplasms, such upper lobe predominance was much more apparent in younger patients.[833] In the upper lobes, the anterior segment is most often affected.[834] Carcinoma most commonly involves the peripheral regions of the lower lobes in patients who have idiopathic pulmonary fibrosis.[835] Some workers have made the same observation in patients who have asbestosis;[200] however, others have not been able to confirm this finding.[200a] Although both squamous cell and small cell carcinomas occur centrally and peripherally, there is clear-cut pre-

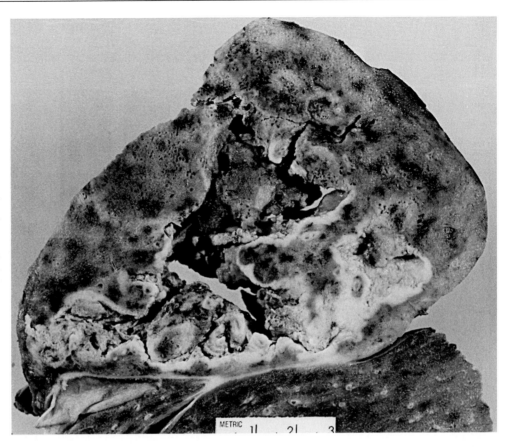

Figure 31–42. Pulmonary Carcinoma—Irregular Shape. A slice of right lung shows a carcinoma with extensive necrosis and cavitation involving much of the upper lobe. The advancing edge of the tumor (indicated by the white tissue) is highly irregular in its outline. The remainder of the lobe is consolidated as a result of obstructive pneumonitis.

dominance in the former location.[836–839] In approximately 50% of cases, adenocarcinoma presents as an isolated peripheral lesion; in the other 50%, it occurs as a peripheral lesion associated with hilar lymphadenopathy or as a central tumor.[839–841] Of tumors that arise in the bronchial tree, most are situated in relation to segmental and lobar branches.[611, 612, 639, 842, 843] Carcinoma arising in the trachea is rare, accounting for less than 1% of cases.[831, 844] Approximately 4% of carcinomas arise in the extreme apex of the upper lobes (Pancoast tumors).[839, 845]

Obstructive Pneumonitis

Radiographic findings secondary to airway obstruction are present in approximately 40% of patients at the time of presentation.[836, 837, 839, 841, 846, 847] The most frequent is related to a combination of pathologic changes that includes atelectasis; bronchiectasis with mucous plugging; and consolidation of lung parenchyma by lipid-laden macrophages, fibrous tissue, and mononuclear inflammatory cells (obstructive pneumonitis). As discussed previously (*see* page 514), these pathologic findings are usually the result of the physical (and perhaps chemical) effects of airway blockage rather than inflammation related to infection.[848] When infection does occur distal to a carcinoma, it most often takes the form of bronchitis or bronchiolitis superimposed on the typical histologic features of obstructive pneumonitis;[848] as a result, the presence of such infection is usually undetectable radiographically, at least in its early stage.

In a review of the radiographic findings in 600 cases of

pulmonary carcinoma, obstructive pneumonitis or atelectasis was identified in 139 of 263 (53%) squamous cell carcinomas, 43 of 114 (38%) small cell carcinomas, 32 of 97 (33%) large cell carcinomas, and 32 of 126 (25%) adenocarcinomas.[847] In another, more recent investigation of 331 patients, obstructive findings were present in 42 of 98 (43%) patients who had squamous cell carcinoma, 43 of 86 (50%) who had small cell carcinoma, 6 of 22 (27%) who had large cell carcinoma, and 36 of 125 (29%) who had adenocarcinoma.[839] The atelectasis is most often segmental or lobar (Fig. 31–43); occasionally an entire lung is affected (Fig. 31–44). Because airway obstruction is usually complete, air cannot pass distally, and an air bronchogram is thus absent; this sign is virtually pathognomonic of an endobronchial obstructing lesion and is clearly important in diagnosis. Bronchi distal to the obstruction are usually dilated and filled with mucus or pus (Fig. 31–45). Occasionally, a tumor is identified as a focal convexity, whereas the interlobar fissure distally is concave as a result of atelectasis, an S-shaped configuration known as the *S sign of Golden* (Fig. 31–46).[849] Obviously that part of the neoplasm that is within the opacity is not visible.

In the majority of patients, obstructive pneumonitis is associated with volume loss; rarely, the obstructed lobe is increased in volume (Fig. 31–47). In some patients—especially those who have had long-standing obstruction and radiotherapy—infectious bronchitis or bronchiolitis is followed by confluent pneumonia with abscess formation. With drainage, one or more cavities may be seen within the obstructed lung parenchyma (Fig. 31–48). Infection can also cause an acute bronchopneumonia, resulting in signs and

Text continued on page 1128

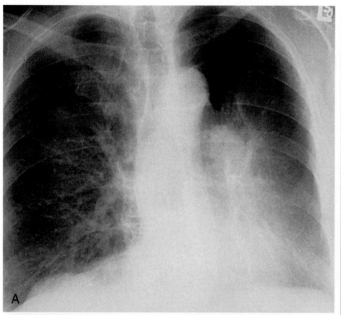

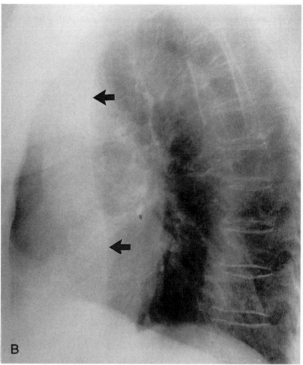

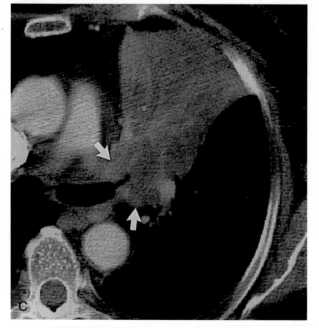

Figure 31–43. Lobar Atelectasis Resulting from Pulmonary Carcinoma. Posteroanterior *(A)* and lateral *(B)* chest radiographs demonstrate left upper lobe atelectasis. Characteristic anterior displacement of the major interlobar fissure *(arrows)* is visible on the lateral radiograph. A contrast-enhanced CT scan *(C)* demonstrates complete obstruction of the left upper lobe bronchus with associated atelectasis and obstructive pneumonitis. A soft tissue tumor can be seen extending anterior and posterior *(arrows)* to the bronchus. Bronchoscopic biopsy demonstrated squamous cell carcinoma. The patient was a 68-year-old woman.

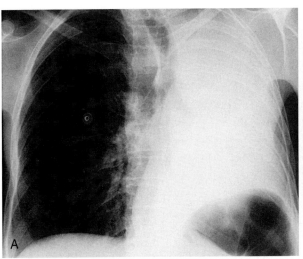

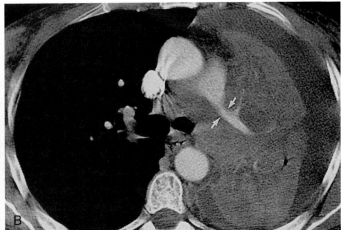

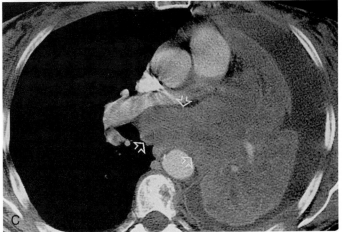

Figure 31–44. Atelectasis and Obstructive Pneumonitis of the Left Lung. A posteroanterior chest radiograph *(A)* shows consolidation and atelectasis of the left lung, mediastinal displacement to the left, and overinflation of the right lung. The marked elevation of the left hemidiaphragm in this patient was the result of phrenic nerve involvement by tumor. A contrast-enhanced CT scan *(B)* at the level of the proximal left main bronchus demonstrates tumor infiltration into the mediastinum and encasement of the left pulmonary artery *(arrows)*. Obstructive pneumonitis and atelectasis of the left lung and a left pleural effusion are also evident. A CT scan at a more caudad level *(C)* shows extensive tumor infiltration of the mediastinum *(open arrows)* with complete obstruction of the left bronchus. The diagnosis of small cell carcinoma was proved by bronchial biopsy.

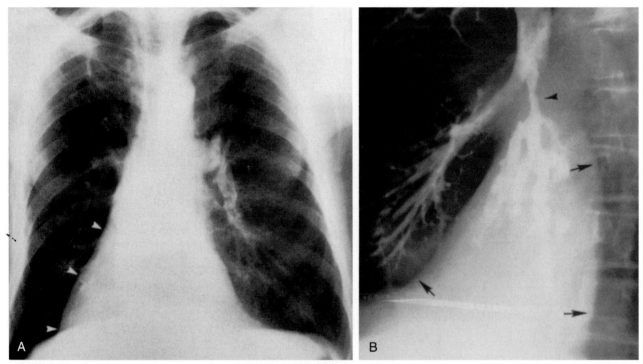

Figure 31–45. Atelectasis of the Right Lower Lobe with Patent Peripheral Bronchi—Pathogenetic Mechanisms in Central Pulmonary Carcinoma. A posteroanterior chest radiograph *(A)* shows a typical pattern of right lower lobe atelectasis *(arrowheads)*. A selective bronchogram in right posterior oblique projection *(B)* reveals circumferential narrowing of the lower lobe bronchus *(arrowhead)* by a biopsy-proven squamous cell carcinoma; contrast medium has entered the dilated lower lobe bronchi, an unusual occurrence because such bronchi either are usually completely obstructed or are distended with mucus or pus. The triangular opacity *(arrows)* distal to the bronchial occlusion represents the consolidated and collapsed lower lobe. This example suggests certain possible consequences of a central obstructing carcinoma: (1) If the tumor causes bronchial dilation and mucopurulent impaction *with little or no surrounding consolidation,* a pattern of mucoid impaction is created; (2) if the accumulation of fluid and macrophages within alveolar air spaces is dominant, volume loss in the lobe may be minimal, and the pattern is one of obstructive pneumonitis; and (3) the fluid and cellular infiltration may not totally compensate for the simultaneous resorption of air, so that a predominantly atelectatic pattern results.

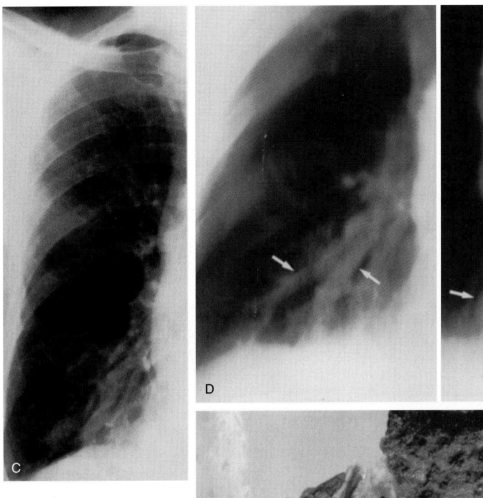

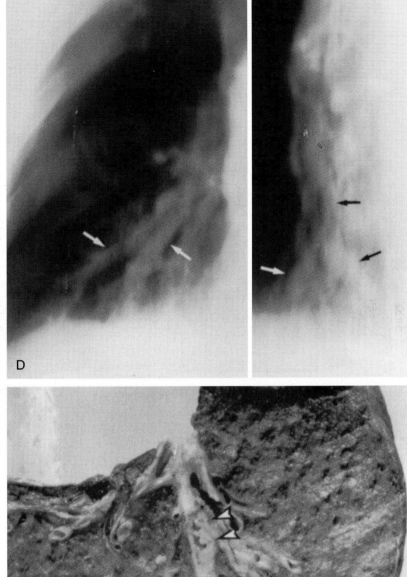

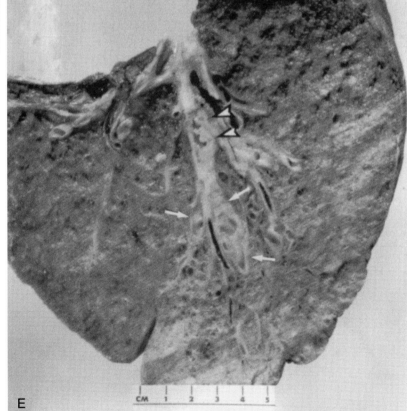

Figure 31–45 *Continued.* The consequences of the first mechanism are illustrated in another patient with a central squamous cell carcinoma *(C)*. A detail view of the right lung from a posteroanterior radiograph shows branching and tubular opacities in the lower lobe, better seen on conventional anteroposterior linear tomograms *(D)*. The "gloved hand" appearance of the dilated bronchi *(arrows)* is consistent with bronchoceles. A sagittal section *(E)* through the resected lower lobe shows an intrabronchial squamous cell carcinoma *(large arrowheads)* and dilated distal bronchi *(arrows)* (on the fresh specimen, the latter were filled with mucopurulent material).

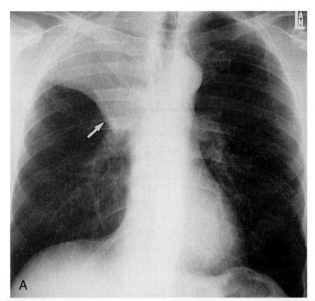

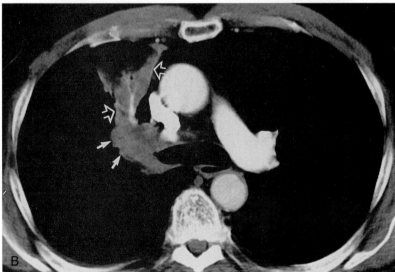

Figure 31–46. S Sign of Golden. An anteroposterior chest radiograph *(A)* in a 67-year-old man demonstrates atelectasis and obstructive pneumonitis of the right upper lobe. The focal convexity in the hilar region *(arrow),* which indicates the location of the tumor, and the concave appearance of the interlobar fissure distally as a result of atelectasis give a configuration that resembles an *S* (the S sign of Golden). A contrast-enhanced CT scan *(B)* demonstrates the central tumor *(straight arrows)* and the atelectatic right upper lobe *(open arrows).* Biopsy showed squamous cell carcinoma.

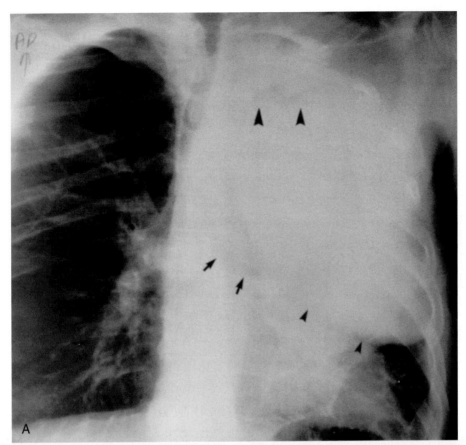

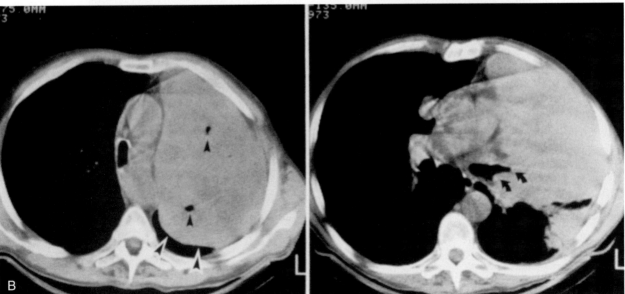

Figure 31–47. Obstructive Pneumonitis of the Left Upper Lobe with Hyperexpansion. A posteroanterior radiograph *(A)* shows a diffuse homogeneous opacity in the left mid and upper hemithorax indicative of massive upper lobe consolidation; a small amount of air is present superiorly *(arrowheads)*. The major fissure *(small arrowheads)* and the left main bronchus *(arrows)* are displaced downward, and the trachea is shifted slightly to the right. CT scans *(B)* through the aortic arch *(left)* and carina *(right)* confirm the features illustrated in *A*. The convex posterior bulge of the major fissure *(large arrowheads)* indicates lobar hyperexpansion. The superior radiolucencies *(small arrowheads)* represent necrotic parenchyma or residual intrapulmonary gas. The left upper lobe bronchus is occluded *(curved arrows)* by a squamous cell carcinoma. The patient was a 58-year-old man.

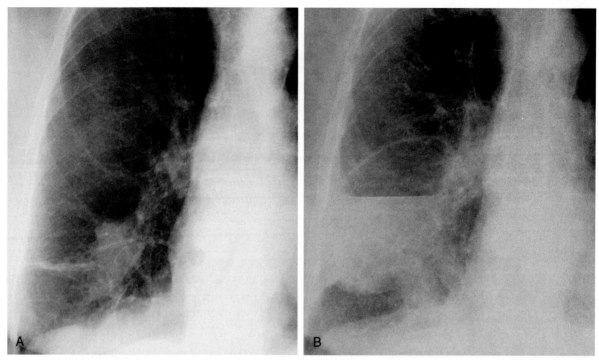

Figure 31–48. Pulmonary Carcinoma with Distal Abscess. A view of the right lung from a posteroanterior chest radiograph *(A)* in an 82-year-old woman shows a right lower lobe mass and focal areas of atelectasis. At bronchoscopy, this was shown to represent a squamous carcinoma. A chest radiograph obtained 5 months later *(B)* demonstrates a large, thin-walled cavity containing an air-fluid level. This cavity was shown to represent a bacterial abscess distal to the carcinoma.

symptoms that may be the first clinical manifestation of the malignancy.

Although obstructive pneumonitis and atelectasis are common manifestations of endobronchial carcinoma, complete endobronchial obstruction may be radiographically occult.[843] In one investigation of 81 completely obstructing endobronchial tumors (involving a main bronchus in 8 [10%], a lobar bronchus in 44 [54%], a segmental bronchus in 27 [33%], and a subsegmental bronchus in 2 [3%]), radiographic signs of bronchial obstruction were present in only 45 (56%) cases;[843] in 23 cases (28%), the chest radiograph was abnormal (hilar mass, solitary nodule, or a focal area of consolidation) but without signs of obstruction, and in 13 cases (16%) it was normal. Radiographic evidence of obstruction was present in 7 of 8 (87%) patients who had obstruction of the main bronchi, in 25 of 44 (57%) of those who had lobar bronchial obstruction, in 11 of 27 (41%) of those who had segmental bronchial obstruction, and in 2 patients who had subsegmental bronchial obstruction.

Even when an obstructing tumor is not apparent on the radiograph, it can usually be seen on dynamic or spiral CT after intravenous administration of a bolus of contrast material or on magnetic resonance (MR) imaging.[850–852] For example, in one retrospective study of 50 patients who had segmental or lobar atelectasis, pulmonary carcinomas causing bronchial obstruction were correctly identified in 24 of 27 (89%) patients on the chest radiograph and in all 27 cases on CT.[850] Although the presence of tumor can usually be inferred from the CT findings, the actual tumor is often difficult to distinguish from the obstructive pneumonitis and atelectasis. The percentage of cases in which such distinction can be made has ranged from 25 to 80 in different studies.[851,]

[853, 854] As indicated, optimal visualization of the tumor in these cases requires the use of an intravenous bolus of contrast material and dynamic or spiral CT (*see* Figs. 31–44 and 31–46);[851, 854] using these techniques, the tumor enhances only slightly, whereas the atelectatic or consolidated lung shows considerable enhancement.

Results of studies of a small number of patients suggest that distinction of carcinoma from obstructive pneumonitis can often be made on T2-weighted spin-echo MR images (Fig. 31–49)[851, 855] or on T1-weighted MR images after intravenous administration of gadolinium.[856, 857] The results of studies comparing MR to CT have been variable: in two series, MR imaging was considered to be superior to CT in the distinction of tumor from obstructive changes,[856, 857] whereas in one it was considered inferior.[851]

Alteration of Regional Lung Volume

Because growth of an endobronchial neoplasm may occur for a considerable period of time before it totally occludes the lumen, it may be associated with no radiographic changes or, rarely, with findings secondary to partial airway obstruction (Fig. 31–50).[858–861] Overinflation of the lung at total lung capacity must be distinguished from air trapping on expiration (resulting in overinflation at residual volume). The former, whether local or general, implies loss of elastic recoil (either reversible, as in asthma, or irreversible, as in emphysema). Such loss of recoil is usually a lengthy process, hardly commensurate with an aggressive condition such as pulmonary carcinoma. In our experience, the volume of lung behind a partly obstructing endobronchial

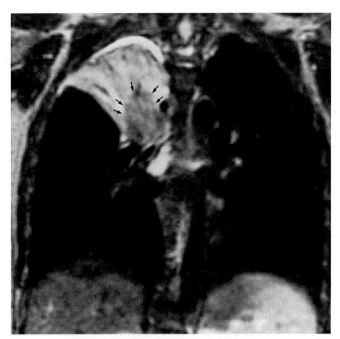

Figure 31–49. Obstructive Pneumonitis and Atelectasis. A coronal spin-echo T2-weighted MR image (TR, 2400; TE, 120) shows right upper lobe atelectasis and obstructive pneumonitis. The obstructing pulmonary carcinoma *(arrows)* has a relatively low signal intensity compared with the consolidated lung. The diagnosis was surgically proven adenocarcinoma.

either from hypoxic vasoconstriction in response to hypoventilation or from compression or invasion of contiguous pulmonary arteries.[860, 861] Air trapping during expiration is a dynamic event resulting from air-flow obstruction as the bronchial caliber reduces adjacent to the endobronchial tumor (Fig. 31–50).

Mucoid Impaction

Occasionally, an obstructing endobronchial carcinoma, most commonly affecting a segmental or subsegmental airway, results in radiographically evident impaction of inspissated secretions (Fig. 31–51).[862–864] Although such mucoid impaction is a frequent pathologic finding in association with atelectasis and obstructive pneumonitis, it obviously is not visible radiographically in these cases. The combination of mucoid impaction and distal air-containing parenchyma requires that there be no infection or obstructive pneumonitis within the lung at the time its airway was obstructed and that there is sufficient collateral ventilation to prevent atelectasis.

Although usually related to squamous cell carcinoma, occasional cases have been described with small cell carcinoma (Fig. 31–52).[865] The abnormality can also be seen in association with a variety of lesions other than pulmonary carcinoma, including metastatic carcinoma, carcinoid tumor, bronchial atresia, and an aspirated foreign body.[866]

lesion is almost invariably reduced at full inspiration. Despite this smaller volume, the opacity of the affected parenchyma typically is *less* than the opposite lung, rather than greater as might be anticipated. This decrease in opacity is caused by a reduction in perfusion (oligemia), resulting

Bronchial Wall Thickening

Pulmonary carcinoma can cause an increase in the thickness of the peribronchial interstitial tissue resulting in increased thickness of the bronchial wall (Fig. 31–53) or in

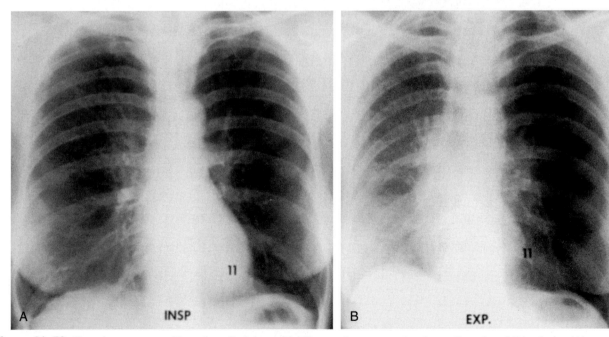

Figure 31–50. Hyperlucency as a Sign of an Endobronchial Tumor. A posteroanterior chest radiograph at full inspiration *(A)* reveals small, barely visible vessels throughout the left lung, reflecting oligemia resulting from hypoxic vasoconstriction. Although the volume of the left lung is slightly reduced, the reduction in blood flow has caused hyperlucency. A radiograph exposed at full expiration *(B)* demonstrates air trapping in the left lung. The patient was a 42-year-old woman who had marked narrowing of the left main bronchus by a pulmonary carcinoma.

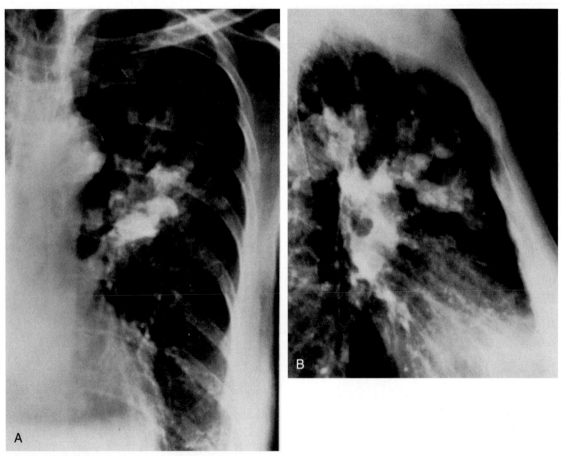

Figure 31–51. Mucoid Impaction Distal to an Obstructing Endobronchial Lesion. Detail views of the left lung from posteroanterior *(A)* and lateral *(B)* chest radiographs reveal broad, finger-like opacities projecting into the anterior segment of the upper lobe. Although these airways are completely obstructed, the peripheral parenchyma is air containing because of collateral ventilation. At bronchoscopy, a squamous cell carcinoma was identified occluding the anterior segmental bronchus. The patient was a 37-year-old woman with a history of one episode of hemoptysis. (Courtesy of Dr. Ken Thomson, Melbourne, Australia.)

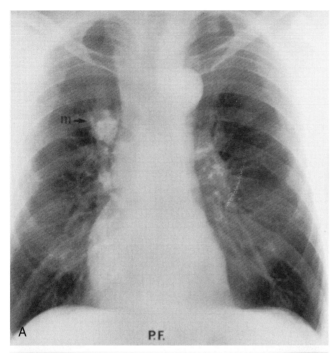

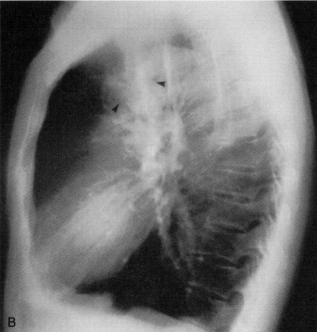

Figure 31–52. Bronchocele Formation Caused by Extension of Pulmonary Carcinoma. Posteroanterior *(A)* and lateral *(B)* chest radiographs reveal a well-defined mass (m) that is intimately related to the right upper hilum; on the lateral projection, the lesion has an obliquely oriented, Y-shaped configuration *(arrowheads)*. The mediastinum is shifted slightly to the right. A CT scan *(C)* shows a sharply marginated, bifurcating opacity (m) that originates in the anterior aspect of the upper hilum and extends into the anterior segmental bronchi *(arrowheads)*. Pathologic examination of the specimen after upper lobectomy disclosed a solid core of tumor cells that extended along dilated anterior segmental bronchi from the more centrally located main tumor. The patient was a 55-year-old man.

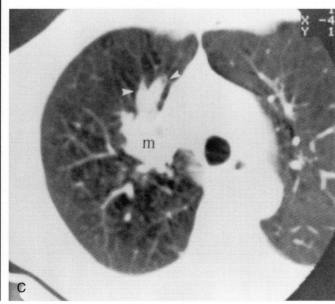

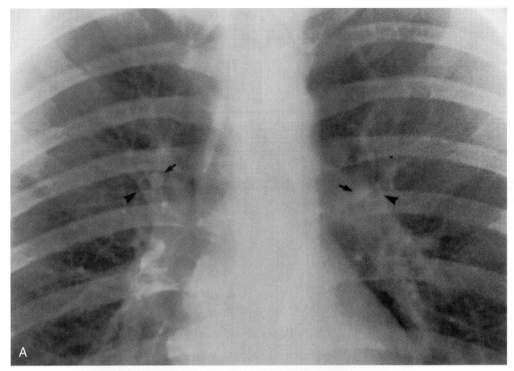

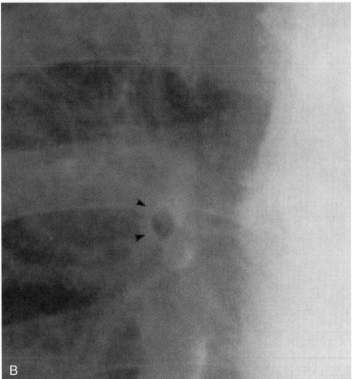

Figure 31–53. Bronchial Cuff Sign in Pulmonary Carcinoma. A detail view *(A)* of the hila from a posteroanterior chest radiograph shows the normal appearance of the anterior segmental bronchi of the upper lobes, possessing a ring-shaped opacity viewed end-on *(arrowheads)*. The homogeneous, opaque arteries *(arrows)* that accompany the bronchi are located medial to the airways; the bronchial walls are effaced where they abut the vessel. Compare this appearance with the sequence of changes that occurred in a 65-year-old patient: A detail view of the right upper hilum from a posteroanterior radiograph *(B)* shows the anterior segmental bronchus *(arrowheads)* to be slightly thickened; the adjacent artery is normal.

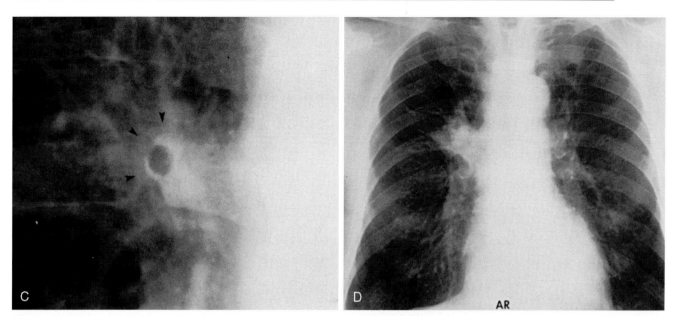

Figure 31–53 *Continued.* Six years later *(C),* there has developed a circumferential cuff of soft tissue around the bronchus *(arrowheads),* and the artery is less well defined superiorly. These features constitute the bronchial cuff sign. Four years later *(D),* the patient presented with typical radiographic signs of an anterior segmental obstructing lesion; the sputum was positive for squamous cell carcinoma.

partial or complete obliteration of its normal curvilinear demarcation. Carcinoma can also extend into the adjacent periarterial interstitial tissue, causing partial or complete obscuration of the vessel.[867] This combination of findings has been demonstrated in the anterior segmental bronchi of the right and left upper lobes and the superior segmental bronchus of the left lower lobe.[867–869] Similar findings may be identified on lateral projection in larger airways, such as the left main or lower lobe bronchus or the intermediate bronchus.

The posterior wall of the intermediate bronchus can be identified on the great majority of lateral radiographs as a vertically oriented linear opacity in continuity with the posterior wall of the trachea and right main bronchus. The wall is visible because of contrast provided by air in the bronchial lumen anteriorly and in lung parenchyma of the azygoesophageal recess posteriorly. In one study of the lateral radiographs of 200 normal subjects, the wall thickness ranged from 0.5 to 3.0 mm (mean, 1.3 mm).[870] In another investigation, disease was invariably present when the wall thickness exceeded 3 mm.[871] In the latter study, 36 patients were identified who had a thickened bronchial wall, 23 caused by left-sided heart failure, 2 by sarcoidosis, and 9 by neoplasm. Of the nine patients who had neoplasia, five had pulmonary carcinoma, the bronchial wall thickening resulting from neoplastic invasion; there were two cases each of lymphoma and metastatic carcinoma. Lobulation of the wall's contour was found to be suggestive of lymph node enlargement rather than edema. Thickening of the wall of the main, lobar, intermediate, or segmental bronchi has also been described as the only abnormality seen on CT in a small number of patients who have pulmonary carcinoma (Fig. 31–54).[872, 873]

Solitary Pulmonary Nodule

There is a wide variation in the criteria for designating a radiologic opacity a solitary nodule, with resultant differ-

ences in radiologic features and prognostic associations. The shape usually is described as round or oval.[874, 875] Although the size has been accepted to vary from 1 to 6 cm in diameter in the past,[874–878] it is more customary today to restrict the maximal diameter to 3 cm,[879–881] larger lesions being designated masses. Reasons for this size limitation include the following: (1) the vast majority of lesions greater than 3 cm in diameter are malignant, whereas a substantial number of those less than 3 cm in diameter prove to be benign;[882, 883] (2) the presence of calcification is helpful only in distinguishing benign from malignant lesions if the lesion measures 3 cm or less in diameter;[883] and (3) pulmonary carcinomas measuring 3 cm or less in diameter are less likely to be associated with mediastinal lymph node metastases[884] and have a better prognosis[885] than larger lesions. For these reasons, we and others prefer to define a solitary pulmonary nodule as a well-circumscribed lesion less than 3.0 cm in diameter within the lung parenchyma unassociated with adenopathy, atelectasis, or pneumonia.[886, 887]

A great variety of conditions may result in solitary pulmonary nodules,[888] as many as 45 being listed in one review.[889] Using clinical and radiographic findings (Table 31–2), the distinction between benign and malignant lesions can often be established with a reasonable degree of confidence, thus helping to make a decision as to whether thoracotomy is warranted. Comparison with previous chest radiographs is of fundamental importance in this process: in many cases, a previous film may show an identical lesion, perhaps overlooked because of the radiographic technique employed or because it was obscured by a rib shadow. Several radiologic signs also aid in differentiating benign and malignant nodules; although some are unquestionably of much greater significance than others, no single sign or group of signs has proved to be absolute in this distinction. Bearing this caveat in mind, it is still possible to make a reasonable determination as to the nature of a particular solitary pulmonary nodule and, at minimum, to suggest what additional investigative procedures might be most rewarding for further clarification.

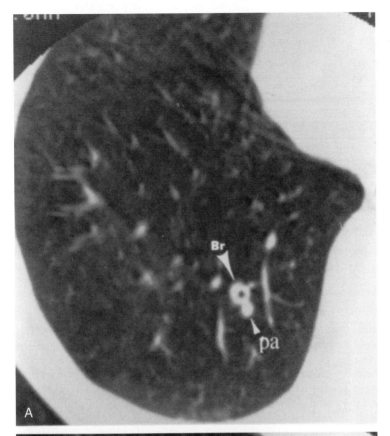

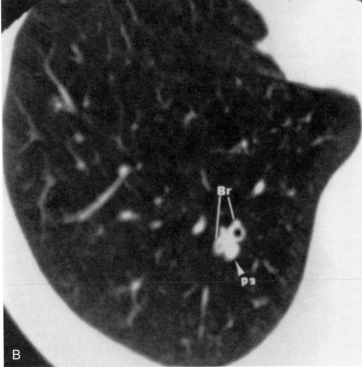

Figure 31–54. Bronchial Cuff Sign—CT Appearance.
CT scans through the right lower lobe (A and B) reveal an eccentrically thickened bronchus (Br) in the posterior portion of the lobe. In B, the contiguous opaque artery (pa) is partly obscured at the divisional point of the airway. Pathologic examination (see Fig. 31–4) demonstrated tumor largely confined to the mucosa and submucosa. (From Foster WL, Roberts L, McLendon RF, Hill RC: Am J Roentgenol 144:906, 1985.)

Table 31–2. CLINICAL AND RADIOLOGIC CRITERIA IN THE DIFFERENTIATION OF BENIGN AND MALIGNANT SOLITARY PULMONARY NODULES

	BENIGN	MALIGNANT
Clinical		
Age	<35 years. Exception is hamartoma	>35 years
Symptoms	Absent	Present
Past history and functional enquiry	High incidence of granuloma in area. Exposure to tuberculosis. Nonsmoker	Diagnosis of primary lesion elsewhere. Smoker. Exposure to carcinogens
Radiographic		
Size	Small (<3 cm in diameter)	Large (>3 cm in diameter)
Location	No predilection except for tuberculosis (upper lobes)	Predominantly upper lobes except for lung metastases
Contour	Margins smooth	Margins spiculated
Calcification	Almost pathognomonic of a benign lesion if laminated, diffuse, or central	Rare, may be eccentric (engulfed granuloma)
Satellite lesions	More common	Less common
Serial studies showing no change over 2 years	Almost diagnostic of benign lesion	Most unlikely
Doubling time	<30 or >490 days	Between these extremes
Computed Tomography		
Calcification	Diffuse or central	Absent or eccentric
Fat	Virtually diagnostic of hamartoma	Absent
Bubble-like lucencies	Uncommon	Common in adenocarcinomas
Enhancement with intravenous contrast material	<15 HU	>25 HU

Experience has shown that it is best to divide solitary nodules into two broad categories for the purposes of differential diagnosis: (1) those that are almost certainly benign, as determined by rigidly defined radiologic signs;[882, 884, 886, 890, 891] and (2) those of indeterminate nature, comprising all other lesions. Thus, the *benign/indeterminate* categorization replaces the more traditional *benign/malignant* distinction. The main reason for this separation is simply that the stringent criteria of benignity are more certain than are the radiologic signs of malignancy. The four features of greatest value in assessing a solitary pulmonary nodule are size, calcification, character of the tumor-lung interface, and doubling time.

Size

As indicated previously, the majority of malignant and the minority of benign solitary pulmonary nodules are 3 cm or greater in diameter; for example, in one study, only 11 (6%) of 176 benign nodules were larger than 3 cm, in contrast to 161 (57%) of 283 primary cancers.[882] In another series, more than 80% of 118 benign nodules measured 1 cm or less, and only 1 of the 36 nodules larger than 3 cm in diameter was benign;[883] by contrast, the diameter of malignant nodules was nearly uniformly distributed in the 1- to 6-cm range, with slightly more than 50% being larger than 2 cm in diameter (18% were ≤ 1 cm).

Clearly, no size criterion allows exclusion of malignancy. In one review of 64 patients who had nodules less than 1 cm in diameter, 38 (57%) were shown to be malignant by video-assisted thoracoscopic biopsy, including 8 which were less than 5 mm in size.[892] The likelihood ratio for malignancy of solitary nodules has been estimated to be 0.52 for those less than 1 cm in diameter, 0.74 for those between 1.1 and 2 cm, 3.7 for those between 2.1 and 3 cm, and 5.2 for those greater than 3 cm.[893] When interpreting these figures, it is important to remember that the likelihood of carcinoma is also strongly influenced by other factors, such as age and smoking history.

Calcification

The presence or absence of calcium is undoubtedly the most important feature that distinguishes benign from malignant nodules.[882, 883, 891, 894] The presence of diffuse, laminated, or central calcification is almost certain evidence of benignity (Fig. 31–55), only rare nodules with these features proving to be malignant (Fig. 31–56).[882, 895–898] The presence of an eccentric calcific opacity in a nodule or mass occasionally represents incorporation of a calcified granuloma within the substance of a carcinoma (Fig. 31–57). Although calcification can be seen on thin-section CT (1- to 3-mm collimation scans) in about 5% to 10% of pulmonary carcinomas,[883, 899, 900] it usually affects tumors greater than 3 cm in diameter; for example, in one study of 39 calcified tumors, only 6 (15%) were smaller than this.[900] The calcification within the pulmonary carcinomas was mild and had not been identified on the original chest radiograph in any case.

Although conventional chest radiographs sometimes reveal convincing evidence of calcification, particularly when this is laminated or "target" in type, definitive examination often requires CT. In one study, thin-section CT was performed on 91 nodules that did not have radiographic evidence of calcification.[901] Criteria for a benign nodule included high attenuation values throughout the nodule or in its center. Twenty of 33 benign lesions as defined by CT and clinical criteria had relatively high CT numbers (≥164 HU), presumably as a result of diffuse calcification; all 58 malignant lesions had comparatively low numbers (mean representative CT number of 92 HU with a standard deviation of 18

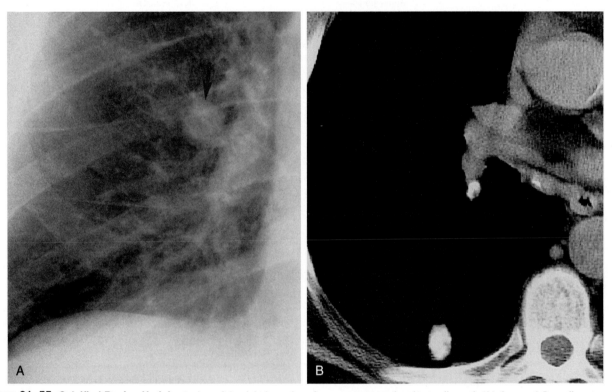

Figure 31–55. Calcified Benign Nodule. A view of the right lower lung from a posteroanterior chest radiograph *(A)* shows a 1.5-cm-diameter nodule *(arrow)*. No calcification is evident on the radiograph. A 7-mm collimation CT scan *(B)* demonstrates diffuse calcification of the nodule and associated calcified right hilar and subcarinal lymph nodes. These features are diagnostic of a granuloma. The patient was a 61-year-old man with a previous diagnosis of histoplasmosis.

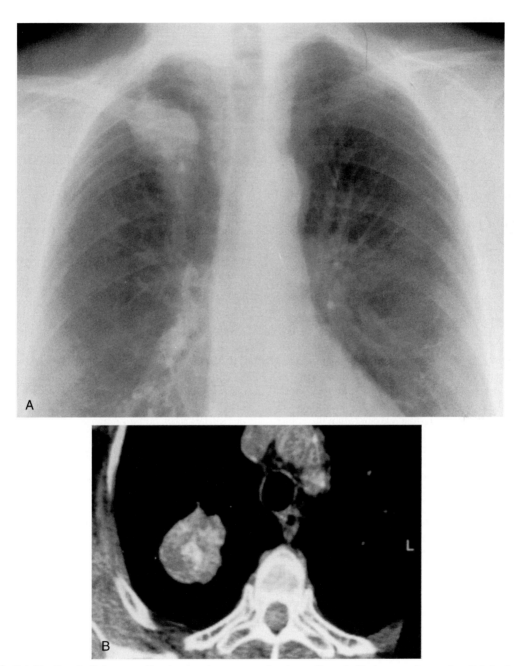

Figure 31–56. Calcification in Pulmonary Carcinoma. A posteroanterior chest radiograph *(A)* shows an elongated, well-defined mass in the apical region of the right upper lobe; no definite calcification is visible within the lesion. A 5-mm collimation CT scan through the upper lobe opacity *(B)* discloses amorphous calcification throughout the lesion. After surgical removal, pathologic examination revealed a highly necrotic carcinoma containing extensive deposits of dystrophic calcium. The patient was a 60-year-old man.

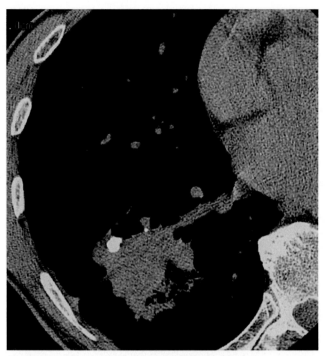

Figure 31–57. Calcification in Pulmonary Carcinoma. An HRCT in a 75-year-old man shows a 4-cm-diameter tumor in the right lower lobe. Focal areas of eccentric calcification are present. At right lower lobectomy, the tumor was shown to be a bronchioloalveolar carcinoma that had engulfed calcified granulomas.

HU). In another study, 176 (63%) of 279 benign nodules had attenuation values of 164 HU or greater throughout the nodule or in its center.[882] In a third investigation in which 200 HU was used as the cut-off criterion for benignity, all 44 nodules that had attenuation values greater than this value were benign;[902] of nodules whose attenuation values were below 200 HU, 96 were malignant, and 37 were benign.

Although the results of these studies suggest that CT attenuation values may be helpful in determining the nature of a pulmonary nodule, there are difficulties in reproducibility of the data between different CT scanners at different institutions.[903, 904] In one study in which a standard phantom was examined on five CT scanners using a variety of conditions that simulated those encountered in routine body CT scanning, a wide range of CT numbers was found for a given tissue type as a result of scanner performance alone;[904] the authors recommended that if absolute CT numbers are to be employed for diagnosis, the user must document that apparatus-related variations are less than the differences in CT number thought to be significant.

Perhaps the most authoritative report to date concerning this issue was a multicenter study in which the use of a special reference phantom enabled CT densitometric measurements to be made independent of variations between scanners and patients.[883] The phantom was standardized to a 1-cm diameter cylinder that had an attenuation of 264 HU. Of 384 nodules not considered to be calcified by radiography or conventional tomography, 118 lesions (31%) proved to be benign; of these, 65 (55%) revealed unsuspected calcification, in 28 by direct inspection of thin-section CT scans at narrow windows and in the remaining 37 by use of the

calibration phantom. Of 229 nodules interpreted as indeterminate on CT, 176 were malignant, and 53 were benign. In only one case was a pulmonary carcinoma interpreted as benign on CT; this was a calcified tumor measuring 3.5 cm in diameter.[883] The authors concluded that thin-section CT aided by a reference phantom in equivocal cases should be an integral part of the diagnostic approach to the solitary pulmonary nodule. In a subsequent investigation, only 2 (3%) of 62 nodules classified as benign using the reference phantom CT were proven to be malignant;[905] one was a 1.5-cm-diameter calcified central carcinoid and the other a 3.5-cm-diameter peripheral pulmonary carcinoma. Using a reference phantom standardized to 185 HU, another group of investigators had a higher number of false-negative diagnoses.[906]

The author of a review in 1994 identified 11 studies in which CT densitometry had been used to evaluate pulmonary nodules.[907] These studies used either the presence of attenuation values with a threshold ranging from 164 to 200 HU to identify the presence of calcification or an internal reference phantom standardized to a given attenuation value (which ranged from 185 to 264 HU in different series). Of 504 nodules denser than the reference, 490 (97%) were benign, and 14 (3%) were malignant. Of 1,109 nodules less dense than the reference, 782 (71%) were malignant, and 327 (29%) were benign. In the vast majority of these cases, the calcification identified on CT was not apparent on conventional radiographs or tomography.

Despite the potential advantages of the use of a reference phantom, it has been all but abandoned in most institutions. Improvements in technology have resulted in scanners that allow more accurate density measurements than those that prompted the development of the CT phantom.[898, 908] Furthermore, use of thin-section CT (1- to 3-mm collimation) allows more common identification of calcification than was possible on conventional CT. For example, in one study of 62 benign nodules, calcification was identified on thin-section CT in 36% of tumors compared with only 12% on standard CT.[905] It cannot be overemphasized that optimal assessment on CT requires the use of a series of thin sections through the nodule. Foci of calcification that are visible on thin-section CT usually have attenuation values of 400 HU or higher.[898, 908] In the absence of such foci, attenuation values of 200 HU or higher can also be considered to represent calcification.[898, 908] Although we and others[898] use HRCT (1-mm collimation reconstructed using a high spatial frequency algorithm) because it may be more sensitive for detecting small amounts of calcium,[898, 908] in some CT scanners, use of this algorithm can result in edge artefacts that may mimic calcification;[909] therefore some radiologists prefer to use a standard or soft tissue reconstruction algorithm.[909]

Other techniques may also be useful for demonstrating the presence of calcification within pulmonary nodules, including dual-energy film subtraction[910] and dual-energy CT.[911–913] Because of a number of limitations, however, these techniques have had limited clinical application. Of greater interest is the use of dual-energy computed radiography. This technique allows a search for a soft tissue nodule on a chest radiograph unobscured by ribs as well as comparison of the density of the nodule with that of calcified structures on another view.[914–918] In one study of 200 patients in which images on single-exposure, dual-energy computed radiography were compared to those on conventional radiography, five independent observers improved their ability to diagnose pulmonary nodules and to characterize the nodules as calcified on dual-energy computed radiography as compared to conventional radiography.[919]

Character of the Nodule-Lung Interface

Pulmonary carcinomas commonly have an irregular spiculated interface (Fig. 31–58). For example, in one study of 283 tumors, 184 (65%) had focal or diffuse spiculation of their margins; 91 (32%) had smooth but lobulated margins; and 8 (3%) had smooth, nonlobulated margins.[882] In another series of 82 carcinomas, 72 (88%) had spiculated margins.[920] Although such spiculation (shagginess of contour) is more common in pulmonary carcinoma, it may also be seen in metastases or benign lesions (Fig. 31–59). In one study of 634 nodules, 50 of 53 (94%) that had diffuse spiculation (corona radiata) and 134 of 165 (81%) with focal spiculation were primary pulmonary carcinomas;[882] by comparison, only 8 of 66 (12%) smoothly marginated, nonlobulated nodules represented primary carcinomas, 6 (1%) being a solitary metastasis and 52 (87%) benign. Lobulation was not helpful in distinguishing benign from malignant lesions. Of 350 smoothly marginated, lobulated lesions, 91 (26%) were primary pulmonary carcinomas, 57 (16%) were metastases, and 202 (58%) were benign. In a review of the literature published by 1993, it was concluded that the

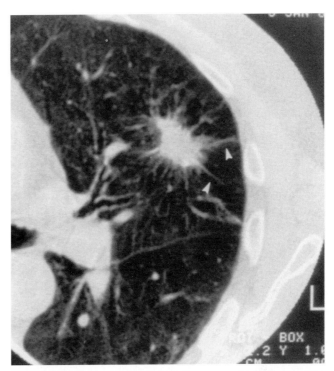

Figure 31–59. Corona Radiata in Exogenous Lipid Pneumonia. A view of the left lung from an HRCT scan demonstrates a nodule that has spiculated margins (arrowheads). At surgery, this was shown to represent lipid pneumonia.

likelihood ratio for malignancy of a nodule that has irregular or spiculated margins is 5.54, the corresponding figures for lobulated or smoothly marginated nodules being 0.74 and 0.30.[893] Radiologic-pathologic correlation has shown that spiculation may reflect the presence of fibrosis in the surrounding parenchyma, direct infiltration of carcinoma into the adjacent parenchyma, or localized lymphangitic spread.[920, 921]

The *tail sign* or pleural tag consists of a linear opacity that extends from a peripheral nodule or mass to the visceral pleura. The tag can represent a strand of fibrous tissue that extends from the nodule to the visceral pleura[920, 922] or can result from inward retraction and apposition of a thickened visceral pleura (Fig. 31–60). As the visceral pleura invaginates, a small quantity of extrapleural fat is drawn into the area, creating the opacity.[923] Pleural tags have been reported on HRCT in 60% to 80% of peripheral pulmonary carcinomas.[920, 924] Although they are most commonly associated with adenocarcinoma,[920, 925, 926] they may be seen with other histologic subtypes;[920, 927] they may also be identified in association with pulmonary metastases[927, 928] and granulomas.[927, 928] As a result of the latter observation, the sign is of limited value in the differentiation of benign from malignant lesions.[927, 928]

Satellite lesions can be present in association with both benign and malignant nodules, although they are much more frequent with the former. When related to carcinoma, they are usually the result of metastasis ("skip lesions") or expansion of one or more peripheral foci of carcinoma contiguous with the main tumor mass; sometimes, they represent a preexistent scar.[929]

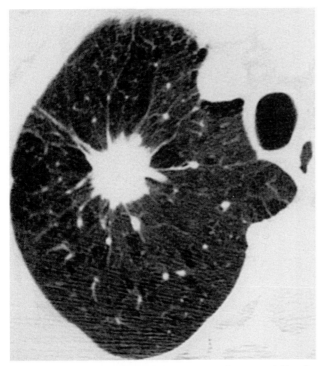

Figure 31–58. Pulmonary Carcinoma with Spiculated Margins. An HRCT in a 62-year-old man demonstrates a 2.5-cm-diameter nodule in the right upper lobe. The nodule has multiple spicules radiating from the lesion into the surrounding parenchyma (corona radiata). The diagnosis was proven adenocarcinoma.

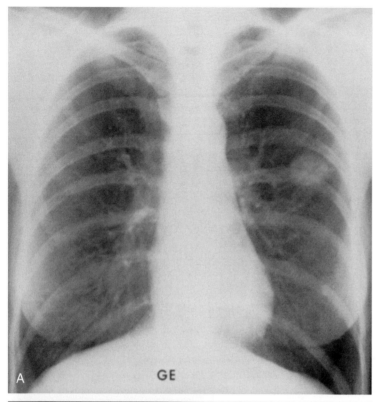

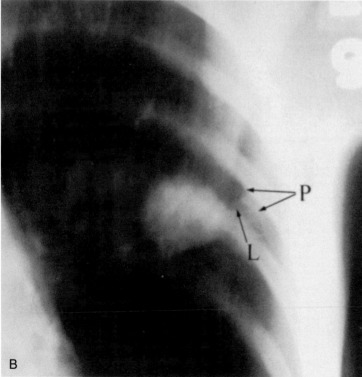

Figure 31–60. Pyramidal Pleural Opacity Associated with a Peripheral Adenocarcinoma. A posteroanterior chest radiograph *(A)* reveals a 3-cm nodule in the left upper lobe. A linear tomogram in anteroposterior projection *(B)* shows the lesion to be homogeneous in density; faint spiculations are present at the lung-tumor interface. A triangular opacity (P) is connected to the mass by a thin line (L).

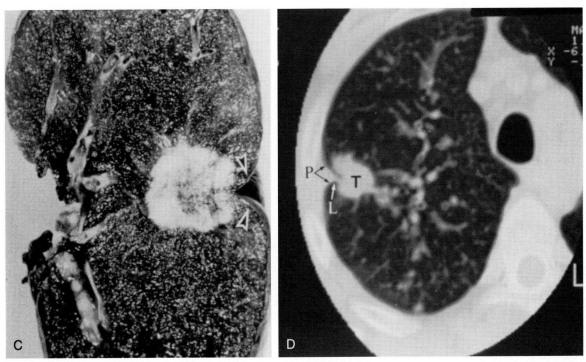

Figure 31–60 *Continued.* After resection of the left upper lobe *(C)*, the lung was sectioned in a coronal plane through the center of the tumor. The visceral pleura *(arrowheads)* is inverted toward the mass. The mechanism by which this opacity is created is considered to be as follows: A potential void created by puckered pleura is filled with a small amount of pleural fluid or extrapleural fat, forming a triangular or pyramidal shadow; the linear opacity relates to apposition of the two opposing (visceral) pleural surfaces. In another patient, a CT scan *(D)* through a right upper lobe nodular adenocarcinoma (T) displays features similar to those already described: A pyramidal pleural opacity (P) is connected to the nodule by a short line (L). CT attenuation from the triangular opacity was +6 HU, consistent with pleural fluid.

Air Bronchogram

On thin-section CT, air bronchograms and air bronchiolograms are seen more commonly in pulmonary carcinomas than in benign nodules (Fig. 31–61).[920, 924, 930] For example, in one review of 132 patients, air bronchograms were identified on thin-section CT in 33 (29%) of 115 pulmonary carcinomas and in only 1 (6%) of 17 benign nodules.[930] The patent airways are frequently tortuous and ectatic.[930, 931] When cut in cross-section, they are seen as focal air collections, usually measuring 5 mm or less in diameter, a finding commonly referred to as *bubble-like lucency* or *pseudocavitation* (Fig. 31–62).[920, 932–934] These lucencies may also result from distended air-filled parenchyma within papillary tumors or, less commonly, from irregular (paracicatricial) emphysema or localized bronchiectasis.[920, 933, 935, 936]

As might be expected, bubble-like lucencies are particularly common in bronchioloalveolar carcinoma; for example, in one review of the findings in 30 patients who had this tumor, they were seen in 18 (60%).[932] In another study, bubble-like lucencies were seen within solitary nodules on thin-section CT in 21 of 85 malignant nodules (25%) and in only 1 (9%) of 11 benign nodules;[920] they were present in 7 (55%) of 13 bronchioloalveolar carcinomas, 9 (31%) of 28 acinar adenocarcinomas, and approximately 10% of squamous carcinomas and large cell carcinomas.

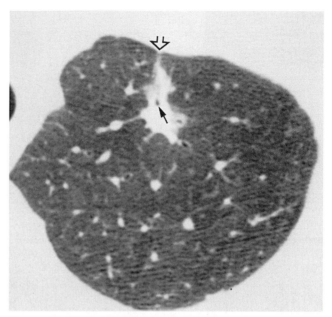

Figure 31–62. Bubble-Like Lucency in Bronchioloalveolar Carcinoma. A view of the left upper lobe from an HRCT scan in a 49-year-old woman demonstrates a 2-cm-diameter spiculated nodule. A small localized area of air density (bubble-like lucency) *(straight arrow)* is present within the nodule. A pleural tag is also present *(open arrow)*. The diagnosis of bronchioloalveolar carcinoma was proved at surgery. Correlation of the HRCT scan with the excised specimen showed that the bubble-like lucency represented a bronchus surrounded by tumor.

Doubling Time

Use of doubling time* in estimating growth rate may be of value in differentiating benign from malignant nodules in individual patients. The concept requires at least two serial chest radiographs showing a roughly spherical lesion whose diameter can be averaged from measurements in at least two planes.[937]

In theory, extrapolation of the data derived from an assessment of doubling time gives an estimate of the time of onset of a cancer.[938–943] Although an unchanging growth rate is assumed in this estimation, perhaps without justification,[944] the results of several studies strongly support this concept.[941–943] Assuming that the original malignant change takes place in a single cell measuring 10 μm^3 and disregarding the effects on volume of apoptosis or tumor necrosis, 20 volume doublings are required to produce a tumor 1 mm in diameter and 30 doublings a tumor 1 cm in diameter (the usual limit of radiographic detection of primary pulmonary carcinoma). Only 10 more volume doublings—40 in all—produce a tumor 10 cm in diameter; most patients die before this occurs. According to this model, 75% of a tumor's lifetime occurs before the lesion is detectable on the chest radiograph. Calculation based on a range of doubling times from 30 to 300 days indicates that the time required for a malignant pulmonary nodule to reach 1 cm in diameter

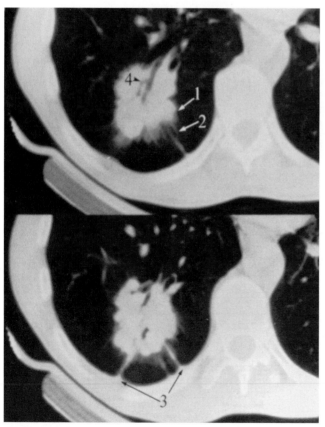

Figure 31–61. Air Bronchogram in Bronchioloalveolar Carcinoma. CT scans through a right lower lobe mass show several signs that strongly favor malignancy: marginal nodulation (1), fine spiculations (2), and pleural retraction (3). An air bronchogram (4) with narrowed, amputated airways suggests a diagnosis of bronchioloalveolar carcinoma, which was proved after surgical excision. The patient was a 55-year-old woman.

---

*Doubling refers to volume, not diameter. Assuming a nodule to be spherical, its diameter must be multiplied by 1.25 to obtain the diameter of a sphere whose volume is double (e.g., the volume of a nodule 2 cm in diameter is doubled by the time its diameter reaches 2.5 cm). Stated another way, a doubling of diameter represents an eightfold increase in volume.

ranges from about 2.5 to more than 25 years.[941] One problem with the radiologic estimation of doubling times is that many pulmonary carcinomas are not spherical, a fact that can lead to considerable overestimation of volume, especially of larger tumors (see Fig. 31–42, page 1121). In addition, hemorrhage into the center of a carcinoma can increase its volume dramatically and put the doubling time within the range usually accepted as denoting benignity (Fig. 31–63).

Despite its limitations, the doubling time concept may be useful in diagnosis. In a study of 218 pulmonary nodules (177 malignant and 41 benign), virtually all those whose doubling time was 7 days or less were benign;[939] similarly, nodules whose volume doubled in 465 days or more were almost always benign. A pulmonary nodule whose rate of growth falls outside these limits must be considered malignant. Perhaps the most useful application of the growth rate principle in assessing solitary nodules is in patients older than 40 years of age, in whom the incidence of malignancy increases markedly. In one study of individuals in this age group, almost every solitary nodule whose doubling time was less than 37 days was benign;[939] of 72 malignant nodules, the slowest growing doubled their volume in 200 days. Other investigators have quoted only slightly different figures.[940, 946, 947] For example, in one series of 67 patients who had pulmonary carcinoma, the doubling time ranged from 30 to 490 days;[941] in another review of 52 cases, it varied from 1 to 14 months.[943] Of pulmonary carcinomas, adenocarcinoma grows most slowly and poorly differentiated carcinomas most rapidly;[942, 943, 946, 948–950] giant cell carcinoma is characterized by extremely rapid growth (Fig. 31–64).

The doubling time provides a more accurate assessment of the nature of a solitary nodule than does simple increase in size. In fact, because benign lesions such as hamartoma and histoplasmoma also may grow slowly,[951, 952] increase in size by itself should not be the sole consideration governing the therapeutic approach to a pulmonary nodule. Absence of growth over a 2-year period is a fairly reliable indicator of benignity.[939, 953, 954] Small changes in size may be difficult to appreciate on the chest radiograph or CT. For example, a 5-mm-diameter nodule increases to only 6-mm diameter after one doubling and to only 8-mm diameter after two doublings. Furthermore, occasional carcinomas have been reported after apparent stability for a period of 2 or more years,[393, 955] and the validity of 2-year stability as an indicator of benignity has been questioned.[956] Despite these limitations, we believe that a 2-year stability can be considered a reasonably reliable criterion for benignity. Carcinomas with longer doubling times tend to have a better prognosis.[957, 958]

Nodule Enhancement

Because the degree of enhancement of a nodule after intravenous administration of contrast material is related to its vascularity and the amount of contrast material that enters the extravascular space,[959, 960] the prominent neovascularity of many malignant nodules makes them more likely to show enhancement than benign tumors.[961] The use of differential nodule enhancement in diagnosis was first reported on conventional tomography,[961] but has since been applied to several radiologic techniques.

Computed Tomography

A number of investigators have provided evidence of the potential usefulness of the measurement of nodule enhancement on thin-section CT.[879, 880, 962, 963] In one study of 163 patients, the median enhancement of 111 malignant nodules was 40 HU (range, 20 to 108 HU) compared to 12 HU (range, −4 to 58 HU) for 52 benign lesions;[962] using 20 HU as the threshold separating malignant from benign nodules, the authors reported a sensitivity of 100%, specificity of 77%, positive predictive value of 90%, and negative predictive value of 100% for the presence of carcinoma (Fig. 31–65). In a prospective study of 107 patients (again using an enhancement of at least 20 HU as a marker for malignancy), the same group of investigators found a 98% sensitivity and a 73% specificity for the diagnosis of carcinoma;[963] the only false-negative result was related to a carcinoma that enhanced 11 HU. Four of 52 malignant neoplasms and 4 of 55 benign nodules had attenuation values between 16 and 24 HU, leading the investigators to consider this range as inconclusive.[963] In another study of 18 cases of pulmonary carcinoma, none enhanced less than 25 HU, whereas the 10 granulomas and 3 of 4 hamartomas enhanced less than 15 HU.[880]

Although the results of these studies are encouraging, it is important to emphasize that they are applicable only to nodules measuring 6 to 30 mm in diameter that have homogeneous attenuation. Furthermore, the technique requires meticulous attention to detail. CT scans should be obtained using 1- to 3-mm collimation, preferentially using spiral technique and reconstruction at 1- to 2-mm intervals. The attenuation is measured in the section closest to the center of the nodule using a region of interest of approximately 60% of the diameter of the nodule. After initial measurement of nodule attenuation on unenhanced scans, iodinated intravenous contrast material is injected for a total dose of 420 mg of iodine per kg at a concentration of 300 mg per ml (100 ml for a 70-kg subject) and a rate of 2 ml/sec. Images are then obtained at 1-, 2-, 3-, and 4-minute intervals, and attenuation values are measured using the identical technique as in the precontrast scan.[963]

One group of investigators examined blood flow patterns of pulmonary nodules after rapid infusion (4 ml/sec) using single-level dynamic CT to acquire clusters of images at 15 and 65 seconds;[964] peak levels of nodule enhancement, time attenuation curves, nodule perfusion, and patterns of contrast enhancement were assessed. The mean peak enhancement of 42 malignant nodules was 42 HU compared to 44 HU for 7 benign inflammatory nodules and 13 HU for 16 benign noninflammatory nodules. Forty (95%) of 42 malignant nodules showed a peak enhancement of 20 HU or more. All the malignant nodules showed measurable enhancement, most commonly in a homogeneous or heterogeneous pattern. Benign nodules showed either no enhancement or peripheral enhancement.

The results of these studies indicate that lack of enhancement or enhancement of less than 15 HU after intravenous administration of contrast material is virtually diagnostic of a benign lesion. The greatest value of nodule enhancement studies is therefore in providing support for conservative follow-up of noncalcified lesions that are con-

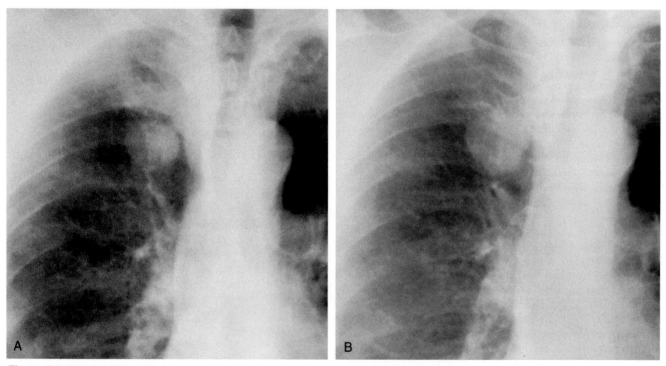

Figure 31–63. Rapid Doubling Time of a Nodular Lung Carcinoma Caused by Hemorrhage. Detail views *(A* and *B)* of the right upper lung from posteroanterior chest radiographs obtained 6 days apart show a well-defined homogeneous mass that has undergone rapid enlargement. Although the sharp definition of the lesion suggests a neoplasm, the rapid increase in size raised the possibility of an infectious cause. After surgical excision, sections showed the lesion to consist of a large cell carcinoma with extensive recent hemorrhage. (Courtesy of Dr. R. Hidvegi, Montreal Chest Hospital Center.)

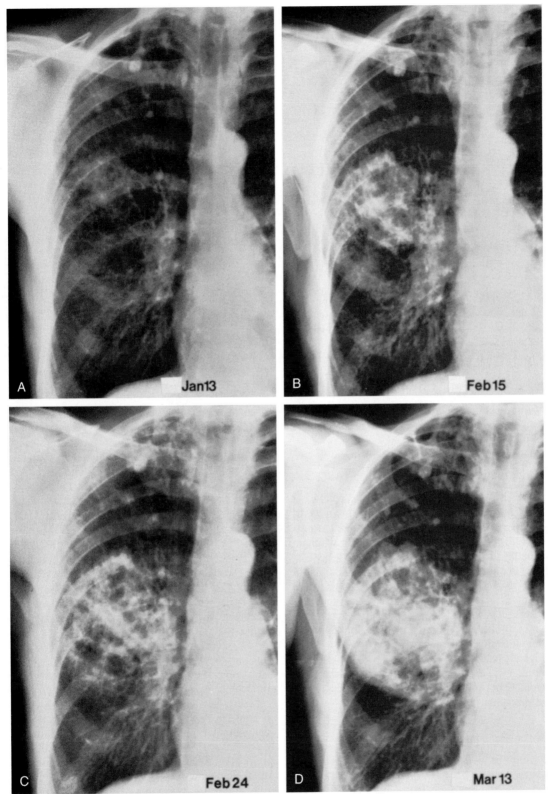

Figure 31–64. Giant Cell Carcinoma of the Right Lower Lobe. Views of the right lung from four sequential radiographs of a 55-year-old asymptomatic man span a period of 2 months. The original examination *(A)* reveals a poorly defined opacity approximately 4 cm in diameter in the midportion of the right lung (situated in the superior segment of the lower lobe); there is obvious enlargement of the right hilum. One month later *(B),* the mass has increased markedly in size and now shows central radiolucencies suggesting cavitation; the right hilum is also larger. Ten days later *(C)* the mass has almost doubled in volume. Two months after the first examination *(D),* the volume of the mass has increased an estimated 20 times. Thoracotomy was performed, and the lesion was found to be unresectable. Histologic examination of biopsy material revealed giant cell carcinoma. The extremely rapid growth observed radiologically is characteristic of this neoplasm. (Courtesy of Dr. John Wrinch, Royal Inland Hospital, Kamloops, British Columbia.)

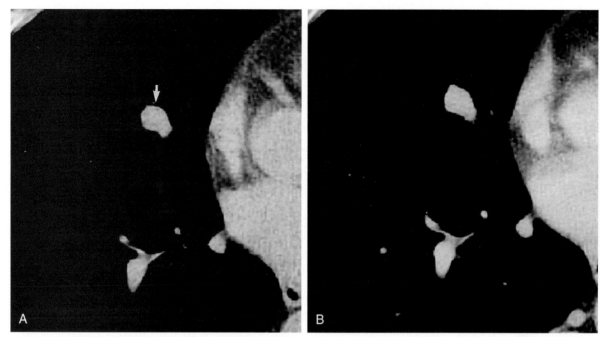

Figure 31–65. Nodule Enhancement in Pulmonary Carcinoma. A view of the right lung from a 3-mm collimation spiral CT scan *(A)* demonstrates a 1.2-cm diameter, noncalcified nodule *(arrow)* in the right middle lobe. A CT scan performed at the same level 2 minutes after intravenous administration of contrast material *(B)* shows marked enhancement of the nodule. The attenuation increased from 10 HU before intravenous contrast administration to 53 HU after contrast administration. At right middle lobectomy, the nodule was shown to represent an adenocarcinoma.

sidered likely to be benign. Because of the number of false-positive examinations, the presence of contrast enhancement is less helpful in diagnosis.

Magnetic Resonance Imaging

MR imaging can also be used to assess enhancement of nodules using intravenous contrast with gadolinium diethylenetriamine penta-acetic acid (DTPA). Preliminary results have shown greater increase in signal intensity of malignant lesions compared with benign ones.[964–966] Adequate assessment of change in signal intensity on MR after administration of contrast material requires the use of sophisticated techniques, such as measurement of enhancement curves showing the percent change in signal intensity during the first transit of a bolus of contrast medium on dynamic snapshot gradient-echo MR images.[964, 965] Because of its greater cost, lower availability, decreased spatial resolution, and, most importantly, inability to identify reliably the presence of calcium, MR imaging plays a limited role in the assessment of the solitary nodule.

Positron-Emission Tomography

Several groups of investigators have assessed the potential use of positron-emission tomography (PET) after intravenous administration of 2-(fluorine-18)-fluoro-2-deoxy-D-glucose ([18]FDG).[945, 967–971a] (The latter is a glucose analogue labeled with a positron emitter ^{18}F; it is transported through the cell membrane and phosphorylated through normal glycolytic pathways, following which it is not metabolized further and remains within the cell.)

In one investigation of 52 patients who had noncalcified nodules, FDG-PET scans were abnormal in 35 of 37 malig-

nant tumors (sensitivity 95%) and 2 of 15 benign ones (specificity 87%).[972] For nodules greater than 1.5 cm in diameter, the sensitivity was 100% and the specificity 67%; for those 1.5 cm or less in diameter, the sensitivity was 83% and the specificity 100%. In another study, FDG-PET scanning was positive in 44 of 47 pulmonary carcinomas (sensitivity 94%) and in 3 of 15 granulomas (specificity 80%);[973] two of the false-negative results were in nodules measuring less than 1 cm in diameter. In a third investigation, FDG-PET scanning was positive in all 82 pulmonary carcinomas (sensitivity 100%) and in 12 of 25 benign nodules (specificity 52%).[971] These studies demonstrate PET imaging to have a high sensitivity and a high negative predictive value, particularly for nodules 1 cm or greater in diameter. The main disadvantages of the technique are limited availability and high cost.

Conventional gamma cameras can be equipped with ultra-high-energy collimators to allow single-photon emission computed tomography (SPECT) imaging. Although this procedure is more readily available, it is inferior to PET imaging in the differentiation of benign from malignant lesions. In one study of 26 patients who had 28 radiologically indeterminate focal pulmonary lesions, 17 of the 21 carcinomas showed FDG uptake on SPECT imaging (sensitivity 81%), whereas none of the 7 benign nodules showed uptake (specificity 100%) (Fig. 31–66);[974] imaging was positive in all 16 carcinomas that were 2 cm in diameter or larger but was negative in 4 of 5 carcinomas smaller than 2 cm in diameter.

Solitary Pulmonary Mass

As discussed previously, the rather arbitrary division of solitary opacities within the lung into two categories, nodules

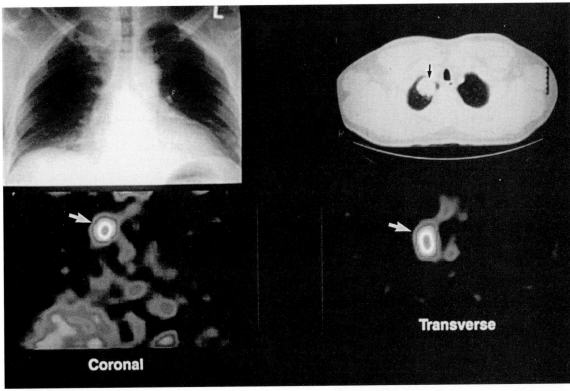

Figure 31–66. **¹⁸FDG SPECT Imaging.** A chest radiograph and CT scan show a 3-cm-diameter right upper lobe nodule *(black arrow)*. Coronal and transverse ¹⁸FDG SPECT images demonstrate increased uptake *(white arrows)*. The diagnosis was surgically proven pulmonary adenocarcinoma. (Courtesy of Dr. Daniel Worsley, Division of Nuclear Medicine, Vancouver General Hospital.)

(measuring ≤ 3 cm in diameter) and masses (measuring > 3 cm in diameter) serves one useful purpose—a mass is much more likely than is a nodule to be malignant. Calcification in a mass does not exclude malignancy as it does in the case of a solitary nodule. For example, in one study of 353 carcinomas, 20 (6%) had calcification evident on CT;[899] 17 of the 20 containing calcification (85%) were greater than 3 cm in diameter. In another investigation, the mean diameter of 39 carcinomas that had calcification identified on CT was 6.2 cm;[900] 33 tumors (85%) were greater than 3 cm in diameter. The calcification in these large tumors may be punctate, chunky, or amorphous in appearance and central, peripheral, or diffuse in distribution (Fig. 31–67).[900] It may be related to psammoma bodies, dystrophic calcification, or incorporation of calcified bronchial cartilage or a focus of prior granulomatous inflammation within the tumor.[714, 900, 975, 976] Although the interface between a mass and contiguous lung can be sharply defined and smooth (e.g., resembling a solitary "cannonball" metastasis), it is much more often ill-defined, a feature that strengthens a suspicion of malignancy. As discussed in the next section, cavitation is a relatively common feature.

Cavitation

The incidence of cavitation in pulmonary carcinoma is about 5% to 15%.[56, 858, 977] Although the complication can occur in tumors of any size, most are greater than 3 cm in diameter.[881] The most common histologic type is squamous cell carcinoma; among 600 carcinomas reported in four studies, it was seen in approximately 7% of 263 squamous cell carcinomas, 4% of 97 large cell carcinomas, 2% of 126 adenocarcinomas, and none of 114 small cell carcinomas.[836, 837, 841, 846] In another investigation of 100 cavitated carcinomas, 82 were squamous cell.[977] Cavity formation was related to three processes: (1) necrosis of the central portion of the neoplasm (77 cases); (2) formation of a lung abscess in an area of obstructive pneumonitis (17 cases); and (3) abscess formation elsewhere in the lungs, presumably as a result of spillover of purulent material from pneumonitis and abscess formation elsewhere (6 cases). The most common locations of the 77 necrotic neoplasms were the posterior segments of the upper lobes and the superior segments of the lower lobes.

Most cavities have an irregular inner surface as a result of variably sized nodules of neoplastic tissue projecting into the cavity and of the patchy nature of the necrosis (Fig. 31–68). The cavities may be central or eccentric and 1 to 10 cm in diameter. The majority have walls 0.5 to 3.0 cm thick. In approximately 3% of cases, the walls are extremely thin, simulating a bulla or bronchogenic cyst (Fig. 31–69).[977] Although some of these may represent bullae or cysts in which the carcinoma has developed,[978–981] others are undoubtedly the result of extensive necrosis of the neoplasm itself (Fig. 31–69). Despite these observations, the vast majority of thin-walled cavities are benign. In a retrospective study of 65 solitary cavities, all those in which the thickest part of the cavity wall was 1 mm were benign;[982] of the

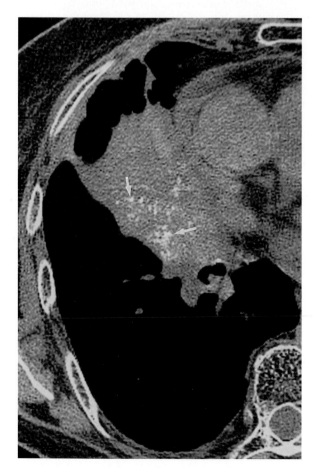

Figure 31–67. Calcification in Pulmonary Carcinoma. An HRCT scan in a 70-year-old woman demonstrates a large mass in the right middle lobe containing numerous small speckled areas of calcification *(arrows)*. The diagnosis of adenocarcinoma was proved at bronchial biopsy.

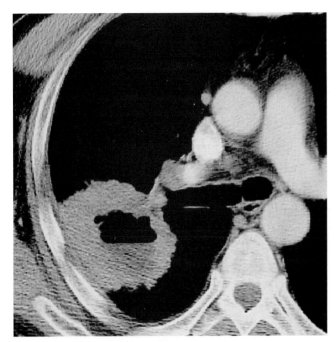

Figure 31–68. Cavitary Pulmonary Carcinoma. A view of the right lung from a contrast-enhanced CT scan in a 56-year-old man shows a 5-cm-diameter cavitated mass in the right upper lobe. The cavity has thick walls and a nodular inner contour characteristic of carcinoma. An air-fluid level within the tumor and right hilar lymphadenopathy are also evident. The diagnosis of squamous cell carcinoma was proved at surgery.

lesions whose thickest measurement was 4 mm or less, 92% were benign; of those that were 5 to 15 mm in their thickest part, benign and malignant lesions were equally divided; and of those in which the cavity wall was more than 15 mm in thickness, 95% were malignant. The authors concluded that measurement of the thickest part of a cavity wall provides a more reliable indication of benignity or malignancy than measurement of the thinnest part.

In a prospective study of 61 additional patients by the same investigators, 19 of 20 cavities (95%) that had a maximal wall thickness of 4 mm or less were benign;[983] of 22 lesions whose greatest wall thickness was 5 to 15 mm (and thus considered to be indeterminate), 16 (73%) were benign and 6 (27%) were malignant. Of the 19 cavities whose wall thickness measured 16 mm or more, 16 (84%) were malignant. From the observations in these two studies, it can be concluded that the vast majority of cavities whose maximal wall thickness is 4 mm or less are benign, whereas those that have a maximal wall thickness of 16 mm or more are malignant.

Air-Space (Pneumonic) Pattern

The air-space pattern of disease is almost entirely restricted to bronchioloalveolar carcinoma (Fig. 31–70). The changes may be local or widely disseminated, the former predominating in 60% to 90% of reported series.[934, 984–986] Some patients in whom the disease appears to be local when first seen have deposits elsewhere in the lungs that can be seen on CT.[981, 987–989] In others, increase in size of the initial tumor is associated with widespread dissemination on radiographs (Fig. 31–71). Radiographic abnormalities range from a hazy increase in density (ground-glass pattern) to dense consolidation and may be seen as an isolated finding or in conjunction with single or multiple nodules.[984–986, 989a]

On CT, this pattern corresponds to areas of ground-glass opacity or consolidation, reflecting the characteristic nondestructive growth of carcinoma on alveolar septa, the presence of secretions in adjacent air spaces, or both. The abnormalities can be focal, measuring from less than 1 cm to several centimeters in diameter (Fig. 31–72), patchy, or nonsegmental;[933, 934, 989, 990] lobar consolidation may occur and be associated with volume loss or lobar expansion.[934, 981, 989, 991] In one study of 42 patients who had bronchioloalveolar carcinoma, 16 (40%) presented with a solitary nodule or mass, 10 (24%) with lobar consolidation, 13 (30%) with multilobar consolidation, and 3 (7%) with diffuse nodules.[992]

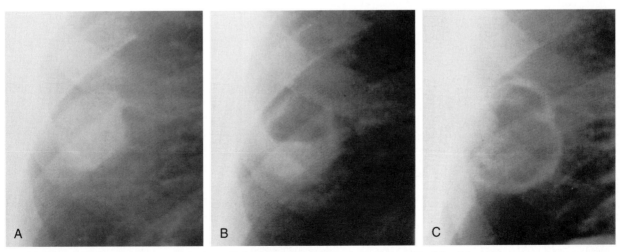

Figure 31–69. Variable Appearance of Cavitary Pulmonary Carcinoma. A detail view *(A)* of the right mid lung zone from a posteroanterior chest radiograph reveals a solitary mass that is homogeneously opaque and sharply marginated, consistent with either a solid or fluid-filled tumor. One month later *(B)*, the lesion has cavitated and now possesses a prominent fluid level that is confined by a 2- to 3-mm-thick wall. Four months later *(C)*, the fluid level has disappeared; the lesion has increased in size and possesses a uniformly thin wall that measures less than 4 mm throughout its circumference. The patient was a 62-year-old man. The lesion was proven squamous cell carcinoma.

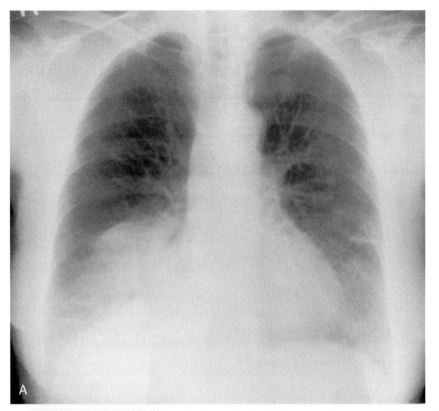

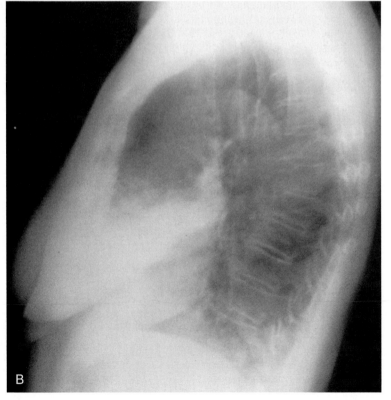

Figure 31–70. Progressive Multicentric Bronchioloalveolar Carcinoma. Posteroanterior *(A)* and lateral *(B)* chest radiographs show bilateral air-space opacities involving the middle lobe and parts of both lower lobes. The middle lobe exhibits the most severe involvement, showing almost complete, homogeneous consolidation except for a faint proximal air bronchogram; the lobe has also lost a little volume.

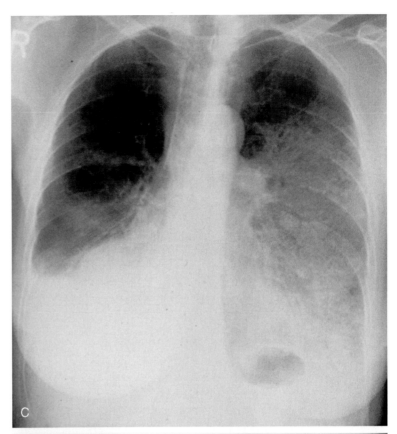

Figure 31–70 *Continued.* One year later, posteroanterior *(C)* and lateral *(D)* radiographs show more extensive consolidation throughout all areas, including both upper lobes. The patient was a 56-year-old woman who died of her disease shortly thereafter; at autopsy, both lungs were extensively involved with bronchioloalveolar carcinoma.

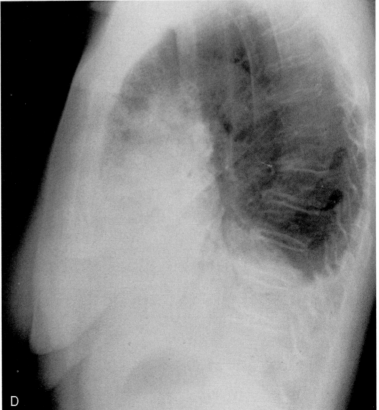

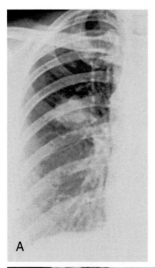

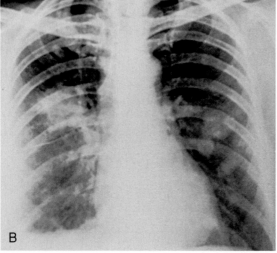

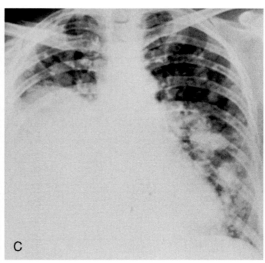

Figure 31–71. Bronchioloalveolar Carcinoma—Solitary Nodule Showing Rapid Growth and Wide Dissemination. A view of the right hemithorax from a posteroanterior radiograph *(A)* shows a solitary mass measuring 4 cm in diameter and possessing a rather indistinctly defined, lobulated contour; the mass is homogeneous in density and contains no calcium. Four months later *(B)*, the mass has increased somewhat in size; in addition, multiple nodular shadows have developed throughout both lungs. Six months later *(C)*, the situation has deteriorated markedly; much of the increase in density in the lower half of the right hemithorax is due to pleural effusion.

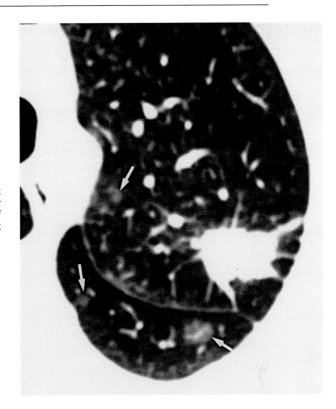

Figure 31–72. Bronchioloalveolar Carcinoma. A view of the left lung from an HRCT scan in a 68-year-old man demonstrates a 3-cm-diameter spiculated nodule in the left upper lobe. Also noted are small focal areas of ground-glass attenuation *(arrows)*. At surgery, the latter areas and the dominant nodule were shown to represent multicentric bronchioloalveolar carcinoma.

Eleven of the 16 nodules or masses (69%) and 13 of the 23 areas of consolidation (56%) were peripherally distributed (Fig. 31–73). Consolidation involving a segment or a complete lobe may simulate acute air-space pneumonia, such as that due to *Streptococcus pneumoniae* (Fig. 31–74).[993] In one investigation of 20 patients who had consolidative bronchioloalveolar carcinoma and 20 who had consolidative infectious pneumonia, findings most suggestive of the former abnormality were nodules (seen in 55% of patients with carcinoma compared with 5% of those with pneumonia) and a peripheral distribution (seen in 70% of patients with carcinoma and 15% with pneumonia).[993a]

Air bronchograms or bronchiolograms and bubble-like lucencies are seen in 50% to 80% of cases on CT.[920, 932] After intravenous administration of contrast material, clear distinction of pulmonary vessels from the relatively low attenuation of the surrounding parenchyma is often present, a finding known as the *CT angiogram sign*.[994] Although this

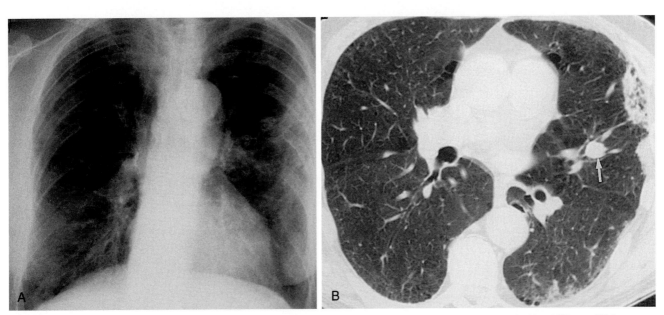

Figure 31–73. Peripheral Consolidation in Bronchioloalveolar Carcinoma. A posteroanterior chest radiograph *(A)* and CT scan *(B)* demonstrate consolidation involving the subpleural regions of the left lung. On the CT scan, a single nodule *(arrow)* can be seen more centrally. At video-assisted thoracoscopic biopsy of the consolidation, this was shown to represent bronchioloalveolar carcinoma.

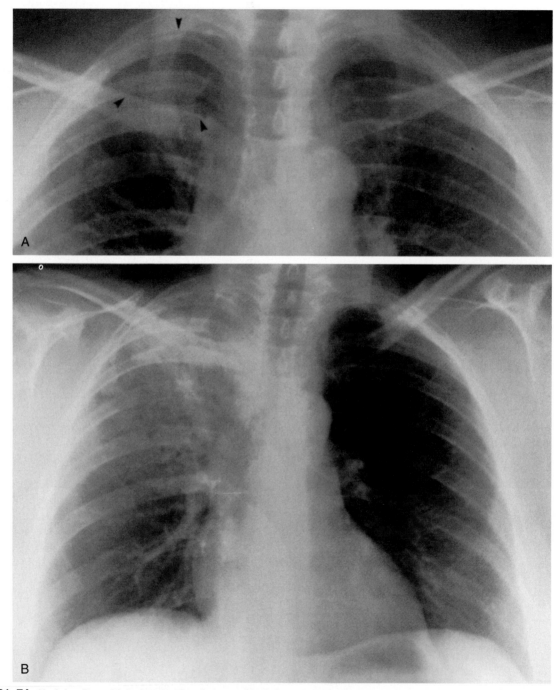

Figure 31–74. Nodular Bronchioloalveolar Carcinoma with Eventual Lobar Involvement. A detail view *(A)* of the lung apices from a posteroanterior chest radiograph reveals a poorly defined mass in the right apex *(arrowheads)*. Three years later *(B)*, most of the upper lobe has become involved. An air bronchogram is present within the consolidated lung.

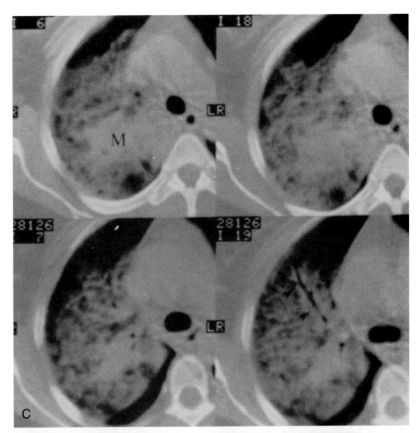

Figure 31–74 *Continued.* A sequence of contiguous CT scans *(C and D)* through the right upper lobe reveals a dominant mass superiorly (M); the air bronchogram *(arrowheads)* is more clearly seen throughout the lobar consolidation. Histologic examination after resection revealed bronchioloalveolar carcinoma. The patient was a 49-year-old woman.

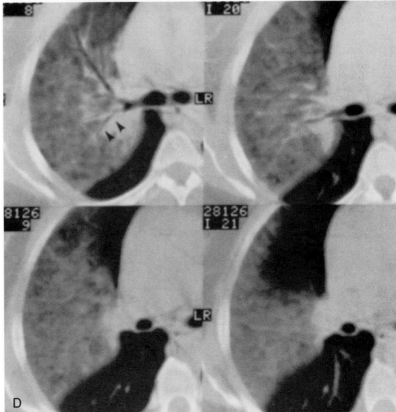

sign was first described in bronchioloalveolar carcinoma, it can also be seen in a variety of other conditions, including obstructive pneumonitis, lymphoma, lipid pneumonia, bacterial pneumonia (Fig. 31–75), pulmonary infarction, and pulmonary edema.[993a, 995–999]

Unusual presentations of bronchioloalveolar carcinoma include origin in a developmental cyst (e.g., bronchogenic cyst or congenital cystic adenomatoid malformation), homogeneous lobar atelectasis without an air bronchogram, and an elongated opacity resembling mucoid impaction.[981, 1000] Occasionally, minute calcific deposits can be identified within the lesion, particularly on CT scans, usually related to psammoma bodies.[976] One patient has been reported in whom calcifications in mediastinal lymph nodes were similar to those in the pulmonary lesion and were subsequently proved to be psammoma bodies situated within nodal metastases.[976]

Hilar Enlargement

Unilateral hilar enlargement may be the earliest radiographic manifestation of pulmonary carcinoma (Fig. 31–76).[56, 858, 859, 1001] It may represent a primary carcinoma that has arisen in a main or lobar bronchus or, more commonly, enlarged bronchopulmonary lymph nodes that are the site of metastases from a primary lesion in adjacent or peripheral parenchyma (Fig. 31–77). Enlargement of hilar lymph nodes by metastases in association with adjacent interstitial and bronchial wall tumor is particularly characteristic of small cell carcinoma; spread of this tumor to contralateral hilar nodes may result in bilateral enlargement.[1002, 1003] Even when too small to enlarge the hilum, a carcinoma is occasionally manifested by increased hilar opacity. The importance of CT in the evaluation of the abnormal hilum and mediastinum cannot be overestimated and is discussed in detail farther on.

Mediastinal Involvement

The mediastinum can be involved by metastases to lymph nodes or by direct invasion from a contiguous neoplasm. In a review of the radiographic presentation in 345 cases, a mediastinal mass or mediastinal lymph node enlargement was seen in 53 of 86 (62%) small cell carcinomas, 45 of 125 (36%) adenocarcinomas, 7 of 22 (32%) large cell carcinomas, and 25 of 98 (26%) squamous carcinomas.[839] Although uncommon, enlargement of mediastinal lymph nodes may be the main or sole abnormality seen radiographically,[56, 858] in which case it usually indicates the presence of small cell carcinoma.[837–839] The chief radiographic sign is mediastinal widening, usually with an undulating or lobulated contour (Fig. 31–78). Involvement of the subcarinal or posterior mediastinal lymph nodes can displace the esophagus[1004–1006] and rarely results in dysphagia (Fig. 31–79); such disease can be revealed by contrast study of the esophagus or, more readily, by CT.

Apical Pulmonary Neoplasms

The superior inlet of the thorax is bounded laterally by the first rib, anteriorly by the first costal cartilage and manubrium, and posteriorly by the head of the first rib and body of the first thoracic vertebra. Most of its area is occupied by the apex of the lung. Neoplasms that arise in this location have been termed *Pancoast tumor*,[1007, 1008] *pulmonary apical tumor*,[1009] *thoracic inlet tumor*, or *superior pulmonary sulcus tumor*;[1010] the last-named is clearly a misnomer because no definite sulcus exists in the extreme lung apex.[1011] The title of Pancoast's 1932 paper was "Superior Pulmonary Sulcus Tumor: Tumor Characterized by Pain, Horner's Syndrome, Destruction of Bone and Atrophy of Hand Muscles."[1008] Since that time, it has become apparent that the majority of patients who have an apical neoplasm fail to fulfill all of the four criteria, and it is now fairly well accepted that the term *Pancoast syndrome* can be applied to any situation in which a neoplasm in the apex of a lung is accompanied by shoulder or arm pain.

Most apical tumors are squamous cell or adenocarcinoma in type; small cell carcinoma occurs rarely.[1116] In early studies, approximately 5% of pulmonary carcinomas were found to arise in the pulmonary apex, with squamous cell

Text continued on page 1161

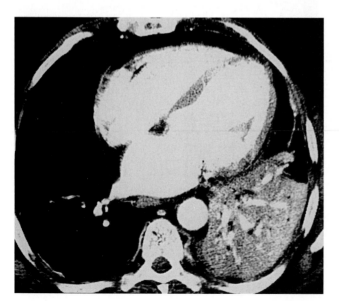

Figure 31–75. CT Angiogram Sign. A contrast-enhanced CT scan demonstrates consolidation in the left lower lobe. The enhanced pulmonary vessels can be clearly identified within the consolidation, a finding known as the *CT angiogram sign*. Although initially considered characteristic of bronchioloalveolar carcinoma, this sign is, in fact, nonspecific. The left lower lobe consolidation in this patient was the result of bacterial pneumonia.

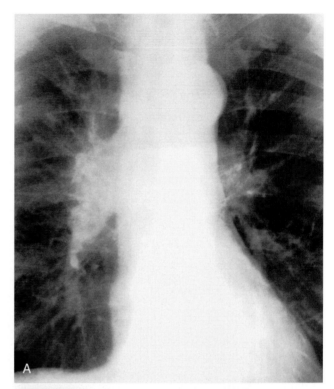

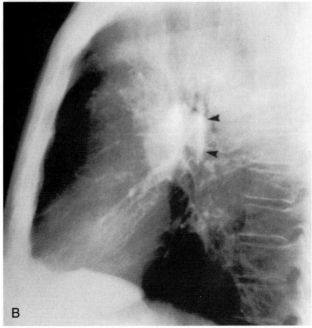

Figure 31–76. Hilar Enlargement. Posteroanterior *(A)* and lateral *(B)* chest radiographs reveal marked asymmetry in the hila, the right being more opaque, larger, and less well defined. Note the abnormally thick intermediate stem line *(arrowheads)* on the lateral view. The patient was a 59-year-old man who had biopsy-proven small cell carcinoma.

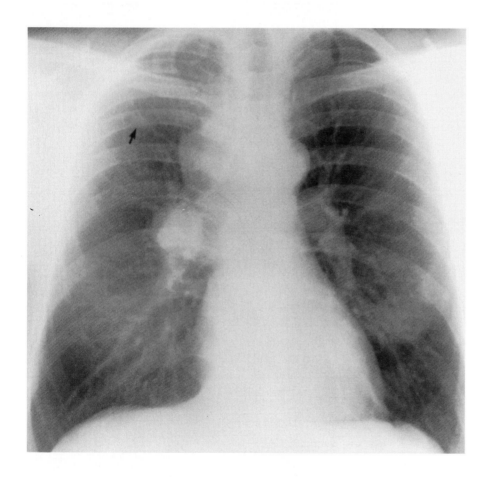

Figure 31–77. Hilar and Mediastinal Lymph Node Metastases from Small Cell Carcinoma. A posteroanterior chest radiograph reveals marked enlargement of the right hilar and paratracheal lymph nodes. The primary was a small cell carcinoma in the right upper lobe *(arrow)*.

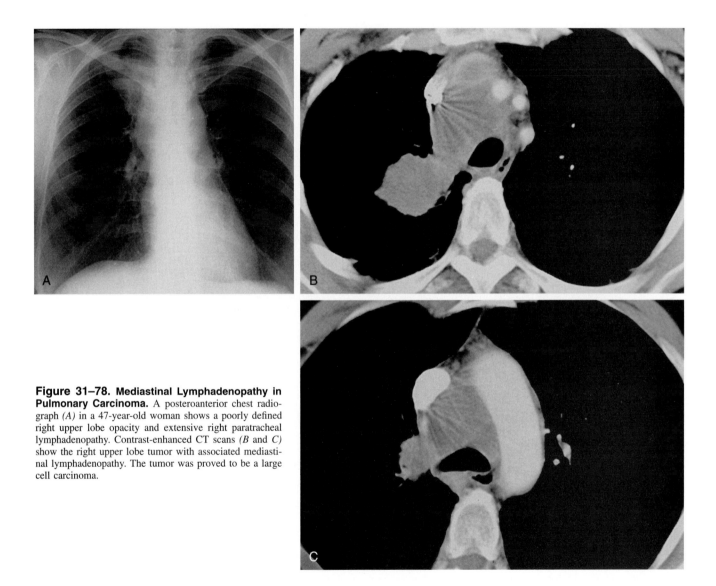

Figure 31–78. Mediastinal Lymphadenopathy in Pulmonary Carcinoma. A posteroanterior chest radiograph *(A)* in a 47-year-old woman shows a poorly defined right upper lobe opacity and extensive right paratracheal lymphadenopathy. Contrast-enhanced CT scans *(B and C)* show the right upper lobe tumor with associated mediastinal lymphadenopathy. The tumor was proved to be a large cell carcinoma.

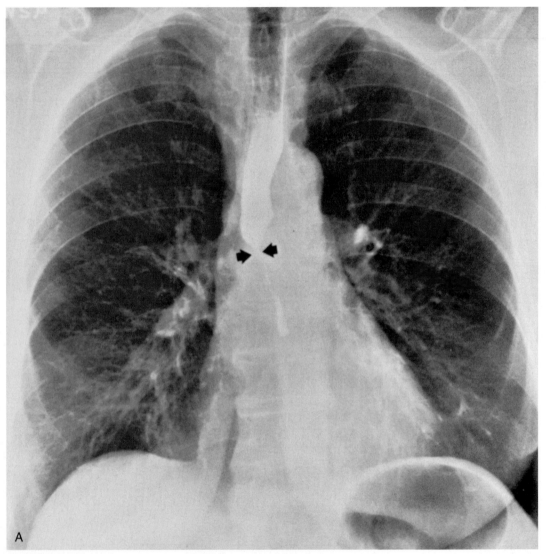

Figure 31–79. Pulmonary Carcinoma First Manifested by Effects on the Esophagus. This 78-year-old woman was admitted to the hospital for investigation of increasing dysphagia over the past several weeks. The chest radiograph *(A)* shows no abnormalities of the lungs or hila; however, the barium swallow reveals an annular constricting lesion of the esophagus at the level of the carina *(arrows)*.

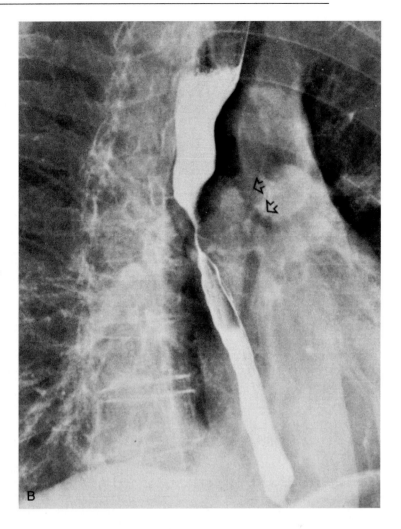

Figure 31–79 *Continued.* In the right anterior oblique projection *(B),* not only is the esophageal stenosis readily identified, but also there is suggestive evidence of narrowing of the left main bronchus *(open arrows)* and blunting of the carinal angle. The diagnosis was proven primary squamous cell carcinoma of the left main bronchus with metastases to carinal and posterior mediastinal lymph nodes, the latter producing circumferential compression of the esophagus.

carcinoma predominating.[836, 837, 841, 846, 847] In a more recent investigation of 345 patients who had newly diagnosed carcinoma, 12 (3.5%) had an apical mass, including 5 of 125 (4%) adenocarcinomas, 4 of 98 (4%) squamous cell carcinomas, and 3 of 86 (3%) small cell carcinomas.[839] In another study of 27 patients who had Pancoast tumors, 21 were adenocarcinomas, 5 were squamous cell carcinomas, 1 was small cell carcinoma, and 1 was anaplastic carcinoma.[1010] In three other series, adenocarcinoma was only slightly more common than squamous cell carcinoma.[1012–1014]

In one study of 29 patients, conventional radiographic findings consisted of an ipsilateral apical cap that measured more than 5 mm in thickness or a 5-mm asymmetry of apical caps on the two sides (55%), an apical mass (45%), and bone destruction (34%) (Fig. 31–80).[1011] Several groups of investigators have shown that CT is superior to radiography in the assessment of these tumors (Fig. 31–81).[1011, 1015–1017] In one investigation in which chest radiographs and transverse, sagittal, and coronal CT images were compared in 17 patients, additional information concerning local tumor extension and metastatic spread was provided by CT in every instance.[1015] Another study involved 50 patients who had 30 malignant and 20 benign abnormalities in the lung apex.[1016] In the malignant group, 20 (66%) patients had pulmonary carcinoma (the majority squamous cell carcinoma and adenocarcinoma), 5 had metastatic cancer, and 5 had

lymphoma. Of the 20 benign abnormalities, 16 (80%) were caused by trauma, cervical spine degenerative disease, neurogenic tumors, or infection. In this comparative study, CT provided substantial additional information beyond the plain radiograph in 17 of the 20 patients who had benign conditions and in 29 of the 30 who had cancer.

The major benefits of CT relate to its ability to identify a tumor mass as distinct from the apical pleural thickening and to assess the presence of bone destruction and invasion of the chest wall and root of the neck. Various investigators, however, have shown significant limitations of CT in the assessment of chest wall invasion, with sensitivities and specificities ranging from 20% to 80%.[1018–1022] These limitations are particularly marked for Pancoast tumors because of the cupola shape of the chest wall in the apical region and because of the presence of beam-hardening artefacts from the adjacent bony structures.

Several workers have shown that MR imaging is superior to CT in the assessment of apical tumors.[1009, 1010, 1023, 1024] The procedure allows direct coronal, sagittal, and oblique imaging that yields excellent anatomic detail of the thoracic inlet and brachial plexus (Fig. 31–82). It also provides better soft tissue differentiation than CT, thus allowing superior depiction of chest wall invasion (which is visualized as disruption of the normal extrapleural fat). Although MR imaging is also superior to CT in the assessment of bone

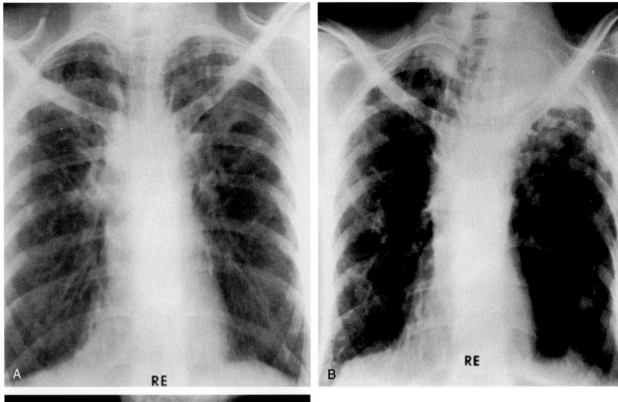

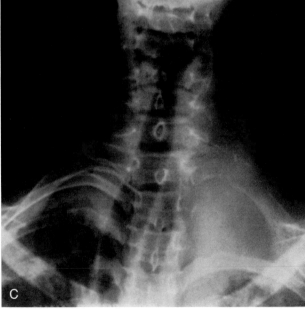

Figure 31–80. Pancoast Tumor Associated with Chronic Sarcoidosis. A posteroanterior chest radiograph *(A)* reveals multiple, poorly defined parenchymal opacities in the upper lobes; the hila are elevated, and the hilar and mediastinal lymph nodes are enlarged. Lymph node biopsy revealed nonnecrotizing granulomas consistent with sarcoidosis. Nine years later *(B)*, a large homogeneous soft tissue opacity had developed over the apex of the left upper lobe. There is evidence of bone destruction in several ribs and vertebrae, seen to better advantage on an overpenetrated view of the thoracic inlet *(C)*. The findings are typical of an apical (Pancoast) neoplasm. Examination of a biopsy specimen showed adenocarcinoma.

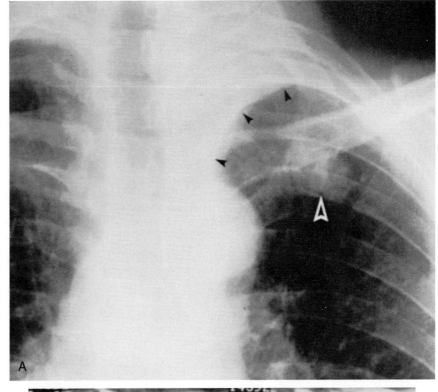

Figure 31–81. Role of CT in the Evaluation of Apical Pulmonary Carcinoma (Pancoast Tumor). A detail view *(A)* of the left upper hemithorax from a posteroanterior chest radiograph shows a broad, curvilinear opacity *(small arrowheads)* over the apex of the left upper lobe. A 2-cm nodule *(large arrowhead),* overlapped by the anterior end of the first and the posterior portion of the fifth ribs, is visible inferiorly; no definite calcification can be identified within the lesion. The trachea is displaced slightly to the right; there is no evidence of bone destruction. In this patient, the distinction between a benign apical pleuroparenchymal plaque and primary peripheral carcinoma is not possible on the evidence provided by the conventional radiograph. Sequential 10-mm CT scans *(B)* through the left apex reveal a plaque of soft tissue superomedially *(white arrowheads)* that hugs the pleural surface at the level of the second and third vertebral bodies. There is minimal bone erosion *(small arrowheads)* in the lateral part of the third vertebral body. The nodule *(large arrowhead)* in the upper lobe is a calcified granuloma (compare the CT density of the lesion to that of the adjacent bones). Transthoracic needle aspiration of the soft tissue plaque disclosed adenocarcinoma. The patient was a 62-year-old man with left shoulder pain.

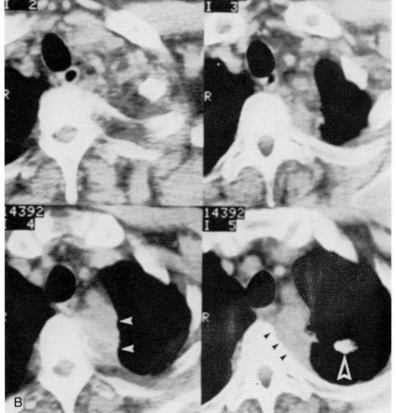

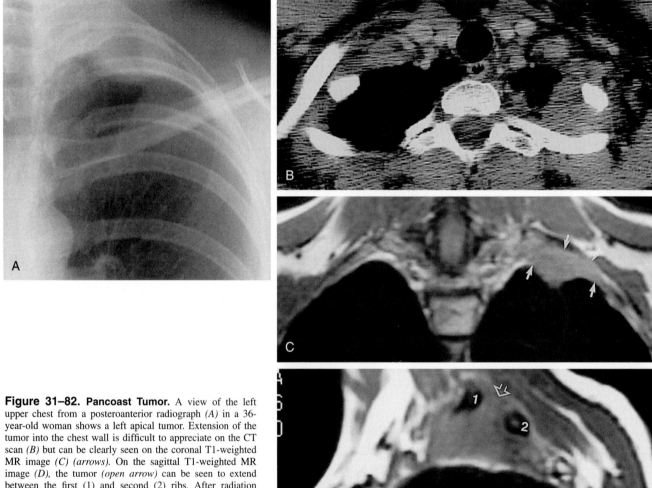

Figure 31–82. Pancoast Tumor. A view of the left upper chest from a posteroanterior radiograph *(A)* in a 36-year-old woman shows a left apical tumor. Extension of the tumor into the chest wall is difficult to appreciate on the CT scan *(B)* but can be clearly seen on the coronal T1-weighted MR image *(C) (arrows)*. On the sagittal T1-weighted MR image *(D),* the tumor *(open arrow)* can be seen to extend between the first (1) and second (2) ribs. After radiation therapy, the patient underwent surgery, and the tumor was shown to be an adenocarcinoma with involvement of the first rib.

marrow involvement, it is inferior in the assessment of rib destruction.[1024] Optimal assessment of the lung apex on MR images requires the use of multiplanar reconstruction and relatively thin sections (5 mm thick) and the use of cardiac gating and both T1-weighted and T2-weighted images.[1010]

Pleural Involvement

Pleural involvement in primary pulmonary carcinoma is not uncommon, effusion having been observed in 8% of patients at presentation in one large series[858] and in 15% in another.[56] It does not invariably denote neoplastic pleural invasion because serous effusion sometimes occurs as a result of lymphatic obstruction by involved mediastinal lymph nodes.[1025] Hemorrhagic effusion, however, nearly always denotes direct tumor invasion. Regardless of the mechanism of its formation, effusion indicates a poor prognosis.[1026]

Although diffuse pleural thickening as a result of malignancy is most often seen with mesothelioma, occasionally a peripheral lung carcinoma presents in an identical fashion (Fig. 31–83).[1027] Such involvement may occur without pleural effusion.[1028] Confident distinction between the two tumors requires pathologic examination.

Spontaneous pneumothorax is an uncommon manifestation of primary pulmonary carcinoma.[1029–1035] The pathogenesis includes direct transgression of the visceral pleural surface by neoplastic cells, perforation into the pleural space by an abscess related to bronchial obstruction, and rupture of a bulla or bleb. Rarely, pneumothorax is the presenting manifestation,[1029, 1031, 1032] sometimes of an occult carcinoma.[1034, 1035]

Chest Wall Involvement

The presence of rib destruction or an obvious chest wall mass on CT allows reliable diagnosis of chest wall invasion;[1018, 1021] however, these findings have a low sensitivity, being present in only 20% to 40% of patients who have this complication.[1018, 1020] Other findings, such as the presence of obtuse angles or focal pleural thickening, are not reliable indicators.[1018–1021] In one series of 47 patients who had peripheral pulmonary carcinomas contacting the pleural surface or chest wall, the presence of an obtuse angle between the mass and the pleura, tumor contact with the pleura over a distance greater than 3 cm, and pleural thickening were associated with a sensitivity of 87% for chest wall invasion;[1019] however, the specificity was only 59%. In this study, the presence of focal chest pain, although not as sensitive as CT, was more specific (94%) in making the diagnosis.

The results of some preliminary studies suggest that detection of parietal pleural and chest wall invasion can be improved by assessing movement of the tumor in relation to the chest wall during expiration.[1036, 1037] In one investigation, spiral CT was performed during deep inspiration and at end expiration in 17 patients who had peripheral pulmonary carcinomas in contact with the chest wall.[1036] Six of the 10 tumors in the middle and lower lobes that showed considerable movement in relation to the chest wall were proved at surgery not to have invaded the parietal pleura. Three lesions

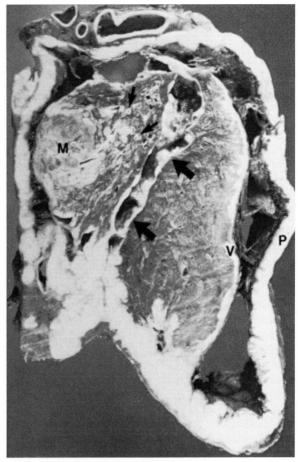

Figure 31–83. Pulmonary Carcinoma Simulating Pleural Mesothelioma. A sagittal section of a left lung and attached pleura shows marked thickening of both visceral (V) and parietal (P) pleura by a solid white tumor. The neoplasm extends into the major fissure *(large arrows)*. This appearance is highly suggestive of diffuse mesothelioma; however, a nodular mass is present in the upper lobe (M) and is associated with fairly extensive lymphangitic spread *(small arrows)*, both features being unusual for mesothelioma. Histologic examination showed the tumor to be a mucin-secreting adenocarcinoma, considered to originate in the upper lobe.

showed no motion in relation to the adjacent chest wall; all had parietal pleural invasion at surgery. The remaining lesion showed no motion and no invasion at surgery; fibrous pleural adhesions related to previous pleuritis were identified at surgery. Induced pneumothorax has also been used in diagnosis of chest wall invasion and mediastinal pleural invasion on CT; a sensitivity of 100% and specificities ranging from 57% to 80% have been reported.[1038, 1039]

Although MR imaging has been shown to be clearly superior to CT in the assessment of chest wall invasion in Pancoast tumors,[1010, 1024] its value in the detection of lateral chest wall invasion is controversial. In one study of 13 patients, it had a negative predictive value of 100%, correctly depicting the lack of chest wall invasion in 9 patients.[1040] In this study, the procedure allowed accurate diagnosis of the presence or absence of chest wall invasion in 9 patients in whom the CT findings were equivocal. In the report of the Radiology Diagnostic Oncology Group trial, however, which included 23 patients who had surgical and pathologic correlation, CT and MR imaging were equivalent in the assessment of chest wall invasion.[1041] The earliest finding of chest wall invasion on MR imaging is disruption of the normal extrapleural fat by soft tissue that has moderate signal intensity on T1-weighted spin-echo images and high signal intensity on T2-weighted imaging (*see* Fig. 31–82).[1046] Inflammatory and neoplastic tissue have similar signal characteristics.[1042–1044]

Disruption of the pleural surface and extension into the chest wall by pulmonary carcinoma can be well assessed by ultrasonography.[1045, 1046] In one study of 120 patients, the procedure allowed correct identification of chest wall invasion in all 19 patients who had invasion proven at surgery (sensitivity 100%) and absence of chest wall invasion in 99 of 101 patients (specificity 98%).[1046]

Bone Involvement

The skeleton may be involved in pulmonary carcinoma either by direct extension to the ribs or vertebrae (Fig. 31–84) or by metastasis to these or other sites (Fig. 31–85). Rib or vertebral destruction is sometimes visible on the chest radiograph but is best depicted on CT. The incidence of bone metastases at the time of death has been reported to range from 10% to 40%.[1047, 1048] Although they are predominantly osteolytic, osteoblastic lesions may occur. In one radiographic analysis of the skeleton in 110 consecutive patients, bone involvement was seen in 38 (35%)—local in 10 cases (destruction of contiguous ribs or spine) and distant in 28.[1049] In 9 of the 38 patients, the metastases were predominantly osteoblastic; in all of these, the cell type was either small cell carcinoma or adenocarcinoma, and there was concomitant bone marrow involvement. None of the 67 patients who had squamous cell or large cell carcinoma showed osteoblastic metastases. The bones most commonly involved are the vertebrae (70%), pelvis (40%), and femora (25%).[1048]

A meta-analysis of seven studies published before 1992 showed that bone metastases were detected at presentation by a combination of clinical, laboratory, and scintigraphic findings in 121 of 633 (21%) patients who had pulmonary carcinoma.[1050] The vast majority of affected patients were symptomatic. Using radionuclide bone scanning as the gold standard, the combination of clinical and laboratory findings in the seven studies had a sensitivity ranging from 79% to 100% (pooled mean, 90%) and a negative predictive value ranging from 70% to 100% (pooled mean, 89%) in excluding bone metastases. A number of conditions, such as proliferative changes related to spondylosis or osteoarthritis, can result in false-positive scans; for example, in one study of 110 patients, 28 (25%) had false-positive bone scans.[1051] Because of the high negative predictive value of the combination of clinical and laboratory findings and the high false-positive rate of radionuclide bone scanning, the latter procedure is not recommended in assessment of asymptomatic patients who have normal laboratory values.[1050, 1051]

Miscellaneous Patterns

Other radiographic signs of pulmonary carcinoma include unilateral diaphragmatic paralysis resulting from phrenic nerve involvement (Fig. 31–86),[56] which should be differentiated from hemidiaphragmatic elevation compensatory to atelectasis and from pseudoelevation of a hemidiaphragm caused by a large infrapulmonary pleural effusion. Paralysis can be caused by malignancy in the absence of symptoms, signs, or other abnormalities on the chest radiograph, as in 5 of 142 patients who had unexplained diaphragmatic paralysis in one series.[1052] Other signs include bilateral parenchymal lesions resulting from contralateral hematogenous metastases[56] and a diffuse or local reticulonodular pattern caused by lymphangitic carcinomatosis.[56, 858]

As discussed previously (*see* page 1118), pulmonary artery invasion by pulmonary carcinoma is commonly seen histologically. If specifically looked for, it can also be detected radiologically in many cases; for example, in one angiographic study of 250 patients, the main pulmonary artery was invaded or compressed in 18% and the lobar and segmental arteries in 53%.[1053] Radiographic manifestations of such involvement are uncommon and include hilar enlargement and pulmonary infarction (Fig. 31–87).[1054–1056] Although most cases of the latter complication are presumably

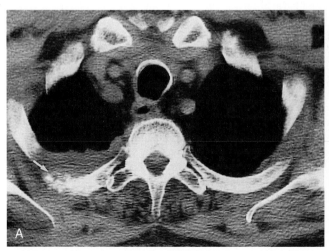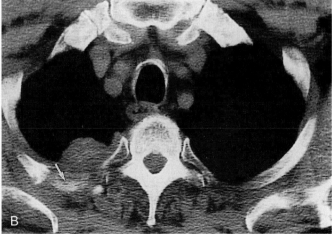

Figure 31–84. Pulmonary Carcinoma with Chest Wall Invasion. CT scans (*A* and *B*) in a 67-year-old man demonstrate a right apical tumor with evidence of chest wall invasion as demonstrated by the partial destruction of the right posterior third rib (*arrows*). The tumor was resected together with the right second, third, and fourth ribs and shown to be a squamous cell carcinoma.

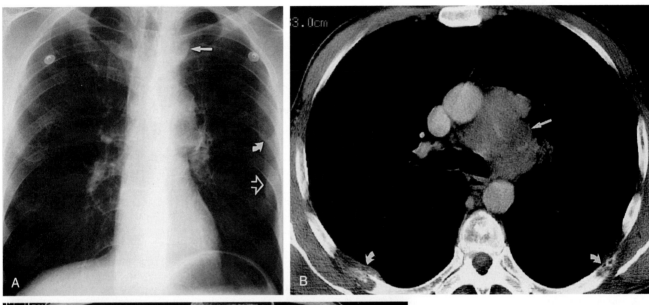

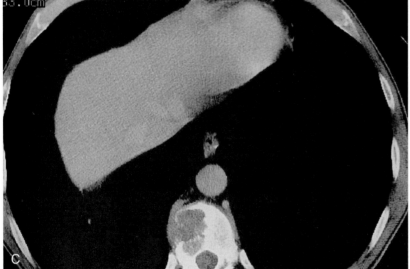

Figure 31–85. Metastatic Pulmonary Carcinoma. A 37-year-old man presented with a 1-month history of weight loss and chest pain. A chest radiograph *(A)* demonstrates localized convexity of the left upper mediastinum *(straight arrow)*, focal irregularity of the left posterior sixth rib *(curved arrow)*, and a focal opacity associated with the anterolateral left fifth rib *(open arrow)*. A contrast-enhanced CT scan *(B)* demonstrates extensive mediastinal lymphadenopathy *(straight arrow)* and lytic rib lesions *(curved arrows)*. A CT scan at a more caudad level *(C)* demonstrates metastasis to a vertebra. The diagnosis was metastatic small cell carcinoma.

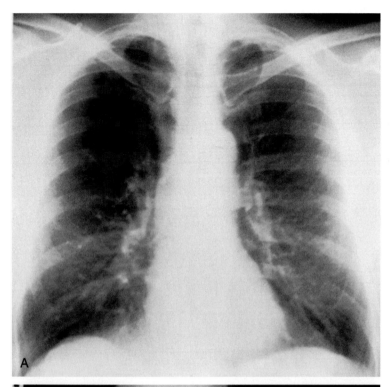

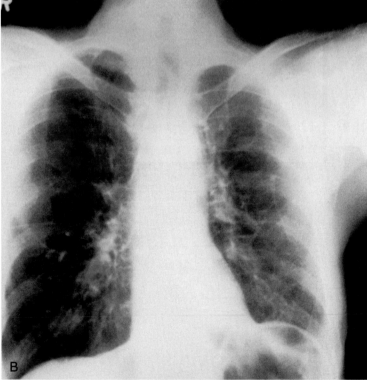

Figure 31–86. Diaphragmatic Paralysis Caused by Pulmonary Carcinoma. A posteroanterior chest radiograph *(A)* is normal. Five years later *(B)*, a plaque of soft tissue had appeared over the apex of the left lung, and enlargement of the mediastinal contour adjacent to the aortic arch had developed; the left hemidiaphragm was elevated. Fluoroscopic examination disclosed paradoxical movement of the left hemidiaphragm attributed to paralysis. Subsequent investigation revealed an apical adenocarcinoma (Pancoast tumor) with mediastinal metastases. The patient was a 56-year-old man.

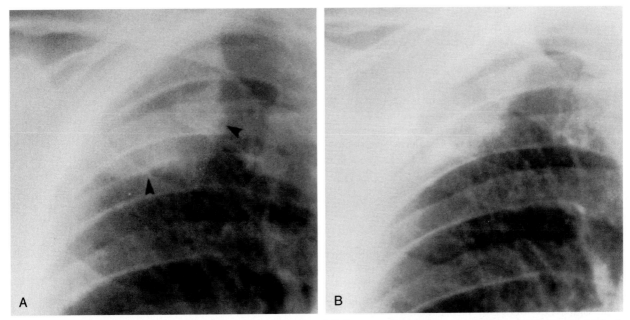

Figure 31–87. Pulmonary Infarction Associated with a Peripheral Pulmonary Carcinoma. A detail view of the right upper lobe from a posteroanterior chest radiograph *(A)* reveals a semilunar opacity *(arrowheads)* adjacent to the visceral pleura over the anterolateral lung. After refusing further investigation, the patient was treated conservatively. Approximately 8 months later *(B),* although the opacity had diminished in size, the upper lobe was excised. Pathologic examination disclosed a peripheral pulmonary carcinoma that was associated with surrounding fibrosis consistent with prior pulmonary infarction.

the result of neoplastic vascular occlusion, it has been postulated that some may also occur secondary to reduction in peripheral blood flow by mechanical and reflex factors.[1055] In one investigation of five patients who had pulmonary carcinoma and who showed radiographic evidence of two opacities, the central one proved to be the carcinoma (four squamous cell) and the peripheral one an infarct;[1056] the authors stressed the importance of performing biopsy on the proximal rather than the distal lesion.

CLINICAL MANIFESTATIONS

Symptoms of pulmonary carcinoma can be the result of local bronchopulmonary disease (e.g., cough and hemoptysis), extension of tumor to adjacent structures (particularly the chest wall and mediastinum), distant metastases (especially to bone, liver, and brain), nonspecific constitutional effects (fatigue, anorexia, and weight loss), and immunologic reactions to or hormone secretion by the tumor (paraneoplastic syndromes). About 10% of patients are asymptomatic when first seen, the diagnosis being suspected initially from an abnormal chest radiograph; rarely, cytologic examination suggests the possibility of carcinoma when performed for screening purposes in an asymptomatic individual.[1057–1062]

Bronchopulmonary Manifestations

The most frequent local symptoms of pulmonary carcinoma are those related to its effects on the airways. Cough, usually mildly productive, is by far the most common of these, occurring in up to 75% of patients.[9, 838, 1063] Because the majority are heavy smokers and have chronic bronchitis,

the cough may not be recognized as a new symptom; instead a change in the character of cough in a patient who has a history of smoking may be the initial feature. Despite this, cough was twice as prevalent among patients who had pulmonary carcinoma in one study as it was in a control group with a similar smoking history.[57] Hemoptysis occurs in about 35% to 50% of patients,[9, 56, 1003, 1064–1066] and may be the only clue to the diagnosis in the patient whose chest radiograph is normal.[1067]

Other airway-related symptoms are less common. Partial or complete obstruction of a bronchus may result in increased shortness of breath or acute symptoms of infection in a region of obstructive pneumonitis. As discussed previously *(see* page 514), many cases of obstructive pneumonitis are sterile, the inflammatory reaction and parenchymal consolidation presumably being related to retained secretions. Secondary infection is likely when there is fever; in one study of 26 consecutive patients who had obstructive pneumonitis, transthoracic needle aspiration yielded organisms in 7 of the 9 who were febrile as compared to 2 of 19 who were not.[1068] A local wheeze may be present when no abnormality is visible on a conventional chest radiograph exposed at full inspiration;[1069–1071] in this circumstance, radiography at maximal expiration may provide useful information by demonstrating local air trapping (the patient should be instructed to expire forcibly).

Neoplasms in the lung periphery seldom cause symptoms, although pain may occur after extension to the pleura.[838, 842] Occasionally a carcinoma is associated with reactivation of tuberculosis, resulting in symptoms that may cause diagnostic confusion.[1071] With the exception of bronchorrhea, the clinical findings in patients who have bronchioloalveolar carcinoma are indistinguishable from those of other pulmonary adenocarcinomas. The results of radiographic surveys suggest that 50% to 70% of patients who have this variety of carcinoma are asymptomatic.[984, 1072] The most common symptom is cough, present in approximately 75% of symptomatic patients. It may be dry or only slightly productive; however, in 20% to 25% of patients, it is associated with expectoration of large quantities of mucoid material, a feature that is highly suggestive of the tumor.[1072–1074] Such bronchorrhea—which may be as much as 4 liters daily—usually indicates extensive lung involvement[1075] and may result in severe hypovolemia and electrolyte depletion.[1076]

Extrapulmonary Intrathoracic Manifestations

Pleura

Involvement of the pleura may be associated with pain on breathing, signs of pleural effusion, and a friction rub. Effusion is more likely to be serous than grossly hemorrhagic; the former appears to be the result of involvement of mediastinal lymph nodes by metastatic carcinoma with secondary lymphatic obstruction, whereas the latter usually results from direct invasion by malignant cells. Because small cell carcinoma is almost always associated with hilar lymph node metastases, it is not surprising that the incidence of pleural effusion is highest with this neoplasm. Spontaneous pneumothorax is uncommon; it usually results from direct pleural invasion by malignant cells, although rupture of a bleb or bulla is an occasional mechanism.[1077] It has also

been noted during regression of small cell carcinoma with chemotherapy.[1078] Spontaneous hemothorax has been reported rarely.[1079]

Mediastinum

Mediastinal disease in carcinoma of the lung is usually caused by the neoplasm itself, either by direct extension from the primary lesion or by lymph node metastases (Fig. 31–88). Nodal enlargement can also be caused by hyperplasia, representing a reaction to either infection in an obstructed region of lung or the carcinoma itself.[1080] The presence *per se* of enlarged nodes or neoplasm in the mediastinum seldom gives rise to symptoms; however, if massive, they may cause a sensation of retrosternal pressure or pain.[1081] Of far greater significance is the effect of a neoplasm on the various structures that reside within the mediastinum, of which the most important are the heart, esophagus, major vessels of the venous and arterial circulation, and nerves.

Heart

Cardiac involvement is more common than is generally realized. For example, in one autopsy study of 205 patients who had pulmonary carcinoma, 98 (48%) were so affected;[1082] arrhythmia was considered to be the direct cause of death in 22. In another autopsy study of 74 cases of pulmonary carcinoma, 23 (31%) had evidence of cardiac or

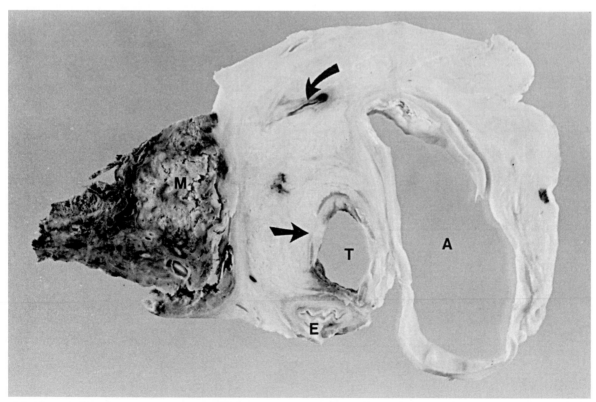

Figure 31–88. Pulmonary Carcinoma with Mediastinal Invasion. A paramediastinal carcinoma (M) in the upper lobe is contiguous with extensive mediastinal tumor. The trachea (T) is somewhat distorted and shows focal infiltration of its wall *(straight arrow)*. The superior vena cava *(curved arrow)* is reduced to a slit and is thrombosed. Although this pattern can result from extension of carcinoma from affected mediastinal lymph nodes, in this case it most likely represents direct spread from the pulmonary primary. A, aortic arch; E, esophagus.

pericardial involvement.[1083] Pericardial infiltration can be caused by direct invasion from a focus of intrapulmonary or mediastinal neoplasm or, more commonly, by retrograde extension of carcinoma along lymphatics from nodal metastases.[1084] The most common complication of such infiltration is effusion; pneumopericardium occurs rarely.[1085]

Effusion often results in signs and symptoms of tamponade. For example, in one series of 51 patients who had pulmonary carcinoma and pericardial involvement, 45 developed this complication;[1086] in 3 patients, tamponade was the initial manifestation of the tumor. Carcinoma is also a relatively common cause of tamponade; for example, in one series of 23 patients who had cardiac tamponade, 8 (35%) were caused by cancer, 7 of which were pulmonary in origin.[1087] In most cases, the cause of the effusion can be identified by cytologic examination of pericardial fluid.[1084, 1086–1089] Cardiac tamponade should be suspected when a patient who has pulmonary carcinoma complains of acute dyspnea and has a thready pulse or pulsus paradoxus, low systolic blood pressure, engorged neck veins, enlarged cardiac silhouette, and total or ventricular electrical alternans.[1089] Superior vena cava syndrome shares some signs and symptoms with tamponade, and it is important not to confuse the two.

Myocardial invasion usually does not cause symptoms; however, when suspected clinically, the invasion may be confirmed with two-dimensional echocardiography[1090, 1091] or transesophageal echocardiography.[1092, 1093] One case has been reported in which myocardial infarction was thought to be secondary to compression of a coronary artery by carcinoma.[1083] Rarely, tumor extends along the pulmonary veins to the left atrium, creating a systolic murmur,[1094] a left atrial mass that simulates myxoma, or both;[1089, 1095] at thoracotomy, a systemic tumor embolus can break loose, with fatal consequences.[1096] Nonbacterial thrombotic endocarditis is another uncommon cardiac complication,[1097] usually associated with adenocarcinoma.

Esophagus

Dysphagia resulting from esophageal involvement is an uncommon presenting symptom of pulmonary carcinoma,[1098] being observed in only 9 (2.2%) of 405 cases in one series.[1099] This low incidence may appear surprising in view of the relative frequency of posterior mediastinal lymph node metastases and the fact that these enlarged nodes commonly relate to the esophagus. Enlarged nodes, however, usually do no more than displace the esophagus, a deformity unlikely to compromise its function significantly. Only when the esophageal wall is invaded by neoplasm is obstruction likely, in which case the primary site is commonly the left main bronchus.

Mediastinal Vessels

Compression or invasion of mediastinal vessels can result in occlusive thrombosis associated with prominent signs and symptoms. The most common vessels to be so affected are the superior vena cava and its major branches. The superior vena cava syndrome consists of edema of the face, neck, and upper extremities; distended neck and arm veins;[1099a] and (sometimes) headache and dizziness.[1066,] [1100, 1101] It is often caused by pulmonary carcinoma;[1102, 1103] for example, in one review of 86 cases, 67 (78%) were caused by malignancy, 45 of which originated in the lung;[1101] all cell types were equally represented. In series of patients who have small cell carcinoma, superior vena cava obstruction has been recognized at the time of diagnosis in about 10% of patients.[1104–1106] In our experience and that of others, obstruction of the superior vena cava does not represent a complication that requires emergency treatment;[1102, 1104, 1107, 1108] however, compression of the trachea or pericardial tamponade may coexist and may require urgent intervention.[1109] Occasionally the axillary or subclavian veins alone are affected, resulting in the appropriate signs in the distribution of the affected venous drainage.[1110]

Although pulmonary arteries within the lungs are often occluded by carcinoma, compression or invasion of their extrapulmonary branches is uncommon and rarely results in clinically significant abnormalities. An unusual case of orthodeoxia has been described in a patient who had a pulmonary carcinoma that completely obstructed the left main bronchus.[1111] When the patient went from the supine to the erect position, the PaO_2 dropped from 62 to 37 mm Hg during air breathing and from 272 to 45 mm Hg during 100% oxygen breathing. After pneumonectomy, the PaO_2 was normal, suggesting that the carcinoma had partly compressed the left pulmonary artery while the patient was recumbent (thus shunting blood to the normal opposite lung) but not while the patient was erect (thus permitting perfusion of the nonventilated lung).

Mediastinal Nerves

Invasion of the recurrent laryngeal nerve can cause hoarseness, and involvement of the vagus nerve can cause dyspnea, particularly in patients who have chronic air-flow obstruction (as so often accompanies pulmonary carcinoma). Although involvement of the phrenic nerve can cause hemidiaphragmatic paresis or paralysis, this usually does not lead to symptoms in the presence of normal ventilatory reserve.

Thoracic Inlet

Tumors of the thoracic inlet almost invariably result in symptoms and signs related to local invasion (Pancoast tumor, *see* page 1156).[1007, 1008, 1112, 1116] Important structures within the superior thoracic inlet are (from front to back) the subclavian and jugular veins, the phrenic and vagus nerves, the subclavian and common carotid arteries, the recurrent laryngeal nerve, the eighth cervical and first thoracic nerves, the sympathetic chain and stellate ganglion, and the first four ribs and upper vertebrae. A Pancoast tumor may involve one or several of these structures, resulting in a variety of signs and symptoms, including pain and weakness of the shoulder and arm, swelling of the arm, and Horner's syndrome.[452, 1113, 1114] The first of these is the most common; in one series of 94 patients who had a Pancoast tumor, pain occurred in 96% and was associated with other signs and symptoms of nervous system involvement in 79%.[1115]

In the vast majority of patients, the symptom complex accompanying a Pancoast tumor is the result of transgression of apical pleura by neoplasm and invasion of local tissues.

It is possible, however, that other mechanisms are involved occasionally, as in a 46-year-old man who presented with a 3-week history of left upper back pain that radiated to the left arm.[1117] Although the pain was gradual in onset, it rapidly became severe; a chest radiograph revealed a left apical mass. To establish a diagnosis before preoperative radiation therapy, a percutaneous needle biopsy was performed, resulting in pneumothorax and retraction of the partly collapsed upper lobe away from the apex of the hemithorax. The neoplasm (which eventually proved to be an adenocarcinoma) was confined to the lung, showing neither adherence to nor invasion of apical parietal pleura. Of major interest was the fact that with the development of pneumothorax, the patient's back and arm pain promptly disappeared. The cause of the pain remained obscure.

Extrathoracic Metastatic Manifestations

Remote metastases develop from spread via the lymphatics and blood vessels[1118] and are usually associated with a previously diagnosed or obvious synchronous pulmonary carcinoma. Occasionally, they are responsible for the initial clinical manifestations in the absence of a radiographically detectable primary lesion. In one series of 67 patients who had metastatic carcinoma in the absence of an apparent primary malignancy, 18 (27%) of the primary neoplasms were eventually found to originate in the lung.[1119] Similarly, in an autopsy review of 387 patients who had pulmonary carcinoma, 28 (7%) were identified in whom the primary pulmonary site was not suspected before death.[1120] In both of these series, symptoms were most often related to bone and central nervous system involvement. In another study of 200 patients who died within 30 days of presumed curative surgery and who underwent autopsy, extrathoracic metastases were present in 48 (24%), including 18 to the adrenal gland and 16 to the liver.[1121]

At autopsy, metastases are almost invariable in patients who have pulmonary carcinoma; for example, in one review of 662 such patients, they were identified in 96%, the incidence being highest with small cell carcinoma and lowest with squamous cell carcinoma.[602] Although metastases can occur in any organ or tissue (e.g., the placenta,[1122] breast,[1123] and skeletal muscle[1124]), the most frequent sites are lymph nodes, liver, adrenal gland, bone, kidney, and brain.[56, 602, 1125–1127] On the basis of a review of four autopsy studies comprising a total of 538 patients and an additional 146 newly described cases, the location and approximate incidence of metastases of small cell carcinoma at autopsy were as follows:[1128] contralateral lung, 25%; mediastinal or hilar lymph nodes, 85%; pleura, 25% to 40%; liver, 60% to 80%; adrenal glands, 40% to 65%; bone marrow, 35% to 60%; brain, 30% to 50%; abdominal lymph nodes, 50% to 60%; and pancreas, 15% to 50%. Other organs and tissues were involved less frequently. There is evidence that radiation or chemotherapy may modify the frequency of metastases in specific sites.[1129]

The frequency and pattern of metastases in patients who have small cell carcinoma have also been studied at the time of diagnosis (pretreatment).[1128] Tumor was found in the bone marrow in 15% to 50% (median, 30%) of patients, in the liver in 15% to 50% (median, 30%), and in the central

nervous system in about 5%. The metastatic pattern of adenocarcinoma is similar to that of small cell carcinoma.[1127, 1130] Although they can also disseminate widely, squamous cell tumors (particularly the better-differentiated forms) not uncommonly remain limited to the thorax, spreading by direct extension into the mediastinum or chest wall and metastasizing only to mediastinal lymph nodes.[1127]

Lymph Nodes

The most common extrapulmonary site of metastatic pulmonary carcinoma is undoubtedly the hilar and mediastinal lymph nodes; the pattern of such metastases is discussed in the section on staging of pulmonary carcinoma (*see* page 1183). Metastasis also occurs frequently to the scalene group of lymph nodes. Contrary to the generally accepted observations made originally by Rouvière,[1131] such dissemination is chiefly ipsilateral from all parts of each lung.[1132–1134] When the carcinoma is advanced, especially in patients who have extensive mediastinal lymph node involvement, spread to periaortic, mesenteric, and other intra-abdominal lymph node groups is also frequent; however, signs and symptoms caused by such spread are usually minimal or absent.

Brain and Spinal Cord

Cerebral metastases have been found at autopsy in 2% to 50% of patients who have pulmonary carcinoma;[602, 1127, 1128, 1135] moreover, the brain is the most common site of metastasis in patients who have non–small cell carcinoma and who have extrathoracic disease at presentation.[1136] In fact, more than one quarter of all autopsy-proven brain metastases have a pulmonary source;[1137] about one third of these are solitary.[1138] In patients who have solitary central nervous system metastases of pulmonary carcinoma, the most common histologic type is adenocarcinoma.[1139] Cerebral metastases are also common in patients who have small cell carcinoma, being discovered at autopsy in 70 (40%) of 177 patients in one series.[1140] In patients who have treated small cell carcinoma, meningeal carcinomatosis is as common a complication as cerebral metastases.[1141–1143]

Symptoms and signs of central nervous system involvement are variable and depend on the specific location of the metastasis. Although most often seen in patients who have known carcinoma, signs and symptoms of cerebral[1138] or cerebellar[1144] lesions occasionally antedate those of the primary tumor.[1145]

In men, metastatic pulmonary carcinoma accounts for the majority of ocular and orbital tumors.[1146] Isolated trigeminal neuropathy caused by pulmonary carcinoma has been reported.[1147] An emergency situation can develop when metastases occur to the spinal cord;[1148, 1149] CT and MR imaging are particularly useful for diagnostic purposes in this area.[1150]

Two rare syndromes associated with malignancy may be misdiagnosed as cerebral metastasis: (1) cerebral infarction resulting from cancer-associated nonbacterial thrombotic endocarditis;[1151] and (2) a slowly progressive neurologic syndrome characterized by apathy, abulia, memory loss, gait ataxia, and corticospinal tract signs.[1152] The latter syndrome tends to develop 2 to 4 years after prophylactic cranial irradiation and systemic chemotherapy in patients who have small cell carcinoma. In one series of six patients,

CT or MR imaging evidence of changes in the periventricular white matter accompanied the syndrome.[1152] As discussed farther on, a number of other paraneoplastic neurologic syndromes can also be confused with metastatic disease during the clinical evaluation of patients.

Bone

Metastatic spread to bone occurs in about 10% to 40% of patients at some time during the course of pulmonary carcinoma.[1148, 1153] More than 20% of patients who have confirmed pulmonary carcinoma have bone pain on initial evaluation; radionuclide bone scans may be abnormal in as many as 40% at this time. Even with this form of examination, false-negative results can occur; for example, in one series of 80 autopsied patients who had had normal technetium-99m scans and skeletal radiographs shortly before death, metastases were detected on macroscopic examination of the vertebrae in 10.[1154] Bone involvement can be associated with hypercalcemia; rarely, this is misinterpreted as a manifestation of primary hyperparathyroidism in patients without detectable abnormality on the chest radiograph.[1155]

Abdominal Viscera

Metastases to intra-abdominal organs are often asymptomatic;[1066] however, involvement of any organ, including the liver, adrenal glands, pancreas, and kidneys, can cause symptoms and signs, sometimes confusing diagnosis.[1156] Small cell carcinoma, in particular, can cause extensive liver metastases with resultant epigastric pain and jaundice and a rapid downhill course that simulates hepatitis;[1157, 1158] hepatic rupture and hemoperitoneum can occur,[1159] and lactic acidosis may develop.[1160, 1161] Even in the absence of these unusual and dramatic manifestations, spread of pulmonary carcinoma to liver is common[1136] and associated with a poor prognosis.[1162]

Jaundice caused by extrahepatic biliary obstruction has been described from pancreatic metastases of small cell carcinoma.[1157, 1163] The same tumor has also been reported to initiate acute pancreatitis, a complication that has been misinterpreted as being caused by gallstones.[1164]

Metastases to the adrenal glands are common and can usually be identified by CT and confirmed if necessary by thin-needle aspiration. Addison's disease is uncommon; however, in one series of 21 patients who had metastatic carcinoma associated with CT evidence of enlarged adrenal glands, 4 had symptomatic adrenal insufficiency.[1165]

Gastrointestinal metastases have been documented in 10% to 15% of patients who have pulmonary carcinoma.[602, 1127, 1135, 1166] Gastric metastases can cause a radiographic appearance of "bull's eye" or "target" lesions.[1168] Small bowel metastases were identified at autopsy in 46 (11%) of 431 patients in one report.[1169] The most common clinical presentation is bleeding and anemia;[1170, 1171] perforation and obstruction can also occur at any level.[1166, 1172]

Extrathoracic Nonmetastatic Manifestations

Constitutional symptoms, such as malaise, weakness, lassitude, fever, and weight loss, are common manifestations of pulmonary carcinoma; for example, in one study of more than 900 patients who had small cell carcinoma, 56% had greater than 10% weight loss at the time of presentation.[1173] Although such constitutional symptoms can be present in the absence of clinical evidence of extrathoracic metastases, in most cases, they are associated with distant spread. In one autopsy study of 85 patients who had small cell carcinoma, the 35 who had had constitutional symptoms had markedly greater tumor burdens and more extensive metastases to bone marrow, liver, and lungs.[1174] Decreased food intake as a result of loss of appetite is an important cause of the weight loss so commonly observed.[1175]

In addition to these relatively nonspecific constitutional manifestations, some patients—particularly those who have small cell carcinoma—have symptoms and signs not directly related to neoplastic infiltration itself.[1173, 1176–1180] These paraneoplastic syndromes are said to occur in up to 10% of patients[1179] and may be seen in the absence of bronchopulmonary symptoms.[1181] The disorders are mediated by hormones or peptides secreted by the tumor or by antitumor antibodies that cross-react with normal tissues.[1173] The clinical manifestations of these syndromes can be considered under several headings, including neuromuscular, cutaneous, skeletal, endocrine or metabolic, hematologic or vascular, and renal.[1179]

Neuromuscular Manifestations

Paraneoplastic neuromuscular syndromes, which are principally associated with pulmonary carcinoma,[1182] usually occur when disease is advanced; however, they occasionally precede detection of the tumor in the lung or are the first sign of tumor recurrence.[1176, 1179] In one series of 280 consecutive cases of early pulmonary carcinoma, they were present in 4 (1.4%).[1183] In some patients, they antedate the diagnosis by as much as 2 to 3 years.[1138, 1183–1185] The neuromyopathy is usually progressive,[1138] but may occur as a single episode or be recurrent.[1184] In some patients, removal of the primary neoplasm has alleviated the neurologic symptoms.[1183, 1186]

Small cell carcinoma is the most common tumor associated with the syndromes,[1183, 1187] which include myopathy, peripheral neuropathy, subacute cerebellar degeneration, encephalomyelopathy, necrotizing myelopathy, intestinal dysmotility, and visual paraneoplastic syndrome.[1179]

Myopathy

Two myopathic syndromes have been associated with pulmonary carcinoma, one simulating myasthenia gravis (Lambert-Eaton myasthenic syndrome) and the other polymyositis. The former differs clinically from true myasthenia gravis by proximal rather than distal involvement of muscle groups in the extremities and by localization in the hip and lower limbs. In addition, ocular and bulbar palsies seldom develop;[1185] peripheral paresthesia, muscle pain, and diminished reflexes are more common and the response to neostigmine is less dramatic.[1188] There is also an important electrophysiologic distinction from myasthenia gravis: the electromyogram in the paraneoplastic syndrome shows amplitude enhancement after 10 to 15 seconds of maximal voluntary contraction or during high-frequency nerve stimulation.[1179] This form of myopathy has been observed in up to 6% of patients who have small cell carcinoma.[1173] Rarely, it is associated with respiratory failure.[1189] The syndrome is related to the development IgG antibodies to a number of voltage-gated calcium channels involved in the release of acetylcholine at motor nerve terminals and to synaptotagmin, a synaptic vesicle protein.[1173, 1179, 1190, 1191]

Malignancy-associated polymyositis is uncommon[1192–1194] and underlying carcinoma is seldom found in the absence of localizing signs and symptoms (*see* page 1465). In one study, there was a sixfold increase in cancer (including pulmonary carcinoma) within 1 year of diagnosis of polymyositis compared with a control population;[1195] no excess cancers were found in the second year of follow-up. Clinical manifestations include muscle tenderness and atrophy.

Peripheral Neuropathy

In most cases, neuropathy is both motor and sensory;[1183, 1186] however, only pain and paresthesia may be noted in the early stages and sensory loss, muscle weakness, and wasting later.[1196] Symptoms may precede the diagnosis of carcinoma by several months.[1179] The neuropathy usually runs a subacute progressive course but may behave in a more indolent fashion.[1197] Degenerative changes can be seen in the dorsal root ganglia and anterior horn cells on histologic examination. In patients who have small cell carcinoma and sensory neuropathy, an antineuronal IgG nuclear antibody (*anti-Hu*) has been found within the neurons of the dorsal root ganglia that also reacts with tumor cells.[1198]

Autonomic neuropathy has been reported in association with giant cell[1199] and small cell carcinoma.[1179, 1191, 1200, 1201] It may be manifested by postural hypotension or intestinal pseudo-obstruction. In the latter abnormality, anti-Hu antibodies directed to the myenteric and submucosal neural plexuses of the jejunum and stomach have been identified.[1179, 1202] Autonomic dysfunction may also have been operative in a patient who had a pulmonary neuroendocrine carcinoma associated with bradycardia and episodic cardiac asystole.[1203] The arrhythmia disappeared after pneumonectomy but recurred months later when metastases developed; at autopsy, no direct neoplastic involvement of the heart was found.

Subacute Cerebellar Degeneration

Subacute cerebellar degeneration is characterized by rapidly progressive ataxia, incoordination, vertigo, nystagmus, and dysarthria. As with other paraneoplastic neuropathies, antibodies have been identified, in this case to cerebellar Purkinje cells.[1204, 1205] Spontaneous remission of the syndrome has been reported before the primary lung tumor was treated.[1206]

Encephalomyelopathy

Cerebral symptoms can develop in the absence of focal neurologic signs and consist chiefly of dementia, euphoria, or a manic-depressive state; somnolence and confusion may alternate with lucid intervals.[1183] The syndrome is usually seen in patients who have anti-Hu antibodies.[1207] One such patient developed episodes of central sleep apnea and subsequent acute respiratory failure.[1208] It is not certain if the anti-Hu antibodies are pathogenic; neuropathologic examination in one patient who had encephalitis showed cerebral infiltration by T cells in the absence of complement or antibody deposition.[1209] Three patients have been described in whom a paraneoplastic encephalomyelitis was the first manifestation of small cell carcinoma;[1201] antiamphiphysin (a synaptic vesicle–related protein) antibodies were identified in each patient.

A syndrome resembling limbic encephalitis has also been described in patients who have small cell carcinoma.[1210, 1211] MR imaging may show distinctive features.[1212] Anti-Hu antibodies have been detected in these cases,[1179] as has an antibody directed to a specific hippocampal antigen in one patient.[1213]

Necrotizing Myelopathy

Necrotizing myelopathy is a rare manifestation of carcinoma that consists of extensive necrosis of the spinal cord, resulting in paralysis and complete sensory loss;[1214] only 22 cases had been described in the English literature by 1984.[1215] Anti-Hu antibodies have been documented in affected patients.[1179]

Visual Paraneoplastic Syndrome

Visual paraneoplastic syndrome, which consists of rapid binocular loss of vision, usually occurs in patients who have small cell carcinoma. Serum antibodies against the photoreceptor protein recoverin may be identified.[1216–1219]

Cutaneous Manifestations

A variety of paraneoplastic skin lesions have been described in association with pulmonary carcinoma, including (1) *hypertrichosis lanuginosa*, an excess growth of fine lanugo hair on the hair-bearing surfaces of the body;[1220–1222] (2) *Bazex's syndrome*, characterized by erythematous-to-plum-colored acral lesions, paronychia, nail dysplasia, and keratoderma (this syndrome is recognized as a specific feature of carcinoma of the upper airways [including the trachea] and upper digestive tract);[1223, 1224] (3) *acanthosis nigricans*, a bilaterally symmetric hyperkeratosis and hyperpigmentation of the skin, affecting chiefly the flexural and intertriginous areas;[1225] (4) *Leser-Trélat sign*, an abnormality characterized by abrupt development of seborrheic keratoses that occurs most commonly in association with adenocarcinoma of the bowel and is considered by some to represent a stage in the development of acanthosis nigricans;[1226, 1227] (5) *subacute cutaneous lupus erythematosus*;[1228] (6) *erythema gyratum repens*, consisting of a marbled erythematous swirling and a thin covering of scale over the trunk, axilla, and groin;[1229, 1230] and (7) *tripe palms*, a rugous thickening of the palms with accentuation of the normal dermal dermatoglyphic ridges.[1231–1233]

Additional cutaneous abnormalities that have been described rarely in patients who have pulmonary carcinoma include pemphigus vegetans,[1234] sarcoid granulomas,[1235] erythema annulare centrifugum,[1236] hyperkeratosis of the palms and soles,[1236] erythroderma, acquired ichthyosis, dermatitis herpetiformis, florid cutaneous papillomatosis, pemphigus vulgaris, pityriasis rotunda, Sweet's syndrome, and vasculitis.[9]

Skeletal Manifestations

Hypertrophic pulmonary osteoarthropathy is an important manifestation of pulmonary disease, carcinoma being by far the most common cause (see page 396). It has been found in about 3% of patients who have pulmonary carcinoma.[1176] It is distinctly uncommon in patients who have small cell carcinoma[1236, 1238] and should suggest the diagnosis of a non–small cell tumor.[1176, 1237, 1239]

The main symptom is deep-seated, burning pain in distal parts of the extremities. Clubbing of the fingers and toes and edema, warmth, and tenderness of the hands, wrists, feet, and lower legs are usually evident. Synovial effusions may develop. Radiography reveals subperiosteal new bone formation, chiefly of the distal bones of the extremities. Because radionuclide bone scanning is a sensitive detector of new bone formation, it may offer a more complete appreciation of the extent of the abnormality than is possible by radiography alone. In one scintigraphic study of 48 cases, a distribution of disease quite different from that usually recognized radiographically was observed.[1240] The proximal and distal portions of each long bone were involved with equal frequency; the mandible and maxilla were affected in 42% of cases, the scapulae in 67%, the patellae in 50%, and the clavicles in 33%. The authors found no difficulty in distinguishing the pattern of hypertrophic osteoarthropathy from that of metastatic disease.

Both the radiographic and the clinical changes in the digits may antedate radiographic visibility of the pulmonary carcinoma, sometimes by as much as 2 years.[1239, 1241] Relief of pain invariably follows resection of the primary tumor and has been reported after simple vagotomy without pulmonary resection;[1242–1244] other features of the syndrome may also be alleviated, albeit usually not to the same extent as pain.[1243] Hypertrophic osteoarthropathy may also occur in association with carcinoma of the upper respiratory tract,[1245, 1246] often in association with metastatic spread to the lung.[1247, 1248]

Endocrine and Metabolic Manifestations

Because neuroendocrine cells containing a variety of polypeptides are normally present within the airway epithelium (see page 10), it is not surprising that neoplastic cells derived from this epithelium contain similar substances; provided that they are of sufficient amount and of appropriate biochemical structure, it is theoretically possible that metabolic changes and clinical signs and symptoms could result from their secretion. The subject of the lung as an endocrine organ and the occurrence of paraneoplastic endocrinopathies associated with pulmonary carcinoma have been reviewed by several authors.[1177, 1179, 1249, 1250] Such endocrinopathies include Cushing's syndrome, carcinoid syndrome, a hyperparathyroid-like picture with hypercalcemia, inappropriate secretion of antidiuretic hormone (ADH) with hyponatremia, secretion of an insulin-like substance with hypoglycemia, excess gonadotropin secretion with gynecomastia, and excess secretion of melanocyte-stimulating hormone with hyperpigmentation of the skin.[1176, 1177, 1179, 1188, 1251] In addition, there appears to be an increased incidence of thyrotoxicosis and diabetes mellitus.[1176]

Criteria for attributing an increased hormone level to a paraneoplastic process include the following:[1179] (1) correlation of fluctuations in hormone concentration with changes in tumor burden associated with therapy or tumor progression; (2) increased hormone concentrations in the tumor compared with adjacent normal tissue; and (3) demonstration of the ability of the tumor cells to synthesize and secrete the hormone or its precursor. Identification of ectopic hormone production in the setting of pulmonary carcinoma is important: it allows for recognition of the cause of particular clinical manifestations, may help in predicting the tissue type of the carcinoma, may serve as a guide to effectiveness of therapy, and may influence the nature of the treatment given the patient.

The overall incidence of endocrinopathy in patients who have pulmonary carcinoma has been estimated to be about 5%[1252] to 12%;[1176] in patients who have small cell carcinoma, it is about 15% to 20%.[1188, 1253] In one series of 85 patients from the Johns Hopkins Hospital, the incidence was 33%.[1174] Such a high rate likely reflects some degree of selection; in an assessment of 75 unselected and untreated patients who had small cell carcinoma in Copenhagen, only 2 were found to have a clinically apparent endocrinopathy.[1254] Similarly, in a study of 604 patients with pulmonary carcinomas of all types in Tokyo, only 10 (1.6%) had a paraneoplastic endocrine syndrome.[1255]

Hormonal assays of pulmonary neoplasms, particularly small cell carcinoma, often reveal peptide production in the absence of clinical or biochemical sequelae of excess hormone.[1255, 1256] Similarly, serum levels of polypeptides that have hormonal activity are not uncommonly raised in asymptomatic patients who have pulmonary carcinoma.[1257, 1258] For example, in one evaluation of 106 patients who had small cell carcinoma, almost half were found to have abnormal control of the secretion of adrenocortical steroids;[1259] however, clinical evidence of an ectopic ACTH syndrome was present in only 2.

Cushing's Syndrome

Benign or malignant neoplasms originating in sites other than the pituitary gland or adrenal cortex were identified in 10% of 232 patients who had Cushing's syndrome associated with hyperplasia of the adrenal cortex in one early study.[1260] Although such tumors have been found in many organs or tissues, including the thymus and sympathetic nervous system,[1260, 1261] the most common is probably the lung.

Rather than direct secretion of corticosteroids, the neoplasm appears to exert its paraneoplastic effects by the production of corticotropin precursors, which either have an ACTH-like action[1262] or are converted to ACTH within the tumor cells.[1179] Occasionally, the syndrome is secondary to production of corticotropin-releasing hormone[1263, 1264] and, rarely, to secretion of a corticotropin-releasing hormone–like substance.[1265] Sophisticated testing has confirmed that the ACTH precursors, pro-ACTH and pro-opiomelanocortin, are the predominant circulating form of hormone in this syndrome.[1262]

Although elevated levels of immunoreactive corticotropin can be detected in the blood of about 50% of patients who have small cell carcinoma[1266] and in a significant number of those who have non–small cell tumors, associated clinical findings are quite unusual. For example, of 840 patients who had small cell carcinoma seen over a 20-year period at a Toronto cancer hospital, only 14 (1.6%) had clinical findings of hyperadrenalism;[1267] in another series of 545 patients, 23 (4.5%) developed the clinical syndrome.[1266] The classic picture of Cushing's syndrome is seldom seen in its entirety. Of 14 patients described in one series, one or more features of Cushing's syndrome were seen in only 8 (57%);[1267] hypokalemia was seen in all 14 and hyperglycemia in 10 (71%). A high rate of infections was also seen, and patients had a particularly poor prognosis. The failure to develop the full-blown syndrome is likely the result of a low rate of conversion of the ACTH precursors to the active hormone and the fact that Cushing's syndrome may take months to years to develop—time not available to patients who have small cell carcinoma.[1177]

Hypokalemia is relatively uncommon in Cushing's disease (pituitary-dependent Cushing's syndrome), but is present in the majority of patients who have Cushing's syndrome caused by ectopic corticotropin secretion.[1266, 1268, 1269] It is an important finding in the recognition of an occult ACTH-producing pulmonary carcinoma during the period when no lesion is apparent on the chest radiograph.[1269] Polyuria is common and is usually ascribed to either the glycosuria or the effect of hypokalemia on the kidneys.

Carcinoid Syndrome

Since the first report in 1960,[1270] several cases of carcinoid syndrome have been reported in patients who have small cell or undifferentiated pulmonary carcinoma.[1271–1274] As with gastrointestinal and pulmonary carcinoid tumors, multiple metastases are usually present in the liver.[1187, 1271, 1272] The neoplasms secrete either 5-hydroxytryptamine[1274, 1275] or 5-hydroxytryptophan,[1272] and the urine contains high levels of 5-hydroxyindoleacetic acid. Symptoms and signs result from excessive secretion of 5-hydroxytryptamine and (probably) from the release of kinins.[1276] As with ACTH, secretion of 5-hydroxytryptamine may be seen without evidence of the clinical syndrome.[1275]

Symptoms include weight loss, anorexia, explosive diarrhea, cutaneous flushing, and tachycardia. The first reported case showed no abnormality on the initial chest radiograph, the diagnosis being made by the demonstration of small cell carcinoma in a liver biopsy specimen.[1270] In another case, the primary lung tumor eventually became visible;[1271] a low serum potassium level and adrenal hyperplasia were found in addition to the manifestations of carcinoid syndrome.

Hyperparathyroid-Like Picture

Pulmonary carcinoma is the most frequent cause of tumor-induced hypercalcemia.[1277] The incidence of the abnormality in patients who have pulmonary carcinoma depends in large measure on the range of values accepted as being normal and on the study design used.[1277, 1278] Thus, in one study in which hypercalcemia was defined as a serum calcium level exceeding 11.5 mg/100 ml on two or more occasions, it was reported in 19 (7%) of 280 consecutive cases of early carcinoma.[1176] In a second, prospective study of 200 patients followed from the time of recognition of pulmonary carcinoma to death, hypercalcemia, defined as

serum calcium levels exceeding 10.5 mg/100 ml on three occasions, was reported in 25 (13%);[1153] 18 had squamous cell carcinoma, 6 had large cell carcinoma, and 1 had adenocarcinoma. Of 55 patients in another series who had pulmonary carcinoma requiring admission to the hospital for management of hypercalcemia 40 (72%) had squamous cell carcinoma;[1279] only 5 had small cell carcinoma. These results are consistent with those of many other reports.[1176, 1277, 1280, 1281]

Many patients who have only a slight increase in serum calcium levels are asymptomatic. Values of 15 to 17 mg/100 ml are commonly associated with drowsiness, hypotonia, polyuria, polydipsia, irritability, constipation, and abdominal pain.[1278, 1282] Altered consciousness or coma may erroneously suggest the presence of cerebral metastases.[1281, 1283] In contrast to many other paraneoplastic manifestations, hypercalcemia has not been associated with clinically occult carcinoma;[1284] instead, its presence is almost invariably associated with advanced disease.[1277, 1284] In the occasional patient in whom hypercalcemia has been associated with resectable disease, surgery has led to its resolution.[1285–1288]

Although it might be logical to attribute hypercalcemia to bone metastases when these are present and to ectopic hormone production when they are not, this would be incorrect in many cases. In one series of 200 patients who had pulmonary carcinoma, 25 developed hypercalcemia;[1153] bone metastases were unassociated with hypercalcemia in most. By comparison, among patients who have pulmonary carcinoma and hypercalcemia, bony metastases can be demonstrated in only half.[1153, 1278, 1279, 1282, 1289]

Several substances are responsible for the hypercalcemia in these patients. A parathyroid hormone–related peptide appears to be the most common, both in patients who have skeletal metastases and in those who do not.[1179, 1277, 1290] This peptide has many of the properties of parathyroid hormone, including the ability to increase bone resorption, the promotion of renal tubular reabsorption of calcium and renal excretion of phosphorus, and the augmentation of urinary excretion of cyclic adenosine monophosphate.[1179] Other substances may be important in some patients. For example, the production of prostaglandin E_2 by pulmonary neoplasms, a well-accepted cause of hypercalcemia in animals, may account for some cases in humans; the association is supported by the finding that serum calcium levels are reduced in some patients after the administration of indomethacin.[1291, 1292] True ectopic parathormone production has been described rarely.[1293] A bone-resorbing lipid indistinguishable from 1,24(R)-dihydroxyvitamin D_3 has also been identified in both tumor and serum in one patient.[1294]

Inappropriate Secretion of Antidiuretic Hormone

The syndrome of inappropriate secretion of ADH (SIADH) includes continuous urinary sodium loss (unassociated with corresponding water loss, despite progressive decrease in serum sodium levels and a urine osmolarity exceeding that of plasma), hyponatremia correctable by restriction of fluid intake, and normal renal and adrenal function. Although a few exceptions have been described,[1251, 1295] the syndrome in patients who have pulmonary carcinoma is largely confined to those who have small cell carcinoma.[1177, 1179, 1295, 1296] As with other paraneoplastic endocrine syndromes, clinical findings are much less common than laboratory abnormalities: although 50% of patients who have small cell carcinoma have elevated levels of ADH in their blood and approximately 10% to 15% have hyponatremia,[1296, 1297] only 1% to 5% have symptoms of SIADH.[1179, 1296]

The qualification "inappropriate" applied to ADH secretion relates to the fact that secretion continues despite reduction in plasma osmolarity. This situation leads to increased reabsorption of free water by the renal tubules under the influence of ADH; because the plasma sodium is diluted and the circulating volume is increased, hyponatremia, in turn, results in decreased aldosterone secretion, presumably because volume receptors inhibit this hormone's secretion by the adrenal glands. With the decrease in aldosterone secretion, the amounts of sodium excreted in the urine are inappropriate to the low plasma sodium concentration, so that the hyponatremia is both depletional and dilutional.[1298, 1299] It has also been suggested that the water retention resulting from ADH secretion produces intracellular hypotonicity, with a subsequent shift of sodium to the intracellular fluid, thus contributing to the hyponatremia.[1300] Bioassay has shown that large amounts of ADH are excreted by the kidneys,[1301] and ADH-like activity has been found in plasma[1295, 1302] and in extracts of neoplasms.[1302, 1303]

When the serum sodium level drops below 120 mEq/liter, symptoms of irritability, confusion, irresponsibility, and weakness appear, all likely caused by the hyponatremia. A sweet taste (dysgeusia) has also been attributed to hyponatremia in some patients.[1304] The chest radiograph is usually unequivocally abnormal; in a minority of patients, the symptoms and the finding of hyponatremia antedate demonstrable radiographic abnormality.[1303, 1305–1307]

Gonadotropin Secretion

Secretion of human chorionic gonadotropin is said to occur by 10% to 15% of all pulmonary carcinomas;[1308] however, clinically evident disease resulting from such secretion is rare. It is associated with Leydig cell hyperplasia, low serum testosterone levels, and increased estradiol production.[1308] Many patients have high serum levels of placental alkaline phosphatase in addition to circulating β-human chorionic gonadotropin and estrogens.[1251, 1308–1310] Although all types of pulmonary carcinoma have been implicated,[1187, 1309–1317] large cell carcinoma appears to be the most common.[1308, 1310, 1318] Affected men can present with testicular atrophy and a high-pitched voice in addition to gynecomastia. False pregnancy has been described in a young woman.[1319] Symptoms and signs may disappear after resection of the primary neoplasm but tend to recur when metastases develop.[1187, 1318] The signs of excess gonadotropin secretion may antedate evidence of the neoplasm.[1314]

Gynecomastia is a common finding in the absence of underlying disease. It has been reported to occur in one third of veterans[1320] and in almost two thirds of 214 hospitalized men;[1321] in these individuals, it is simply a physical finding that correlates to some extent with age and the amount of body fat. Given the rarity with which gynecomastia is the result of pulmonary carcinoma, it is more appropriate to search first for other causes, such as certain drugs.[1177]

Calcitonin Secretion

The most common polypeptide hormone produced by pulmonary neoplasms may be calcitonin;[1322, 1323] for example, in two series, levels of this substance were elevated in both serum and urine in 90% of patients.[1324, 1325] The biochemical abnormality does not cause symptoms; however, levels determined by radioimmunoassay have been used as markers of response to therapy or recurrence of neoplasm.[1323, 1325, 1326] There is evidence that the calcitonin is not directly produced by the tumor in some patients.[1327]

Miscellaneous Hormones and Enzymes

One case has been reported in which pulmonary squamous cell carcinoma was associated with hypoglycemia;[1187] the abnormality was relieved after removal of the primary neoplasm. Much more frequently, this hormonal syndrome accompanies mesenchymal neoplasms;[1286] in the thorax, the vast majority of these are solitary fibrous tumor of pleura (*see* page 2828). Insulin-like growth factor–binding protein-2 is secreted by some patients who have small cell carcinoma;[1328] in some, this is associated with abnormal glucose homeostasis.

Increased levels of somatostatin have been reported occasionally in patients who have pulmonary carcinoma;[1329–1331] diabetes mellitus, steatorrhea, and cholelithiasis may result. In one series of 21 consecutive untreated patients who had pulmonary carcinoma, elevated prolactin levels were found in 7;[1332] 4 had squamous cell carcinoma. Pulmonary carcinomas have also been associated with increased serum levels of α-fetoprotein,[1333] gastrin, estrogens,[1334] amylase, and alkaline phosphatase.[1335–1339]

Vascular and Hematologic Manifestations

Migratory thrombophlebitis, thromboembolism, and various hematologic disorders, including purpura and anemia, have all been described in association with pulmonary carcinoma.

Thrombosis

Although a much more frequent complication of carcinoma of the pancreas, thrombophlebitis has been well documented in cases of pulmonary carcinoma.[1225, 1340–1342] The process is typically migratory, occurs in unusual sites, and tends to be resistant to anticoagulant therapy. Rarely, it is extensive and involves virtually all veins.[1341] The complication is seen most often with adenocarcinoma.[1342] An unusual form of paraneoplastic thrombosis, often misinterpreted as metastatic disease, is primary cerebral venous thrombosis.[1343] Nonbacterial thrombotic endocarditis has also been described in some patients who have pulmonary carcinoma, again usually adenocarcinoma.[1086]

The incidence of deep venous thrombosis and pulmonary thromboembolism also is excessive in patients who have pulmonary carcinoma. In one study of 77 patients undergoing thoracotomy, 20 (26%) had thromboembolic events during their hospitalization (mostly deep venous thrombosis);[1344] thromboembolism was more common in patients who had pulmonary carcinoma (15 of 59) than in those who had benign or metastatic disease (0 of 18). Most of the patients who had thromboembolism had adenocarcinoma (11 of 25 versus 4 of 34). The risk of thromboembolism was greater with more advanced tumor stage and more extensive lung resection. These findings are likely explained by the subtle procoagulant state found in many patients who have pulmonary carcinoma, especially those who have metastatic disease. High serum levels of thrombin–antithrombin III complexes,[1345, 1346] *d*-dimer fragments, and plasmin–alpha$_2$-antitrypsin complex[1346] characterize this state. Coexistent thrombocytosis may be an additional factor (*see* farther on). Patients who have advanced malignancy have also been reported to have "thrombosis-inducing activity." In one study of 73 patients who had Stage IIIb or IV non–small cell carcinoma, 41 (56%) demonstrated such activity;[1347] disseminated intravascular coagulation and adult respiratory distress syndrome were terminal complications.

Leukocytosis

Some degree of neutrophilic leukocytosis and lymphocytopenia may occur with any neoplasm that secretes ACTH; in fact, some investigators have found persistent lymphocytopenia to be a useful diagnostic clue to the presence of pulmonary carcinoma.[1348] A leukemoid reaction of polymorphonuclear neutrophils (white blood cell count of $\geq$ 50,000/mm^3) can be associated with a variety of carcinomas, particularly of the lung.[1349–1353] It tends to be a late phenomenon, usually being manifested shortly before death. The abnormality does not appear to be related to any pathologic finding, including necrosis or neutrophil infiltration of the tumor.[1361] One group of investigators found an especially frequent association with large cell carcinoma.[1353] Assay of serum or the tumor itself occasionally reveals the presence of colony-stimulating factor.[1354–1356]

Peripheral eosinophilia is seen occasionally, usually in association with squamous cell or large cell carcinoma;[1352, 1353, 1357–1360] the leukocytosis can reach levels of greater than 100,000/mm^3, 25% to 75% of the cells being eosinophils. Extracts of the tumors may contain eosinophilic chemotactic factor, eosinophil colony-stimulating factor, or both.[1349, 1350, 1352, 1358–1362]

Thrombocytosis

An elevated platelet count is common; for example, in one investigation, the abnormality was noted in 32% of 1,165 patients who had pulmonary carcinoma compared with only 6% of 550 patients who had benign lung disease.[1363] Thrombocytosis was more common in patients who had more advanced tumor stage and correlated with poor survival, even after controlling for stage. After lung resection, the thrombocytosis frequently resolved in the postoperative period.

Purpura and Anemia

In one series of 280 patients, anemia (equally divided between microcytic and normocytic) was present in 22 (8%), hemoglobin values being below 10.0 g/100 ml.[1176] The anemia is most often the result of an impaired erythroid marrow

response to erythropoietin, perhaps compounded by insufficient erythropoietin production.[1364] Anemic patients given erythropoietin have a favorable response.[1365] Anemia may also develop secondary to increased hemolysis,[1225, 1366] bone marrow aplasia,[1366a] iron deficiency, chemotherapy, bone marrow infiltration, and erythrocyte aplasia.[1179] Hemolysis has been found by some investigators to have a particular association with giant cell carcinoma.[1366]

Thrombocytopenia and fibrinolytic purpura are relatively rare complications of pulmonary carcinoma.[1225, 1367] The former may result from neoplastic replacement of bone marrow, marrow depression caused by chemotherapy,[1368] or (occasionally) an immune process.[1369] Two patients have been described who presented with Henoch-Schönlein purpura in association with squamous cell carcinoma.[1370] Other rare vascular and hematologic paraneoplastic manifestations of pulmonary carcinoma include pancytopenia with hypercellular bone marrow and macrocytic anemia,[1371] a disorder similar to myelofibrosis,[1372] and digital necrosis.[1373]

Renal Manifestations

Glomerulonephritis has long been recognized as a paraneoplastic syndrome, sometimes in association with pulmonary carcinoma. In most cases, nephritis is membranous in type;[1374, 1375] minimal change nephropathy has also been reported.[1376, 1377] Nephrotic syndrome, regressing with therapy directed at the cancer, has been seen in a patient who had small cell carcinoma.[1378] Renal failure related to the production of a paraneoplastic paraprotein has been described in a patient who had metastatic squamous cell carcinoma.[1379] Rarely, small cell carcinoma has been associated with a syndrome of marked renal phosphate wasting.[1380, 1381]

INVESTIGATION OF THE PATIENT WHO HAS PULMONARY CARCINOMA

The patient who has radiographic or clinical evidence suggestive of pulmonary carcinoma requires three distinct lines of investigation. First, it is necessary to establish the diagnosis, including a determination of the specific histologic classification. Second, because surgical excision is currently the best method of treating a pulmonary neoplasm for cure, it is necessary to establish resectability or unresectability by a process of staging. Third, the ability of the patient to tolerate the anticipated surgery must be evaluated. The first two of these are discussed in this chapter.

Because considerable variability exists in the natural history of the different histologic types of pulmonary carcinoma and in the extent of disease when the patient is first seen, the investigative protocol should ideally be tailored to the specific presentation of each patient. Nevertheless, we have found it desirable to develop an approach to the diagnostic and staging workup that is organized along fairly precise lines. Procedures performed at various stages of the investigation should result in the highest yield of pertinent information at the lowest cost and obviate the performance of other procedures unlikely to result in useful information. It is clear, however, that investigative protocols vary somewhat from institution to institution, depending on the expertise and preferences of local physicians and the availability of specific equipment. The approaches that we present here are those that we have found successful and that appear valid on the strength of information gleaned from many reports in the literature.

Clinical Considerations

Although there are no specific clinical features of pulmonary carcinoma, the association of certain symptoms and signs with radiographic evidence of a pulmonary abnormality is sometimes virtually diagnostic. For example, a complaint of shoulder and arm pain in association with a lesion at the apex of a lung or a history of the recent onset of clubbing or hypertrophic osteoarthropathy associated with a peripheral spiculated pulmonary mass almost invariably indicates the presence of carcinoma. Hemoptysis associated with a pulmonary mass is also highly suggestive of malignancy; however, hemoptysis in association with a normal chest radiograph is seldom caused by pulmonary carcinoma in the absence of certain specific risk factors, such as smoking history or older age.[1382–1385] Similarly, when the chest radiograph is normal, a localized wheeze may indicate the presence of pulmonary carcinoma. There is a tendency by some physicians to disregard the diagnosis of pulmonary carcinoma in nonsmokers; however, in an assessment of the reasons for missed diagnosis in patients in whom pulmonary carcinoma was found at autopsy, one group of investigators concluded that reliance on the well-accepted association of smoking and cancer might be a significant cause for misdiagnosis in the nonsmoking population.[1386, 1387]

Laboratory Considerations

Routine Cytology

Cytologic examination of sputum, bronchial washings and brushings, bronchoalveolar lavage fluid, and pleural fluid is a well-established method of diagnosis in patients who have suspected carcinoma (*see* page 339). Briefly, the sensitivity of sputum cytology has been found to be about 65% and the specificity 99%.[1388] Washings and brushings performed during bronchoscopy are complementary, but in such a small number of cases that the routine performance of both procedures is questionable.[1389–1391] As might be expected, positive cytologic diagnoses are made more often with central than with peripheral neoplasms and with large than with small tumors.[1392–1396]

In general, the cytologic diagnosis has been found to agree with the histologic diagnosis in about 40% to 80% of large cell carcinomas, 75% to 85% of adenocarcinomas, 85% to 95% of squamous cell carcinomas, and 90% to 95% of small cell carcinomas.[1392, 1394, 1398, 1399] Most importantly, the distinction between small cell and non–small cell carcinoma can be made with confidence in the vast majority of cases. Bronchoalveolar lavage can also be useful, particularly for peripheral tumors that are not visualized endoscopically; in this situation, it yields a positive diagnosis in approximately 65% to 70% of patients.[1400, 1401] Most authors report a sensitivity of about 50% for the cytologic diagnosis of malignancy in pleural effusions.[1402–1404] As with

sputum and bronchial washing specimens, repeated examinations are likely to increase the yield of positive diagnosis.[1402]

When considering cytologic diagnosis, the possibility of a false-positive finding must always be borne in mind (although the incidence of such cases is $< 1\%$ in most laboratories). Malignant cells can originate from the upper digestive tract; although these are almost always squamous cell in type, rare cases of small cell carcinoma of the esophagus[1406] and larynx[1407] have been reported. Conversely, misdiagnosis is possible when an occult carcinoma of the lung is responsible for the shedding of malignant cells in a patient who has a lesion of the esophagus.[1408]

Tumor Markers

Many substances have been identified that are produced by a carcinoma or by host cells in response to it.[534] They can be measured in a variety of specimens, including serum,[1409–1413] tissue,[1414, 1415] pleural fluid,[1416] sputum,[1417] and bronchoalveolar lavage fluid.[1418–1420] Their utility in diagnosis,[1409, 1411–1413, 1419, 1421–1424] staging,[1412, 1425, 1426] distinction of tissue type,[1410, 1416, 1427] separation of primary from metastatic disease,[1415, 1428, 1429] prognostication,[1430–1436] predicting chemotherapy responsiveness,[1437] and follow-up[1421, 1424, 1438–1441] has been explored in a vast number of investigations. A major potential role for these biomarkers in the diagnosis of pulmonary carcinoma is the enhancement of the sensitivity of sputum analysis compared to cytology for screening purposes.[1442] Markers that have been investigated for this purpose include oncogenes such as P53 and K-*ras*.[1443, 1444] The evaluation of any gene or gene product in sputum has not yet had sufficient sensitivity or specificity for detection of early carcinoma to allow for its use in screening.[1443] Another molecule that is currently being evaluated for potential benefit in the early detection of pulmonary carcinoma in prospective trials is a ribonucleoprotein detected by monoclonal antibody reaction.[1443]

Numerous substances have been evaluated in the serum to determine if their measurement is helpful in distinguishing benign from malignant lung lesions.[1409, 1421, 1423] The cytokeratin fragment 19 (CYFRA 21-1) shows some promise in this respect,[1409, 1411, 1421, 1422, 1424] although its precise value has not yet been determined. (Measurement of the same substance in bronchoalveolar lavage fluid has not been found useful because of a lack of specificity.[1420]) No serum marker has been found to have sufficient sensitivity or specificity for the early diagnosis of pulmonary carcinoma to allow for its use as a screening tool.[1445] Tumor markers might be useful in distinguishing malignant pleural effusions caused by non–small cell carcinoma from those caused by small cell carcinoma and could conceivably help avoid more aggressive intervention for diagnosis in patients who have metastatic disease;[1416] however, prospective evaluation of this approach is still required.

Biochemical procedures are of little value in the diagnosis of pulmonary carcinoma. Several investigators, however, have found that serum lactate dehydrogenase levels are increased when metastases are present and when neoplasm recurs after resection.[1446–1448] Liver enzyme elevation may be a clue to metastases to the liver, whereas hyponatremia or hypercalcemia should raise the possibility of a paraneoplastic phenomenon and give some indication of tissue type.

Radiologic Considerations

Radiography

Although the diagnosis of pulmonary carcinoma depends on examination of tissue or cells obtained by a variety of different biopsy techniques, the *presence* of a potentially malignant lesion is usually identified on conventional chest radiographs. The value of the lateral radiograph in the detection of pulmonary carcinoma is controversial. In a retrospective review of posteroanterior and lateral radiographs of 78 patients who had proven pulmonary carcinoma (in 27 of whom the cancer was initially undetected) and 10,597 patients in whom radiographs had been obtained for any reason, in no instance was a lesion detected on the lateral view only.[1449] However, other investigators have concluded that the lateral radiograph is helpful in determining the presence of carcinoma: for example, in one study, this view was considered to be decisive in recognizing the presence of pulmonary carcinoma in 33 (20%) of 168 patients.[1450] In another investigation of 78 patients who had pulmonary carcinoma detected on screening chest radiography, the tumor was seen only on the lateral view in 2 (3%);[1451] in an additional 4 (5%), it was better seen on the lateral than on the frontal view. In a third series of 27 patients in whom the pulmonary carcinoma had been missed on the chest radiograph prospectively but could be identified in retrospect, the lateral radiograph (which was available for 23 patients) revealed the missed lesion better than the posteroanterior view in 4 (17%).[1452] As a result of the findings of these studies, we and others recommend the use of both posteroanterior and lateral projections for pulmonary carcinoma screening.[1451, 1452]

Failure of a radiologist or pulmonary physician to detect a pulmonary carcinoma that is evident on the chest radiograph in retrospect is relatively common. This failure has been best demonstrated in studies in which screening chest radiographs were performed in individuals known to be at high risk for pulmonary carcinoma. In one of these, chest radiographs were performed at 4-month intervals and interpreted by more than one observer with awareness that the images were from high-risk individuals.[1453] The investigators found that lesions initially missed could be seen in retrospect in 45 of 50 (90%) of individuals who developed a peripheral pulmonary carcinoma and in 12 of 16 (75%) who had a perihilar tumor. In another study of 105 carcinomas, 57 (54%) were identified retrospectively on previous radiographs.[1454] These missed carcinomas are not necessarily small; only 5 (19%) of 27 initially missed tumors in one study measured less than 1 cm in diameter, and 8 (31%) measured more than 2 cm in diameter.[1452] The reasons for missing these tumors include partial obscuration by overlying bony structures, poorly defined margins, and failure to compare the radiographs with a sequence of previous radiographs rather than with only the most recent previous examination.[1452]

Review of previous films is important not only in the detection of primary tumors, but also to provide comparison of the hila and mediastinum for possible node enlargement. In the case of a solitary pulmonary nodule, comparison also permits estimation of doubling time.

Computed Tomography

CT plays a major role in the differentiation of benign from malignant nodules and in the staging of pulmonary carcinoma (*see* further on). As discussed in greater detail previously (*see* page 1133), several findings have been shown to have a high degree of specificity for detecting benign lesions. A number of investigators have shown that a nodule that measures less than 3 cm in diameter, has homogeneous attenuation, and does not enhance or enhances less than 15 HU after intravenous administration of contrast material has an approximately 99% probability of being benign.[879, 880, 962] Furthermore, a nodule less than 3 cm in diameter that has diffuse or central calcification occupying more than 10% of its cross-sectional area or that contains focal areas of fat attenuation on thin-section CT is almost certainly benign.[882, 883, 890, 907] CT is also helpful in confirming the presence of lung nodules suspected on radiographs and in distinguishing nodules from chest wall abnormalities or focal scars. In one study of 362 consecutive patients who were referred to a thoracic surgery center for evaluation of suspected pulmonary carcinoma based on findings on the chest radiograph, 44 (12%) had findings categorized as definitely benign on CT, including normal CT, calcified granuloma, and focal scar.[884]

Although CT is clearly superior to chest radiography in the detection of lung lesions, pulmonary carcinomas also may be missed on CT.[1397, 1455, 1456] For example, one group identified 14 patients in whom a total of 15 pulmonary carcinomas had been overlooked on CT.[1455] The indications for CT included further evaluation of a lung nodule seen on the chest radiograph in six patients, hemoptysis in four, and miscellaneous causes in four. Ten of the 15 missed tumors (67%) were endobronchial, 2 were solitary nodules, 1 was a local peripheral area of consolidation, and 1 was a focus of pleural-based thickening. Eleven of the missed tumors were located in a lower lobe. The lesions ranged from 0.2 to 2 cm in diameter (mean, 1.2 cm). In another review of nine patients, the largest missed lesion measured 8 mm in diameter.[1456] A study using three-dimensional computer-simulated nodules measuring 1 to 7 mm in diameter showed that experienced radiologists were able to detect 62% of the nodules; the sensitivity for nodules less than 3 mm in diameter was 48% and that for nodules less than 1.5 mm in diameter was 1%.[1457]

Magnetic Resonance Imaging

MR imaging plays an important role in the assessment of metastatic pulmonary carcinoma, particularly to the brain and adrenals (*see* farther on). It also is an important ancillary imaging modality in the assessment of patients who have questionable chest wall or mediastinal invasion on CT.

Scintigraphy

Perfusion scintigraphy is helpful in predicting postoperative pulmonary function. After quantitative assessment of regional lung perfusion, the postoperative FEV_1 can be predicted by multiplying the preoperative FEV_1 by the percentage of perfusion to the lung that will remain after surgery.[1458] The method is most accurate to determine residual function after pneumonectomy, although it can also be used (albeit with less accuracy) for lobectomy.[1459] In one study of 41 patients, the mean error of perfusion lung scintigraphy in predicting the postlobectomy FEV_1 was approximately 20%.[1459]

Preliminary studies suggest that thallium-201 scintigraphy using SPECT technique may be helpful in the assessment of primary pulmonary carcinomas and mediastinal lymph nodes.[1042, 1460–1462] In one study of 113 patients, the procedure was superior to CT in staging mediastinal involvement with non–small cell carcinoma, with a sensitivity of 76% and a specificity of 92% compared to 62% and 80% for CT.[1463] Further studies are required to assess the potential use of the technique.

Although scintigraphy has traditionally played a limited role in the diagnosis and staging of pulmonary carcinoma, this is changing rapidly with the advent of PET. PET cameras have a much higher resolution and a greater sensitivity to low levels of radiation than SPECT cameras. Several investigators have shown that FDG-PET imaging can be helpful in the distinction of benign from malignant pulmonary nodules[968–972] and in the staging of metastases to hilar and mediastinal lymph nodes (*see* farther on). Furthermore, PET imaging can also demonstrate unsuspected lesions in the contralateral lung,[1464] as well as metastases to lymph nodes, brain, bone, adrenals, liver, pelvis, and skin.[1465–1467] PET imaging also has a high sensitivity and specificity in the detection of recurrent pulmonary carcinoma; in five studies, which included a total of 219 patients, the procedure allowed detection of 135 of 139 cases of recurrent carcinoma (sensitivity 97%) and was falsely positive in 15 of 80 cases (specificity 81%).[1468–1472] (The sensitivity of CT in these patients was 67% and the specificity 85%.) The capability for whole-body imaging using PET and its high diagnostic accuracy have the potential of leading to a rapid change in the approach to the diagnosis and staging of pulmonary carcinoma, in monitoring response to treatment, and in the assessment of tumor recurrence. The main limitations of the procedure are its high cost and the need for access to a cyclotron for production of ^{18}F-deoxyglucose.

Staging

Schemes for Staging

Staging is a procedure by which the nature and extent of the spread of a neoplasm are determined to establish specific therapy and prognosis for the individual patient and to provide a standard by which various therapeutic regimens can be compared. Because a combination of clinical, radiographic, laboratory, and pathologic investigations can be used to stage a particular cancer, different staging systems have been developed.

The most widely used scheme for staging non–small cell carcinoma of the lung is the TNM classification initially outlined in 1972 by the Union Internationale Contre le Cancer (UICC) and the American Joint Committee on Cancer (AJCC) Staging and End Results Reporting.[1473] A variety of alterations in this scheme have been made over the years to better group patients with similar prognosis and treatment options. The most recent revision was approved by the AJCC and the UICC and published in 1997.[1474] An accompanying article outlines refinements made in regional lymph node classification.[1475] Whether all the changes are useful has been questioned,[1167] and it is likely that further refinements will be made. Specific properties of each of the T, N, and M subtypes as defined by this revision are shown in Table 31–3. The various combinations of T, N, and M that define different stages are depicted in Table 31–4. A more detailed discussion of stage in relation to prognosis is given on page 1198.

Patients who have small cell carcinoma are frequently staged in a simple fashion into two categories: (1) *limited* disease, defined as carcinoma confined to a tolerable radiation port; depending on the investigators, this has included regional mediastinal and supraclavicular lymph nodes with or without the presence of pleural effusion; and (2) *extensive* disease, in which carcinoma has extended beyond these limits.[534, 1476] Alternative staging systems using various combinations of anatomic, radiologic, and clinical data[1477–1479] have also been described and are discussed further in the section on prognosis (*see* page 1199).

Methods of Staging

The approach to staging varies with the individual patient and the particular carcinoma and should be tailored to the presenting clinical, radiographic, and bronchoscopic findings. For example, patients who have a central lesion (either obstructing or nonobstructing) usually require mediastinoscopy for evaluation of lymph nodes, whereas this procedure is not indicated in patients who have a solitary pulmonary nodule unassociated with radiologic evidence of abnormality of the ipsilateral hilum or mediastinum.

Staging is often subdivided into clinical, imaging, surgical, and pathologic phases; although these terms are not always precisely defined, by and large they depict an increasingly precise data spectrum of initial clinical presentation, followed by noninvasive and (if necessary) invasive investigative procedures and finally by surgical or autopsy findings. Although the last-named are usually considered the "gold standard," pathologic assessment is also subject to different levels of sophistication; for example, the detection of visceral pleural invasion may be apparent only with the use of elastic tissue stains,[804] and lymph node or bone marrow metastases may be evident only after application of the polymerase chain reaction (PCR)[1405] or monoclonal antibodies.[1480, 1481] An illustration of the potential importance of the latter test is provided by a study of 72 patients who had non–small cell carcinoma that had been staged as N0 by standard histologic examination.[1480] Application of a monoclonal antibody (Ber-Ep4) to frozen tissue sections of lymph nodes sampled at the time of surgery showed isolated tumor cells in 11 of the 72 cases (15%); patients who had such micrometastases were found to have a significantly shorter disease-free survival than immunopathologically documented node-negative patients.

Although it is important to base staging on the best objective criteria, there is nevertheless a close correlation between symptoms and signs and positive findings on CT, MR imaging, and radionuclide scanning, especially when these studies are directed toward the detection of extensive disease.[1482, 1483] The following sections discuss the investigative protocols that apply to each of the T, N, and M parameters of the staging system.

Table 31-3. TNM DESCRIPTORS

PRIMARY TUMOR (T)

TX Primary tumor cannot be assessed or tumor proven by the presence of malignant cells in sputum or bronchial washings but not visualized by imaging or bronchoscopy

T0 No evidence of primary tumor

Tis Carcinoma *in situ*

T1 Tumor ≤3 cm in greatest dimension, surrounded by lung or visceral pleura, without bronchoscopic evidence of invasion more proximal than the lobar bronchus* (i.e., not in the main bronchus)

T2 Tumor with any of the following features of size or extent
>3 cm in greatest dimension
Involves main bronchus, ≥2 cm distal to the carina
Invades the visceral pleura
Associated with atelectasis or obstructive pneumonitis that extends to the hilar region but does not involve the entire lung

T3 Tumor of any size that directly invades any of the following: chest wall (including superior sulcus tumors), diaphragm, mediastinal pleura, parietal pericardium; or tumor in the main bronchus <2 cm distal to the carina but without involvement of the carina; or associated atelectasis or obstructive pneumonitis of the entire lung

T4 Tumor of any size that invades any of the following: mediastinum, heart, great vessels, trachea, esophagus, vertebral body, carina; or tumor with a malignant pleural or pericardial effusion,† or with satellite tumor nodule(s) within the ipsilateral primary-tumor lobe of the lung

REGIONAL LYMPH NODES (N)

NX Regional lymph nodes cannot be assessed

N0 No regional lymph node metastasis

N1 Metastasis to ipsilateral peribronchial and/or ipsilateral hilar lymph nodes and intrapulmonary nodes involved by direct extension of the primary tumor

N2 Metastasis to ipsilateral mediastinal and/or subcarinal lymph node(s)

N3 Metastasis to contralateral mediastinal, contralateral hilar, ipsilateral or contralateral scalene, or supraclavicular lymph node(s)

DISTANT METASTASIS (M)

MX Presence of distant metastasis cannot be assessed

M0 No distant metastasis

M1 Distant metastasis present‡

---

*The uncommon superficial tumor of any size with its invasive component limited to the bronchial wall, which may extend proximal to the main bronchus, is also classified T1.

†Most pleural effusions associated with lung cancer are due to tumor. There are a few patients, however, in whom multiple cytopathologic examinations of pleural fluid show no tumor. In these cases, the fluid is nonbloody and is not an exudate. When these elements and clinical judgment dictate that the effusion is not related to the tumor, the effusion should be excluded as a staging element, and the patient's disease should be staged T1, T2, or T3. Pericardial effusion is classified according to the same rules.

‡Separate metastatic tumor nodule(s) in the ipsilateral nonprimary tumor lobe(s) of the lung also are classified M1.

From Mountain CF: Revisions in the international system for staging lung cancer. Chest 111:1710, 1997.

T (Primary Tumor)

Radiography. Of the criteria that define the T categories in the most recent TNM classification, most are established during the initial diagnostic workup. For example, conventional chest radiographs reveal the size of the lesion in patients in whom it is circumscribed and the degree of associated atelectasis or obstructive pneumonitis in the presence of airway obstruction. In the latter situation, bronchoscopy documents the proximal extent of the neoplasm. The chest radiograph also establishes the presence or absence of pleural effusion, the exception being the situation in which atelectasis or obstructive pneumonitis of a lower lobe obscures its presence.

In some cases, extrapulmonary spread may also be evident without the results of special investigations. For example, direct extension of a neoplasm into the chest wall may be established by radiographic evidence of destruction of ribs or vertebrae or clinical evidence of a palpable mass. Evidence of invasion of the mediastinum may be suggested by marked elevation of a hemidiaphragm caused by phrenic nerve paralysis or by clinical signs of superior vena cava syndrome or laryngeal paralysis.[1484] Paramediastinal lesions sometimes displace or narrow the tracheal air column, thereby providing convincing radiographic evidence of mediastinal invasion. In the absence of signs such as these, conventional radiography is generally unreliable in detecting invasion of the chest wall, diaphragm, or mediastinum, and it is necessary to resort to CT or MR imaging for such evaluation.[884, 1041, 1485–1489]

Computed Tomography. CT can reliably detect invasion of the mediastinum, provided that major mediastinal vessels or bronchi are surrounded by tumor (Fig. 31–89).[1488] However, a tumor that abuts but does not obviously invade the mediastinum cannot be considered as invasive, even when there is obliteration of the fat plane between the mediastinum

Table 31-4. STAGE GROUPING—TNM SUBSETS*

STAGE	TNM SUBSET
0	Carcinoma *in situ*
IA	T1N0M0
IB	T2N0M0
IIA	T1N1M0
IIB	T2N1M0
	T3N0M0
IIIA	T3N1M0
	T1N2M0
	T2N2M0
	T3N2M0
IIIB	T4N0M0
	T4N1M0
	T4N2M0
	T1N3M0
	T2N3M0
	T3N3M0
	T4N3M0
IV	Any T Any N M1

*Staging is not relevant for occult carcinoma, designated TXN0M0.
From Mountain CF: Revisions in the international system for staging lung cancer. Chest 111:1710, 1997.

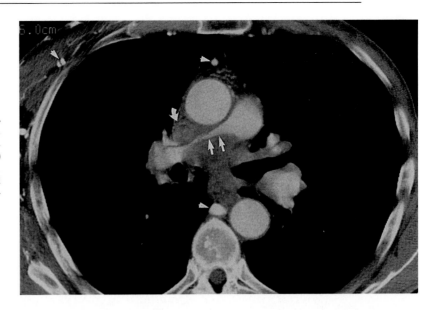

Figure 31–89. Unresectable Pulmonary Carcinoma. A contrast-enhanced CT scan demonstrates extensive mediastinal involvement by tumor with encasement of the right pulmonary artery *(straight arrows)* and obstruction of the superior vena cava *(curved arrow).* Note collateral venous circulation in the chest wall and mediastinum *(arrowheads).* The diagnosis was biopsy-proven large cell carcinoma.

and the tumor mass.[1488] CT criteria suggesting that a tumor abutting the mediastinum is likely to be resectable (albeit possibly minimally invasive) include (1) less than 3 cm contact between the tumor and the adjacent mediastinum; (2) less than 90 degrees circumferential contact between the tumor and the aorta; and (3) the presence of fat between the tumor and the adjacent mediastinal structures.[1490] Carcinomas that involve the tracheal carina or that surround, encase, or abut more than 180 degrees of the aorta, main or proximal portion of the right or left pulmonary arteries, or esophagus are likely to be extensively invasive and unresectable.[884, 1491]

The detection of a T4 status is considered one of the main indications for use of CT in the staging of pulmonary carcinoma.[1492] For example, in one study of 275 patients, CT scans demonstrated surgically unresectable tumors (T4) in 34 patients (12%).[884] In another, prospective investigation of 250 patients, only 2 underwent thoracotomy and were found to have T4 disease undetected by CT.[1041] Although tumors that abut the mediastinum for less than 3 cm are generally resectable and those that encase major mediastinal vessels or bronchi are unresectable, there are no reliable criteria to predict resectability of tumors that abut the mediastinum for more than 3 cm but are not associated with major mediastinal extension (Fig. 31–90).[1493, 1494] In one study of 90 patients who underwent CT and thoracotomy, only 11 of 17 mediastinal structures distorted by adjacent tumor (65%) and 5 of 7 central vessels with apparent intraluminal tumor (71%) were shown to be involved at thoracotomy.[1493] Greater than 90-degree contact of tumor with a mediastinal structure had a sensitivity of 40% (10 of 25 structures) and a specificity of 99% (752 of 760 structures) in the detection of mediastinal tumor invasion. All seven structures with more than 180 degrees of contact with the tumor were involved (specificity 100%); however, the sensitivity was only 28%. The authors excluded from the study 48 patients who had clearly unresectable disease because of advanced local extension (T4 lesions) as well as 60 patients who had positive mediastinoscopic examinations.

Magnetic Resonance Imaging. MR imaging is superior to CT in the demonstration of the pericardium, cardiac chambers, and mediastinal vessels; it also does not require intravenous contrast administration.[857, 1495, 1496] Disruption of the normal 2- to 3-mm low signal intensity of the pericardium is suggestive of pericardial infiltration, although this does not necessarily preclude complete surgical resection (Fig. 31–91). Coronal images are particularly helpful in the assessment of tumor extension into the subcarinal region, aortopulmonary window, and superior vena cava.[857, 1041, 1043, 1495] Disadvantages of MR imaging include lower spatial resolution and artefacts as a result of cardiac and respiratory motion.

The benefit of MR imaging over CT in the overall assessment of mediastinal invasion is controversial. In two studies, MR imaging was found to be slightly more accurate than CT in the diagnosis of mediastinal invasion.[857, 1041] In one of these studies (which involved 170 patients who had non–small cell carcinoma [including 30 who had T3 or T4 tumors]), however, there was no significant difference in the overall diagnostic accuracy of CT and MR imaging;[1041] the sensitivity of CT and MR imaging was 63% and 56% and the specificity 84% and 80% for distinguishing T3 and T4 tumors from less extensive pulmonary carcinomas. As with CT, the main limitation of MR imaging is the inability to distinguish tumor invasion of mediastinal fat from inflammatory changes.[856, 1496]

N (Lymph Nodes)

Hilar (N1), ipsilateral (N2), or contralateral (N3) mediastinal lymph node metastases are often present at the time of initial diagnosis of pulmonary carcinoma. The identification of affected nodes is important, both in determining which patients are candidates for potentially curative resection and in predicting prognosis. Assessment of the presence of lymph node involvement on radiography, CT, and MR imaging is based on nodal enlargement. This approach necessarily entails a degree of inaccuracy, because normal-sized nodes can contain metastases and enlarged nodes may be only hyperplastic. Furthermore, there has been considerable controversy concerning the accepted normal range in size of mediastinal lymph nodes as well as their classification *(see*

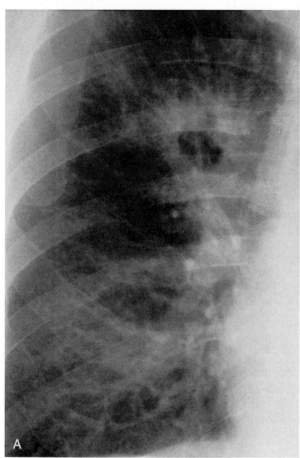

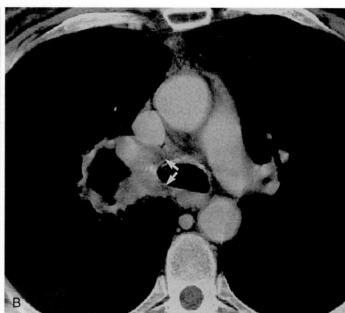

Figure 31–90. Resectable (T3) Pulmonary Carcinoma. A view of the right lung from an anteroposterior chest radiograph *(A)* reveals a 4-cm-diameter cavitated mass in the right upper lobe. A contrast-enhanced CT scan *(B)* demonstrates the mass as well as soft tissue extension anterior and posterior *(arrows)* to the right main bronchus. The diagnosis of squamous cell carcinoma was confirmed at bronchoscopy. The patient was a 60-year-old man who presented with hemoptysis. The tumor (stage IIIa) was completely resected at pneumonectomy.

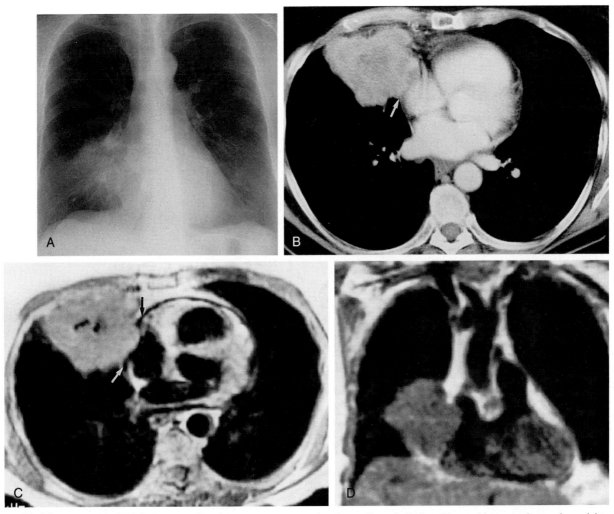

Figure 31–91. Resectable (T3) Pulmonary Carcinoma. A posteroanterior chest radiograph *(A)* in a 62-year-old woman shows a large right middle lobe tumor abutting the heart. A contrast-enhanced CT scan *(B)* shows local thickening of the pericardium *(arrow)* and focal mediastinal invasion. The extent of mediastinal invasion, however, cannot be reliably assessed on the CT image. A transverse, cardiac-gated, spin-echo MR image *(C)* better demonstrates the pericardium *(arrows)* and the focal extension of tumor as well as focal compression of the right atrium. A coronal MR image *(D)* better demonstrates the relationship of the tumor with the right atrium. Neither the CT nor the MR images allow definite diagnosis or exclusion of invasion of the right atrium. At surgery, this was shown to be a resectable (T3) squamous cell carcinoma with focal pericardial invasion, which compressed the right atrium but did not involve the right atrial wall (stage IIb pulmonary carcinoma).

page 184). The following represent the most widely accepted criteria for radiologic assessment.

1. Lymph nodes should be classified according to a standardized lymph node map. One of the most accepted schemas was that advocated by the American Thoracic Society (*see* page 184).[1497] This classification had a number of deficiencies, however, including the absence of a specific designation for hilar lymph nodes; as a result, some authors included the right tracheobronchial (10R) and left peribronchial (10L) nodes as mediastinal nodes[1498] and others as hilar nodes.[1499] The more recently described lymph node map adopted by the American Joint Committee on Cancer (AJCC) and the UICC includes position 10 nodes as hilar

lymph nodes (Fig. 31–92 and Table 31–5) and is the preferred scheme at the present time.[1475]

2. The most reliable and practical measurement of lymph node size on CT is its short-axis diameter (i.e., the shortest diameter on the cross-sectional image); this parameter correlates better than the long-axis diameter with the node volume and is less influenced by the spatial orientation of the node.[1501, 1502] Although some authors have suggested the use of various nodal size criteria specific for each mediastinal nodal station,[1503, 1504] for practical reasons we and others consider a diameter greater than 10 mm in short axis as abnormal regardless of nodal station.[907, 1042]

3. Factors that facilitate visualization of mediastinal lymph nodes are the presence of mediastinal fat, use of

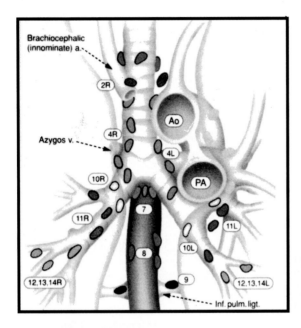

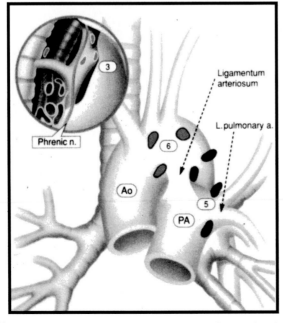

Superior Mediastinal Nodes

● **1** Highest Mediastinal

● **2** Upper Paratracheal

◑ **3** Pre-vascular and Retrotracheal

◑ **4** Lower Paratracheal
    (including Azygos Nodes)

N_2 = single digit, ipsilateral
N_3 = single digit, contralateral or supraclavicular

Aortic Nodes

● **5** Subaortic (A-P window)

● **6** Para-aortic (ascending
    aorta or phrenic)

Inferior Mediastinal Nodes

◑ **7** Subcarinal

◑ **8** Paraesophageal
    (below carina)

● **9** Pulmonary Ligament

N_1 Nodes

○ **10** Hilar

● **11** Interlobar

◑ **12** Lobar

◑ **13** Segmental

◑ **14** Subsegmental

Figure 31–92. Regional Lymph Node Stations for Lung Cancer Staging. (From Mountain CF, Dresler CM: Regional lymph node classification for lung cancer staging. Chest 111:1719, 1997.)

Table 31–5. LYMPH NODE MAP DEFINITIONS

NODAL STATION	ANATOMIC LANDMARKS
N2 nodes—all N2 nodes lie within the mediastinal pleural envelope	
1 Highest mediastinal nodes	Nodes lying above a horizontal line at the upper rim of the brachiocephalic (left innominate) vein where it ascends to the left, crossing in front of the trachea at its midline
2 Upper paratracheal nodes	Nodes lying above a horizontal line drawn tangential to the upper margin of the aortic arch and below the inferior boundary of No. 1 nodes
3 Prevascular and retrotracheal nodes	Prevascular and retrotracheal nodes may be designated 3A and 3P; midline nodes are considered to be ipsilateral
4 Lower paratracheal nodes	The lower paratracheal nodes on the right lie to the right of the midline of the trachea between a horizontal line drawn tangential to the upper margin of the aortic arch and a line extending across the right main bronchus at the upper margin of the upper lobe bronchus and contained within the mediastinal pleural envelope; the lower paratracheal nodes on the left lie to the left of the midline of the trachea between a horizontal line drawn tangential to the upper margin of the aortic arch and a line extending across the left main bronchus at the level of the upper margin of the left upper lobe bronchus, medial to the ligamentum arteriosum and contained within the mediastinal pleural envelope
	Researchers may wish to designate the lower paratracheal nodes as No. 4s (superior) and No. 4i (inferior) subsets for study purposes; the No. 4s nodes may be defined by a horizontal line extending across the trachea and drawn tangential to the cephalic border of the azygos vein; the No. 4i nodes may be defined by the lower boundary of No. 4s and the lower boundary of No. 4, as described above
5 Subaortic (aortopulmonary window)	Subaortic nodes are lateral to the ligamentum arteriosum or the aorta or left pulmonary artery and proximal to the first branch of the left pulmonary artery and lie within the mediastinal pleural envelope
6 Para-aortic nodes (ascending aorta or phrenic)	Nodes lying anterior and lateral to the ascending aorta and the aortic arch or the innominate artery, beneath a line tangential to the upper margin of the aortic arch
7 Subcarinal nodes	Nodes lying caudal to the carina of the trachea but not associated with the lower lobe bronchi or arteries within the lung
8 Paraesophageal nodes (below carina)	Nodes lying adjacent to the wall of the esophagus and to the right or left of the midline, excluding subcarinal nodes
9 Pulmonary ligament nodes	Nodes lying within the pulmonary ligament, including those in the posterior wall and lower part of the inferior pulmonary vein
N1 nodes—all N1 nodes lie distal to the mediastinal pleural reflection and within the visceral pleura	
10 Hilar nodes	Proximal lobar nodes, distal to the mediastinal pleural reflection and the nodes adjacent to the bronchus intermedius on the right; radiographically the hilar shadow may be created by enlargement of both hilar and interlobar nodes
11 Interlobar nodes	Nodes lying between the lobar bronchi
12 Lobar nodes	Nodes adjacent to the distal lobar bronchi
13 Segmental nodes	Nodes adjacent to the segmental bronchi
14 Subsegmental nodes	Nodes around the subsegmental bronchi

From Mountain CF, Dresler CM: Regional lymph node classification for lung cancer staging. Chest 111:1720, 1997.

intravenous contrast material, and thinner CT sections. Intravenous contrast material is particularly helpful in the distinction of the truncus anterior from a right paratracheal lymph node and in the assessment of the aortopulmonary window region, where the superior aspect of the main pulmonary artery may be misinterpreted as an enlarged lymph node on scans performed without intravenous contrast material. Despite these advantages, we believe that intravenous contrast material is not routinely required for the assessment of mediastinal nodes when using spiral CT technique and 5- to 7-mm collimation scans. In one study of 79 patients, 5-mm collimation scans without the use of intravenous contrast material allowed identification of more nodes than 10-mm-thick sections with intravenous contrast material.[1505]

Computed Tomography. Assessment of hilar lymph nodes requires the use of intravenous injection of contrast material and dynamic incremental[1506] or spiral CT (Fig. 31–93).[1507, 1508] It has been suggested that assessment of these nodes can be improved by evaluating the appearance of the margins of peribronchovascular hypoattenuated areas rather than measuring nodal short-axis diameter.[1508] In one study of seven inflated and fixed lung specimens, the interfaces of such hypoattenuated areas with the adjacent parenchyma were concave or straight in 95% of normal nodes (183 of 193 contact sites) and convex in 95% of abnormal nodes (54 of 57 contact sites).[1508] Using the criterion of convexity, the authors demonstrated that the sensitivity of CT for detecting abnormal hilar lymph nodes in 95 patients who had pulmonary carcinoma was 87% and the specificity 83% (compared with 50% sensitivity and 80% specificity for nodal size criteria).[1508]

Although there is no question that CT is superior to chest radiography in the detection of mediastinal lymph node metastases (Fig. 31–94), the specificity for the diagnosis is slightly less.[1041, 1454, 1509, 1510] For example, in one study of 418 patients, the sensitivity and specificity of chest radiography were 40% and 99%; for the same group, CT had a sensitivity and a specificity of 84%.[1510] In another investigation of 170 patients, the sensitivity and specificity of radiography were 9% and 92%, whereas the corresponding figures for CT were 52% and 69%.[1509] Thus, appreciation of mediastinal lymph

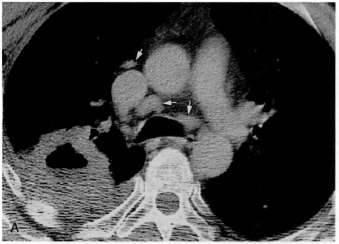

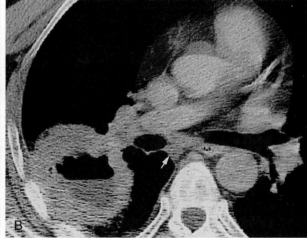

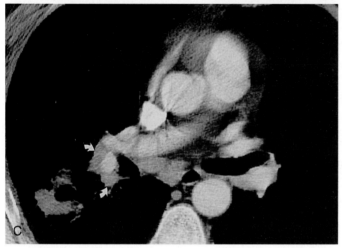

Figure 31–93. Value of Contrast Enhancement. CT scans performed without intravenous contrast material *(A and B)* demonstrate a 5-cm-diameter cavitated tumor in the right lung. Mediastinal nodes *(arrows)* can be identified without the use of intravenous contrast material as soft tissue opacities surrounded by fat. The CT scan at the level of the right hilum *(B)* does not allow adequate assessment of hilar and interlobar nodes. After intravenous administration of contrast material *(C)*, the enlarged right hilar nodes *(curved arrows)* can be readily distinguished from the interlobar pulmonary artery. The patient was a 56-year-old man who had surgically proven squamous cell carcinoma with involvement of the right hilar (10) lymph nodes. The mediastinal nodes did not contain carcinoma.

node enlargement on radiography almost invariably indicates the presence of metastatic carcinoma.

As the results of the previous studies suggest, there has been considerable variability in the reported sensitivity and specificity of CT in the assessment of mediastinal nodal metastases; although several groups have demonstrated a sensitivity greater than 85%,[1511–1515] others have reported values from 40% to 70%.[1401, 1509, 1516, 1517] This variability is related to several factors, including different size criteria for abnormal lymph nodes, different patient populations studied, use of a per-patient versus a per–nodal station analysis, interobserver variability, and differences in the diagnostic "gold standard."

Absence of Uniform Size Criteria. Some investigators have used 5-, 10-, or 15-mm long-axis diameter measurements and others 10-mm short-axis diameter measurements. The diagnostic accuracy of various nodal measurement criteria was assessed in one study of 151 patients in whom mediastinal nodal metastases were present in 56 (37%).[1518] The sensitivity of a long-axis measurement greater than 5 mm was 95%; corresponding figures for measurements greater than 10 mm and 15 mm were 79% and 61%, whereas the sensitivity of a short-axis measurement greater than 10 mm was 61%. The specificities were 23%, 65%, 93%, and 93%. As indicated previously, the majority of radiologists

now use 10 mm in short axis as the upper limit of normal for mediastinal nodes.

Different Patient Populations. In this context, the qualifier "different" refers both to the character of the population under study and to its size, a number of series involving relatively few patients (≤50). The prevalence of nodal metastases is related to the T stage of the tumor. For example, in one study of 159 patients, of whom 60 had mediastinal nodal metastases, the prevalence of nodal metastases was 22% in 46 patients who had T1 lesions, 42% in 81 patients who had T2 lesions, and 50% in 32 patients who had T3 carcinoma.[884] The sensitivity of CT in the detection of these metastases was 40% for T1 lesions, 56% for T2 lesions, and 87% for T3 lesions. The specificity decreased from 97% for T1 lesions to 83% for T2 lesions and 69% for T3 lesions. The decreased specificity of CT in T2 and T3 lesions is presumably related to the increased likelihood of hyperplastic nodes secondary to postobstructive pneumonitis and atelectasis.[1516, 1519]

As might be expected, the significance of enlarged mediastinal lymph nodes is also influenced by the presence of previous granulomatous disease. In general, studies from regions that have a lower incidence of granulomatous diseases, such as the West Coast of Canada,[884, 1518, 1521] Europe,[1503] or Japan,[1504] have been associated with a relatively

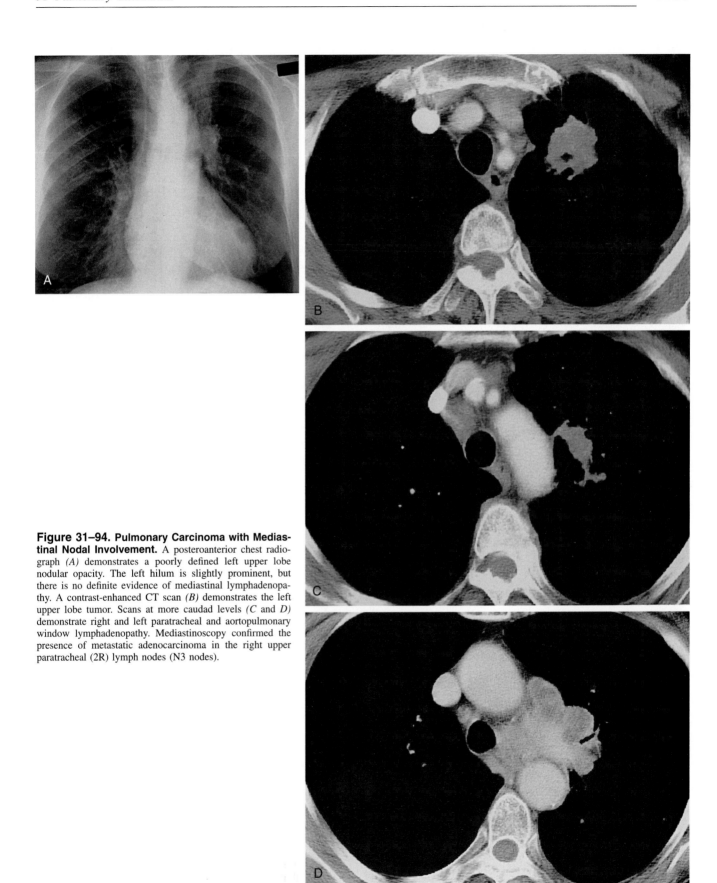

Figure 31–94. Pulmonary Carcinoma with Mediastinal Nodal Involvement. A posteroanterior chest radiograph *(A)* demonstrates a poorly defined left upper lobe nodular opacity. The left hilum is slightly prominent, but there is no definite evidence of mediastinal lymphadenopathy. A contrast-enhanced CT scan *(B)* demonstrates the left upper lobe tumor. Scans at more caudad levels *(C* and *D)* demonstrate right and left paratracheal and aortopulmonary window lymphadenopathy. Mediastinoscopy confirmed the presence of metastatic adenocarcinoma in the right upper paratracheal (2R) lymph nodes (N3 nodes).

high CT specificity for metastases (80% to 90%). By contrast, the majority of studies from the United States, particularly those from regions where infections such as histoplasmosis are relatively common, have been associated with lower specificities (50% to 70%).[1041, 1516, 1517]

Per-Patient Versus Per–Nodal Station Analysis. In a per-patient analysis, a CT examination is considered to be a true positive if it shows an enlarged lymph node in a patient who has mediastinal lymph node metastases, regardless of whether the node that contains tumor is interpreted as being in the same nodal station as that identified on CT. On a per–nodal station assessment, the CT examination is considered as being truly positive only if it shows an enlarged node in the same nodal station in which metastatic lymph node involvement is present pathologically.

As might be expected, the sensitivity of CT on a per-patient analysis is higher than that on a per–nodal station analysis.[884, 1518, 1521] In one study of 151 patients who underwent preoperative mediastinoscopy and thorough mediastinal exploration at surgery, the authors tried to match nodal stations as assessed on CT with those assessed at surgery using the American Thoracic Society nodal map.[1518] The sensitivity of CT on a per-patient basis was 79%. Tumor was absent, however, in the enlarged nodal stations as classified on CT but considered to be present at surgery in an adjacent nodal station that had normal-sized nodes at CT in 7 of 44 patients (16%); thus, the sensitivity on a per–nodal station basis was 66%. Although tumor involvement may have been present in normal-sized rather than enlarged nodes, it is perhaps more likely that the difference was due to difficulties in determining precisely the location of the involved nodes. In another investigation in which 362 nodal stations were sampled at mediastinoscopy or thoracotomy in 104 patients who had T1 pulmonary carcinoma, the sensitivity of CT on a per-patient basis was 59%, whereas the sensitivity on a per–nodal station basis was 41%.[1521] When adjacent nodal stations were included in the analysis (i.e., when it was assumed that the CT findings were positive whenever a node identified at surgery was in the same or in an adjacent nodal station), the sensitivity increased to 59%.

Interobserver Variability. Several workers have shown that there is considerable interobserver variability in determining mediastinal nodal status on CT. For example, in one study of 147 patients, of whom 68 were shown to have mediastinal node metastases at mediastinoscopy or thoracotomy, the sensitivity of CT for four independent observers was 40%, 62%, 63%, and 69%, and the specificity was 91%, 65%, 79%, and 61%.[1522] The sensitivities for individual nodal stations were lower, ranging from 14% to 48%. In a second study, the average agreement rates between four expert observers ranged from 58% to 90% (average kappa statistics between 0.40 and 0.60).[1523] Agreement varies with individual nodal stations; in one study of 50 patients, interobserver agreement between four radiologists as assessed by the kappa statistic was 0.68 for right superior mediastinal (2R, 4R, 10R) nodes, 0.28 for left superior mediastinal nodes (2L, 4L, 10L), 0.54 for aortopulmonary nodes (5, 6), and 0.58 for subcarinal nodes (7).[1498] The intraobserver and interobserver agreement is similar for contrast-enhanced and non–contrast-enhanced CT.[1500] The interobserver variability on MR imaging is similar to that on CT.[1523]

"Gold Standard." Differences in the methods for confirming or ruling out the presence of mediastinal lymph node metastases clearly influence the sensitivity and specificity of diagnosis. For example, the average sensitivity of CT in the detection of mediastinal lymph node metastases was 93% in 3 studies in which only selective node sampling was performed, 78% in 23 studies in which all visible or palpable nodes were biopsied, and 83% in 8 studies in which "complete" nodal dissection was performed.[1524]

Although there is considerable variability in the reported accuracy of CT in the diagnosis of mediastinal lymph node metastases, the authors of a meta-analysis of 42 studies published between 1980 and 1988 concluded that the sensitivity was 83% and the specificity was 81%, on a per-patient basis.[1524] These figures are similar to those of a prospective multicenter Canadian Lung Oncology Group study of mediastinal nodal metastases, in which CT was found to have a sensitivity of 78% and a specificity of 69%.[1525] The authors of the latter study also assessed the cost-effectiveness of CT. The study was prospective and included 685 patients, 342 of whom were randomly assigned to have mediastinoscopy for preoperative staging and 343 to have CT. Patients who underwent CT proceeded to mediastinoscopy if they had any mediastinal nodes greater than 10 mm in short-axis diameter or directly to thoracotomy if all nodes were 10 mm or less in diameter. The primary end point, chosen before the beginning of the study, was thoracotomy without cure (defined as patients who had unresectable disease at the time of thoracotomy, patients who underwent incomplete resections, or patients in whom recurrent disease developed within 3 years). The percentage of patients who had positive N2 nodes at thoracotomy was similar in the CT and mediastinoscopy groups (23%). Overall, the number of thoracotomies without cure was virtually the same in the two groups (103 of 343 [30%] in the CT group and 109 of 342 [32%] in the mediastinoscopy group). The number of thoracotomies in patients who had benign disease was also lower in the CT group (4 of 20, 20%) than in the mediastinoscopy group (12 of 25, 48%). The CT strategy therefore produced the same number of or fewer unnecessary thoracotomies than mediastinoscopy in all patients and was also less expensive. These results suggest that CT rather than mediastinoscopy should be performed in all patients who are suspected to have pulmonary carcinoma. Patients who are still considered to have carcinoma after CT and who have normal-sized nodes may proceed directly to thoracotomy.[1525] Because of the relative lack of specificity of enlarged nodes detected by CT alone, biopsy is usually required to confirm the presence of metastases.

Positive nodes missed on CT are less likely to be associated with extracapsular spread of tumor than nodes larger than 1 cm in diameter.[1526–1528] Furthermore, patients who have metastasis to normal-sized nodes are more likely to have negative results at mediastinoscopy and to have the affected nodes discovered only at subsequent thoracotomy. There is evidence that patients who have microscopic metastases discovered at the time of thoracotomy have an improved survival rate if the primary tumor and the involved mediastinal nodes are resected.[1526, 1527]

Magnetic Resonance Imaging. As with CT, MR imaging relies on size criteria to identify nodal abnormalities and therefore is comparable to it in the assessment of mediastinal nodal metastasis.[1041, 1529–1532] MR imaging has the advantage of allowing ready distinction of mediastinal vessels from nodes without the need for intravenous contrast administration; in addition, it has the ability of imaging directly in the sagittal and coronal planes, which can be particularly helpful in the assessment of the aortopulmonary window and subcarinal region.[1043, 1533] MR imaging has a lower spatial resolution than CT, however, and adjacent small nodes may be misinterpreted as a single enlarged node.[1531, 1534] Moreover, because calcification may not be apparent on MR imaging, enlarged calcified nodes may be classified as malignant.[1535] The results of a preliminary study suggest that the accuracy of MR imaging diagnosis may be improved with the use of intravenous contrast material.[1536] In this study, nine patients who had pulmonary carcinoma underwent dynamic MR imaging after intravenous administration of gadoterade meglumine. Mediastinal nodes involved with tumor demonstrated marked enhancement, whereas anthracotic nodes and nodes containing granulomas showed only minimal enhancement.

Positron Emission Tomography. Although CT and MR rely on the anatomic assessment of nodes, PET is primarily a physiologic imaging technique that relies on a biochemical difference between normal and neoplastic cells. Mediastinal nodes containing carcinoma have been shown to have increased uptake and accumulation of FDG, a glucose analogue labeled with the positron emitter ^{18}F. Several groups have shown that PET is superior to CT in the assessment of mediastinal nodal metastases.[1537–1539a] In one study of 42 patients in which 62 nodal stations (40 hilar, 22 mediastinal) were surgically sampled, the sensitivity and specificity for hilar lymph node station metastases using PET were 73% and 76% compared with 27% and 86% for CT.[1537] For mediastinal node station metastasis, the sensitivity and specificity using PET were 92% and 100% compared with 58% and 80% for CT. In another study of 99 patients, the sensitivity and specificity for the diagnosis of N2 disease were 83% and 94% for PET compared with 63% and 73% for CT.[1538]

In a third, prospective study of 50 patients who had potentially resectable non–small cell pulmonary carcinoma, the sensitivity and specificity of CT were 67% and 59% compared with 67% and 97% for PET.[1539] Enlarged mediastinal lymph nodes on CT were found in 23 patients, only 10 of whom had metastatic carcinoma at pathologic examination. Twenty-seven patients did not have enlarged mediastinal lymph nodes; metastatic carcinoma was found in 5. PET was positive in 11 cases (correct in 10). In 39 cases, there was no suspicion of metastatic carcinoma on PET scans; 5 of these had carcinoma at pathologic staging. At a second reading, the PET images were correlated with the CT findings to allow more precise localization of the hot spots. This assessment changed the conclusion as to the presence of carcinoma in four patients. The combination of PET and CT was positive for N2 disease in 15 patients, and this was correct in 14. In 35 patients, there was no suspicion of metastatic carcinoma; only one of them had disease pathologically. Therefore the sensitivity of PET combined with CT was 93%, and the specificity was 97%. The authors concluded that PET and CT were complementary because visual correlation with the anatomic information on CT improved the reader's ability to discriminate between hilar and mediastinal lymph nodes on PET imaging.

M (Distant Metastases)

Imaging techniques are of great importance in the investigation of patients who have possible extrathoracic metastases. The most widely used are CT (to demonstrate metastases to the adrenal glands and liver), MR imaging (to assess the brain and adrenals), and radionuclide scans (to identify skeletal metastases). The use of these techniques in the identification of metastases should be considered in the context of the clinical picture. For example, in patients who have non–small cell carcinoma, brain CT and radionuclide scanning of bone are indicated only if there is clinical or laboratory evidence of metastatic disease. Such evidence includes not only organ-specific signs and symptoms (liver enlargement, bone pain), but also nonspecific symptoms of anorexia, weight loss, and fatigue.

In one study of 309 patients who had non–small cell carcinoma in an early stage (T1 or T2, N0 or N1), routine bone, brain, and liver scans or bone scan and abdominal and brain CT were done before anticipated surgery.[1540] Only 1 of the 472 studies (0.2%) revealed an unexpected metastasis; all other metastatic disease detected was associated with clinical signs and symptoms or abnormal biochemical profiles. In a 1995 meta-analysis of 25 studies that addressed the issue of the appropriateness of preoperative evaluation of metastatic disease, the authors concluded that a negative clinical evaluation had a high negative predictive value (consistently exceeding 90%) for finding occult metastases by bone scan and CT evaluation of the brain and abdomen.[1541] These values were even more impressive (>97%) when an expanded clinical evaluation, which included consideration of constitutional symptoms, was used. Although some investigators have reported occult brain metastases in asymptomatic individuals, especially those who have adenocarcinoma,[1542, 1543] such findings must be balanced against the significant number of false-positive brain CT scans[1541] and low cost-effectiveness.[1544] In general, head CT without clinical evidence of metastases is unwarranted.[1050, 1055]

Computed Tomography. Because the adrenal glands are common sites for metastatic pulmonary carcinoma and because of the ease of examination, most radiologists extend the chest CT to include the adrenal glands in patients who have a pulmonary tumor.[884, 1545] In one study of 110 patients who had pulmonary carcinoma (cell type not specified), adrenal masses were identified in 11 (10%);[1485] in 5 of these, the adrenal glands were the only apparent site of metastases. An even higher yield of positive results has been obtained in a study of 65 patients who had small cell carcinoma and who underwent upper abdominal CT scanning, in which metastases to the liver or adrenal glands were identified in 16 (25%).[1487] In a retrospective review of CT studies of the abdomen performed in 72 patients who had small cell carcinoma, the authors found that of the 44 patients with extensive disease (beyond the confines of one hemithorax), 26 (59%) had CT evidence of one or more sites of metastatic disease.

When interpreting the results of CT scans, it is important to remember that a normal scan does not rule out adrenal metastases; for example, in one study in which biopsies were performed on 43 adrenal glands in patients who had small cell carcinoma and morphologically normal glands at CT, 5 (17%) of the 29 biopsy specimens that had adequate cellular material showed metastatic carcinoma.[1546] On the other hand, the majority of adrenal lesions do not represent metastases. For example, in an investigation of 330 patients who had non–small cell carcinoma, of whom 32 had adrenal masses on CT and 25 had biopsy, only 8 (32%) had metastasis;[1547] the other 17 (68%) had an adrenal adenoma or hyperplasia. The latter abnormalities measure 3 mm or larger in diameter and are relatively common, having been demonstrated in 3% of 7,437 autopsies in one study.[1548] Their incidence increases with age, being found in about 5% of patients 60 to 70 years old.[1548, 1549] The best criteria to differentiate a metastasis from a nonfunctioning adenoma are the size of the lesion and its attenuation coefficient on unenhanced CT scans.[1550] Lesions 1 cm or less in diameter are most likely to be adenomas, whereas those 3 cm or larger are usually metastases (Fig. 31–95). In one study, the use of a threshold of 0 HU for attenuation of the adrenal mass on an unenhanced CT scan allowed diagnosis of a benign adrenal mass with a sensitivity of 47% and a specificity of 100%, whereas the use of a threshold of 10 HU was associated with a sensitivity of 79% and a specificity of 96%.[1550] In another study, a threshold of 16.5 HU was associated with a sensitivity of 100% and a specificity of 95% for the diagnosis of a nonfunctioning adenoma.[1551] Similar results were reported using a threshold of 18 HU.[1552] The sensitivity and specificity of CT are obviously influenced by the density threshold used for distinguishing benign from malignant adrenal lesions. One group of investigators analyzed the results derived from 10 studies that included a total of 272 benign and 223 malignant adrenal lesions.[1555] The sensitivity for detecting a benign adrenal lesion ranged from 47% at a threshold of 2 HU to 88% at a threshold of 20 HU; the specificity ranged from 100% at a threshold of 2 HU to 84% at a threshold of 20 HU.

Although evaluation of the adrenals on CT can easily be done without the use of intravenous contrast material, assessment of the liver requires the use of a bolus of intravenous contrast material and careful timing of its injection and subsequent imaging.[1553] Furthermore, small benign hepatic lesions (<1.5 cm in diameter) are commonly present in the liver. For example, in one study of 1,454 consecutive contrast-enhanced abdominal CT scans, 17% showed small lesions, 80% of which were benign.[1554] In the same study, 51% of hepatic lesions in the 107 patients who had pulmonary carcinoma were shown to be benign. The vast majority of these lesions are cysts; because these are much more readily assessed using ultrasound, we do not routinely perform CT of the liver when evaluating patients who have pulmonary carcinoma.

Magnetic Resonance Imaging. Several groups have assessed the diagnostic accuracy of MR imaging in the detection of adrenal metastases and in their distinction from adrenal adenomas. The results of initial studies showed considerable overlap between the MR signal characteristics of malignant and benign adrenal lesions on conventional spin-echo and gradient recalled echo images.[1556–1560] More recent studies in which more sophisticated techniques have been employed, however, have shown an improved ability to identify adenomas and to distinguish them from metastases.[1561–1563] On spin-echo MR images performed using fat-saturation technique, adrenal adenomas have a characteristic hyperintense rim;[1561] in one study of 48 patients, this sign was seen in 26 of 28 (92%) adenomas and in only 1 of 20 (5%) metastases.[1561] The distinction between adenomas and metastases can also be made in the majority of cases using fast spin-echo and chemical shift MR imaging.[1562, 1563]

Scintigraphy. Scintigraphy is considerably more sensitive than conventional radiography in the detection of skeletal metastases.[1564, 1565] In one prospective study of 146 patients who had potentially resectable non–small cell pulmonary carcinoma, bone scanning detected metastases in 5 (3.4%).[1566] Because metastases are rarely seen in asymptomatic patients and because false-positive scans are common, routine radionuclide studies are not indicated for asymptomatic patients who have non–small cell carcinoma and a normal biochemical examination.[1050]

Positron Emission Tomography. The potential role of [18]FDG PET imaging in the detection of distal metastases has generated considerable interest. In one prospective investigation of 27 patients who had pulmonary carcinoma and a total of 33 adrenal masses identified on CT, FDG uptake was increased in 25 adrenal masses, 23 (92%) of which were proved to represent metastatic carcinoma;[1566a] uptake was normal in the 8 benign lesions. Another group of investigators performed a prospective evaluation of whole-body PET imaging for staging pulmonary carcinoma in 99 patients.[1538] PET imaging showed previously unsuspected distal metastases in 11 patients (11%); there were no false-positive diagnoses. Normal PET findings were present in 19 patients (19%) who had distal abnormalities on CT; in only one of these

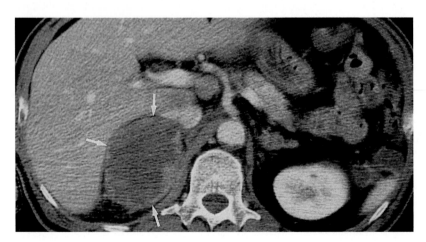

Figure 31–95. Adrenal Metastasis. A contrast-enhanced CT scan in a 69-year-old man demonstrates a 6-cm-diameter inhomogeneous right adrenal mass *(arrows)*. The diagnosis of metastatic adenocarcinoma was proved by ultrasound-guided biopsy. The primary tumor was a 2-cm-diameter left upper lobe pulmonary carcinoma.

was the PET result falsely negative. This ability of PET imaging to demonstrate metastases not apparent on CT has been confirmed by other investigators.[1566b,c]

INVESTIGATION OF SPECIFIC RADIOGRAPHIC PATTERNS

The diagnostic approach to the patient who has pulmonary carcinoma, particularly with respect to the presence or absence of mediastinal lymph node metastases, depends in large measure on the initial radiographic appearance—the solitary pulmonary nodule or mass with or without associated adenopathy, the obstructing endobronchial lesion, or the central nonobstructing lesion. The approaches to investigation outlined in this section are meant to provide general guidelines only; specific circumstances and individual preferences may lead to legitimate deviation from these recommendations.

Solitary Pulmonary Nodule

As discussed previously (*see* page 1133), the solitary pulmonary nodule is generally defined as a well-circumscribed lesion less than 3 cm in diameter within the lung parenchyma,[9, 1567, 1568] without associated adenopathy, atelectasis, or pneumonia.[886, 887] Comparison with previous radiographs is an essential first step in establishing whether the lesion is new or has grown or not grown over time. Nodules that have shown no growth over at least a 2-year period can generally be considered benign.[9] In most circumstances, a new nodule should be considered malignant. The second step is to determine the presence or absence of calcification, a judgment that can sometimes be made with confidence from the chest radiograph; if not, thin-section CT is the logical next step. The presence of diffuse, laminated, or popcorn calcification or central calcification involving more than 10% of the cross-sectional area of the nodule means that malignancy is unlikely and that observation only is appropriate.[1569] The presence of calcification can usually be assessed by visual assessment alone. In questionable cases, it may be considered present when the nodule has an attenuation value of 200 HU or greater.[898] Localized areas of fat attenuation are virtually diagnostic of a hamartoma.[890] A nodule can also be considered almost certainly benign if it has homogeneous density and shows no enhancement or enhancement of less than 15 HU after intravenous administration of contrast material.[962, 963] In the absence of any of these features, the nodule should be considered to be of indeterminate origin.

In most surgical series, the incidence of malignancy in such indeterminate nodules is approximately 40%; in some, it is considerably less.[1570] These figures suggest that surgical intervention could be avoided in the majority of patients. The risk for malignancy increases with age of the patient, smoking history, significant exposure to occupational carcinogens, history of previous malignancy, certain radiologic features (*see* page 1133), and increasing size of the nodule.[9, 893, 1571] For example, in one series in which the average patient was a 63-year-old man who had a 2.5-cm-diameter nodule, more than 90% of indeterminate nodules that were

resected in the 1990s were malignant;[1572] this reflected the prior identification of many benign lesions by CT scanning. In a review of studies in which CT densitometry was combined with other CT parameters, misclassification of malignant lesions occurred in only 12 of 359 (3.3%) cases.[1569] PET scanning can identify malignancy in lung nodules as small as 1 cm in diameter with a high degree of accuracy.[945, 969, 1573–1576] In one study, the likelihood ratio for malignancy in a solitary pulmonary nodule that had an abnormal PET scan was 7.11, with a normal scan having a likelihood ratio of only 0.06; a positive scan was able to distinguish benign from malignant lesions with more accuracy than any standard criteria.[1573] The test, however, is expensive and available only in a few specialized centers. In the absence of an early and significant smoking history, malignancy is uncommon in patients younger than 35 years old, and most such patients can be followed expectantly.

A variety of additional tests can be considered to determine the nature of an indeterminant nodule. Fiberoptic bronchoscopy has little role; although it can establish a diagnosis of malignancy, it cannot exclude it[1567] and, as a result, is unlikely to alter any decision regarding the advisability of surgery. In one review of 33 patients who underwent bronchoscopy for a solitary nodule, not a single procedure uncovered findings that precluded surgery and potentially curative resection in the absence of constitutional symptoms, hemoptysis, or focal wheeze.[1577] Similarly, cytologic examination of sputum specimens or samples obtained by transthoracic needle aspiration is unlikely to be cost-effective or to alter decision making in this setting[1578, 1578a] except in special situations, such as residence in a geographic region in which a relatively high proportion of specific benign diagnoses might be expected (e.g., areas where coccidioidomycosis is endemic).

Decision making regarding various management options in a patient who has a solitary pulmonary nodule can be difficult. The physician's and the patient's choices are influenced by the probability of malignancy in any given context. That "guesstimates" of the presence or absence of malignancy can often be correct was shown in a study in which computerized Bayesian algorithms using a total of 44 preoperative clinical and radiologic factors were used to categorize pulmonary lesions as either benign or malignant.[1579] The model correctly identified 96 of 100 lesions; its sensitivity for identifying malignancy was 98% and its specificity 87%. Using decision analysis algorithms to determine the best approach to the initial management of solitary pulmonary nodules, one group of investigators compared the average life expectancy of patients who had noncalcified solitary pulmonary nodules managed by immediate surgery, biopsy followed by surgery or observation depending on the result of the biopsy, or observation alone.[891] In patients in whom the probability of malignancy was high according to Bayes' theorem, immediate surgery was associated with a longer average life expectancy. Observation was associated with a longer life expectancy in patients who had a low probability for malignancy, and biopsy as an initial procedure proved the preferable course in patients who had an intermediate probability of malignancy. The difference in anticipated survival between the strategies was small, however, and the authors suggested that patients should be encouraged to participate in decision making.

The cost-effectiveness of various management strategies has also been calculated, using simulations of different patient risk-taking attitudes.[1580] In patients willing to take risk, invasive strategies were the most cost-effective; for cautious patients, expectant waiting was the most cost-effective strategy. In our experience, the most difficult management decisions concern the patient with indeterminate nodules of intermediate malignant risk who has significant comorbid conditions, especially chronic obstructive pulmonary disease. In such patients, the risks of both thoracotomy and invasive diagnostic investigations are increased. Our approach is influenced by patient preference under these conditions; however, expectant waiting is often the route followed.

Mediastinal exploration for nodal metastases before resectional surgery is not necessary for patients who have solitary pulmonary nodules and whose CT scans fail to show nodes greater than 1 cm in diameter (*see* page 1190). On the one hand, the prevalence of metastatic carcinoma in this setting, as assessed by mediastinoscopy, is low;[1581] on the other, patients in this group might benefit from surgical resection despite the presence of pathologically confirmed metastases in the ipsilateral mediastinum.[1582, 1583]

Peripheral Nodule or Mass with Suspected Hilar or Mediastinal Adenopathy

In the situation of a peripheral nodule or mass with suspected hilar or mediastinal adenopathy, the physician is dealing with the possibility of metastases in lymph nodes situated in the hilum alone, the mediastinum alone, or both. (Mediastinal nodes can be involved by metastatic carcinoma in the absence of hilar involvement because lesions located proximal to the origin of segmental bronchi can drain via lymphatic channels that communicate directly with the mediastinum.[1584]) In the absence of evidence for distant metastases, patients who have radiographic signs of hilar or mediastinal lymphadenopathy usually require CT evaluation. This can detect small metastases in the lung not visible on radiographs, small pleural effusions, and liver and adrenal metastases. Refined information regarding the size and location of enlarged lymph nodes can provide a guide to site of biopsy and choice of biopsy procedure.[1583] As discussed previously, the specificity of CT scanning for the identification of malignancy in the mediastinum is imperfect (about 80% to 90% in cases in which a node diameter of $\leq$ 1 cm is considered to indicate benignity).[1585] This deficiency is especially evident in the presence of obstructive pneumonitis, in which situation hyperplastic lymph nodes are common.[9] Thus, biopsy confirmation is required both to confirm the presence of malignancy in enlarged nodes and to identify extension of tumor to lymph nodes of normal size.[1586, 1587] The sensitivity of CT scanning for the detection of lymph node metastases is about 80%.[1585] The utility of the various techniques that have been developed for biopsy of lymph nodes in the mediastinum is discussed in Chapter 15 (*see* page 366).

When there is radiologic evidence of hilar or mediastinal lymph node enlargement, bronchoscopy is usually performed.[1590] If a lesion is endoscopically visible, a tissue diagnosis can be obtained in more than 90% of cases. For more peripheral lesions, bronchoalveolar lavage of the in-

volved lung segment confirms a diagnosis of carcinoma in 33%[1591] to 65%[1592] of cases. Transbronchial needle aspiration of mediastinal lymph nodes increases the diagnostic yield of bronchoscopy as well as providing information for staging (*see* page 347).[1593–1599]

Lobar or Segmental Atelectasis or a Hilar Mass with Normal Lungs

Bronchoscopy plays a valuable role in patients who have radiographic patterns of lobar or segmental atelectasis or a hilar mass with normal lungs, not only in diagnosis, but also in staging. If the lesion proves to be T3 on bronchoscopy (proximal growth demonstrably < 2.0 cm distal to the carina), it is probably unresectable; however, it is still desirable to establish the extent of mediastinal disease for purposes of treatment planning. If bronchoscopic biopsy or cytology has established the tumor to be small cell carcinoma, it can be assumed that the lesion is unresectable in the vast majority of patients. Similar considerations apply to the evaluation of the mediastinum as for peripheral lesions.

In patients who have non–small cell carcinoma, most pleural effusions that are discovered during the course of the initial investigation are related to metastases to pleura.[1474] The recovery of malignant cells from pleural fluid of patients who have proven pulmonary carcinoma is generally regarded as evidence of inoperability.[1600] Because the effusions may be the result of pneumonia or other pathology, however, it is incumbent on the physician to obtain confirmation of diagnosis (provided that there are no other signs of unresectability).

CYTOLOGIC AND RADIOLOGIC SCREENING FOR PULMONARY CARCINOMA

Ignoring the potential impact of smoking prevention measures and acknowledging that smoking cessation efforts were less than uniformly successful, it was thought in the early 1970s that screening programs to detect early pulmonary carcinoma were the best hope to reduce mortality from the disease.[1601] The results of studies of the usefulness of screening cytology to identify *early* carcinoma were disappointing. In one investigation of male cigarette smokers 45 years old or older carried out at the Mayo Clinic, Johns Hopkins University Hospitals, and Memorial Sloan–Kettering Cancer Center over a 6-year period, more than 30,000 men were randomly assigned to two cohorts;[1057–1062] one received annual chest radiographs only, and the other had annual chest radiographs plus 4-monthly sputum cytology evaluation (at the Mayo Clinic, films were obtained at 4-monthly intervals). Although cytologic screening was found to result in earlier detection of pulmonary carcinoma, the length of survival and mortality were the same in the two groups. Based on the results of these and other studies, mass screening for the early detection of pulmonary carcinoma has been abandoned.[1602, 1603]

The hypothesis offered to explain the apparent contradiction of earlier detection and unchanged mortality was that squamous cell carcinomas discovered by cytologic examination alone were slow growing and likely to remain localized until identified by radiographic examination. Although there is some evidence to support such a conclusion,[1604] it is unlikely that patients who had screening-detected carcinoma would never have come to medical attention or would have died of causes other than pulmonary carcinoma. A systematic review of the causes of death in patients who had Stage I carcinoma identified in three National Institutes of Health trials cited previously and who did not undergo surgery because of refusal or because of severe comorbidity revealed that most of those patients died of pulmonary carcinoma;[1601] only 2 of 45 survived 5 years compared with a 5-year survival of 70% in the patients who had Stage I carcinoma and who underwent surgical resection. Similarly a randomized, prospective screening of a high-risk population of 6,364 men was carried out in Czechoslovakia in which the control group consisted of individuals in whom cancer was discovered on the basis of symptoms, incidental chest radiographs, or at autopsy.[1605] The screened group was found to have both earlier diagnosis and longer survival.

In another large study reported from Japan, the efficacy of screening by chest radiography was compared with that of radiography plus sputum cytology.[1606] Cytology for screening was confined to high-risk groups, such as smokers exposed to occupational carcinogens.[1607, 1608] Among the 148 carcinomas detected by sputum cytology, 132 were squamous cell carcinoma, 116 (78%) were unassociated with radiographic abnormalities, and 90 (61%) were Stage 0 or Stage I after resection; 47 were less than 10 mm in diameter. By contrast, only 166 of 432 tumors (38%) detected radiographically were Stage I after resection, and only 4 patients had tumors less than 10 mm in diameter.

Although screening programs have largely been abandoned because of their failure to reduce mortality from pulmonary carcinoma, as in the study from Japan,[1606] the results of both the Mayo Clinic[1057] and Czechoslovakia trials[1605] demonstrate that carcinomas identified by radiographic screening are associated with a lower stage, an increased likelihood of resectability, and a longer survival compared with carcinomas diagnosed in unscreened populations. Despite these features, the mortality was the same in the two groups because there was a higher incidence of carcinoma in the screened one than in the control one.[1602] Because mortality is an indisputable end point, it had been assumed that other end points, such as stage distribution, resectability, survival, and cancer incidence, were somehow subject to confounding biases, such as lead time or overdiagnosis bias.[1602]

These concerns have been addressed in a reanalysis of the data derived from randomized, controlled trials of screening efficacy.[1602] Although the implied conclusion of the authors of this report is that the mortality comparisons are biased, their explanation for this conclusion can be questioned. The hypothesis that there was insufficient randomization to account for confounding risk factors for pulmonary carcinoma distinct from tobacco smoke, such as diet, genetic factors, and occupational carcinogens (i.e., that the screened and control groups were not the same) seems improbable, given the large number of patients in these trials. Further studies are required to settle the issue of the efficacy of screening for detection of carcinoma in high-risk individuals, including its cost-effectiveness. In our own practice, we consider it prudent to obtain annual chest radiographs in smokers and former smokers for the development of pulmonary carcinoma, particularly those who have a heavy smoking history and/or an occupational risk.

It has also been suggested that spiral CT be used in mass screening for peripheral pulmonary carcinomas in individuals at high risk.[1609, 1610] In one study in which posteroanterior and lateral radiographs and low-dose (50 mA) spiral CT scans were performed every 6 months over an 18-month period in 1,369 individuals, peripheral carcinomas were detected in 15 of 3,457 (0.43%) examinations on CT and in 4 (0.12%) examinations on chest radiography;[1609] 14 of the 15 carcinomas (93%) were Stage I. In another investigation of 5,437 individuals who underwent screening for pulmonary carcinoma by chest radiography, further workup was required in 230 because of abnormal findings.[1610] Of 221 patients who had spiral CT as a second step, 110 had abnormalities confirmed on CT, whereas the remaining 111 had normal examinations. In 66 of the 110 patients (60%), the same abnormality was visible on CT as on radiography; in the other 44 (40%), the abnormality seen on the radiograph was not recognized on CT, but another abnormality was incidentally noted, including 37 benign lesions and 7 pulmonary carcinomas. Further studies are required to determine the cost-effectiveness of low-dose spiral CT in the screening of selected individuals at high risk for developing pulmonary carcinoma.

In a third investigation of 5,483 individuals who had undergone annual chest radiography and cytologic assessment of sputum, low-dose spiral CT demonstrated abnormalities confirmed to represent carcinoma in 19 patients.[1588] The detection rate with CT was 0.48% compared with 0.03% to 0.05% for standard mass assessments done previously in the same population. Another group of investigators compared the effectiveness of low-dose (20-mA) to that of conventional-dose (200-mA) CT in the detection of pulmonary nodules.[1589] Lowering the x-ray dose reduced the detectability of peripheral nodules and nodules separated from blood vessels; however, there was no significant difference in the detection rates of nodules as small as 3 mm in diameter on low-dose as compared with conventional-dose CT.

PROGNOSIS AND NATURAL HISTORY

Pulmonary carcinoma is one of the most important human neoplasms, not only because of its frequency, but also because of its dismal prognosis: overall, only about 10% to 15% of patients survive 5 years or longer.[534] The 5-year survival varies from virtually nil for patients who have radiographically apparent mediastinal lymph node metastases or whose neoplasm arises in a main bronchus[1474] to about 65% for asymptomatic patients who have peripheral nodules and no lymph node metastases.[1474, 1475] In general hospitals, the incidence of unresectability of non–small cell carcinoma ranges from 80% to 85%, including the 5% of cases in which this is determined at thoracotomy.[1611, 1612] In several large series, operative mortality has ranged from about 1% to 6%;[1611, 1613, 1614] older patients now experience results similar to[1615–1617] or only slightly worse[1618] than those of younger patients.

The survival of patients who have pulmonary carcinoma

depends on a variety of factors, some so closely interrelated that it is virtually impossible to assess their relative importance. Many can be divided into factors inherent to the host and those attributable to the neoplasm itself. The latter can be further considered in three major categories: (1) *pathologic factors*, the most important of which is histologic classification; (2) *anatomic factors*, of which tumor stage is paramount; and (3) *clinical factors*, which relate particularly to cancer-related symptoms and whether they are local or systemic and recent or prolonged. A variety of additional factors, such as tumor ploidy and the presence of biologic markers in serum or tumor tissue, have also been considered by some investigators to influence prognosis. Although each of these factors is discussed individually, it must be borne in mind that the complexity of their interrelationships necessitates their overall consideration in every patient.

Influence of Host Factors

Race, sex, and age have relatively minor prognostic influence in patients who have pulmonary carcinoma compared to tumor stage and histology, patient performance status, and burden of comorbid disease. However, although not extensively analyzed by multivariate analysis, most investigators have shown an improved survival in women.[1476, 1619-1629] Age has a more clear-cut (albeit not necessarily independent) influence. The prognosis is poor in patients who are younger than 40 years old,[1630, 1631] an observation likely related to the fact that they tend to present with tumors of advanced stage.[1631, 1632] A poor prognosis is also seen in the elderly, possibly because of the prevalence of comorbid disease[1627, 1629] and possibly because of the use of less aggressive therapy.[1633] In fact, some investigators have found that the survival of patients over the age of 70 who undergo lung resection is similar to that of younger patients.[1634] Despite shortened survival times, elderly patients appear to have relatively slower tumor growth and less metastatic disease.[1633, 1635, 1636]

Few workers have evaluated survival according to race. Results have been conflicting, some investigators finding it not to be a factor in prognosis[1637] and others to have a significant role (whites faring worse than other groups, at least with respect to small cell carcinoma[1638]). In one study of 92,182 patients who had pulmonary carcinoma demonstrated in hospital cancer registries in the United States in 1992, representing about 55% of all lung cancers in that country, the prognosis of African Americans was found to be especially poor.[1639] Whether this finding was the result of more aggressive disease or to socioeconomic factors, such as access to health care, is not certain; however, African Americans were less likely to undergo resection than were non-Hispanic whites, despite the fact that both groups had similar stage distribution.

Influence of Histologic Classification

Although there can be little doubt that the histologic classification of a tumor is correlated with both natural history and prognosis, the degree of correlation and its significance relative to other factors are difficult to determine precisely from a review of the literature. This difficulty is the result of a number of methodologic factors, including (1) intraobserver and interobserver variability in the diagnosis of specific tumor types; (2) deficiencies in some studies of a precise determination of stage; and (3) an absence in many studies of an assessment of which factors other than histologic classification independently predict prognosis. Conclusions as to the influence of tumor type on prognosis must be made with these points in mind. In fact, in some studies, tumor type has been found to exert no statistically significant independent influence on prognosis once the effect of stage is accounted for.[1640] Despite these reservations, several general statements are applicable.

Squamous Cell Carcinoma

Squamous cell carcinoma tends to remain localized to the thorax more than other cell types and thus causes death more frequently by local complications.[602, 1127, 1641] For example, in a review of 303 non–small cell carcinomas less than 3 cm in diameter, adenocarcinomas were more likely to involve regional lymph nodes at the time of presentation than squamous cell carcinomas.[1642] Most investigators have found a better prognosis, stage-for-stage, for squamous cell carcinoma than for adenocarcinoma or large cell carcinoma,[1626, 1643-1647] even when locally advanced tumor is treated with identical courses of radiation therapy.[1648] For example, in one study of 313 patients who underwent resection, 63 of whom had Stage II cancer, no patient who had adenocarcinoma survived 5 years compared to a 46% survival in patients who had squamous cell carcinoma.[1649] Other investigators, however, have found no substantial difference in survival between the two types of tumor.[1627, 1650] Histologic grade is also related to prognosis.[1651, 1652] High proliferation activity as determined by DNA flow cytometry was associated with poor survival in one study of 171 patients who underwent resection for squamous cell carcinoma.[1653] A better prognosis for diploid than aneuploid cell tumors has also been found by a number of workers (*see* page 356).[1653a-c]

Although as a group their survival time is undoubtedly better, even patients with *in situ* or minimally invasive squamous cell carcinoma have a guarded prognosis.[615, 1654, 1655] In one study of 54 such patients, all of whom underwent resection of tumor after its being localized by bronchoscopy within months of positive cytology results, 90% survived 5 years;[1654] subsequently, 5 died of the original neoplasm, and 12 developed second primary carcinomas. In another study of 47 patients who had occult carcinomas treated by resection, none recurred after 2 months to 20 years;[1655] however, 21 (45%) patients developed a second carcinoma, 15 of which were primary in the lung. In a smaller series of 16 patients, the outcome was more dismal;[1656] 14 were dead 10 years after the initial diagnosis, including 7 from malignancy (local recurrence, metastases from the original tumor, or a second primary carcinoma). Others have documented a more favorable experience: in a study of 27 patients who had early cancer treated in Japan, the 10-year survival was 92%;[1657] only 1 patient died of a second primary lung cancer 6 years after initial resection.

Small Cell Carcinoma

Small cell carcinoma is a fast-growing neoplasm and, in most cases, spread has occurred beyond the thorax at the time of diagnosis.[1658] Although many tumors show a response to chemotherapy, this is often incomplete and of short duration. The overall median survival is about 6 to 10 months,[1658] and 5-year survival rates range from only 1% to 5%.[1659–1666] As might be expected, a better prognosis is associated with limited as opposed to extensive disease,[1667] with demonstrable response to chemotherapy, and with surgical excision of a solitary pulmonary nodule in the absence of hilar or mediastinal node involvement.[1668] (With respect to the last of these situations, in some instances of long-term survival associated with a diagnosis of small cell carcinoma, pathologic reappraisal has resulted in a change of diagnosis, usually to atypical carcinoid tumor.[1669]) A worse prognosis and a poorer response to therapy have been found by some investigators for combined (large cell/small cell) carcinoma compared to the classic form.[653–655, 1670] A biologic basis for these clinical observations has been found in experiments with tumor cell lines.[1671–1673]

Patients who have prolonged survival after a diagnosis of small cell carcinoma are at increased risk of developing a second malignancy, just as often acute leukemia as pulmonary carcinoma.[1660, 1674–1677] For example, in a follow-up study of 578 patients who had small cell carcinoma at the U.S. National Cancer Institute, 15 developed 16 second pulmonary carcinomas;[1678] 2 others developed a carcinoma of the upper airway. The cumulative actuarial risk of developing a second primary carcinoma 16 years after initial diagnosis was 69%. Smoking cessation after successful therapy is associated with a significant reduction in risk for development of a second lung carcinoma in this population.[1679, 1680]

Adenocarcinoma

Although some investigators have shown the prognosis for adenocarcinoma and large cell carcinoma to be similar,[1641, 1643, 1644] others have found the prognosis for adenocarcinoma to be more favorable,[1626] particularly in the absence of lymph node involvement.[1645, 1646] These observations may be related to the inclusion of peripheral bronchioloalveolar carcinoma, a subtype that has a relatively good 5-year survival when resected at the solitary nodule stage;[1625, 1681, 1682] for example, in one study of 12 patients who underwent lobectomy for such a tumor, the overall 5-year survival was 75%.[1681] This survival rate may reflect the slow growth of this tumor; in another series of 12 patients, the mean doubling time was 300 days.[1683] Survival beyond 5 years, however, does not necessarily represent cure; recurrence has occasionally been reported as long as 20 years after resection of the primary tumor.[1684] The distinction between nodular and diffuse forms of bronchioloalveolar carcinoma is of considerable prognostic importance, survival being much better in the former;[708a, 1685] a number of investigators have also found a poorer prognosis in patients who have mucinous as opposed to nonmucinous tumors.[708a]

In one study of 236 patients who underwent resection of adenocarcinomas of less than 2-cm diameter, prognosis was determined in large part by the histology of the tumor.[1686] Those who had bronchioloalveolar carcinoma, unassociated with fibroblastic proliferation, had no lymph node metastases and 100% 5-year survival; by contrast, patients who had poorly differentiated adenocarcinoma, papillary adenocarcinoma, or acinar adenocarcinoma had a less favorable prognosis. In another study of 137 consecutive patients with Stage I and II adenocarcinoma who underwent surgical resection, those who had bronchioloalveolar carcinoma had the longest median survival (44 months).[1687] Histologic grade,[1688, 1689] the pattern of local tissue invasion,[1690] the presence or absence of a papillary pattern,[685a] and the presence of a continuous as opposed to a discontinuous basement membrane adjacent to tumor cells[1690] have also been found to be prognostic factors.

Large Cell Carcinoma

The prognosis of large cell carcinoma is generally poor;[1628, 1650, 1691] however, this is not always the case if resection is accomplished for cure,[1691] particularly in low-stage tumors.[1645] There is also evidence that patients who have a lymphoepithelioma-like subtype may have a better prognosis than those who have other histologic types of large cell tumor.[450] Regardless of tissue histology, the prognosis of patients who have advanced non–small cell carcinoma is dismal.[1692] Even among terminally ill patients who have advanced disease admitted to a hospice, patients who have adenocarcinoma and squamous cell carcinoma have been found to live longer than patients who have large cell tumors.[1693]

Adenosquamous Carcinoma

Because the number of well-documented cases of adenosquamous carcinoma is small, prognostic statements are difficult to make with confidence. Some investigators have found them to possess a behavior and prognosis similar to other forms of non–small cell carcinoma;[767] however, others have found evidence of a more aggressive behavior.[768, 1694] For example, in one series of 44 patients who underwent resection, only 7 survived 5 years.[1695] In another study of 127 patients, only 10% of patients presented solely with local disease;[1696] however, the 5-year survival in that group was 62%.

Carcinomas with Pleomorphic, Sarcomatoid, or Sarcomatous Elements

As might be expected, endobronchial carcinosarcomas, especially when unassociated with parenchymal extension, appear to have a better prognosis than do predominantly intraparenchymal forms;[783, 785, 788] in occasional cases, prolonged survival and even cure have followed resection.[788] Despite this, of 23 cases reviewed in the literature between 1951 and 1977 (of which 19 were resectable), the 1-year survival rate was only 36%.[791] Both endobronchial tumors accompanied by parenchymal invasion and peripheral parenchymal lesions tend to behave in an aggressive fashion, with local invasion of contiguous structures, widespread metastases, and (frequently) rapid death. Pleomorphic carcinomas also tend to be aggressive and are associated with a poor prognosis; the 5-year survival in one study of 69 patients who had adequate follow-up was only 12%.[708] Similarly, patients who have giant cell carcinoma have a uniformly dismal prognosis.

Influence of Stage

One of the most important factors determining the prognosis of patients with pulmonary carcinoma is the anatomic extent of disease at the time of presentation as defined by the TNM staging system.[1474, 1625, 1650, 1697–1702] Mountain[1474] analyzed 5,319 cases of histologically proven carcinoma of the lung according to the 1996 revision of the TNM classification. Patients were included only if their tumors had been diagnosed 5 or more years earlier and if follow-up information was available either up to the time of death or to survival for at least 5 years. Assessment by stage, as determined both clinically and pathologically, revealed a clear relationship between the anatomic extent of the carcinoma and survival (Tables 31–6 to 31–8 and Fig. 31–96). Favorable factors were identified for both early-stage and late-stage disease. As might be expected, the accuracy in predicting prognosis is improved when staging is done on the basis of pathologic criteria rather than clinical or radiologic criteria.[9, 1474, 1697]

The size of the primary neoplasm was of particular importance in early-stage disease; in the absence of metastases to regional lymph nodes, T1 tumors were associated with a 5-year survival of 61%, compared to 38% for T2 tumors. This important difference in prognosis was responsible for the division of stage I into IA and IB.[1703] The prognostic significance of tumor size has also been found by other investigators;[1704, 1704a] for example, in a study of 59 patients who had resected peripheral lesions measuring 2 cm or less in diameter, CT evidence of mediastinal lymph node metastases was found in none.[1704] As might be expected from these findings, tumor volume is also an important prognostic indicator across all stages: risk of death has been found to increase by almost 25% per doubling of tumor volume in Stage I and II non–small cell carcinoma.[1705]

The importance of distinguishing staging accomplished clinically and radiographically from that established pathologically has been emphasized by many investigators. The term "Will Rogers phenomenon" has been used to describe

Table 31–6. CLINICAL (TOP) AND PATHOLOGIC (BOTTOM) STAGE IA AND STAGE IB BY cTNM (TOP) AND pTNM (BOTTOM) SUBSET

	MONTHS AFTER TREATMENT (CUMULATIVE PERCENT SURVIVING)				
	12 (%)	24 (%)	36 (%)	48 (%)	60 (%)
cTNM					
cT1N0M0 (n = 687)	91	79	71	67	61
cT2N0M0 (n = 1,189)	72	54	46	41	38
pTNM					
pT1N0M0 (n = 511)	94	86	80	73	67
pT2N0M0 (n = 549)	87	76	67	62	57

From Mountain CF: Revisions in the international system for staging lung cancer. Chest 111:1710, 1997.

Table 31–7. CLINICAL (TOP) AND SURGICAL-PATHOLOGIC (BOTTOM) STAGE IIA AND STAGE IIB BY cTNM (TOP) AND pTNM (BOTTOM) SUBSET

	MONTHS AFTER TREATMENT (CUMULATIVE PERCENT SURVIVING)				
	12 (%)	24 (%)	36 (%)	48 (%)	60 (%)
cTNM					
cT1N1M0 (n = 29)	79	49	38	34	34
cT2N1M0 (n = 250)	61	42	34	26	24
cT3N0M0 (n = 107)	55	37	31	27	22
pTNM					
pT1N1M0 (n = 76)	89	70	64	61	55
pT2N1M0 (n = 288)	78	56	47	42	39
pT3N0M0 (n = 87)	76	55	47	40	38

From Mountain CF: Revisions in the international system for staging lung cancer. Chest 111:1710, 1997.

the impact of a change in stage on prognosis.[1701] When patients in a more favorable stage are downgraded ("migrate") to a poorer-prognosis stage because of the application of more refined and accurate diagnostic methods, the survival in both groups improves without any change in overall outcome. The impact on survival of pathologic staging as compared to clinical staging can be seen in Tables 31–6 and 31–7. Patients having definitive pathologic staging are indicated by the prefix *p*, whereas clinically staged patients are identified by *c*. The importance of this distinction is intuitively apparent. It can be expected, for example, that bulky mediastinal adenopathy identified radiologically will be associated with a worse prognosis than the involvement of the same nodes by a small focus of carcinoma identified in a resected surgical specimen. A more specific example of this effect is provided by patients who have N2 disease

Table 31–8. CLINICAL STAGE IIIB AND STAGE IV BY cTNM SUBSET

	MONTHS AFTER TREATMENT (CUMULATIVE PERCENT SURVIVING)				
	12 (%)	24 (%)	36 (%)	48 (%)	60 (%)
cTNM					
cT4N0-1-2M0 (n = 458)	37	15	10	8	7
cAny T N3M0 (n = 572)	32	11	6	4	3
cAny T Any N M1 (n = 1,427)	20	5	2	2	1

From Mountain CF: Revisions in the international system for staging lung cancer. Chest 111:1710, 1997.

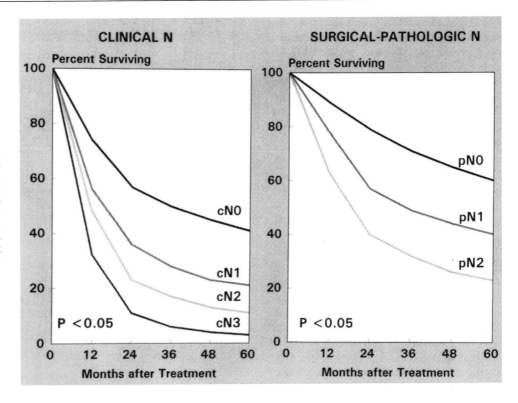

Figure 31–96. Survival from Pulmonary Carcinoma According to Lymph Node Status. Survival curves of patients stratified according to clinical and pathologic evidence of lymph node metastases. (From Mountain CF, Dresler CM: Regional lymph node classification for lung cancer staging. Chest 111:1718, 1997.)

that is clinically recognizable or is identified by standard radiography, transbronchial needle biopsy, or mediastinoscopy, in whom the 5-year survival rate is only 2%, even when aggressive surgical resection is attempted.[1699, 1706] By contrast, when N2 disease requires thoracotomy for identification, the resectability rate is higher, and the 5-year survival rate varies from about 15% to 30%.[1699, 1706–1708] The extrapolation of the relatively favorable results of aggressive surgical approaches in patients in the latter group to those in the former is thus inappropriate. The presence of metastases in lymph nodes is usually a marker of systemic disease and is associated with a poor prognosis; successful surgical resection can be accomplished in the small minority of patients in whom Stage III disease is apparent at thoracotomy only.[1707]

The latest revision of the TNM staging system defines T3 tumors as those that invade the chest wall, mediastinum, or proximal portion of the main bronchus but are surgically resectable by conventional criteria. T4 lesions are generally not resectable. Despite the advanced nature of T3 tumors, 5-year survival has been attained in a small number of patients, in sharp contrast to the dismal prognosis of patients who have T4 lesions. It is likely, however, that there is important heterogeneity with respect to prognostic features even in patients who have Stage IIIB and IV cancers; for example, in one study of 84 patients who had satellite nodules (T4) and underwent resection (N0 to N2), the 5-year survival was 22%, in contrast to the 7% survival of all patients with T4 lesions.[1709] At one extreme was a group of 15 patients who had isolated intrapulmonary metastases of well-differentiated adenocarcinoma without evidence of vascular or lymphatic invasion histopathologically;[1710] all had an excellent prognosis, whereas none of the other 35 patients survived 5 years. Similar results have been documented by another group of investigators.[1710a] It has also been shown that tumors that are

classified as T3 by virtue of direct chest wall invasion have a better prognosis than those whose T3 designation is determined by invasion of mediastinal structures, the brachial plexus, or the proximal portion of the main bronchus.[1702, 1711]

The prognosis of patients in the various TNM groups relates largely to non–small cell carcinoma. As indicated previously, patients who have small cell carcinoma are usually divided simply into those with limited and those with extensive disease; as might be expected, the former typically survive longer.[1629, 1712] Among patients who have limited disease, those who have apparently resectable disease appear to have a better prognosis; for example, about 25% of 56 such patients survived more than 5 years in one series.[1713] Prognosis is also linked to the number and location of metastatic sites.[1476] Particularly bad sites from a prognostic point of view are the liver[1714] and bone marrow.[1715] When the brain is the sole site of metastatic disease, survival is similar to that of patients who have limited disease.[1716] When the bone marrow is involved (as occurs in about 30% of cases[1128]), survival time is appreciably shortened when thrombocytopenia develops.[1715]

Influence of Clinical Factors

The clinical manifestations of pulmonary carcinoma and its functional effects are also important prognostic factors.[1697] The performance status of the patient is the best overall measure of these effects;[1717–1721] however, performance status can be affected by a variety of influences, each of which could have prognostic importance individually. A sophisticated staging system has been developed by Feinstein and Wells[1477] for defining and evaluating clinical features of prognostic importance in patients who have pulmonary carcinoma. Such "clinical-severity" staging has a prognostic importance independent of TNM staging, so that their combined use allows a more refined estimate of prognosis than the use of either alone. Although this clinical staging system has not been widely applied, consideration of its components is important for two reasons: (1) it calls attention to important prognostic factors that are not considered in TNM staging or in any measure of performance status; and (2) it allows for selection and comparison of comparable patient groups in therapeutic trials.[1477]

According to Feinstein's system, clinical findings are assessed for symptom pattern, severity, and comorbidity. The first of these refers to whether symptoms are the result of lung involvement by tumor (e.g., cough), of systemic effects of tumor (e.g., weight loss), or of metastatic disease (e.g., mediastinal versus distant). An index of symptom severity was developed for each pattern (e.g., quantitation of weight loss), and the prognosis of significant comorbid conditions, such as severe congestive heart failure, was estimated. Using these variables, a composite "clinical-severity" system of five stages was developed. Stage A included patients who were asymptomatic or had transient primary symptoms only. In Stage B, patients had systemic or persistent primary symptoms only. Stage C patients had regional symptoms (such as Horner's syndrome or chest wall pain) or major weight loss. Stage D patients had symptoms related to distant metastases, extreme weight loss, or severe dyspnea. Stage E patients had severe tumor effects or significant comorbidity. When this staging system was combined with TNM staging, each system showed important prognostic gradients independent of the other, underscoring the importance of considering the elements that make up both.

A variety of other factors were incorporated in this staging system, including chronometry (time from first cancer symptom to first treatment intervention), iatropy (the immediate reason the patient sought attention), histologic tumor type, anemia, sex, age, and cigarette smoking. Women had better survival than men for each of the "clinical-severity" stages. Patients in the long chronometry group (>6 months) survived longer than those in the short one. In the interests of simplicity, these factors were not used in the final analysis. None of the other variables had a consistent effect across all stages.

Miscellaneous Factors

Although the TNM and Feinstein clinical staging systems clearly separate patients into different prognostic groups, considerable variability in survival exists among individual patients within any TNM or clinical stage.[1722] As indicated, some of this variability is probably related to the histologic type of tumor. In addition, a large number of studies, generally in small groups of patients, have been conducted in an attempt to relate survival to the presence or absence of particular biologic markers or to their levels in serum or tumor tissue.[1722] For most of these studies, it remains to be determined whether the conclusions reached will be confirmed in larger investigations in which better-established clinical prognostic factors have been used for analysis.

In one review, these biomarkers (the "biologic prophets of cancer cell aggression") were classified into three categories—those reflecting aberrant gene expression, tumor-associated antigens, and others (including tumor cell DNA content, growth factors, and indices of tumor cell proliferation).[1722] Some of these have been found to have a role in monitoring disease status and response to therapy in a limited number of patients.[1421, 1442, 1723] If such markers were also able to identify surgically resected patients at high risk of relapse, independent of anatomic and clinical stage, investigational adjuvant therapies could be applied in an efficient fashion.

An unfavorable prognosis has been associated with the expression of a number of oncogenes by the carcinoma (including members of the *ras* family,[532, 1431, 1724, 1725] *myc* family,[531] c-*erb*B-3,[1726] and c-*erb*B-2,[539, 544]) as well as with abnormalities in the P53[551, 552, 1727–1730] and *Rb* suppressor genes.[547] Other oncogene abnormalities, such as expression of *bcl*-2, have been associated with a more favorable prognosis in some investigations[1731] but not others.[1731a] One group attempted to determine if the use of multiple markers might have greater predictive power than any single marker;[1731b] unfortunately, identification of mutations in a number of oncogenes and of abnormal expression of P53 was not found to be useful prognostically, independent of TNM stage.

Tumor-associated antigens that have been associated with a poorer prognosis include the cytokeratin marker CYFRA 21-1,[1426, 1434] CA 125,[1430, 1433, 1435, 1732] squamous cell carcinoma antigen,[1732] tissue polypeptide antigen,[1425, 1436] CEA,[1430, 1732–1733a] KP16D3 (a monoclonal antibody recognizing a protein associated with mucin-nonproducing papillary adenocarcinoma),[1734] motility-related protein-1 (MRP-1/CD9) and other members of the transmembrane-4 gene superfamily,[1735, 1735a] and certain blood group precursor antigens.[1736] By contrast, preservation of expression of blood group antigen A by tumor cells in A-positive or AB-positive patients seems to be an important favorable prognostic factor in non–small cell carcinoma.[1737]

Other biologic markers or tumor characteristics that have been associated with an adverse prognosis include (1) high levels of plasmin-alpha$_2$-plasmin inhibitor complex;[1738] (2) a high tumor proliferative activity as determined by Ki-67 immunostaining,[1739] mitotic count,[1740] polo-like kinase expression,[1741] transferrin receptor expression (in adenocarcinoma),[1742] and tumor DNA content assessed by flow cytometry (*see* page 356);[1743–1745] (3) the expression in tumor tissue of certain growth factors such as transforming growth factor beta-1;[1746, 1746a] (4) increased immunohistochemical expression of cathepsin B,[1747] soluble interleukin-2 receptors,[1748, 1749] and neuron-specific enolase[1748] in tumor tissue; (5) expression of embryonal neural cell adhesion molecule in Stage I non–small cell carcinoma;[1750, 1751] (6) evidence of enhanced tumor angiogenesis[1752, 1752a] or vascular invasion;[1740, 1753] (7) higher levels of polymorphonuclear leukocyte elastase in tumor cells;[1753a] (8) absence of an inflammatory reaction involving macrophages and eosinophils[814–816] and presence of one involving neutrophils;[661] (9) reduced expression of tumor-produced e-cadherin;[1753b] (10) elevated serum lactate dehydrogenase in patients who have non–small cell tumors;[1753c] (11) elevated serum intercellular adhesion molecule (ICAM)-1;[1753d] and (12) evidence for enhanced apoptosis.[1730, 1754] A host of other factors, generally with inconsistent impact on prognosis, have been outlined in a detailed review of the subject.[1697]

Spontaneous Regression of Pulmonary Carcinoma

Spontaneous regression of cancer of any type is rare.[1755] Only 176 cases that satisfied criteria of adequate documentation and histologic confirmation could be found in one extensive review.[1755] More than 50% of these cases occurred in four types of cancer: renal cell carcinoma, neuroblastoma, malignant melanoma, and choriocarcinoma. Rare cases of well-documented spontaneous regression of primary pulmonary carcinoma have been described.[1756–1759] Of particular interest was a report of four patients who had small cell carcinoma associated with a paraneoplastic peripheral neuropathy.[1760, 1761]

MULTIPLE PRIMARY CARCINOMAS OF THE LUNG

The criteria used to make a diagnosis of an independent carcinoma as opposed to recurrence of or metastasis from an initial neoplasm can be complex and vary from investigator to investigator.[1762] It seems reasonable to conclude, however, that tumors are separate primary lesions if they have a different histologic appearance or, if this is the same, that there is a disease-free interval of at least 2 years or the presence of tumors in different lobes without extrapulmonary metastases or evidence of carcinoma in common lymphatics.[1763] In some cases, it is impossible to determine with certainty the true nature of an apparent second primary lesion.

The incidence of multiple primary pulmonary carcinomas varies with the criteria used to define them and with the techniques used to establish the diagnosis. In one review of 12,685 cases of pulmonary carcinoma reported in the English language literature from 1931 to 1984, 382 instances of multiple carcinomas were found, an incidence of 1.7%.[1762] Other investigators have reported figures ranging from 0.2% to 4.3%.[1764–1772] These figures refer chiefly to cases in which the additional tumor has become clinically or radiologically apparent during the patient's life; there is no doubt that the incidence figures would be much higher if unrecognized tumors discovered by the pathologist in surgically excised or autopsy specimens were included in the estimates. For example, in one series of 69 consecutive patients who had pulmonary carcinoma and in whom the bronchial tree was examined carefully, occult neoplasms were identified in 3 (4.3%).[1773] In another investigation of 62 resected specimens of pulmonary adenocarcinoma, 12 (19%) were considered to have two or more independent foci of malignancy.[1774] In a third study, 2% of 1,029 surgical specimens from patients who underwent resectional lung surgery between 1979 and 1985 contained a second primary carcinoma.[1775]

Careful autopsy studies have been similarly revealing. For example, one group of investigators examined numerous sections from the tracheobronchial tree of 258 patients who had died of pulmonary carcinoma.[1776] Using strict microscopic and gross criteria, they found at least nine patients (3.5%) who had one or more invasive carcinomas in addition to the one that was clinically apparent. In a similar study, the airways of 210 uranium miners were compared with a control group of nonminers who had pulmonary carcinoma (all patients having smoked cigarettes).[1776] Carcinoma *in situ* was observed in 96% of the miners and 92% of the nonminers; in addition, 32% of the miners and 22% of the nonminers were considered to have one or more foci of early invasive carcinoma.[363] The increased incidence in autopsy series is undoubtedly attributable to the poor prognosis associated with most lung cancers: many patients die before the second tumor has grown sufficiently to produce clinical or radiographic manifestations.

Multiple primary carcinomas of the lung can develop synchronously (usually defined as the presence of two tumors at the time of or closely after initial diagnosis) or metachronously (the second cancer appearing after a time interval, usually $\geq$ 12 months).[1777] The latter constitute at least two thirds of multiple pulmonary neoplasms[1762, 1763, 1766, 1778] and on average are recognized 4 to 5 years after the first primary.[1763, 1779] It has been estimated that patients who undergo "curative resection" for a pulmonary carcinoma have a 10% to 15% chance of developing a second lung neoplasm.[1780] For those patients who are resectable and operable, survival after resection of the second tumor has been reported to be 30% or more after 5 years and 20% or more after 10 years.[1781–1784]

Squamous cell carcinoma is the most common histologic type seen in patients who have multiple tumors, the most frequent combinations being squamous/squamous (33 of 108 synchronous and 73 of 137 metachronous in one series[1770]), squamous/small cell, and squamous/adenocarcinoma.[1762, 1770, 1771] When synchronous carcinomas develop in the context of fibrotic lung disease, some workers have found them more likely to be of small cell type.[1785] In the majority of patients, only two cancers are present; however, three lesions are not rare.[1764, 1781, 1782, 1786–1788] Synchronous primary carcinomas should be distinguished from foci of atypical adenomatous hyperplasia, which can be found in the surgical specimens of up to 10% of patients who have adenocarcinoma (*see* page 1108).[1789]

OTHER NEOPLASMS ASSOCIATED WITH PULMONARY CARCINOMA

Patients who have pulmonary carcinoma are at increased risk for the development of carcinoma elsewhere, especially in the head and neck.[1790–1793] The association of these neoplasms is likely a result of the influence of tobacco smoke on the epithelium at the different sites. This risk seems to be particularly important for supraglottic tumors (RR = 32.6), especially multicentric supraglottic tumors in the first 2 years of follow-up (RR = 62.5).[1794] A smaller but increased risk for pulmonary carcinoma has also been described following the diagnosis of other smoking-related tumors, such as those of the uterine cervix[1795, 1796] or urinary bladder.[1797] Patients who have chronic lymphocytic leukemia[1798–1800] or who smoke and who have received thoracic irradiation for Hodgkin's disease[1801] or breast carcinoma also have an increased incidence of pulmonary carcinoma.[1802–1804]

In one series of 5,643 patients who had pulmonary carcinoma, 85 (1.5%) also had primary malignancies of the upper airway;[1790] in 70 of these, the head and neck primary was clinically apparent before the lung tumor. In another series of 1,450 patients who had upper airway carcinoma, 61 (4.1%) also had pulmonary carcinoma;[1791] in 60 of these, the pulmonary tumor was detected after the upper airway lesion, with a mean diagnostic interval of about 6 years. In another group of 377 patients who had squamous cell carcinoma of the floor of the mouth, squamous cell carcinoma subsequently developed in the upper respiratory and digestive tracts in 58 and in the lungs in 24.[1792] Some of these lower respiratory tract lesions may have represented metastases—as in 15 of the 55 malignancies involving the lung and the head and neck in one series.[1805] In one review of 927 cases of multiple primary neoplasms of the head and neck and the lung reported in the English literature, 90% of the pulmonary carcinomas were squamous cell in type.[1806] Although the authors of this review noted an increasing number of reports of non–squamous cell carcinoma, a striking predominance of squamous cell carcinoma was also documented in a more recent report of 114 multiple tumors.[1807]

The frequency of multiple primary "aerodigestive" tract malignancies in patients who have laryngeal carcinoma has prompted some authorities to advocate periodic bronchoesophagoscopy and chest radiography in follow-up of this high-risk group.[1808, 1809] In a 3-year prospective study of 286 patients who had a tracheostomy after laryngectomy for cancer, a diagnosis of pulmonary carcinoma was made on fiberoptic bronchoscopy in 36 (12%), 6 of whom had a normal chest radiograph.[1810] However, others have not been able to confirm the usefulness of this approach; in a 34-month follow-up of 170 patients who had laryngeal carcinoma, only two tumors were discovered solely by bronchoscopy.[1811]

In the diagnostic workup of a possible pulmonary carcinoma, malignant cells from head and neck sites may be present in sputum and lead to an erroneous conclusion regarding the primary site. The distinction between a primary pulmonary carcinoma and a solitary metastasis from an upper airway carcinoma also may be difficult. Because of the relatively frequent association of the two forms of tumor, this is not an uncommon problem. An important differential diagnostic clue is the presence of cervical lymph node enlargement, because systemic metastases from an upper airway tumor are often preceded by metastases to this site. In the absence of this finding, a solitary lung lesion most likely represents a second primary tumor. Some patients who have small cell carcinoma and who survive for a considerable time after intensive chemotherapy develop acute leukemia;[1812] as in patients with other malignancies in whom this occurs, it is likely that this is related to the effects on the bone marrow of the chemotherapy itself.[1812]

REFERENCES

1. Travis WD, Colby TV, Corrin B, et al, and Collaborators from 14 Countries: World Health Organization Pathology Panel: World Health Organization. Histological Typing of Lung and Pleural Tumors: International Histological Classification of Tumors, 3rd ed, Berlin, Springer-Verlag. In press.
2. Parkin DM: Trends in lung cancer incidence worldwide. Chest 96:5, 1989.
3. Travis WD, Lubin J, Ries L, et al: United States lung carcinoma incidence trends—declining for most histologic types among males, increasing among females. Cancer 77:2464, 1996.
4. Rozenberg S, Liebens F, Kroll M, et al: Principal cancers among women: Breast, lung and colorectal. Int J Fertil Menopausal Stud 41:166, 1996.
5. Ernster VL: Female lung cancer. Annu Rev Public Health 17:97, 1996.
6. Kabat GC: Recent developments in the epidemiology of lung cancer. Semin Surg Oncol 9:73, 1993.
7. Beckett WS: Epidemiology and etiology of lung cancer. Clin Chest Med 14:1, 1993.
8. Samet JM: The epidemiology of lung cancer. Chest 103:20, 1993.
9. American Thoracic Society/European Respiratory Society: Pretreatment evaluation of nonsmall-cell lung cancer. Am J Respir Crit Care Med 156:320, 1997.
10. Shopland DR: Tobacco use and its contribution to early cancer mortality with a special emphasis on cigarette smoking. Environ Health Perspect 8:131, 1995.
11. Beckett WS: Epidemiology and etiology of lung cancer. Clin Chest Med 14:1, 1993.
12. Schwartz AG, Swanson GM: Lung carcinoma in African Americans and whites: A population-based study in metropolitan Detroit, Michigan. Cancer 79:45, 1997.
13. Harris RE, Zang EA, Anderson JI, et al: Race and sex differences in lung cancer risk associated with cigarette smoking. Int J Epidemiol 22:592, 1993.
14. Cole P, Rodu B: Declining cancer mortality in the United States. Cancer 78:2045, 1996.
15. Fry WA, Menck HR, Winchester DP: The National Cancer Data Base report on lung cancer. Cancer 77:1947, 1996.
16. Stanley K, Stjernswärd: Lung cancer—a worldwide health problem. Chest 96:1, 1989.
17. Lopez-Abente G, Pollan M, de la Iglesia P, et al: Characterization of the lung cancer epidemic in the European Union (1970–1990). Cancer Epidemiol Biomarkers Prev 4:813, 1995.
18. Kennedy A: Relationship between cigarette smoking and histological type of lung cancer in women. Thorax 28:204, 1973.
19. Andrews JL Jr, Bloom S, Balogh K, et al: Lung cancer in women: Lahey Clinic experience, 1957–1980. Cancer 55:2894, 1985.
20. Weiss W: Cigarette smoking and lung cancer trends—a light at the end of the tunnel? Chest 111:1414, 1997.
21. Zang EA, Wynder EL: Differences in lung cancer risk between men and women: Examination of the evidence. J Natl Cancer Inst 88:183, 1996.
22. Engeland A, Haldorsen T, Andersen A, et al: The impact of smoking habits on lung cancer risk: 28 years' observation of 26,000 Norwegian men and women. Cancer Causes Control 7:366, 1996.
23. Risch HA, Howe GR, Jain M, et al: Are female smokers at higher risk for lung cancer than male smokers? Am J Epidemiol 138:281, 1993.
24. Engeland A: Trends in the incidence of smoking-associated cancers in Norway, 1954–93. Int J Cancer 68:39, 1996.
25. Peto R, Lopez AD, Boreham J, et al: Mortality from smoking worldwide. Br Med Bull 52:12, 1996.
26. Peto R, Lopez AD, Boreham J, et al: Mortality from tobacco in developed countries: Indirect estimation from national vital statistics. Lancet 339:1268, 1992.
27. Charloux A, Quoix E, Wolkove N, et al: The increasing incidence of lung adenocarcinoma: Reality or artefact? A review of the epidemiology of lung adenocarcinoma. Int J Epidemiol 26:14, 1997.
28. Caldwell CJ, Berry CL: Is the incidence of primary adenocarcinoma of the lung increasing? Virchows Arch 429:359, 1996.
29. Perng DW, Perng RP, Kuo BI, et al: The variation of cell type distribution in lung cancer: A study of 10,910 cases at a medical center in Taiwan between 1970 and 1993. Jpn J Clin Oncol 26:229, 1996.
30. Wynder EL, Muscat JE: The changing epidemiology of smoking and lung cancer histology. Environ Health Perspect 8:143, 1995.
31. Kabat GC: Aspects of the epidemiology of lung cancer in smokers and nonsmokers in the United States. Lung Cancer 15:1, 1996.
32. Moolgavkar SH, Dewanji A, Luebeck G: Cigarette smoking and lung cancer: Reanalysis of the British doctors' data. J Natl Cancer Inst 81:415, 1989.
33. Cangemi V, Volino P, D'Andrea N, et al: Lung cancer in young patients. Panminerva Med 38:1, 1996.
34. van Loon AJ, Brug J, Goldbohm RA: Differences in cancer incidence and mortality among socio-economic groups. Scand J Soc Med 23:110, 1995.
35. Mansson J, Marklund B, Bengtsson C, et al: Differences in cancer incidence between parts with different socio-economic structure within a Swedish big-city area. Neoplasma 42:149, 1995.
36. van Loon AJ, Goldbohm RA, van den Brandt PA: Lung cancer: Is there an association with socioeconomic status in the Netherlands? J Epidemiol Commun Health 49:65, 1995.
37. Engholm G, Palmgren F, Lynge E: Lung cancer, smoking, and environment: A cohort study of the Danish population. BMJ 312:1259, 1996.
38. van Lon AJ, Goldbohm RA, Kant IJ, et al: Socioeconomic status and lung cancer incidence in men in the Netherlands: Is there a role for occupational exposure? J Epidemiol Commun Health 51:24, 1997.
39. Stevens RG, Moolgavkar SH: A cohort analysis of lung cancer and smoking in British males. Am J Epidemiol 119:624, 1984.
40. Kristein MM: 40 years of U.S. cigarette smoking and heart disease and cancer mortality rates. J Chronic Dis 37:317, 1984.
41. Samet JM, Wiggins CL, Humble CG, et al: Cigarette smoking and lung cancer in New Mexico. Am Rev Respir Dis 137:1110, 1988.
42. Bartecchi CE, MacKenzie TD, Schrier RW: The human costs of tobacco use. N Engl J Med 907:330, 1994.
43. Friedman GD, Dales LG, Ury HK: Mortality in middle-aged smokers and nonsmokers. N Engl J Med 300:213, 1979.
44. Auerbach O, Garfinkel L, Parks VR: Scar cancer of the lung: Increase over a 21 year period. Cancer 43:636, 1979.
45. Redmond DE Jr: Tobacco and cancer: The first clinical report, 1761. N Engl J Med 282:18, 1970.
46. Reagan R, DeBakey ME, Hanlon CR, et al: Memorial tribute. J Thorac Cardiovasc Surg 84:1, 1982.
47. Ochsner A, DeBakey ME: Primary pulmonary malignancy: Treatment by total pneumonectomy: Analysis of 79 collected cases and presentation of 7 personal cases. Surg Gynecol Obstet 68:435, 1939.
48. Ochsner A, DeBakey ME: Carcinoma of the lung. Arch Surg 42:209, 1941.
49. Tylecote FE: Cancer of the lungs. Lancet 2:256, 1927.
50. Barbone F, Bovenzi M, Cavallieri F, et al: Cigarette smoking and histologic type of lung cancer in men. Chest 112:1474, 1997.
51. Hill AB: The environment and disease: Association and causation. Proc R Soc Med 58:295, 1965.
52. Guyatt GH, Newhouse MT: Are active and passive smoking harmful? Determination of causation. Chest 445:88, 1985.
53. Wynder EL, Lemon FR: Cancer, coronary artery disease and smoking: A preliminary report on differences in incidence between Seventh-Day Adventists and others. Calif Med 89:267, 1958.
54. Lemon FR, Walden RT: Death from respiratory system disease among Seventh-Day Adventist men. JAMA 198:117, 1966.
55. Rele JR: Demographic approach to the problem of the connection between lung cancer and smoking. Br J Prev Soc Med 14:181, 1960.
56. Cohen, S, Hossain SA: Primary carcinoma of the lung: A review of 417 histologically proved cases. Dis Chest 49:67, 1966.
57. Boucot KR, Cooper DA, Weiss W, et al: Cigarettes, cough, and cancer of the lung. JAMA 196:985, 1966.
58. Kabat GC, Wynder EL: Lung cancer in nonsmokers. Cancer 53:1214, 1984.
59. Ockene JK, Kuller LH, Svendsen KH, et al: The relationship of smoking cessation to coronary heart disease and lung cancer in the Multiple Risk Factor Intervention Trial. Am J Public Health 80:954, 1990.
60. Fletcher CM, Horn D: Smoking and health. Presented at World Health Assembly, Geneva, May 17th, 1970. National Clearinghouse for Smoking and Health Bulletin, June, 1970.
61. Osann KE, Anton-Culver H, Kurosaki T, et al: Sex differences in lung cancer risk associated with cigarette smoking. Int J Cancer 54:44, 1993.
62. Carbone D: Smoking and cancer. Am J Med 93:1a, 1992.
63. Thun MJ, Day-Lally CA, Calle EE, et al: Excess mortality among cigarette smokers: Changes in a 20-year interval. Am J Public Health 1223:85, 1995.
64. Mori W, Sakai R: A study on chronologic change of the relationship between cigarette smoking and lung cancer based on autopsy diagnosis. Cancer 54:1038, 1984.
65. Waldron I: The contribution of smoking to sex differences in mortality. Public Health Rep 101:163, 1986.
66. Mori W, Sakai R: A study on chronologic change of the relationship between cigarette smoking and lung cancer based on autopsy diagnosis. Cancer 54:1038, 1984.
67. Lubin JH, Blot WJ, Berring F, et al: Patterns of lung cancer risk according to type of cigarette smoked. Int J Cancer 33:569, 1984.
68. Peto R: Influence of dose and duration of smoking on lung cancer rates. In Zaridge D, Peto R (eds): Tobacco: A Major International Health Hazard. IARC Scientific Publication No. 74. Lyons, International Agency for Cancer Research, 1986, pp 23–33.
69. Hammond EC: Smoking in relation to the death rates of one million men and women. Natl Cancer Inst Monogr 19:127, 1966.
70. Wynder EL, Mabuchi K, Beattie EJ Jr: The epidemiology of lung cancer: Recent trends. JAMA 213:2221, 1970.
71. Samet JM: Editorial: The 1990 report of the Surgeon General: The health benefits of smoking cessation. Am Rev Respir Dis 142:993, 1990.
72. Siegfried JM, DeMichele AA, Hunt JD, et al: Expression of mRNA for gastrin-releasing peptide receptor by human bronchial epithelial cells. Am J Respir Crit Care Med 156:358, 1997.
73. Tong L, Spitz MR, Fuefer JJ, et al: Lung carcinoma in former smokers. Cancer 78:1004, 1996.
74. Benhamou S, Benhamou E, Auquier A, et al: Differential effects of tar content, type of tobacco and use of a filter on lung cancer risk in male cigarette smokers. Int J Epidemiol 23:437, 1994.

75. Tobin MJ, Sackner MA: Monitoring smoking patterns of low and high tar cigarettes with inductive plethysmography. Am Rev Respir Dis 126:258, 1982.

76. Kuller LH, Ockene JR, Meillahn E, et al: Cigarette smoking and mortality. MRFIT Research Group. Prev Med 20:638, 1991.

77. Fielding JE, Phenow KJ: Health effects of involuntary smoking. N Engl J Med 319:1452, 1988.

78. Smith GD, Phillips AN: Passive smoking and health: Should we believe Philip Morris's "experts"? BMJ 313:929, 1996.

79. Office of Health and Environmental Assessment and Office of Research and Development: Respiratory Effects of Passive Smoking: Lung Cancer and Other Disorders. Washington, DC, U.S. Environmental Protection Agency, 1992.

80. Heath CW Jr: Passive smoking: Environmental tobacco smoke and lung cancer. Lancet 341:526, 1993.

81. Weiss ST: Editorial: Passive smoking and lung cancer. Am Rev Respir Dis 133:1, 1986.

82. Wigle DT, Collishaw NE, Kirkbride J, et al: Deaths in Canada from lung cancer due to involuntary smoking. Can Med Assoc J 136:945, 1987.

83. Akiba S, Kato H, Blot WJ: Passive smoking and lung cancer among Japanese women. Cancer Res 46:4804, 1986.

84. Dalager NA, Williams Pickle L, Mason TJ, et al: The relation of passive smoking to lung cancer. Cancer Res 46:4808, 1986.

85. Sandler DP, Everson RB, Wilcox AJ: Passive smoking in adulthood and cancer risk. Am J Epidemiol 121:37, 1985.

86. Hirayama T: Cancer mortality in nonsmoking women with smoking husbands based on a large-scale cohort study in Japan. Prev Med 13:680, 1984.

87. Humble CG, Samet JM, Pathak DR: Marriage to a smoker and lung cancer risk. Am J Public Health 77:598, 1987.

88. Garpinkel L, Auerbach D, Joubert L: Involuntary smoking and lung cancer: A case control study. J Natl Cancer Inst 75:463, 1985.

89. Pershagen G, Grubec Z, Svensson C: Passive smoking and lung cancer in Swedish women. Am J Epidemiol 125:17, 1987.

90. Nyberg F, Agrenius V, Svartengren K, et al: Environmental tobacco smoke and lung cancer in nonsmokers: Does time since exposure play a role? Epidemiology 9:301, 1998.

91. Cardenas VM, Thun MJ, Austin H, et al: Environmental tobacco smoke and lung cancer mortality in the American Cancer Society's Cancer Prevention Study. Cancer Causes Control 8:57, 1997.

92. Miller GH, Golish JA, Cox CE, et al: Women and lung cancer: A comparison of active and passive smokers with nonexposed nonsmokers. Cancer Detect Prev 18:421, 1994.

93. Tredaniel J, Boffetta P, Saracci R, et al: Exposure to environmental tobacco smoke and risk of lung cancer: The epidemiological evidence. Eur Respir J 7:1877, 1994.

94. Fontham ET, Correa P, Reynolds P: Environmental tobacco smoke and lung cancer in nonsmoking women: A multicenter study. JAMA 271:1752, 1994.

94a. Wells AJ: Lung cancer from passive smoking at work. Am J Public Health 88:1025, 1998.

94b. Nyberg F, Agudo A, Boffetta P, et al: A European validation study of smoking and environmental tobacco smoke exposure in nonsmoking lung cancer cases and controls. Cancer Causes Control 9:173, 1998.

95. Janerich DT, Thompson D, Varela LR, et al: Lung cancer and exposure to tobacco in the household. N Engl J Med 323:632, 1990.

96. Wang FL, Love EJ, Liu N, et al: Childhood and adolescent passive smoking and the risk of female lung cancer. Int J Epidemiol 23:223, 1994.

97. Wu AH, Fontham ET, Reynolds P, et al: Family history of lung cancer among lifetime nonsmoking women in the United States. Am J Epidemiol 143:535, 1996.

98. Burns DM: Cigarette smoking. In Aisner J, Arriagada R, Green MR, et al (eds): Comprehensive Textbook of Thoracic Oncology. Baltimore, Williams & Wilkins, 1996.

99. Rockey EE, Speer FD, Thompson SA, et al: Experimental study on effect of cigarette smoke condensate on bronchial mucosa. JAMA 182:1094, 1962.

100. Harris RJC, Negroni G: Production of lung carcinomas in C57BL mice exposed to a cigarette smoke and air mixture. BMJ 4:637, 1967.

101. Stanton MF, Miller E, Wrench C, et al: Experimental induction of epidermoid carcinoma in the lungs of rats by cigarette smoke condensate. J Natl Cancer Inst 49:867, 1972.

102. Auerbach O, Stout AP, Hammond EC, et al: Changes in bronchial epithelium in relation to cigarette smoking and in relation to lung cancer. N Engl J Med 265:253, 1961.

103. Auerbach O, Stout AP, Hammond EC, et al: Bronchial epithelium in former smokers. N Engl J Med 267:119, 1962.

104. Auerbach O, Hammond EC, Garfinkel L: Changes in bronchial epithelium in relation to cigarette smoking, 1955–1960 versus 1970–1977. N Engl J Med 300:381, 1979.

105. Plamenac P, Nikulin A, Pikula B, et al: Cytologic changes of the respiratory tract as a consequence of air pollution and smoking. Acta Cytol 23:449, 1979.

106. Band PR, Feldstein M, Saccomanno G: Reversibility of bronchial marked atypia: Implication for chemoprevention. Cancer Detect Prev 9:157, 1986.

107. Hecht SS, Carmella SG, Murphy SE, et al: A tobacco-specific lung carcinogen in the urine of men exposed to cigarette smoke. N Engl J Med 329:1543, 1993.

108. Coultas DB, Howard CA, Peake GT, et al: Salivary cotinine levels and involuntary tobacco smoke exposure in children and adults in New Mexico. Am Rev Respir Dis 136:305, 1987.

109. Witschi H, Espiritu I, Peake JL, et al: The carcinogenicity of environmental tobacco smoke. Carcinogenesis 18:575, 1997.

110. Trichopoulos D, Mollo F, Tomatis L, et al: Active and passive smoking and pathological indicators of lung cancer risk in an autopsy study. JAMA 268:1697, 1992.

111. Agapitos E, Mollo F, Tomatis L, et al: Epithelial, possibly precancerous, lesions of the lung in relation to smoking, passive smoking, and socio-demographic variables. Scand J Soc Med 24:259, 1996.

112. Whitesell PL, Drage CW: Occupational lung cancer. Mayo Clin Proc 68:183, 1993.

113. Steenland K, Loomis D, Shy C, et al: Review of occupational lung carcinogens. Am J Ind Med 29:474, 1996.

114. International Agency for Research on Cancer: IARC Monographs on the Evaluation of Carcinogenic Risk to Humans: Overall Evaluation of Carcinogenicity: An Updating of IARC Monographs Volumes 1 to 42 (Suppl 7). Lyons, International Agency for Research on Cancer, 1987.

115. Kjuus H, Langard S, Skjaerven R: A case-referent study of lung cancer, occupational exposures and smoking: III. Etiologic fraction of occupational exposures. Scand J Work Environ Health 12:210, 1986.

116. Vineis P, Thomas T, Hayes RB, et al: Proportion of lung cancers in males, due to occupation, in different areas of the USA. Int J Cancer 42:851, 1988.

117. Doll R, Peto R: The causes of cancer: Quantitative estimates of avoidable risks of cancer in the United States today. J Natl Cancer Inst 66:1191, 1981.

118. Pastorino U, Berrino F, Gervasio A: Proportion of lung cancers due to occupational exposure. Int J Cancer 33:231, 1984.

119. Kvale G, Bielke E, Heuch I: Occupational exposure and lung cancer risk. Int J Cancer 37:185, 1986.

120. Castleman BI: Asbestos and cancer: History and public policy. Br J Ind Med 48:427, 1991.

121. McDonald JC: Asbestos and lung cancer: Has the case been proven? Chest 78(Suppl):374, 1980.

122. Sluis-Cremer GK: The relationship between asbestosis and bronchial cancer. Chest 78(Suppl):380, 1980.

123. McDonald JC, Liddell FDK, Dufresne A, et al: The 1891–1920 birth cohort of Quebec chrysotile miners and millers: Mortality 1976–88. Br J Ind Med 50:1073, 1993.

124. McDonald JC, McDonald AD: Epidemiology of asbestos-related lung cancer. In Asbestos-Related Malignancy. Orlando, Grune & Stratton, 1986.

125. Selikoff JJ, Churg J, Hammond EC: Asbestos exposure and neoplasia. JAMA 188:22, 1964.

126. Webster I: Asbestosis. S Afr Med J 38:870, 1964.

127. Wagner JC, Sleggs CA, Marchand P: Diffuse pleural mesothelioma and asbestos exposure in the north western Cape Province. Br J Ind Med 7:260, 1960.

128. Hourihane D O'B, Lessof L, Richardson PC: Hyaline and calcified pleural plaques as an index of exposure to asbestos: A study of radiological and pathological features of 100 cases with a consideration of epidemiology. BMJ 1:1069, 1966.

129. Hourihane D O'B: A biopsy series of mesotheliomata, and attempts to identify asbestos within some of the tumors. Ann N Y Acad Sci 132:647, 1965.

130. Freundlich IM, Greening RR: Asbestosis and associated medical problems. Radiology 89:224, 1967.

131. Hourihane D O'B: The pathology of mesotheliomata and an analysis of their association with asbestos exposure. Thorax 19:268, 1964.

132. Enticknap JB, Smither WJ: Peritoneal tumours in asbestosis. Br J Ind Med 21:20, 1964.

133. Editorial: Asbestosis and malignant disease. N Engl J Med 72:590, 1965.

134. Elmes PC, McCaughey WTE, Wade OL: Diffuse mesothelioma of the pleura and asbestos. BMJ 1:350, 1965.

135. Elwood PC, Cochrane AL: A follow-up study of workers from an asbestos factory. Br J Ind Med 21:304, 1964.

136. Doll R: Mortality from lung cancer in asbestos workers. Br J Ind Med 12:81, 1955.

137. Williams W: Asbestosis and lung cancer. Arch Environ Health 10:44, 1965.

138. Hardy HL: Asbestos related disease. Am J Med Sci 250:381, 1965.

139. Enterline P, DeCoufle P, Henderson V: Respiratory cancer in relation to occupational exposures among retired asbestos workers. Br J Ind Med 30:162, 1973.

140. Blair H, Walrath J, Rogot B: Mortality patterns among U.S. veterans by occupation: I. Cancer. J Natl Cancer Inst 75:1039, 1985.

141. Botha JL, Irwig LM, Strebel PM: Excess mortality from stomach cancer, lung cancer, and asbestosis and/or mesothelioma in crocidolite mining districts in South Africa. Am J Epidemiol 123:30, 1986.

142. Baker JE, Reutens DC, Graham DF, et al: Morphology of bronchogenic carcinoma in workers formerly exposed to crocidolite at Wittenoom Gorge in Western Australia. Int J Cancer 37:547, 1986.

143. Newhouse ML, Berry G, Wagner JC: Mortality of factory workers in east London 1933–80. Br J Ind Med 42:4, 1985.

144. McDonald AD, Fry JS, Woolley AJ, et al: Dust exposure and mortality in an American chrysotile asbestos friction products plant. Br J Ind Med 41:151, 1984.

145. Finkelstein MM: Mortality among employees of an Ontario asbestos-cement factory. Am Rev Respir Dis 129:754, 1984.

146. Alies-Fatin AM, Valleron AJ: Mortality of workers in a French asbestos cement factory 1940–82. Br J Ind Med 42:219, 1985.

147. Zoloth S, Michaels D: Asbestos disease in sheet metal workers: The results of a proportional mortality analysis. Am J Ind Med 7:315, 1985.

148. Selikoff IJ, Churg J, Hammond EC: Classics in oncology: Asbestos exposure and neoplasia. CA Cancer J Clin 34:48, 1984.

149. Selikoff IJ, Hammond EC, Seidman S: Latency of asbestos disease among insulation workers in the United States and Canada. Cancer 46:2736, 1980.

150. Bjot WJ, Harrington JM, Toledo A, et al: Lung cancer after employment in shipyards during World War II. N Engl J Med 299:620, 1978.

151. Sanden A, Naslund P-E, Jarvholm B: Mortality in lung and gastrointestinal cancer among shipyard workers. Int Arch Occup Environ Health 55:277, 1985.

152. Hasan PM, Nash G, Kazemi H: Asbestos exposure and related neoplasia: The 28 year experience of a major urban hospital. Am J Med 65:649, 1978.

153. Ohlson CG, Klaesson B, Hogstedt C: Mortality among asbestos-exposed workers in a railroad workshop. Scand J Work Environ Health 10:283, 1984.

154. Martischnio KM, Newell DJ, Barnsley WC, et al: Unsuspected exposure to asbestos and bronchogenic carcinoma. BMJ 1:746, 1977.

155. Kjuus H, Skjaerven R, Langard S, et al: A case-referent study of lung cancer, occupational exposures and smoking: II. Role of asbestos exposure. Scand J Work Environ Health 12:203, 1986.

156. Whitwell F, Newhouse ML, Bennett DR: A study of the histological cell types of lung cancer in workers suffering from asbestosis in the United Kingdom. Br J Ind Med 31:298, 1976.

157. Roggli VL, Pratt PC, Brody AR: Asbestos content of lung tissue in asbestos associated diseases: A study of 110 cases. Br J Ind Med 43:18, 1986.

158. Auerbach O, Garfinkel L, Parks VR, et al: Histologic type of lung cancer and asbestos exposure. Cancer 54:3017, 1984.

159. Becklake MR: Asbestos-related diseases of the lung and other organs: Their epidemiology and implications for clinical practice. Am Rev Respir Dis 114:187, 1976.

160. Whitesell PL, Drage CW: Occupational lung cancer. Mayo Clin Proc 68:183, 1993.

161. Talcott JA, Thurber WA, Kantor AF, et al: Asbestos-associated diseases in a cohort of cigarette-filter workers. N Engl J Med 321:1220, 1989.

162. McDonald AD, Fry JS, Wooley AJ, et al: Dust exposure and mortality in an American factory using crysotile, amosite, and crocidolite in mainly textile manufacture. Br J Ind Med 40:368, 1983.

163. Weill H, Hughes J, Waggenspack C: Influence of dose and fiber type on respiratory malignancy risk in asbestos cement manufacturing. Am Rev Respir Dis 120:345, 1979.

164. Stovin PGI, Partidge P: Pulmonary asbestos and dust content in East Africa. Thorax 37:185, 1982.

165. Albin M, Johansson L, Pooley FD, et al: Mineral fibres, fibrosis, and asbestos bodies in lung tissue from deceased asbestos cement workers. Br J Ind Med 47:767, 1990.

166. McDonald JC, Liddell FDK, Gibbs GW, et al: Dust exposure and mortality in chrysotile mining, 1910–75. Br J Ind Med 37:11, 1980.

167. Wagner JC, Mondrieff CB, Coles R, et al: Correlations between fibre content of the lungs and disease in naval stockyard workers. Br J Ind Med 43:391, 1986.

168. Hughes JM, Weill H, Hammad YY: Mortality of workers employed in two asbestos cement manufacturing plants. Br J Ind Med 44:161, 1987.

169. Becklake MR: Asbestos-related disease of the lungs and pleura: Current clinical issues. Am Rev Respir Dis 126:187, 1982.

170. Leading article: Asbestos pollution and pleural plaques. Med J Austral 1:444, 1981.

171. Mossman BT: Editorial: Mechanisms of asbestos carcinogenesis and toxicity: The amphibole hypothesis revisited. Br J Ind Med 50:673, 1993.

172. Davis JM, McDonald JD: Editorial: Low level exposure to asbestos: Is there a cancer risk? Br J Ind Med 45:505, 1988.

173. Zhu H, Wang Z: Study of occupational lung cancer in asbestos factories in China. Br J Ind Med 50:1039, 1993.

174. Cheng WN, Kong J: A retrospective mortality cohort study of chrysotile asbestos products workers in Tianjin 1972–1987. Environ Res 59:271, 1992.

175. de Klerk NH, Musk AW, Armstrong BK, et al: Smoking, exposure to crocidolite, and the incidence of lung cancer and asbestosis. Br J Ind Med 48:412, 1991.

176. McDonald JC: Asbestos and lung cancer: Has the case been proven? Chest 78(Suppl):374, 1980.

177. Surgeon General of the United States: Asbestos exposed workers. *In* The Health Consequences of Smoking: Cancer and Chronic Lung Disease in the Workplace. U.S. Department of Health and Human Services. Washington, DC, U.S. Government Printing Office, 1985, p 228.

178. Hammond EC, Selikoff IJ, Seidman H: Asbestos exposure, cigarette smoking and death rates. Ann N Y Acad Sci 330:473, 1979.

179. Selikoff IJ, Bader RA, Bader ME, et al: Asbestosis and neoplasia. Am J Med 42:487, 1967.

180. Selikoff IJ, Hammond EC: Asbestos and smoking (editorial). JAMA 242:458, 1979.

181. Berry G, Newhouse ML, Turok M: Combining effect of asbestos exposure and smoking on mortality from lung cancer in factory workers. Lancet 2:476, 1972.

182. Miller AB: Lung cancer. Can Lung Assoc Bull 59:3, 1980.

183. Enterline FE: Attributability in the face of uncertainty. Chest 78(Suppl):377, 1980.

184. McDonald JC, Liddell FDK, Gibbs GW, et al: Dust exposure and mortality in chrysotile mining. 1910–75. Br J Ind Med 37:11, 1980.

185. Juntonen J, Huuskonen MS, Matikainen E, et al: Asbestosis, the nervous system and cancer. Ann Acad Med Singapore 13(2 Suppl):353, 1984.

186. Parkes W: Occupational Lung Disorders. 2nd Ed. London, Butterworths, 1985.

187. Warnock ML, Isenberg W: Asbestos burden and the pathology of lung cancer. Chest 89:20, 1986.

188. Jones RN, Hughes JM, Weill H: Asbestos exposure, asbestosis and asbestos-attributable lung cancer. Thorax 51:S9, 1996.

189. Egilman D, Reinert A: Lung cancer and asbestos exposure: Asbestosis is not necessary. Am J Ind Med 30:398, 1996.

190. Churg A: Asbestos, asbestosis, and lung cancer. Mod Pathol 6:509, 1993.

191. Warnock ML, Isenberg W: Asbestos burden and the pathology of lung cancer. Chest 89:20, 1986.

192. Sluis-Cremer GK, Bezuidenhout BN: Relation between asbestosis and bronchial cancer in amphibole asbestos miners. Br J Ind Med 46:537, 1989.

193. Kipen HM, Lilis R, Suzuki Y, et al: Pulmonary fibrosis in asbestos insulation workers with lung cancer: A radiological and histopathological evaluation. Br J Ind Med 44:96, 1987.

194. Hughes JM, Weill H: Asbestosis as a precursor of asbestos related lung cancer: Results of a prospective mortality study. Br J Ind Med 48:229, 1991.

195. Sluis-Cremer GK, Bezuidenhout BN: Relation between asbestosis and bronchial cancer in amphibole asbestos miners. Br J Ind Med 46:537, 1989.

196. Wilkinson P, Hansell DM, Janssens J, et al: Is lung cancer associated with asbestos exposure when there are no small opacities of the chest radiograph? Lancet 345:1074, 1995.

197. Liddell FDK, McDonald JC: Radiological findings as predictors of mortality in Quebec asbestos workers. Br J Ind Med 37:257, 1980.

198. Becklake MR: Asbestos related fibrosis of the lungs (asbestosis) and pleura. *In* Fishman AP (ed): Update: Pulmonary Diseases and Disorders. New York, McGraw Hill, 1982, p 167.

199. Wagner JC, Berry G, Skidmore JW, et al: The effects of inhalation of asbestos in rats. Br J Cancer 29:252, 1974.

200. Karjalainen A, Anttila S, Heikkila L, et al: Lobe of origin of lung cancer among asbestos-exposed patients with or without diffuse interstitial fibrosis. Scand J Work Environ Health 19:102, 1993.

200a. Lee BW, Wain JC, Kelsey KT, et al: Association of cigarette smoking and asbestos exposure with location and histology of lung cancer. Am J Respir Crit Care Med 157:748, 1998.

201. Browne K: A threshold for asbestos related lung cancer. Br J Ind Med 43:556, 1986.

202. Browne K: Editorial: Asbestos related malignancy and the Cairns hypothesis. Br J Ind Med 48:73, 1991.

203. Janssen YMW, Heintz NH, Marsh JP, et al: Induction of c-fos and c-jun proto-oncogenes in target cells of the lung and pleura by carcinogenic fibers. Am J Respir Cell Mol Biol 1:522, 1994.

204. Rom WN, Travis WD, Brody AR: Cellular and molecular basis of the asbestos-related diseases. Am Rev Respir Dis 143:408, 1991.

205. Al Jarad N, Macey M, Uthayakumar S, et al: Lymphocyte subsets in subjects exposed to asbestos: Changes in circulating natural killer cells. Br J Ind Med 49:811, 1992.

206. Ginnis LC, Ryu JH, Rogol PR, et al: Natural killer cell activity in cigarette smokers and asbestos workers. Am Rev Respir Dis 131:831, 1985.

207. Robinson BWS: Asbestos and cancer: Human natural killer cell activity is suppressed by asbestos fibers but can be restored by recombinant interleukin-2. Am Rev Respir Dis 139:897, 1989.

208. Weiss W: Asbestos-related pleural plaques and lung cancer. Chest 103:1854, 1993.

209. Järup L, Pershagen G: Arsenic exposure, smoking, and lung cancer in smelter workers—a case-control study. Am J Epidemiol 134:545, 1991.

210. Taylor PR, Qiao YL, Schatzkin A, et al: Relation of arsenic exposure to lung cancer among tin miners in Yunnan Province, China. Br J Ind Med 46:881, 1989.

211. Enterline PE, Marsh GM, Esmen NA, et al: Some effects of cigarette smoking, arsenic, and SO2 on mortality among U.S. copper smelter workers. J Occup Med 29:831, 1987.

212. Blair A, Grauman DJ, Lubin JH, et al: Lung cancer and other causes of death among licensed pesticide applicators. J Natl Cancer Inst 71:31, 1983.

213. Stubbs HA, Harris J, Spear RC: A proportionate mortality analysis of California agricultural workers, 1978–1979. Am J Ind Med 6:305, 1984.

214. Ott MG, Holder BB, Gordon HL: Respiratory cancer and occupational exposure to arsenicals. Arch Environ Health 29:250, 1974.

215. Bulatti B, Kriebel D, Geddes M, et al: A case control study of lung cancer in Florence, Italy: I. Occupational risk factors. J Epidemiol Commun Health 39:244, 1985.

216. Wingren G, Axelson O: Mortality pattern in a glass producing area in SE Sweden. Br J Ind Med 42:411, 1985.

217. Kasper ML, Schoenfield L, Strom RL, et al: Hepatic angiosarcoma and bronchioloalveolar carcinoma induced by Fowler's solution. JAMA 252:3407, 1984.

218. Doll R: Occupational lung cancer: A review. Br J Ind Med 16:181, 1959.

219. Bidstrup PL: Use of radiology in the early detection of lung cancer as an industrial disease. Br J Radiol 37:337, 1964.

220. Delarue NC: A review of some important problems concerning lung cancer: Part I. Considerations of epidemiology, etiology, and pathogenesis. Can Med Assoc J 84:1374, 1961.

221. Doll R: Cancer of the lung and nose in nickel workers. Br J Ind Med 15:217, 1958.

222. Williams WJ: The pathology of the lungs in five nickel workers. Br J Ind Med 15:235, 1958.

223. Chovil A, Sutherland RB, Halliday M: Respiratory cancer in a cohort of nickel sinter plant workers. Br J Ind Med 38:327, 1981.

224. Roberts RS, Julian JA, Muir DC, et al: Cancer mortality associated with the high-temperature oxidation of nickel subsulfide. IARC Sci Publ 53:23, 1984.

225. Andersen A, Berge SR, Engeland A, et al: Exposure to nickel compounds and

smoking in relation to incidence of lung and nasal cancer among nickel refinery workers. Occup Environ Med 53:708, 1996.

226. Rafnsson V, Gunnarsdottir H, Kiilunen M: Risk of lung cancer among masons in Iceland. Occup Environ Med 54:184, 1997.

227. Kim S, Iwai Y, Fujino M, et al: Chromium-induced pulmonary cancer. Acta Pathol Jpn 35:643, 1985.

228. Mancuso TF: Chromium as an industrial carcinogen: Part I. Am J Ind Med 31:129, 1997.

229. Rosenman KD, Stanbury M: Risk of lung cancer among former chromium smelter workers. Am J Ind Med 29:491, 1996.

230. Davies JM: Lung cancer mortality among workers making lead chromate and zinc chromate pigments at three English factories. Br J Ind Med 41:158, 1984.

231. Nishivama H, Yano H, Nishiwaki Y, et al: Lung cancer in chromate workers: Analysis of 17 cases. Jpn J Clin Oncol 15:489, 1985.

232. Ohsaki Y, Abe S, Kimura K, et al: Lung cancer in Japanese chromate workers. Thorax 33:372, 1978.

233. Hayes RB, Sheffet A, Spirtas R: Cancer mortality among a cohort of chromium pigment workers. Am J Ind Med 16:127, 1989.

234. Sorahan T, Burges DC, Waterhouse JA: A mortality study of nickel/chromium platers. Br J Ind Med 44:250, 1987.

235. Langard S: Role of chemical species and exposure characteristics in cancer among persons occupationally exposed to chromium compounds. Scand J Work Environ Health 1:81, 1993.

236. Axelsson G, Rylander R, Schmidt A: Mortality and incidence of tumours among ferrochromium workers. Br J Ind Med 37:121, 1980.

237. Langard S, Andersen AA, Gylseth B: Incidence of cancer among ferrochromium and ferrosilicon workers. Br J Ind Med 37:114, 1980.

237a. Sorahan T, Burges DC, Hamilton L, et al: Lung cancer mortality in nickel/chromium platers, 1946–95. Occup Environ Med 55:236, 1998.

238. Becker N, Claude J, Frentzel-Bevme R: Cancer risk of arc welders exposed to fumes containing chromium and nickel. Scand J Work Environ Health 11:75, 1985.

239. Abe S, Ohsaki Y, Kimura K, et al: Chromate lung cancer with special reference to its cell type and relation to the manufacturing process. Cancer 49:783, 1982.

240. Tsuneta Y, Ohsaki Y, Kimura K, et al: Chromium content of lungs of chromate workers with lung cancer. Thorax 35:294, 1980.

241. Ishikawa Y, Nakagawa K, Satoh Y, et al: Characteristics of chromate workers' cancers, chromium lung deposition and precancerous bronchial lesions: An autopsy study. Br J Cancer 70:160, 1994.

242. McDonald JD: Silica, silicosis and lung cancer. Br J Ind Med 46:289, 1989.

243. Pairon JD, Brochard P, Jaurand MC, et al: Silica and lung cancer: A controversial issue. Eur Respir J 4:730, 1991.

244. Goldsmith DF: Silica exposure and pulmonary cancer. *In* Savnet JM (ed): Epidemiology of Lung Cancer. New York, Marcel Dekker, 1994.

245. Hill AB: The environment and disease: Association or causation? Proc R Soc Med 58:295, 1965.

246. Holland LM: Crystalline silica and lung cancer: A review of recent experimental evidence. Regul Toxicol Pharmacol 12:224, 1990.

247. Weill H, McDonald JC: Exposure to crystalline silica and risk of lung cancer: The epidemiological evidence. Thorax 51:97, 1996.

248. International Agency for Research on Cancer: IARC Monographs on the Evaluation of Carcinogenic Risks to Humans—Silica, Some Silicates, Coal Dust and Para-aramid Fibrils. Monograph 68. Lyons, International Agency for Research on Cancer, 1996.

249. Simonato L, Fletcher AC, Saracci R, et al: Occupational exposure to silica and cancer risk. IARC Sci Publ 97:124, 1990.

250. Kurppa K, Gudbergsson H, Hannunkari I, et al: Lung cancer among silicotics in Finland. *In* Goldsmith DF, Winn DM, Shy CM (eds): Silica, Silicosis and Cancer: Controversy in Occupational Medicine. New York, Praeger, 1986, p 311.

251. Finkelstein M, Liss GM, Krammer F, et al: Mortality among workers receiving compensation awards for silicosis in Ontario 1940–85. Br J Ind Med 44:588, 1987.

252. Chia SE, Chia KS, Phon WH, et al: Silicosis and lung cancer among Chinese granite workers. Scand J Work Environ Health 17:170, 1991.

253. Carta P, Cocco PL, Casula D: Mortality from lung cancer among Sardinian patient with silicosis. Br J Ind Med 48:122, 1991.

254. Amandus HE, Castellan RM, Shy C, et al: Reevaluation of silicosis and lung cancer in North Carolina dusty trades workers. Br J Ind Med 22:147, 1992.

255. Amandus H, Costello J: Silicosis and lung cancer in U.S. metal miners. Arch Environ Health 46:82, 1991.

256. Chiyotani K, Saito K, Okubo T, et al: Lung cancer risk among pneumoconiosis patients in Japan, with special reference to silicotics. IARC Sci Publ 97:95, 1990.

257. Tornling G, Hogstedt C, Westerholm P: Lung cancer incidence among Swedish ceramic workers with silicosis. IARC Sci Publ 97:113, 1990.

258. Ng TP, Chan SL, Lee J: Mortality of a cohort of men in a silicosis register: Further evidence of an association with lung cancer. Am J Ind Med 17:163, 1990.

259. Infante-Rivard C, Armstrong B, Petitclerc M, et al: Lung cancer mortality and silicosis in Quebec, 1938–85. Lancet 2:1504, 1989.

260. Neuberger M, Kundi M: Occupational dust exposure and cancer mortality—results of prospective cohort study. IARC Sci Publ 97:65, 1990.

261. Siemiatycki J, Gerin M, Dewar R, et al: Silica and cancer associations from a multicancer occupational exposure case-referent study. IARC Sci Publ 97:29, 1990.

262. Checkoway H, Heyer NJ, Demers PA, et al: Mortality among workers in the diatomaceous earth industry. Br J Ind Med 50:586, 1993.

263. Costello J, Graham WG: Vermont granite workers' mortality study. Am J Ind Med 13:483, 1988.

264. Hnizdo E, Sluis-Cremer GK, Abramowitz JA: Emphysema type in relation to silica dust exposure in South African gold miners. Am Rev Respir Dis 143:1241, 1991.

265. Steenland K, Brown D: Mortality study of gold miners exposed to silica and nonasbestiform amphibole minerals: An update with 14 more years of follow-up. Am J Ind Med 27:217, 1995.

266. Thomas TL: Lung cancer mortality among pottery workers in the United States. IARC Sci Publ 97:75, 1990.

267. Thomas TL, Stewart PA: Mortality from lung cancer and respiratory disease among pottery workers exposed to silica and talc. Am J Epidemiol 125:35, 1987.

268. Chen SY, Hayes RB, Liang SR, et al: Mortality experience of haematite mine workers in China. Br J Ind Med 47:175, 1990.

269. Finkelstein MM: Radiographic abnormalities and the risk of lung cancer among workers exposed to silica dust in Ontario. Can Med Assoc J 152:37, 1995.

270. Carta P, Cocco P, Picchiri G: Lung cancer mortality and airways obstruction among metal miners exposed to silica and low levels of radon daughters. Am J Ind Med 25:489, 1994.

271. McLaughlin JK, Chen JQ, Dosemeci M, et al: A nested case-control study of lung cancer among silica exposed workers in China. Br J Ind Med 49:167, 1993.

272. Knizdo E, Sluis-Cremer GK: Silica exposure, silicosis, and lung cancer: A mortality study of South African gold miners. Br J Ind Med 48:53, 1991.

273. Tossavainen A: Estimated risk of lung cancer attributable to occupational exposures in iron and steel foundries. IARC Sci Publ 104:363, 1990.

274. Perera FP, Hemminki K, Young TL, et al: Detection of polycyclic aromatic hydrocarbon-DNA adducts in white blood cells of foundry workers. Cancer Res 48:2288, 1988.

275. Moulin JJ, Wild P, Mantout B, et al: Mortality from lung cancer and cardiovascular diseases among stainless-steel producing workers. Cancer Causes Control 4:75, 1993.

276. Sherson D, Iversen E: Mortality among foundry workers in Denmark due to cancer and respiratory and cardiovascular diseases. *In* Goldsmith DF, Winn DM, Shy CM (eds): Silica, Silicosis and Cancer: Controversy in Occupational Medicine. New York, Praeger, 1986, p 403.

277. Simonato L, Moulin JJ, Javelaud B, et al: A retrospective mortality study of workers exposed to arsenic in a gold mine and refinery in France. Am J Ind Med 25:625, 1994.

278. Kusiak RA, Springer J, Ritchie AC, et al: Carcinoma of the lung in Ontario gold miners: Possible aetiological factors. Br J Ind Med 48:808, 1991.

279. Lynge E, Kurppa K, Kristofersen L, et al: Occupational groups potentially exposed to silica dust: A comparative analysis of cancer mortality and incidence based on the Nordic occupational mortality and cancer incidence registers. IARC Sci Publ 97:7, 1990.

280. Mehnert WH, Stanecek W, Mohner M, et al: A mortality study of a cohort of slate quarry workers in the German Democratic Republic. IARC Sci Publ 97:55, 1990.

281. Guenel P, Hojberg G, Lynge E: Cancer incidence among Danish stone workers. Scand J Work Environ Health 15:265, 1989.

282. Forastiere R, Lagorio S, Michelozzi P, et al: Silica, silicosis and lung cancer among ceramic workers: A case-referent study. Am J Ind Med 10:363, 1986.

283. Axelson O: Editorial: Confounding from smoking in occupational epidemiology. Br J Ind Med 46:505, 1989.

284. Winter PD, Gardner MJ, Fletcher AC, et al: A mortality follow-up study of pottery workers: Preliminary findings on lung cancer. IARC Sci Publ 97:83, 1990.

285. Zambon P, Simonato L, Mastrangelo G, et al: Mortality of workers compensated for silicosis during the period 1959–1963 in the Veneto region of Italy. Scand J Work Environ Health 13:118, 1987.

286. Cocco PL, Carta P, Flore V, et al: Lung cancer mortality among female mine workers exposed to silica. J Occup Med 36:894, 1994.

287. Lawler AB, Mandel JS, Schuman LM, et al: A retrospective cohort mortality study of iron ore (hematite) miners in Minnesota. J Occup Med 27:507, 1985.

288. Figueroa WG, Raszkowski R, Weiss W: Lung cancer in chloromethyl methyl ether workers. N Engl J Med 288:1096, 1973.

289. Gowers DS, DeFonso LR, Schaffer P, et al: Incidence of respiratory cancer among workers exposed to chloromethyl-ethers. Am J Epidemiol 137:31, 1993.

290. McCallum RI, Woolley V, Petrie A: Lung cancer associated with chloromethyl methyl ether manufacture: An investigation at two factories in the United Kingdom. Br J Ind Med 40:384, 1983.

291. Weiss W, Moser RL, Auerbach O: Lung cancer in chloromethyl ether workers. Am Rev Respir Dis 120:1031, 1979.

292. Wada N: Toxic gas and lung cancer. Jpn J Chest Dis 6:308, 1962.

293. Wada S, Miyanishi M, Nishimoto Y, et al: Mustard gas as a cause of respiratory neoplasia in man. Lancet 1:1161, 1968.

294. Nishimoto Y, Yamakido M, Ishioka S, et al: Epidemiological studies of lung cancer in Japanese mustard gas workers. Princess Takamatsu Symp 18:95, 1987.

295. Easton DF, Peto J, Doll R: Cancers of the respiratory tract in mustard gas workers. Br J Ind Med 45:652, 1988.

296. Tokuoka S, Hayashi Y, Inai K, et al: Early cancer and related lesions in the bronchial epithelium of former workers of mustard gas factory. Acta Pathol Jpn 36:533, 1986.

297. Tokuoka S, Hayashi Y, Inai K, et al: Early cancer and related lesions in the bronchial epithelium in former workers of mustard gas factory. Acta Pathol Jpn 36:533, 1986.

298. International Agency for Research on Cancer: IARC Monographs on Some Metals and Metallic Compounds. Monograph 23. Lyons, International Agency for Research on Cancer, 1980.

299. Ward E, Okun A, Ruder A, et al: A mortality study of workers at seven beryllium processing plants. Am J Ind Med 22:885, 1992.

300. Steenland K, Ward E: Lung cancer incidence among patients with beryllium disease: A cohort mortality study. J Natl Cancer Inst 83:1380, 1991.

301. International Agency for Research on Cancer: IARC Monographs on Polynuclear Aromatic Compounds, Part 3, Industrial Exposures in Aluminum Production, Coal Gasification, Coke Production, and Iron and Steel Founding. Monograph 34. Lyons, International Agency for Research on Cancer, 1984.

302. International Agency for Research on Cancer: IARC Monographs on Overall Evaluation of Carcinogenicity: An Updating of IARC Monographs 1–42 (Suppl 7). Lyons, International Agency for Research on Cancer, 1987.

303. International Agency for Research on Cancer: IARC Monographs on Polynuclear Aromatic Compounds, Part 4, Bitumens, Coal-Tars and Derived Products, Shale-Oils, and Soots. Monograph 35. Lyons, International Agency for Research on Cancer, 1985.

304. Parent ME, Siemiatycki J, Renaud G: Case-control study of exposure to carbon black in the occupational setting and risk of lung cancer. Am J Ind Med 30:285, 1996.

305. International Agency for Research on Cancer: IARC Monographs on Diesel and Gasoline Engine Exhausts and Some Nitrosamines. Monograph 46. Lyons, International Agency for Research on Cancer, 1989.

306. Costantino JP, Redmond CK, Beardon A: Occupationally related cancer risk among coke oven workers: 30 years of follow-up. J Occup Environ Med 37:597, 1995.

307. Xu Z, Brown LM, Pan GW, et al: Cancer risks among iron and steel workers in Anshan, China: Part II. Case-control studies of lung and stomach cancer. Am J Ind Med 30:7, 1996.

308. Swaen GMH, Slangen JJM, Volovics A, et al: Mortality of coke plant workers in the Netherlands. Br J Ind Med 48:130, 1991.

309. Hurley JF, Archibald RM, Collings PL, et al: The mortality of coke workers in Britain. Am J Ind Med 4:691, 1983.

310. Madison R, Afifi AA, Mittman C: Respiratory impairment in coke oven workers: Relationship to work exposure and bronchial inflammation detected by sputum cytology. J Chronic Dis 37:167, 1984.

311. Bertrand JP, Chau N, Patris A, et al: Mortality due to respiratory cancers in the coke oven plants of the Lorraine coalmining industry (Houilleres du Bassin de Lorraine). Br J Ind Med 44:559, 1987.

312. Ronneberg A, Andersen A: Mortality and cancer morbidity in workers from an aluminum smelter with prebaked carbon anodes: Part II. Cancer morbidity. Occup Environ Med 52:250, 1995.

313. Armstrong B, Tremblay C, Baris D, et al: Lung cancer mortality and polynuclear aromatic hydrocarbons: A case-cohort study of aluminum production workers in Arvida, Quebec, Canada. Am J Epidemiol 139:250, 1994.

314. Finkelstein MM: Lung cancer among steelworkers in Ontario. Am J Ind Med 26:549, 1994.

315. Parkes HG, Vevs CA, Waterhouse JAH, et al: Cancer mortality in the British rubber industry. Br J Ind Med 39:209, 1982.

316. Delzell E, Monson RR: Mortality among rubber workers: VII. Aerospace workers. Am J Ind Med 6:265, 1984.

317. Evanoff BA, Gustavsson P, Hogstedt C: Mortality and incidence of cancer in a cohort of Swedish chimney sweeps: An extended follow-up study. Br J Ind Med 50:450, 1993.

318. Nakanishi Y, Chen S, Inutsuka S, et al: Possible role of indoor environment and coal combustion emission in lung carcinogenesis in Fuyuan County, China. Neoplasma 44:69, 1997.

319. Cohen AJ, Pope CA 3rd: Lung cancer and air pollution. Environ Health Perspect 8:219, 1995.

320. Pfluger DH, Minder CE: A mortality study of lung cancer among Swiss professional drivers: Accounting for the smoking related fraction by a multivariate approach. Soz Praventivmed 39:372, 1994.

321. Borgia P, Forastiere F, Rapiti E, et al: Mortality among taxi drivers in Rome: A cohort study. Am J Ind Med 25:507, 1994.

322. Emmelin A, Nystrom L, Wall S: Diesel exhaust exposure and smoking: A case-referent study of lung cancer among Swedish dock workers. Epidemiology 4:237, 1993.

323. Garshik E, Schenker MB, Muñoz A, et al: A retrospective cohort study of lung cancer and diesel exhaust exposure in railroad workers. Am Rev Respir Dis 137:820, 1988.

323a. Hansen J, Raaschou-Nielsen O, Olsen JH: Increased risk of lung cancer among different types of professional drivers in Denmark. Occup Environ Med 55:115, 1998.

324. Muscat JE: Carcinogenic effects of diesel emissions and lung cancer: The epidemiologic evidence is not causal. J Clin Epidemiol 49:891, 1996.

325. Muscat JE, Wynder EL: Diesel engine exhaust and lung cancer: An unproven association. Environ Health Perspect 103:812, 1995.

325a. Bhatia R, Lopipero P, Smith AH: Diesel exhaust exposure and lung cancer. Epidemiology 9:84, 1998.

326. Sorahan T, Lister A, Gilthorpe MS, et al: Mortality of copper cadmium alloy workers with special reference to lung cancer and nonmalignant diseases of the respiratory system, 1946–92. Occup Environ Med 52:804, 1995.

327. Sorahan T: Mortality from lung cancer among a cohort of nickel cadmium battery workers. Br J Ind Med 44:803, 1987.

328. Stayner L, Smith R, Thun M, et al: A dose-response analysis and quantitative assessment of lung cancer risk and occupational cadmium exposure. Ann Epidemiol 2:177, 1992.

329. Lamm SH, Parkinson M, Anderson M, et al: Determinants of lung cancer risk among cadmium-exposed workers. Ann Epidemiol 3:195, 1992.

330. Kazantzis G, Lam TH, Sullivan KR: Mortality of cadmium-exposed workers: A five-year update. Scand J Work Environ Health 14:220, 1988.

331. International Agency for Research on Cancer: IARC Monographs on Beryllium, Cadmium, Mercury and Exposures in the Glass Manufacturing Industry. Monograph 58. Lyons, International Agency for Research on Cancer, 1993.

332. Frank AL: The epidemiology and etiology of lung cancer. Clin Chest Med 3:219, 1982.

333. Dvorackova I: Aflatoxin inhalation and alveolar cell carcinoma. BMJ 1:691, 1976.

334. Sorahan T, Cathcart M: Lung cancer mortality among workers in a factory manufacturing chlorinated toluenes: 1961–84. Br J Ind Med 46:425, 1989.

335. Wagoner JK: Toxicity of vinyl chloride and polyvinyl chloride: A critical review. Environ Health Perspect 52:61, 1983.

336. Simonato L, Fletcher AC, Cherrie J, et al: Updating lung cancer mortality among a cohort of man-made mineral fibre production workers in seven European countries. Cancer Lett 30:18, 1986.

337. Stayner LT, Meinhardt T, Lemen R, et al: A retrospective cohort mortality study of a phosphate fertilizer production facility. Arch Environ Health 40:133, 1985.

338. Checkoway H, Mathew RM, Hickey JL, et al: Mortality among workers in the Florida phosphate industry: II. Cause-specific mortality relationships with work areas and exposures. J Occup Med 27:893, 1985.

339. Blair A, Stewart P, O'Berg M, et al: Mortality among industrial workers exposed to formaldehyde. J Natl Cancer Inst 76:1071, 1986.

340. Sterling TD, Weinkam JJ: Mortality from respiratory cancers (including lung cancer) among workers employed in formaldehyde industries. Am J Ind Med 25:593, 1994.

341. Hughson WG, Fedoruk MJ: Occupational and environmental causes of lung cancer and esophageal cancer. In Aisner J, Arriagada R, Green MR, et al (eds): Comprehensive Textbook of Thoracic Oncology. Baltimore, Williams & Wilkins, 1996.

342. Muller J: Radiation as a lung carcinogen. Chest 89(Suppl):312S, 1986.

343. Whittemore AS, McMillan A: Lung cancer mortality among U.S. uranium miners: A reappraisal. J Natl Cancer Inst 71:489, 1983.

344. Roscoe RJ, Deddens JA, Salvan A, et al: Mortality among Navajo uranium miners. Am J Public Health 85:535, 1995.

345. Tirmarche M, Raphalen A, Allin F, et al: Mortality of a cohort of French uranium miners exposed to relatively low radon concentrations. Br J Cancer 67:1090, 1993.

346. Finkelstein MM: Clinical measures, smoking, radon exposure, and risk of lung cancer in uranium miners. Occup Environ Med 53:697, 1996.

347. Morrison HI, Semenciw RM, Mao Y, et al: Cancer mortality among a group of fluorspar miners exposed to radon progeny. Am J Epidemiol 128:1266, 1988.

347a. Morrison HI, Villeneuve PJ, Lubin JH, et al: Radon-progeny exposure and lung cancer risk in a cohort of Newfoundland fluorspar miners. Radiat Res 150:58, 1998.

348. Solli HM, Andersen A, Strandon E, et al: Cancer incidence among workers exposed to radon and thoron daughters at a niobium mine. Scand J Work Environ Health 11:7, 1985.

349. Radford ER, Renard KG: Lung cancer in Swedish iron miners exposed to low doses of radon daughters. N Engl J Med 310:1485, 1984.

350. Jorgensen HS: Lung cancer among underground workers in the iron ore mine of Kiruna based on thirty years of observation. Ann Acad Med Singapore 13(Suppl):371, 1984.

351. Cocco PL, Carta P, Belli S, et al: Mortality of Sardinian lead and zinc miners: 1960–88. Occup Environ Med 51:674, 1994.

352. Xuan XZ, Lubin JH, Li JY, et al: A cohort study in southern China of tin miners exposed to radon and radon decay products. Health Phys 64:120, 1993.

353. Loomis DP, Wolf SH: Mortality of workers at a nuclear materials production plant at Oak Ridge, Tennessee 1947–1990. Am J Ind Med 29:131, 1996.

354. Khokhriakov VF, Romanov SA: Estimation of the temporal distribution and dose dependency of lung cancers among workers of nuclear fuel reprocessing plants. Health Phys 71:83, 1996.

355. International Agency for Research on Cancer: IARC Monographs on the Evaluation of Carcinogenic Risk to Humans: Man-made Mineral Fibres and Radon. Monograph 43. Lyons, International Agency for Research on Cancer, 1988.

356. Howe GR, Nair RC, Newcombe HB, et al: Lung cancer mortality (1950–80) in relation to radon daughter exposure in a cohort of workers at the Eldorado Beaverlodge uranium mine. J Natl Cancer Inst 77:357, 1986.

357. Sevc J, Tomasek L, Kunz E, et al: A survey of the Czechoslovak follow-up of lung cancer mortality in uranium miners. Health Phys 64:355, 1993.

358. Woodward A, Roder D, McMichael AJ, et al: Radon daughter exposures at the Radium Hill uranium mine and lung cancer rates among former workers, 1952–87. Cancer Causes Control 2:213, 1991.

359. Roscoe RJ, Steenland K, Halperin WE, et al: Lung cancer mortality among nonsmoking uranium miners exposed to radon daughters. JAMA 262:629, 1989.

360. Muggenburg BA, Guilmette RA, Mewhinney JA, et al: Toxicity of inhaled plutonium dioxide in beagle dogs. Radiat Res 145:361, 1996.

361. Gilbert ES, Cross FT, Dagle GE: Analysis of lung tumor risks in rats exposed to radon. Radiat Res 145:350, 1996.

362. Edling C, Kling H, Axelson O: Radon in homes: A possible cause of lung cancer. Scand J Work Environ Health 10:25, 1984.

363. Auerbach O, Saccomanno G, Kuschner M, et al: Histologic findings in the tracheobronchial tree of uranium miners and nonminers with lung cancer. Cancer 42:483, 1979.

364. Archer VE: Enhancement of lung cancer by cigarette smoking in uranium and other miners. Carcinog Compr Surv 8:23, 1985.

365. Steenland K: Age specific interactions between smoking and radon among United States uranium miners. Occup Environ Med 51:192, 1994.

366. Archer VE, Saccomanno G, Jones JH: Frequency of different histologic types of bronchogenic carcinoma as related to radiation exposure. Cancer 34:2056, 1974.

367. Saccomanno G, Auerbach O, Kuschner M, et al: A comparison between the localization of lung tumours in uranium miners and in nonminers from 1947 to 1991. Cancer 77:1278, 1996.

368. Kusiak RA, Ritchie AC, Muller J, et al: Mortality from lung cancer in Ontario in uranium miners. Br J Ind Med 50:920, 1993.

369. Samet JM: Radon and lung cancer. J Natl Cancer Inst 81:745, 1989.

370. Lubin JH, Boice JD Jr, Edling C, et al: Lung cancer in radon-exposed miners and estimation of risk from indoor exposure. J Natl Cancer Inst 87:817, 1995.

371. Lubin JH, Tomasek L, Edling C, et al: Estimating lung cancer mortality rates from residential radon using data for low exposures of miners. Radiat Res 147:126, 1997.

372. Puskin JS, Nelson CB: EPA's perspective on risks from residential radon exposure. JAPCA 39:915, 1989.

373. Yesner R: Pathogenesis and pathology. Clin Chest Med 14:17, 1993.

374. Pershagen G, Akerblom G, Axelson O, et al: Residential radon exposure and lung cancer in Sweden. N Engl J Med 330:159, 1994.

375. Ennemoser O, Ambach W, Brunner P, et al: Unusual high radon exposure in homes and lung cancer. Lancet 344:127, 1994.

376. Engeland A, Green BM, Haldorsen T, et al: Residential radon exposure and lung cancer—an epidemiological study of Norwegian municipalities. Int J Cancer 58:1, 1994.

377. Lubin JH, Liang Z, Hrubec Z, et al: Radon exposure in residences and lung cancer among women: Combined analysis of three studies. Cancer Causes Control 5:114, 1994.

378. Auvinen A, Makelainen I, Hakama M, et al: Indoor radon exposure and risk of lung cancer: A nested case-control study in Finland. J Natl Cancer Inst 88:966, 1996.

379. Letourneau EG, Krewski D, Coi NW, et al: Case-control study of residential radon and lung cancer in Winnipeg, Manitoba, Canada. Am J Epidemiol 140:310, 1994.

380. Neuberger JS: Residential radon exposure and lung cancer: An overview of published studies. Cancer Detect Prev 15:435, 1991.

381. Lubin JH, Boice JD Jr, Samet JM: Errors in exposure assessment, statistical power and the interpretation of residential radon studies. Radiat Res 144:329, 1995.

382. Stidley CA, Samet JM: Assessment of ecologic regression in the study of lung cancer and indoor radon. Am J Epidemiol 139:312, 1994.

383. Lagarde F, Pershagen G, Akerblom G, et al: Residential radon and lung cancer in Sweden: Risk analysis accounting for random error in the exposure assessment. Health Phys 72:269, 1997.

384. Warner KE, Mendez D, Courant PN: Toward a more realistic appraisal of the lung cancer risk from radon: The effects of residential mobility. Am J Public Health 86:1222, 1996.

385. Lubin JGH, Boice JD Jr: Lung cancer risk from residential radon: Meta-analysis of eight epidemiologic studies. J Natl Cancer Inst 89:49, 1997.

386. Wanebo CK, Johnson KG, Sato K, et al: Lung cancer following atomic radiation. Am Rev Respir Dis 98:778, 1968.

387. Cihak RW, Ishimaru T, Steer A, et al: Lung cancer at autopsy in A-bomb survivors and controls, Hiroshima and Nagasaki, 1961–1970. Cancer 33:1580, 1974.

388. Land CE, Shimosato Y, Saccomanno G, et al: Radiation-associated lung cancer: A comparison of the histology of lung cancer in uranium miners and survivors of the atomic bombings of Hiroshima and Nagasaki. Radiat Res 134:234, 1993.

389. List AF, Doll DC, Greco FA: Lung cancer in Hodgkin's disease: Association with previous radiotherapy. J Clin Oncol 3:215, 1985.

390. Oliphant L, McFadden RG: Lung cancer following therapy for Hodgkin's disease. Can Med Assoc J 132:533, 1985.

391. Wiernik PH, Sklarin NT, Dutcher JP, et al: Adjuvant radiotherapy for breast cancer as a risk factor for the development of lung cancer. Med Oncol 11:121, 1994.

392. Inskip PD, Stovall M, Flannery JT: Lung cancer risk and radiation dose among women treated for breast cancer. J Natl Cancer Inst 86:983, 1994.

393. Neugut AI, Robinson E, Lee WC, et al: Lung cancer after radiation therapy for breast cancer. Cancer 71:3054, 1993.

394. Hod I, Herz A, Zimber A: Pulmonary carcinoma (Jaagsiekte) of sheep: Ultra-structural study of early and advanced tumor lesions. Am J Pathol 86:545, 1977.

395. Perk K, Hod I: Sheep lung carcinoma: An endemic analogue of a sporadic human neoplasm. J Natl Cancer Inst 69:747, 1982.

396. Hecht SJ, Sharp JM, Demartini JC: Retroviral aetiopathogenesis of ovine pulmonary carcinoma: A critical appraisal. Br Vet J 152:395, 1996.

397. Palmarini M, Cousens C, Dalziel RG, et al: The exogenous form of Jaagsiekte retrovirus is specifically associated with a contagious lung cancer of sheep. J Virol 70:1618, 1996.

398. Palmarini M, Dewar P, De las Heras M, et al: Epithelial tumour cells in the lungs of sheep with pulmonary adenomatosis are major sites of replication for Jaagsiekte retrovirus. J Gen Virol 76:2731, 1995.

399. Heimann HL, Samuel E: Pulmonary adenomatosis. S Afr Med J 27:934, 1953.

400. Tsumuraya M, Kodama T, Kameya T, et al: Light and electron microscopic analysis of intranuclear inclusions in papillary adenocarcinoma of the lung. Acta Cytol 25:523, 1981.

401. Steinberg BM, Topp WC, Schneider PS, et al: Laryngeal papillomavirus infection during clinical remission. N Engl J Med 308:1261, 1983.

402. Dallimore NS: Squamous bronchial carcinoma arising in a case of multiple juvenile papillomatosis. Thorax 40:797, 1985.

403. Schnadio VJ, Clark WD, Clegg TJ, et al: Invasive papillomatosis and squamous carcinoma complicating juvenile laryngeal papillomatosis. Arch Otolaryngol Head Neck Surg 112:966, 1986.

404. Soini Y, Nuorva K, Kamel D, et al: Presence of human papillomavirus DNA and abnormal p53 protein accumulation in lung carcinoma. Thorax 51:887, 1996.

405. Hirayasu T, Iwamasa T, Kamada Y, et al: Human papillomavirus DNA in squamous cell carcinoma of the lung. J Clin Pathol 49:810, 1996.

406. Kinoshita I, Dosaka Akita H, Shindoh M, et al: Human papillomavirus type 18 DNA and E6-E7 mRNA are detected in squamous cell carcinoma and adenocarcinoma of the lung. Br J Cancer 71:344, 1995.

407. Shamanin V, Delius H, de Villiers EM: Development of a broad spectrum PCR assay for papillomavirus and its application in screening lung cancer biopsies. J Gen Virol 75:1149, 1994.

408. Welt A, Hummel M, Niedobitek G, et al: Human papillomavirus infection is not associated with bronchial carcinoma: Evaluation by in situ hybridization and the polymerase chain reaction. J Pathol 181:276, 1997.

409. Carey FA, Salter DM, Kerr KM, et al: An investigation into the role of human papillomavirus in endobronchial papillary squamous tumours. Respir Med 84:445, 1990.

410. Wong MP, Chung LP, Yuen ST, et al: In situ detection of Epstein-Barr virus in non–small cell lung carcinomas. J Pathol 177:233, 1995.

411. Pittaluga S, Wong MP, Chung LP, et al: Clonal Epstein-Barr virus in lymphoepi-thelioma-like carcinoma of the lung. Am J Surg Pathol 17:678, 1993.

412. Chan JK, Hui PK, Tsang WY, et al: Primary lymphoepithelioma-like carcinoma of the lung: A clinicopathologic study of 11 cases. Cancer 76:413, 1995.

413. Conway EJ, Hudnall SD, Lazarides A, et al: Absence of evidence for an etiologic role for Epstein-Barr virus in neoplasms of the lung and pleura. Mod Pathol 9:491, 1996.

414. Raeburn C, Spencer H: A study of the origin and development of lung cancer. Thorax 8:1, 1953.

415. Raeburn C, Spencer H: Lung scar cancers. Br J Tuberc 51:237, 1957.

416. Auerbach O, Garfinkel L, Parks VR: Scar cancer of the lung: Increase over a 21 year period. Cancer 43:636, 1979.

417. Lamb D: Histological classification of lung cancer. Thorax 39:161, 1984.

418. Berkheiser SW: Pulmonary infarction associated with lung cancer. Dis Chest 47:36, 1965.

419. Limas C, Japaze H, Garcia-Bunuel R: "Scar" carcinoma of the lung. Chest 59:219, 1971.

420. Strauss FH, Dordal E, Kappas A: The problem of pulmonary scar tumors. Arch Pathol 76:693, 1964.

421. Blake JM: Primary carcinoma of the bronchus associated with foreign body. Am Rev Tuberc 47:109, 1943.

422. Kitagawa M: Autopsy study of lung cancer with special reference to scar cancer. Acta Pathol 15:199, 1965.

423. Berkheiser SW: Bronchiolar proliferation and metaplasia associated with bron-chiectasis, pulmonary infarcts, and anthracosis. Cancer 12:499, 1959.

424. Madri JA, Carter D: Scar cancers of the lung: Origin and significance. Hum Pathol 15:625, 1984.

425. McDonnell L, Long JP: Lung scar cancer—a reappraisal. J Clin Pathol 34:996, 1981.

426. Kung ITM, Lui IOL, Loke SL, et al: Pulmonary scar cancer: A pathologic reappraisal. Am J Surg Pathol 9:391, 1985.

427. Shimosato Y, Hashimoto T, Kodama T, et al: Prognostic implications of fibrotic focus (scar) in small peripheral lung cancers. Am J Surg Pathol 4:365, 1980.

428. Barsky SH, Huang SJ, Bhuta S: The extracellular matrix of pulmonary scar carcinomas is suggestive of a desmoplastic origin. Am J Pathol 124:412, 1986.

429. El-Torky M, Giltman LI, Dabbous M: Collagens in scar carcinoma of the lung. Am J Pathol 121:322, 1985.

430. Dubeau L, Fraser RS: Long-term effects of pulmonary shrapnel injury. Arch Pathol Lab Med 108:407, 1984.

431. Jackson D, Greenberg SD, Howell JP: Pulmonary scar carcinoma: A case with two primaries. Cancer 54:361, 1984.

432. Turner-Warwick M, Lebowitz M, Burrows B, et al: Cryptogenic fibrosing alveolitis and lung cancer. Thorax 35:496, 1980.

433. Twersky J, Twersky N, Lehr C: Scleroderma and carcinoma of the lung. Clin Radiol 27:203, 1976.

434. Roumm AD, Medsger TA Jr: Cancer and systemic sclerosis: An epidemiologic study. Arthritis Rheum 28:1336, 1985.

435. Lee FI, Brain AT: Chronic diffuse interstitial pulmonary fibrosis and rheumatoid arthritis. Lancet 2:693, 1962.

436. Mellemkjaer L, Linet MS, Gridley G, et al: Rheumatoid arthritis and cancer risk. Eur J Cancer 32:1753, 1996.

437. Webb WR, Goodman PC: Fibrosing alveolitis in patients with neurofibro-matosis. Radiology 122:289, 1977.

438. De Scheerder T, Elinck W, Van Rentergham D, et al: Desquamative interstitial

pneumonia and scar cancer of the lung complicating generalised neurofibromatosis. Eur J Respir Dis 65:623, 1984.

439. Kuhara H, Wakabayashi T, Kishimoto H, et al: Lung cancer and chronic interstitial pneumonia associated with systemic sarcoidosis. Acta Pathol Jpn 35:199, 1985.

440. Noone PG, O'Brian DS, Luke D, et al: Adenocarcinoma of the lung in association with chronic sarcoidosis. Ir Med J 86:27, 1993.

441. Kuhara H, Wakabayashi T, Kishimoto H, et al: Synchronous bilateral double primary lung cancer associated with diffuse interstitial fibrosing pneumonitis (DIFP). Acta Pathol Jpn 34:617, 1984.

442. Fraire AE, Greenberg SD: Carcinoma and diffuse interstitial fibrosis of lung. Cancer 31:1078, 1972.

443. Meyer EC, Liebow AA: Relationship of interstitial pneumonia, honeycombing and atypical epithelial proliferation to cancer of the lung. Cancer 18:322, 1965.

444. Kawai T, Yakumaru K, Suzuki M, et al: Diffuse interstitial pulmonary fibrosis and lung cancer. Acta Pathol Jpn 37:11, 1987.

445. Lee HJ, Im JG, Ahn JM, et al: Lung cancer in patients with idiopathic pulmonary fibrosis: CT findings. J Comput Assist Tomogr 20:979, 1996.

446. Mizushima Y, Kobayashi M: Clinical characteristics of synchronous multiple lung cancer associated with idiopathic pulmonary fibrosis. Chest 108:1272, 1995.

447. Nishikawa A, Furukawa F, Imazawa T, et al: Cell proliferation in lung fibrosis-associated hyperplastic lesions. Hum Exp Toxicol 14:701, 1995.

448. Khalil N, O'Connor RN, Flanders KC, et al: TGF-beta 1, but not TGF-beta 2 or TGF-beta 3, is differentially present in epithelial cells of advanced pulmonary fibrosis: An immunohistochemical study. Am J Respir Cell Mol Biol 14:131, 1996.

449. Bohlmeyer T, Le TN, Shroyer AL, et al: Detection of human papillomavirus in squamous cell carcinomas of the lung by polymerase chain reaction. Am J Respir Cell Mol Biol 18:265, 1998.

450. Chen F-F, Yan J-J, Lai W-W, et al: Epstein-Barr virus–associated nonsmall cell lung carcinoma: Undifferentiated "lymphoepithelioma-like" carcinoma as a distinct entity with better prognosis. Cancer 82:2334, 1998.

451. Bobrowitz ID, Elkin M, Evans JC, et al: Effect of direct irradiation on the course of pulmonary tuberculosis (using cancerocidal doses). Dis Chest 40:397, 1961.

452. Woodruff CE, Barrett RJ, Champan PT, et al: Carcinoma of the chest with bone destruction. Am Rev Respir Dis 93:442, 1966.

453. Lee BW, Wain JC, Kelsey KT, et al: Association between diet and lung cancer location. Am J Respir Crit Care Med 158:1197, 1998.

454. Murasawa K, Altmann V: Primary lung cancer and pulmonary tuberculosis: A study based on 570 postmortem examinations. Sea View Hosp Bull 17:37, 1958.

455. Greenberg SD, Jenkins DE, Bahar D, et al: Co-existence of carcinoma and tuberculosis of the lung. Am Rev Respir Dis 90:67, 1964.

456. Kreuzer M, Kreienbrock L, Gerken M, et al: Risk factors for lung cancer in young adults. Am J Epidemiol 147:1028, 1998.

457. Holden HM, Quinlan JJ, Hiltz JE: Co-existing pulmonary tuberculosis and bronchogenic carcinoma: A report of 15 cases. Can Med Assoc J 93:1306, 1965.

458. Lazo BG, Feiner LL, Seriff NS: A study of routine cytologic screening of sputum for cancer in 800 men consecutively admitted to a tuberculosis service. Chest 65:646, 1974.

459. Wu AH, Fontham ET, Reynolds P, et al: Previous lung disease and risk of lung cancer among lifetime nonsmoking women in the United States. Am J Epidemiol 141:1023, 1995.

460. Alavanja MCR, Brownson RC, Boice JD, et al: Preexisting lung disease and lung cancer among nonsmoking women. Am J Epidemiol 136:623, 1992.

461. Vesterinen E, Pukkala E, Timonen T, et al: Cancer incidence among 78,000 asthmatic patients. Int J Epidemiol 22:976, 1993.

462. Campbell AH, Lee EJ: The relationship between lung cancer and chronic bronchitis. Br J Dis Chest 57:113, 1963.

463. Rimington J: Smoking, chronic bronchitis, and lung cancer. BMJ 2:373, 1971.

464. Lange P, Nyboe J, Appleyard M, et al: Ventilatory function and chronic mucus hypersecretion as predictors of death from lung cancer. Am Rev Respir Dis 141:613, 1990.

465. Islam SS, Schottenfeld D: Declining FEV1 and chronic productive cough in cigarette smokers: A 25-year prospective study of lung cancer incidence in Tecumseh, Michigan. Cancer Epidemiol Biomarkers Prev 3:289, 1994.

466. Nomura A, Stemmermann GN, Chyou PH, et al: Prospective study of pulmonary function and lung cancer. Am Res Respir Dis 144:307, 1991.

467. Tockman MS, Anthonisen NR, Wright EC, et al: Airways obstruction and the risk for lung cancer. Ann Intern Med 106:512, 1987.

468. Harper P, Oren A, Mohsenifar Z, et al: Obstructive airway disease as a risk factor for asbestos-associated malignancy. J Occup Environ Med 28:82, 1986.

469. Zulueta JJ, Bloom SM, Rozansky MI, et al: Lung cancer in patients with bullous disease. Am J Respir Crit Care Med 154:519, 1996.

470. Levesque MA, D'Costa M, Spratt EH, et al: Quantitative analysis of p53 protein in non–small cell lung cancer and its prognostic value. Int J Cancer 79:494, 1998.

471. Wu X, Zhao Y, Kemp BL, et al: Chromosome 5 aberrations and genetic predisposition to lung cancer. Int J Cancer 79:490, 1998.

472. Hennekens CH, Buring JE, Peto R: Antioxidant vitamins—benefits not yet proved. N Engl J Med 330:1080, 1994.

473. Koo LC: Diet and lung cancer 20+ years later: More questions than answers? Int J Cancer 10:22, 1997.

474. Lei YX, Cai WC, Chen YZ, et al: Some lifestyle factors in human lung cancer: A case-control study of 792 lung cancer cases. Lung Cancer 14:121, 1996.

475. Fraser GE, Beeson WL, Phillips RL: Diet and lung cancer in California Seventh-Day Adventists. Am J Epidemiol 133:683, 1991.

476. Mayne ST, Janerich DT, Greenwald P, et al: Dietary beta carotene and lung cancer risk in U.S. nonsmokers. J Natl Cancer Inst 86:33, 1994.

477. Ocke MC, Bueno-de-Mesquita HB, Feskens EJ: Repeated measurements of vegetables, fruits, beta-carotene and vitamins C and E in relation to lung cancer. The Zutphen study. Am J Epidemiol 145:358, 1997.

478. Rylander R, Axelsson G, Andersson L, et al: Lung cancer, smoking and diet among Swedish men. Lung Cancer 14:75, 1996.

479. Le Marchand L, Hankin JH, Bach F, et al: An ecological study of diet and lung cancer in the South Pacific. Int J Cancer 63:18, 1995.

480. Mayne ST, Janerich DT, Greenwald P, et al: Dietary beta carotene and lung cancer risk in U.S. nonsmokers. J Natl Cancer Inst 86:33, 1994.

481. Knekt P: Vitamin E and smoking and the risk of lung cancer. Ann N Y Acad Sci 686:280, 1993.

482. Dorgan JF, Ziegler RG, Schoenberg JB, et al: Race and sex differences in associations of vegetables, fruits, and carotenoids with lung cancer risk in New Jersey. Cancer Causes Control 4:273, 1993.

483. Pisani P, Berrino F, Macaluso M, et al: Carrots, green vegetables and lung cancer: A case-control study. Int J Epidemiol 15:463, 1986.

484. Bond GG, Thompson FE, Cook RR: Dietary vitamin A and lung cancer: Results of a case-control study among chemical workers. Nutr Cancer 9:109, 1987.

485. Wald N, Idle M, Boreham J, et al: Low serum vitamin A and subsequent risk of cancer. Lancet 2:813, 1980.

486. Chung FL, Morse MA, Eklind KI, et al: Inhibition of tobacco-specific nitrosamine-induced lung tumorigenesis by compounds derived from cruciferous vegetables and green tea. Ann N Y Acad Sci 686:186, 1993.

487. Anonymous: The effect of vitamin E and beta carotene on the incidence of lung cancer and other cancers in male smokers. N Engl J Med 330:1029, 1994.

488. Omenn GS, Goodman GE, Thornquist MD, et al: Effects of a combination of beta carotene and vitamin A on lung cancer and cardiovascular disease. N Engl J Med 334:1150, 1996.

489. Verhoeven DT, Goldbohm RA, van Poppel G, et al: Epidemiological studies on brassica vegetables and cancer risk. Cancer Epidemiol Biomarkers Prev 5:733, 1996.

490. Castonguay A: Pulmonary carcinogenesis and its prevention by dietary polyphenolic compounds. Ann N Y Acad Sci 686:177, 1993.

491. Ziegler RG, Mayne ST, Swanson CA: Nutrition and lung cancer. Cancer Causes Control 7:157, 1996.

492. Hinds MW, Kolonel LN, Hankin JH, et al: Dietary cholesterol and lung cancer risk in a multiethnic population in Hawaii. Int J Cancer 32:727, 1983.

493. Heilbrun LK, Nomura AM, Stemmermann GN: Dietary cholesterol and lung cancer risk among Japanese men in Hawaii. Am J Clin Nutr 39:375, 1984.

494. Wu Y, Zheng W, Sellers TA, et al: Dietary cholesterol, fat, and lung cancer incidence among older women: The Iowa Women's Health Study (United States). Cancer Causes Control 5:395, 1994.

495. Chyou PH, Nomura AM, Stemmermann GN, et al: Lung cancer: A prospective study of smoking, occupation and nutrient intake. Arch Environ Health 48:69, 1993.

496. De Stefani E, Fontham ET, Chen V, et al: Fatty foods and the risk of lung cancer: A case-control study from Uruguay. Int J Cancer 71:760, 1997.

497. Deneo-Pellegrini H, De Stefani E, Ronco A, et al: Meat consumption and risk of lung cancer: A case-control study from Uruguay. Lung Cancer 14:195, 1996.

498. Alavanja MC, Brownson RC, Benichou J: Estimating the effect of dietary fat on the risk of lung cancer in nonsmoking women. Lung Cancer 14:63, 1996.

499. Wynder EL, Hebert JR, Kabat GC: Association of dietary fat and lung cancer. J Natl Cancer Inst 79:631, 1987.

500. Hirvonen A: Genetic factors in individual responses to environmental exposures. J Occup Environ Med 37:37, 1995.

501. Ogawa H, Kato I, Tominaga S: Family history of cancer among cancer patients. Jpn J Cancer Res 76:113, 1985.

502. Lynch HT, Kimberling WJ, Markvicka SE, et al: Genetics and smoking-associated cancers: A study of 485 families. Cancer 57:1640, 1986.

503. Goltman TE, Hassinger DD, Mulvihill JJ: Familial respiratory tract cancer: Opportunities for research and prevention. JAMA 247:1020, 1982.

504. Harnden DG: Familial susceptibility to cancer (editorial). BMJ 286:1531, 1983.

505. Sellers TA, Doi WL, Elston RC, et al: Increased familial risk for nonlung cancer among relatives of lung cancer patients. Am J Epidemiol 126:237, 1987.

506. Tokuhata GK: Familial factors in human lung cancer and smoking. Am J Public Health 54:24, 1964.

507. Odi WL, Elston RC, Chen VW, et al: Increased familial risk for lung cancer. J Natl Cancer Inst 76:217, 1986.

508. Samet JM, Humble CG, Pathak DR: Personal and family history of respiratory disease and lung cancer risk. Am Rev Respir Dis 134:466, 1986.

509. Sellers TA, Bailey-Wilson JE, Potter JD, et al: Effect of cohort differences in smoking prevalence on models of lung cancer susceptibility. Genet Epidemiol 9:261, 1992.

510. Horwitz RI, Smaldone LF, Viscoli CM: An ecogenetic hypothesis for lung cancer in women. Arch Intern Med 148:2609, 1988.

511. Osann KE: Lung cancer in women: The importance of smoking, family history of cancer, and medical history of respiratory disease. Cancer Res 51:4893, 1991.

512. Bartsch H, Petruzzelli S, De Flora S, et al: Carcinogen metabolism in human lung tissues and the effect of tobacco smoking: Results from a case-control multicenter study on lung cancer patients. Environ Health Perspect 98:119, 1992.

513. Geneste O, Camus AM, Castegnaro M, et al: Comparison of pulmonary DNA adduct levels, measured by 32P-postlabelling and aryl hydrocarbon hydroxylase activity in lung parenchyma of smokers and ex-smokers. Carcinogenesis 12:1301, 1991.

514. Yoshikawa M, Arashidani K, Kawamoto T, et al: Aryl hydrocarbon hydroxylase activity in human lung tissue: In relation to cigarette smoking and lung cancer. Environ Res 65:1, 1994.

515. Kawajiri K, Eguchi H, Nakachi K, et al: Association of CYP1A1 germ line polymorphisms with mutations of the p53 gene in lung cancer. Cancer Res 56:72, 1996.

516. Okada T, Kawashima K, Fukushi S, et al: Association between a cytochrome P450 CYP1A1 genotype and incidence of lung cancer. Pharmacogenetics 4:333, 1994.

517. Hirvonen A, Husgafvel-Pursiainen K, Anttila S, et al: PCR-based CYP2D6 genotyping for Finnish lung cancer patients. Pharmacogenetics 3:19, 1993.

518. Xu X, Kelsey KT, Wiencke JK, et al: Cytochrome P450 CYP1A1 MspI polymorphism and lung cancer susceptibility. Cancer Epidemiol Biomarkers Prev 5:687, 1996.

519. El-Zein RA, Zwischenberger JB, Abdel-Rahman SZ, et al: Polymorphism of metabolizing genes and lung cancer histology: Prevalence of CYP2E1 in adeno-carcinoma. Cancer Lett 112:71, 1997.

520. Oyama T, Kawamoto T, Mizoue T, et al: Cytochrome P450 2E1 polymorphism as a risk factor for lung cancer: In relation to p53 gene mutation. Anticancer Res 17:583, 1997.

521. Bouchardy C, Benhamou S, Dayer P: The effect of tobacco on lung cancer risk depends on CYP2D6 activity. Cancer Res 56:251, 1996.

522. Crespi CL, Penman BW, Gelboin HV, et al: A tobacco smoke-derived nitrosa-mine, 4-(methylnitrosamino)-1-(3-pyridyl)-1-butanone, is activated by multiple human cytochrome P450s including the polymorphic human cytochrome P4502D6. Carcinogenesis 12:1197, 1991.

523. Agundez JA, Martinez C, Ladero JM, et al: Debrisoquine oxidation genotype and susceptibility to lung cancer. Clin Pharmacol Ther 55:10, 1994.

524. Puchetti V, Faccini GB, Micciolo R, et al: Dextromethorphan test for evaluation of congenital predisposition to lung cancer. Chest 105:449, 1994.

525. Bartsch H, Hietanen E: The role of individual susceptibility in cancer burden related to environmental exposure. Environ Health Perspect 3:569, 1996.

526. Nakajima T, Elovaara E, Anttila S, et al: Expression and polymorphism of glutathione S-transferase in human lungs: Risk factors in smoking-related lung cancer. Carcinogenesis 16:707, 1995.

527. Seidegard J, Pero RW, Markowitz MM, et al: Isoenzyme(s) of glutathione transferase (class Mu) as a marker for the susceptibility to lung cancer: A follow-up study. Carcinogenesis 11:33, 1990.

528. Miller YE, Franklin WA: Molecular events in lung carcinogenesis. Hematol Oncol Clin North Am 11:215, 1997.

529. Minna JD: The molecular biology of lung cancer pathogenesis. Chest 103:449, 1993.

530. Salgia R, Skarin AT: Molecular abnormalities in lung cancer. J Clin Oncol 16:1207, 1998.

531. Testa JR, Liu Z, Feder M, et al: Advances in the analysis of chromosome alterations in human lung carcinomas. Cancer Genet Cytogenet 95:20, 1998.

532. Devereux TR, Taylor JA, Barrett JC: Molecular mechanisms of lung cancer—interaction of environmental and genetic factors. Chest 109:14, 1996.

533. Hamm RD: Occupational cancer in the oncogene era. Br J Ind Med 47:217, 1990.

534. Filderman AE, Matthay RA: Bronchogenic carcinoma. In Bone RC, Dantzker DR, George RB, et al (eds): Pulmonary and Critical Care Medicine. St. Louis, Mosby, 1997.

535. Anderson MLM, Spandidos DA: Oncogenes and onco-suppressor genes in lung cancer. Respir Med 87:413, 1993.

536. Lorenz J, Friedberg T, Paulus R, et al: Oncogene overexpression in nonsmall-cell lung cancer tissue: Prevalence and clinicopathological significance. Clin Invest 72:156, 1994.

537. Slebos RJC, Kibbelaar RE, Dalesio O, et al: K-Ras oncogene activation as a prognostic marker in adenocarcinoma of the lung. N Engl J Med 323:561, 1990.

538. Kashii T, Mizushima Y, Lima CE, et al: Studies on clinicopathological features of lung cancer patients with K-ras/p53 gene alterations: Comparison between younger and older groups. Oncology 52:219, 1995.

539. Kern JA, Schwartz DA, Nordberg JE, et al: P185neu expression in human lung adenocarcinomas predicts shortened survival. Cancer Res 50:5184, 1990.

540. Pezzella F, Turley H, Kuzu I, et al: bcl-2 protein in nonsmall-cell lung carci-noma. N Engl J Med 329:690, 1993.

541. Kitagawa Y, Wong F, Lo P, et al: Overexpression of Bcl-2 and mutations in p53 and K-ras in resected human non–small cell lung cancers. Am J Respir Cell Mol Biol 15:45, 1996.

542. Szabo E, Riffe ME, Steinberg SM, et al: Altered cJUN expression: An early event in human lung carcinogenesis. Cancer Res 56:305, 1996.

543. Guinee DG Jr, Travis WD, Trivers GE, et al: Gender comparisons in human lung cancer: Analysis of p53 mutations, anti-p53 serum antibodies and C-erbB-2 expression. Carcinogenesis 16:993, 1995.

544. Yu CJ, Shun CT, Yang PC, et al: Sialomucin expression is associated with erbB-2 oncoprotein overexpression, early recurrence, and cancer death in non-small-cell lung cancer. Am J Respir Crit Care Med 155:1419, 1997.

545. Kern JA, Filderman AE: Oncogenes and growth factors in human lung cancer. Clin Chest Med 14:31, 1993.

546. Weintraub SJ: Inactivation of tumor suppressor proteins in lung cancer. Am J Respir Cell Mol Biol 15:150, 1996.

547. Xu HJ, Quinlan DC, Davidson AG, et al: Altered retinoblastoma protein expression and prognosis in early-stage nonsmall-cell lung carcinoma. J Natl Cancer Inst 86:695, 1994.

548. Lung ML, Wong MP, Skaanild MT, et al: p53 mutations in non–small cell lung carcinomas in Hong Kong. Chest 109:718, 1996.

549. Nuorva K, Soini Y, Kamel D, et al: Concurrent p53 expression in bronchial dysplasias and squamous cell lung carcinomas. Am J Pathol 142:725, 1993.

550. Boers JE, Ten Velde GPM, Thunnissen FBJM: p53 in squamous metaplasia: A marker for risk of respiratory tract carcinoma. Am J Respir Crit Care Med 153:411, 1996.

551. Ebina M, Steinberg SM, Mulshine JL, et al: Relationship of p53 overexpression and up-regulation of proliferating cell nuclear antigen with the clinical course of non–small cell lung cancer. Cancer Res 54:2496, 1994.

552. Fujino M, Dosaka-Akita H, Harada M, et al: Prognostic significance of p53 and ras p21 expression in non–small cell lung cancer. Cancer 76:2457, 1995.

553. Woll PJ: Growth factors and lung cancer. Thorax 46:924, 1991.

554. Yamaguchi K, Imanishi KI, Maruno K, et al: Lung cancer and autocrine growth factors. Chest 96:29, 1989.

555. Minna JD: Genetic events in the pathogenesis of lung cancer. Chest 96:17, 1989.

556. Sundaresan V, Heppell-Parton A, Coleman N, et al: Somatic genetic changes in lung cancer and precancerous lesions. Ann Oncol 1:27, 1995.

557. Merlo A, Gabrielson E, Mabry M, et al: Homozygous deletion on chromosome 9p and loss of heterozygosity on 9q, 6p, and 6q in primary human small cell lung cancer. Cancer Res 54:2322, 1994.

558. Pastorino U, Sozzi G, Miozzo M, et al: Genetic changes in lung cancer. J Cell Biochem 17(Suppl):237, 1993.

559. Shiseki M, Kohno T, Nishikawa R, et al: Frequent allelic losses on chromo-somes 2q, 18q, and 22q in advanced non–small cell lung carcinoma. Cancer Res 54:5643, 1994.

560. Savage AM, Pritchard JAV, Deeley TJ, et al: Immunological state of patients with carcinoma of the bronchus before and after radiotherapy. Thorax 35:500, 1980.

561. Anthony HM, Madsen KE, Mason MK, et al: Lung cancer, immune status, histopathology and smoking: Is oat cell carcinoma lymphodependent? Br J Dis Chest 75:40, 1981.

562. Giuliano AE, Rangel D, Golub SH, et al: Serum-mediated immunosuppression in lung cancer. Cancer 43:917, 1979.

563. Brugarolas A, Takita H: Immunologic status in lung cancer. Chest 64:427, 1973.

564. Pisani RJ: Bronchogenic carcinoma: Immunologic aspects. Mayo Clin Proc 68:386, 1993.

565. Kurosawa S, Matsuzaki G, Harada M, et al: Early appearance and activation of natural killer cells in tumor-infiltrating lymphoid cells during tumor develop-ment. Eur J Immunol 23:1029, 1993.

566. Feo Figarella F, Morillo F, Blanca I, et al: Failure of cell-mediated effector mechanisms in lung cancer. J Natl Cancer Inst 73:1, 1984.

567. Fujisawa T, Yamaguchi Y: Autologous tumor killing activity as a prognostic factor in primary resected non–small cell carcinoma of the lung. Cancer 79:474, 1997.

568. Weissler JC, Nicod LP, Toews GB: Pulmonary natural killer cell activity is reduced in patients with bronchogenic carcinoma. Am Rev Respir Dis 135:1353, 1987.

569. Tollerud DJ, Clark JW, Morris Brown L, et al: Association of cigarette smoking with decreased numbers of circulating natural killer cells. Am Rev Respir Dis 139:194, 1989.

570. Kimura H, Yamaguchi Y: Adjuvant immunotherapy with interleukin 2 and lymphokine-activated killer cells after noncurative resection of primary lung cancer. Lung Cancer 13:31, 1995.

571. LeFever A, Funahashi A: Lymphokine-activated killer cell activity in lung cancer. Chest 99:292, 1991.

572. Melis M, Spatafora M, Melodia A, et al: ICAM-1 expression by lung cancer cell lines: Effects of upregulation by cytokines on the interaction with LAK cells. Eur Respir J 9:1831, 1996.

573. Ferrarini M, Heltai S, Pupa SM, et al: Killing of laminin receptor-positive human lung cancers by tumor infiltrating lymphocytes bearing gamma delta (+) T-cell receptors. J Natl Cancer Inst 88:436, 1996.

574. Takenoyama M, Yasumoto K, Harada M, et al: Expression of activation-related molecules on regional lymph node lymphocytes in human lung cancer. Immunobiology 195:140, 1996.

575. Fujisawa T, Yamaguchi Y: Autologous tumor killing activity as a prognostic factor in primary resected non–small cell carcinoma of the lung. Cancer 79:474, 1997.

576. Meta M, Ponte M, Guastella M, et al: Detection of oligoclonal T lymphocytes in lymph nodes draining from advanced nonsmall-cell lung cancer. Cancer Immunol Immunother 40:235, 1995.

577. Kubota M, Kagamimori S, Yokoyama K, et al: Reduced killer cell activity of lymphocytes from patients with asbestosis. Br J Ind Med 42:276, 1985.

578. Takeo S, Yasumoto K, Nagashima A, et al: Role of tumor-associated macro-phages in lung cancer. Cancer Res 46:3179, 1986.

579. Venkataraman M, Rao DS, Levin RD, et al: Suppression of B-lymphocyte function by T-lymphocytes in patients with advanced lung cancer. J Natl Cancer Inst 74:37, 1985.

580. Jansen HM, The TH, de Gast GC, et al: The primary immune response of patients with different stages of squamous-cell bronchial carcinoma. Thorax 33:755, 1978.

581. Bousquet J, Pujol JL, Barneon G, et al: Skin test reactivity in patients suffering from lung and breast cancer. J Allergy Clin Immunol 87:1066, 1991.

582. McDuffie HH, Cockcroft DW, Talebi Z, et al: Lower prevalence of positive atopic skin tests in lung cancer patients. Chest 93:241, 1988.

583. Winter SF, Sekido Y, Minna JD, et al: Antibodies against autologous tumor cell proteins in patients with small-cell lung cancer: Associated with improved survival. J Natl Cancer Inst 85:2012, 1993.

584. Marchesani W: Über den primären bronchialkrebs. Frankfurter Pathol 30:158, 1924.

585. Muller K-M: Histological classification and histogenesis of lung cancer. Eur J Respir Dis 65:4, 1984.

586. Kreyberg L, in collaboration with Liebow AA, Euhlinger EA: Histological Typing of Lung Tumors. Issued by World Health Organization, International Reference Center for the Histological Definition and Classification of Lung Tumors, Geneva, 1967.

587. Yesner R, Gerstl B, Auerbach O: Application of the World Health Organization classification of lung carcinoma to biopsy material. Ann Thorac Surg 1:33, 1965.

588. Matthews MJ: Panel report: Morphologic classification of bronchogenic carcinoma. Cancer Chemother Rep 4:299, 1973.

589. Kreyberg L: International histological classification of tumours. In Histological Typing of Lung Tumours. Geneva, World Health Organization, 1981.

590. Roth JA: Molecular events in lung cancer. Lung Cancer 12(Suppl):3, 1995.

591. Sobin LH: The histologic classification of lung tumors: The need for a double standard. Hum Pathol 14:1020, 1983.

592. Nash G: The diagnosis of lung cancer in the 80s: Will routine light microscopy suffice? Hum Pathol 14:1021, 1983.

593. Dunnill MS, Gatter KC: Cellular heterogeneity in lung cancer. Histopathology 10:461, 1986.

594. Elema JD, Kenning WM: The use of electron microscopy for the diagnosis of cancer in bronchial biopsies. Hum Pathol 19:304, 1988.

595. Gatter KC, Dunnill MS, Pulford KA, et al: Human lung tumours: A correlation of antigenic profile with histological type. Histopathology 9:805, 1985.

596. Reinila A, Dammert K: An attempt to use the WHO typing in the histological classification of lung carcinomas. Acta Pathol Microbiol Scand 82:783, 1974.

597. Hirsch FR, Matthews MJ, Yesner R: Histopathologic classification of small cell carcinoma of the lung. Cancer 50:1360, 1982.

598. Roggli VL, Vollmer RT, Greenberg SD, et al: Lung cancer heterogeneity: A blinded and randomized study of 100 consecutive cases. Hum Pathol 16:569, 1985.

599. Vollmer RT, Ogden L, Crissman JD: Separation of small-cell from nonsmall-cell lung cancer. Arch Pathol Lab Med 108:792, 1984.

600. Wagenaar SS: Preliminary results of the pathological review of a small cell lung cancer trial (EORTC 08825). Eur J Respir Dis 70:63, 1987.

601. Fraire AE, Johnson EH, Yesner R, et al: Prognostic significance of histopathologic subtype and stage in small cell lung cancer. Hum Pathol 23:520, 1992.

602. Auerbach O, Garfinkel L, Parks VR: Histologic type of lung cancer in relation to smoking habits, year of diagnosis and sites of metastases. Chest 67:382, 1975.

603. Feinstein AR, Gelfman NA, Yesner R, et al: Observer variability in the histopathologic diagnosis of lung cancer. Am Rev Respir Dis 101:671, 1970.

604. Haratake J, Horie A, Tokudome S, et al: Inter- and intra-pathologist variability in histologic diagnoses of lung cancer. Acta Pathol Jpn 37:1053, 1987.

605. Cox JD, Yesner R, Mietlowski W, et al: Influence of cell type on failure pattern after irradiation for locally advanced carcinoma of the lung. Cancer 44:94, 1979.

606. Jacques J, Hill DP, Shier KJ, et al: Appraisal of the World Health Organization classification of lung tumours. Can Med Assoc J 122:897, 1980.

607. Thomas JStJ, Lamb D, Ashcroft T, et al: How reliable is the diagnosis of lung cancer using small biopsy specimens? Report of a UKCCCR* Lung Cancer Working Party. Thorax 48:1135, 1993.

608. Chuang MT, Marchevsky A, Teirstein AS, et al: Diagnosis of lung cancer by fibreoptic bronchoscopy: Problems in the histological classification of non–small cell carcinomas. Thorax 39:175, 1984.

609. Yoshida Y: A correlation between mutation of the p53 gene and histological heterogeneity in differentiated adenocarcinomas of the lung, with reference to stepwise progression and metastatic ability. Hiroshima J Med Sci 43:13, 1994.

610. Yoneda K, Boucher LD: Bronchial epithelial changes associated with small cell carcinoma of the lung. Hum Pathol 24:1180, 1993.

611. Lisa JR, Trinidad S, Rosenblatt MB: Site of origin, histogenesis, and cytostructure of bronchogenic carcinoma. Am J Clin Pathol 44:375, 1965.

612. Melamed MR, Zaman MB, Flehinger BJ, et al: Radiologically occult in situ and incipient invasive epidermoid lung cancer: Detection by sputum cytology in a survey of asymptomatic cigarette smokers. Am J Surg Pathol 1:5, 1977.

613. Nagamoto N, Saito Y, Sato M, et al: Clinicopathological analysis of 19 cases of isolated carcinoma in situ of the bronchus. Am J Surg Pathol 17:1234, 1993.

614. Nagamoto N, Saito Y, Suda H, et al: Relationship between length of longitudinal extension and maximal depth of transmural invasion and roentgenographically occult squamous cell carcinoma of the bronchus (nonpolypoid type). Am J Surg Pathol 13:11, 1989.

615. Dulmet-Brender E, Jaubert F, Huchon G: Exophytic endobronchial epidermoid carcinoma. Cancer 57:1358, 1986.

616. Carter D: Squamous cell carcinoma of the lung: An update. Semin Diagn Pathol 2:226, 1985.

617. Carter D: Pathology of early squamous cell carcinoma of the lungs. Pathol Annu 13:131, 1978.

618. Hind CRK: Lobar infiltration by squamous cell carcinoma. Thorax 35:633, 1980.

619. Sidhu GS: The ultrastructure of malignant epithelial neoplasms of the lung. Pathol Annu 17:235, 1982.

620. Edwards C, Carlile A: Poorly differentiated squamous carcinoma of the bronchus: A light and electron microscopic study. J Clin Pathol 39:284, 1986.

621. Dingemans KP, Mooi WJ: Ultrastructure of squamous cell carcinoma of the lung. Pathol Annu 19:249, 1984.

622. Saba SR, Espinoza CG, Richman AV, et al: Carcinomas of the lung: An ultrastructural and immunocytochemical study. Am J Clin Pathol 80:6, 1983.

623. McDowell EM, McLaughlin JS, Merenyl DK, et al: The respiratory epithelium. V. Histogenesis of lung carcinomas in the human. J Natl Cancer Inst 61:587, 1978.

624. Heard BE, Dewar A: Squamous cell carcinoma of bronchus: Polypoid granules and mitochondrial densities found by electron microscopy. Diagn Histopathol 5:189, 1982.

625. Ilardi CF, Faro JC: Localization of parathyroid hormone-like substance in squamous cell carcinomas. Arch Pathol Lab Med 109:752, 1985.

626. Banks-Schlegel SP, McDowell EM, Wilson TS, et al: Keratin proteins in human lung carcinomas. Am J Pathol 114:273, 1984.

627. Schlegel R, Banks-Schlegel S, McLeod JA, et al: Immunoperoxidase localization of keratin in human neoplasms. Am J Pathol 101:41, 1980.

628. Harach HR, Skinner M, Gibbs AR: Biological markers in human lung carcinoma: An immunopathological study of six antigens. Thorax 38:937, 1983.

629. Bensch KG, Corrin B, Pariente R, et al: Oat-cell carcinoma of the lung: Its origin and relationship to bronchial carcinoid. Cancer 22:1163, 1968.

630. Tischler AS, Dichter MA, Biales B: Electrical excitability of oat cell carcinoma. J Pathol 122:153, 1977.

631. Clark RK, Miettinen M, Leij L, et al: Terminally differentiated derivatives of pulmonary small cell carcinomas may contain neurofilaments. Lab Invest 53:243, 1985.

632. Moss F, Bobrow LG, Sheppard MN, et al: Expression of epithelial and neural antigens in small cell and non–small cell lung carcinoma. J Pathol 149:103, 1986.

633. Sorenson GD, Pettengill OS, Brinck-Johnsen T, et al: Hormone production by cultures of small-cell carcinoma of the lung. Cancer 47:1289, 1981.

634. Gould VE, Warren WH, Memoli VA: Neuroendocrine neoplasms of the lung. In Becker KL, Gazdar AF (eds): The Endocrine Lung in Health and Disease. Philadelphia, WB Saunders, 1984, p 406.

635. McDowell EM, Trump BF: Pulmonary small cell carcinoma showing tripartite differentiation in individual cells. Hum Pathol 12:286, 1981.

636. Churg A, Johnston WH, Stulbarg M: Small cell squamous and mixed small cell squamous–small cell anaplastic carcinomas of the lung. Am J Surg Pathol 4:255, 1980.

637. Said JW, Vimadalal S, Nash G, et al: Immunoreactive neuron-specific enolase, bombesin, and chromogranin as markers for neuroendocrine lung tumors. Hum Pathol 16:236, 1985.

638. McDowell EM, Wilson TS, Trump BF: Atypical endocrine tumors of the lung. Arch Pathol Lab Med 105:20, 1981.

639. Carter D: Small-cell carcinoma of the lung. Am J Surg Pathol 7:787, 1983.

640. Yesner R: Small cell tumors of the lung. Am J Surg Pathol 7:775, 1983.

641. Kreisman H, Wolkove N, Quoix E: Small cell lung cancer presenting as a solitary pulmonary nodule. Chest 101:225, 1992.

642. Gephardt GN, Grady KJ, Ahmad M, et al: Peripheral small cell undifferentiated carcinoma of the lung: Clinicopathologic features of 17 cases. Cancer 61:1002, 1988.

643. Hirsch FR, Matthews MJ, Aisner S, et al: Histopathologic classification of small cell lung cancer. Cancer 62:973, 1988.

644. Terasaki T, Kameya T, Nakajima T, et al: Interconversion of biological characteristics of small cell lung cancer depending on culture conditions. Gann 75:1089, 1984.

645. Vollmer RT: The effect of cell size on the pathologic diagnosis of small and large cell carcinomas of the lung. Cancer 50:1380, 1982.

646. Nomori H, Shimosato Y, Kodama T, et al: Subtypes of small cell carcinoma of the lung: Morphometric, ultrastructural, and immunohistochemical analyses. Hum Pathol 17:604, 1986.

647. Bepler G, Neumann K, Holle R, et al: Clinical relevance of histologic subtyping in small cell lung cancer. Cancer 64:74, 1989.

648. Davenport RD: Diagnostic value of crush artefact in cytologic specimens: Occurrence in small cell carcinoma of the lung. Acta Cytol 34:502, 1990.

649. Tsubota YT, Kawaguchi T, Hoso T, et al: A combined small cell and spindle cell carcinoma of the lung: Report of a unique case with immunohistochemical and ultrastructural studies. Am J Surg Pathol 16:1108, 1992.

650. Mangum MD, Greco FA, Hainsworth JD, et al: Combined small-cell and nonsmall-cell lung cancer. J Clin Oncol 7:607, 1989.

651. Yoneda K, Boucher LD: Bronchial epithelial changes associated with small cell carcinoma of the lung. Hum Pathol 24:1180, 1993.

652. Gazdar AF, Carney DN, Nau MM, et al: Characterization of variant subclasses of cell lines derived from small cell lung cancer having distinctive biochemical, morphological, and growth properties. Cancer Res 45:2924, 1985.

653. Hirsch FR, Osterlind K, Hansen HH: The prognostic significance of histopathologic subtyping of small cell carcinoma of the lung according to the classification of the World Health Organization. Cancer 52:2144, 1983.

654. Vollmer RT, Birch R, Ogden L, et al: Subclassification of small cell cancer of the lung: The Southeastern Cancer Study Group experience. Hum Pathol 16:247, 1985.

655. Radice PA, Matthews MJ, Ihde DC, et al: The clinical behavior of "mixed"

small cell/large cell bronchogenic carcinoma compared to "pure" small cell subtypes. Cancer 50:2894, 1982.

656. Bégin P, Sahai S, Wang N-S: Giant cell formation in small cell carcinoma of the lung. Cancer 52:1875, 1983.

657. Sehested M, Hirsch FR, Osterlind K, et al: Morphologic variations of small cell lung cancer: A histopathologic study of pretreatment and posttreatment specimens in 104 patients. Cancer 57:804, 1986.

658. Kasimis BS, Wuerker RB, Hunt JD, et al: Relationship between changes in the histologic subtype of small cell carcinoma of the lung and the response to chemotherapy. Am J Clin Oncol 9:318, 1986.

659. Brereton HD, Mathews MM, Costa J, et al: Mixed anaplastic small-cell and squamous-cell carcinoma of the lung. Ann Intern Med 88:805, 1978.

660. Abeloff MD, Eggleston JC, Mendelsohn G, et al: Changes in morphologic and biochemical characteristics of small cell carcinoma of the lung. Am J Med 66:757, 1979.

661. Bellocq A, Antoine M, Flahault A, et al: Neutrophil alveolitis in bronchioloalveolar carcinoma: Induction by tumor-derived interleukin-8 and relation to clinical outcome. An J Pathol 152:83, 1998.

662. Vollmer RT, Shelburne JD, Iglehart JD: Intercellular junctions and tumor stage in small cell carcinoma of the lung. Hum Pathol 18:22, 1986.

663. Fisher ER, Palekar A, Paulson JD: Comparative histopathologic, histochemical, electron microscopic and tissue culture studies of bronchial carcinoids and oat cell carcinomas of lung. Am J Clin Pathol 69:165, 1978.

664. Tateishi R, Horai T, Hattori S: Demonstration of argyrophil granules in small cell carcinoma of the lung. Virchows Arch [Pathol Anat] 377:203, 1978.

665. Hattori S, Matsuda M, Tateishi R, et al: Oat-cell carcinoma of the lung: Clinical and morphological studies in relation to its histogenesis. Cancer 30:1014, 1972.

666. Mooi WJ, Dingemans KP, Van Zandwijk N: Prevalence of neuroendocrine granules in small cell lung cancer: Usefulness of electron microscopy in lung cancer classification. J Pathol 149:41, 1986.

667. Hage E, Hansen M, Hirsch FR: Electron microscopic sub-classification of small cell carcinoma of the lung. Acta Pathol Jpn 33:671, 1983.

668. Nomori H, Shimosato Y, Kodama T, et al: Subtypes of small cell carcinoma of the lung: Morphometric, ultrastructural, and immunohistochemical analyses. Hum Pathol 17:604, 1986.

669. Yoshida Y, Mori M, Sonoda T, et al: Ultrastructural, immunohistochemical, and biochemical studies on amylase and ACTH producing lung cancer. Virchows Arch [Pathol Anat] 408:163, 1985.

670. Guinee D, Fishback NF, Koss MN, et al: Diagnostic utility of immunohistochemistry in small cell lung carcinoma in transbronchial and open lung biopsies. Am J Clin Pathol 102:406, 1994.

671. Travis WD, Linnoila RI, Tsokos MG, et al: Neuroendocrine tumors of the lung with proposed criteria for large-cell neuroendocrine carcinoma: An ultrastructural, immunohistochemical, and flow cytometric study of 35 cases. Am J Surg Pathol 15:529, 1991.

672. Michels S, Swanson PE, Robb JA, et al: Leu-7 in small cell neoplasms: An immunohistochemical study with ultrastructural correlations. Cancer 60:2958, 1987.

673. Korkolopoulou P, Oates J, Crocker J, et al: p53 expression in oat and nonoat small cell lung carcinomas: Correlations with proliferating cell nuclear antigen. J Clin Pathol 46:1093, 1993.

674. Fukayama M, Hayashi Y, Koike M, et al: Human chorionic gonadotropin lung and lung tumors. Lab Invest 55:433, 1986.

675. Asa SL, Kovacs K, Vale W, et al: Immunohistologic localization of corticotropin-releasing hormone in human tumors. Am J Clin Pathol 87:327, 1987.

676. Manning JT Jr, Spjut HJ, Tschen JA: Bronchioloalveolar carcinoma: The significance of two histopathologic types. Cancer 54:525, 1984.

677. Schraufnagel D, Peloquin A, Paré JAP, et al: Differentiating bronchioloalveolar carcinoma from adenocarcinoma. Am Rev Respir Dis 125:74, 1982.

678. Edwards CW: Pulmonary adenocarcinoma: Review of 106 cases and proposed new classification. J Clin Pathol 40:125, 1987.

679. Rossmann P, Vortel V: Pulmonary metastases imitating alveolar-cell carcinoma. J Pathol Bacteriol 81:313, 1961.

680. Rosenblatt MB, Lisa JR, Collier F: Primary and metastatic bronchiolo-alveolar carcinoma. Dis Chest 52:147, 1967.

681. Ogata T, Endo K: Clara cell granules of peripheral lung cancers. Cancer 54:1635, 1984.

682. Kimula Y: A histochemical and ultrastructural study of adenocarcinoma of the lung. Am J Surg Pathol 2:253, 1978.

683. Bedrossian CWM, Weilbaecher DG, Bentinck DC, et al: Ultrastructure of human bronchioloalveolar cell carcinoma. Cancer 36:1399, 1975.

684. Rainio P, Sutinen S, Sutinen SH: Histological subtypes or grading of pulmonary adenocarcinoma. Acta Pathol Microbiol Immunol Scand 91:227, 1983.

685. Edwards CW: Alveolar carcinoma: A review. Thorax 39:166, 1984.

685a. Silver SA, Askin FB: True papillary carcinoma of the lung: A distinct clinicopathologic entity. Am J Surg Pathol 21:43, 1997.

686. Bolen JW, Thorning D: Histogenetic classification of pulmonary carcinomas. In Sommers SC, Rosen PP (eds): Pathology Annual, Vol. 77, Norwalk, CT, Appleton-Century-Crofts, 1982.

687. Singh G, Katyal SL, Torikata C: Carcinoma of type II pneumocytes. Am J Pathol 102:195, 1981.

688. Dermer GB: Origin of bronchioloalveolar carcinoma and peripheral bronchial adenocarcinoma. Cancer 49:881, 1982.

689. Greenberg SD, Smith MN, Spjut HJ: Bronchiolo-alveolar carcinoma: Cell of origin. Am J Clin Pathol 63:153, 1975.

690. Sidhu GS, Forrester EM: Glycogen-rich Clara cell-type bronchiolo-alveolar carcinoma. Cancer 40:2209, 1977.

691. Nakamura M, Itoh K, Honda Y, et al: A case of bronchioloalveolar carcinoma. Cancer 52:861, 1983.

692. Morningstar WA, Hassan MO: Bronchiolo-alveolar carcinoma with nodal metastases. Am J Surg Pathol 3:273, 1979.

693. Espinoza CG, Balis JU, Saba SR, et al: Ultrastructural and immunohistochemical studies of bronchiolo-alveolar carcinoma. Cancer 54:2182, 1984.

694. Dermer GB: Autoradiography of cellular glycoproteins reveals histogenesis of bronchogenic adenocarcinomas. Cancer 47:2000, 1981.

695. Kodama T, Shimosato Y, Koide T, et al: Endobronchial polypoid adenocarcinoma of the lung. Am J Surg Pathol 8:845, 1984.

696. Sheffield EA, Addis BJ, Corrin B, et al: Epithelial hyperplasia and malignant change in congenital lung cysts. J Clin Pathol 40:612, 1987.

697. Prichard MG, Brown PJE, Sterrett GF: Bronchioloalveolar carcinoma arising in longstanding lung cysts. Thorax 39:545, 1984.

698. Bennett DE, Sasser WF, Ferguson TB: Adenocarcinoma of the lung in men. Cancer 23:431, 1969.

699. Higashiyama M, Doi O, Kodama K, et al: Extramammary Paget's disease of the bronchial epithelium. Arch Pathol Lab Med 115:185, 1991.

700. Dixon AY, Moran JF, Wesselius LJ, et al: Pulmonary mucinous cystic tumor: Case report with review of the literature. Am J Surg Pathol 17:722, 1993.

701. Sfrensen JB, Hirsch FR, Olsen J: The prognostic implication of histopathologic subtyping of pulmonary adenocarcinoma according to the classification of the World Health Organization: An analysis of 259 consecutive patients with advanced disease. Cancer 62:361, 1988.

702. Sfrensen JB, Olsen JE: Prognostic implications of histopathologic subtyping in patients with surgically treated stage I or II adenocarcinoma of the lung. J Thorac Cardiovasc Surg 97:245, 1989.

703. Scroggs MW, Roggli VL, Fraire AE, et al: Eosinophilic intracytoplasmic globules in pulmonary adenocarcinomas: A histochemical, immunohistochemical, and ultrastructural study of six cases. Hum Pathol 20:845, 1989.

704. Kish JK, Ro JY, Ayala AG, et al: Primary mucinous adenocarcinoma of the lung with signet-ring cells: A histochemical comparison with signet-ring cell carcinomas of other sites. Hum Pathol 20:1097, 1989.

705. Katzenstein A-LA, Prioleau PG, Askin FB: The histologic spectrum and significance of clear-cell change in lung carcinoma. Cancer 45:943, 1980.

706. Edwards C, Carlile A: Clear cell carcinoma of the lung. J Clin Pathol 38:880, 1985.

707. Adachi H, Aki T, Yoshida H, et al: Combined choriocarcinoma and adenocarcinoma of the lung. Acta Pathol Jpn 39:147, 1989.

708. Fishback NF, Travis WD, Moran CA, et al: Pleomorphic (spindle/giant cell) carcinoma of the lung: A clinicopathologic correlation of 78 cases. Cancer 73:2936, 1994.

708a. Dumont P, Gasser B, Rougé C, et al: Bronchoalveolar carcinoma: Histopathologic study of evolution in a series of 105 surgically treated patients. Chest 113:391, 1998.

709. Clayton F: Bronchioloalveolar carcinomas. Cancer 57:1555, 1986.

710. Ohori NP, Yousem SA, Griffin J, et al: Comparison of extracellular matrix antigens in subtypes of bronchioloalveolar carcinoma and conventional pulmonary adenocarcinoma: An immunohistochemical study. Am J Surg Pathol 16:675, 1992.

711. Nakanishi K, Kawai T, Suzuki M: Large intracytoplasmic body in lung cancer compared with Clara cell granule. Am J Clin Pathol 88:472, 1987.

712. Unterman DH, Reingold IM: The occurrence of psammoma bodies in papillary adenocarcinoma of the lung. Am J Clin Pathol 57:297, 1972.

713. London SB, Winter WJ: Calcification within carcinoma of the lung: Report of a case with isolated pulmonary nodule. Arch Intern Med 94:151, 1954.

714. Gupta PK, Verma K: Calcified (psammoma) bodies in alveolar cell carcinoma of the lung. Acta Cytol 16:59, 1972.

715. Silverman JF, Finley JL, Park HK, et al: Psammoma bodies and optically clear nuclei in bronchiolo-alveolar cell carcinoma: Diagnosis by fine needle aspiration biopsy with histologic and ultrastructural confirmation. Diagn Cytopathol 1:205, 1985.

716. Oka S, Konno J, Suzuki S: Differential diagnosis of solitary round shadow of the lung. Jpn J Chest Dis 22:361, 1963.

717. Kay S: Morphologic aspects of nuclear bodies in a case of bronchiolar-alveolar carcinoma of the lung. Hum Pathol 8:224, 1977.

718. Sheppard MN, Thurlow NP, Dewar A: Amphicrine differentiation in bronchioloalveolar cell carcinoma. Ultrastruct Pathol 18:437, 1994.

719. Tsao M-S, Fraser RS: Primary pulmonary adenocarcinoma with enteric differentiation. Cancer 68:1754, 1991.

720. Lovzowski CT, Hajdu SI: Cytology and immunocytochemistry of bronchioloalveolar carcinoma. Acta Cytol 31:717, 1987.

721. Tao LC, Weisbrod GL, Pearson FG, et al: Cytologic diagnosis of bronchioloalveolar carcinoma by fine-needle aspiration biopsy. Cancer 57:1565, 1986.

722. Zaman SS, van Hoeven KH, Slott S, et al: Distinction between bronchioloalveolar carcinoma and hyperplastic pulmonary proliferations: A cytologic and morphometric analysis. Diagn Cytopathol 16:396, 1997.

723. Auger M, Katz RL, Johnston DA: Differentiating cytological features of bronchioloalveolar carcinoma from adenocarcinoma of the lung in fine-needle aspirations: A statistical analysis of 27 cases. Diagn Cytopathol 16:253, 1997.

723a. Saleh HA, Haapaniemi J, Khatib G, et al: Bronchioloalveolar carcinoma: Diagnostic pitfalls and immunocytochemical contribution. Diagn Cytopathol 18:301, 1998.

724. Miller RR: Bronchioloalveolar cell adenomas. Am J Surg Pathol 14:904, 1990.

725. Carey FA, Wallace WAH, Fergusson RJ, et al: Alveolar atypical hyperplasia in association with primary pulmonary adenocarcinoma: A clinicopathological study of 10 cases. Thorax 47:1041, 1992.

726. Mori M, Tezuka F, Chiba R, et al: Atypical adenomatous hyperplasia and adenocarcinoma of the human lung: Their heterology in form and analogy in immunohistochemical characteristics. Cancer 77:665, 1996.

727. Nakayama H, Noguchi M, Tsuchiya R, et al: Clonal growth of atypical adenomatous hyperplasia of the lung: Cytofluorometric analysis of nuclear DNA content. Mod Pathol 3:314, 1990.

728. Ohshima S, Shimizu Y, Takahama M: Detection of c-Ki-ras gene mutation in paraffin sections of adenocarcinoma and atypical bronchioloalveolar cell hyperplasia of human lung. Virchows Arch 424:129, 1994.

729. Yokozaki M, Kodama T, Yokose T, et al: Differentiation of atypical adenomatous hyperplasia and adenocarcinoma of the lung by use of DNA ploidy and morphometric analysis. Mod Pathol 9:1156, 1996.

729a. Nakanishi K, Hiroi S, Kawai T, et al: Argyrophilic nucleolar-organizer region counts and DNA status in bronchioloalveolar epithelial hyperplasia and adenocarcinoma of the lung. Hum Pathol 29:235, 1998.

730. Sterner DJ, Mori M, Roggli V, et al: Prevalence of pulmonary atypical alveolar cell hyperplasia in an autopsy population: A study of 100 cases. Mod Pathol 10:469, 1997.

731. Herrera GA, Alexander CB, DeMoraes HP: Ultrastructural subtypes of pulmonary adenocarcinoma. Chest 84:581, 1983.

731a. Albertine KH, Steiner RM, Radack DM, et al: Analysis of cell type and radiographic presentation as predictors of the clinical course of patients with bronchioloalveolar cell carcinoma. Chest 113:997, 1998.

732. Grove A: Amylase in lung carcinomas: An ultrastructural and immunohistochemical study of two adenocarcinomas, and a review of the literature. APMIS 102:135, 1994.

733. Rainio P, Sutinen S, Vaananen R: A scanning and transmission electron microscopic study of pulmonary adenocarcinoma with histological correlation. Acta Pathol Microbiol Immunol Scand [A] 90:463, 1982.

734. Sun NCJ, Edgington TD, Carpentier CL, et al: Immunohistochemical localization of carcinoembryonic antigen (CEA), CEA-S, and nonspecific cross-reacting antigen (NCA) in carcinomas of lung. Cancer 52:1632, 1983.

735. Ghosh AK, Gatter KC, Dunnill MS, et al: Immunohistological staining of reactive mesothelium, mesothelioma, and lung carcinoma with a panel of monoclonal antibodies. J Clin Pathol 40:19, 1987.

736. Ramaekers F, Huysmans A, Moesker O, et al: Monoclonal antibody to keratin filaments, specific for glandular epithelia and their tumors. Lab Invest 49:353, 1983.

737. Muijen GNP, Ruiter DJ, Van Leeuwen C, et al: Cytokeratin and neurofilament in lung carcinomas. Am J Pathol 116:363, 1984.

738. Kitinya JN, Sueishi K, Tanaka K, et al: Immunoreactivity of surfactant-apoprotein in adenocarcinomas, large cell and small cell carcinomas of the lung. Acta Pathol Jpn 36:1271, 1986.

739. Mizutani Y, Nakajima T, Morinaga S, et al: Immunohistochemical localization of pulmonary surfactant apoproteins in various lung tumors. Cancer 61:532, 1988.

740. Linnoila RI, Jensen SM, Steinberg SM, et al: Peripheral airway cell marker expression in non–small cell lung carcinoma: Association with distinct clinicopathologic features. Am J Clin Pathol 97:233, 1992.

741. Khoor A, Whitsett JA, Stahlman MT, et al: Expression of surfactant protein B precursor and surfactant protein B mRNA in adenocarcinoma of the lung. Mod Pathol 10:62, 1997.

742. Upton MP, Hirohashi S, Tome Y, et al: Expression of vimentin in surgically resected adenocarcinomas and large cell carcinomas of lung. Am J Surg Pathol 10:560, 1986.

743. Kondi-Paphitis A, Addis BJ: Secretory component in pulmonary adenocarcinoma and mesothelioma. Histopathology 10:1279, 1986.

744. Singh G, Scheithauer BW, Katyal SL: The pathobiologic features of carcinomas of type II pneumocytes: An immunocytologic study. Cancer 57:994, 1986.

745. Visscher DW, Zarbo RJ, Trojanowski JQ, et al: Neuroendocrine differentiation in poorly differentiated lung carcinomas: A light microscopic and immunohistologic study. Mod Pathol 3:508, 1990.

746. Linnoila RI, Mulshine JL, Steinberg SM, et al: Neuroendocrine differentiation in endocrine and nonendocrine lung carcinomas. Am J Clin Pathol 90:641, 1988.

747. Ollayos CW, Riordan GP, Rushin JM: Estrogen receptor detection in paraffin sections of adenocarcinoma of the colon, pancreas, and lung. Arch Pathol Lab Med 118:630, 1994.

748. Horie A, Ohta M: Ultrastructural features of large cell carcinoma of the lung with reference to the prognosis of patients. Hum Pathol 12:423, 1981.

749. Auerbach O, Frasca JM, Parks VR, et al: A comparison of World Health Organization (WHO) classification of lung tumors by light and electron microscopy. Cancer 50:2079, 1982.

750. Mennemeyer R, Hammar SP, Bauermeister DE, et al: Cytologic, histologic and electron microscopic correlations in poorly differentiated primary lung carcinoma. Acta Cytol 23:297, 1979.

751. Churg A: The fine structure of large cell undifferentiated carcinoma of the lung. Hum Pathol 9:143, 1978.

752. Hammond ME, Sause WT: Large cell neuroendocrine tumors of the lung: Clinical significance and histopathologic definition. Cancer 56:1624, 1985.

753. Yesner R: Large cell carcinoma of the lung. Semin Diagn Pathol 2:255, 1985.

754. Ritter JH, Boucher LD, Wick MR: Peripheral pulmonary adenocarcinoma with bronchioloalveolar features: Immunophenotypes correlate with histologic patterns. Mod Pathol 11:566, 1998.

755. Schulte MA, Ramzy I, Greenberg SD: Immunocytochemical characterization of large-cell carcinomas of the lung: Role, limitations and technical considerations. Acta Cytol 35:175, 1991.

756. Ishida T, Kaneko S, Tateishi M, et al: Large cell carcinoma of the lung: Prognostic implications of histopathologic and immunohistochemical subtyping. Am J Clin Pathol 93:176, 1990.

757. Banerjee SS, Eyden BP, Wells S, et al: Pseudoangiosarcomatous carcinoma: A clinicopathological study of seven cases. Histopathology 21:13, 1992.

758. Yamamato T, Yazawa T, Ogata T, et al: Clear cell carcinoma of the lung: A case report and review of the literature. Lung Cancer 10:101, 1993.

759. Moro D, Brichon PY, Brambilla E, et al: Basaloid bronchial carcinoma: A histologic group with a poor prognosis. Cancer 73:2734, 1994.

760. Brambilla E, Moro D, Veale D, et al: Basal cell (basaloid) carcinoma of the lung: A new morphologic and phenotypic entity with separate prognostic significance. Hum Pathol 23:993, 1992.

761. Arnould L, Drouot F, Fargeot P, et al: Hepatoid carcinoma of the lung: Report of a case of an unusual α-fetoprotein-producing lung tumor. Am J Surg Pathol 21:1113, 1997.

762. Ishikura H, Kanda M, Ito M, et al: Hepatoid adenocarcinoma: A distinctive histologic subtype of α-fetoprotein-producing lung carcinoma. Virchows Arch A Path Anat Histopathol 417:73, 1990.

763. Nasu M, Soma T, Fukushima H, et al: Hepatoid carcinoma of the lung with production of α-fetoprotein and abnormal prothrombin: An autopsy case report. Mod Pathol 10:1054, 1997.

764. Butler AE, Colby TV, Weiss L, et al: Lymphoepithelioma-like carcinoma of the lung. Am J Surg Pathol 13:632, 1989.

765. Onizuka M, Doi M, Mitsui K, et al: Undifferentiated carcinoma with prominent lymphocytic infiltration (so-called lymphoepithelioma) in the trachea. Chest 98:236, 1990.

766. Fitzgibbons PL, Kern WH: Adenosquamous carcinoma of the lung: A clinical and pathologic study of seven cases. Hum Pathol 16:463, 1985.

767. Ishida T, Kaneko S, Yokoyama H, et al: Adenosquamous carcinoma of the lung: Clinicopathologic and immunohistochemical features. Am J Clin Pathol 97:678, 1992.

768. Takamori S, Noguchi M, Morinaga S, et al: Clinicopathologic characteristics of adenosquamous carcinoma of the lung. Cancer 67:649, 1991.

769. Alvarez-Fernandez E: Alveolar trapping in pulmonary carcinomas. Diagn Histopathol 5:59, 1982.

770. Carter D, Eggleston JC: Atlas of Tumor Pathology: Tumors of the Lower Respiratory Tract. 2nd ed. Washington, DC, Armed Forces Institute of Pathology, 1980.

771. Addis BJ, Corrin B: Pulmonary blastoma, carcinosarcoma and spindle-cell carcinoma: An immunohistochemical study of keratin intermediate filaments. J Pathol 147:291, 1985.

772. Suster S, Huszar M, Herczeg E: Spindle cell squamous carcinoma of the lung: Immunocytochemical and ultrastructural study of a case. Histopathology 11:871, 1987.

773. Humphrey PA, Scroggs MW, Roggli VL, et al: Pulmonary carcinomas with a sarcomatoid element: An immunocytochemical and ultrastructural analysis. Hum Pathol 19:155, 1988.

774. Matsui K, Kitagawa M, Miwa A: Lung carcinoma with spindle cell components: Sixteen cases examined by immunohistochemistry. Hum Pathol 23:1289, 1992.

775. Berho M, Moran CA, Suster S: Malignant mixed epithelial/mesenchymal neoplasms of the lung. Semin Diagn Pathol 12:123, 1995.

776. Attanoos RL, Papagiannis A, Suttinont P, et al: Pulmonary giant cell carcinoma: Pathological entity or morphological phenotype? Histopathology 32:225, 1998.

777. Holst VA, Finkelstein S, Colby TV, et al: p53 and K-ras mutational genotyping in pulmonary carcinosarcoma, spindle cell carcinoma, and pulmonary blastoma: Implications for histogenesis. Am J Surg Pathol 21:801, 1997.

778. Humphrey PA, Scroggs MW, Roggli VL, et al: Pulmonary carcinomas with a sarcomatoid element: An immunocytochemical and ultrastructural analysis. Hum Pathol 19:155, 1988.

779. Nappi O, Glasner SD, Swanson PE, et al: Biphasic and monophasic sarcomatoid carcinomas of the lung: A reappraisal of "carcinosarcomas" and "spindle-cell carcinomas." Am J Clin Pathol 102:331, 1994.

780. Ro JY, Chen JL, Lee JS, et al: Sarcomatoid carcinoma of the lung: Immunohistochemical and ultrastructural studies of 14 cases. Cancer 69:376, 1992.

781. Wick MR, Ritter JH, Humphrey PA: Sarcomatoid carcinomas of the lung: A clinicopathologic review. Am J Clin Pathol 108:40, 1997.

782. Barson AJ, Jones AW, Lodge KV: Pulmonary blastoma. J Clin Pathol 21:480, 1968.

783. Stackhouse EM, Harrison EG Jr, Ellis FH Jr: Primary mixed malignancies of lung: Carcinosarcoma and blastoma. J Thorac Cardiovasc Surg 57:385, 1969.

784. McCann MP, Fu Y-S, Kay S: Pulmonary blastoma: A light and electron microscopic study. Cancer 38:789, 1976.

785. Roth JA, Elguezabal A: Pulmonary blastoma evolving into carcinosarcoma: A case study. Am J Surg Pathol 2:407, 1978.

786. Cohen-Salmon D, Michel RP, Wang NS, et al: Pulmonary carcinosarcoma and carcinoma: Report of a case studied by electron microscopy, with critical review of the literature. Ann Pathol 5:115, 1985.

787. Davis MP, Eagan RT, Weiland LH, et al: Carcinosarcoma of the lung: Mayo Clinic experience and response to chemotherapy. Mayo Clin Proc 59:598, 1984.

788. Bergmann M, Ackerman LV, Kemler RL: Carcinosarcoma of the lung: Review of the literature and report of two cases treated by pneumonectomy. Cancer 4:919, 1951.

789. Drury RAB, Stirland RM: Carcino-sarcomatous tumours of the respiratory tract. J Pathol Bacteriol 77:543, 1959.

790. Rainosek DE, Ro JY, Ordonez NG, et al: Sarcomatoid carcinoma of the lung: A case with atypical carcinoid and rhabdomyosarcomatous components. Am J Clin Pathol 102:360, 1994.

791. Ludwigsen E: Endobronchial carcinosarcoma: A case with osteosarcoma of pulmonary invasive part, and a review with respect to prognosis. Virchows Arch [Pathol Anat Histol] 373:293, 1977.

792. Prive L, Tellem M, Meranze DR, et al: Carcinosarcoma of the lung. Arch Pathol 72:119, 1961.

793. Zimmerman KG, Sobonya RE, Payne CM: Histochemical and ultrastructural features of an unusual pulmonary carcinosarcoma. Hum Pathol 12:1046, 1981.

794. Huszar M, Herczeg E, Lieberman Y, et al: Distinctive immunofluorescent labeling of epithelial and mesenchymal elements of carcinosarcoma with antibodies specific for different intermediate filaments. Hum Pathol 15:532, 1984.

795. Chaudhuri MR: Bronchial carcinosarcoma. J Thorac Cardiovasc Surg 61:319, 1971.

796. Herman DL, Bullock WK, Waker JK: Giant cell adenocarcinoma of the lung. Cancer 19:1337, 1966.

797. Nash AD, Stout AP: Giant cell carcinoma of the lung. Cancer 11:369, 1958.

798. Wang N-S, Seemayer TA, Ahmed MN, et al: Giant cell carcinoma of the lung. Hum Pathol 7:3, 1976.

799. Nonomura A, Saito K, Kono N, et al: Cytoplasmic hyalins resembling Mallory's alcoholic hyalins in pulmonary carcinoma cells. Acta Pathol Jpn 36:1669, 1986.

800. Ginsberg SS, Buzaid AC, Stern H, et al: Giant cell carcinoma of the lung. Cancer 70:606, 1992.

801. Addis BJ, Dewar A, Thurlow NP: Giant cell carcinoma of the lung—immuno-histochemical and ultrastructural evidence of dedifferentiation. J Pathol 155:231, 1988.

802. Yoshimoto T, Higashino K, Hada T, et al: A primary lung carcinoma producing alpha-fetoprotein, carcinoembryonic antigen, and human chorionic gonadotropin: Immunohistochemical and biochemical studies. Cancer 60:2744, 1987.

803. Pääkkö P, Risteli J, Risteli L, et al: Immunohistochemical evidence that lung carcinomas grow on alveolar basement membranes. Am J Surg Pathol 14:464, 1990.

804. Gallagher B, Urbanski SJ: The significance of pleural elastica invasion by lung carcinomas. Hum Pathol 21:512, 1990.

805. Neyazaki T, Ikeda M, Mitsui K, et al: Angioarchitecture of pulmonary malignancies in humans. Cancer 26:1246, 1970.

806. Zielinski KW, Kulig A, Zielinski J: Morphology of the microvascular bed in primary human carcinomas of lung. Pathol Res Pract 178:369, 1984.

807. Zielinski KW, Kulig A: Morphology of the microvascular bed in primary human carcinomas of lung. Pathol Res Pract 178:243, 1984.

808. Muller K-M, Meyer-Schwickerath M: Bronchial arteries in various stages of bronchogenic carcinoma. Pathol Res Pract 163:34, 1978.

809. Milne ENC: Circulation of primary and metastatic pulmonary neoplasms. Am J Roentgenol 100:603, 1967.

810. Kolin A, Koutoulakis T: Invasion of pulmonary arteries by bronchial carcinomas. Hum Pathol 18:1165, 1987.

811. Roberts TE, Hasleton PS, Musgrove C, et al: Vascular invasion in non–small cell lung carcinoma. J Clin Pathol 45:591, 1992.

812. Macchiarini P, Fontanini G, Dulmet E, et al: Angiogenesis: An indicator of metastasis in non–small cell lung cancer invading the thoracic inlet. Ann Thorac Surg 57:1534, 1994.

813. Svennevig J-L, Holter J: The local cell response to human lung carcinomas. Acta Pathol Microbiol Scand 89:147, 1981.

814. Kolb E, Muller E: Local responses in primary and secondary human lung cancers: II. Clinical correlations. Br J Cancer 40:410, 1979.

815. Di Paola M, Bertolotti A, Colizza S, et al: Histology of bronchial carcinoma and regional lymph nodes as putative immune response of the host to the tumor. J Thorac Cardiovasc Surg 73:531, 1977.

816. Kayser K, Bulzebruck H, Ebert W, et al: Local tumor inflammation, lymph node metastasis, and survival of operated bronchus carcinoma patients. J Natl Cancer Inst 77:77, 1986.

817. Furukawa T, Watanabe S, Kodama T, et al: T-zone histiocytes in adenocarcinoma of the lung in relation to postoperative prognosis. Cancer 56:2651, 1985.

818. Nakajima T, Kodama T, Tsumuraya M, et al: S-100 protein-positive Langerhans cells in various human lung cancers, especially in peripheral adenocarcinomas. Virchows Arch 407:177, 1985.

819. Hammar S, Bockus D, Remington F, et al: The widespread distribution of Langerhans cells in pathologic tissues: An ultrastructural and immunohistochemical study. Hum Pathol 17:894, 1986.

820. Kolin A, Hiruki T: Palisading granulomas associated with lung cancer. Arch Pathol Lab Med 114:697, 1990.

821. Kayser K, Toomes H, Vollhaber H-H, et al: Tumour volume and macroscopic growth pattern of bronchogenic carcinoma. Virchows Arch [A] 405:387, 1985.

822. Kundel HL, Revesz G: Lesion conspicuity, structured noise, and film reader error. Am J Roentgenol 126:1233, 1976.

823. Woodring JH: Pitfalls in the radiologic diagnosis of lung cancer. Am J Roentgenol 154:1165, 1990.

824. Newell RR, Garneau R: The threshold visibility of pulmonary shadows. Radiology 56:409, 1951.

825. Kundel HL: Predictive value and threshold detectability of lung tumors. Radiology 139:25, 1981.

826. Garland LH: Bronchial carcinomas: Lobar distribution of lesions in 250 cases. Calif Med 94:7, 1961.

827. Lee SH, Ts'O TOT: Histological typing of lung cancers in Hong Kong. Br J Cancer 17:37, 1963.

828. Miyaji T, Tada S, Sando H, et al: Morphology of carcinoma of the lung, with specific reference to its histologic classification. Jpn J Chest Dis 19:381, 1960.

829. Hood RH Jr, Campbell DC Jr, Dooley BN, et al: Bronchogenic carcinoma in young people. Dis Chest 48:469, 1965.

830. Macfarlane JCW, Doughty BJ, Crosbie WA: Carcinoma of the lung: An analysis of 362 cases diagnosed and treated in one year. Br J Dis Chest 56:57, 1962.

831. Kyttä J, Pulkkinen K, Koskinen O: Endoscopic aspects of bronchogenic carcinoma. Ann Chir Gynaecol Fenn 51:361, 1962.

832. Ioannou J, Prétet S: Aspects endoscopiques du cancer bronchique: Confrontation topographique, radiologique et anatomopathologique. [Bronchoscopic aspects of bronchogenic carcinoma: Topographic, radiologic and anatomo-pathologic correlation.] Rev Tuberc 28:585, 1964.

833. Byers TE, Vena JE, Rzepka TF: Predilection of lung cancer for the upper lobes: An epidemiologic inquiry. J Natl Cancer Inst 72:1271, 1984.

834. Lisa JR, Trinidad S, Rosenblatt MB: Site of origin, histogenesis, and cytostructure of bronchogenic carcinoma. Am J Clin Pathol 44:375, 1965.

835. Lee HJ, Im JG, Ahn JM, et al: Lung cancer in patients with idiopathic pulmonary fibrosis: CT findings. J Comput Assist Tomogr 20:979, 1996.

836. Byrd RB, Miller WE, Carr DT, et al: The roentgenographic appearance of squamous cell carcinoma of the bronchus. Mayo Clin Proc 43:327, 1968.

837. Byrd RB, Miller WE, Carr DT, et al: The roentgenographic appearance of small cell carcinoma of the bronchus. Mayo Clin Proc 43:337, 1968.

838. Chute CG, Greenberg ER, Baron J, et al: Presenting conditions of 1539 population-based lung cancer patients by cell type and stage in New Hampshire and Vermont. Cancer 56:2107, 1985.

839. Quinn D, Gianlupi A, Broste S: The changing radiographic presentation of bronchogenic carcinoma with reference to cell types. Chest 110:1474, 1996.

840. Woodring JH, Stelling CB: Adenocarcinoma of the lung: A tumor with changing pleomorphic character. Am J Roentgenol 140:657, 1983.

841. Lehar TJ, Carr DT, Miller WE, et al: Roentgenographic appearance of bronchogenic adenocarcinoma. Am Rev Respir Dis 96:245, 1967.

842. Gupta AK, Pryce DM, Blenkinsopp WK: Pre-operative length of history and tumour size in central and peripheral bronchial carcinomata. Thorax 20:398, 1965.

843. Shure D: Radiographically occult endobronchial obstruction in bronchogenic carcinoma. Am J Med 91:19, 1991.

844. Ranke EJ, Presley SS, Holinger PH: Tracheogenic carcinoma. JAMA 182:519, 1962.

845. Laval P, Payan H, Bonneau H, et al: Cancer de l'apex pulmonaire. [Cancer of the pulmonary apex.] J Fr Med Chir Thorac 17:231, 1963.

846. Byrd RB, Miller WE, Carr DT, et al: The roentgenographic appearance of large cell carcinoma of the bronchus. Mayo Clin Proc 43:333, 1968.

847. Byrd RB, Carr DT, Miller WE, et al: Radiographic abnormalities in carcinoma of the lung as relation to histological cell type. Thorax 24:573, 1969.

848. Burke M, Fraser RS: Obstructive pneumonitis: A pathologic and pathogenetic reappraisal. Radiology 166:699, 1988.

849. Golden R: The effect of bronchostenosis upon the roentgen-ray shadows in carcinoma of the bronchus. Am J Roentgenol Radiat Ther 13:21, 1925.

850. Woodring JH: Determining the cause of pulmonary atelectasis: A comparison of plain radiography and CT. Am J Roentgenol 150:757, 1988.

851. Tobler J, Levitt RG, Glazer HS, et al: Differentiation of proximal bronchogenic carcinoma from post-obstructive lobar collapse by magnetic resonance imaging: Comparison with computed tomography. Invest Radiol 22:538, 1987.

852. Molina PL, Hiken JN, Glazer HS: Imaging evaluation of obstructive atelectasis. J Thorac Imaging 11:176, 1996.

853. Khouri MB, Godwin JD, Halvorsen RA: CT of lobar collapse. Invest Radiol 20:708, 1985.

854. Onitsuka H, Tsukuda M, Araki A, et al: Differentiation of central lung tumor from postobstructive lobar collapse by rapid sequence computed tomography. J Thorac Imaging 6:28, 1991.

855. Herold CJ, Kuhlman JE, Zerhouni EA: Pulmonary atelectasis: Signal patterns with MR imaging. Radiology 178:715, 1991.

856. Stiglbauer R, Schurawitzki H, Klepetko W: Contrast-enhanced MR imaging for the staging of bronchogenic carcinoma: Comparison with CT and histopathologic staging—preliminary results. Clin Radiol 44:293, 1991.

857. Kameda K, Adachi S, Kono M: Detection of T-factor in lung cancer using magnetic resonance imaging and computed tomography. J Thorac Imaging 3:73, 1988.

858. Emerson GL, Emerson MS, Sherwood CE: The natural history of carcinoma of the lung. J Thorac Cardiovasc Surg 37:291, 1959.

859. Rigler LG: The roentgen signs of carcinoma of the lung. Am J Roentgenol 74:415, 1955.

860. Secker-Walker RH, Provan JL, Jackson JA, et al: Lung scanning in carcinoma of the bronchus. Thorax 26:23, 1971.

861. Fraser HS, MacLeod WM, Garnett ES, et al: Lung scanning in the preoperative assessment of carcinoma of the bronchus. Am Rev Respir Dis 101:349, 1970.

862. Felson B: Mucoid impaction (inspissated secretions) in segmental bronchial obstruction. Radiology 133:9, 1976.

863. Woodring JH, Bernady MO, Loh FK: Mucoid impaction of the bronchi. Australas Radiol 29:234, 1995.

864. Woodring JH: Unusual radiographic manifestations of lung cancer. Radiol Clin North Am 28:599, 1990.
865. Aronberg DJ, Sagel SS, Jost RG, et al: Oat cell carcinoma manifesting as a bronchocele. Am J Roentgenol 132:23, 1979.
866. Felson B: Mucoid impaction (inspissated secretions) in segmental bronchial obstruction. Radiology 133:9, 1979.
867. Genereux GP: Unusual intrathoracic manifestations of bronchogenic carcinoma. In Margulis AR, Gooding CA (eds): Diagnostic Radiology. San Francisco, University of California, 1977, pp 553–584.
868. Spizarny DL, Cavanaugh B: The anterior bronchus sign: A new clue to hilar abnormality. Am J Roentgenol 145:265, 1986.
869. Littleton JT, Durizch ML: Sectional Imaging Methods: A Comparison. Baltimore, University Park Press, 1983, p 161.
870. Proto A, Speckman JM: The left lateral radiograph of the chest. Med Radiogr Photogr 55:30, 1979.
871. Schnur MJ, Winkler B, Austin JHM: Thickening of the posterior wall of the bronchus intermedius. Radiology 139:551, 1981.
872. Foster WL, Roberts L, McLendon RE, et al: Localized peribronchial thickening: A CT sign of occult bronchogenic carcinoma. Am J Roentgenol 144:906, 1985.
873. Saida Y, Kujiraoka Y, Akaogi E, et al: Early squamous cell carcinoma of the lung: CT and pathologic correlation. Radiology 201:61, 1996.
874. Walske BR: The solitary pulmonary nodule: A review of 217 cases. Dis Chest 49:302, 1966.
875. Davis DW, Peabody JW Jr, Katz S: The solitary pulmonary nodule: A ten-year study based on 215 cases. J Thorac Cardiovasc Surg 32:728, 1956.
876. Edwards WM, Cox RS Jr, Garland LH: The solitary nodule (coin lesion) of the lung: An analysis of 52 consecutive cases treated by thoracotomy and a study of preoperative diagnostic accuracy. Am J Roentgenol 88:1020, 1962.
877. Phillips T, Hanson A: The problem of circumscribed lung opacities. Br J Dis Chest 56:17, 1962.
878. Steele JD: The solitary pulmonary nodule: Report of a cooperative study of resected asymptomatic solitary pulmonary nodules in males. J Thorac Cardiovasc Surg 46:21, 1963.
879. Swensen SJ, Morin RL, Schueler BA, et al: Solitary pulmonary nodule: CT evaluation of enhancement with iodinated contrast material—a preliminary report. Radiology 182:343, 1992.
880. Yamashita K, Matsunobe S, Tsuda T: Intratumoral necrosis of lung carcinoma: A potential pitfall in incremental dynamic computed tomography analysis of solitary nodules? J Thorac Imaging 12:181, 1997.
881. Mack MJ, Hazebrigg SR, Landreneau RJ, et al: Thoracoscopy for the diagnosis of the indeterminate solitary pulmonary nodule. Ann Thorac Surg 56:825, 1993.
882. Siegelman SS, Khouri NF, Leo FP, et al: Solitary pulmonary nodules: CT assessment. Radiology 160:307, 1986.
883. Zerhouni EA, Stitik FP, Siegelman SS, et al: CT of the pulmonary nodule—a cooperative study. Radiology 160:319, 1986.
884. Primack SL, Lee KS, Logan PM, et al: Bronchogenic carcinoma: Utility of CT in the evaluation of patients with suspected lesions. Radiology 193:795, 1994.
885. Mountain CF: Revisions in the International System for Staging Lung Cancer. Chest 111:1710, 1997.
886. Midthun DE, Swensen SJ, Jett JR: Approach to the solitary pulmonary nodule. Mayo Clin Proc 68:378, 1993.
887. Khouri NF, Meziane MA, Zerhouni EA, et al: The solitary pulmonary nodule—assessment, diagnosis and management. Chest 91:127, 1987.
888. Godwin JD: The solitary pulmonary nodule. Radiol Clin North Am 21:709, 1983.
889. Bateson EM: An analysis of 155 solitary lung lesions illustrating the differential diagnosis of mixed tumours of the lung. Clin Radiol 16:51, 1965.
890. Siegelman SS, Khouri NF, Scott WW, et al: Pulmonary hamartoma: CT findings. Radiology 160:313, 1986.
891. Cummings SR, Lillington GA, Richard RJ: Managing solitary pulmonary nodules: The choice of strategy is a "close call." Am Rev Respir Dis 134:453, 1986.
892. Munden RF, Pugatch RD, Liptay MJ, et al: Small pulmonary lesions detected at CT: Clinical importance. Radiology 202:105, 1997.
893. Gurney JW: Determining the likelihood of malignancy in solitary pulmonary nodules with Bayesian analysis: Part I. Theory. Radiology 186:405, 1993.
894. Sagel SS: The solitary pulmonary nodule: Role of CT. Am J Roentgenol 147:26, 1986.
895. McLendon RE, Roggli VL, Foster WL Jr, et al: Carcinoma of the lung with osseous stromal metaplasia. Arch Pathol Lab Med 109:1051, 1985.
896. Kyser PL, McComb BL, Bennett WF: CT evidence of calcification within a small cell carcinoma of the lung. Comput Radiol 10:107, 1986.
897. Goldstein MS, Rush M, Johnson P, et al: A calcified adenocarcinoma of the lung with very high CT numbers. Radiology 150:785, 1984.
898. Webb WR: Radiologic evaluation of the solitary pulmonary nodule. Am J Roentgenol 154:701, 1990.
899. Mahoney MC, Shipley RT, Corcoran HL, et al: CT demonstration of calcification in carcinoma of the lung. Am J Roentgenol 154:255, 1990.
900. Grewal RG, Austin JHM: CT demonstration of calcification in carcinoma of the lung. J Comput Assist Tomogr 18:867, 1994.
901. Siegelman SS, Zerhouni EA, Leo FP, et al: CT of the solitary pulmonary nodule. Am J Roentgenol 135:1, 1980.
902. Proto AV, Thomas SR: Pulmonary nodules studied by computed tomography. Radiology 156:149, 1985.
903. Godwin JD, Speckman JM, Fram EK, et al: Distinguishing benign from malignant pulmonary nodules by computed tomography. Radiology 144:349, 1982.

904. Levi C, Gray JE, McCullough EC, et al: The unreliability of CT numbers as absolute values. Am J Roentgenol 139:443, 1982.
905. Khan A, Herman PG, Vorwerk P, et al: Solitary pulmonary nodules: Comparison of classification with standard, thin-section, and reference phantom CT. Radiology 179:477, 1991.
906. Swensen SJ, Harms GF, Morin RL, et al: CT evaluation of solitary pulmonary nodules. Am J Roentgenol 156:925, 1991.
907. Colice GL: Chest CT for known or suspected lung cancer. Chest 106:1538, 1994.
908. Im J-G, Gamsu G, Birnberg FA, et al: CT densitometry of pulmonary nodules in a frozen human thorax. Am J Roentgenol 150:61, 1988.
909. Swensen SJ, Morin RL, Aughenbaugh GL, et al: CT reconstruction algorithm selection in the evaluation of solitary pulmonary nodules. J Comput Assist Tomogr 19:932, 1995.
910. Brody WR, Cassel DM, Sommer FG, et al: Dual-energy projection radiography: Initial clinical experience. Am J Roentgenol 137:201, 1981.
911. Cann CE, Gamsu G, Birnberg FA, et al: Quantification of calcium in solitary pulmonary nodules using single- and dual-energy CT. Radiology 145:493, 1982.
912. Bhalla M: Use of dual kVp to assess solitary pulmonary nodules. J Comput Assist Tomogr 19:44, 1995.
913. Higashi Y, Nakamura H, Matsumoto T, et al: Dual-energy computed tomographic diagnosis of pulmonary nodules. J Thorac Imaging 9:31, 1994.
914. Fraser RG, Hickey NM, Niklason LT, et al: Calcification in pulmonary nodules: Detection with dual-energy digital radiography. Radiology 160:595, 1986.
915. Ishigaki T, Sakuma S, Horikowa Y, et al: One-shot dual-energy subtraction imaging. Radiology 161:271, 1986.
916. Oestman JW, Green R, Rhea JT, et al: "Single-exposure" dual energy digital radiography in the detection of pulmonary nodules and calcifications. Invest Radiol 24:517, 1989.
917. Ho JT, Kruger RA: Comparison of dual-energy and conventional chest radiography for nodule detection. Invest Radiol 24:861, 1989.
918. Ergun DL, Mistretta CA, Brown DE, et al: Single-exposure dual-energy computed radiography: Improved detection and processing. Radiology 174:243, 1990.
919. Kelcz F, Zink FE, Peppler WW, et al: Conventional chest radiography vs dual-energy computed radiography in the detection and characterization of pulmonary nodules. Am J Roentgenol 162:271, 1994.
920. Zwirewich CV, Vedal S, Miller RR, Müller NL: Solitary pulmonary nodule: High-resolution CT and radiologic-pathologic correlation. Radiology 179:469, 1991.
921. Heitzman ER: The Lung: Radiologic-Pathologic Correlations. 2nd ed. St. Louis, CV Mosby, 1984.
922. Shapiro R, Wilson GL, Yesner R, et al: A useful roentgen sign in the diagnosis of localized bronchioloalveolar carcinoma. Am J Roentgenol 114:516, 1972.
923. Sone S, Sakai F, Takashima S, et al: Factors affecting the radiologic appearance of peripheral bronchogenic carcinomas. J Thorac Imaging 12:159, 1997.
924. Kuriyama K, Tateishi R, Doi O, et al: CT-pathologic correlation in small peripheral lung cancers. Am J Roentgenol 149:1139, 1987.
925. Fletcher CM, Horn D: Smoking and health. Presented at World Health Assembly, Geneva, May 17, 1970. National Clearing House for Smoking and Health Bulletin, June, 1970.
926. Schraufnagel DE, Peloquin A, Paré JAP, et al: Differentiating bronchioloalveolar carcinoma from adenocarcinoma. Am Rev Respir Dis 125:74, 1982.
927. Webb WR: The pleural tail sign. Radiology 127:309, 1978.
928. Hill CA: "Tail" signs associated with pulmonary lesions: Critical reappraisal. Am J Roentgenol 139:311, 1982.
929. Heitzman ER, Markarian B, Raasch BN, et al: Pathways of tumor spread through the lung: Radiologic correlations with anatomy and pathology. Radiology 144:3, 1982.
930. Kui M, Templeton PA, White CS, et al: Evaluation of the air bronchogram sign on CT in solitary pulmonary lesions. J Comput Assist Tomogr 20:983, 1996.
931. Gaeta M, Barone M, Russi EG, et al: Carcinomatous solitary pulmonary nodules: Evaluation of the tumor-bronchi relationship with thin-section CT. Radiology 187:535, 1993.
932. Kuhlman JE, Fishman EK, Kuhajda FP, et al: Solitary bronchioloalveolar carcinoma: CT criteria. Radiology 167:379, 1988.
933. Adler B, Padley S, Miller RR, Müller NL: High-resolution CT of bronchioloalveolar carcinoma. Am J Roentgenol 159:275, 1992.
934. Lee KS, Kim Y, Han J, et al: Bronchioloalveolar carcinoma: Clinical, histopathologic, and radiologic findings. Radiographics 17:1345, 1997.
935. Wong JSL, Weisbrod GL, Chamberlain D, et al: Bronchioloalveolar carcinoma and the air bronchogram sign: A new pathologic explanation. J Thorac Imaging 9:141, 1994.
936. Weisbrod GL, Chamberlain D, Herman SJ: Cystic change (pseudocavitation) associated with bronchioloalveolar carcinoma: A report of four patients. J Thorac Imaging 10:106, 1995.
937. Garland LH: The rate of growth and natural duration of primary bronchial cancer. Am J Roentgenol 96:604, 1966.
938. Collins VP, Loeffler RK, Tivey H: Observations on growth rates of human tumors. Am J Roentgenol 76:988, 1956.
939. Nathan MH, Collins VP, Adams RA: Differentiation of benign and malignant pulmonary nodules by growth rate. Radiology 79:221, 1962.
940. Weiss W, Boucot KR, Cooper DA: The survival of men with measurable proved lung cancer in relation to growth rate. Am J Roentgenol 98:404, 1966.
941. Steele JD, Buell P: Asymptomatic solitary pulmonary nodules, host survival, tumor size, and growth rate. J Thorac Cardiovasc Surg 65:140, 1973.

942. Chahinian P: Relationship between tumor doubling time and anatomoclinical features in 50 measurable pulmonary cancers. Chest 61:340, 1972.

943. Weiss W: Peripheral measurable bronchogenic carcinoma: Growth rate and period of risk after therapy. Am Rev Respir Dis 103:198, 1971.

944. Smithers DW: Clinical assessment of growth-rate in human tumours. Clin Radiol 19:113, 1968.

945. Erasmus JJ, McAdams HP, Patz EF Jr, et al: Thoracic FDG PET: State of the art. RadioGraphics 18:5, 1998.

946. Garland LH, Coulson W, Wollin E: The rate of growth and apparent duration of untreated primary bronchial carcinoma. Cancer 16:694, 1963.

947. Wolff G: Die Bedeutung der verdoppelungs zeit für die Differentialdiagnose von Rundherden. [The significance of the growth doubling time for the differential diagnosis of coin lesions.] Fortschr Roentgenstr 101:366, 1964.

948. Spratt JS Jr, Spjut HJ, Roper CL: The frequency distribution of the rates of growth and the estimated duration of primary pulmonary carcinomas. Cancer 16:687, 1963.

949. Weiss W, Boucot KR, Cooper D: Survival of men with peripheral lung cancer in relation to histological characteristics and growth rate. Am Rev Respir Dis 98:75, 1968.

950. Weiss W, Boucot KR, Cooper DA: Growth rate in the detection and prognosis of bronchogenic carcinoma. JAMA 198:1246, 1966.

951. Jensen JG, Schiodt T: Growth conditions of hamartoma of the lung: A study based on 22 cases operated on after radiographic observation for from one to 18 years. Thorax 13:233, 1958.

952. Weisel W, Glicklich M, Landis FB: Pulmonary hamartoma, an enlarging neoplasm. Arch Surg 71:128, 1955.

953. Good CA: Management of patient with solitary mass in lung. Chic Med Soc Bull 55:893, 1953.

954. Good CA, Wilson TW: The solitary circumscribed pulmonary nodule: Study of seven hundred five cases encountered roentgenologically in a period of three and one-half years. JAMA 166:210, 1958.

955. Bennett DE, Sasser WF, Ferguson TB: Adenocarcinoma of the lung in men. Cancer 23:431, 1969.

956. Yankelevitz DF, Henschke CI: Does 2-year stability imply that pulmonary nodules are benign? Am J Roentgenol 168:325, 1997.

957. Weiss W: Tumor doubling time and survival of men with bronchogenic carcinoma. Chest 65:3, 1974.

958. Mizuno T, Masaoka A, Ichimura H: Comparison of actual survivorship after treatment with survivorship predicted by actual tumor-volume doubling time from tumor diameter at first observation. Cancer 53:2716, 1984.

959. Kormano M, Dean PB: Extravascular contrast material: The major component of contrast enhancement. Radiology 121:379, 1976.

960. Newhouse JH, Murphy RX Jr: Tissue distribution of soluble contrast: Effect of dose variation and changes with time. Am J Roentgenol 136:463, 1981.

961. Littleton JT, Durizch ML, Moeller G, et al: Pulmonary masses: Contrast enhancement. Radiology 177:861, 1990.

962. Swensen SJ, Brown LR, Colby TV, et al: Pulmonary nodules: CT evaluation of enhancement with iodinated contrast material. Radiology 194:393, 1995.

963. Swensen SJ, Brown LR, Colby TV, et al: Lung nodule enhancement at CT: Prospective findings. Radiology 201:447, 1996.

964. Zhang M, Kono M: Solitary pulmonary nodules: Evaluation of blood flow patterns with dynamic CT. Radiology 205:471, 1997.

965. Kono M, Adachi S, Kusumoto M, et al: Clinical utility of Gd-DTPA-enhanced magnetic resonance imaging in lung cancer. J Thorac Imaging 8:18, 1993.

966. Guckel C, Schnabel K, Deimling M, et al: Solitary pulmonary nodules: MR evaluation of enhancement patterns with contrast-enhanced dynamic snapshot gradient-echo imaging. Radiology 200:681, 1996.

967. Kubota K, Matsuzawa T, Fujiwara T, et al: Differential diagnosis of lung tumor with positron emission tomography: A prospective study. J Nucl Med 31:1927, 1990.

968. Gupta NC, Frank AR, Dewan NA: Solitary pulmonary nodules: Detection of malignancy with PET with 2-[F18] fluoro-2-deoxy-D-glucose. Radiology 184:441, 1992.

969. Patz EF, Lowe VJ, Hoffman JM, et al: Focal pulmonary abnormalities: Evaluation with F-18 fluorodeoxyglucose PET scanning. Radiology 188:487, 1993.

970. Duhaylongsod FG, Lowe VJ, Patz EF, et al: Detection of primary and recurrent lung cancer by means of F-18 fluorodeoxyglucose positron emission tomography. J Thorac Cardiovasc Surg 110:130, 1995.

971. Sazon DAD, Siverio SM, Soo Hoo GW, et al: Fluorodeoxyglucose-positron emission tomography in the detection and staging of lung cancer. Am J Respir Crit Care Med 153:417, 1996.

971a. Lowe VJ, Fletcher JW, Gobar L, et al: Prospective investigation of positron emission tomography in lung nodules. J Clin Oncol 16:1075, 1998.

972. Dewan NA, Shehan CJ, Reeb SD, et al: Likelihood of malignancy in a solitary pulmonary nodule: Comparison of Bayesian analysis and results of FDG-PET scan. Chest 112:416, 1997.

973. Scott WJ, Schwabe JL, Gupta NC, et al: Positron emission tomography of lung tumours and mediastinal lymph nodes using [18F] fluorodeoxyglucose. Ann Thorac Surg 58:698, 1994.

974. Worsley DF, Celler A, Adam MJ, et al: Pulmonary nodules: Differential diagnosis using 18 F-fluorodeoxyglucose single-photon emission computed tomography. Am J Roentgenol 168:771, 1997.

975. Nakata H, Hirakata K, Watanabe H, et al: Lung cancer associated with punctate calcification: CT and histological correlation. Radiat Med 15:91, 1997.

976. Mallens WMC, Nijuis-Heddes JMA, Bakker W: Calcified lymph node metastases in bronchioloalveolar carcinoma. Radiology 161:103, 1986.

977. Chaudhuri MR: Primary pulmonary cavitating carcinomas. Thorax 28:354, 1973.

978. Peabody J Jr, Katz S, Davis EW: Bronchial carcinoma arising in a lung cyst. Am J Roentgenol 77:1048, 1957.

979. Goldstein MJ, Snider GL, Liberson M, et al: Bronchogenic carcinoma and giant bullous disease. Am Rev Respir Dis 97:1062, 1968.

980. Peabody JW Jr, Rupnick EJ, Hanner JM: Bronchial carcinoma masquerading as a thin-walled cyst. Am J Roentgenol 77:1051, 1957.

981. Huang D, Weisbrod GL, Chamberlain DW: Unusual radiologic presentations of bronchioloalveolar carcinoma. J Can Assoc Radiol 37:94, 1986.

982. Woodring JH, Fried AM, Chuang VP: Solitary cavities of the lung: Diagnostic implications of cavity wall thickness. AJR 135:1269, 1980.

983. Woodring JH, Fried AM: Significance of wall thickness in solitary cavities of the lung: A follow-up study. Am J Roentgenol 140:473, 1983.

984. Fitzpatrick HF, Miller RE, Edgar MS Jr, et al: Bronchiolar carcinoma of the lung: A review of 33 patients. J Thorac Cardiovasc Surg 42:310, 1961.

985. Donaldson JC, Kaminsky DB, Elliott RC: Bronchiolar carcinoma: Report of 11 cases and review of the literature. Cancer 41:250, 1978.

986. Hill CA: Bronchioloalveolar carcinoma: A review. Radiology 150:15, 1984.

987. Muggia FM, Shervu L: Lung cancer: Diagnosis and metastatic sites. Semin Oncol 1:217, 1974.

988. Metzger RA, Mulhern CB Jr, Arger PH, et al: CT differentiation of solitary from diffuse bronchioloalveolar carcinoma. J Comput Assist Tomogr 5:830, 1981.

989. Zwirewich CV, Miller RR, Müller NL: Multicentric adenocarcinoma of the lung: CT-pathologic correlation. Radiology 176:185, 1990.

989a. Gaeta M, Caruso R, Barone M, et al: Ground-glass attenuation in nodular bronchioloalveolar carcinoma: CT patterns and prognostic value. J Comput Assist Tomogr 22:215, 1998.

990. Jang HJ, Lee KS, Kwon OJ, et al: Bronchioloalveolar carcinoma: Focal area of ground-glass attenuation at thin-section CT as an early sign. Radiology 199:485, 1996.

991. Epstein DM, Gefter WB, Miller WT: Lobar bronchioloalveolar cell carcinoma. Am J Roentgenol 139:463, 1982.

992. Trigaux JP, Genevois PA, Goncette L, et al: Bronchioloalveolar carcinoma: Computed tomography findings. Eur Respir J 9:9, 1996.

993. Epstein DM, Gefter WB, Miller WT: Lobar bronchioloalveolar cell carcinoma. Am J Roentgenol 139:463, 1982.

993a. Aquino SL, Chiles C, Halford P: Distinction of consolidative bronchioloalveolar carcinoma from pneumonia: Do CT criteria work? Am J Roentgenol 171:359, 1998.

994. Im JG, Han MC, Yu EJ, et al: Lobar bronchioloalveolar carcinoma: "Angiogram sign" on CT scans. Radiology 176:749, 1990.

995. Walykey MM: And what is your sign (letter)? Radiology 178:894, 1991.

996. Schuster MR, Scanlan KA: "CT angiogram sign" (letter). Radiology 181:903, 1991.

997. Senac JP, Bousquet C, Giron JM, et al: "Angiogram sign": Semiotic value in 60 cases (abstract). Radiology 185(P):243, 1992.

998. Vincent JM, Ng YY, Norton AJ, et al: CT "angiogram sign" in primary pulmonary lymphoma. J Comput Assist Tomogr 16:829, 1992.

999. Murayama S, Onitsuka H, Murakami J, et al: "CT angiogram sign" in obstructive pneumonitis and pneumonia. J Comput Assist Tomogr 17:609, 1993.

1000. Prichard MG, Brown PJ, Sterrett GF: Bronchioloalveolar carcinoma arising in long standing lung cysts. Thorax 39:545, 1984.

1001. Boucot KR, Cooper DA, Weiss W, et al: Appearance of first roentgenographic abnormalities due to lung cancer. JAMA 190:1103, 1964.

1002. Richardson RL, Weiss RB: Small cell carcinoma of the lung presenting as bilateral hilar adenopathy. South Med J 70:763, 1977.

1003. Selby HM, Luomanen R, Sherman RS: The x-ray appearance of oat-cell cancer of the lung. Radiology 81:817, 1963.

1004. Fleischner FG: The esophagus and mediastinal lymphadenopathy in bronchial carcinoma. Radiology 58:48, 1952.

1005. Fleischner FG, Sachsse E: Retrotracheal lymphadenopathy in bronchial carcinoma, revealed by the barium-filled esophagus. Am J Roentgenol 90:792, 1963.

1006. Lennard TWJ, Lennard AL, Elliot MJ: Barium swallow as an aid to preoperative assessment in patients with bronchogenic carcinoma. Br J Clin Pract 36:138, 1982.

1007. Pancoast HK: Importance of careful roentgen ray investigations of apical chest tumors. JAMA 83:1407, 1924.

1008. Pancoast HK: Superior pulmonary sulcus tumor: Tumor characterized by pain, Horner's syndrome, destruction of bone and atrophy of hand muscles. JAMA 99:1391, 1932.

1009. Freundlich IM, Chasen MH, Varma DGK: Magnetic resonance imaging of pulmonary apical tumors. J Thorac Imaging 11:210, 1996.

1010. Heelan RT, Demas BE, Caravelli JF, et al: Superior sulcus tumors: CT and MR imaging. Radiology 170:637, 1989.

1011. O'Connel RS, McLoud TC, Wilkins EW: Superior sulcus tumor: Radiographic diagnosis and workup. Am J Roentgenol 140:25, 1983.

1012. Stanford W, Barnes RP, Tucker AR: Influence of staging in superior sulcus (Pancoast) tumors of the lung. Ann Thorac Surg 29:406, 1980.

1013. Anderson TM, Moy PM, Holmes EC, et al: Factors affecting survival in superior sulcus tumors. J Clin Oncol 4:1598, 1986.

1014. Shahian DM, Neptune WB, Ellis FH Jr: Pancoast tumors: Improved survival with preoperative and postoperative radiotherapy. Ann Thorac Surg 43:32, 1987.

1015. Hamlin DJ, Burgener FA: CT, including sagittal and coronal reconstruction, in the evaluation of pancoast tumors. CT 6:43, 1982.

1016. Takasugi JE, Godwin JD, Halvorsen RE, et al: Computed tomographic evaluation of lesions in the thoracic apex. Invest Radiol 20:260, 1985.

1017. Webb WR, Jeffrey RB, Godwin JD: Thoracic computed tomography in superior sulcus tumors. CT 5:361, 1981.

1018. Scott IR, Müller NL, Miller RR, et al: Resectable stage III lung cancer: CT, surgical, and pathologic correlation. Radiology 166:75, 1988.

1019. Glazer HS, Duncan-Meyer J, Aronberg DJ, et al: Pleural and chest wall invasion in bronchogenic carcinoma: CT evaluation. Radiology 157:191, 1985.

1020. Pennes DR, Glazer GM, Wimbish KJ, et al: Chest wall invasion by lung cancer: Limitations of CT evaluation. Am J Roentgenol 144:507, 1985.

1021. Pearlberg JL, Sandler MA, Beute GH, et al: Limitations of CT in evaluation of neoplasms involving chest wall. J Comput Assist Tomogr 11:290, 1987.

1022. Ratto GB, Piacenza G, Frola C, et al: Chest wall involvement by lung cancer: Computed tomographic detection and results of operation. Ann Thorac Surg 51:182, 1991.

1023. Takasugi J, Rapoport S, Shaw C: Superior sulcus tumors: The role of imaging. J Thorac Imaging 4:41, 1989.

1024. McLoud TC, Filon RB, Edelman RR, et al: MR imaging of superior sulcus carcinoma. J Comput Assist Tomogr 13:233, 1989.

1025. Meyer PC: Metastatic carcinoma of the pleura. Thorax 21:437, 1966.

1026. Brinkman GL: The significance of pleural effusion complicating otherwise operable bronchogenic carcinoma. Dis Chest 36:152, 1959.

1027. Leung AN, Müller NL, Miller RR: CT in differential diagnosis of diffuse pleural disease. Am J Roentgenol 154:487, 1990.

1028. Murayama S, Murakami J, Yoshimitsu K, et al: CT diagnosis of pleural dissemination without pleural effusion in primary lung cancer. Radiat Med 14:117, 1996.

1029. Laurens RG Jr, Pine JR, Honig EG: Spontaneous pneumothorax in primary cavitating lung carcinoma. Radiology 146:295, 1983.

1030. Hyde L, Hyde CI: Rare occurrence of simultaneous pneumothorax and lung cancer. JAMA 239:1421, 1978.

1031. Yusuf MF, Luria SB, Marjani MA, et al: Spontaneous pneumothorax as a presenting feature of primary lung carcinoma. Conn Med 42:210, 1977.

1032. Steinhauslin CA, Cuttat JF: Spontaneous pneumothorax: A complication of lung cancer? Chest 88:709, 1985.

1033. Ayres JG, Pitcher DW, Rees PJ: Pneumothorax associated with primary bronchial carcinoma. Br J Dis Chest 74:180, 1980.

1034. Yeung K-Y, Bonnet JD: Bronchogenic carcinoma presenting as spontaneous pneumothorax: Case reports with review of literature. Cancer 39:2286, 1977.

1035. Watt AG: Occult carcinoma of the lung presenting as spontaneous pneumothorax. Med J Aust 2:277, 1978.

1036. Shirakawa T, Fukuda K, Miyamoto Y, et al: Parietal pleural invasion in lung masses: Evaluation with CT performed during deep inspiration and expiration. Radiology 192:809, 1994.

1037. Murata K, Takahashi M, Mori M, et al: Chest wall and mediastinal invasion by lung cancer: Evaluation with multisection expiratory dynamic CT. Radiology 191:251, 1994.

1038. Watanabe A, Shimokata K, Saka H, et al: Chest CT combined with artificial pneumothorax: Value in determining origin and extent of tumor. Am J Roentgenol 156:707, 1991.

1039. Yokoi K, Mori K, Miyazawa N, et al: Tumor invasion of the chest wall and mediastinum in lung cancer: Evaluation with pneumothorax CT. Radiology 181:147, 1991.

1040. Haggar AM, Pearlberg JL, Froelich JW, et al: Chest-wall invasion by carcinoma of the lung: Detection by MR imaging. Am J Roentgenol 148:1075, 1987.

1041. Webb WR, Gatsonis C, Zerhouni EA, et al: CT and MR imaging in staging non–small cell bronchogenic carcinoma: Report of the Radiologic Diagnostic Oncology Group. Radiology 178:705, 1991.

1042. Quint LE, Francis IR, Wahl RL, et al: Preoperative staging of nonsmall-cell carcinoma of the lung: Imaging methods. Am J Roentgenol 164:1349, 1995.

1043. Gefter WB: Magnetic resonance imaging in the evaluation of lung cancer. Semin Roentgenol 25:73, 1990.

1044. Webb WR, Sostman HD: MR imaging of thoracic disease: Clinical uses. Radiology 182:621, 1992.

1045. Sugana Y, Kobayashi H, Kitamura S, et al: Ultrasonographic evaluation of pleural and chest wall invasion of lung cancer. Chest 94:1271, 1988.

1046. Susuki N, Saitoh T, Kitamura S: Tumor invasion of the chest wall in lung cancer: Diagnosis with U.S. Radiology 187:39, 1993.

1047. Lamay P, Anthoine D, Rebeix G, et al: Ostéoses et myéloses cancéreuses d'origine bronchique. [Metastatic lesions of bone and bone marrow in bronchogenic carcinoma.] Rev Tuberc 29:401, 1965.

1048. Clain A: Secondary malignant disease of bone. Br J Cancer 19:15, 1965.

1049. Napoli LD, Hansen HH, Muggia FM, et al: The incidence of osseous involvement in lung cancer, with special reference to the development of osteoblastic changes. Radiology 108:17, 1973.

1050. Silvestri GA, Littenberg B, Colice GL: The clinical evaluation for detecting metastatic lung cancer: A meta-analysis. Am J Respir Crit Care Med 152:225, 1995.

1051. Michel F, Soler M, Imhof E, et al: Initial staging of non–small cell lung cancer: Value of routine radioisotope bone scanning. Thorax 46:469, 1991.

1052. Piehler JM, Pairolero PC, Gracey DR, et al: Unexplained diaphragmatic paralysis: A harbinger of malignant disease? J Thorac Cardiovasc Surg 84:861, 1982.

1053. Steinberg I, Finby N: Great vessel involvement in lung cancer: Angiocardiographic report on 250 consecutive proved cases. Am J Roentgenol 81:807, 1959.

1054. Hanbury WJ, Cureton RJR, Simon G: Pulmonary infarcts associated with bronchogenic carcinoma. Thorax 9:304, 1954.

1055. Held BT, Siegelman SS: Pulmonary infarction secondary to bronchogenic carcinoma. Am J Roentgenol 120:145, 1974.

1056. Marriott AE, Weisbrod G: Bronchogenic carcinoma associated with pulmonary infarction. Radiology 146:593, 1982.

1057. Fontana RS, Sanderson DR, Taylor WF, et al: Early lung cancer detection: Results of the initial (prevalence) radiologic and cytologic screening in the Mayo Clinic study. Am Rev Respir Dis 130:561, 1984.

1058. Frost JK, Ball WC Jr, Levin ML, et al: Early lung cancer detection: Results of the initial (prevalence) radiologic and cytologic screening in the Johns Hopkins study. Am Rev Respir Dis 130:549, 1984.

1059. Flehinger BJ, Melamed MR, Zaman MB, et al: Early lung cancer detection: Results of the initial (prevalence) radiologic and cytologic screening in the Memorial Sloan-Kettering study. Am Rev Respir Dis 130:555, 1984.

1060. Melamed MR, Flehinger BJ, Zaman MB, et al: Screening for early lung cancer: Results of the Memorial Sloan-Kettering study in New York. Chest 86:44, 1984.

1061. Screening (lung cancer). Chest 89(4 Suppl):324S, 1986.

1062. Melamed MR, Flehinger BJ, Zaman MB: Impact of early detection on the clinical course of lung cancer. Surg Clin North Am 67:909, 1987.

1063. Lee JJ, Lin RLM, Chen CH, et al: Clinical manifestations of bronchogenic carcinoma. J Formos Med Assoc 91:146, 1992.

1064. Le Roux BT: Bronchial carcinoma. Thorax 23:136, 1968.

1065. Boucot K, Cooper DA, Weiss W: The Philadelphia pulmonary neoplasm research project: An interim report. Ann Intern Med 54:363, 1961.

1066. Patel AM, Peters SG: Clinical manifestations of lung cancer. Mayo Clin Proc 68:273, 1993.

1067. Santiago SM, Lehrman S, Williams AJ: Bronchoscopy in patients with haemoptysis and normal chest roentgenograms. Br J Dis Chest 81:186, 1987.

1068. Liaw YS, Yang PC, Wu ZG, et al: The bacteriology of obstructive pneumonitis: A prospective study using ultrasound-guided transthoracic needle aspiration. Am J Respir Crit Care Med 149:1648, 1994.

1069. Lerner MA, Rosbash H, Frank HA, et al: Radiologic localization and management of cytologically discovered bronchial carcinoma. N Engl J Med 264:480, 1961.

1070. Woolner LB, Andersen HA, Bernatz PE: "Occult" carcinoma of the bronchus: A study of 15 cases of in situ or early invasive bronchogenic carcinoma. Dis Chest 37:278, 1960.

1071. Snider GL, Placik B: The relationship between pulmonary tuberculosis and bronchogenic carcinoma: A topographic study. Am Rev Respir Dis 99:229, 1969.

1072. Greco RJ, Steiner RM, Goldman S, et al: Bronchoalveolar cell carcinoma of the lung. Ann Thorac Surg 41:652, 1986.

1073. Roelsen E, Lund T, Søndergaard T, et al: Primary alveolar carcinomatosis (carcinoma) of the lung (so-called pulmonary adenomatosis or alveolar cell tumor): A review and report of 12 cases. Acta Med Scand 163:367, 1959.

1074. Knudson RJ, Hatch HB, Mitchell WT, et al: Unusual cancer of the lung: II. Bronchiolar carcinoma of the lung. Dis Chest 48:628, 1965.

1075. Marcq M, Galy P: Bronchioloalveolar carcinoma: Clinicopathologic relationships, natural history, and prognosis in 29 cases. Am Rev Respir Dis 107:621, 1973.

1076. Homma H, Kira S, Takahashi Y, et al: A case of alveolar cell carcinoma accompanied by fluid and electrolyte depletion through production of voluminous amounts of lung liquid. Am Rev Respir Dis 111:857, 1975.

1077. Heimlich HJ, Rubin M: Spontaneous pneumothorax as a presenting feature of primary carcinoma of the lung. Dis Chest 27:457, 1955.

1078. O'Connor BM, Ziegler P, Spaulding MB: Spontaneous pneumothorax in small cell lung cancer. Chest 102:628, 1992.

1079. Chou S-H, Cheng Y-J, Kao E-L, et al: Spontaneous haemothorax: An unusual presentation of primary lung cancer. Thorax 48:1185, 1993.

1080. Liebow AA: Pathology of carcinoma of the lung as related to the roentgen shadow. Am J Roentgenol 74:383, 1955.

1081. Stevens AE: Mediastinal pain in bronchial carcinoma. Lancet 1:1230, 1963.

1082. Sobel M, Rodman T, Pastor BH: The incidence and clinical significance of cardiac involvement in bronchogenic carcinoma. Am J Med Sci 240:739, 1960.

1083. Tamura A, Matsubara O, Yoshimura N, et al: Cardiac metastasis of lung cancer: A study of metastatic pathways and clinical manifestations. Cancer 70:437, 1992.

1084. Fraser RS, Viloria JB, Wang N-S: Cardiac tamponade as a presentation of extracardiac malignancy. Cancer 45:1697, 1980.

1085. Harris RD, Kostiner AI: Pneumopericardium associated with bronchogenic carcinoma. Chest 67:115, 1975.

1086. Okamoto H, Shinkai T, Yamakido M, et al: Cardiac tamponade caused by primary lung cancer and the management of pericardial effusion. Cancer 71:93, 1993.

1087. Haskell RJ, French WJ: Cardiac tamponade as the initial presentation of malignancy. Chest 88:70, 1985.

1088. Gilkey S, Reyes CV: Cardiac tamponade in lung cancer. J Surg Oncol 28:301, 1985.

1089. Gilbert I, Henning RJ: Adenocarcinoma of the lung presenting with pericardial tamponade: Report of a case and review of the literature. Heart Lung 14:83, 1985.

1090. Corris PA, Kertes PJ, Jennings K, et al: Detection of occult cardiac invasion by two dimensional echocardiography in patients with bronchial carcinoma. Thorax 41:138, 1986.

1091. Weg IL, Mehra S, Azueta V, et al: Cardiac metastasis from adenocarcinoma of the lung: Echocardiographic-pathologic correlation. Am J Med 80:108, 1986.

1092. Lee TM, Chen MF, Liau CS, et al: Role of transesophageal echocardiography in the management of metastatic tumours invading the left atrium. Cardiology 88:214, 1997.

1093. Lynch M, Balk MA, Lee RB, et al: Role of transesophageal echocardiography in the management of patients with bronchogenic carcinoma invading the left atrium. Am J Cardiol 76:1101, 1995.

1094. Onuigbo WIB: Direct extension of cancer between pulmonary veins and the left atrium. Chest 62:444, 1972.

1095. Al-Hillawi AH, Hayward R, Johnson NMcI, et al: Lung cancer masquerading as atrial myxoma. Thorax 38:870, 1983.

1096. Miranda AL, Rufilanchas JJ, Juffe A, et al: Direct extension of bronchogenic carcinoma through the pulmonary veins: Surgical implications. Chest 68:123, 1975.

1097. Fujishima S, Okada Y, Irie K, et al: Multiple brain infarction and hemorrhage by nonbacterial thrombotic endocarditis in occult lung cancer—a case report. Angiology 45:161, 1994.

1098. Dines DE: Dysphagia—symptom of bronchogenic carcinoma. Dis Chest 55:1, 1969.

1099. Stankey RM, Roshe J, Sogocio RM: Carcinoma of the lung and dysphagia. Dis Chest 55:13, 1969.

1099a. Hirschmann JV, Raugi GJ: Dermatologic features of the superior vena cava syndrome. Arch Dermatol 128:953, 1992.

1100. Maddox A-M, Valdivieso M, Lukeman J, et al: Superior vena cava obstruction in small cell bronchogenic carcinoma: Clinical parameters and survival. Cancer 52:2165, 1983.

1101. Parish JM, Marschke RF Jr, Dines DE, et al: Etiologic considerations in superior vena cava syndrome. Mayo Clin Proc 56:407, 1981.

1102. Schraufnagel DE, Hill R, Leech JA, et al: Superior vena caval obstruction: Is it a medical emergency? Am J Med 70:1169, 1981.

1103. Conlan AA, Pool R, Louridas G, et al: Superior vena caval obstruction in urban blacks: A report of 82 cases. S Afr Med J 64:827, 1983.

1104. Sculier JP, Evans WK, Feld R, et al: Superior vena caval obstruction syndrome in small cell lung cancer. Cancer 57:847, 1986.

1105. Wurschmidt F, Bunemann H, Heilmann HP: Small cell lung cancer with and without superior vena cava syndrome: A multivariate analysis of prognostic factors in 408 cases. Int J Radiat Oncol Biol Phys 33:77, 1995.

1106. Urban T, Lebeau B, Chastang C, et al: Superior vena cava syndrome in small-cell lung cancer. Arch Intern Med 153:384, 1993.

1107. Gauden SJ: Superior vena cava syndrome induced by bronchogenic carcinoma: Is this an oncological emergency? Australas Radiol 37:363, 1993.

1108. Yellin A, Rosen A, Reichert N, et al: Superior vena cava syndrome—the myth—the facts. Am Rev Respir Dis 141:1114, 1990.

1109. King JW, Walsh TE: Variable intrathoracic upper airway obstruction due to non–small cell lung cancer: Palliation using physiologic and mechanical stenting. Chest 89:896, 1986.

1110. Mason BA: Axillary-subclavian vein occlusion in patients with lung neoplasms. Cancer 48:1886, 1981.

1111. Gacad G, Akhtar N, Cohn JN: Orthostatic hypoxemia in a patient with bronchogenic carcinoma. Arch Intern Med 134:1113, 1974.

1112. Spengler DM, Kirsh MM, Kaufer H: Orthopaedic aspects and early diagnosis of superior sulcus tumor of lung (Pancoast). J Bone Joint Surg Am 55:1645, 1973.

1113. Simon H, Moon A: Pitfalls in the diagnosis of Pancoast tumor. Radiology 82:235, 1964.

1114. Woodruff CE, Steininger WJ: Intrathoracic squamous cell carcinoma, central and peripheral. Am Rev Respir Dis 91:363, 1965.

1115. Hepper NGG, Herskovic T, Witten DM, et al: Thoracic inlet tumors. Ann Intern Med 64:979, 1966.

1116. Johnson DH, Hainsworth JD, Greco FA: Pancoast's syndrome and small cell lung cancer. Chest 82:602, 1982.

1117. Rockoff SD: Apical lung cancer masquerading as a Pancoast tumor. Am J Roentgenol 139:163, 1982.

1118. Onuigbo WIB: Some pathological data on 2,000 adenocarcinomas and squamous cell carcinomas of the lung. Br J Cancer 17:1, 1963.

1119. Osteen RT, Kopf G, Wilson RE: In pursuit of the unknown primary. Am J Surg 135:494, 1978.

1120. Clary CF, Michel RP, Wang N-S, et al: Metastatic carcinoma. Cancer 51:362, 1983.

1121. Matthews MJ, Kanhouwa S, Peckren J, et al: Frequency of residual and metastatic tumor in patients undergoing curative surgical resection in lung cancer. Chem Rep 4:63, 1973.

1122. Jones EM: Placental metastases from bronchial carcinoma. BMJ 2:491, 1969.

1123. Kelly C, Henderson D, Corris P: Breast lumps: Rare presentation of oat cell carcinoma of lung. J Clin Pathol 41:171, 1988.

1124. Sridhar KS, Rao RK, Kunhardt B: Skeletal muscle metastases from lung cancer. Cancer 59:1530, 1987.

1125. Onuigbo WIB: Centrifugal metastasis in lung cancer. Br J Dis Chest 55:86, 1961.

1126. Warren S, Gates O: Lung cancer and metastasis. Arch Pathol 78:467, 1964.

1127. Berge T, Toremalm NG: Bronchial cancer—a clinical and pathological study. Scand J Respir Dis 56:109, 1975.

1128. Hirsch FR: Histopathologic Classification and Metastatic Pattern of Small Cell Carcinoma of the Lung. Copenhagen, Munksgaard, 1983.

1129. De La Monte SM, Hutchins GM, Moore GW: Altered metastatic behavior of small cell carcinoma of the lung after chemotherapy and radiation. Cancer 61:2176, 1988.

1130. Yesner R, Carter D: Pathology of carcinoma of the lung. Clin Chest Med 3:257, 1982.

1131. Rouvière H: Anatomy of the Human Lymphatic System. (Translated by Tobias MJ). Ann Arbor, Edwards, 1938.

1132. Baird JA: The pathways of lymphatic spread of carcinoma of the lung. Br J Surg 52:868, 1965.

1133. Onuigbo WIB: Contralateral cervical node metastases in lung cancer. Thorax 17:201, 1962.

1134. Shields TW: An evaluation of bronchogenic carcinoma in scalene lymph nodes. Union Internationalis Contra Cancrum Acta 15:508, 1959.

1135. Warren S, Gates O: Lung cancer and metastasis. Arch Pathol 78:467, 1964.

1136. Quint LE, Tummala S, Brisson LJ, et al: Distribution of distant metastases from newly diagnosed non–small cell lung cancer. Ann Thorac Surg 62:246, 1996.

1137. O'Neill BP, Buckner JC, Coffey RJ, et al: Brain metastatic lesions. Mayo Clin Proc 69:1062, 1994.

1138. Brain L: The neurological complications of neoplasms. Lancet 1:179, 1963.

1139. Salvati M, Cervoni L, Delfini R: Solitary brain metastases from nonoat cell lung cancer: Clinical and prognostic features. Neurosurg Rev 19:221, 1996.

1140. Burgess RE, Burgess VF, Dibella NJ: Brain metastasis in small cell carcinoma of the lung. JAMA 242:2084, 1979.

1141. Balducci L, Little DD, Khansur T, et al: Carcinomatous meningitis in small cell lung cancer. Am J Med Sci 287:31, 1984.

1142. Rosen ST, Aisner J, Makuch RW, et al: Carcinomatous leptomeningitis in small cell lung cancer: A clinicopathologic review of the National Cancer Institute experience. Medicine 61:45, 1982.

1143. Aroney RS, Dalley DN, Chan WK, et al: Meningeal carcinomatosis in small cell carcinoma of the lung. Am J Med 71:26, 1981.

1144. Weisberg LA: Solitary cerebellar metastases: Clinical and computed tomographic correlations. Arch Neurol 42:336, 1985.

1145. Andrews RJ, Gluck DS, Konchinergi RH: Surgical resection of brain metastases from lung cancer. Acta Neurochir (Wien) 138:382, 1996.

1146. Dunaway RL: Ptosis as the presenting sign of orbital involvement from metastatic bronchogenic carcinoma. Am J Optom Physiol Opt 62:908, 1985.

1147. Delaney P, Khoa N, Saini N: Isolated trigeminal neuropathy: An unusual complication of carcinoma of the lung. JAMA 237:2522, 1977.

1148. Murphy KC, Feld R, Evans WK, et al: Intramedullary spinal cord metastases from small cell carcinoma of the lung. J Clin Oncol 1:99, 1983.

1149. Nori D, Sundaresan N, Bains M, et al: Bronchogenic carcinoma with invasion of the spine: Treatment with combined surgery and perioperative brachytherapy. JAMA 248:2491, 1982.

1150. Wang A-M, Lewis ML, Rumbaugh CL, et al: Spinal cord or nerve root compression in patients with malignant disease: CT evaluation. CT 8:420, 1984.

1151. Rogers LR, Cho ES, Kempin S, et al: Cerebral infarction from nonbacterial thrombotic endocarditis: Clinical and pathological study including the effects of anticoagulation. Am J Med 83:746, 1987.

1152. So NK, O'Neill BP, Frytak S, et al: Delayed leukoencephalopathy in survivors with small cell lung cancer. Neurology 37:1198, 1987.

1153. Bender RA, Hansen H: Hypercalcemia in bronchogenic carcinoma, a prospective study of 200 patients. Ann Intern Med 80:205, 1974.

1154. Covelli HD, Zaloznik AJ, Shekitka KM, et al: Evaluation of bone pain in carcinoma of the lung: Role of the localized false-negative scan. JAMA 244:2625, 1980.

1155. Keim LW, Hoffman PF: Bilateral symmetrical metastases to the clavicular heads from bronchogenic carcinoma simulating primary hyperparathyroidism. Chest 66:99, 1974.

1156. Sinclair DJ, Gravelle IH: Abdominal presentation of bronchogenic carcinoma. Br J Radiol 40:441, 1967.

1157. Johnson DH, Hainsworth JD, Greco FA: Extrahepatic biliary obstruction caused by small-cell lung cancer. Ann Intern Med 102:487, 1985.

1158. McGuire BM, Cherwitz DL, Rabe KM, et al: Small-cell carcinoma of the lung manifesting as acute hepatic failure. Mayo Clin Proc 72:133, 1997.

1159. Mittleman RE: Hepatic rupture due to metastatic lung carcinoma. Am J Clin Pathol 88:506, 1987.

1160. Sheriff DS: Lactic acidosis and small cell carcinoma of the lung. Postgrad Med J 62:297, 1986.

1161. Rice K, Schwartz SH: Lactic acidosis with small cell carcinoma: Rapid response to chemotherapy. Am J Med 79:501, 1985.

1162. Hilsenbeck SG, Raub WA Jr, Sridhar KS: Prognostic factors in lung cancer based on multivariate analysis. Am J Clin Oncol 16:301, 1993.

1163. Howe HR Jr, Hansen HJ, Albertson DA: Metastatic oat cell carcinoma of the lung producing extrahepatic bile duct obstruction. South Med J 78:1398, 1985.

1164. Allan SG, Bundred N, Eremin O, et al: Acute pancreatitis in association with small cell lung carcinoma: Potential pitfall in diagnosis and management. Postgrad Med J 61:643, 1985.

1165. Seidenwurm DJ, Elmer EB, Kaplan LM, et al: Metastases to the adrenal glands and the development of Addison's disease. Cancer 54:552, 1984.

1166. Antler AS, Ough Y, Pitchumoni CS, et al: Gastrointestinal metastases from malignant tumors of the lung. Cancer 49:170, 1982.

1167. Ginsberg RJ: Continuing controversies in staging NSCLC: An analysis of the revised 1997 staging system. Oncology 12:51, 1998.

1168. Rubin SA, Davis M: "Bull's eye" or "target" lesions of the stomach secondary to carcinoma of the lung. Am J Gastroenterol 80:67, 1985.

1169. Belcher JR: The changing pattern of bronchial carcinoma. Br J Dis Chest 81:87, 1987.

1170. Hsu CC, Chen JJ, Changchien CS: Endoscopic features of metastatic tumors in the upper gastrointestinal tract. Endoscopy 28:249, 1996.

1171. Jarry O, Vincent M, van Sraaten L, et al: Intestinal metastasis of pulmonary cancers: Apropos of 2 cases. Rev Pneumol Clin 46:283, 1990.
1172. Quayle AR, Holt S, Clark RG: Jejunal perforation secondary to metastatic bronchogenic carcinoma. Postgrad Med J 61:163, 1985.
1173. Eisen T, Hickish T, Smith IE, et al: Small-cell lung cancer. Lancet 345:1285, 1995.
1174. de la Monte SM, Hutchins GM, Moore GW: Paraneoplastic syndromes and constitutional symptoms in prediction of metastatic behavior of small cell carcinoma of the lung. Am J Med 77:851, 1984.
1175. Lindsey AM, Piper BF: Anorexia and weight loss: Indicators of cachexia in small cell lung cancer. Nutr Cancer 7:65, 1985.
1176. Rassam JW, Anderson G: Incidence of paramalignant disorders in bronchogenic carcinoma. Thorax 30:86, 1975.
1177. Eisenberg H: Endocrine manifestations of lung cancer. Semin Respir Med 9:414, 1988.
1178. Marchioli CC, Graziano SL: Paraneoplastic syndromes associated with small cell lung cancer. Chest Surg Clin North Am 7:65, 1997.
1179. Patel AM, Davila DG, Peters SG: Paraneoplastic syndromes associated with lung cancer. Mayo Clin Proc 68:278, 1993.
1180. Schiller JH, Jones JC: Paraneoplastic syndromes associated with lung cancer. Curr Opin Oncol 5:335, 1993.
1181. Pate JW, Campbell RE, Hughes FA: Unsuspected bronchogenic carcinoma. Dis Chest 37:56, 1960.
1182. Greene JG, Divertie M, Matthew B, et al: Small cell carcinoma of lung: Observations on four patients including one with a myasthenic syndrome. Arch Intern Med 122:333, 1968.
1183. Morton DL, Itabashi HH, Grimes DF: Nonmetastatic neurological complications of bronchogenic carcinoma: The carcinomatous neuromyopathies. J Thorac Cardiovasc Surg 51:14, 1966.
1184. Holt GW: Idiopathic neuropathy in cancer: A first sign in multiple system syndromes associated with malignancy. Am J Med Sci 242:93, 1961.
1185. Barontini F, Maurri S, Marini P: Total extrinsic ophthalmoplegia as only paraneoplastic sign two years before x-ray diagnosis of bronchial carcinoma. Ital J Neurol Sci 6:441, 1985.
1186. Boruchow I, Sanders V, Pabico R, et al: Peripheral neuropathy in bronchogenic carcinoma. Arch Intern Med 110:461, 1962.
1187. Daughtry DG, Chesney JG, Spear HC, et al: Unexplained systemic manifestations of malignant lung tumors. Dis Chest 52:632, 1967.
1188. Eagan RT, Maurer LH, Forcier RJ, et al: Small cell carcinoma of the lung: Staging, paraneoplastic syndromes, treatment, and survival. Cancer 33:527, 1974.
1189. Gracey DR, Southorn PA: Respiratory failure in Lambert-Eaton myasthenic syndrome. Chest 91:716, 1987.
1190. Lennon VA, Kryzer TJ, Griesmann GE, et al: Calcium-channel antibodies in the Lambert-Eaton syndrome and other paraneoplastic syndromes. N Engl J Med 332:1467, 1995.
1191. Johnston I, Lang BM, Leys K, et al: Heterogeneity of calcium channel autoantibodies detected using a small-cell lung cancer line derived from a Lambert-Eaton myasthenic syndrome patient. Neurology 44:334, 1994.
1192. Rose AL, Walton JN: Polymyositis: A survey of 89 cases with particular reference to treatment and prognosis. Brain 89:747, 1966.
1193. Winkelmann RK, Mulder DW, Lambert EH, et al: Course of dermatomyositis-polymyositis: Comparison of untreated and cortisone-treated patients. Mayo Clin Proc 43:545, 1968.
1194. Benbassat J, Gefel D, Larholt K, et al: Prognostic factors in polymyositis/dermatomyositis: A computer-assisted analysis of ninety-two cases. Arthritis Rheum 28:249, 1985.
1195. Chow WH, Gridley G, Mellemjaer L, et al: Cancer risk following polymyositis and dermatomyositis: A nationwide cohort study in Denmark. Cancer Causes Control 6:9, 1995.
1196. Siemsen JK, Meister L: Bronchogenic carcinoma associated with severe orthostatic hypotension. Ann Intern Med 58:669, 1963.
1197. Graus F, Bonaventura I, Uchuya M, et al: Indolent anti-Hu-associated paraneoplastic sensory neuropathy. Neurology 44:2258, 1994.
1198. Graus F, Elkon KB, Cordon-Cardo C, et al: Sensory neuronopathy and small cell lung cancer: Antineuronal antibody that also reacts with the tumor. Am J Med 80:45, 1986.
1199. Rudd AG, Nicholas D, Hodkinson HM: Autonomic neuropathy and hypertrophic osteoarthropathy in association with malignancy. Br J Dis Chest 79:396, 1985.
1200. Schuffler MD, Baird HW, Fleming CR, et al: Intestinal pseudo-obstruction as the presenting manifestation of small-cell carcinoma of the lung: A paraneoplastic neuropathy of the gastrointestinal tract. Ann Intern Med 98:129, 1983.
1201. Dropcho EJ: Antiamphiphysin antibodies with small-cell lung carcinoma and paraneoplastic encephalomyelitis. Ann Neurol 39:659, 1996.
1202. Simpson DA, Pawlak AM, Tegmeyer L, et al: Paraneoplastic intestinal pseudo-obstruction, mononeuritis multiplex, and sensory neuropathy/neuronopathy. J Am Osteopath Assoc 96:125, 1996.
1203. Maier HC, Sommers SC: Neuroendocrine carcinoma of lung associated with bradycardia and episodic cardiac asystole. Ann Thorac Surg 41:560, 1986.
1204. Greenlee JE, Lipton HL: Anticerebellar antibodies in serum and cerebrospinal fluid of a patient with oat cell carcinoma of the lung and paraneoplastic cerebellar degeneration. Ann Neurol 19:82, 1986.
1205. Dhib-Jalbut S, Liwnicz BH: Immunocytochemical binding of serum IgG from a patient with oat cell tumor and paraneoplastic motoneuron disease to normal

human cerebral cortex and molecular layer of cerebellum. Acta Neuropath 69:96, 1986.
1206. Eekhof JL: Remission of a paraneoplastic cerebellar syndrome. Clin Neurol Neurosurg 87:133, 1985.
1207. Sekido Y, Bader SA, Carbone DP, et al: Molecular analysis of the HuD gene encoding a paraneoplastic encephalomyelitis antigen in human lung cancer cell lines. Cancer Res 54:4988, 1994.
1208. Ball JA, Warner T, Reid P, et al: Central alveolar hypoventilation associated with paraneoplastic brain-stem encephalitis and anti-Hu antibodies. J Neurol 241:561, 1994.
1209. Panegyres PK, Reading MC, Esiri MM: The inflammatory reaction of paraneoplastic ganglionitis and encephalitis: An immunohistochemical study. J Neurol 240:93, 1993.
1210. Brennan LV, Craddock PR: Limbic encephalopathy as a nonmetastatic complication of oat cell lung cancer: Its reversal after treatment of the primary lung lesion. Am J Med 75:518, 1983.
1211. Delsedime M, Cantello R, Durelli L, et al: A syndrome resembling limbic encephalitis, associated with bronchial carcinoma, but without neuropathological abnormality: A case report. J Neurol 231:165, 1984.
1212. Kalkman PH, Allan S, Birchall IW: Magnetic resonance imaging of limbic encephalitis. Can Assoc Radiol J 44:121, 1993.
1213. Sakai K, Gofuku M, Kitagawa Y, et al: A hippocampal protein associated with paraneoplastic neurologic syndrome and small cell lung carcinoma. Biochem Biophys Res Commun 199:1200, 1994.
1214. Mancall EL, Rosales RK: Necrotizing myelopathy associated with visceral carcinoma. Brain 87:639, 1964.
1215. Ojeda VJ: Necrotizing myelopathy associated with malignancy: A clinicopathologic study of two cases and literature review. Cancer 53:1115, 1984.
1216. Matsubara S, Yamaji Y, Fujita T, et al: Cancer-associated retinopathy syndrome: A case of small cell lung cancer expressing recoverin immunoreactivity. Lung Cancer 14:265, 1996.
1217. Thirkill CE: Lung cancer-induced blindness. Lung Cancer 14:253, 1996.
1218. Adamus G, Guy J, Schmied JL, et al: Role of anti-recoverin autoantibodies in cancer-associated retinopathy. Invest Ophthalmol Vis Sci 34:2626, 1993.
1219. Thirkill CE, Keltner JL, Tyler NK, et al: Antibody reactions with retina and cancer-associated antigens in 10 patients with cancer-associated retinopathy. Arch Ophthalmol 111:931, 1993.
1220. Knowling MA, Meakin JW, Hradsky NS, et al: Hypertrichosis lanuginosa acquisita associated with adenocarcinoma of the lung. Can Med Assoc J 126:1308, 1982.
1221. Shee CD, Graham VAL: Acquired hypertrichosis lanuginosa and carcinoma of the bronchus. Thorax 36:153, 1981.
1222. Hovenden AL: Acquired hypertrichosis lanuginosa associated with malignancy. Arch Intern Med 147:2013, 1987.
1223. Witkowski JA, Parish LC: Bazex's syndrome: Paraneoplastic acrokeratosis. JAMA 248:2883, 1982.
1224. Jacobsen FK, Abildtrup N, Laursen SO, et al: Acrokeratosis paraneoplastica (Bazex's syndrome). Arch Dermatol 120:502, 1984.
1225. Knowles JH, Smith LH Jr: Extrapulmonary manifestations of bronchogenic carcinoma. N Engl J Med 262:505, 1960.
1226. Doll DC, McCagh MF, Welton WA: Sign of Leser-Trélat. JAMA 238:236, 1977.
1227. Hattori A, Umegae Y, Kataki S, et al: Small cell carcinoma of the lung with Leser-Trélat sign. Arch Dermatol 118:1017, 1982.
1228. Brenner S, Golan H, Gat A, et al: Paraneoplastic subacute cutaneous lupus erythematosus: Report of a case associated with cancer of the lung. Dermatology 194:172, 1997.
1229. Rojo Sanchez S, Suarez Fernandez R, de Eusebio Murillo E, et al: Erythema gyratum repens: Another case of a rare disorder but no new insight into pathogenesis. Dermatology 193:336, 1996.
1230. Caux F, Lebbe C, Thomine E, et al: Erythema gyratum repens: Case studies with immunofluorescence, immunoelectron microscopy and immunohistochemistry. Br J Dermatol 131:102, 1994.
1231. Mullans EA, Cohen PR: Tripe palms: A cutaneous paraneoplastic syndrome. South Med J 89:626, 1996.
1232. Cohen PR: Hypertrophic pulmonary osteoarthropathy and tripe palms in a man with squamous cell carcinoma of the larynx and lung: Report of a case and review of cutaneous paraneoplastic syndromes associated with laryngeal and lung malignancies. Am J Clin Oncol 16:268, 1993.
1233. Requena L, Aguilar A, Renedo G, et al: Tripe palms: A cutaneous marker of internal malignancy. J Dermatol 22:491, 1995.
1234. Bastiaens MT, Zwan NV, Verschueen GL, et al: Three cases of pemphigus vegetans: Induction by enalapril—association with internal malignancy. Int J Dermatol 33:168, 1994.
1235. Conejo-Mir JS, Casals M, Garciandia C, et al: Cutaneous sarcoid granulomas with oat cell carcinoma of the lung. Dermatology 191:59, 1995.
1236. Monsieur I, Meysman M, Noppen M, et al: Non-small-cell lung cancer with multiple paraneoplastic syndromes. Eur Respir J 8:1231, 1995.
1237. Yacoub MH: Relation between the histology of bronchial carcinoma and hypertrophic pulmonary osteoarthropathy. Thorax 20:537, 1965.
1238. Fujishita T, Mizushima Y, Yoshida Y, et al: A case of small cell carcinoma of the lung associated with hypertrophic pulmonary osteoarthropathy. Tumori 82:259, 1996.
1239. Semple T, McCluskie RA: Generalized hypertrophic osteoarthropathy in association with bronchial carcinoma: A review based on 24 cases. BMJ 1:754, 1955.
1240. Ali A, Tetalman MR, Fordham EW, et al: Distribution of hypertrophic pulmonary osteoarthropathy. Am J Roentgenol 134:771, 1980.

1241. Berman B: Pulmonary hypertrophic osteoarthropathy. Arch Intern Med 112:947, 1963.

1242. Huckstep RL, Bodkin PE: Vagotomy in hypertrophic pulmonary osteoarthropathy associated with bronchial carcinoma. Lancet 2:343, 1958.

1243. Court P, Binet J-P, Lemoine G, et al: Syndrome de Pierre Marie-Bamberger et cancer du poumon: (à propos de 12 interventions dont 2 vagotomies). [Pierre Marie-Bamberger syndrome (hypertrophic pulmonary osteoarthropathy) and cancer of the lung: 12 surgical interventions, including 2 vagotomies.] J Fr Med Chir Thorac 18:69, 1964.

1244. Greenfield GB, Schorsch HA, Shkolnik A: The various roentgen appearances of pulmonary hypertrophic osteoarthropathy. Am J Roentgenol 101:927, 1967.

1245. Shapiro M: Hypertrophic osteoarthropathy. AMA Arch Intern Med 98:700, 1956.

1246. Papavasiliou CG: Pulmonary metastases from cancer of the nasopharynx associated with hypertrophic osteoarthropathy. Br J Radiol 36:680, 1963.

1247. Liu RS, Chen YK, Yen SH, et al: Hypertrophic pulmonary osteoarthropathy in nasopharyngeal carcinoma: An early sign of pulmonary metastasis. Nucl Med Commun 16:785, 1995.

1248. Daly BD: Thoracic metastases from nasopharyngeal carcinoma presenting as hypertrophic pulmonary osteoarthropathy: Scintigraphic and CT findings. Clin Radiol 50:545, 1995.

1249. Becker KL, Gazdar AF (eds): The Endocrine Lung in Health and Disease. Philadelphia, WB Saunders, 1984.

1250. Havemann K, Sorenson G, Gropp C (eds): Peptide Hormones in Lung Cancer. Recent Results Cancer Res 99, 1985.

1251. Gomez-Uria A, Pazianos AG: Syndromes resulting from ectopic hormone-producing tumors. Med Clin North Am 59:431, 1975.

1252. Leading article: Endocrine abnormalities in bronchial carcinoma. BMJ 4:5, 1968.

1253. Lokich JJ: The frequency and clinical biology of the ectopic hormone syndromes of small cell carcinoma. Cancer 50:2111, 1982.

1254. Hansen M, Hammer M, Hummer L: Diagnostic and therapeutic implications of ectopic hormone production in small cell carcinoma of the lung. Thorax 35:101, 1980.

1255. Abe K, Kameya T, Yamaguchi K, et al: Hormone-producing lung cancers: Endocrinologic and morphologic studies. In Becker KL, Gazdar AF (eds): The Endocrine Lung in Health and Disease. Philadelphia, WB Saunders, 1984, p 549.

1256. Imura H, Matsukura S, Yamamoto H, et al: Studies on ectopic ACTH-producing tumors: II. Clinical and biochemical features of 30 cases. Cancer 35:430, 1975.

1257. Lichter I, Sirett NE: Serial measurement of plasma cortisol in lung cancer. Thorax 30:91, 1975.

1258. Hatch HB Jr, Segaloff A, Ochsner A: Adrenocortical function in bronchogenic carcinoma: Study of 100 patients. Ann Surg 161:645, 1965.

1259. Bondy PK, Gilby ED: Endocrine function in small cell undifferentiated carcinoma of the lung. Cancer 50:2147, 1982.

1260. Riggs BL Jr, Sprague RG: Association of Cushing's syndrome and neoplastic disease: Observations in 232 cases of Cushing's syndrome and review of literature. Arch Intern Med 108:841, 1961.

1261. Hemley SD, Arida EJ, Finby N: Cushing's syndrome associated with bronchogenic carcinoma. Radiology 80:1061, 1963.

1262. Stewart PM, Gibson S, Crosby SR, et al: ACTH precursors characterize the ectopic ACTH syndrome. Clin Endocrinol (Oxf) 40:199, 1994.

1263. Auchus RJ, Mastorakos G, Friedman TC, et al: Corticotropin-releasing hormone production by a small cell carcinoma in a patient with ACTH-dependent Cushing's syndrome. J Endocrinol Invest 17:447, 1994.

1264. Suda T, Tozawa F, Dobashi I, et al: Corticotropin-releasing hormone, proopiomelanocortin, and glucocorticoid receptor gene expression in adrenocorticotropin-producing tumors in vitro. J Clin Invest 92:2790, 1993.

1265. Boon ES, Leers MP, Tjwa MK: Ectopic Cushing's syndrome in a patient with squamous cell carcinoma of the lung due to CRF-like production. Monaldi Arch Chest Dis 49:19, 1994.

1266. Shepherd FA, Laskey J, Evans WK, et al: Cushing's syndrome associated with ectopic corticotropin production and small-cell lung cancer. J Clin Oncol 10:21, 1992.

1267. Delisle L, Boyer MJ, Warr D, et al: Ectopic corticotropin syndrome and small-cell carcinoma of the lung: Clinical features, outcome, and complications. Arch Intern Med 153:746, 1993.

1268. Jex RK, van Heerden JA, Carpenter PC, et al: Ectopic ACTH syndrome: Diagnostic and therapeutic aspects. Am J Surg 149:276, 1985.

1269. Findling JW, Tyrrell JB: Occult ectopic secretion of corticotropin. Arch Intern Med 146:929, 1986.

1270. Williams ED, Azzopardi JG: Tumours of the lung and the carcinoid syndrome. Thorax 15:30, 1960.

1271. Azzopardi JG, Bellau AR: Carcinoid syndrome and oat-cell carcinoma of the bronchus. Thorax 20:393, 1965.

1272. Gowenlock AH, Platt DS, Campbell ACP, et al: Oat-cell carcinoma of the bronchus secreting 5-hydroxytryptophan. Lancet 1:304, 1964.

1273. Kinloch JD, Webb JM, Eccleston D, et al: Carcinoid syndrome associated with oat-cell carcinoma of bronchus. BMJ 1:1533, 1965.

1274. Majcher SJ, Lee ER, Reingold IM, et al: Carcinoid syndrome in bronchogenic carcinoma. Arch Intern Med 117:57, 1966.

1275. Parish DJ, Crawford N, Spencer AT: The secretion of 5-hydroxytryptamine by a poorly-differentiated bronchial carcinoma. Thorax 19:62, 1964.

1276. Leading article: Pharmacology of the carcinoid syndrome. Lancet 1:404, 1968.

1277. Takai E, Yano T, Iguchi H, et al: Tumor-induced hypercalcemia and parathyroid hormone-related protein in lung carcinoma. Cancer 78:1384, 1996.

1278. Carey VCI: The incidence of hypercalcemia in association with bronchogenic carcinoma. Am Rev Respir Dis 93:584, 1966.

1279. Campbell JH, Ralston S, Boyle IT, et al: Symptomatic hypercalcaemia in lung cancer. Respir Med 85:223, 1991.

1280. Stuart-Harris R, Ahern V, Danks JA, et al: Hypercalcaemia in small cell lung cancer: Report of a case associated with parathyroid hormone-related protein (PTHrP). Eur J Cancer 29:1601, 1993.

1281. Strickland NJ, Bold AM, Medd WE: Bronchial carcinoma with hypercalcaemia simulating cerebral metastases. BMJ 3:590, 1967.

1282. Locks MO: Incidence of hypercalcemia in patients with proved carcinoma of the lung. Lancet 82:165, 1962.

1283. Carey VCI: Hypercalcemia and bronchial carcinoma. Am Rev Respir Dis 85:258, 1962.

1284. Coggeshall J, Merrill W, Hande K, et al: Implications of hypercalcemia with respect to diagnosis and treatment of lung cancer. Am J Med 80:325, 1986.

1285. Connor TB, Thomas WC Jr, Howard JE: The etiology of hypercalcemia associated with lung carcinoma. J Clin Invest 35:697, 1956.

1286. Lipsett MB (moderator): Clinical Staff Conference National Cancer Institute (National Institutes of Health): Humoral syndromes associated with nonendocrine tumors. Ann Intern Med 61:733, 1964.

1287. Taylor DM, Siemsen AW: Bronchogenic carcinoma simulating hyperparathyroidism. Arch Intern Med 115:67, 1965.

1288. Tanaka H, Kobayashi S, Masaoka A, et al: Hypercalcemia induced by parathyroid hormone-related protein from lung cancer tissue. Chest 100:1451, 1991.

1289. Myers WPL: Hypercalcemia in neoplastic disease. AMA Arch Surg 80:308, 1960.

1290. Segura Dominguez A, Andrade Olivie MA, Rodriguez Sousa T, et al: Plasma parathyroid hormone related-protein levels in patients with cancer, normocalcemic and hypercalcemic. Clin Chim Acta 244:163, 1996.

1291. Sherwood LM: The multiple causes of hypercalcemia in malignant disease. N Engl J Med 303:1412, 1980.

1292. Robertson RP: Prostaglandins and hypercalcemia of cancer. Med Clin North Am 65:845, 1981.

1293. Nielsen PK, Rasmussen AK, Feldt-Rasmussen U, et al: Ectopic production of intact parathyroid hormone by a squamous cell lung carcinoma in vivo and in vitro. J Clin Endocrinol Metab 81:3793, 1996.

1294. Shigeno C, Yamamoto I, Dokoh S, et al: Identification of 1,24(R)-Dihydroxyvitamin D3-like bone resorbing lipid in a patient with cancer-associated hypercalcemia. J Clin Endocrinol Metab 61:761, 1985.

1295. Johnson BE, Chute JP, Rushin J, et al: A prospective study of patients with lung cancer and hyponatremia of malignancy. Am J Respir Crit Care Med 156:1669, 1997.

1296. List AF, Hainsworth JD, Davis BW, et al: The syndrome of inappropriate secretion of antidiuretic hormone (SIADH) in small-cell lung cancer. J Clin Oncol 4:1191, 1986.

1297. Gross AJ, Steinberg SM, Reilly JG, et al: Atrial natriuretic factor and arginine vasopressin production in tumor cell lines from patients with lung cancer and their relationship to serum sodium. Cancer Res 53:67, 1993.

1298. Schwartz WB, Tassel D, Bartter FC: Further observations on hyponatremia and renal sodium loss probably resulting from inappropriate secretion of antidiuretic hormone. N Engl J Med 262:743, 1960.

1299. Ross EJ: Hyponatremic syndromes associated with carcinoma of the bronchus. QJM 32:297, 1963.

1300. Kaye M: An investigation into the cause of hyponatremia in the syndrome of inappropriate secretion of antidiuretic hormone. Am J Med 41:910, 1966.

1301. Thorn NA, Transbøl I: Hyponatremia and bronchogenic carcinoma associated with renal excretion of large amounts of antidiuretic material. Am J Med 35:257, 1963.

1302. Bower BF, Mason DM, Forsham PH, et al: Bronchogenic carcinoma with inappropriate antidiuretic activity in plasma and tumor. N Engl J Med 271:934, 1964.

1303. Amatruda TT Jr, Mulrow PJ, Gallagher JC, et al: Carcinoma of the lung with inappropriate antidiuresis: Demonstration of antidiuretic-hormone-like activity in tumor extract. N Engl J Med 269:544, 1963.

1304. Panayiotou H, Small SC, Hunter JH, et al: Sweet taste (dysgeusia): The first symptoms of hyponatremia in small cell carcinoma. Arch Intern Med 155:1325, 1995.

1305. Taylor HC, Fallon MD, Velasco ME: Oncogenic osteomalacia and inappropriate antidiuretic hormone secretion due to oat-cell carcinoma. Ann Intern Med 101:786, 1984.

1306. Cohen IM, Warren SE, Skowsky WR: Occult pulmonary malignancy in syndrome of inappropriate ADH secretion with normal ADH levels. Chest 86:929, 1984.

1307. Coyle S, Penney MD, Masters PW, et al: Early diagnosis of ectopic arginine vasopressin secretion. Clin Chem 39:152, 1993.

1308. Metz SA, Weintraub B, Rosen SW, et al: Ectopic secretion of chorionic gonadotropin by a lung carcinoma: Pituitary gonadotropin and subunit secretion and prolonged chemotherapeutic remission. Am J Med 65:325, 1978.

1309. Braunstein GD, Vaitukaitis JL, Carbone PP, et al: Ectopic production of human chorionic gonadotropin by neoplasms. Ann Intern Med 78:39, 1973.

1310. Charles MA, Claypool R, Schaaf M, et al: Lung carcinoma associated with production of three placental proteins: Ectopic human chorionic gonadotropin, human chorionic somatomammotropin, and placental alkaline phosphatase. Arch Intern Med 132:427, 1973.

1311. Fusco FD, Rosen SW: Gonadotropin-producing anaplastic large-cell carcinomas of the lung. N Engl J Med 275:507, 1966.
1312. Camiel MR, Benninghoff DL, Alexander LL: Gynecomastia associated with lung cancer. Dis Chest 52:445, 1967.
1313. Faiman C, Colwell JA, Ryan RJ, et al: Gonadotropin secretion from a bronchogenic carcinoma: Demonstration by radioimmunoassay. N Engl J Med 277:1395, 1967.
1314. Rosen SW, Becker CE, Schlaff S, et al: Ectopic gonadotropin production before clinical recognition of bronchogenic carcinoma. N Engl J Med 279:640, 1968.
1315. Cottrell JC, Becker KL, Matthews MJ, et al: The histology of gonadotropin-secreting bronchogenic carcinoma. Am J Clin Pathol 52:720, 1969.
1316. Cottrell JC, Becker KL, Moore CF: Immunofluorescent studies in gonadotropin-secreting bronchogenic carcinoma. Am J Clin Pathol 50:422, 1968.
1317. Fairlamb D, Boesen E: Gynaecomastia associated with gonadotropin-secreting carcinoma of the lung. Postgrad Med J 53:269, 1977.
1318. Dailey JE, Marcuse PM: Gonadotropin secreting giant cell carcinoma of the lung. Cancer 24:388, 1969.
1319. Byrd RP, Byrd RP Jr, Roy TM: False pregnancy: An unusual paraneoplastic syndrome associated with bronchogenic neoplasm. J Ky Med Assoc 91:510, 1993.
1320. Carlson HE: Current concepts: Gynecomastia. N Engl J Med 303:795, 1980.
1321. Niewoehner CB, Nuttal FQ: Gynecomastia in a hospitalized male population. Am J Med 77:633, 1984.
1322. Milhaud G, Calmette C, Taboulet J, et al: Hypersecretion of calcitonin in neoplastic conditions. Lancet 1:462, 1974.
1323. Silva OL, Becker KL, Primack A, et al: Increased serum calcitonin levels in bronchogenic cancer. Chest 69:495, 1976.
1324. Krauss S, Macy S, Ichiki AT: A study of immunoreactive calcitonin (CT), adrenocorticotropic hormone (ACTH), and carcinoembryonic antigen (CEA) in lung cancer and other malignancies. Cancer 47:2485, 1981.
1325. Becker KL, Nash DR, Silva OL, et al: Urine calcitonin levels in patients with bronchogenic carcinoma. JAMA 243:670, 1980.
1326. Williams GA: Elevated plasma calcitonin as a marker for bronchogenic carcinoma. Chest 69:451, 1976.
1327. Kelley MJ, Becker KL, Rushin JM, et al: Calcitonin elevation in small cell lung cancer without ectopic production. Am J Respir Crit Care Med 149:183, 1994.
1328. Reeve JG, Morgan J, Clark PM, et al: Insulin-like growth factor (IGF) and IGF binding proteins in growth hormone dysregulation and abnormal glucose tolerance in small cell lung cancer patients. Eur J Cancer 31:1455, 1995.
1329. Ghose RR, Gupta SK: Oat cell carcinoma of bronchus presenting with somatostatinoma syndrome. Thorax 36:550, 1981.
1330. Sano T, Saito H, Yamasaki R, et al: Immunoreactive somatostatin and calcitonin in pulmonary neuroendocrine tumor. Cancer 57:64, 1986.
1331. Jackson JA, Raju BU, Fachnie JD, et al: Malignant somatostatinoma presenting with diabetic ketoacidosis. Clin Endocrinol 26:609, 1987.
1332. Davis S, Proper S, May PB, et al: Elevated prolactin levels in bronchogenic carcinoma. Cancer 44:676, 1979.
1333. Okunaka T, Kato H, Konaka C, et al: Primary lung cancer producing α-fetoprotein. Ann Thorac Surg 53:151, 1992.
1334. Bhatavdekar JM, Patel DD, Chikhlikar PR, et al: Levels of circulating peptide and steroid hormones in men with lung cancer. Neoplasma 41:101, 1994.
1335. Katayama S, Ikeuchi M, Kanazawa Y, et al: Amylase-producing lung cancer: Case report and review of the literature. Cancer 48:2499, 1981.
1336. Pfeffer JM, Stovin PGI: Tumour production of alkaline phosphatase in a patient with giant-cell carcinoma of bronchus. Thorax 33:261, 1978.
1337. Grove A: Amylase in lung carcinomas: An ultrastructural and immunohistochemical study of two adenocarcinomas, and a review of the literature. APMIS 102:135, 1994.
1338. Seyama K, Nukiwa T, Takahashi K, et al: Amylase mRNA transcripts in normal tissue and neoplasms: The implication of different expressions of amylase isogenes. J Cancer Res Clin Oncol 120:213, 1994.
1339. Lenler-Petersen P, Grove A, Brock A, et al: Alpha-amylase in resectable lung cancer. Eur Respir J 7:941, 1994.
1340. Barden RP: Para-endocrine syndromes associated with carcinoma of the lung. Am J Roentgenol 100:626, 1967.
1341. Lowe WC, Tassy F: Massive venous thrombosis and carcinoma of the lung. Am Rev Respir Dis 95:980, 1967.
1342. Byrd RB, Divertie MB, Spittell JA Jr: Bronchogenic carcinoma and thromboembolic disease. JAMA 202:1019, 1967.
1343. Hickey WF, Garnick MB, Henderson IC, et al: Primary cerebral venous thrombosis in patients with cancer—a rarely diagnosed paraneoplastic syndrome: Report of three cases and review of the literature. Am J Med 73:740, 1982.
1344. Ziomek S, Read RC, Tobler HG, et al: Thromboembolism in patients undergoing thoracotomy. Ann Thorac Surg 56:223, 1993.
1345. Tricerri A, Vangeli M, Errani AR, et al: Plasma thrombin-antithrombin complexes, latent coagulation disorders and metastatic spread in lung cancer: A longitudinal study. Oncology 53:455, 1996.
1346. Gabazza EC, Taguchi O, Yamakami T, et al: Evaluating prethrombotic state in lung cancer using molecular markers. Chest 103:196, 1993.
1347. Ogino H, Hayashi S, Kawasaki M, et al: Association of thrombosis-inducing activity (TIA) with fatal hypercoagulable complications in patients with lung cancer. Chest 105:1683, 1994.
1348. McMahon LJ, Thomson SP, Nugent CA, et al: Persistent lymphocytopenia as a diagnostic feature of bronchogenic carcinoma. Chest 78:583, 1980.
1349. Anger B, Bockman R, Andreeff M, et al: Characterization of two newly established human cell lines from patients with large-cell anaplastic lung carcinoma. Cancer 50:1518, 1982.
1350. Okabe T, Fujisawa M, Kudo H, et al: Establishment of a human colony-stimulating factor-producing cell line from an undifferentiated large cell carcinoma of the lung. Cancer 54:1024, 1984.
1351. McKee LC Jr: Excess leukocytosis (leukemoid reactions) associated with malignant diseases. South Med J 78:1475, 1985.
1352. Slungaard A, Ascensao J, Zanjani E, et al: Pulmonary carcinoma with eosinophilia: Demonstration of a tumor-derived eosinophilopoietic factor. N Engl J Med 309:778, 1983.
1353. Ascensao JL, Oken MM, Ewing SL, et al: Leukocytosis and large cell lung cancer: A frequent association. Cancer 60:903, 1987.
1354. Suda T, Miura Y, Mizoguchi H, et al: A case of lung cancer associated with granulocytosis and production of colony-stimulating activity by the tumour. Br J Cancer 41:980, 1980.
1355. Furihata M, Sonobe H, Iwata J, et al: Lung squamous cell carcinoma producing both parathyroid hormone-related peptide and granulocyte stimulating factor. Pathol Int 46:376, 1996.
1356. Adachi N, Yamaguchi K, Morikawa T, et al: Constitutive production of multiple colony-stimulating factors in patients with lung cancer associated with neutrophilia. Br J Cancer 69:125, 1994.
1357. Remacle P, Bruart J, Hemmeghien C: Bronchial cancer and hypereosinophilia. Eur Respir J 1:191, 1988.
1358. Kodama T, Takada K, Kameya T, et al: Large cell carcinoma of the lung associated with marked eosinophilia: A case report. Cancer 54:2313, 1984.
1359. Knox AJ, Johnson CE, Page RL: Eosinophilia associated with thoracic malignancy. Br J Dis Chest 80:92, 1986.
1360. Goetzl EJ, Tashjian AH Jr, Rubin RH, et al: Production of a low molecular weight eosinophil polymorphonuclear leukocyte factor by anaplastic squamous cell carcinomas of human lung. J Clin Invest 61:770, 1978.
1361. Wasserman SI, Goetz EJ, Ellman L, et al: Tumor-associated eosinophilotactic factor. N Engl J Med 290:420, 1974.
1362. Kodama T, Takada K, Kameya T, et al: Large cell carcinoma of the lung associated with marked eosinophilia. Cancer 54:2313, 1984.
1363. Pedersen LM, Milman N: Prognostic significance of thrombocytosis in patient with primary lung cancer. Eur Respir J 9:1826, 1996.
1364. Dowlati A, R'Zik S, Fillet G, et al: Anaemia of lung cancer is due to impaired erythroid marrow response to erythropoietin stimulation as well as relative inadequacy of erythropoietin production. Br J Haematol 97:297, 1997.
1365. Ludwig H, Sundal E, Pecherstorfer M, et al: Recombinant human erythropoietin for the correction of cancer associated anemia with and without concomitant cytotoxic chemotherapy. Cancer 76:2319, 1995.
1366. Flanagan P, Roeckel IE: Giant cell carcinoma of the lung: Anatomic and clinical correlation. Am J Med 36:214, 1964.
1366a. Entwistle CC, Fentem PH, Jacobs A: Red-cell aplasia with carcinoma of the bronchus. BMJ 2:1504, 1964.
1367. Goldstein J, Hart J: Pruritus and purpura as unusual symptoms in carcinoma of the bronchus. Tubercle 40:119, 1959.
1368. Silvis SE, Turkbas N, Doscherholmen A: Thrombocytosis in patients with lung cancer. JAMA 211:1852, 1970.
1369. Brodie GN, Bliss D, Firkin BG: Thrombocytopenia and carcinoma. BMJ 1:540, 1970.
1370. Cairns SA, Mallick NP, Lawler W, et al: Squamous cell carcinoma of bronchus presenting with Henoch-Schönlein purpura. BMJ 2:474, 1978.
1371. Raz I, Shinar E, Polliack A: Pancytopenia with hypercellular bone marrow—a possible paraneoplastic syndrome in carcinoma of the lung: A report of three cases. Am J Hematol 16:403, 1984.
1372. McIllmurray MB, Ryrie DR, Fletcher J: Carcinoma of the lung presenting with a myeloproliferative disorder: A report of two patients. Postgrad Med J 53:702, 1977.
1373. Petri M, Fye KH: Digital necrosis: A paraneoplastic syndrome. J Rheumatol 12:800, 1985.
1374. Higgins MR, Randall RE Jr, Still WJS: Nephrotic syndrome with oat-cell carcinoma. BMJ 3:450, 1974.
1375. Vincent FM: Paraneoplastic central nervous system and renal syndromes: Simultaneous occurrence in a patient with bronchogenic carcinoma. JAMA 240:862, 1978.
1376. Moorthy AV: Minimal change glomerular disease: A paraneoplastic syndrome in two patients with bronchogenic carcinoma. Am J Kidney Dis 3:58, 1983.
1377. Singer CR, Boulton-Jones JM: Minimal change nephropathy associated with anaplastic carcinoma of bronchus. Postgrad Med J 62:213, 1986.
1378. Boon ES, Vrid AA, Nieuwhot C, et al: Small cell lung cancer with paraneoplastic nephrotic syndrome. Eur Respir J 7:1192, 1994.
1379. Safadi R, Gotsman O, Friedlaender M, et al: Renal failure, paraproteinemia, and lung squamous cell carcinoma. Ren Fail 19:495, 1997.
1380. Shaker JL, Brickner RC, Divgi AB, et al: Case report: Renal phosphate wasting, syndrome of inappropriate antidiuretic hormone, and ectopic corticotropin production in small cell carcinoma. Am J Med Sci 310:38, 1995.
1381. Robin N, Gill G, van Heyningen C, et al: A small cell bronchogenic carcinoma associated with tumoral hypophosphataemia and inappropriate antidiuresis. Postgrad Med J 70:746, 1994.
1382. Jackson CV, Savage PJ, Quinn DL: Role of fiberoptic bronchoscopy in patients with hemoptysis and a normal chest roentgenogram. Chest 87:142, 1985.
1383. Poe RH, Israel RH, Martin MG, et al: Utility of fiberoptic bronchoscopy in patients with hemoptysis and a nonlocalizing chest roentgenogram. Chest 93:68, 1988.

1384. Lederle FA, Nichol KL, Parenti CM: Bronchoscopy to evaluate hemoptysis in older men with nonsuspicious chest roentgenograms. Chest 95:1043, 1989.

1385. O'Neil KM, Lazarus AA: Hemoptysis: Indications for bronchoscopy. Arch Intern Med 151:171, 1991.

1386. McFarlane MJ, Feinstein AR, Wells CK: Necropsy evidence of detection bias in the diagnosis of lung cancer. Arch Intern Med 146:1695, 1986.

1387. McFarlane MJ, Feinstein AR, Wells CK: Clinical features of lung cancers discovered as a postmortem "surprise." Chest 90:520, 1986.

1388. Böcking A, Biesterfeld S, Chatelain R, et al: Diagnosis of bronchial carcinoma on sections of paraffin-embedded sputum: Sensitivity and specificity of an alternative to routine cytology. Acta Cytol 36:37, 1992.

1389. Naryshkin S, Daniels J, Young NA: Diagnostic correlation of fiberoptic bronchoscopic biopsy and bronchoscopic cytology performed simultaneously. Diagn Cytopathol 8:119, 1992.

1390. Bender BL, Cherock M-A, Sotos SN: Effective use of bronchoscopy and sputa in the diagnosis of lung cancer. Diagn Cytopathol 1:183, 1985.

1391. Matsuda M, Horai T, Nakamura S, et al: Bronchial brushing and bronchial biopsy: Comparison of diagnostic accuracy and cell typing reliability in lung cancer. Thorax 41:475, 1986.

1392. Ng ABP, Horak GC: Factors significant in the diagnostic accuracy of lung cytology in bronchial washing and sputum samples: II. Sputum samples. Acta Cytol 27:397, 1983.

1393. Rosa UW, Prolla JC, da Silva Gastal E: Cytology in diagnosis of cancer affecting the lung: Results in 1,000 consecutive patients. Chest 63:203, 1973.

1394. Ng ABP, Horak GC: Factors significant in the diagnostic accuracy of lung cytology in bronchial washing and sputum samples: I. Bronchial washings. Acta Cytol 27:391, 1983.

1395. Clee MD, Sinclair DJM: Assessment of factors influencing the result of sputum cytology in bronchial carcinoma. Thorax 36:143, 1981.

1396. Raab SS, Hornberger J, Raffin T: The importance of sputum cytology in the diagnosis of lung cancer. Chest 112:937, 1997.

1397. Rozenshtein A, White CS, Austin JHM, et al: Incidental lung carcinoma detected at CT in patients selected for lung volume reduction surgery to treat severe pulmonary emphysema. Radiology 207:487, 1998.

1398. Risse EKJ, van't Hof MA, Laurini RN, et al: Sputum cytology by the Saccomanno method in diagnosing lung malignancy. Diagn Cytopathol 1:286, 1985.

1399. Johnston WW, Frable WJ: Cytopathology of the respiratory tract: A review. Am J Pathol 84:371, 1976.

1400. Pirozynski M: Bronchoalveolar lavage in the diagnosis of peripheral, primary lung cancer. Chest 102:372, 1992.

1401. Lidner J, Radio SJ, Robbins RA, et al: Bronchoalveolar lavage in the diagnosis of disseminated lung tumors. Acta Cytol 31:796, 1987.

1402. Light RW, Erozan YS, Ball WC Jr: Cells in pleural fluid: Their value in differential diagnosis. Arch Intern Med 132:854, 1973.

1403. Naylor B, Schmidt RW: The case for exfoliative cytology of serous effusions. Lancet 1:711, 1964.

1404. Dewald GW, Hicks GA, Dines DE, et al: Cytogenetic diagnosis of malignant pleural effusions: Culture methods to supplement direct preparations in diagnosis. Mayo Clin Proc 57:488, 1982.

1405. Salerno CT, Frizelle S, Niehans GA, et al: Detection of occult micrometastases in non–small cell lung carcinoma by reverse transcriptase–polymerase chain reaction. Chest 113:1526, 1998.

1406. Ho KJ, Herrera GA, Jones JM, et al: Small cell carcinoma of the esophagus: Evidence for a unified histogenesis. Hum Pathol 15:460, 1984.

1407. Fertilo A: Oat cell carcinoma of the larynx. Ann Otol 83:254, 1974.

1408. Faling LJ, Haesaert SP, Schimmel EM: Occult bronchogenic carcinoma masquerading as esophageal cancer: Case reports with recommendations for a change in reporting esophageal cytology. Arch Intern Med 140:489, 1980.

1409. Pastor A, Menendez R, Cremades MJ, et al: Diagnostic value of SCC, CEA and CYFRA 21.1 in lung cancer: A Bayesian analysis. Eur Respir J 10:603, 1997.

1410. Paone G, De Angelis G, Portalone L, et al: Validation of an algorithm able to differentiate small-cell lung cancer (small cell carcinoma) from non–small cell lung cancer (non–small cell carcinoma) patients by means of a tumour marker panel: Analysis of the errors. Br J Cancer 75:448, 1997.

1411. Berzinec P, Zuffova H, Letkovicova M, et al: Serum tumor marker CYFRA 21-1 in the diagnostics of squamous cell lung cancer—comparison with CEA. Neoplasma 43:159, 1996.

1412. Giovanella L, Ceriani L, Bandera M, et al: Evaluation of the serum markers CEA, NSE, TPS and CYFRA 21.1 in lung cancer. Int J Biol Markers 10:156, 1995.

1413. Plebani M, Basso D, Navaglia F, et al: Clinical evaluation of seven tumour markers in lung cancer diagnosis: Can any combination improve the results? Br J Cancer 72:170, 1995.

1414. Han AC, Peralta-Soler A, Knudsen KA, et al: Differential expression of N-cadherin in pleural mesotheliomas and E-cadherin in lung adenocarcinomas in formalin-fixed, paraffin-embedded tissues. Hum Pathol 28:641, 1997.

1415. Hirano T, Fujioka K, Franzn B, et al: Relationship between TA01 and TA02 polypeptides associated with lung adenocarcinoma and histocytological features. Br J Cancer 75:978, 1997.

1416. Paone G, De Angelis G, Greco S, et al: Carcinoembryonic antigen, tissue polypeptide antigen and neuron-specific enolase pleural levels used to classify small-cell and nonsmall-cell lung cancer patients by discriminant analysis. J Cancer Res Clin Oncol 122:499, 1996.

1417. Scott F, Cuttitta F, Treston AM, et al: Prospective trial evaluating immunocytochemical-based sputum techniques for early lung cancer detection: Assays for promotion factors in the bronchial lavage. J Cell Biochem 17(Suppl):175, 1993.

1418. Sanguinetti CM, Riccioni G, Marchesani F, et al: Bronchoalveolar lavage fluid level of carcinoembryonic antigen in the diagnosis of peripheral lung cancer. Monaldi Arch Chest Dis 50:177, 1995.

1419. Jacobson DR, Fishman CL, Mills NE: Molecular genetic tumor markers in the early diagnosis and screening of nonsmall-cell lung cancer. Ann Oncol 3:3, 1995.

1420. Trevisani L, Putinati S, Sartori S et al: Cytokeratin tumor marker levels in bronchial washing in the diagnosis of lung cancer. Chest 109:104, 1986.

1421. Huang MS, Jong SB, Tsai MS, et al: Comparison of cytokeratin fragment 19 (CYFRA 21-1), tissue polypeptide antigen (TPA) and carcinoembryonic antigen (CEA) as tumour markers in bronchogenic carcinoma. Respir Med 91:135, 1997.

1422. Rapellino M, Niklinski J, Pecchio F, et al: CYFRA 21-1 as a tumour marker for bronchogenic carcinoma. Eur Respir J 8:407, 1995.

1423. Bergman B, Brezicka FT, Engstrom CP, et al: Clinical usefulness of serum assays of neuron-specific enolase, carcinoembryonic antigen and CA-50 antigen in the diagnosis of lung cancer. Eur J Cancer 29:198, 1993.

1424. Lai RS, Hsu HH, Lu JY, et al: CYFRA 21-1 enzyme-linked immunosorbent assay—evaluation as a tumor marker in non–small cell lung cancer. Chest 109:995, 1996.

1425. Buccheri G, Ferrigno D: The tissue polypeptide antigen serum test in the preoperative evaluation of non–small cell lung cancer: Diagnostic yield and comparison with conventional staging methods. Chest 107:471, 1995.

1426. Wieskopf B, Demangeat C, Purohit A, et al: CYFRA 21-1 as a biologic marker of non–small cell lung cancer. Chest 108:163, 1995.

1427. Paone G, De Angelis G, Munno R, et al: Discriminant analysis on small cell lung cancer and non–small cell lung cancer by means of NSE and CYFRA-21.1. Eur Respir J 8:1136, 1995.

1428. Nicholson AG, McCormick CJ, Shimosato Y, et al: The value of PE-10, a monoclonal antibody against pulmonary surfactant, in distinguishing primary and metastatic lung tumours. Histopathology 27:57, 1995.

1429. Itoh K, Natori H, Suzuki A, et al: Differentiation of primary or metastatic lung carcinoma by phospholipid analysis: A new approach for lung carcinoma differentiation. Cancer 57:1350, 1986.

1430. Diez M, Torres A, Maestro ML, et al: Prediction of survival and recurrence by serum and cytosolic levels of CEA, CA125 and SCC antigens in resectable nonsmall-cell lung cancer. Br J Cancer 73:1248, 1996.

1431. Kanters SD, Lammers JW, Voest EE: Molecular and biological factors in the prognosis of non–small cell lung cancer. Eur Respir J 8:1389, 1995.

1432. Seregni E, Botti C, Bogni A, et al: Tumour marker evaluation in patients with lung cancer. Scand J Clin Lab Invest 221(Suppl):67, 1995.

1433. Diez M, Gomez A, Hernando F, et al: Serum CEA, CA125, and SCC antigens and tumor recurrence in resectable non–small cell lung cancer. Int J Biol Markers 10:5, 1995.

1434. Pujol JL, Grenier J, Parrat E, et al: Cytokeratins as serum markers in lung cancer: A comparison of CYFRA 21-1 and TPS. Am J Respir Crit Care Med 154:725, 1996.

1435. Diez M, Torres A, Pollan M, et al: Prognostic significance of serum CA 125 antigen assay in patients with non–small cell lung cancer. Cancer 1:1368, 1994.

1436. Buccheri G, Ferrigno D: Prognostic value of the tissue polypeptide antigen in lung cancer. Chest 101:1287, 1992.

1437. Graziano SL, Mazid R, Newman N, et al: The use of neuroendocrine immunoperoxidase markers to predict chemotherapy response in patients with nonsmall-cell lung cancer. J Clin Oncol 7:1398, 1989.

1438. Takada M, Kusunoki Y, Masuda N, et al: Pro-gastrin-releasing peptide (31-98) as a tumour marker of small-cell lung cancer: Comparative evaluation with neuron-specific enolase. Br J Cancer 73:1227, 1996.

1439. Buccheri G, Ferrigno D: Monitoring lung cancer with tissue polypeptide antigen: An ancillary, profitable serum test to evaluate treatment response and posttreatment disease status. Lung Cancer 13:155, 1995.

1440. Paone G, De Angelis G, Pallotta G, et al: Evaluation of the response to chemotherapy in patients affected with small cell lung cancer using discriminate analysis: A preliminary report. Q J Nucl Med 39:140, 1995.

1441. Jorgensen LG, Osterlind K, Hansen HH, et al: Serum neuron-specific enolase (S-NSE) in progressive small–cell lung cancer (small–cell carcinoma). Br J Cancer 70:759, 1994.

1442. Strauss GM, Skarin AT: Use of tumor markers in lung cancer. Hematol Oncol Clin North Am 8:507, 1994.

1443. Mulshine JL, Zhou J, Treston AM, et al: New approaches to the integrated management of early lung cancer. Hematol Oncol Clin North Am 11:235, 1997.

1444. Mao L, Hruban RH, Boyle JO, et al: Detection of oncogene mutations in sputum precedes diagnosis of lung cancer. Cancer Res 54:1634, 1994.

1445. Ferrigno D, Buccheri G, Biggi A: Serum tumour markers in lung cancer: History, biology and clinical applications. Eur Respir J 7:186, 1994.

1446. Wróblewski F: The significance of alternations in lactic dehydrogenase activity of body fluids in the diagnosis of malignant tumors. Cancer 12:27, 1959.

1447. Hinton JM: Serum lactate dehydrogenase in bronchial carcinoma. Thorax 20:198, 1965.

1448. Gold JA: Serum enzymes in bronchogenic carcinoma and other pulmonary diseases. Dis Chest 39:62, 1961.

1449. Forrest JV, Sagel SS: The lateral radiograph for early diagnosis of lung cancer. Radiology 131:309, 1979.

1450. Tala E: Carcinoma of the lung: A retrospective study with special reference to the pre-diagnosis period and roentgenographic signs. Acta Radiol Diagn 268(Suppl):1, 1967.

1451. Stitik FP, Tockman MS: Radiographic screening in the early detection of lung cancer. Radiol Clin North Am 16:347, 1978.

1452. Austin JHM, Romney BM, Goldsmith LS: Missed bronchogenic carcinoma: Radiographic findings in 27 patients with a potentially resectable lesion evident in retrospect. Radiology 182:115, 1992.

1453. Muhm JR, Miller WE, Fontana RS, et al: Lung cancer detected during a screening program using four-month chest radiographs. Radiology 148:609, 1983.

1454. Heelan RT, Flehinger BJ, Melamed MR, et al: Non-small-cell lung cancer: Results of the New York screening program. Radiology 151:289, 1984.

1455. White CS, Romney BM, Mason AC, et al: Primary carcinoma of the lung overlooked at CT: Analysis of findings in 14 patients. Radiology 199:109, 1996.

1456. Gurney JW: Missed lung cancer at CT: Imaging findings in nine patients. Radiology 199:117, 1996.

1457. Naidich DP, Rusinek H, McGuinness G, et al: Variables affecting pulmonary nodule detection with computed tomography: Evaluation with three-dimensional computer simulation. J Thorac Imaging 8:291, 1993.

1458. Boysen PG, Harris JO, Block AJ, et al: Prospective evaluation for pneumonectomy using perfusion scanning: Follow-up beyond one year. Chest 80:163, 1981.

1459. Giordano A, Calcagni ML, Meduri G, et al: Perfusion lung scintigraphy for the prediction of postlobectomy residual pulmonary function. Chest 111:1542, 1997.

1460. Matsuno S, Tanabe M, Kawasaki Y, et al: Effectiveness of planar image and single photon emission tomography of thallium-201 compared with gallium-67 in patients with primary lung cancer. Eur J Nucl Med 19:86, 1992.

1461. Ishibashi M, Honda N, Yoshioka F, et al: Validation of single-photon emission computed tomography (SPECT) using thallium-201 in patients with lung cancer. Kurume Med J 38:87, 1991.

1462. Duman Y, Burak Z, Erdem S, et al: The value and limitations of ^{201}Tl scintigraphy in the evaluation of lung lesions and post-therapy follow-up of primary lung carcinoma. Nucl Med Commun 14:446, 1993.

1463. Yokoi K, Okuyama A, Mori K, et al: Mediastinal lymph node metastasis from lung cancer: Evaluation with Tl-201 SPECT—comparison with CT. Radiology 192:813, 1994.

1464. Chinn R, Ward R, Keyes JW, et al: Mediastinal staging of nonsmall-cell cancer with positron emission tomography. Am J Respir Crit Care Med 152:2090, 1995.

1465. Rege SD, Hoh CK, Glaspy JA, et al: Imaging of pulmonary mass lesions with whole-body positron emission tomography and fluorodeoxyglucose. Cancer 72:82, 1993.

1466. Lewis P, Griffin S, Marsden P, et al: Whole-body 18-F-fluorodeoxyglucose positron emission tomography in preoperative evaluation of lung cancer. Lancet 344:1265, 1994.

1467. Erasmus JJ, Patz EF Jr, McAdams HP, et al: Evaluation of adrenal masses in patients with bronchogenic carcinoma using 18F-fluorodeoxy-glucose positron emission tomography. Am J Roentgenol 168:1357, 1997.

1468. Duhaylongsod FG, Lowe VJ, Patz EF, et al: Detection of primary and recurrent lung cancer by means of F-18 fluorodeoxyglucose positron emission tomography. J Thorac Cardiovasc Surg 110:130, 1995.

1469. Hubner KF, Buonocore E, Singh SK, et al: Characterization of chest masses by FDG positron emission tomography. Clin Nucl Med 20:293, 1995.

1470. Patz EF, Lowe VJ, Hoffman JM, et al: Persistent or recurrent bronchogenic carcinoma: Detection with PET and 2-[F-18]-fluoro-2-deoxy-D-glucose. Radiology 191:379, 1994.

1471. Frank A, Lefkowitz D, Jaeger S, et al: Decision logic for retreatment of asymptomatic lung cancer recurrence based on PET findings. Int J Radiat Oncol Biol Phys 32:1495, 1995.

1472. Inoue T, Kim EE, Komaki R, et al: Detecting recurrent or residual lung cancer with FDG-PET. J Nucl Med 36:788, 1995.

1473. TNM Classification of Malignant Tumors. Joint Publication of International Union Against Cancer and American Joint Committee on Cancer Staging and End Results Reporting. Geneva, 1972.

1474. Mountain CF: Revisions in the international system for staging lung cancer. Chest 111:1710, 1997.

1475. Mountain CF, Dresler CM: Regional lymph node classification for lung cancer staging. Chest 111:1718, 1997.

1476. Abrams J, Doyle LA, Aisner J: Staging, prognostic factors, and special considerations in small cell lung cancer. Semin Oncol 15:261, 1988.

1477. Feinstein AR, Wells CK: A clinical-severity staging system for patients with lung cancer. Medicine 69:1, 1990.

1478. Feinstein AR: A new staging system for cancer and reappraisal of "early" treatment and "cure" by radical surgery. N Engl J Med 279:747, 1968.

1479. Carbone PP, Frost JK, Feinstein AR, et al: Lung cancer: Perspectives and prospects. Ann Intern Med 73:1003, 1970.

1480. Passlick B, Izbicki JR, Kubuschok B, et al: Immunohistochemical assessment of individual tumor cells in lymph nodes of patients with nonsmall-cell lung cancer. J Clin Oncol 12:1827, 1994.

1481. Beiske K, Myklebust AT, Aamdal S, et al: Detection of bone marrow metastases in small cell lung cancer patients: Comparison of immunologic and morphologic methods. Am J Pathol 141:531, 1992.

1482. Bone RC, Balk R: Staging of bronchogenic carcinoma. Chest 82:473, 1982.

1483. White DM, McMahon LJ, Denny WF: Usefulness outcome in evaluating the utility of nuclear scans of the bone, brain, and liver in bronchogenic carcinoma patients. Am J Med Sci 283:114, 1982.

1484. Robbins HM, Sweet ME, Jefferson SE, et al: The determination of resectability of lung cancer by fiberoptic bronchoscopy. Arch Intern Med 141:649, 1981.

1485. Ekholm S, Albrechtsson U, Kugelberg J, et al: Computed tomography in preoperative staging of bronchogenic carcinoma. CT 4:763, 1980.

1486. Kagan AR, Steckel RJ: Pulmonary mass in a smoker: Preoperative imaging for staging of lung cancer. Am J Roentgenol 136:739, 1981.

1487. Hirleman MT, Yiu-Chiu VS, Chiu LC, et al: The resectability of primary lung carcinoma: A diagnostic staging review. CT 4:146, 1980.

1488. Baron RL, Levitt RG, Sagel SS, et al: Computed tomography in the preoperative evaluation of bronchogenic carcinoma. Radiology 145:727, 1982.

1489. Gamsu G, Webb WR, Sheldon P, et al: Nuclear magnetic resonance imaging of the thorax. Radiology 147:473, 1983.

1490. Glazer HS, Kaiser LR, Anderson DJ, et al: Indeterminate mediastinal invasion in bronchogenic carcinoma: CT evaluation. Radiology 173:37, 1989.

1491. Gay SB, Black WB, Armstrong P, et al: Chest CT of unresectable lung cancer. Radiographics 8:735, 1988.

1492. Epstein DM, Stephenson LW, Gefter WB, et al: Value of CT in the preoperative assessment of lung cancer: A survey of thoracic surgeons. Radiology 161:423, 1986.

1493. Herman SJ, Winton TL, Weisbrod GL, et al: Mediastinal invasion by bronchogenic carcinoma: CT signs. Radiology 190:841, 1994.

1494. White PG, Adams H, Crane MD, et al: Preoperative staging of carcinoma of the bronchus: Can computed tomographic scanning reliably identify stage III tumors? Thorax 49:951, 1994.

1495. Weinreb JC, Naidich DP: Thoracic magnetic resonance imaging. Clin Chest Med 12:33, 1991.

1496. Mayr B, Lenhard M, Fink U, et al: Preoperative evaluation of bronchogenic carcinoma: Value of MR in T- and N-staging. Eur J Radiol 14:245, 1992.

1497. Tisi GM, Friedman PH, Peters RM, et al: American Thoracic Society: Clinical staging of primary lung cancer. Am Rev Respir Dis 127:659, 1983.

1498. Guyatt GH, Lefcoe M, Walter S, et al: Interobserver variation in the computed tomographic evaluation of mediastinal lymph node size in patients with potentially resectable lung cancer. Chest 107:116, 1995.

1499. Arita T, Kuramitsu T, Kawamura M, et al: Bronchogenic carcinoma: Incidence of metastases to normal sized lymph nodes. Thorax 50:1267, 1995.

1500. Cascade PN, Gross BH, Kazerooni EA, et al: Variability in the detection of enlarged mediastinal lymph nodes in staging lung cancer: A comparison of contrast-enhanced and unenhanced CT. Am J Roentgenol 170:927, 1998.

1501. Quint LE, Glazer GM, Orringer MB, et al: Mediastinal lymph node detection and sizing at CT and autopsy. Am J Roentgenol 147:469, 1986.

1502. Glazer GM, Gross BH, Quint LE, et al: Normal mediastinal lymph nodes: Number and size according to the American Thoracic Society mapping. Am J Roentgenol 144:261, 1985.

1503. Buy JN, Ghossain MA, Poirson F, et al: Computed tomography of mediastinal lymph nodes in non–small cell lung cancer: A new approach based on the lymphatic pathway of tumor spread. J Comput Assist Tomogr 12:545, 1988.

1504. Ikezoe J, Kadowaki K, Morimoto S, et al: Mediastinal lymph node metastases from non–small cell bronchogenic carcinoma: Reevaluation with CT. J Comput Assist Tomogr 14:340, 1990.

1505. Haramati LB, Cartagena AM, Austin JHM: CT evaluation of mediastinal lymphadenopathy: Non-contrast 5-mm versus post-contrast 10-mm sections. J Comput Assist Tomogr 19:375, 1995.

1506. Glazer GM, Francis IR, Gebarski K, et al: Dynamic incremental computed tomography in evaluation of the pulmonary hila. J Comput Assist Tomogr 7:59, 1983.

1507. Remy-Jardin M, Duyck P, Remy J, et al: Hilar lymph nodes: Identification with spiral CT and histologic correlation. Radiology 196:387, 1995.

1508. Shimoyama K, Murata K, Takahashi M, et al: Pulmonary hilar lymph node metastases from lung cancer: Evaluation based on morphology at thin-section, incremental, dynamic CT. Radiology 203:187, 1997.

1509. McKenna RJ Jr, Libshitz HI, Mountain CE, et al: Roentgenographic evaluation of mediastinal nodes for preoperative assessment in lung cancer. Chest 88:206, 1985.

1510. Lewis JW, Pearlberg JL, Beaute GH, et al: Can computed tomography of the chest stage lung cancer? Yes and no. Ann Thorac Surg 49:591, 1990.

1511. Daly BD, Pugatch RD, Gale ME, et al: Computed tomography, an effective technique for mediastinal staging in lung cancer. J Thorac Cardiovasc Surg 88:486, 1984.

1512. Lewis JW Jr, Madrazo BL, Gross SC, et al: The value of radiographic and computed tomography in the staging of lung carcinoma. Ann Thorac Surg 34:553, 1982.

1513. Baron RL, Levitt RG, Sagel SS, et al: Computed tomography in the preoperative evaluation of bronchogenic carcinoma. Radiology 145:727, 1982.

1514. Osbourne DR, Korobkin M, Ravin CE, et al: Comparison of plain radiography, conventional tomography, and computed tomography in detecting intrathoracic lymph node metastases from lung cancer. Radiology 142:157, 1982.

1515. Glazer GM, Orringer MB, Gross BH, et al: The mediastinum in non–small cell lung cancer: CT-surgical correlation. Am J Roentgenol 142:1101, 1984.

1516. Libshitz HI, McKenna RJ Jr: Mediastinal lymph node size in lung cancer. Am J Roentgenol 143:715, 1984.

1517. McLoud TC, Bourgouin PM, Greenberg RW, et al: Bronchogenic carcinoma: Analysis of staging in the mediastinum with CT by correlative lymph node mapping and sampling. Radiology 182:319, 1992.

1518. Staples CA, Müller NL, Miller RR, et al: Mediastinal nodes in bronchogenic carcinoma: Comparison between CT and mediastinoscopy. Radiology 167:367, 1988.

1519. Hirleman MR, Yiu-Chiu VS, Chiu LC, et al: The resectability of primary lung carcinoma: A diagnostic staging review. CT 4:146, 1980.

1520. Barakos JA, Brown JJ, Higgins CB: MR imaging of secondary cardiac and paracardiac lesions. Am J Roentgenol 153:47, 1989.

1521. Seely JM, Mayo JR, Miller RR, et al: T1 lung cancer: Prevalence of mediastinal nodal metastases and diagnostic accuracy of CT. Radiology 186:129, 1993.

1522. Bollen ECM, Goei R, Hof-Grootenboer BE, et al: Interobserver variability and accuracy of computed tomographic assessment of nodal status in lung cancer. Ann Thorac Surg 58:158, 1994.

1523. Webb WR, Sarin M, Zerhouni EA, et al: Interobserver variability in CT and MR staging of lung cancer. J Comput Assist Tomogr 17:841, 1993.

1524. Dales RA, Stark RM, Raman S: Computed tomography to stage lung cancer: Approaching a controversy using meta-analysis. Am Rev Respir Dis 141:1096, 1990.

1525. Guyatt DH, Cook DJ, Walter S: The Canadian Lung Oncology Group. Investigation for mediastinal disease in patients with apparently operable lung cancer. Ann Thorac Surg 60:1382, 1995.

1526. Bergh NP, Schersten T: Bronchogenic carcinoma: A follow-up study of a surgically treated series with special reference to the prognostic significance of lymph node metastases. Acta Chir Scand 347(Suppl):1, 1965.

1527. Pearson FG, DeLarue NC, Ilves R, et al: Significance of positive superior mediastinal nodes identified at mediastinoscopy in patients with resectable cancer of the lung. J Thorac Cardiovasc Surg 83:11, 1982.

1528. Gross BH, Glazer GM, Orringer MB, et al: Bronchogenic carcinoma metastatic to normal-sized lymph nodes: Frequency and significance. Radiology 166:71, 1988.

1529. Martini N, Heelan R, Westcott J, et al: Comparative merits of conventional, computed tomographic, and magnetic resonance imaging in assessing mediastinal involvement in surgically confirmed lung carcinoma. J Thorac Cardiovasc Surg 90:639, 1985.

1530. Grenier P, Dubray B, Carette MF, et al: Preoperative thoracic staging of lung cancer: CT and MR evaluation. Diagn Intervent Radiol 1:23, 1989.

1531. Musset D, Grenier P, Carette MF, et al: Primary lung cancer staging: Prospective comparative study of MR imaging with CT. Radiology 160:607, 1986.

1532. Poon PY, Bronskill MJ, Henkelman RM, et al: Mediastinal lymph node metastases from bronchogenic carcinoma: Detection with MR imaging and CT. Radiology 162:651, 1987.

1533. Batra P, Brown K, Steckel RJ, et al: MR imaging of the thorax: A comparison of axial, coronal and sagittal imaging planes. J Comput Assist Tomogr 12:75, 1988.

1534. Webb WR, Gamsu G, Stark DD, et al: Magnetic resonance imaging of the normal and abnormal pulmonary hila. Radiology 152:89, 1984.

1535. Levitt RG, Glazer HS, Roper CL, et al: Magnetic resonance imaging of mediastinal and hilar masses: Comparison with CT. Am J Roentgenol 145:9, 1985.

1536. Laissy JP, Gay-Depassier P, Soyer P, et al: Enlarged mediastinal lymph nodes in bronchogenic carcinoma: Assessment with dynamic contrast-enhanced MR imaging. Radiology 191:263, 1994.

1537. Patz EF, Lowe VJ, Goodman PC, et al: Thoracic nodal staging with PET imaging with [18]FDG in patients with bronchogenic carcinoma. Chest 108:1617, 1995.

1538. Valk PE, Pounds TR, Hopkins DM, et al: Staging non–small cell lung cancer by whole-body positron emission tomographic imaging. Ann Thorac Surg 60:1573, 1995.

1539. Vansteenkiste JF, Stroobants SG, De Leyn PR, et al: Mediastinal lymph node staging with FDG-PET scan in patients with potentially operable non–small cell lung cancer: A prospective analysis of 50 cases. Chest 112:1480, 1997.

1539a. Boiselle PM, Patz EF Jr, Vining DJ, et al: Imaging of mediastinal lymph nodes: CT, MR, and FDG PET. RadioGraphics 18:1061, 1998.

1540. Ichinose Y, Hara N, Ohta M, et al: Preoperative examination to detect distant metastasis is not advocated for asymptomatic patients with stages 1 and 2 non–small cell lung cancer—preoperative examination for lung cancer. Chest 96:1104, 1989.

1541. Silvestri GA, Littenberg B, Colice GL: The clinical evaluation for detecting metastatic lung cancer: A meta-analysis. Am J Respir Crit Care Med 152:225, 1995.

1542. Ferrigno D, Buccheri G: Cranial computed tomography as a part of the initial staging procedures for patients with nonsmall-cell lung cancer. Chest 106:1025, 1994.

1543. Mintz BJ, Tuhrim S, Alexander S, et al: Intracranial metastases in the initial staging of bronchogenic carcinoma. Chest 86:849, 1984.

1544. Colice GL, Birkmeyer JD, Black WC, et al: Cost-effectiveness of head CT in patients with lung cancer without clinical evidence of metastases. Chest 108:1264, 1995.

1545. Webb WR, Golden JA: Imaging strategies in the staging of lung cancer. Clin Chest Med 12:133, 1991.

1546. Pagani JJ: Normal adrenal glands in small cell lung carcinoma: CT-guided biopsy. Am J Roentgenol 140:949, 1983.

1547. Oliver TW Jr, Bernardino ME, Miller JI, et al: Isolated adrenal masses in nonsmall-cell bronchogenic carcinoma. Radiology 153:217, 1984.

1548. Commons RR, Callaway CP: Adenomas of the adrenal cortex. Arch Intern Med 81:37, 1948.

1549. Dunnick NR, Korobkin M, Francis I: Adrenal radiology: Distinguishing benign from malignant adrenal masses. Am J Roentgenol 167:861, 1996.

1550. Lee MJ, Hahn PF, Papanicolaou N, et al: Benign and malignant adrenal masses: CT distinction with attenuation coefficients, size, and observer analysis. Radiology 179:415, 1991.

1551. van Erkel AR, van Gils APG, Lequin M, et al: CT and MR distinction of adenomas and nonadenomas of the adrenal gland. J Comput Assist Tomogr 18:432, 1994.

1552. Korobkin M, Brodeur FJ, Yutzy GG, et al: Differentiation of adrenal adenomas from nonadenomas using CT attenuation values. Am J Roentgenol 166:531, 1996.

1553. Silverman PM, O'Malley J, Tefft MC, et al: Conspicuity of hepatic metastases on helical CT: Effect of different time delays between contrast administration and scanning. Am J Roentgenol 164:619, 1995.

1554. Jones EC, Chezmar JL, Nelson RC, et al: The frequency and significance of small (≤ 15 mm) hepatic lesions detected by CT. Am J Roentgenol 158:535, 1992.

1555. Boland GWL, Lee MJ, Gazelle GS, et al: Characterization of adrenal masses using unenhanced CT: An analysis of the CT literature. Am J Roentgenol 171:201, 1998.

1556. Reinig JW, Doppman JL, Dwyer AJ, et al: Distinction between adrenal adenomas and adrenal metastases using MR imaging. J Comput Assist Tomogr 9:898, 1985.

1557. Reinig JW, Doppman JL, Dwyer AJ, et al: Adrenal masses differentiated by MR. Radiology 158:81, 1986.

1558. Chang A, Glazer HS, Lee JKT, et al: Adrenal gland: MR imaging. Radiology 163:123, 1987.

1559. Burt M, Heelan RT, Coit D, et al: Prospective evaluation of unilateral adrenal masses in patients with operative nonsmall-cell lung cancer: Impact of magnetic resonance imaging. J Thorac Cardiovasc Surg 107:584, 1994.

1560. Reinig JW, Stutley JE, Leonhardt CM, et al: Differentiation of adrenal masses with MR imaging: Comparison of techniques. Radiology 192:41, 1994.

1561. Ichikawa T, Ohtomo K, Uchiyama G, et al: Adrenal adenomas: Characteristic hyperintense rim sign on fat-saturated spin-echo MR images. Radiology 193:247, 1994.

1562. Korobkin M, Lombardi TJ, Aisen AM, et al: Characterization of adrenal masses with chemical shift and gadolinium-enhanced MR imaging. Radiology 197:411, 1995.

1563. Schwartz LH, Panicek DM, Koutcher JA, et al: Adrenal masses in patients with malignancy: Prospective comparison of echo-planar, fast spin-echo, and chemical shift MR imaging. Radiology 197:421, 1995.

1564. Hooper RG, Beechler CR, Johnson MC: Radioisotope scanning in the initial staging of bronchogenic carcinoma. Am Rev Respir Dis 118:279, 1978.

1565. Donato AT, Ammerman EG, Sullesta O: Bone scanning in the evaluation of patients with lung cancer. Ann Thorac Surg 27:300, 1979.

1566. Salvatierra A, Baamonde C, Llamas JM, et al: Extrathoracic staging of bronchogenic carcinoma. Chest 97:1052, 1990.

1566a. Erasmus JJ, Patz EF Jr, McAdams HP, et al: Evaluation of adrenal masses in patients with bronchogenic carcinoma using ^{18}F-fluorodeoxyglucose positron emission tomography. Am J Roentgenol 168:1357, 1997.

1566b. Lewis P, Griffin S, Marsden P, et al: Whole-body ^{18}F-fluorodeoxyglucose positron emission tomography in preoperatiave evaluation of lung cancer. Lancet 344:1265, 1994.

1566c. Bury T, Dowlati A, Paulus P, et al: Evaluation of the solitary pulmonary nodule by positron emission tomography imaging. Eur Resp J 9:410, 1996.

1567. Chechani V: Bronchoscopic diagnosis of solitary pulmonary nodules and lung masses in the absence of endobronchial abnormality. Chest 109:620, 1996.

1568. Lillington GA, Caskey CI: Evaluation and management of solitary and multiple pulmonary nodules. Clin Chest Med 14:111, 1993.

1569. Colice GL: Chest CT for known or suspected lung cancer. Chest 106:1538, 1994.

1570. Lillington GA, Cummings SR: Decision analysis approaches in solitary pulmonary nodules. Semin Respir Med 10:227, 1989.

1571. Cummings SR, Lillington GA, Richard RJ: Estimating the probability of malignancy in solitary pulmonary nodules: A Bayesian approach. Am Rev Respir Dis 134:449, 1986.

1572. Rubins JB, Bloomfield H: Temporal trends in the prevalence of malignancy in resected solitary pulmonary lesions. Chest 109:100, 1996.

1573. Dewan NA, Shehan CJ, Reeb SD, et al: Likelihood of malignancy in a solitary pulmonary nodule—comparison of Bayesian analysis and results of FDG-PET scan. Chest 112:416, 1997.

1574. Dewan NA, Gupta NC, Redepenning LS, et al: Diagnostic efficacy of PET-FDG imaging in solitary pulmonary nodules—potential role in evaluation and management. Chest 104:997, 1993.

1575. Dewan NA, Reeb SD, Gupta NC, et al: PET-FDG imaging and transthoracic needle lung aspiration biopsy in evaluation of pulmonary lesions—a comparative risk-benefit analysis. Chest 108:441, 1995.

1576. Sazon DAD, Santiago SM, Soo Hoo GW, et al: Fluorodeoxyglucose-positron emission tomography in the detection and staging of lung cancer. Am J Respir Crit Care Med 153:417, 1996.

1577. Goldberg SK, Walkenstein MD, Steinbach A, et al: The role of staging bronchoscopy in the preoperative assessment of a solitary pulmonary nodule. Chest 104:94, 1993.

1578. Goldberg-Kahn B, Healy JC, Bishop JW: The cost of diagnosis—a comparison of four different strategies in the workup of solitary radiographic lung lesions. Chest 111:870, 1997.

1578a. Larscheid RC, Thorpe PE, Scott WJ: Percutaneous transthoracic needle aspiration biopsy. Chest 114:704, 1998.

1579. Edwards FH, Schaefer PS, Callahan S, et al: Bayesian statistical theory in the preoperative diagnosis of pulmonary lesions. Chest 92:888, 1987.

1580. Raab SS, Hornberger J: The effect of a patient's risk-taking attitude on the cost effectiveness of testing strategies in the evaluation of pulmonary lesions. Chest 111:1583, 1997.

1581. Kaplan DK: Mediastinal lymph node metastases in lung cancer: Is size a valid criterion? Thorax 47:332, 1992.

1582. Pearson M: Is CT scanning essential in the pre-operative assessment of lung cancer? Respir Med 83:93, 1989.

1583. Little AG, Stitik FP: Clinical staging of patients with non–small cell lung cancer. Chest 97:1431, 1990.

1584. Riquet M, Hidden G, Debesse B: Direct lymphatic drainage of lung segments to the mediastinal nodes—an anatomic study of 260 adults. J Thorac Cardiovasc Surg 97:623, 1989.

1585. Dales RE, Stark RM, Raman S: Computed tomography to stage lung cancer—approaching a controversy using meta-analysis. Am Rev Respir Dis 141:1096, 1990.

1586. Arita T, Matsumoto T, Kuramitsu T, et al: Is it possible to differentiate malignant mediastinal nodes from benign nodes by size? Chest 110:1004, 1996.

1587. Karmy-Jones R, Vallieres E, Lewis JW, et al: Investigation of patients with apparently inoperable lung cancer. Can Respir J 3:309, 1996.

1588. Sone S, Takashima S, Li F, et al: Mass screening for lung cancer with mobile spiral computed tomography scanner. Lancet 351:1242, 1998.

1589. Rusinek H, Naidich DP, McGuinness G, et al: Pulmonary nodule detection: Low-dose versus conventional CT. Radiology 209:243, 1998.

1590. Burgher LW, Jones FL, Patterson JR, et al: Guidelines for fiberoptic bronchoscopy in adults. Am Rev Respir Dis 136:1066, 1987.

1591. De Gracia J, Bravo C, Miravitlles M, et al: Diagnostic value of bronchoalveolar lavage in peripheral lung cancer. Am Rev Respir Dis 147:649, 1993.

1592. Pirozynski M: Bronchoalveolar lavage in the diagnosis of peripheral, primary lung cancer. Chest 102:372, 1992.

1593. Harrow EM, Wang K-P: The staging of lung cancer by bronchoscopic transbronchial needle aspiration. Chest Surg Clin North Am 6:223, 1996.

1594. Wang KP: Flexible transbronchial needle aspiration biopsy for histologic specimens. Chest 88:860, 1995.

1595. Utz JP, Patel AM, Edell ES: The role of transcarinal needle aspiration in the staging of bronchogenic carcinoma. Chest 104:1012, 1993.

1596. Harrow E, Halber M, Hardy S, et al: Bronchoscopic and roentgenographic correlates of a positive transbronchial needle aspiration in the staging of lung cancer. Chest 100:1592, 1991.

1597. Wilsher ML, Gurley AM: Transtracheal aspiration using rigid bronchoscopy and a rigid needle for investigating mediastinal masses. Thorax 51:197, 1996.

1598. Vansteenkiste J, Lacquet LM, Demedts M, et al: Transcarinal needle aspiration biopsy in the staging of lung cancer. Eur Respir J 7:265, 1994.

1599. Shure D, Fedullo PF: Transbronchial needle aspiration in diagnosis of submucosal and peribronchial bronchogenic carcinoma. Chest 88:49, 1985.

1600. Maier HC: Surgical treatment (of pulmonary carcinoma). In Mayer E, Maier HC (eds): Pulmonary Carcinoma: Pathogenesis, Diagnosis, and Treatment. New York, New York University Press, 1956, p 298.

1601. Flehinger BJ, Melamed MR: Current status of screening for lung cancer. Chest Surg Clin North Am 4:1, 1994.

1602. Strauss GM, Gleason RE, Sugarbaker DJ: Screening for lung cancer—another look: A different view. Chest 111:754, 1997.

1603. Eddy DM: Screening for lung cancer. Ann Intern Med 111:232, 1989.

1604. Hakama M, Holli K, Visakorpi T, et al: Low biological aggressiveness of screen-detected lung cancers may indicate over-diagnosis. Int J Cancer 66:6, 1996.

1605. Kubik A, Polak J: Lung cancer detection: Results of a randomized prospective study in Czechoslovakia. Cancer 57:2427, 1986.

1606. Saito Y, Takahashi S, Usuda K, et al: Detection of early cancer by lung cancer screening. Nippon Rinsho 54:1410, 1996.

1607. Kobusch AB, Simard A, Feldstein M, et al: Pulmonary cytology in chrysotile asbestos workers. J Chronic Dis 37:599, 1984.

1608. Frost JK, Ball WC Jr, Levin ML, et al: Sputum cytopathology: Use and potential in monitoring the workplace environment by screening for biological effects of exposure. J Occup Med 28:692, 1986.

1609. Kaneko M, Eguchi K, Ohmatsu H, et al: Peripheral lung cancer: Screening and detection with low-dose spiral CT versus radiography. Radiology 201:798, 1996.

1610. Mori K, Tominaga K, Hirose T, et al: Utility of low-dose helical CT as a second step after plain chest radiography for mass screening for lung cancer. J Thorac Imaging 12:173, 1997.

1611. Shields TW: Surgical therapy for carcinoma of the lung. Clin Chest Med 14:121, 1993.

1612. Malmberg R, Bergman B, Branehog I, et al: Lung cancer in West Sweden 1976–1985: A study of trends and survival with special reference to surgical treatment. Acta Oncol 35:185, 1996.

1613. Wada H, Tanaka F, Yanagihara K, et al: Time trends and survival after operations for primary lung cancer from 1976 through 1990. J Thorac Cardiovasc Surg 112:349, 1996.

1614. Shah R, Sabanathan S, Richardson J, et al: Results of surgical treatment of stage I and II lung cancer. J Cardiovasc Surg (Torino) 37:169, 1996.

1615. Shirakusa T, Tsutsui M, Iriki N, et al: Results of resection for bronchogenic carcinoma in patients over the age of 80. Thorax 44:189, 1989.

1616. Roxburgh JC, Thompson J, Goldstraw P. Hospital mortality and long-term survival after pulmonary resection in the elderly. Ann Thorac Surg 51:800, 1991.

1617. Ishida T, Yokoyama H, Kaneko S, et al: Long-term results of operation for non–small cell lung cancer in the elderly. Ann Thorac Surg 50:919, 1990.

1618. Massard G, Moog R, Wihlm JM, et al: Bronchogenic cancer in the elderly: Operative risk and long-term prognosis. Thorac Cardiovasc Surg 44:40, 1996.

1619. Maki E, Feld R: Prognostic factors in patients with non–small cell lung cancer: A critique of the world literature. Lung Cancer 7:27, 1991.

1620. O'Connell JP, Kris MG, Gralla RJ, et al: Frequency and prognostic importance of pretreatment clinical characteristics in patients with advanced non–small cell lung cancer treated with combination chemotherapy. J Clin Oncol 4:1604, 1986.

1621. Hespanhol V, Queiroga H, Magalhaes A, et al: Survival predictors in advanced non–small cell lung cancer. Lung Cancer 13:253, 1995.

1622. Palomares MR, Sayre JW, Shekar KC, et al: Gender influence on weight-loss pattern and survival of nonsmall-cell lung cancer patients. Cancer 78:2119, 1996.

1623. Ries LA: Influence of extent of disease, histology, and demographic factors on lung cancer survival in the SEER population-based data. Semin Surg Oncol 10:21, 1994.

1624. Johnson BE, Steinberg SM, Phelps R, et al: Female patients with small cell lung cancer live longer than male patients. Am J Med 85:194, 1988.

1625. Williams DE, Pairolero PC, Davis CS, et al: Survival of patients surgically treated for Stage I lung cancer. J Thorac Cardiovasc Surg 82:70, 1981.

1626. Gail MH, Eagan RT, Feld R, et al: Prognostic factors in patients with resected stage 1 non–small cell lung cancer. Cancer 54:1802, 1984.

1627. Rossing TH, Rossing RG: Survival in lung cancer. Am Rev Respir Dis 126:771, 1982.

1628. Finkelstein DM, Ettinger DS, Ruckdischel JC: Long-term survivors in metastatic nonsmall-cell lung cancer: An Eastern Cooperative Oncology Group Study. J Clin Oncol 4:702, 1986.

1629. Osterlind K, Andersen PK: Prognostic factors in small cell lung cancer: Multivariate model based on 778 patients treated with chemotherapy with or without irradiation. Cancer Res 46:4189, 1986.

1630. Green LS, Fortoul TI, Ponciano G, et al: Bronchogenic cancer in patients under 40 years old—the experience of a Latin American country. Chest 104:1477, 1993.

1631. Antkowiak JG, Regal AM, Takita H: Bronchogenic carcinoma in patients under age 40. Ann Thorac Surg 47:391, 1989.

1632. Nugent WC, Edney MT, Hammerness PG, et al: Non-small cell lung cancer at the extremes of age: Impact on diagnosis and treatment. Ann Thorac Surg 63:193, 1997.

1633. Lee-Chiong TL Jr, Matthay RA: Lung cancer in the elderly patient. Clin Chest Med 14:453, 1993.

1634. Massard G, Moog R, Wihlm JM, et al: Bronchogenic cancer in the elderly: Operative risk and long-term prognosis. Thorac Cardiovasc Surg 44:40, 1996.

1635. Ershler WB, Socinski MA, Greene CJ: Bronchogenic cancer, metastases, and aging. J Am Geriatr Soc 31:673, 1983.

1636. O'Rourke MA, Feussner JR, Feigl P, et al: Age trends of lung cancer stage at diagnosis: Implications for lung cancer screening in the elderly. JAMA 258:921, 1987.

1637. Lipford EH III, Eggleston JC, Lillemoe KD, et al: Prognostic factors in surgically resected limited-stage, non–small cell carcinoma of the lung. Am J Surg Pathol 8:357, 1984.

1638. Nomura A, Kolonel L, Rellahan W, et al: Racial survival patterns for lung cancer in Hawaii. Cancer 48:1265, 1981.

1639. Fry WA, Menck HR, Winchester DP: The national cancer data base report on lung cancer. Cancer 77:1947, 1996.

1640. Fraire AE, Roggli VL, Vollmer RT, et al: Lung cancer heterogeneity: Prognostic implications. Cancer 60:370, 1987.

1641. Stanley K, Cox JD, Petrovich Z, et al: Patterns of failure in patients with inoperable carcinoma of the lung. Cancer 47:2725, 1981.

1642. Tateishi M, Fukuyama Y, Hamatake M, et al: Characteristics of non–small cell lung cancer 3 cm or less in diameter. J Surg Oncol 59:251, 1995.

1643. Mountain CF, Carr DT, Anderson WAD: A system for the clinical staging of lung cancer. Am J Roentgenol 120:130, 1974.

1644. Huhti E, Sutinen S, Saloheimo M: Survival among patients with lung cancer: An epidemiologic study. Am Rev Respir Dis 124:13, 1981.

1645. Rubinstein I, Baum GL, Kalter Y, et al: The influence of cell type and lymph node metastases on survival of patients with carcinoma of the lung undergoing thoracotomy. Am Rev Respir Dis 119:253, 1979.

1646. Girling DJ, Stott H, Stephens RJ, et al: Fifteen-year follow-up of all patients in a study of postoperative chemotherapy for bronchial carcinoma. Br J Cancer 52:867, 1985.

1647. Cangemi V, Volpino P, D'Andrea N, et al: Results of surgical treatment of stage IIIA non–small cell lung cancer. Eur J Cardiothorac Surg 9:352, 1995.

1648. Coen V, Van Lannncker M, De Neve W, et al: Prognostic factors in locoregional non–small cell lung cancer treated with radiotherapy. Am J Clin Oncol 18:111, 1995.

1649. Shah R, Sabanathan S, Richardson J, et al: Results of surgical treatment of stage I and II lung cancer. J Cardiovasc Surg (Torino) 37:169, 1996.

1650. Lipford EH III, Eggleston JC, Lillemoe KD, et al: Prognostic factors in surgically resected limited-stage, non–small cell carcinoma of the lung. Am J Surg Pathol 8:357, 1984.

1651. Ichinose Y, Yano T, Asoh H, et al: Prognostic factors obtained by a pathologic examination in completely resected nonsmall-cell lung cancer: An analysis in each pathologic stage. J Thorac Cardiovasc Surg 110:601, 1995.

1652. Bernardi D del C, Capelozzi VL, Takagaki TY, et al: Usefulness of morphometric evaluation of histopathologic slides in predicting long-term outcome of patients with squamous cell carcinoma of the lung: A preliminary report. Chest 107:614, 1995.

1653. Visakorpi T, Holli K, Hakama M: High cell proliferation activity determined by DNA flow cytometry and prognosis in epidermoid lung carcinoma. Acta Oncol 34:605, 1995.

1653a. Sahin AA, Ro JY, El-Naggar AK, et al: Flow cytometric analysis of the DNA content of non–small cell lung cancer: Ploidy as a significant prognostic indicator in squamous cell carcinoma of the lung. Cancer 65:530, 1990.

1653b. Filderman AE, Silvestri GA, Gatsonis C, et al: Prognostic significance of tumor proliferative fraction and DNA content in stage I non–small cell lung cancer. Am Rev Respir Dis 146:707, 1992.

1653c. Carey FA, Prasad US, Walker WS, et al: Prognostic significance of tumor deoxyribonucleic acid content in surgically resected small cell carcinoma of lung. J Thorac Cardiovasc Surg 103:1214, 1992.

1654. Cortese DA, Pairolero PC, Bergstralh EJ, et al: Roentgenographically occult lung cancer: A ten-year experience. J Thorac Cardiovasc Surg 86:373, 1983.

1655. Martini N, Melamed MR: Occult carcinomas of the lung. Ann Thorac Surg 30:215, 1980.

1656. Mason MK, Jordan JW: Outcome of carcinoma in situ and early invasive carcinoma of the bronchus. Thorax 37:453, 1982.

1657. Watanabe Y, Shimizu J, Oda M, et al: Early hilar lung cancer: Its clinical aspect. J Surg Oncol 48:75, 1991.

1658. Blanke CD, Johnson DH: Treatment of small cell lung cancer. Semin Thorac Cardiovasc Surg 9:101, 1997.

1659. Huhti E, Sutinen S, Saloheimo M: Survival among patients with lung cancer: An epidemiologic study. Am Rev Respir Dis 124:13, 1981.

1660. Osterlind K, Hansen HH, Hansen M, et al: Mortality and morbidity in long-term surviving patients treated with chemotherapy with or without irradiation for small-cell lung cancer. J Clin Oncol 4:1044, 1986.

1661. Van Wyk CE, Tucker RD: Survival rates in undifferentiated small-cell carcinoma of the bronchus: A review and 2 case reports. S Afr Med J 65:307, 1984.

1662. Vogelsang GV, Abeloff MD, Ettinger DS, et al: Long-term survivors of small cell carcinoma of the lung. Am J Med 79:49, 1985.

1663. Hansen M, Hansen HH, Dombernowsky P: Long-term survival in small cell carcinoma of the lung. JAMA 244:247, 1980.

1664. Johnson BE, Ihde DC, Bunn PA, et al: Patients with small-cell lung cancer treated with combination chemotherapy with or without irradiation: Data on potential cures, chronic toxicities, and late relapses after a five- to eleven-year follow-up. Ann Intern Med 103:430, 1985.

1665. Pallares C, Bastus R, Lopez JJ, et al: Long-term survival in small cell carcinoma of the lung. Eur J Cancer Clin Oncol 23:541, 1987.

1666. Skarin AT: Analysis of long-term survivors with small-cell lung cancer. Chest 103:440, 1993.

1667. Johnson BE: Concurrent approaches to combined chemotherapy and chest radiotherapy for the treatment of patients with limited stage small cell lung cancer. Lung Cancer 1:281, 1994.

1668. Urschel JD: Surgical treatment of peripheral small cell lung cancer. Chest Surg Clin North Am 7:95, 1997.

1669. Kron IL, Harman PK, Mills SE, et al: A reappraisal of limited stage undifferentiated carcinoma of the lung: Does stage I small cell undifferentiated carcinoma exist? J Thorac Cardiovasc Surg 84:734, 1982.

1670. Radice PA, Matthews MJ, Ihde DC, et al: The clinical behavior of "mixed" small cell/large cell bronchogenic carcinoma compared to "pure" small cell subtypes. Cancer 50:2894, 1982.

1671. Shtivelman E: A link between metastasis and resistance to apoptosis of variant small cell lung carcinoma. Oncogene 14:2167, 1997.

1672. Linnoila RI: Spectrum of neuroendocrine differentiation in lung cancer cell lines featured by cytomorphology, markers, and their corresponding tumors. J Cell Biochem 24(Suppl):92, 1996.

1673. Levin NA, Brzoska P, Gupta N, et al: Identification of frequent novel genetic alterations in small cell lung carcinoma. Cancer Res 54:5086, 1994.

1674. Craig J, Powell B, Muss HB, et al: Second primary bronchogenic carcinoma after small cell carcinoma: Report of two cases and review of the literature. Am J Med 76:1013, 1984.

1675. Volk SA, Mansour RF, Gandara DR, et al: Morbidity in long-term survivors of small cell carcinoma of the lung. Cancer 54:25, 1984.

1676. Yu PP, Waxman JS, Chahinian AP, et al: Acute myelogenous leukemia following complete remission of small cell carcinoma of the lung. Med Pediatr Oncol 14:100, 1986.

1677. Chak LY, Sikic BI, Tucker MA, et al: Increased incidence of acute nonlymphocytic leukemia following therapy in patients with small cell carcinoma of the lung. J Clin Oncol 2:385, 1984.

1678. Johnson BE, Linnoila RI, Williams JP, et al: Risk of second aerodigestive cancers increases in patients who survive free of small cell lung cancer for more than 2 years. J Clin Oncol 13:101, 1995.

1679. Richardson GE, Tucker MA, Venzon DJ, et al: Smoking cessation after successful treatment of small-cell lung cancer is associated with fewer smoking-related second primary cancers. Ann Intern Med 119:383, 1993.

1680. Kawahara M, Ushijima S, Kamimori T, et al: Second primary tumours in more than 2-year disease-free survivors of small cell lung cancer in Japan: The role of smoking cessation. Br J Cancer 78:409, 1998.

1681. Munnell ER, Dilling E, Grantham RN, et al: Reappraisal of solitary bronchiolar (alveolar cell) carcinoma of the lung. Ann Thorac Surg 25:289, 1978.

1682. Horie A, Kotoo Y, Ohta M, et al: Relation of fine structure to prognosis for papillary adenocarcinoma of the lung. Hum Pathol 15:870, 1984.

1683. Heikkila L, Mattila P, Harjula A, et al: Tumour growth rate and its relationship to prognosis in bronchiolo-alveolar and pulmonary adenocarcinoma. Ann Chir Gynaecol 74:210, 1985.

1684. Coslett HB, Teja K, Sutula TP: Meningeal carcinomatosis 21 years following bronchiolo-alveolar carcinoma: Diagnosis by cisternal CSF examination. Cancer 49:173, 1982.

1685. Dumont P, Gasser B, Rougé C, et al: Bronchoalveolar carcinoma—histopathologic study of evolution in a series of 105 surgically treated patients. Chest 113:391, 1998.

1686. Noguchi M, Morikawa A, Kawasaki M, et al: Small adenocarcinoma of the lung: Histologic characteristics and prognosis. Cancer 75:2844, 1995.

1687. Sorensen JB, Olsen JE: Prognostic implications of histopathologic subtyping in patients with surgically treated stage I or II adenocarcinoma of the lung. J Thorac Cardiovasc Surg 97:245, 1989.

1688. Matsui K, Kitagawa M, Sugiyama S, et al: Distribution pattern of the basement membrane components is one of the significant prognostic correlates in peripheral lung adenocarcinomas. Hum Pathol 26:186, 1995.

1689. Harpole DH Jr, Herndon JE 2nd, Wolfe WG, et al: A prognostic model of recurrence and death in stage I non–small cell lung cancer utilizing presentation, histopathology, and oncoprotein expression. Cancer Res 55:51, 1995.

1690. Watanabe N, Nakajima I, Abe S, et al: Staining pattern of type IV collagen and prognosis in early stage adenocarcinoma of the lung. J Clin Pathol 47:613, 1994.

1691. Mitchell DM, Morgan PGM, Ball JB: Prognostic features of large cell anaplastic carcinoma of the bronchus. Thorax 35:118, 1980.

1692. Hespanhol V, Queiroga H, Magalhaes A, et al: Survival predictors in advanced non–small cell lung cancer. Lung Cancer 13:253, 1995.

1693. Schonwetter RS, Robinson BE, Ramirez G: Prognostic factors for survival in terminal lung cancer patients. J Gen Intern Med 9:366, 1994.

1694. Naunheim KS, Taylor JR, Skosey C, et al: Adenosquamous lung carcinoma: Clinical characteristics, treatment and prognosis. Ann Thorac Surg 44:462, 1987.

1695. Shimizu J, Oda M, Hayashi Y, et al: A clinicopathologic study of resected cases of adenosquamous carcinoma of the lung. Chest 109:989, 1996.

1696. Sridhar KS, Bounassi MJ, Raub W, et al: Clinical features of adenosquamous lung carcinoma in 127 patients. Am Rev Respir Dis 142:19, 1990.

1697. Buccheri G, Ferrigno D: Prognostic factors in lung cancer: Tables and comments. Eur Respir J 7:1350, 1994.

1698. Watanabe Y, Hayashi Y, Shimizu J, et al: Mediastinal nodal involvement and the prognosis of non–small cell lung cancer. Chest 100:422, 1991.

1699. Shields TW: The significance of ipsilateral mediastinal lymph node metastasis (N2 disease) in non–small cell carcinoma of the lung. J Thorac Cardiovasc Surg 99:48, 1990.

1700. Miller JD, Gorenstein LA, Patterson GA: Staging: The key to rational management of lung cancer. Ann Thorac Surg 53:170, 1992.

1701. Feinstein AR, Sosin DM, Wells CK: The Will Rogers phenomenon—stage migration and new diagnostic techniques as a source of misleading statistics for survival in cancer. N Engl J Med 312:1604, 1985.

1702. Detterbeck FC, Socinski MA: IIb or not IIB: The current question in staging non–small cell lung cancer. Chest 112:229, 1997.

1703. Padilla J, Calvo V, Penalver JC, et al: Surgical results and prognostic factors in early non–small cell lung cancer. Ann Thorac Surg 63:324, 1997.

1704. Daly BD Jr, Faling LJ, Bite G, et al: Mediastinal lymph node evaluation by computed tomography in lung cancer: An analysis of 345 patients grouped by TNM staging, tumor size, and tumor location. J Thorac Cardiovasc Surg 94:664, 1987.

1704a. Inoue K, Sato M, Fujimura S, et al: Prognostic assessment of 1310 patients with non–small cell lung cancer who underwent complete resection from 1980 to 1993. J Thorac Cardiovasc Surg 116:407, 1998.

1705. Jefferson MF, Pendleton N, Faragher EB, et al: "Tumour volume" as a predictor of survival after resection on nonsmall-cell lung cancer (NSCLC). Br J Cancer 74:456, 1996.

1706. van Klaveren RJ, Festen J, Otten HJAM, et al: Prognosis of unsuspected but completely resectable N2 non–small cell lung cancer. Ann Thorac Surg 56:300, 1993.

1707. Sabanathan S, Richardson J, Mearns AJ, et al: Results of surgical treatment of stage III lung cancer. Eur J Cardiothorac Surg 8:183, 1994.

1708. Riquet M, Manac'h D, Saab M, et al: Factors determining survival in resected N2 lung cancer. Eur J Cardiothorac Surg 9:300, 1995.

1709. Deslauriers J, Brisson J, Cartier R, et al: Carcinoma of the lung—evaluation of satellite nodules as a factor influencing prognosis after resection. J Thorac Cardiovasc Surg 97:504, 1989.

1710. Nakajima J, Furuse A, Oka T, et al: Excellent survival in a subgroup of patients with intrapulmonary metastasis of lung cancer. Ann Thorac Surg 61:158, 1996.

1710a. Yano M, Arai T, Inagaki K, et al: Intrapulmonary satellite nodule of lung cancer as a T factor. Chest 114:1305, 1998.

1711. Mountain CF: The biological operability of stage III non–small cell lung cancer. Ann Thorac Surg 40:60, 1985.

1712. Postmus PE, Sleijfer DT, Meinesz AF, et al: No response improvement after sequential chemotherapy for small cell lung cancer. Eur J Respir Dis 68:279, 1986.

1713. Prasad US, Naylor AR, Walker WS, et al: Long term survival after pulmonary resection for small cell carcinoma of the lung. Thorax 44:784, 1989.

1714. Mulshine JL, Makuch RW, Johnston-Early A, et al: Diagnosis and significance of liver metastases in small cell carcinoma of the lung. J Clin Oncol 2:733, 1984.

1715. Hirsch FR, Hansen HH: Bone marrow involvement in small cell anaplastic carcinoma of the lung: Prognostic and therapeutic aspects. Cancer 46:206, 1980.

1716. Kochhar R, Frytak S, Shaw EG: Survival of patients with extensive small-cell lung cancer who have only brain metastases at initial diagnosis. Am J Clin Oncol 20:125, 1997.

1717. Sorensen JB, Badsberg JH: Prognostic factors in resected stages I and II adenocarcinoma of the lung. J Thorac Cardiovasc Surg 99:218, 1990.

1718. Wigren T, Oksanen H, Kellokumpu-Lehtinen P: A practical prognostic index for inoperable nonsmall-cell lung cancer. J Cancer Res Clin Oncol 123:259, 1997.

1719. Vansteenkiste JF, De Leyn PR, Deneffe GJ, et al: Survival and prognostic factors in resected N2 non–small cell lung cancer: A study of 140 cases. Leuven Lung Cancer Group. Ann Thorac Surg 63:1441, 1997.

1720. Takigawa N, Segawa Y, Okahara M, et al: Prognostic factors for patients with advanced non–small cell lung cancer: Univariate and multivariate analyses including recursive partitioning and amalgamation. Lung Cancer 15:67, 1996.

1721. Buccheri G, Ferrigno D, Tamburini M: Karnofsky and ECOG performance status scoring in lung cancer: A prospective, longitudinal study of 536 patients from a single institution. Eur J Cancer 32:1135, 1996.

1722. Mountain CF: New prognostic factors in lung cancer—biologic prophets of cancer cell aggression. Chest 108:246, 1995.

1723. Osaki T, Mitsudomi T, Oyama T, et al: Serum level and tissue expression of c-erb-2 protein in lung adenocarcinoma. Chest 108:157, 1995.

1724. Slebos RJC, Kibbelaar RE, Dalesio O, et al: K-Ras oncogene activation as a prognostic marker in adenocarcinoma of the lung. N Engl J Med 323:561, 1990.

1725. Cho JY, Kim JH, Lee YH, et al: Correlation between K-ras gene mutation and prognosis of patients with non–small cell lung carcinoma. Cancer 79:462, 1997.

1726. Yi ES, Harclerode D, Gondo M, et al: High c-erbB-3 protein expression is associated with shorter survival in advanced non–small cell lung carcinoma. Mod Pathol 10:142, 1997.

1727. van Zandwijk N, Mooi WJ, Rodenhuis S: Prognostic factors in non–small cell carcinoma: Research experiences. Lung Cancer 1:27, 1995.

1728. Fontanini G, Vignati S, Lucchi M, et al: Neoangiogenesis and p53 protein in lung cancer: Their prognostic role and their relation with vascular endothelial growth factor (VEGF) expression. Br J Cancer 75:1295, 1997.

1729. Dalquen P, Sauter G, Torhorst J, et al: Nuclear p53 overexpression is an independent prognostic parameter in node-negative non–small cell lung carcinoma. J Pathol 178:53, 1996.

1730. Tormanen U, Eerola AK, Rainio P, et al: Enhanced apoptosis predicts shortened survival in non–small cell lung carcinoma. Cancer Res 55:5595, 1995.

1731. Higashiyama M, Doi O, Kodama K, et al: bcl-2 oncoprotein in surgically resected non–small cell lung cancer: Possibly favorable prognostic factor in association with low incidence of distant metastasis. J Surg Oncol 64:48, 1997.

1731a. Fleming MV, Guinee DG Jr, Chu WS, et al: BCL-2 immunohistochemistry in a surgical series of non–small cell lung cancer patients. Hum Pathol 29:60, 1998.

1731b. Greatens TM, Niehans GA, Rubins JB, et al: Do molecular markers predict survival in non–small cell lung cancer? Am J Respir Crit Care Med 157:1093, 1998.

1732. Diez M, Torres A, Maestro ML, et al: Prediction of survival and recurrence by serum and cytosolic levels of CEA, CA125 and SCC antigens in resectable nonsmall-cell lung cancer. Br J Cancer 73:1248, 1996.

1733. Yoshimasu T, Miyoshi S, Maebeya S, et al: Analysis of the early postoperative serum carcinoembryonic antigen time-course as a prognostic tool for bronchogenic carcinoma. Cancer 79:1533, 1997.

1733a. Rubins JB, Dunitz J, Rubins HB, et al: Serum carcinoembryonic antigen as an adjunct to preoperative staging of lung cancer. J Thorac Cardiovasc Surg 116:412, 1998.

1734. Suehiro T, Ishida T, Sugio K, et al: Monoclonal antibody KP16D3 as a prognostic marker in stage I lung adenocarcinoma. J Surg Oncol 54:51, 1993.

1735. Higashiyama M, Doi O, Kodama K, et al: Immunohistochemically detected expression of motility-related protein-1 (MRP-1/CD9) in lung adenocarcinoma and its relation to prognosis. Int J Cancer 74:205, 1997.

1735a. Adachi M, Taki T, Konishi T, et al: Novel staging protocol for non–small cell lung cancers according to MRP-1/CD9 and KAI1/CD82 gene expression. J Clin Oncol 16:1397, 1998.

1736. Miyake M, Taki T, Hitomi S, et al: Correlation of expression of H/Ley/Leb antigens with survival in patients with carcinoma of the lung. N Engl J Med 327:14, 1992.

1737. Lee JS, Ro JY, Sahin A, et al: Expression of blood-group antigen A—a favorable prognostic factor in nonsmall-cell lung cancer. N Engl J Med 324:1084, 1991.

1738. Taguchi O, Gabazza EC, Yoshida M, et al: High plasma level of plasmin-alpha 2-plasmin inhibitor complex is predictor of poor prognosis in patients with lung cancer. Clin Chim Acta 244:69, 1996.

1739. Viberti L, Papotti M, Abbona GC, et al: Value of Ki-67 immunostaining in preoperative biopsies of carcinomas of the lung. Hum Pathol 28:189, 1997.

1740. Macchiarini P, Fontanini G, Hardin MJ, et al: Blood vessel invasion by tumor cells predicts recurrence in completely resected T1 N0 M0 nonsmall-cell lung cancer. J Thorac Cardiovasc Surg 106:80, 1993.

1741. Wolf G, Elez R, Doermer A, et al: Prognostic significance of polo-like kinase (PLK) expression in non–small cell lung cancer. Oncogene 14:543, 1997.

1742. Kondo K, Noguchi M, Mukai K, et al: Transferrin receptor expression in adenocarcinoma of the lung as a histopathologic indicator of prognosis. Chest 97:1367, 1990.

1743. Carey FA, Prasad US, Walker WS, et al: Prognostic significance of tumor deoxyribonucleic acid content in surgically resected small-cell carcinoma of lung. J Thorac Cardiovasc Surg 103:1214, 1992.

1744. Filderman AE, Silvestri GA, Gatsonis C, et al: Prognostic significance of tumor proliferative fraction and DNA content in stage I non–small cell lung cancer. Am Rev Respir Dis 148:707, 1992.

1745. Salvati F, Teodori L, Gagliardi L, et al: DNA flow cytometric studies of 66 human lung tumors analyzed before treatment—prognostic implications. Chest 96:1092, 1989.

1746. Takanami I, Tanaka F, Hashizume T, et al: Roles of the transforming growth factor beta 1 and its type I and II receptors in the development of a pulmonary adenocarcinoma: Results of an immunohistochemical study. J Surg Oncol 64:262, 1997.

1746a. Bennett WP, el-Deiry WS, Rush WL, et al: p21waf1/cip1 and transforming growth factor beta-1 protein expression correlate with survival in non–small cell lung cancer. Clin Cancer Res 4:1499, 1998.

1747. Sukoh N, Abe S, Ogura S, et al: Immunohistochemical study of cathepsin B: Prognostic significance in human lung cancer. Cancer 74:46, 1994.

1748. Sarandakou A, Poulakis N, Rizos D, et al: Soluble interleukin-2 receptors (sIL-2R) and neuron specific enolase (NSE) in small cell lung carcinoma. Anticancer Res 13:173, 1993.

1749. Buccheri G, Marino P, Preatoni A, et al: Soluble interleukin 2 receptor in lung cancer—an indirect marker of tumor activity? Chest 99:1433, 1991.

1750. Kwa HB, Verheijen MG, Litvinov SV, et al: Prognostic factors in resected non–small cell lung cancer: An immunohistochemical study of 39 cases. Lung Cancer 16:35, 1996.

1751. Pujol JL, Simony J, Demoly P, et al: Neural cell adhesion molecule and prognosis of surgically resected lung cancer. Am Rev Respir Dis 148:1071, 1993.

1752. Fontanini G, Lucchi M, Vignati S, et al: Angiogenesis as a prognostic indicator of survival in nonsmall-cell lung carcinoma: A prospective study. J Natl Cancer Inst 89:881, 1997.

1752a. Shibusa T, Shijubo N, Abe S: Tumor angiogenesis and vascular endothelial growth factor expression in stage I lung adenocarcinoma. Clin Cancer Res 4:1483, 1998.

1753. Brechot JM, Chevret S, Charpentier MC, et al: Blood vessel and lymphatic vessel invasion in resected non–small cell lung carcinoma: Correlation with TNM stage and disease free and overall survival. Cancer 78:2111, 1996.

1753a. Yamashita JI, Tashiro K, Yoneda S, et al: Local increase in polymorphonuclear leukocyte elastase is associated with tumor invasiveness in non–small cell lung cancer. Chest 109:1328, 1996.

1753b. Sulzer MA, Leers MP, Van Noord JA, et al: Reduced E-cadherin expression is associated with increased lymph node metastasis and unfavorable prognosis in non–small cell lung cancer. Am J Respir Crit Care Med 157:1319, 1998.

1753c. Stokkel MP, van Eck-Smit BL, Zwinderman AH, et al: Pretreatment serum lactate dehydrogenase as additional staging parameter in patients with small cell lung carcinoma. J Cancer Res Clin Oncol 124:215, 1998.

1753d. De Vita F, Infusino S, Auriemma A, et al: Circulating levels of soluble intercellular adhesion molecule-1 in non–small cell lung cancer patients. Oncology Reports 5:393, 1998.

1754. Komaki R, Fujii T, Perkins P, et al: Apoptosis and mitosis as prognostic factors in pathologically staged N1 non–small cell lung cancer. Int J Radiat Oncol Biol Phys 36:601, 1996.

1755. Everson TC, Cole WH: Spontaneous Regression of Cancer: A Study and Abstract of Reports in the World Medical Literature and of Personal Communications Concerning Spontaneous Regression of Malignant Disease. Philadelphia, WB Saunders, 1966.

1756. Blades B, McCorkle RG Jr: A case of spontaneous regression of an untreated bronchiogenic carcinoma. J Thorac Cardiovasc Surg 27:415, 1954.

1757. Sutton M, Pratt-Johnson JH: Spontaneous regression of carcinoma of bronchus. Clin Radiol 21:256, 1970.

1758. Gautam HP: Spontaneous regression and metachronous contralateral occurrence of bronchial carcinoma. Am Rev Respir Dis 103:275, 1971.

1759. Sperduto P, Vaezy A, Bridgman A, et al: Spontaneous regression of squamous cell lung carcinoma with adrenal metastasis. Chest 94:887, 1988.

1760. Darnell RB, DeAngelis LM: Regression of small-cell lung carcinoma in patients with paraneoplastic neuronal antibodies. Lancet 341:21, 1993.

1761. Zaheer W, Friedland ML, Cooper EB, et al: Spontaneous regression of small cell carcinoma of lung associated with severe neuropathy. Cancer Invest 11:306, 1993.

1762. Bewtra C: Multiple primary bronchogenic carcinomas, with a review of the literature. J Surg Oncol 25:207, 1984.

1763. Rosengart TK, Martini N, Ghosn P, et al: Multiple primary lung carcinomas: Prognosis and treatment. Ann Thorac Surg 52:773, 1991.

1764. Verhagen AFTM, Tavilla G, van de Wal HJCM, et al: Multiple primary lung cancers. Thorac Cardiovasc Surg 42:40, 1994.

1765. Ribet M, Dambron P: Multiple primary lung cancers. Eur J Cardiothorac Surg 9:231, 1995.

1766. Antakli T, Schaefer RF, Rutherford JE, et al: Second primary lung cancer. Ann Thorac Surg 59:863, 1995.

1767. Caceres J, Felson B: Double primary carcinomas of the lung. Radiology 102:45, 1972.

1768. Hughes RK, Blades B: Multiple primary bronchogenic carcinoma. J Thorac Cardiovasc Surg 41:421, 1961.

1769. von Ott A, Titscher R: Das primäre Doppelkarzinom der Lunge. [Primary double carcinoma of the lung.] Fortschr Geb Roentgstr Nuklearmed 110:793, 1969.

1770. Bower SL, Choplin RH, Muss HB: Multiple primary bronchogenic carcinomas of the lung. Am J Roentgenol 140:253, 1983.

1771. Wu SC, Lin ZQ, Xu CW, et al: Multiple primary lung cancers. Chest 92:892, 1987.
1772. Stark P: Multiple independent bronchogenic carcinomas. Radiology 145:599, 1982.
1773. Lundgren R: Bilateral bronchial carcinoma. Br J Dis Chest 78:201, 1984.
1774. Miller RR, Nelems B, Evans KG, et al: Glandular neoplasia of the lung: A proposed analogy to colonic tumors. Cancer 61:1009, 1988.
1775. Carey FA, Donnelly SC, Walker WS, et al: Synchronous primary lung cancers: Prevalence in surgical material and clinical implications. Thorax 48:344, 1993.
1776. Auerbach O, Stout AP, Hammond EC, et al: Multiple primary bronchial carcinomas. Cancer 20:699, 1967.
1777. Coffman B, Crum E, Forman WB: Two primary carcinomas of the lung: Adenocarcinoma and a metachronous squamous cell carcinoma: A case report and a review of the literature. Cancer 51:124, 1983.
1778. Treasure T, Belcher JR: Prognosis of peripheral lung tumours related to size of the primary. Thorax 36:5, 1981.
1779. Chung TS: Multiple primary carcinomas of the lung. J Surg Oncol 24:124, 1983.
1780. Little AG, DeMeester TR, Ferguson MK, et al: Modified stage 1 (T1N0M0, T2N0M0) non–small cell lung cancer: Treatment results, recurrence patterns, and adjuvant immunotherapy. Surgery 100:621, 1986.
1781. Mathisen DJ, Jensik RJ, Faber LP, et al: Survival following resection for second and third primary lung cancers. J Thorac Cardiovasc Surg 88:502, 1984.
1782. Jensik RJ, Faber LP, Kittle CF, et al: Survival following resection for 2nd primary bronchogenic carcinoma. J Thorac Cardiovasc Surg 82:658, 1981.
1783. Pommier RF, Vetto JT, Lee JT, et al: Synchronous non–small cell lung cancers. Am J Surg 171:521, 1996.
1784. Angeletti CA, Mussi A, Janni A, et al: Second primary lung cancer and relapse: Treatment and follow-up. Eur J Cardiothorac Surg 9:607, 1995.
1785. Mizushima Y, Kobayashi M: Clinical characteristics of synchronous multiple lung cancer associated with idiopathic pulmonary fibrosis: A review of Japanese cases. Chest 108:1272, 1995.
1786. Motohiro A, Matsumoto T, Ienaga S: Synchronous growth of triple lung cancer. Surg Today 25:1054, 1995.
1787. Jung-Legg Y, McGowan SE, Sweeney KG, et al: Synchronous triple malignant tumors of the lung: A case report of bronchial carcinoid, small cell carcinoma, and adenocarcinoma of the right lung. Am J Clin Pathol 85:96, 1986.
1788. Paul SM, Bacharach B: Three synchronous bilateral lung tumors: A case report. J Surg Oncol 34:253, 1987.
1789. Logan PM, Miller RR, Evans K, et al: Bronchogenic carcinoma and coexistent bronchioloalveolar cell adenomas—assessment of radiologic detection and follow-up in 28 patients. Chest 109:713, 1996.
1790. Marks PH, Schechter FG: Multiple primary carcinomas of the head, neck, and lung. Ann Thorac Surg 33:324, 1982.
1791. Yellin A, Hill LR, Benfield JR: Bronchogenic carcinoma associated with upper aerodigestive cancers. J Thorac Cardiovasc Surg 91:674, 1986.
1792. Tepperman BS, Fitzpatrick PJ: Second respiratory and upper digestive tract cancers after oral cancer. Lancet 2:547, 1981.

1793. Shibuya H, Hisamitsu S, Shiori S, et al: Multiple primary cancer risk in patients with squamous cell carcinoma of the oral cavity. Cancer 60:3083, 1987.
1794. Silvestri F, Bussani R, Cosatti C, et al: High relative risk of a second pulmonary cancer in patients affected by laryngeal cancer: Differences by specific site of occurrence and lung cancer histotype. Laryngoscope 104:222, 1994.
1795. Bergfeldt K, Einhorn S, Rosendahl I, et al: Increased risk of second primary malignancies in patients with gynecological cancer: A Swedish record-linkage study. Acta Oncol 34:771, 1995.
1796. Engeland A, Bjorge T, Haldorsen T, et al: Use of multiple primary cancers to indicate associations between smoking and cancer incidence: An analysis of 500,000 cancer cases diagnosed in Norway during 1953–93. Int J Cancer 70:401, 1997.
1797. Salminen E, Pukkala E, Teppo L, et al: Risk of second cancers among lung cancer patients. Acta Oncol 34:165, 1995.
1798. Mellemgaard A, Geisler CH, Storm HH: Risk of kidney cancer and other second solid malignancies in patients with chronic lymphocytic leukemia. Eur J Haematol 53:218, 1994.
1799. Bertoldero G, Scribano G, Podda L, et al: Occurrence of second neoplasms in chronic lymphocytic leukemia: Experience at Padua Hospital between 1979 and 1991. Ann Hematol 69:195, 1994.
1800. Rahal PS, Cornelius V: Oat cell carcinoma of the lung in patients with CLL. J Ky Med Assoc 92:183, 1994.
1801. van Leeuwen FE, Klokman WJ, Stovall M, et al: Roles of radiotherapy and smoking in lung cancer following Hodgkin's disease. J Natl Cancer Inst 87:1530, 1995.
1802. Wiernik PH, Sklarin NT, Dutcher JP, et al: Adjuvant radiotherapy for breast cancer as a risk factor for the development of lung cancer. Med Oncol 11:121, 1994.
1803. Inskip PD, Stovall M, Flannery JT: Lung cancer risk and radiation dose among women treated for breast cancer. J Natl Cancer Inst 86:983, 1994.
1804. Neugut AI, Murray T, Santos J, et al: Increased risk of lung cancer after breast cancer radiation therapy in cigarette smokers. Cancer 73:1615, 1994.
1805. Lefor AT, Bredenberg CE, Kellman RM, et al: Multiple malignancies of the lung and head and neck: Second primary tumor or metastasis? Arch Surg 121:265, 1986.
1806. Lyons MF, Redmond J III, Covelli H: Multiple primary neoplasia of the head and neck and lung: The changing histopathology. Cancer 57:2193, 1986.
1807. Massard G, Wihlm JM, Ameur S, et al: Association of bronchial and pharyngolaryngeal malignancies: A reappraisal. Eur J Cardiothorac Surg 10:397, 1996.
1808. Shons AR, McQuarrie DG: Multiple primary epidermoid carcinomas of the upper aerodigestive tract. Arch Surg 120:1007, 1985.
1809. Lundgren J, Olofsson J: Multiple primary malignancies in patients treated for laryngeal carcinoma. J Otolaryngol 15:145, 1986.
1810. Rodriguez E, Castella J, Puzo C, et al: Lung cancer in patients with tracheostomy due to cancer of the larynx. Respiration 46:323, 1984.
1811. Rachmat L, Vreeburg GC, de Vries N, et al: The value of twice yearly bronchoscopy in the workup and follow-up of patients with laryngeal cancer. Eur J Cancer 29:1096, 1993.
1812. Markman M, Pavy MD, Abeloff MD: Acute leukemia following intensive therapy for small-cell carcinoma of the lung. Cancer 50:672, 1982.

Neuroendocrine Neoplasms

As discussed in Chapter 1 (*see* page 10), a small number of cells that contain neurosecretory granules and a variety of polypeptide hormones are present in the normal tracheobronchial epithelium. Several types of pulmonary neoplasm show ultrastructural and immunohistochemical features similar to these neuroendocrine (NE) cells. Although it has been hypothesized that these tumors are derived directly from NE cells,[1] it has also been proposed that they originate in a primitive "stem" or "indifferent" cell that for unknown reasons differentiates in an NE direction.[2, 3] Finally, although seemingly unlikely, some investigators have suggested that occasional pulmonary neuroendocrine tumors may be derived from cells of the peripheral nervous system.[4] Whatever their histogenesis, the vast majority of these tumors have morphologic and/or immunohistochemical features that enable them to be separated from other pulmonary neoplasms, and they can conveniently be discussed together.

The tumors that can be included in this group are varied and the terminology applied to them is somewhat confusing. Most observers believe that carcinoid tumor, both the typical and atypical types, is the prime example of pulmonary NE neoplasm. Some also consider small cell carcinoma to be of the same ilk and believe it to represent the most undifferentiated end of a spectrum of NE cell tumors.[2, 5, 6] Although there is some logic in this viewpoint, we prefer to consider small cell carcinoma separately because of its genetic differences[7] and its closer clinical and epidemiologic association with the other common forms of pulmonary carcinoma. In addition to these well-recognized neuroendocrine tumors, some large cell carcinomas histologically resemble carcinoid tumor and show ultrastructural and immunohistochemical evidence of NE differentiation; some investigators believe that these tumors should be considered in a separate category

(so-called large cell NE carcinoma, *see* page 1246).[8] Finally, some large cell carcinomas lack specific differentiation on light microscopy but have immunohistochemical and/or ultrastructural evidence of NE differentiation that might theoretically be included in the general group of NE tumors.[8–10]

CARCINOID TUMOR

Pulmonary carcinoid tumor is a low-grade malignant neoplasm believed to be derived from surface or glandular epithelium of the conducting or transitional airways. It is uncommon, accounting for only about 0.5% to 2.5% of all pulmonary neoplasms.[11–15] On the basis of histologic and cytologic features, tumors can be divided into two fairly distinct clinicopathologic types: typical and atypical.[16] The latter represent about 10% to 20% of pulmonary carcinoid tumors in most series.[16–18]

Carcinoid tumor has also been known as "bronchial adenoma," a generic term used to refer to adenoid cystic and mucoepidermoid carcinoma, as well as carcinoid tumor.[19] There are several reasons why this terminology is inappropriate. Despite its low-grade malignant potential, pulmonary carcinoid tumor is clearly capable of metastasizing and causing death; in addition, although it can show focal evidence of glandular differentiation, the predominant proliferating cell is NE in type. The designation adenoma (benign glandular neoplasm) is thus clearly inaccurate. Second, as discussed in more detail elsewhere (*see* page 1251), both adenoid cystic carcinoma and mucoepidermoid carcinoma are believed to be derived from tracheobronchial glandular epithelium and to be analogous to salivary gland tumors; although central bronchial carcinoid tumors may also originate in glandular epithelium, they possess no morphologic counterpart in the salivary gland and, by inference, no common histogenetic basis. Thus, apart from the common features of relatively good prognosis and proximal intraluminal growth (at least for central carcinoids), these neoplasms share little in common. The term "bronchial adenoma" is therefore both inaccurate and misleading with respect to these three neoplasms and should be used only in relation to a discussion of the history of medicine.

Overall, there appears to be a slight female preponderance;[11–13, 20] however, some investigators have found that patients with atypical tumors are more frequently men.[21, 22] The mean age at diagnosis is between 40 and 60,[13, 15, 23–26] centrally located tumors and typical forms tending to become manifested earlier than peripheral or atypical ones.[27, 28] The tumor is the most common primary pulmonary neoplasm in children and adolescents.[29–31] In some studies, the incidence has been found to be higher in white individuals than African Americans.[13, 32]

The etiology and pathogenesis of most carcinoid tumors are unclear. Although many patients with atypical tumors have a history of cigarette smoking, no association has been found between this habit and the more common typical tumor. In addition, there is no clear link of either form of tumor with other agents known to be associated with pulmonary carcinoma. Chronic inhalation of chrysotile or crocidolite asbestos fibers by rats has been shown to result in a proliferation of NE cells;[33] however, since asbestos workers do not appear to have an increased incidence of carcinoid tumor relative to the nonexposed population, the significance of this experimental observation is not clear. Although administration of several carcinogenic nitroso compounds to hamsters has been shown to result in an increase in the number of neuroepithelial bodies and the number of cells per neuroepithelial body,[2] neoplasms that subsequently develop are not composed of NE cells.

Although mutations in the *p53* gene have been found in some typical and atypical carcinoid tumors,[34, 35] some workers have found these to be infrequent.[36] In one investigation of 20 carcinoid tumors (10 typical and 10 atypical), no evidence of point mutations in the Ki-*ras* gene was found.[37] Similarly, retinoblastoma gene inactivation appears to be uncommon.[48]

Pathologic Characteristics

Typical Carcinoid Tumor

Typical carcinoid tumors account for 80% to 90% of all cases of carcinoid tumor. The majority of these (about 80% to 85%) appear to arise in a lobar, segmental, or proximal subsegmental bronchus; most of the remainder are located in the lung periphery, often without a clear airway association on gross examination. Rare examples occur in the trachea.[38] Tumors arising in proximal bronchi generally measure from 1 to 4 cm in diameter; because they are less likely to be associated with symptoms, peripheral tumors tend to be somewhat larger.[39] Multiple tumors (usually pe-

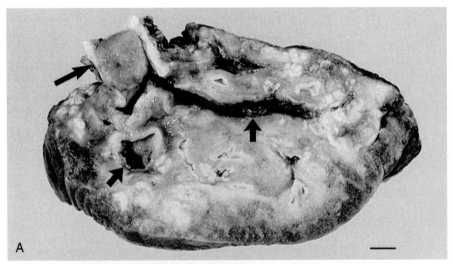

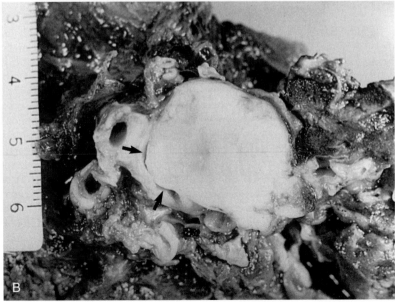

Figure 32–1. Central Carcinoid Tumor. A small round fleshy tumor *(long arrow)* completely fills the lumen of a middle lobe bronchus *(A)*. Distal airways *(short arrows)* are ectatic and the parenchyma is the site of obstructive pneumonitis. *(Bar, 5 mm.)* A larger but still well defined tumor from another patient *(B)* fills the lumen of a segmental bronchus *(arrows)* and expands into the surrounding parenchyma to produce an "iceberg" appearance.

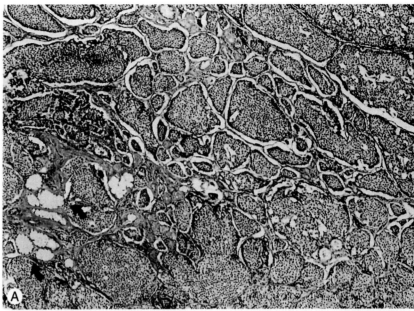

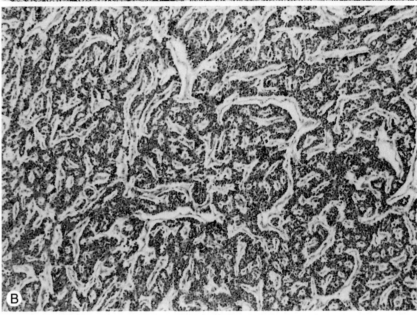

Figure 32–2. Carcinoid Tumor. Sections from two tumors show nests *(A)* and trabeculae *(B)* of uniform cells separated by a prominent but delicate vascular stroma. Note the remnants of a bronchial gland surrounded by neoplasm *(arrows),* a consequence of its local infiltrative properties. (*A* and *B,* ×60.)

ripheral) occur occasionally.[39] Although some bronchus-associated tumors are predominantly or entirely intraluminal (Fig. 32–1),[1] many extend both within the airway lumen and outside the bronchial wall (Fig. 32–1). In these cases, the bulk of the tumor may be located in the surrounding lung parenchyma, only a small amount being intraluminal, an appearance that has given rise to the designation "iceberg tumor." Most tumors have well-defined "pushing" margins; rarely, a neoplasm displays a more aggressive appearance such as vascular invasion or extension into the mediastinum.[40] The cut surface of the tumor is often yellow to tan and frequently somewhat fleshy. Focal areas of apparent hemorrhage may be seen, but necrosis is absent. The lung parenchyma distal to tumors arising in a proximal bronchus often shows obstructive pneumonitis (Fig. 32–1).[25, 41]

Histologically, typical carcinoid tumors have well-defined, generally smooth margins and may be separated from the overlying airway epithelium or adjacent lung tissue by a thin layer of compressed connective tissue.[1, 42] In airway-associated tumors, the epithelium is usually intact and often shows squamous metaplasia; occasionally it is ulcerated. A variety of histologic patterns can be seen, the most common consisting of sheets (insular pattern), trabeculae, or small nests of cells separated by a thin fibrovascular stroma (Fig. 32–2); more than one pattern is commonly present in an individual tumor. In some cases (particularly in peripheral tumors), the neoplastic cells have a spindle shape and are grouped in small nests, which gives a somewhat whorled appearance (Fig. 32–3). This pattern can be confused with a mesenchymal neoplasm such as fibrous histiocytoma, hemangiopericytoma, or leiomyoma.[39, 43, 44] Focal glandular differentiation is also not uncommon, and individual cells and intercellular lumens sometimes contain a periodic acid–Schiff (PAS) or mucicarmine-positive substance.[1, 40] Occa-

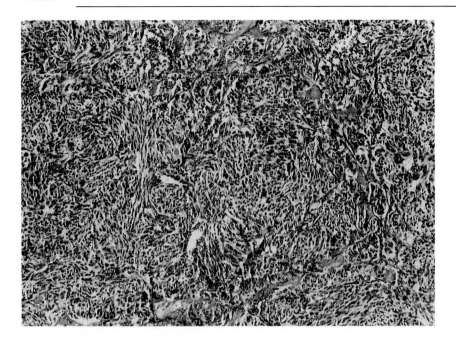

Figure 32–3. Peripheral ("Spindle Cell") Carcinoid Tumor. Interconnecting sheets and fascicles of cells possess a prominent spindle appearance. Ultrastructural examination showed numerous neurosecretory granules. (×70.)

sionally, evidence of glandular differentiation is extensive, which has led some authors to use the term *adenocarcinoid* tumor.[45]

Other histologic patterns include papillary (sometimes with sclerosis), follicular (resembling thyroid gland), and interstitial (in which the tumor spreads within alveolar septa and is covered by alveolar epithelial cells). Rare examples have also been reported of neoplasms that have evidence of other forms of epithelial differentiation, including Clara cell, Type II pneumocyte, and signet-ring cell.[46, 47] Tumorlets or foci of intraepithelial NE cell hyperplasia may be seen elsewhere in the lung, particularly in association with peripheral tumors (*see* page 1243).[39]

The cytoplasm of individual tumor cells is usually moderate in amount and lightly eosinophilic or clear. Occasionally, it is more abundant, strongly eosinophilic, and finely granular (oncocytic); this appearance is caused by the presence of numerous intracytoplasmic mitochondria, as in oncocytes in other situations.[49–51] An appearance resembling acinic cells can also be present.[52] Exceptionally, tumors are pigmented and show ultrastructural evidence of melanin production, either in the tumor cells themselves or in adjacent stromal cells.[53–55] Cell nuclei in all histologic variants are oval or round and show mild pleomorphism, finely stippled chromatin, and small nucleoli (Fig. 32–4); mitotic figures are scarce or absent.

Although the fibrovascular stroma separating tumor cell nests is usually thin, it may become quite thick and contain hyalinized collagen. Foci of bone formation, either in the thickened stroma (Fig. 32–5) or in adjacent cartilage plates, are not uncommon and may be quite extensive.[56] Although the pathogenesis of this metaplasia is unknown, it has been suggested that it may be related to local release of calcitonin by the tumor.[42] Deposits of amyloid are also present in the stroma occasionally;[57] in at least some of these cases they are probably related to the production and local release of NE substances by the tumor.[58] In one exceptional case, a tumor was associated with foci of extramedullary hematopoiesis.[59]

Silver stains such as the Grimelius stain may reveal minute, intracytoplasmic granules that correspond to the neurosecretory granules seen ultrastructurally (*see* Fig. 32–4); the frequency and extent of positive reactions vary greatly with the staining method,[60] and a negative result does not exclude the diagnosis. Staining of tissue sections embedded in glycol methacrylate with PAS–lead hematoxylin has been reported to identify the granules reliably.[61] As a result of their greater sensitivity, immunohistochemical studies are now more commonly used to identify NE differentiation.[62–64] Among the most useful antibodies are those directed to chromogranin, synaptophysin, and Leu-7.[65, 66] It should be remembered, however, that the specificity of the reactions to these substances has been questioned; for example, in one investigation of 47 histologically non-NE tumors (including 26 adenocarcinomas, 10 squamous cell carcinomas, and 11 large cell carcinomas), 81% were found to exhibit positivity for one or more of synaptophysin, chromogranin, Leu-7, or neuron-specific enolase.[67] Some investigators have found NE-specific protein reticulons (endoplasmic reticulum–associated protein complex) to be a more sensitive marker of NE differentiation than chromogranin or synaptophysin.[68]

Many specific NE substances can also be identified immunohistochemically in carcinoid tumors.[27, 62, 69] Serotonin, gastrin-releasing peptide (bombesin),[70, 71] pancreatic polypeptide, vasoactive intestinal polypeptide, and leu-enkephalin have been found most frequently; other substances include adrenocorticotropic hormone (ACTH),[72] calcitonin and calcitonin gene–related peptide,[73] antidiuretic hormone, corticotropin-releasing hormone,[74] growth hormone–releasing factor,[75] somatostatin, and the tachykinins substance P and neurokinin A.[76] Most tumors display reactivity for more than one substance, typically in a heterogeneous fashion.[62] Occasional cases have been reported in which different histologic appearances corresponded to the presence of different intracytoplasmic peptides.[71]

A variety of other substances have also been immunohistochemically identified in carcinoid tumors. The α-subunit

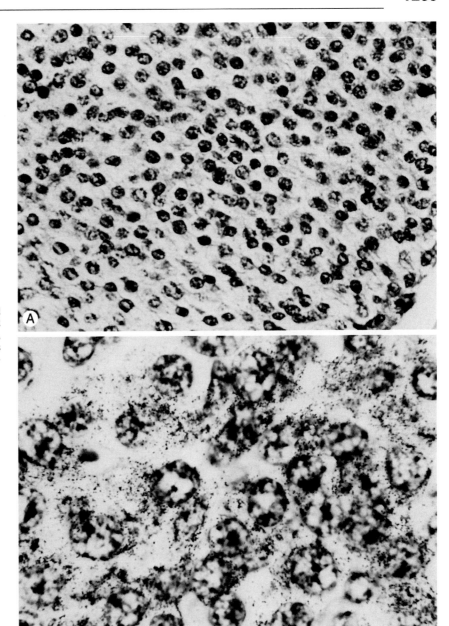

Figure 32–4. Carcinoid Tumor. A magnified view *(A)* of a nest of cells illustrated in Figure 32–2 shows uniform round to oval nuclei, small nucleoli, ample cytoplasm, and no mitotic figures. Grimelius silver stain *(B)* reveals numerous minute intracytoplasmic granules. *(A, ×600; B, ×1,500.)*

of human chorionic gonadotropin was identified in 27 (49%) of 55 tumors in one study;[77] although staining for the β-subunit is also occasionally positive,[78] in most instances there is no reaction.[77] Neuron-specific enolase[79-81] and carcinoembryonic antigen (CEA)[82] positivity have been found in many tumors; however, both of these markers are seen in a significant number of non-NE tumors and their use in diagnosis is questionable.[67, 69] Human neurofilament subunits and glial fibrillary acidic protein have also been demonstrated in some tumors.[83, 84] As might be expected, more sensitive analysis using *in situ* hybridization for specific gene products is able to document evidence for the production of NE substances in an even greater number of cases than immunohistochemistry.[85]

Ultrastructurally, carcinoid tumors are composed of uniform cells surrounded by basal laminae and joined by well-developed intercellular junctions (Fig. 32–6).[62, 81, 86] Elon-gated cell processes are frequent and may show complex interdigitation. Glandular lumens with apical microvilli are also common. As a rule, neurosecretory granules (membrane-bound granules with an electron-dense core surrounded by a clear halo) are abundant. Most range from 150 to 300 μm in diameter; occasionally, they are much larger.[3] Pleomorphic granules similar to those seen in carcinoid tumors of the gastrointestinal tract have been identified rarely.[3, 87] Granule structure can vary between different tumors[81, 86] and between different cells in the same tumor,[3, 71] thus suggesting that there may be a structural correlate to the different reactions found on immunohistochemical examination. Intermediate filaments are occasionally quite numerous and arranged in aggregates to form an intracytoplasmic "inclusion body."[88] In one case, intracytoplasmic lamellar inclusions similar to those seen in Type II pneumocytes were identified within tumor cells, raising the possibil-

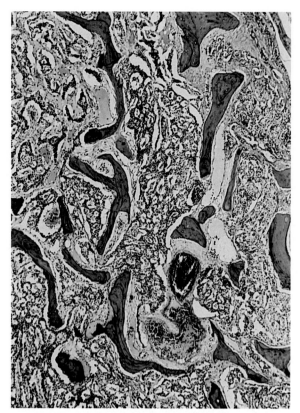

Figure 32–5. Carcinoid Tumor: Ossification. A section of a typical carcinoid tumor shows a trabecular pattern of neoplastic cells with several irregularly shaped spicules of mature bone within the fibrous stroma. (×52.)

ity that the neoplasm might have been showing both NE and pneumocytic differentiation.[89] Rare tumors show evidence of melanocytic, schwannian, or NE differentiation.[90]

The histologic diagnosis of typical carcinoid tumor in resected specimens is usually straightforward. Despite the fairly characteristic morphologic features, however, small tissue samples obtained by bronchoscopic or transthoracic needle biopsy may be difficult to distinguish from small cell carcinoma, especially in the presence of crush artefact. Reported examples of misdiagnosis in such cases are not uncommon,[91, 92] and it seems reasonable for both the pathologist and clinician to seriously question the diagnosis of small cell carcinoma in any nonsmoking individual under 45 years of age; similarly, the diagnosis of small cell carcinoma should be reconsidered in any patient who survives 5 years or longer.[93, 94] These statements apply particularly in situations in which the radiologic features are atypical for small cell carcinoma, such as the presence of a solitary pulmonary nodule or the absence of hilar/mediastinal lymph node enlargement. Difficulty in histologic diagnosis may also be experienced on frozen sections.[95]

Atypical Carcinoid Tumor

As indicated previously, some pulmonary tumors that have an overall architectural pattern similar to that of typical carcinoid tumor also show certain histologic and cytologic features suggestive of an aggressive nature.[16, 17, 21, 22, 28, 96] Although these tumors may represent one end of a continuum of NE neoplasms rather than a separate entity, to under-

line their more ominous prognosis they have been designated "atypical carcinoid tumor."[16] (The terms *Kulchitsky cell carcinoma [Grade II]*[97] and *well-differentiated [low-grade] neuroendocrine carcinoma*[2, 62] have also been applied to this histologic subtype.)

As defined by Arrigoni and colleagues, the term *atypical* should be applied to a histologically recognizable carcinoid tumor when one or more of the following features are present:[16] (1) increased mitotic activity, consisting of at least 5 to 10 mitoses per 10 high-power fields (some investigators believe that a greater mitotic rate indicates an even more aggressive neoplasm, designated large cell NE carcinoma[8] [*see* page 1246]); (2) nuclear pleomorphism and hyperchromasia associated with prominent nucleoli and an increased nuclear/cytoplasmic ratio; (3) areas of increased cellularity associated with loss of typical architecture; and (4) necrosis.

Although some investigators have suggested that atypical carcinoid tumors are more frequently peripheral,[96, 98] most have found a similar incidence in peripheral and central locations.[6, 17, 99] They tend to be somewhat larger than the typical form. Although many are well delimited at their periphery, infiltration into adjacent lung can occur. By definition, the atypical variety shows a low-power organoid pattern suggestive of carcinoid tumor (Fig. 32–7). Individual cells show a varying degree of nuclear atypia, and mitotic figures and foci of necrosis are common.[62, 96] Rarely, other forms of histologic differentiation (such as sarcomatous) are found in addition to NE.[100]

Neurosecretory granules, demonstrated by either histochemical[101] or ultrastructural analysis,[62] are usually present in smaller numbers and are of smaller size than those in typical carcinoid tumors. Immunohistochemical staining for various nonspecific NE markers (e.g., chromogranin and synaptophysin) is usually positive;[22, 62] no significant difference in reaction between this form and typical carcinoid tumor has been found.[28] As might be expected from the histologic features and behavior, p53 and bcl-2 overexpression is more likely to be present in atypical than typical carcinoid tumors.[102]

Radiologic Manifestations

Radiologic manifestations depend largely on the location of the tumor. Since 80% to 85% are located centrally in major or segmental bronchi, evidence of bronchial obstruction is the most common radiographic finding. In most cases the obstruction is complete, with peripheral atelectasis and obstructive pneumonitis. Thus, the characteristic radiographic pattern consists of a homogeneous increase in density confined precisely to a lobe or to one or more segments, usually with considerable loss of volume (Fig. 32–8). Segmental atelectasis and pneumonitis may show periodic exacerbations and remissions, presumably reflecting intermittent relief of the obstruction. Recurrent infection distal to the neoplasm can result in bronchiectasis (Fig. 32–9) and lung abscesses. Occasionally, retention of mucus in airways leads to mucoid impaction unaccompanied by atelectasis.

When the carcinoid tumor only partially occludes a bronchus, the reduction in ventilation of affected parenchyma can result in hypoxic vasoconstriction and a reduction in lung volume; the oligemia can constitute a subtle but highly suggestive sign of the presence of an endobronchial

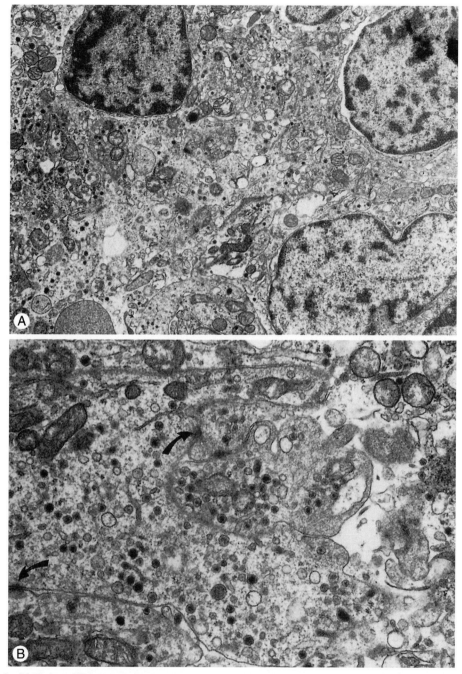

Figure 32–6. Carcinoid Tumor: Ultrastructure. A low-power photomicrograph *(A)* shows three fairly uniform nuclei and abundant cytoplasm containing numerous neurosecretory granules. A higher-power view *(B)* of several cell processes reveals intercellular junctions *(arrows)* and neurosecretory granules. The latter have well-defined limiting membranes and contain a central electron-dense core surrounded by a thin, lucent halo. (*A*, ×17,000; *B*, ×38,300.)

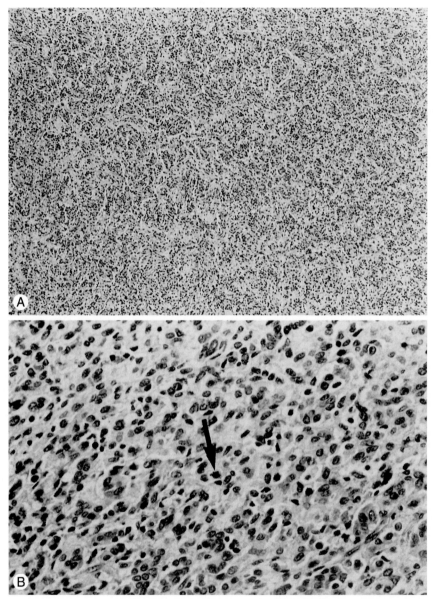

Figure 32–7. Atypical Carcinoid Tumor. A section from a 3-cm endobronchial neoplasm *(A)* shows small nests of cells with numerous interspersed blood vessels suggestive of a carcinoid tumor. However, a magnified view *(B)* shows a greater degree of pleomorphism than is seen in typical carcinoid tumor and in addition reveals occasional mitotic figures *(arrow)* (compare with Figure 32–4, page 1233). A Grimelius stain showed the presence of moderate numbers of neurosecretory granules. (*A*, ×60; *B*, ×350.) (Courtesy of the Canadian Reference Centre for Cancer Pathology, Ottawa.)

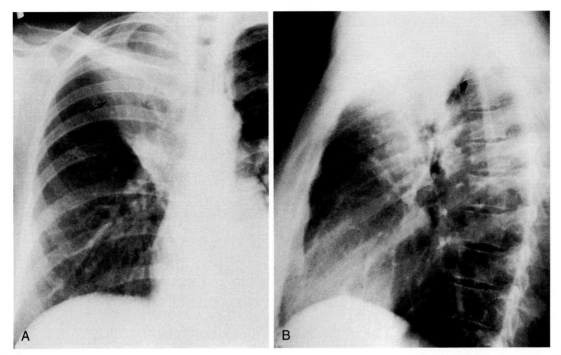

Figure 32–8. Carcinoid Tumor. Views of the right hemithorax from posteroanterior *(A)* and lateral *(B)* radiographs demonstrate a roughly triangular shadow of homogeneous density occupying the superomedial portion of the right lung. The inferolateral border of the shadow is formed by the upwardly displaced minor fissure *(arrow* in *A)* and the posterior border of the anteriorly displaced major fissure *(arrow* in *B).* This shadow represents combined consolidation and atelectasis of the right upper lobe secondary to an endobronchial carcinoid tumor. The patient was a 30-year-old woman.

lesion and should lead to a recommendation for bronchoscopy (Fig. 32–10).[103] This phenomenon has been well illustrated in reported cases in which carcinoid tumors arising in main bronchi caused expiratory air trapping and a marked reduction in perfusion of whole lungs.[104, 105]

Peripheral carcinoid tumors appear radiologically as solitary nodules (Fig. 32–11). They are usually homogeneous in density, sharply defined, round or oval, and slightly lobulated.[106, 107] The majority measure 1 to 3 cm in diameter,[108, 109] although they may become as large as 10 cm.[107, 110]

CT may be helpful in assessing these neoplasms, particularly centrally placed tumors likely to cause deformity of a contiguous bronchial air column *(see* Fig. 32–10). The procedure is also useful in assessing the presence and extent of local invasion, particularly when histologic examination of a biopsy specimen has revealed atypical features. Because bronchial carcinoid tumors are very vascular, marked enhancement may be seen following intravenous administration of contrast medium.[111, 112] Marked signal enhancement can also be demonstrated by using ultrafast contrast-enhanced magnetic resonance (MR) imaging with a gradient-echo sequence (Turbo-Flash).[113] Small carcinoid tumors may be difficult to distinguish from pulmonary vessels on CT, but can be readily identified on MR imaging;[114] the tumors have signal intensity similar to that of muscle on T1-weighted spin-echo images, a moderately bright signal on T2-weighted spin-echo images, and very bright signal on short–inversion time inversion-recovery (STIR) images. Tumors usually do not show increased metabolic activity on ^{18}F-fluorodeoxyglucose (FDG) positron-emission tomography and thus cannot be distinguished from benign lesions by this technique.[114a]

Despite the fairly common demonstration of bone within carcinoid tumors pathologically, ossification is seldom visible on the chest radiograph;[115, 116] for example, in one review of 72 patients it was documented in only 3 (4%).[117] However, the abnormality can be identified on CT in approximately 30% of cases (Fig. 32–12).[108, 118] Ossification is more common in central than in peripheral tumors: in two studies it was identified in 3 of 5 (60%)[108] and 7 of 18 (39%)[118] central carcinoids and in only 1 of 7 (14%) and 1 of 13 (8%) peripheral tumors. The pattern of calcification is variable and may include small or large, smooth or irregular, and central, eccentric, or peripheral foci.[108, 118] Occasionally, an endobronchial tumor is so extensively ossified that it mimics broncholithiasis.[119]

Osseous metastases, which may be revealed by a radiographic bone survey, develop in few cases; although it has been emphasized that they are frequently osteoblastic (usually in patients with carcinoid syndrome),[120, 121] in one series of 99 patients only 8 had osseous metastases and all were lytic (1 patient had combined lytic and blastic features).[32] Metastases from carcinoid tumors to bones and the liver may also be identified by using radionuclide scanning with an iodine-labeled somatostatin analogue (^{123}I-octreotide) *(see* farther on).

Atypical carcinoid tumors tend to be larger than typical tumors (Fig. 32–13), sometimes attaining a huge size.[122] They are also more commonly associated with hilar and mediastinal lymph node enlargement.[123–125] In a study comparing the radiologic findings in 10 patients with typical carcinoid tumors and 10 with atypical forms, the average size of the former was 1.8 ± 0.7 cm as compared with 3.9 ± 1.3 cm for the latter;[124] lymph node enlargement was present in 1 of 10 typical and 4 of 10 atypical tumors. In one investigation of the radiographic appearances of 32

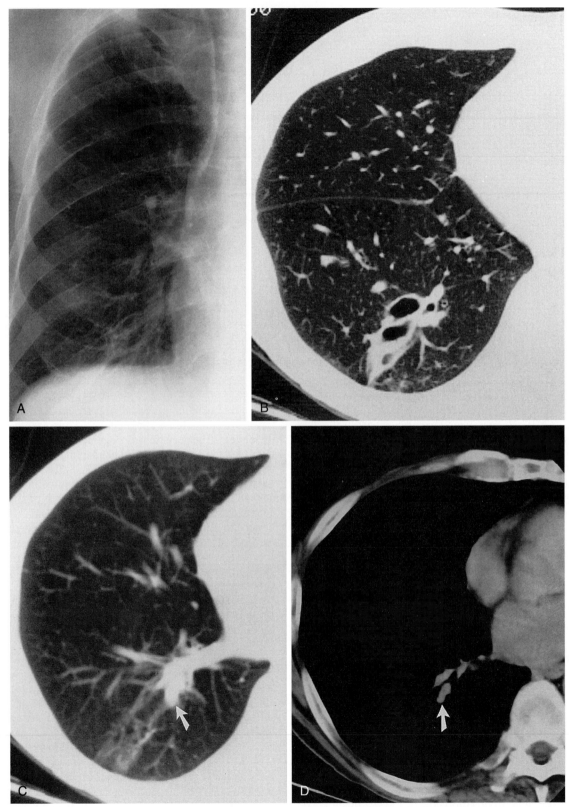

Figure 32–9. Carcinoid Tumor with Distal Bronchiectasis. A view of the right lung from a posteroanterior chest radiograph *(A)* shows focal areas of atelectasis and pneumonitis in the right lower lobe. HRCT *(B)* demonstrates a focal area of bronchiectasis in the lateral basal segment. Conventional CT scans *(C and D)* demonstrate a localized soft tissue lesion in the lateral basal segmental bronchus *(arrows)*. The patient was a 66-year-old man with a history of recurrent right lower lobe pneumonia. The diagnosis of typical carcinoid was made at bronchoscopy and confirmed at surgery.

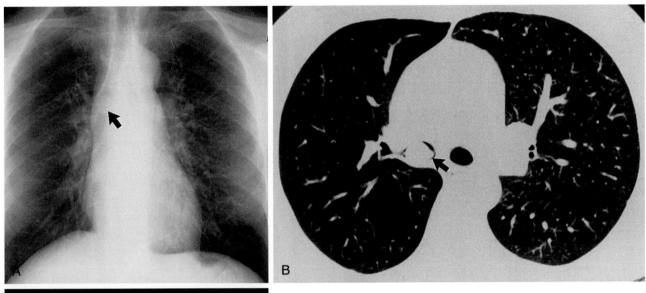

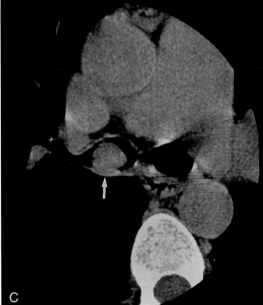

Figure 32–10. Central Carcinoid Tumor—Partial Airway Obstruction with Hypoxic Vasoconstriction. A posteroanterior chest radiograph *(A)* in a 48-year-old woman demonstrates a tumor in the right main bronchus *(arrow)*. The right lung is slightly smaller than the left and shows decreased vascularity. HRCT *(B)* confirms the presence of intraluminal tumor in the right main bronchus *(arrow)*; decreased vascularity and decreased attenuation of the right lung in comparison to the left lung are evident, presumably as a result of reflex vasoconstriction. Soft tissue windows *(C)* demonstrate focal thickening of the posterior wall of the right main bronchus *(arrow)*; there is no evidence of extrabronchial extension. The diagnosis of typical carcinoid tumor was made at bronchoscopy and confirmed at surgery.

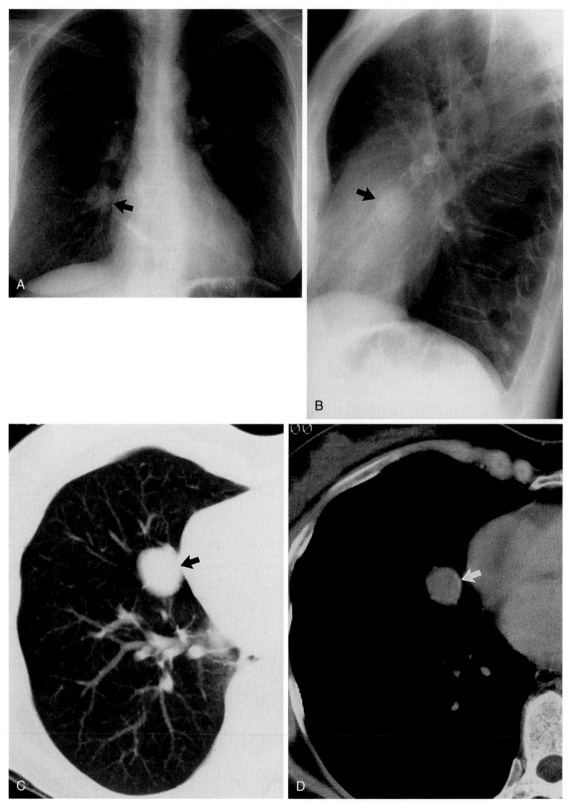

Figure 32–11. Peripheral Carcinoid Tumor. Posteroanterior *(A)* and lateral *(B)* chest radiographs in a 59-year-old woman demonstrate a 2.5-cm smoothly marginated nodule in the right middle lobe *(arrows)*. CT scans *(C* and *D)* essentially confirm the radiographic findings *(arrows)*. A diagnosis of typical carcinoid tumor was proved at surgery.

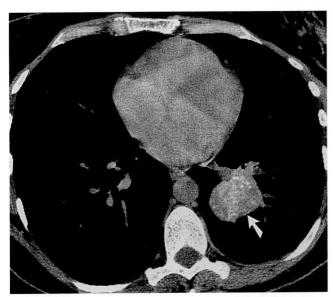

Figure 32–12. Calcified Carcinoid Tumor. An HRCT scan in a 41-year-old woman demonstrates a 4-cm-diameter mass in the left lower lobe *(arrow)*. Numerous small areas of calcification can be seen within the tumor. The diagnosis of typical carcinoid tumor was confirmed at surgery.

atypical carcinoid tumors, the most frequent finding—present in 21 patients—was a round or ovoid peripheral mass 1.5 to 10 cm in diameter.[123] Fifteen of these masses showed slight to marked lobulation; although some were smoothly bordered, others exhibited a spiculated margin (Fig. 32–14). Other patterns that were seen less commonly included a multilobulated mass, a thin-walled cavity, lobar atelectasis without a demonstrable mass, a mediastinal mass, and a hilar mass.

Clinical Manifestations

It is not rare to find a carcinoid tumor at autopsy of a patient who has not complained of symptoms during life;[101] most of these tumors are peripheral in location. By contrast, the majority of central carcinoid tumors give rise to symptoms and signs as a result of bronchial obstruction.[92, 126] The former include cough, expectoration, fever, and chest pain; hemoptysis occurs in 30% to 50% of cases.[92, 127, 128] Some patients have symptoms simulating asthma.[105] Physical signs depend on the degree of obstruction, the size of the bronchus obstructed, and whether infection has developed. The percussion note may be dull, and breath sounds may be decreased over a segment, a lobe, or an entire lung; crackles and even a friction rub may be heard when infection is present. Massive atelectasis is reflected in the clinical signs of loss of volume, such as mediastinal shift.

Although carcinoid tumors typically contain one or more immunoreactive NE products, clinical signs and symptoms related to their presence are distinctly uncommon. In most cases, extensive metastatic disease is necessary before they appear,[129–131] possibly reflecting the need for adequate tumor bulk to produce sufficient amounts of active hormone. Uncommonly, a small tumor is associated with paraneoplastic clinical manifestations, usually Cushing's syndrome.[132, 133]

Most patients have a single syndrome; occasionally, symptoms can be attributed to more than one ectopically produced substance.[134] As with small cell carcinoma, serum levels of various tumor-related immunoreactive polypeptides are not uncommonly elevated in the absence of clinical signs and symptoms. For example, in one study of 33 consecutive patients with carcinoid tumor, only 4 of whom showed clinically overt acromegaly, the diurnal mean serum growth hormone levels were significantly higher than in control subjects, and over a third of the patients had levels in a range similar to those of acromegalic patients without carcinoid tumor.[135]

Cushing's syndrome is the most common paraneoplastic manifestation;[27, 133, 136] in fact, carcinoid tumor has been said to be the most frequent cause of the paraneoplastic form of the syndrome.[137] ACTH has been found in assays of tumor tissue, including material obtained by transthoracic needle aspiration.[138] As indicated previously, the syndrome may occur in the absence of metastases and with a very small primary tumor (sometimes unrecognizable radiographically).[133] Some patients have had bilateral adrenalectomy for presumed adrenal adenoma only to have persistence of symptoms followed many years later by appearance of the primary pulmonary tumor.[139, 140] There is evidence that tumors associated with the syndrome may behave in a more aggressive fashion than the usual carcinoid tumor despite having "typical" histologic features.[141]

Regardless of the name of the tumor, carcinoid syndrome is uncommon,[142] with relatively recent reviews documenting an incidence ranging from 0% to 3%.[12, 41, 143] Symptoms and signs consist of flushing, fever, nausea and vomiting, diarrhea, hypotension, wheezing, and respiratory distress.[144, 145] Heart murmurs develop in a few cases as a result of endocardial damage caused by polypeptides such as 5-hydroxytryptamine. Such murmurs may be restricted to the left side of the heart when the polypeptides enter the

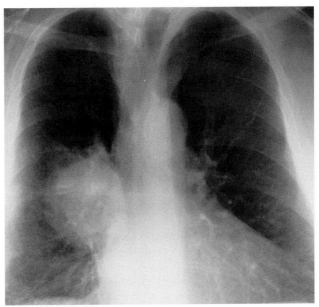

Figure 32–13. Atypical Carcinoid Tumor. A chest radiograph in a 64-year-old man demonstrates a 6-cm-diameter mass in the right lower lobe. At surgery the patient also had right hilar lymph node metastases.

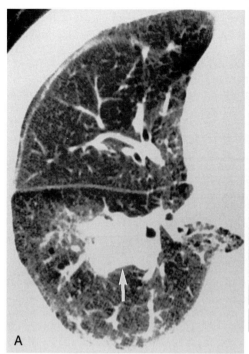
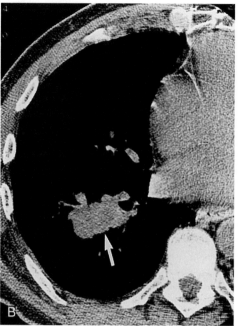

Figure 32–14. Atypical Carcinoid Tumor. CT scans *(A and B)* in a 61-year-old man demonstrate a 3-cm-diameter lobulated tumor in the right lower lobe *(arrows)*. A diagnosis of atypical carcinoid tumor was made at surgery.

pulmonary veins from the lungs.[144] Those cases in which the polypeptides emanate from hepatic metastases show the effects of right-sided cardiac involvement similar to what occurs with abdominal carcinoid tumors.[146]

Acromegaly is a more common manifestation of pulmonary carcinoid tumors than carcinoid syndrome. It appears to be caused most often by tumor-related growth hormone–releasing factor acting directly on the pituitary;[135, 147, 148] however, immunochemical demonstration of growth hormone in some tumors suggests that the release of this substance itself may be the cause in some patients.[149] Other syndromes related to ectopic hormone production include Zollinger-Ellison syndrome[70] and hyperinsulinemia.[131] Occasional cases of pulmonary carcinoid tumor have been associated with endocrine neoplasia or hyperplasia elsewhere in the body, an association that has been considered to be part of the multiple endocrine neoplasia syndrome.[150, 151]

Laboratory Findings and Diagnosis

In the investigation of carcinoid tumors, there is sometimes hesitancy in performing bronchoscopic biopsy because of the highly vascular nature of the lesions and the attendant risk of bleeding. For example, in one series of 69 patients seen over a 20-year period, there were 6 cases of severe hemorrhage following bronchial biopsy.[128] However, other investigators have encountered no serious problems from hemorrhage following biopsy with either rigid[41] or flexible[126] bronchoscopes. Our own inclination is generally to perform biopsy with appropriate precautions to control bleeding. Rarely, symptoms of carcinoid syndrome have followed tumor biopsy.[152, 153] The typical bronchoscopic appearance is that of a smooth-surfaced vascular tumor that partially or completely obstructs the airway lumen.

Cytologic examination of sputum or bronchial washings

and brushings is usually unrewarding as a result of the intact bronchial epithelium overlying most proximal tumors;[154] occasionally, sufficient cells are available for diagnosis.[155] Obviously, transthoracic needle aspiration is more likely to yield cells suitable for cytologic interpretation.[156–158] Although the diagnosis should be suggested in these cases by cellular regularity and bland nuclear features, occasional tumors present diagnostic problems, especially the peripheral spindle cell and atypical variants. The greatest difficulty lies in the differentiation of carcinoid tumor from small cell carcinoma[156, 159] and in distinguishing typical from atypical forms.[160] The cytologic findings have been described in detail for both typical[161] and atypical tumors.[94, 162] Using an image analysis technique, one group of investigators has shown that nuclear DNA content increases from typical to atypical carcinoid tumors to small cell carcinoma.[163] In one morphometric investigation, no significant difference in nuclear size was found between small cell carcinoma and carcinoid tumor.[164]

Cytogenetic analyses of carcinoid tumors are few and do not permit definite diagnostic conclusions. In one investigation of six cases, two of the four typical tumors had a normal karyotype;[165] abnormalities in the remaining two typical tumors and the two atypical forms were not uniform.

Laboratory tests are occasionally helpful, particularly in confirming paraneoplastic syndromes. The diagnosis of carcinoid syndrome can be confirmed by demonstrating large amounts of 5-hydroxyindoleacetic acid (5-HIAA) and 5-hydroxytryptamine (serotonin) in the urine. In some patients, urinary levels of 5-HIAA are normal and serotonin levels are elevated.[166] Intraoperative measurement of ACTH in pulmonary vessels by radioimmunoassay has been reported to be beneficial in identifying occult carcinoid tumors and ensuring adequate surgical excision.[167] Pulmonary carcinoid tumors, as well as NE tumors in other organs, have also been shown to be associated with elevated serum levels of chromogranin A and the α-subunit of glycoprotein hormones.[168]

The diagnosis has been confirmed in some cases by using somatostatin receptor scintigraphy.[137, 140, 169] Carcinoid tumors, similar to other NE tumors such as pancreatic islet cell tumors, have cell membrane receptors with a high affinity for the neuroregulatory peptide somatostatin.[170, 171] The results of preliminary investigations indicate that use of a radiolabeled somatostatin analogue (^{123}I-octreotide) allows the identification of both primary and metastatic tumors not seen with other radionuclide agents such as metaiodobenzylguanidine (^{123}I-MIBG).[170, 172]

Prognosis and Natural History

Typical Carcinoid Tumors

The prognosis of typical carcinoid tumors is excellent, adequate surgical excision resulting in cure in the vast majority of patients.[173] In one series of 203 patients, regional lymph node metastases were found in the operative specimens in only 11 cases (5.4%);[154] 71% of all patients were alive at 5 years (although it is not clear from the authors' discussion how many of the patients died as a result of the neoplasm). In another study of 62 patients who had typical carcinoid tumors, only 3 had regional lymph node metastases in the operative specimen;[17] in none of the remaining 59 patients did metastases develop in a follow-up period ranging from 3½ to 20 years. Other investigators have reported 10-year survival rates of about 90% to 95% (many patients probably dying of causes unrelated to the tumor itself);[15, 24, 92, 101, 174, 175] in fact, some have found 5- or 10-year survival rates of virtually 100%,[24, 26] even in the presence of lymph node metastases.[173, 175a] Even with more distant metastases, typical carcinoid tumors may be very slowly growing and permit prolonged survival for many years;[91, 143] in fact, because of the relatively slow growth, recurrence of tumor may occur many years after apparently curative resection, so follow-up must be prolonged.[92, 176] As might be expected from the preceding discussion, relatively conservative local therapies such as segmentectomy,[173] sleeve resection,[177] and Nd-YAG laser treatment[173, 178] have generally been found to be associated with a good outcome.

Despite those excellent statistics overall, it is clear that occasional histologically typical carcinoid tumors are associated with more concerning behavior. For example, in one retrospective investigation of 79 patients, the presence of an aggressive tumor (defined as one showing extension to the carina, involvement of regional lymph nodes, and/or vascular invasion) was found to be associated with a 5-year survival rate of approximately 50%;[184] 18% of these "aggressive" tumors were classified as typical according to standard histologic criteria. As with pulmonary carcinoma, a variety of clinical and pathologic investigations have been undertaken to document criteria by which those typical tumors that will metastasize can be distinguished from those that will not. Unfortunately, no single criterion or combination of criteria have been identified that can differentiate tumors with metastatic potential with a reasonable degree of certainty in an individual patient. In one epidemiologic study, patients who had a family history of cancer were found to

be more prone to the development of metastases;[179] among 67 patients without metastatic carcinoid tumor at diagnosis, the risk of distant metastasis by 5 years was 40% in patients who had a positive family history of cancer as compared with only 6% in those whose relatives were unaffected. Some workers have found evidence that larger tumors or tumors associated with Cushing's syndrome are more likely to be associated with lymph node metastases[141, 180] and to have a worse prognosis.[141, 181, 182] There is also some evidence that the basic architectural pattern of metastatic tumors (insular, trabecular, glandular, or mixed) may be of some value in predicting survival.[129] Positive antibody staining of tumor cells for CEA has been found by some investigators to be closely associated with treatment failure.[183]

Several flow cytometric studies have been performed in an attempt to relate tumor DNA content to histologic type and prognosis.[182, 185, 186, 186a] Aneuploidy is common in both typical and atypical types (approximately 20% to 40% of the former and 50% to 85% of the latter).[182, 186a, 187] Although the results of some of these studies have suggested that aneuploidy is associated with a poorer prognosis,[182, 187] this association has not been clearly shown to have predictive value independent of histologic type; in particular, it has not been shown that typical carcinoid tumors that are aneuploid are more likely to behave in an aggressive fashion. Despite these findings, some investigators have found evidence that the degree of proliferative activity of a tumor as measured by the immunohistochemical reaction to Ki-67 correlates strongly with survival.[188]

Atypical Carcinoid Tumors

In contrast to typical carcinoid tumor, tumors that have atypical histologic features have a significantly worse prognosis;[22, 28, 96, 97] approximately 50% to 70% of patients have lymph node metastases at the time of initial evaluation,[16, 189] and the 5-year survival rate is on the order of 40% to 70%, depending on the stage at diagnosis.[97, 126, 174, 175, 182, 190]

PULMONARY TUMORLETS AND NEUROENDOCRINE CELL HYPERPLASIA

The term *pulmonary tumorlet* refers to a minute, somewhat nodular proliferation of airway NE cells that extends beyond the epithelium into the adjacent wall or lung parenchyma. The term *neuroendocrine cell hyperplasia* is meant to describe a purely intraepithelial proliferation of the same cells. Although either abnormality may be identified in otherwise normal lung, evidence of concomitant pulmonary disease is frequent, the most common associated conditions being bronchiectasis and carcinoid tumor itself.[191, 192] For example, in one series of 102 patients with bronchiectasis who were subjected to surgical resection, tumorlets were identified in 20;[193] in another review of 25 patients with peripheral carcinoid tumors, 19 were found to have foci of NE cell hyperplasia.[194] Both abnormalities can also be seen in association with foci of parenchymal fibrosis caused by a variety of etiologies such as chronic abscess or tuberculosis.[191, 195, 196] Tumorlets have been reported rarely in association with congenital adenomatoid malformation,[197] intralobar sequestration,[198] and diffuse panbronchiolitis.[199]

The fundamental nature of these NE cell proliferations is somewhat controversial. The multiplicity of tumorlets and their frequent association with pulmonary fibrosis and bronchiectasis suggest that they represent a hyperplastic response to nonspecific airway injury. Their invariable small size when found in these circumstances certainly argues against autonomous growth; in fact, if the latter were the case, an increased incidence of carcinoid tumors would be expected in patients with bronchiectasis, and there is no evidence of such an association. The exceptional case of a tumorlet remaining essentially stationary in size over a 12-year period also supports their nonneoplastic nature.[200]

On the other hand, the occasional presence of tumorlets in otherwise normal lung and their morphologic resemblance and occasional association with carcinoid tumor imply that at least some are neoplastic and in fact represent minute peripheral carcinoid tumors.[201, 202] The rare reports of regional lymph node deposits[192, 203–205] and radiographic evidence of an increase in size over time[206] support this hypothesis. It is clear that at some point all carcinoid tumors must be of small size, and it is only reasonable to expect that the occasional case of a solitary tumorlet represents such an early form. In addition, as indicated previously, pathologic studies of the excised lungs from some patients with carcinoid tumor have shown multiple foci of intraepithelial NE cell proliferation (Fig. 32–15).[194, 208] The presence of such disease, as well as the multiplicity of some tumorlets, is reminiscent of the neoplastic field effect seen in other tissues such as urothelium. In light of these observations, it is probably appropriate to consider both tumorlets and NE cell hyperplasia as representing two forms of disease—one, a relatively localized hyperplastic reaction to pulmonary injury that does not progress, and the other a more diffuse abnormality of NE cells that is often associated with frank neoplasia.

Tumorlets range in size from minute, microscopic foci to well-defined, grossly identifiable nodules measuring several millimeters in diameter. (A precise size distinction between a hyperplastic and neoplastic proliferation is not possi-

ble; however, a nodule greater than 5 mm should probably be considered a small carcinoid tumor.) They are most often found adjacent to small bronchioles but can occur in the bronchial wall or the subpleural parenchyma;[191, 210] when associated with an area of parenchymal fibrosis, the relationship to an airway may not be apparent. They are frequently multiple[191, 193] and, occasionally, virtually innumerable.[211]

Histologically, they consist of nests of oval to spindle-shaped cells that contain a small to moderate amount of eosinophilic cytoplasm (Fig. 32–16).[191, 201, 212] Fibrovascular tissue separates individual cell nests and is usually greater in amount than generally seen in carcinoid tumor. The nests themselves may be situated entirely within peribronchial or peribronchiolar interstitial tissue or may project into the airway lumen or surrounding alveolar air spaces and parenchymal interstitium. Cellular nuclear features are bland and resemble those of typical carcinoid tumor. Sustentacular (Langerhans') cells are commonly admixed.[213] Ultrastructural examination reveals neurosecretory granules,[201, 202, 210, 212] and immunohistochemical studies show the presence of polypeptides similar to those in carcinoid tumor.[194, 199]

Continuity of the main portion of the tumorlet with the overlying bronchial or bronchiolar epithelium has been demonstrated in many cases;[199, 210, 212] in this instance, the basal epithelial layer of the airway is usually expanded by a cellular proliferation identical to the tumorlet itself. Such foci of NE cell hyperplasia can also be seen in the absence of recognizable tumorlets, particularly in cases associated with an obvious carcinoid tumor. In some of these cases, partial or complete bronchiolar obliteration by fibrous tissue can also be seen.[208, 211]

Pulmonary tumorlets are usually found in older individuals,[201] although to some extent this probably reflects the presence of coexistent lung disease and the fact that in many cases the lesions are discovered at autopsy. A distinct female preponderance ranging from 65% to 80% has been noted by some investigators.[191, 194, 201] Because of their minute size, they are not usually apparent on the radiograph or CT

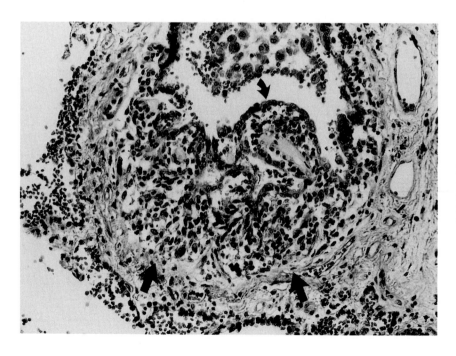

Figure 32–15. Neuroendocrine Cell Hyperplasia. A cluster of hyperplastic neuroendocrine cells is present between the lamina propria *(straight arrows)* and the epithelium *(curved arrow)* of this small bronchiole. Elsewhere in the lobe (resected for a peripheral carcinoid tumor), several small tumorlets were identified. (×200.)

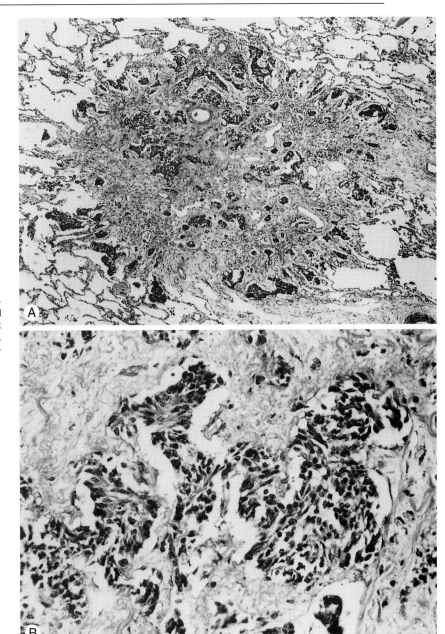

Figure 32–16. Pulmonary Tumorlet. Haphazardly arranged nests *(A)* of cells are situated within fibrous tissue and lung parenchyma adjacent to a small bronchus (not illustrated on this section). A magnified view *(B)* shows clusters of fairly uniform, oval- to spindle-shaped cells. (*A,* ×40; *B,* ×250.)

scan; however, several cases have been reported in which numerous tumorlets increased sufficiently in size to be visible as minute nodules (Fig. 32–17).[206, 211, 214, 215]

In most cases, no clinical manifestations can be attributed to the tumorlets themselves. However, cough and progressive dyspnea associated with obstructive pulmonary function changes have been reported in some patients.[194, 208, 211] The characteristic growth within and around small airways, focally associated with significant luminal obliteration by fibrous tissue or the NE cells themselves, is presumably involved in the pathogenesis of these findings;[194, 208, 211] rarely, the airway narrowing is extensive enough to cause respiratory failure.[215] Cushing's syndrome is another rare consequence of tumorlets/NE cell hyperplasia.[206]

The vast majority of pulmonary tumorlets behave in a benign fashion. The rare cases that have been associated with regional lymph node metastases[192, 204, 205] presumably represent true, minute carcinoid tumors and have not developed evidence of further disease during follow-up. When associated with carcinoid tumors, the prognosis depends on the behavior of the latter rather than the tumorlets or the extent of NE cell hyperplasia. The exception is the occasional patient who has extensive disease as a result of obliterative bronchiolitis, in whom a significant obstructive deficit may develop.[208, 215] Rarely, fragments of tumorlet are seen in bronchial biopsy specimens or cytology smears,[191] in which case they may be misinterpreted as undifferentiated pulmonary carcinoma.

MISCELLANEOUS PULMONARY TUMORS SHOWING NEUROENDOCRINE DIFFERENTIATION

As indicated previously, the extent and severity of cytologic and architectural atypia vary with different carcinoid

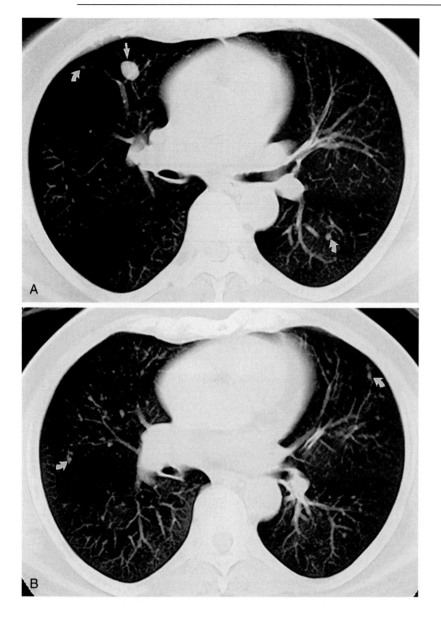

Figure 32–17. Carcinoid Tumor Associated with Tumorlets and Neuroendocrine Cell Hyperplasia. CT scans *(A* and *B)* demonstrate a 1.5-cm-diameter nodule in the right middle lobe *(straight arrow)*, as well as several smaller nodules in both lungs *(curved arrows)*. Following a right middle lobectomy, the largest nodule was shown to represent a carcinoid tumor and the smaller nodules, tumorlets. Multiple foci of neuroendocrine cell hyperplasia were also evident and were associated with obstruction of several bronchioles. The patient was a 69-year-old woman with a history of shortness of breath. Pulmonary function tests showed an FEV_1/FVC ratio of 0.53 and a residual volume/total lung capacity ratio of 0.56, but no impairment in gas transfer. (Courtesy of Dr. R. McLean, Royal Alexandria Hospital, Edmonton, Canada.)

tumors. To maintain some semantic clarity, we believe that the term *atypical carcinoid* should be restricted to tumors that possess a focally recognizable NE (organoid) architecture but also display an increased mitotic rate, necrosis, and/or cytologic atypia. In addition to neoplasms that fulfill these criteria, some investigators have proposed an additional subtype of NE tumor ("large cell neuroendocrine carcinoma") that resembles atypical carcinoid tumor but has a higher mitotic rate (greater than 10 mitoses per 10 high-power fields), more extensive necrosis, and more severe cytologic atypia.[8, 207, 216] There is evidence that tumors with these histologic features follow a more aggressive course than do atypical carcinoid tumors as defined earlier.[8, 207] It is possible that these various histologic subtypes represent a spectrum of differentiation, with large cell NE carcinoma occupying a position between atypical carcinoid tumor and small cell carcinoma. In fact, one study of interobserver reproducibility in the diagnosis of NE lung tumors revealed discrepant diagnoses in 11 (22%) of 50 cases of large cell neuroendocrine carcinoma (2 considered to be atypical carcinoid tumor

and 9 small cell carcinoma).[209] Nevertheless, there is evidence that large and small cell carcinomas have molecular genetic features that differ from those of carcinoid tumors,[7, 217] and it is possible that additional investigation may further justify separate classification.

In addition to tumors that have an organoid (NE) morphology, some large cell carcinomas lack this architectural feature but have immunohistochemical and/or ultrastructural evidence of NE differentiation.[9, 10, 218–222] These tumors have been termed *large cell neuroendocrine tumors* or *atypical endocrine tumors* and have also been considered by some to represent a form of neoplasia intermediate between small cell carcinoma and typical carcinoid tumor. Some of these neoplasms also possess squamous and glandular features;[9, 222] as a result, it is not entirely clear whether they simply represent an expression of multiple forms of differentiation known to occur in pulmonary malignancy or whether they are part of a spectrum of NE neoplasia beginning with carcinoid tumor. Whatever the case, their biologic behavior in general is significantly worse than that of carcinoid tumors, including the atypical form.[10, 219, 220]

REFERENCES

1. Salyer DC, Salyer WR, Eggleston JC: Bronchial carcinoid tumors. Cancer 36:1522, 1975.
2. Gould VE, Linnoila I, Memoli VA, et al: Biology of disease. Neuroendocrine components of the bronchopulmonary tract: Hyperplasias, dysplasias, and neoplasms. Lab Invest 49:519, 1983.
3. McDowell EM, Sorokin SP, Hoyt RF Jr, et al: An unusual bronchial carcinoid tumor: Light and electron microscopy. Hum Pathol 12:338, 1981.
4. El-Salhy M, Lundqvist M, Wilander E: Bronchial carcinoids and phaeochromocytomas. Acta Pathol Microbiol Immunol Scand 94:229, 1986.
5. Fisher ER, Palekar A, Paulson JD: Comparative histopathologic, histochemical, electron microscopic and tissue culture studies of bronchial carcinoids and oat cell carcinomas of lung. Am J Clin Pathol 69:165, 1978.
6. Paladugu RR, Benfield JR, Pak HY, et al: Bronchopulmonary Kulchitzky cell carcinomas. Cancer 55:1303, 1985.
7. Przygodzki RM, Finkelstein SD, Langer JC, et al: Analysis of p53, K-ras-2, and C-raf-1 in pulmonary neuroendocrine tumors. Correlation with histological subtype and clinical outcome. Am J Pathol 148:1531, 1996.
8. Travis WD, Linnoila RI, Tsokos MG, et al: Neuroendocrine tumors of the lung with proposed criteria for large-cell neuroendocrine carcinoma. An ultrastructural, immunohistochemical, and flow cytometric study of 35 cases. Am J Surg Pathol 15:529, 1991.
9. McDowell EM, Wilson TS, Trump BF: Atypical endocrine tumors of the lung. Arch Pathol Lab Med 105:20, 1981.
10. Neal MH, Kosinski R, Cohen P, et al: Atypical endocrine tumors of the lung: A histologic, ultrastructural, and clinical study of 19 cases. Hum Pathol 17:1264, 1986.
11. de Lima R: Bronchial adenoma. Chest 77:81, 1980.
12. Paladugu RR, Benfield JR, Pak HY, et al: Bronchopulmonary Kulchitzky cell carcinomas: A new classification scheme for typical and atypical carcinoids. Cancer 55:1303, 1985.
13. Godwin JD II: Carcinoid tumors. An analysis of 2837 cases. Cancer 36:560, 1975.
14. Berge T, Linell F: Carcinoid tumours. Frequency in a defined population during a 12-year-period. Acta Pathol Microbiol Scand 84:322, 1976.
15. Harpole DH Jr, Feldman JM, Buchanan S, et al: Bronchial carcinoid tumors: A retrospective analysis of 126 patients. Ann Thorac Surg 54:50, 1992.
16. Arrigoni MG, Woolner LB, Bernatz PE: Atypical carcinoid tumors of the lung. J Cardiovasc Thorac Surg 64:413, 1972.
17. Lawson RM, Ramanathan L, Hurley G, et al: Bronchial adenoma: Review of an 18-year experience at the Brompton Hospital. Thorax 31:245, 1976.
18. Wilkins EW, Grillo HC, Moncure AC, et al: Changing times in surgical management of bronchopulmonary carcinoid tumor. Ann Thorac Surg 38:339, 1984.
19. Leading article: Bronchial adenoma. BMJ 282:252, 1981.
20. Dah QC, Hybarger CP, Geist R, et al: Carcinoids associated with multiple endocrine neoplasia syndromes. Am J Surg 54:142, 1987.
21. Torre M, Barberis M, Barbieri B, et al: Typical and atypical bronchial carcinoids. Respir Med 83:305, 1989.
22. Valli M, Fabris GA, Dewar A, et al: Atypical carcinoid tumour of the lung: A study of 33 cases with prognostic features. Histopathology 24:363, 1994.
23. Pock-Steen OC: Bronchial adenoma. Acta Radiol 51:266, 1959.
24. McCaughan BC, Martini N, Bains MS: Bronchial carcinoids: Review of 124 cases. J Thorac Cardiovasc Surg 89:8, 1985.
25. Brandt B III, Heintz SE, Rose EF, et al: Bronchial carcinoid tumors. Ann Thorac Surg 38:63, 1984.
26. Akiba T, Naruke T, Kondo H, et al: Carcinoid tumor of the lung: Clinicopathological study of 32 cases. Jpn J Clin Oncol 22:92, 1992.
27. Bosman FT, de la Riviere AB, Giard RW, et al: Amine and peptide hormone production by lung carcinoid: A clinicopathological and immunocytochemical study. J Clin Pathol 37:931, 1984.
28. Grote TH, Macon WR, Davis B, et al: Atypical carcinoid of the lung. A distinct clinicopathologic entity. Chest 93:370, 1988.
29. Wellons HA Jr, Eggleston P, Golden GT, et al: Bronchial adenoma in childhood. Two case reports and review of literature. Am J Dis Child 130:301, 1976.
30. Hartman GE, Shochat SJ: Primary pulmonary neoplasms of childhood: A review. Ann Thorac Surg 36:108, 1983.
31. Wang LT, Wilkins EW Jr, Bode HH: Bronchial carcinoid tumors in pediatric patients. Chest 103:1426, 1993.
32. Giustra PE, Stassa G: The multiple presentations of bronchial adenomas. Radiology 93:1013, 1969.
33. Johnson NF, Wagner JC, Wills HA: Endocrine cell proliferation in the rat lung following asbestos inhalation. Lung 158:221, 1980.
34. Hiyama K, Hasegawa K, Ishioka S, et al: An atypical carcinoid tumor of the lung with mutations in the p53 gene and the retinoblastoma gene. Chest 104:1606, 1993.
35. Roncalli M, Doglioni C, Springall DR, et al: Abnormal p53 expression in lung neuroendocrine tumors. Diagnostic and prognostic implications. Diagn Mol Pathol 1:129, 1992.
36. Lohmann DR, Fesseler B, Putz B, et al: Infrequent mutations of the p53 gene in pulmonary carcinoid tumors. Cancer Res 53:5797, 1993.
37. Wagner SN, Muller R, Boehm J, et al: Neuroendocrine neoplasms of the lung are not associated with point mutations at codon 12 of the Ki-ras gene. Virchows Arch 63:325, 1993.
38. Briselli M, Mark GJ, Grillo HC: Tracheal carcinoids. Cancer 42:2870, 1978.
39. Ranchod M, Levine GD: Spindle-cell carcinoid tumors of the lung. A clinicopathologic study of 35 cases. Am J Surg Pathol 4:315, 1980.
40. Markel SF, Abell MR, Haight C, et al: Neoplasms of bronchus commonly designated as adenomas. Cancer 17:590, 1964.
41. Hurt R, Bates M: Carcinoid tumours of the bronchus: A 33 year experience. Thorax 39:617, 1984.
42. Cooney T, Sweeney EC, Luke D: Pulmonary carcinoid tumours: A comparative regional study. J Clin Pathol 32:1100, 1979.
43. Craig ID, Finley RJ: Spindle-cell carcinoid tumor of lung. Cytologic, histopathologic and ultrastructural features. Acta Cytol 26:495, 1982.
44. Churg A: Large spindle cell variant of peripheral bronchial carcinoid tumor. Arch Pathol Lab Med 101:216, 1977.
45. Nguyen G, Shnitka TK: Aspiration biopsy cytology of adenocarcinoid tumor of the bronchial tree. Acta Cytol 31:726, 1987.
46. Wise WS, Bonder D, Aikawa M, et al: Carcinoid tumor of lung with varied histology. Am J Surg Pathol 6:261, 1982.
47. Mark EJ, Quay SC, Dickersi GR: Papillary carcinoid tumor of the lung. Cancer 48:316, 1981.
48. Gouyer V, Gazzéri S, Bolon I, et al: Mechanism of retinoblastoma gene inactivation in the spectrum of neuroendocrine lung tumors. Am J Respir Cell Mol Biol 18:188, 1998.
49. Sklar JL, Churg A, Bensch KG: Oncocytic carcinoid tumor of the lung. Am J Surg Pathol 4:287, 1980.
50. Scharifker D, Marchevsky A: Oncocytic carcinoid of lung: An ultrastructural analysis. Cancer 47:530, 1981.
51. Kuwahara T, Maruyama K, Mochizuki S, et al: Oncocytic carcinoid of the lung: An ultrastructural observation. Acta Pathol Jpn 34:355, 1984.
52. Miura K, Morinaga S, Horiuchi M, et al: Bronchial carcinoid tumor mimicking acinic cell tumor. Acta Pathol Jpn 38:523, 1988.
53. Cebelin MS: Melanocytic bronchial carcinoid tumor. Cancer 46:1843, 1980.
54. Grazer R, Cohen SM, Jacobs JB, et al: Melanin-containing peripheral carcinoid of the lung. Am J Surg Pathol 6:73, 1982.
55. Gal AA, Koss MN, Hochholzer L, et al: Pigmented pulmonary carcinoid tumor. An immunohistochemical and ultrastructural study. Arch Pathol Lab Med 117:832, 1993.
56. Kinney FJ, Kovarik JL: Bone formation in bronchial adenoma. Am J Clin Pathol 44:52, 1965.
57. Al-Kaisi N, Abdul-Karim FW, Mendelsohn G, et al: Bronchial carcinoid tumor with amyloid stroma. Arch Pathol Lab Med 112:211, 1988.
58. Abe Y, Utsunomiya H, Tsutsumi Y: Atypical carcinoid tumor of the lung with amyloid stroma. Acta Pathol Jpn 42:286, 1992.
59. Lara JF, Rosen PP: Extramedullary hematopoiesis in a bronchial carcinoid tumor. An unusual complication of agnogenic myeloid metaplasia. Arch Pathol Lab Med 114:1283, 1990.
60. Smith DM Jr, Haggitt RC: A comparative study of generic stains for carcinoid secretory granules. Am J Surg Pathol 7:61, 1983.
61. Hoyt RF, Sorokin SP, McDowell EM, et al: Periodic acid–Schiff–lead hematoxylin as a marker for the endocrine phenotype in human lung tumors. Arch Pathol Lab Med 110:943, 1986.
62. Gould VE, Linnoila RI, Memoli VA, et al: Neuroendocrine cells and neuroendocrine neoplasms of the lung. Pathol Annu 18:287, 1983.
63. Bostwick DG, Bensch KG: Gastrin releasing peptide in human neuroendocrine tumors. J Pathol 147:237, 1985.
64. Yang K, Ulich T, Taylor I, et al: Pulmonary carcinoids. Immunohistochemical demonstration of brain-gut peptides. Cancer 52:819, 1983.
65. Gould VE, Wiedenmann B, Lee I, et al: Synaptophysin expression in neuroendocrine neoplasms as determined by immunocytochemistry. Am J Pathol 126:243, 1987.
66. Martin JME, Maung RT: Differential immunohistochemical reactions in carcinoid tumors. Hum Pathol 18:941, 1987.
67. Loy TS, Darkow GVD, Quesenberry JT: Immunostaining in the diagnosis of pulmonary neuroendocrine carcinomas. An immunohistochemical study with ultrastructural correlations. Am J Surg Pathol 19:173, 1995.
68. Senden NH, Timmer ED, de Bruine A, et al: A comparison of NSP-reticulons with conventional neuroendocrine markers in immunophenotyping of lung cancers. J Pathol 182:13, 1997.
69. Addis BJ, Hamid Q, Ibrahim NBN, et al: Immunohistochemical markers of small cell carcinoma and related neuroendocrine tumours of the lung. J Pathol 153:137, 1987.
70. Lewin KJ, Layfield L, Cheng L: Disseminated bombesin-producing carcinoid tumor of pulmonary origin. Am J Surg Pathol 9:129, 1985.
71. Tamai S, Kameya T, Yamaguchi K, et al: Peripheral lung carcinoid tumor producing predominantly gastrin-releasing peptide (GRP). Cancer 52:273, 1983.
72. Ghatei MA, Stratton MR, Allen JM, et al: Co-secretion of calcitonin gene–related peptide, gastrin-releasing peptide and ACTH by a carcinoid tumour metastasizing to the cerebellum. Postgrad Med J 63:123, 1987.
73. Tsutsumi Y: Immunohistochemical analysis of calcitonin and calcitonin gene–related peptide in human lung. Hum Pathol 20:896, 1989.
74. Asa SL, Kovacs K, Vale W, et al: Immunohistologic localization of corticotropin-releasing hormone in human tumors. Am J Clin Pathol 87:327, 1987.

75. Carroll DG, Delahunt JW, Teaque CA, et al: Resolution of acromegaly after removal of a bronchial carcinoid shown to secrete growth hormone releasing factor. Aust N Z J Med 17:63, 1987.

76. Bishop AE, Hamid QA, Adams C, et al: Expression of tachykinins by ileal and lung carcinoid tumors assessed by combined in situ hybridization, immunocyto-chemistry, and radioimmunoassay. Cancer 63:1129, 1989.

77. Heitz PU, von Herbay G, Klöppel G, et al: The expression of subunits of human chorionic gonadotropin (hCG) by nontrophoblastic, nonendocrine, and endocrine tumors. Am J Clin Pathol 88:467, 1987.

78. Fukayama M, Hayashi Y, Koike M, et al: Human chorionic gonadotropin lung and lung tumors. Lab Invest 55:433, 1986.

79. Said JW, Vimadalal S, Nash G, et al: Immunoreactive neuron-specific enolase, bombesin, and chromogranin as markers for neuroendocrine lung tumors. Hum Pathol 16:236, 1985.

80. Sheppard MN, Corrin B, Bennett MH, et al: Immunocytochemical localization of neuron specific enolase in small cell carcinomas and carcinoid tumours of the lung. Histopathology 8:171, 1984.

81. Hage E: Histochemistry and fine structure of bronchial carcinoid tumours. Virchows Arch 361:121, 1973.

82. Bishopric GA, Ordonez NG: Carcinoembryonic antigen in primary carcinoid tumors of the lung. Cancer 58:1316, 1986.

83. Christen B, Trojanowski JQ, Pietra GG: Immunohistochemical demonstration of phosphorylated and nonphosphorylated forms of human neurofilament subunits in human pulmonary carcinoids. Hum Pathol 18:997, 1987.

84. Doglioni C, Barbareschi M, Balercia G, et al: Atypical lung carcinoid with GFAP immunoreactive cells. Pathol Res Pract 189:83, 1993.

85. Black M, Carey FA, Farquharson MA, et al: Expression of the pro-opiomelano-cortin gene in lung neuroendocrine tumours: In situ hybridization and immuno-histochemical studies. J Pathol 169:329, 1993.

86. Capella C, Gabrielli M, Polak JM, et al: Ultrastructural and histological study of 11 bronchial carcinoids. Evidence for different types. Virchows Arch 381:313, 1979.

87. Hosoda S, Nakamura W, Suzuki H, et al: A bronchial carcinoid having low serotonin concentration. Arch Pathol 90:320, 1970.

88. Berger G, Berger F, Bejui F, et al: Bronchial carcinoid with fibrillary inclusion related to cytokeratins: An immunohistochemical and ultrastructural study with subsequent investigation of 12 foregut APUDomas. Histopathology 8:245, 1984.

89. Geller SA, Gordon RE: Peripheral spindle-cell carcinoid tumor of the lung with type II pneumocyte features. An ultrastructural study with comments on possible histogenesis. Am J Surg Pathol 8:145, 1984.

90. Carlson JA, Dickersin GR: Melanotic paraganglioid carcinoid tumor: A case report and review of the literature. Ultrastruct Pathol 17:353, 1993.

91. Berendsen HH, Postmus PE, Edens ET, et al: Irresectable bronchial carcinoid with a 32 year natural history. Eur J Respir Dis 68:151, 1986.

92. Hurt R, Bates M: Carcinoid tumours of the bronchus: A 33 year experience. Thorax 39:617, 1984.

93. Kron IL, Harman PK, Mills SE, et al: A reappraisal of limited stage undifferenti-ated carcinoma of the lung: Does stage I small cell undifferentiated carcinoma exist? J Thorac Cardiovasc Surg 84:734, 1982.

94. Jordan AG, Predmore L, Sullivan MM, et al: The cytodiagnosis of well-differen-tiated neuroendocrine carcinoma. A clinicopathologic entity. Acta Cytol 31:464, 1987.

95. Sheppard MN: Nuclear pleomorphism in typical carcinoid tumours of the lung: Problems in frozen section interpretation. Histopathology 30:478, 1997.

96. Mills SE, Cooper PH, Walker RA, et al: Atypical carcinoid tumor of the lung. A clinicopathologic study of 17 cases. Am J Surg Pathol 6:643, 1982.

97. Paladugu RR, Benfield JR, Pak HY, et al: Bronchopulmonary Kulchitzky cell carcinomas. A new classification scheme for typical and atypical carcinoids. Cancer 55:1303, 1985.

98. Mark EJ, Ramirez JF: Peripheral small-cell carcinoma of the lung resembling carcinoid tumor. Arch Pathol Lab Med 109:263, 1985.

99. McCaughan BC, Martini N, Baines MS: Bronchial carcinoids. J Thorac Cardio-vasc Surg 89:8, 1985.

100. Rainosek DE, Ro JY, Ordonez NG, et al: Sarcomatoid carcinoma of the lung. A case with atypical carcinoid and rhabdomyosarcomatous components. Am J Clin Pathol 102:360, 1994.

101. Blondal T, Grimelius L, Nou E, et al: Argyrophil carcinoid tumors of the lung: Incidence, clinical study, and follow-up of 46 patients. Chest 78:840, 1980.

102. Coppola D, Clarke M, Landreneau R, et al: Bcl-2, p53, CD44, and CD44v6 isoform expression in neuroendocrine tumors of the lung. Mod Pathol 9:484, 1996.

103. Chaudhuri TK, Chaudhuri TK, Schapiro RL, et al: Abnormal lung perfusion in a patient with bronchial adenoma. Chest 62:110, 1972.

104. McGuinnis EJ, Lull RJ: Bronchial adenoma causing unilateral absence of pulmo-nary perfusion. Radiology 120:367, 1976.

105. Wynn SR, O'Connell EJ, Frigas E, et al: Exercise-induced "asthma" as a presentation of bronchial adenoma. Ann Allergy 57:139, 1986.

106. Bluth I: A note on the roentgen features of bronchial adenoma of the peripheral type. Radiology 68:193, 1957.

107. Good CA, Harrington SW: Asymptomatic bronchial adenoma. Proc Mayo Clin 28:577, 1953.

108. Magid D, Siegelman SS, Eggleston JC, et al: Pulmonary carcinoid tumors: CT assessment. J Comput Assist Tomogr 13:244, 1989.

109. Harpole DH Jr, Feldman JM, Buchanan S, et al: Bronchial carcinoid tumors: A retrospective analysis of 126 patients. Ann Thorac Surg 54:50, 1992.

110. Markel SF, Abell MR, Haight C, et al: Neoplasms of bronchus commonly designated as adenomas. Cancer 17:590, 1964.

111. Aronchick JM, Wexler JA, Christen B, et al: Computed tomography of bronchial carcinoid. J Comput Assist Tomogr 10:71, 1986.

112. Davis SD, Zirn JR, Govoni AF, et al: Peripheral carcinoid tumor of the lung: CT diagnosis. Am J Roentgenol 155:1185, 1990.

113. Douek PC, Simoni L, Revel D, et al: Diagnosis of bronchial carcinoid tumor by ultrafast contrast-enhanced MR imaging. Am J Roentgenol 163:563, 1994.

114. Doppman JL, Pass HI, Nieman LK, et al: Detection of ACTH-producing bron-chial carcinoid tumors: MR imaging vs CT. Am J Roentgenol 156:39, 1991.

114a. Erasmus JJ, McAdams HP, Patz EF Jr, et al: Evaluation of primary pulmonary carcinoid tumors using FDG PET. Am J Roentgenol 170:1369, 1998.

115. Troupin R: Ossifying bronchial carcinoid: A case report. Am J Roentgenol 104:808, 1968.

116. Heimburger IL, Kilman JW, Battersby JS: Peripheral bronchial adenomas. J Thorac Cardiovasc Surg 52:542, 1966.

117. Lawson RM, Ramanathan L, Hurley G, et al: Bronchial adenoma: Review of an 18-year experience at the Brompton Hospital. Thorax 31:245, 1976.

118. Zwiebel BR, Austin JHM, Grimes MM: Bronchial carcinoid tumors: Assessment with CT of location and intratumoral calcification in 31 patients. Radiology 179:483, 1991.

119. Shin MS, Berland LL, Myers JL, et al: CT demonstration of an ossifying bronchial carcinoid simulating broncholithiasis. Am J Roentgenol 153:51, 1989.

120. Thomas BM: Three unusual carcinoid tumours, with particular reference to osteoblastic bone metastases. Clin Radiol 19:221, 1968.

121. Hyman GA, Wells J: Bronchial carcinoid with osteoblastic metastases. Cases with carcinoid syndrome. Arch Intern Med 114:541, 1964.

122. Sheppard BB, Follette DM, Meyers FJ: Giant carcinoid tumor of the lung. Ann Thorac Surg 63:851, 1997.

123. Choplin RH, Kawamoto EH, Dyer RB, et al: Atypical carcinoid of the lung: Radiographic features. Am J Roentgenol 146:665, 1986.

124. Forster BB, Müller NL, Miller RR, et al: Neuroendocrine carcinomas of the lung: Clinical, radiologic, and pathologic correlation. Radiology 170:441, 1989.

125. Müller NL, Miller RR: Neuroendocrine carcinomas of the lung. Semin Roent-genol 25:96, 1990.

126. Rea F, Binda R, Spreafico G, et al: Bronchial carcinoids: A review of 60 patients. Ann Thorac Surg 47:412, 1989.

127. Bower G: Bronchial adenoma: A review of twenty-eight cases. Am Rev Respir Dis 92:558, 1965.

128. Todd TR, Cooper JD, Weissberg D, et al: Bronchial carcinoid tumors: 20 years' experience. J Thorac Cardiovasc Surg 79:532, 1980.

129. Johnson LA, Lavin P, Moertel CG, et al: Carcinoids: The association of histologic growth pattern and survival. Cancer 51:882, 1983.

130. Smith RA: Bronchial carcinoid tumours. Thorax 24:43, 1969.

131. Shames JM, Dhurandhar NR, Blackard WG: Insulin-secreting bronchial carcinoid tumor with widespread metastases. Am J Med 44:632, 1968.

132. DeStephano DB, Lloyd RV, Schteingart DE: Cushing's syndrome produced by a bronchial carcinoid tumor. Case studies. Hum Pathol 15:890, 1984.

133. Doppman JL, Nieman L, Miller D, et al: Ectopic adrenocorticotropic hormone syndrome: Localization studies in 28 patients. Radiology 172:115, 1989.

134. Amann ST, Myers MA, Cicale MJ: Severe diarrhea and Cushing's syndrome from an atypical bronchial carcinoid. South Med J 87:855, 1994.

135. Oberg K, Norheim I, Wide L: Serum growth hormone in patients with carcinoid tumours: Basal levels and response to glucose and thyrotrophin releasing hor-mone. Acta Endocrinol 109:13, 1985.

136. Isawa T, Okubo K, Konno K, et al: Cushing's syndrome caused by recurrent malignant bronchial carcinoid. Case report with 12 years' observation. Am Rev Respir Dis 108:1200, 1973.

137. Oliaro A, Filosso PL, Casadio C, et al: Bronchial carcinoid associated with Cushing's syndrome. J Cardiovasc Surg 36:511, 1995.

138. Doppman JL, Loughlin T, Miller DL, et al: Identification of ACTH-producing intrathoracic tumors by measuring ACTH levels in aspirated specimens. Radiol-ogy 163:501, 1987.

139. Boscaro M, Merola G, Sonino N, et al: Evidence for ectopic ACTH production years after bilateral adrenalectomy for Cushing's syndrome: In vivo and in vitro studies. J Endocrinol Invest 8:417, 1985.

140. Iser G, Pfohl M, Dorr U, et al: Ectopic ACTH secretion due to a bronchopulmo-nary carcinoid localized by somatostatin receptor scintigraphy. Clin Invest 72:887, 1994.

141. Shrager JB, Wright CD, Wain JC, et al: Bronchopulmonary carcinoid tumors associated with Cushing's syndrome: A more aggressive variant of typical carci-noid. J Thorac Cardiovasc Surg 114:367, 1997.

142. Andler M, Scheuer PJ, Watt PJ: 5-Hydroxytryptophan–secreting bronchial carci-noid tumour. Lancet 2:1067, 1961.

143. Bertelsen S, Aasted A, Lund C, et al: Bronchial carcinoid tumours: A clinicopath-ologic study of 82 cases. Scand J Thorac Cardiovasc Surg 19:105, 1985.

144. Melmon K, Sjoerdsma A, Mason D: Distinctive clinical and therapeutic aspects of the syndrome associated with bronchial carcinoid tumors. Am J Med 39:568, 1965.

145. Escovitz WE, Reingold IM: Functioning malignant bronchial carcinoid with Cushing's syndrome and recurrent sinus arrest. Ann Intern Med 54:1248, 1961.

146. Tanaka M, Matsubara O, Takemura T, et al: Cardiovascular lesion of carcinoid syndrome. An autopsy case of bronchial carcinoid. Acta Pathol Jpn 34:201, 1984.

147. Saeed uz Zafar M, Mellinger RC, Fine G, et al: Acromegaly associated with a bronchial carcinoid tumor: Evidence for ectopic production of growth hormone-releasing activity. J Clin Endocrinol Metab 48:66, 1979.

148. Scheithauer BW, Carpenter PC, Bloch B, et al: Ectopic secretion of a growth hormone–releasing factor: Report of a case of acromegaly with bronchial carcinoid tumor. Am J Med 76:605, 1984.

149. Dabek JT: Bronchial carcinoid tumour with acromegaly in two patients. J Clin Endocrinol Metab 38:329, 1974.

150. Cooney T, Benediktsson H, Mukai K: Immunohistochemical evaluation of a complex endocrinopathy. Am J Surg Pathol 4:491, 1980.

151. Nakhoul F, Kerner H, Levin M, et al: Carcinoid tumor of the lung and type-1 multiple endocrine neoplasia associated with persistent hypercalcemia: A case report. Miner Electrolyte Metab 20:107, 1994.

152. Karmy-Jones R, Vallieres E: Carcinoid crisis after biopsy of a bronchial carcinoid. Ann Thorac Surg 56:1403, 1993.

153. Sukumaran M, Wilkinson ZS, Christianson L: Acute carcinoid syndrome: A complication of flexible bronchoscopy. Ann Thorac Surg 34:702, 1982.

154. Okike N, Bernatz PE, Woolner LB: Carcinoid tumors of the lung. Ann Thorac Surg 22:270, 1976.

155. Nguyen GK: Cytopathology of pulmonary carcinoid tumors in sputum and bronchial brushings. Acta Cytol 39:1152, 1995.

156. Suen KC, Quenville NF: Fine needle aspiration cytology of uncommon thoracic lesions. Am J Clin Pathol 75:803, 1981.

157. Anderson C, Ludwig ME, O'Donnell M, et al: Fine needle aspiration cytology of pulmonary carcinoid tumors. Acta Cytol 34:505, 1990.

158. Collins BT, Cramer HM: Fine needle aspiration cytology of carcinoid tumors. Acta Cytol 40:695, 1996.

159. Kyriakos M, Rockoff SD: Brush biopsy of bronchial carcinoid—a source of cytologic error. Acta Cytol 16:261, 1972.

160. Frierson HF Jr, Covell JL, Mills SE: Fine needle aspiration cytology of atypical carcinoid of the lung. Acta Cytol 31:471, 1987.

161. Gephardt GN, Belovich DM: Cytology of pulmonary carcinoid tumors. Acta Cytol 26:434, 1982.

162. Frierson HF Jr, Covell JL, Mills SE: Fine needle aspiration cytology of atypical carcinoid of the lung. Acta Cytol 31:471, 1987.

163. Larismont D, Kiss R, De Launoit Y, et al: Characterization of the morphonuclear features and DNA ploidy of typical and atypical carcinoids and small cell carcinomas of the lung. Am J Clin Pathol 94:378, 1990.

164. Gottlieb C, Kini S, Feingold M: Cytomorphometric analysis of small cell neoplasms of the lung from specimens obtained via bronchoscopy. Anal Quant Cytol Histol 14:41, 1992.

165. Johansson M, Heim S, Mandahl N, et al: Cytogenetic analysis of six bronchial carcinoids. Cancer Genet Cytogenet 66:33, 1993.

166. Feldman JM: Urinary serotonin in the diagnosis of carcinoid tumors. Clin Chem 32:840, 1986.

167. Raff H, Shaker JL, Seifert PE, et al: Intraoperative measurement of adrenocorticotropin (ACTH) during removal of ACTH-secreting bronchial carcinoid tumors. J Clin Endocrinol Metab 80:1036, 1995.

168. Nobels FR, Kwekkeboom DJ, Coopmans W, et al: Chromogranin A as serum marker for neuroendocrine neoplasia: Comparison with neuron-specific enolase and the alpha-subunit of glycoprotein hormones. J Clin Endocrinol Metab 82:2622, 1997.

169. Kalkner KM, Janson ET, Nilsson S, et al: Somatostatin receptor scintigraphy in patients with carcinoid tumors: Comparison between radioligand uptake and tumor markers. Cancer Res 55(Suppl 23):5801, 1995.

170. Kvols LK, Brown ML, O'Connor MK, et al: Evaluation of a radiolabeled somatostatin analog (I-123 octreotide) in the detection and localization of carcinoid and islet cell tumors. Radiology 187:129, 1993.

171. Reubi JC, Kvols LK, Nagorney DM, et al: Detection of somatostatin receptors in surgical and percutaneous needle biopsy samples of carcinoids and islet cell carcinomas. Cancer Res 50:5969, 1990.

172. Bomanji J, Ur E, Mather S, et al: A scintigraphic comparison of iodine-123-metaiodobenzylguanidine and an iodine-labeled somatostatin analog (Tyr-3-octreotide) in metastatic carcinoid tumors. J Nucl Med 33:1121, 1992.

173. Schreurs AJ, Westermann CJ, van den Bosch JM, et al: A twenty-five-year follow-up of ninety-three resected typical carcinoid tumors of the lung. J Thorac Cardiovasc Surg 104:1470, 1992.

174. DeCaro LF, Paladugu R, Benfield JR, et al: Typical and atypical carcinoids within the pulmonary APUD tumor spectrum. J Thorac Cardiovasc Surg 86:528, 1983.

175. Attar S, Miller JE, Hankins J, et al: Bronchial adenoma: A review of 51 patients. Ann Thorac Surg 40:126, 1985.

175a. Ducrocq X, Thomas P, Massard G, et al: Operative risk and prognostic factors of typical bronchial carcinoid tumors. Ann Thorac Surg 65:1410, 1998.

176. Bernstein C, McGoey J, Lertzman M: Recurrent bronchial carcinoid tumor. Chest 95:693, 1989.

177. Schepens MA, Van Schil PE, Knaepen PJ, et al: Late results of sleeve resection for typical bronchial carcinoids. Eur J Cardiothorac Surg 8:118, 1994.

178. Sutedja TG, Schreurs AJ, Vanderschueren RG, et al: Bronchoscopic therapy in patients with intraluminal typical bronchial carcinoid. Chest 107:556, 1995.

179. Perkins P, Lee JR, Kemp BL, et al: Carcinoid tumors of the lung and family history of cancer. J Clin Epidemiol 50:705, 1997.

180. Thunnissen FBJM, Van Eijk J, Baak JPA, et al: Bronchopulmonary carcinoids and regional lymph node metastases. A quantitative pathologic investigation. Am J Pathol 132:119, 1988.

181. Hajdu SI, Winawer SJ, Myers WPL: Carcinoid tumors. A study of 204 cases. Am J Clin Pathol 61:521, 1974.

182. El-Naggar AK, Ballance W, Abdul Karim FW, et al: Typical and atypical bronchopulmonary carcinoids. A clinicopathologic and flow cytometric study. Am J Clin Pathol 95:828, 1991.

183. Bishopric GA Jr, Ordonez NG: Carcinoembryonic antigen in primary carcinoid tumors of the lung. Cancer 58:1316, 1986.

184. Perkins P, Kemp BL, Putnam JB Jr, et al: Pretreatment characteristics of carcinoid tumors of the lung which predict aggressive behavior. Am J Clin Oncol 20:285, 1997.

185. Kujari H, Joensuu H, Klemi P, et al: A flow cytometric analysis of 23 carcinoid tumors. Cancer 61:2517, 1988.

186. Yousem SA, Taylor SR: Typical and atypical carcinoid tumors of lung: A clinicopathologic and DNA analysis of 20 tumors. Mod Pathol 3:502, 1990.

186a. Jackson-York GL, Davis BH, Warren WH, et al: Flow cytometric DNA content analysis in neuroendocrine carcinoma of the lung: Correlation with survival and histologic subtype. Cancer 68:374, 1991.

187. Padberg B-C, Woenckhaus J, Hilger G, et al: DNA cytophotometry and prognosis in typical and atypical bronchopulmonary carcinoid tumors. Am J Surg Pathol 20:815, 1996.

188. Bohm J, Koch S, Gais P, et al: Prognostic value of MIB-1 in neuroendocrine tumours of the lung. J Pathol 178:402, 1996.

189. Marty-Ane CH, Costes V, Pujol JL, et al: Carcinoid tumors of the lung: Do atypical features require aggressive management? Ann Thorac Surg 59:78, 1995.

190. Lequaglie C, Patriarca C, Cataldo I, et al: Prognosis of well-differentiated neuroendocrine carcinoma of the lung. Chest 100:1053, 1991.

191. Whitwell F: Tumourlets of the lung. J Pathol Bacteriol 70:529, 1955.

192. Cureton RJR, Hill IM: Malignant change in bronchiectasis. Thorax 10:131, 1955.

193. Cunningham GJ, Nassau E, Walter JB: The frequency of tumour-like formations in bronchiectatic lungs. Thorax 13:64, 1958.

194. Miller RR, Müller NL: Neuroendocrine cell hyperplasia and obliterative bronchiolitis in patients with peripheral carcinoid tumors. Am J Surg Pathol 19:653, 1995.

195. Prior JT: Minute peripheral pulmonary tumors. Observations on their histogenesis. Am J Pathol 29:703, 1953.

196. King LS: Atypical proliferation of bronchiolar epithelium. AMA Arch Pathol 58:59, 1954.

197. Chen KT: Congenital cystic adenomatoid malformation of the lung and pulmonary tumorlets in an adult. J Surg Oncol 30:106, 1985.

198. Pelosi G, Zancanaro C, Sbabo L, et al: Development of innumerable neuroendocrine tumorlets in pulmonary lobe scarred by intralobar sequestration. Immunohistochemical and ultrastructural study of an unusual case. Arch Pathol Lab Med 116:1167, 1992.

199. Watanabe H, Kobayashi H, Honma K, et al: Diffuse panbronchiolitis with multiple tumorlets. Acta Pathol Jpn 35:1221, 1985.

200. MacMahon HE, Werch J, Sorger K: Tumorlet of bronchus with a 12 year follow-up. Arch Pathol 83:359, 1967.

201. Churg A, Warnock ML: Pulmonary tumorlet. A form of peripheral carcinoid. Cancer 37:1469, 1976.

202. Bonikos DS, Archibald R, Bensch KG: On the origin of the so-called tumorlets of the lung. Hum Pathol 17:461, 1976.

203. D'Agati VD, Perzin KH: Carcinoid tumorlets of the lung with metastasis to a peribronchial lymph node. Cancer 55:2472, 1985.

204. Spain DM, Parsonnet V: Multiple origin of minute bronchiolargenic carcinomas. Report of a case. Cancer 4:277, 1951.

205. D'Agati VD, Perzin KH: Carcinoid tumorlets of the lung with metastasis to a peribronchial lymph node: Report of a case and review of the literature. Cancer 55:2472, 1985.

206. Rodgers-Sullivan RF, Weiland LH, Palumbo PJ, et al: Pulmonary tumorlets associated with Cushing's syndrome. Am Rev Respir Dis 117:799, 1978.

207. Jiang S-X, Kameya T, Shoji M, et al: Large cell neuroendocrine carcinoma of the lung: A histologic and immunohistochemical study of 22 cases. Am J Surg Pathol 22:526, 1998.

208. Aguayo SM, Miller YE, Waldron JA Jr, et al: Brief report: Idiopathic diffuse hyperplasia of pulmonary neuroendocrine cells and airways disease. N Engl J Med 327:1285, 1992.

209. Travis WD, Gal AA, Colby TV, et al: Reproducibility of neuroendocrine lung tumor classification. Hum Pathol 29:272, 1998.

210. Torikata C, Kawai T, Yakumaru K, et al: Histopathological studies on the tumourlet of the lung with special reference to the cytogenesis of proliferating cells. Acta Pathol Jpn 25:539, 1975.

211. Miller MA, Mark GJ, Kanarek D: Multiple peripheral pulmonary carcinoids and tumorlets of carcinoid type, with restrictive and obstructive lung disease. Am J Med 65:373, 1978.

212. Ranchod M: The histogenesis and development of pulmonary tumorlets. Cancer 39:1135, 1977.

213. Resl M, Kral B, Simek J, et al: S-100 protein positive (sustentacular) cells in pulmonary carcinoid tumorlets: A quantitative study of 24 cases. Pathol Res Pract 192:414, 1996.

214. Bennett GL, Chew FS: Pulmonary carcinoid tumorlets. Am J Roentgenol 162:568, 1994.

215. Brown MJ, English J, Müller NL: Bronchiolitis obliterans due to neuroendocrine hyperplasia: High-resolution CT-pathologic correlation. Am J Roentgenol 168:1561, 1997.

216. Dresler CM, Ritter JH, Patterson GA, et al: Clinical-pathologic analysis of 40 patients with large cell neuroendocrine carcinoma of the lung. Ann Thorac Surg 63:180, 1997.

217. Rusch VW, Klimstra DS, Venkatraman ES: Molecular markers help characterize neuroendocrine lung tumors. Ann Thorac Surg 62:798, 1996.

218. Mooi WJ, Zandwijk N, Dingemans KP, et al: The "grey area" between small cell and nonsmall cell lung carcinomas. Light and electron microscopy versus clinical data in 14 cases. J Pathol 149:49, 1986.

219. Hammond ME, Sause WT: Large cell neuroendocrine tumors of the lung. Cancer 56:1624, 1985.

220. Wick MR, Berg LC, Hertz MI: Large cell carcinoma of the lung with neuroendo-crine differentiation. A comparison with large cell "undifferentiated" pulmonary tumors. Am J Clin Pathol 97:796, 1992.

221. Linnoila RI, Mulshine JL, Steinberg SM, et al: Neuroendocrine differentiation in endocrine and nonendocrine lung carcinomas. Am J Clin Pathol 90:641, 1988.

222. Neal MH, Kosinski R, Cohen P, et al: Atypical endocrine tumors of the lung: A histologic, ultrastructural, and clinical study of 19 cases. Hum Pathol 17:1264, 1986.

CHAPTER 33

Neoplasms of Tracheobronchial Glands

GENERAL CHARACTERISTICS

The observations that the morphology of the tracheobronchial mucous glands is similar to that of the oropharyngeal salivary glands and that neoplasms with an identical histologic appearance occur in both locations have led to the belief that a group of pulmonary tumors are derived from the glands themselves. They can thus be designated *tracheobronchial gland tumors* (although some pathologists consider the nonhistogenic term *salivary-like* to be more appropriate[1]). Whatever their histogenesis, their histologic pattern, characteristic growth into the lumen of central airways, lack of association with cigarette smoking, and much better overall prognosis than neoplasms of surface airway epithelium, warrant their consideration as a distinct group. As discussed previously (*see* page 1229), inclusion of some of these tumors under the term *bronchial adenoma* is both confusing and inaccurate and is a practice that should be regarded as of historic interest only.

The tumors are quite uncommon, probably accounting for no more than 0.1% to 0.2% of all tracheobronchial tumors;[2, 3] the majority are either adenoid cystic or mucoepidermoid carcinoma, the other varieties being exceptionally rare. Over a 50-year period at the Mayo Clinic, 20 cases of adenoid cystic and 12 cases of mucoepidermoid carcinoma were seen; during the same period, there were 236 typical and 30 atypical carcinoid tumors.[4] Presumably because the concentration of mucous glands is greatest in the trachea and proximal bronchi, these are the most common sites of origin.

The diagnosis should be considered in anyone who has radiographic or endoscopic evidence of a polypoid intraluminal mass in the trachea or major bronchi. Although clinical features are not specific, a history of adult-onset "asthma" that has increased in severity despite adequate therapy should alert one to the possibility of a central obstructing lesion.

The dyspnea occasioned by these neoplasms has been said to be frequently paroxysmal and to occur most often at night or when the patient is recumbent.[5]

It is worth stressing that the presence of these tumors on standard posteroanterior and lateral chest radiographs is all too frequently overlooked, the tracheal air column constituting a "blind area" for many radiologists. We have seen one patient who had been followed for 4 years with a clinical diagnosis of asthma in whom a tracheal mucoepidermoid carcinoma was finally identified (Fig. 33–1); in fact, the tumor was clearly visible on several radiographs obtained during the 4 years of observation. Endotracheal neoplasms are frequently missed because of radiographic underexposure;[6] for this reason, the high-kilovoltage technique described in Chapter 13 (*see* page 302), which obviates this technical deficiency, is strongly recommended as standard technique. CT scanning is also indicated in suspicious cases; in one study of 35 patients who had focal or diffuse lesions of the trachea or main bronchi, the abnormalities were detected on the chest radiograph in 23 (66%) compared with 33 patients (94%) on CT.[7]

It is worth reiterating that the site of origin of a tracheal neoplasm strongly influences the clinical presentation. Since the intrathoracic portion of the trachea dilates on inspiration and narrows on expiration, a lesion arising in this segment will be characterized clinically by expiratory airway obstruction, often simulating asthma, and radiographically by expiratory air trapping. Conversely, the cervical portion of the trachea narrows on inspiration and dilates on expiration, so that symptoms and signs of expiratory airway obstruction are lacking. A further indicator is the timing of a wheeze; with an intrathoracic tumor, this will occur on expiration and with a cervical one it will be evident on inspiration. Because of these differences, clinical awareness of a lesion in the cervical location develops much later, enhancing the potential for local extension of the neoplasm.

A variety of histologically distinct tracheobronchial gland neoplasms have been described, including adenoid cystic carcinoma, mucoepidermoid carcinoma, acinic cell carcinoma, pleomorphic adenoma, oncocytoma, and mucous gland adenoma. A single case has been reported of a peripheral lung nodule that possessed light microscopic and ultrastructural features suggestive of myoepithelioma.[8] Although the authors suggested that it was analogous to similar neoplasms that occur in salivary glands, whether such a tumor

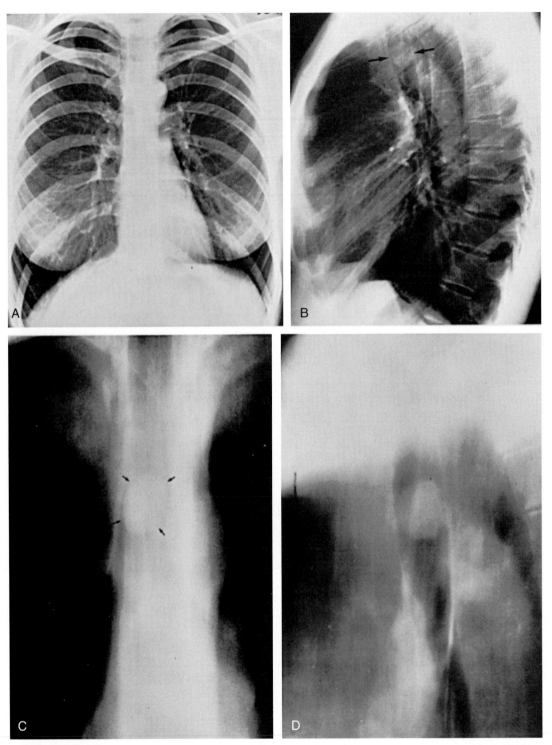

Figure 33–1. Mucoepidermoid Carcinoma. At the time of the radiograph illustrated in *A*, this 32-year-old woman presented with a 4-year history of sporadic attacks of acute shortness of breath that had been diagnosed and treated by her family physician as spasmodic asthma. A number of radiographic examinations of the chest during this period had been interpreted as normal. This posteroanterior radiograph reveals mild to moderate overinflation of both lungs, consistent with a diagnosis of asthma. However, note that the mediastinum is intolerably underexposed, to a point at which the tracheal air column is not visible. In lateral projection *(B)*, a smooth, sharply demarcated mass can be identified in the plane of the tracheal air column *(arrows)*. Tomographic sections of the mediastinum in anteroposterior *(C)* and lateral *(D)* projections show the mass to lie within the trachea approximately 3 cm proximal to the carina *(arrows in C)*. The mass is almost completely occluding the tracheal air column. Following resection, the patient experienced an uneventful recovery. This case illustrates graphically the often repeated observation that the tracheal air column tends to be a "blind area" for many radiologists. (Courtesy of Dr. Michael Lefcoe, Victoria Hospital, London, Ontario.)

represents a separate entity or simply part of a spectrum of pleomorphic adenoma is debatable. Two cases of mixed epithelial-myoepithelial tumors (hypothesized to arise from the glandular duct region) have also been reported.[9, 10] Finally, a single case has been documented of an intrabronchial tumor that possibly arose from mucous glands and that was composed of a mixture of mucus-secreting, ciliated, oncocytic, and clear cells.[11] Rarely, obstruction of the glandular collecting duct can result in dilation of distal acini and a grossly recognizable "tumor" (mucocele); we have seen one such lesion that measured 3 cm in diameter and that arose in the lower trachea of a patient with cystic fibrosis.

Tracheobronchial gland tumors need to be distinguished from an unusual condition termed *mucoid pseudotumor*.[12, 13] In this abnormality, a focal accumulation of thick, tenacious mucus adheres to the tracheal or proximal bronchial wall, creating a hemispheric opacity that closely mimics a primary or secondary malignant neoplasm; although the deposits are generally small, some measure 2 cm in their largest diameter.[13] The nonneoplastic nature of the condition can be confirmed by its disappearance on a subsequent study or upward migration of the mucous plug following an episode of vigorous coughing.

SPECIFIC TUMORS

Adenoid Cystic Carcinoma

Adenoid cystic carcinoma (cylindroma) is a distinctive neoplasm characterized by local infiltrative growth and a variable but frequently prolonged clinical course. Although precise figures are difficult to obtain, it is clearly the most common subtype of tracheobronchial gland tumor, probably accounting for 75% to 80% of reported cases. Approximately 80% arise with about equal frequency in the trachea and main bronchi;[14, 15] approximately 10% to 15% develop in the lung periphery.[16] Although adenoid cystic carcinoma forms an extremely small proportion of primary neoplasms arising in the bronchi, its relative incidence in the trachea is much higher where, with squamous cell carcinoma, it comprises the vast majority of primary tumors.[2, 3, 5, 17] Within the trachea, most tumors arise in the lower or upper third, with a tendency to originate at the lateral and posterolateral wall near the junction of the cartilaginous and membranous portions.[3, 5, 18]

Most tumors are discovered in middle age; the mean age in two series of 16 and 38 patients was 51 and 45 years, respectively.[19, 20] There is no sex predominance.[5, 14, 18] The etiology is unknown. In series in which histories were adequate, cigarette smoking has not been associated.[1, 18] One case has been reported in which an endotracheal tumor was discovered in an 18-year-old patient who had received radiation therapy 10 years previously for an "enlarged thymus."[18]

Pathologically, adenoid cystic carcinoma characteristically grows into the airway lumen, forming a smooth-surfaced, somewhat polypoid tumor (Fig. 33–2); occasionally, growth is circumferential and annular. Submucosal extension, sometimes to a considerable distance from the main tumor, is not uncommon;[14, 21] cases involving the entire trachea or extending from the lung periphery to the proximal

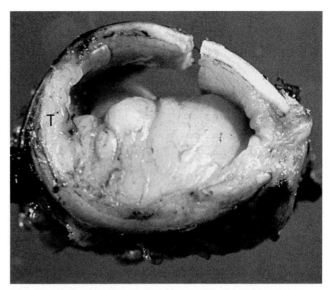

Figure 33–2. Adenoid Cystic Carcinoma. A magnified view of a cross section of the mid-portion of the trachea shows a somewhat lobulated tumor almost completely obstructing the lumen. The surface of the neoplasm is smooth, suggesting that it is composed of intact tracheal epithelium. Although tumor is present in the lateral tracheal wall (T), it does not appear to extend into the adjacent soft tissue.

bronchi have been reported.[22] The overlying tracheobronchial epithelium is usually intact, although it may ulcerate. Cut sections of the tumor typically reveal a white to tan surface without evidence of necrosis or hemorrhage.

The histologic appearance is identical to that of salivary gland tumors, consisting most commonly of rather uniform cells with relatively little cytoplasm arranged in well-defined nests of variable size (Fig. 33–3).[14, 19, 21, 23] The nests frequently have a cribriform pattern in which the cells are separated by well-defined cystic spaces containing a mucinous substance that stains strongly with alcian blue and weakly with periodic acid–Schiff (PAS);[24] occasionally, the intercellular material has a homogeneous, eosinophilic (hyalinized) appearance. Trabecular and solid histologic patterns can also be seen.[19] Mitotic activity and necrosis are seldom observed. The tumor may extend directly into and destroy cartilage, and perineural invasion is frequent. Ultrastructurally, neoplastic cells show evidence of both epithelial differentiation (with true gland formation) and myoepithelial differentiation (with prominent cytoplasmic filaments and abundant basal laminae);[24] such findings may be helpful in the distinction from basaloid carcinoma.[25] Immunohistochemical reactions to low-molecular-weight keratin, actin, and vimentin are usually positive;[1, 19] that for protein S-100 is variable.

The conventional radiographic features of adenoid cystic carcinoma consist of an endotracheal or endobronchial lobulated, polypoid or smooth, hemispheric mass that encroaches on the airway lumen to a variable degree (Fig. 33–4).[26, 27] Since approximately 75% of the tracheal lumen must be narrowed before dyspnea becomes evident,[26] the tumors are apt to be disturbingly large by the time the diagnosis is made. Circumferential involvement may result in a radiographic appearance resembling tracheal stenosis.[27] Rarely, a tumor presents as a solitary nodule (Fig. 33–5).

CT is superior to chest radiography in demonstrating

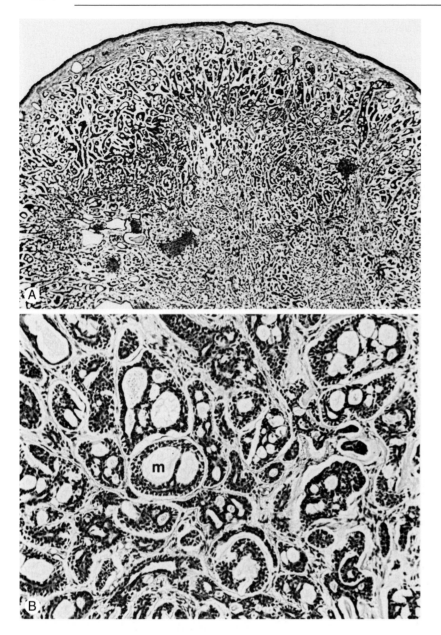

Figure 33–3. Adenoid Cystic Carcinoma. A section from a tracheal tumor shows *(A)* an intact surface epithelium overlying a clearly infiltrating neoplasm. A magnified view *(B)* reveals well-defined nests of tumor cells, many of which possess a prominent cribriform pattern *(arrow)*. Numerous cystic spaces, some containing lightly stained mucinous material (m), are present within the nests. *(A,* ×20; *B,* ×150.)

the presence of tracheal tumors and is particularly helpful in assessing the presence of extraluminal extent and mediastinal invasion (Fig. 33–6; *see also* Fig. 33–4).[7, 28] In one study of six patients who were evaluated by CT scanning, extratracheal extension of tumor was demonstrated in all six;[29] however, the investigators indicated that CT tended to underestimate the longitudinal extent of the tumor (because of partial volume averaging and the tendency of the tumor to infiltrate beneath the mucosa), an important caveat to bear in mind considering the advances in tracheal resection and carinal reconstructive surgery.[30] Assessment of tracheal abnormalities can be greatly improved with the use of thin-section (3- to 5-mm-collimation scans) and spiral CT, which allows continuous data acquisition and results in high-quality multiplanar reconstructions and improved spatial resolution over conventional CT.[31, 32]

Clinical features are similar to those of other tumors that show predominantly intraluminal growth, consisting of cough, hoarseness, hemoptysis, dyspnea, wheeze, and recur-

rent pneumonitis. As with other proximal airway tumors, a history of "asthma" is not uncommon,[5] sometimes progressing in severity despite therapy. Occasionally, a tumor arising in the upper trachea extends anteriorly and presents as a "thyroid" nodule.[33, 34] A case has been reported in which the presenting signs and symptoms were those of Pancoast's syndrome.[35]

Endoscopy typically reveals a smooth-surfaced, sometimes lobulated tumor partly or completely occluding the airway lumen. Cytologic diagnosis from bronchial washing specimen has been reported but is rare.[36, 37] Pathologic diagnosis may be difficult with the small and sometimes partly crushed biopsy fragments obtained by endoscopy, in which case the tumor may be confused with poorly differentiated carcinoma.[38] A single case has been reported of a patient who had an elevated serum level of the cancer-associated antigen CA19-9.[39]

The clinical course is often prolonged, and the overall prognosis is much better than that of the more common

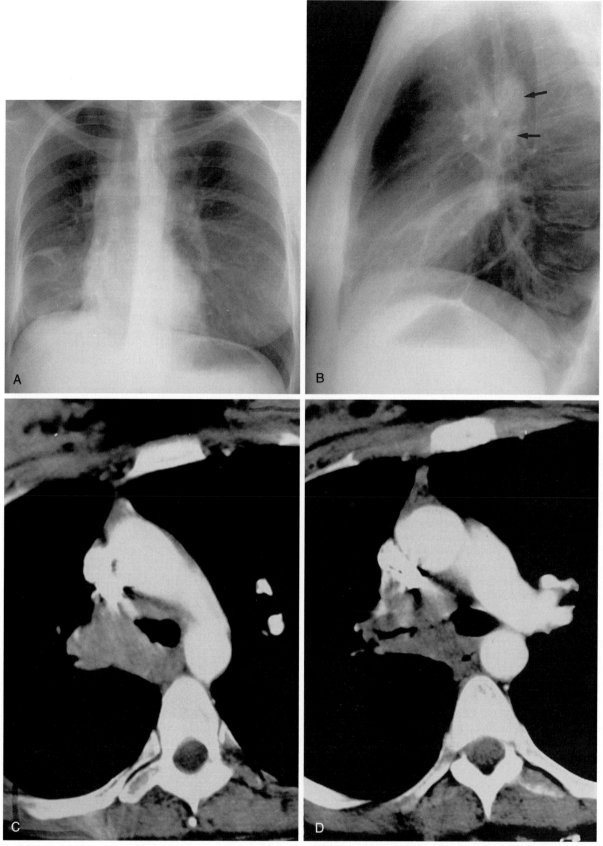

Figure 33–4. Adenoid Cystic Carcinoma. A 27-year-old man presented with progressive shortness of breath. Posteroanterior and lateral chest radiographs *(A* and *B)* demonstrate areas of atelectasis in the right lower and middle lobes. The lateral radiograph also shows thickening of the posterior wall of the distal trachea and right main bronchus *(arrows).* Contrast-enhanced CT scans *(C* and *D)* demonstrate circumferential tumor at the level of the tracheal carina and right main and right upper lobe bronchi associated with narrowing of the lumen. Focal extension into the left main bronchus is also evident.

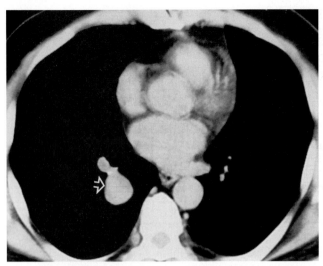

Figure 33–5. Adenoid Cystic Carcinoma. A CT scan in a 64-year-old man demonstrates a smoothly marginated 2-cm-diameter nodule *(arrow)* in the right lower lobe. Note homogeneous enhancement with intravenous contrast medium.

forms of pulmonary carcinoma.[2, 5, 40] Although approximately 50% of patients described in the older literature either died of the neoplasm or developed recurrent disease,[15] the more sophisticated diagnostic and therapeutic techniques available currently may be expected to result in cure in a higher proportion of cases, especially when the tumor is relatively small. For example, the overall 5-year survival rate in one relatively recent review was 80%.[2] In another series of 65 patients, the 5- and 10-year survival rates, respectively, were 73% and 57%.[41] In a third review of 32 patients seen over a 32-year period (1963 to 1995), of whom 16 underwent complete, potentially curative resection and 16 underwent partial resection (residual tumor at the airway margin on final pathologic examination), mean survival was approximately 10 years in the former group and 7.5 years in the latter.[20] An association between histologic type and both behavior and prognosis (the solid pattern tending to grow predominantly extraluminally and to be more likely to metastasize) has been suggested by some,[42] but not all,[19] investigators. No association of prognosis with nuclear organizer region (AgNOR) counts was documented in one study.[43]

Distant metastases are relatively uncommon, and death is usually the result of local recurrence and intrathoracic complications.[18, 23, 44] Because of the rather slow tumor growth, patients must be followed for a considerable period before the final outcome is established; death from recurrent disease has been documented up to 30 years after the initial discovery of the tumor.[5]

Mucoepidermoid Carcinoma

After adenoid cystic carcinoma, mucoepidermoid carcinoma is probably the most common form of tracheobronchial gland neoplasm;[45–47] despite this, only seven cases (two tracheal and five bronchial) were identified in one series during the same period as 4,250 primary pulmonary carcinomas (a proportion of only 0.16%).[48] A review of the files of the Armed Forces Institute of Pathology (AFIP) published

in 1987 revealed 58 cases.[46] Tumors can occur from childhood to old age; in the AFIP series, the average age of people with low-grade tumors was 35 years and with high-grade forms, 45 years.[46] A substantial number are discovered in people younger than 20 years of age.[46, 49] Although some authors have documented a male-to-female predominance,[45] others have found the reverse to be true.[46]

The precise histogenesis is uncertain. In the salivary gland, the tumor is believed to arise from the glandular duct;[45] however, since there is not a precise morphologic correlation between salivary and tracheobronchial glandular ducts, an origin from the latter is not certain. Little is known concerning etiology; although a history of cigarette smoking has been noted by some authors,[50] it has been absent in other series.[45]

The lesion is usually said to occur in two forms:[21, 45, 46] (1) a low-grade tumor with minimal nuclear pleomorphism, few mitotic figures, and a benign clinical course; and (2) a neoplasm showing more atypical cytologic features and a relatively aggressive course. Although there is good clinico-pathologic evidence confirming the existence of the former type, whether or not the latter is a separate entity has been questioned.[45] The main reason for this is its histologic similarity with mixed pulmonary carcinomas (such as adenosquamous carcinoma), which undoubtedly are much more common. Although it is certainly possible that some cases reported as high-grade mucoepidermoid carcinoma are better considered adenosquamous carcinoma,[51, 52] the ultrastructural and light microscopic similarities of some high- and low-grade tumors and the occasional reports of the coexistence of both histologic patterns in the same tumor [21, 53, 54] suggest that both are real entities.[45, 46] Perhaps because of the difficulty of confident diagnosis, the reported incidence of the

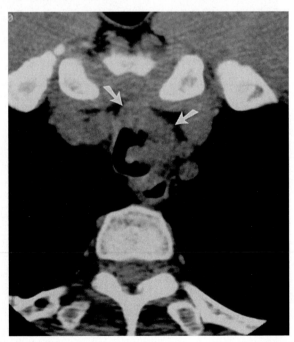

Figure 33–6. Adenoid Cystic Carcinoma of the Trachea. A 3-mm-collimation CT scan performed without intravenous contrast agent demonstrates an endotracheal tumor with extensive involvement of the tracheal wall and extension into the adjacent mediastinum *(arrows).* The patient was a 36-year-old man. The tumor was completely resected.

high-grade variant is considerably less than that of the low-grade form.[45, 46]

Most tumors are situated in the main or lobar bronchi;[46, 50] uncommonly, they involve the lung periphery or the trachea, in the latter site usually in a supracarinal location.[53, 55] Most grow within the airway lumen and produce a polypoid mass with an intact or occasionally ulcerated surface epithelium; peripheral extension within the bronchial lumen occurs sometimes.[56] Low-grade tumors are often confined to the bronchial wall; by contrast, the high-grade form not uncommonly extends into the peribronchial interstitium or adjacent lung parenchyma.

Histologically, low-grade mucoepidermoid carcinoma is composed of uniform cells arranged in sheets or trabeculae that are either solid or contain well-defined cystlike spaces (Fig. 33–7).[1, 21, 45, 46, 56] Individual cells are polygonal or columnar and have cytoplasm that is typically either vacuo-lated and mucus containing or rather homogeneous and eosinophilic (intermediate cells); rarely, they have an oxyphilic or clear appearance.[46, 57] Intermediate cells are arranged in a sheetlike "epidermoid" fashion. Evidence of true squamous differentiation, such as individual cell keratinization and intercellular bridge formation, can be seen but is infrequent; keratin pearl formation is typically absent. The intimate association of mucus-secreting and epidermoid cells is responsible for the designation "mucoepidermoid." Nuclear pleomorphism is mild, and mitotic figures are sparse or absent. A papillary variant of the tumor has been described.[58] Although high-grade mucoepidermoid carcinoma has an overall pattern similar to that of the low-grade form, it shows areas of cytologic atypia, relatively frequent mitoses, and foci of necrosis.[46]

The radiologic appearance depends on tumor location, size, and presence or absence of obstructive pneumonitis. In

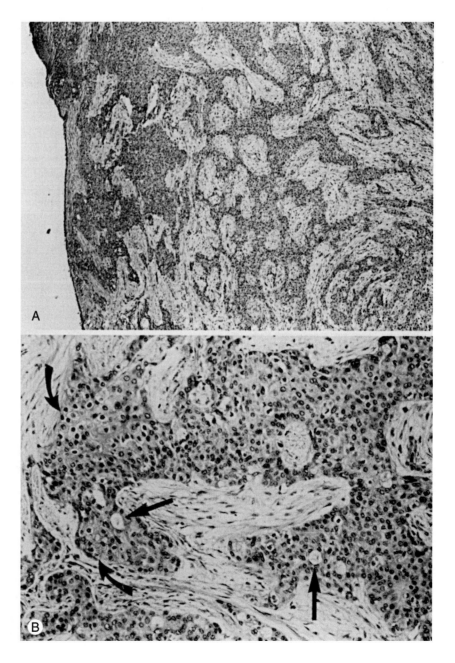

Figure 33–7. Low-Grade Mucoepidermoid Carcinoma. A section of a polypoid tumor of the right main bronchus from a 30-year-old woman *(A)* shows anastomosing sheets of cells in a fibroblastic stroma. At higher magnification *(B)*, focal clusters of cells with more abundant cytoplasm and well-defined borders can be identified, representing an epidermoid appearance *(curved arrows)*. Small glandular spaces containing mucin *(straight arrows)* are also present. Note the lack of necrosis and mitotic figures and uniformity of cell nuclei. The tumor was closely excised by sleeve resection; there was no evidence of recurrence or metastases at follow-up 15 years later. *(A, ×44; B, ×170.)*

the AFIP review of 58 cases, radiographs showed a solitary nodule or mass in 41 and parenchymal consolidation in 16;[46] in 1 patient, the radiograph was considered to be normal. The radiographic appearance of low- and high-grade forms was similar. Less commonly, the tumors involve the trachea rather than the bronchi and present as a polypoid intraluminal nodule on the radiograph and CT (see Fig. 33–1).[28] As with adenoid cystic carcinoma, CT scanning allows better assessment of intraluminal tumor as well as the extent of involvement of the tracheal wall and mediastinum (Fig. 33–8).[7, 28]

As might be expected, symptoms are related predominantly to intraluminal growth and include cough, hemoptysis, wheeze, recurrent pneumonia, and fever.[45] A history of "asthma" can be obtained in some patients.[59]

Low-grade tumors are typically slow growing; provided they are surgically resectable, the prognosis is usually excellent, with no evidence of local recurrence or metastases, even when treated with relatively conservative sleeve resection.[46, 47] Despite this, occasional patients develop widespread metastases and death,[60, 61] sometimes with only limited invasion at the primary bronchial site.[62] Behavior of the high-grade form, although worse than that of low-grade tumors, appears to be better than the more common forms of pulmonary carcinoma; of 13 patients with follow-up in the AFIP series, 8 were alive without evidence of disease at an average of 48 months after surgery.[46]

Acinic Cell Carcinoma

Acinic cell carcinoma is a rare pulmonary neoplasm; in a review published in 1992 only nine cases were identified.[63] Histologically, the tumor is composed of polygonal cells arranged in acini, small nests, sheets, or tubulopapillary formations. The cells contain abundant, finely granular, PAS-positive, diastase-resistant cytoplasm. Electron microscopic examination reveals intracytoplasmic membrane-bound granules similar to zymogen granules of the normal salivary gland. The tumor has been reported in the trachea,[64] bronchi,[65] and lung periphery without clear airway association.[66] Because of its rarity and varied histologic appearance, it can be confused with several other pulmonary neoplasms, including oncocytic carcinoid tumor, granular cell tumor, and clear cell tumor.[1] Ultrastructural and immunohistochemical investigations should enable confident distinction between them.

Patients may present with clinical and radiologic features of airway obstruction or with an asymptomatic solitary pulmonary nodule.[1] Salivary gland acinic cell tumors behave as low-grade neoplasms, recurrence and extension usually being local and metastases exceptional. Although the number and follow-up period of reported tracheobronchial tumors are small, there is nothing to suggest a different behavior in this location.[63]

Pleomorphic Adenoma

Pleomorphic adenoma (mixed tumor) arising in the lung is also a rare form of tracheobronchial gland tumor.[21, 67–69] Histologic appearances are similar to those of the more common salivary gland neoplasms, consisting of an epithelial component that forms sheets or small glandlike structures and a myoepithelial component that is frequently associated with a myxomatous stroma and that sometimes undergoes cartilaginous transformation.[70] Because the histologic pattern is often quite variable in a particular tumor, considerable difficulty can be encountered in making the diagnosis with small biopsy fragments.[71]

Most tumors occur in the trachea or proximal bronchi and cause signs and symptoms as a result of luminal obstruction; however, some are located in the lung periphery, apparently unassociated with an airway.[70, 72] The majority are well circumscribed, show minimal cytologic atypia, and have few mitoses. Although local recurrences have occasionally been reported,[73] metastases are generally absent; however, some

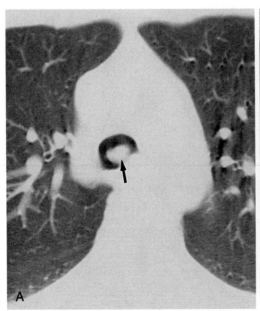

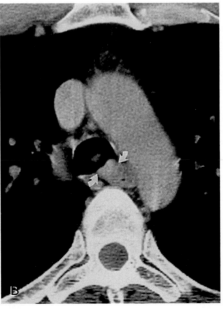

Figure 33–8. Mucoepidermoid Carcinoma of the Trachea. Five-millimeters-collimation CT scans *(A and B)* at the level of the aortic arch demonstrate an endotracheal tumor *(straight arrows)* associated with thickening of the posterolateral wall of the trachea *(curved arrow).* At surgery, the tumor was shown to be an exophytic mucoepidermoid carcinoma primarily involving the membranous trachea. The patient was a 44-year-old man who presented with hemoptysis.

tumors have a more aggressive pathologic appearance, in which case metastases and death can occur.[70, 74]

Oncocytoma

An oncocytoma (oxyphilic adenoma) is a benign neoplasm composed of cells that have a central, compact nucleus and abundant granular eosinophilic cytoplasm caused by the presence of numerous mitochondria.[75, 76] Individual or small clusters of cells with identical features (termed *oncocytes*) are sometimes present in both glandular and ductal portions of the normal tracheobronchial gland (*see* page 14),[77] and it has been hypothesized that the neoplasm may have its origin in these structures.[78] Since some carcinoid tumors,[44, 79] mucoepidermoid carcinomas,[46, 57] and mucous gland adenomas[80] can show focal (and at times extensive) oncocytic change, thorough tissue sampling as well as electron-microscopic studies must be performed before a tumor can be confidently designated an oncocytoma.

Well-documented pulmonary oncocytomas have been reported rarely.[75, 76, 78, 81–83] Most have had an origin in a proximal bronchus; one has been reported in a parenchymal location unrelated to an identifiable airway.[78] Although all have behaved in an indolent fashion, local tissue infiltration and lymph node metastases have been documented in one case.[82]

Mucous Gland Adenoma

Mucous gland adenoma (bronchial cystadenoma) is an uncommon tumor that histologically resembles the mucus-secreting component of the tracheobronchial gland.[21, 84–86] The majority arise within main, lobar, or segmental bronchi, although one case has been reported in which a solitary parenchymal nodule presumably arose in a subsegmental bronchus.[87] One group identified 41 previously reported cases and documented 10 more in a 1995 review.[84]

Grossly, the tumor usually projects into the bronchial lumen as a smooth-surfaced obstructing mass; the cut surface may show multiple small cystic spaces that have a mucoid appearance. Microscopically, the neoplasm consists of numerous irregularly arranged, tubular or dilated glands lined by a single layer of columnar (occasionally flattened) mucus-secreting cells;[84] oncocytic, clear, and ciliated cells are seen occasionally.[80] Cytologic atypia, mitotic figures, and necrosis are absent. The glands may be seen to connect to the surface epithelium by short ducts.[21] In some cases, papillary projections of the surface epithelium overlie the adenomatous mass.[84, 88]

Radiologic and clinical features are nonspecific and usually reflect airway obstruction. The tumor appears to be truly benign, neither recurrence after surgical excision nor metastases having been reported.

REFERENCES

1. Moran CA: Primary salivary gland–type tumors of the lung. Semin Diagn Pathol 12:106, 1995.
2. Gelder CM, Hetzel MR: Primary tracheal tumours: A national survey. Thorax 48:688, 1993.
3. Howard DJ, Haribhakti VV: Primary tumours of the trachea: Analysis of clinical features and treatment results. J Laryngol Otol 108:230, 1994.
4. Conlan AA, Payne WS, Woolner LB, et al: Adenoid cystic carcinoma (cylindroma) and mucoepidermoid carcinoma of the bronchus: Factors affecting survival. J Thorac Cardiovasc Surg 76:369, 1978.
5. Houston HE, Payne WS, Harrison EG Jr, et al: Primary cancers of the trachea. Arch Surg 99:132, 1969.
6. Janower ML, Grillo HC, MacMillan AS Jr, et al: The radiological appearance of carcinoma of the trachea. Radiology 96:39, 1970.
7. Kwong JS, Adler BD, Padley SPG, et al: Diagnosis of diseases of the trachea and main bronchi: Chest radiography versus CT. Am J Roentgenol 161:519, 1993.
8. Strickler JG, Hegstrom J, Thomas MJ, et al: Myoepithelioma of the lung. Arch Pathol Lab Med 111:1082, 1987.
9. Horinouchi H, Ishihara T, Kawamura M, et al: Epithelial myoepithelial tumour of the tracheal gland. J Clin Pathol 46:185, 1993.
10. Nistal M, Garcia-Viera M, Martinez-Garcia C, et al: Epithelial-myoepithelial tumor of the bronchus. Am J Surg Pathol 18:421, 1994.
11. Akhtar M, Young I, Reyes F: Bronchial adenoma with polymorphous features. Cancer 33:1572, 1974.
12. Karasick S, Karasick S, Lally JF: Mucoid pseudotumors of the tracheobronchial tree in two cases. Am J Roentgenol 132:459, 1979.
13. Westra D: Mucus plugs—phantom tumors of the major air passages: The tomographic appearances. Fortschr Geb Rontgenstr Nuklearmed 112:428, 1975.
14. Reid JD: Adenoid cystic carcinoma (cylindroma) of the bronchial tree. Cancer 5:685, 1952.
15. Enterline HT, Schoenberg HW: Carcinoma (cylindromatous type) of trachea and bronchi and bronchial adenoma: A comparative study. Cancer 7:663, 1954.
16. Gallagher CG, Stark R, Teskey J, et al: Atypical manifestations of pulmonary adenoid cystic carcinoma. Br J Dis Chest 80:396, 1986.
17. Olmedo G, Rosenberg M, Fonseca R: Primary tumors of the trachea: Clinicopathologic features and surgical results. Chest 81:701, 1982.
18. Hajdu SI, Huvos AG, Goodner JT, et al: Carcinoma of the trachea: Clinicopathologic study of 41 cases. Cancer 25:1448, 1970.
19. Moran CA, Suster S, Koss MN: Primary adenoid cystic carcinoma of the lung: A clinicopathologic and immunohistochemical study of 16 cases. Cancer 73:1390, 1994.
20. Maziak DE, Todd TR, Keshavjee SH, et al: Adenoid cystic carcinoma of the airway: Thirty-two-year experience. J Thorac Cardiovasc Surg 112:1522, 1996.
21. Spencer H: Bronchial mucous gland tumors. Virchows Arch [Pathol Anat Histol] 383:101, 1979.
22. Inoue H, Iwashita A, Kanegae H, et al: Peripheral pulmonary adenoid cystic carcinoma with substantial extension to the proximal bronchus. Thorax 46:147, 1991.
23. Markel SF, Abell MR: Adenocystic basal cell carcinoma of the trachea. J Thorac Cardiovasc Surg 48:211, 1964.
24. Lawrence JB, Mazur MT: Adenoid cystic carcinoma: A comparative pathologic study of tumors in salivary gland, breast, lung, and cervix. Hum Pathol 13:916, 1982.
25. Hewan-Lowe K, Dardick I: Ultrastructural distinction of basaloid-squamous carcinoma and adenoid cystic carcinoma. Ultrastruct Pathol 19:371, 1995.
26. Cleveland RH, Nice CM, Ziskind J: Primary adenoid cystic carcinoma (cylindroma) of the trachea. Radiology 122:597, 1977.
27. McCarthy MJ, Rosado-de-Christenson ML: Tumors of the trachea. J Thorac Imag 10:180, 1995.
28. Kwong JS, Müller NL, Miller RR: Diseases of the trachea and main-stem bronchi: Correlation of CT with pathologic findings. RadioGraphics 12:645, 1992.
29. Spizarny DL, Shepard J-AO, McLoud TC, et al: CT of adenoid cystic carcinoma of the trachea. Am J Roentgenol 146:1129, 1986.
30. Bueno R, Wain JC, Wright CD, et al: Bronchoplasty in the management of low-grade airway neoplasms and benign bronchial stenoses. Ann Thorac Surg 62:824, 1996.
31. Naidich DP: Helical computed tomography of the thorax. Radiol Clin North Am 32:759, 1994.
32. Newmark GM, Conces DJ Jr, Kopecky KK: Spiral CT evaluation of the trachea and bronchi. J Comput Assist Tomogr 18:552, 1994.
33. Zirkin HJ, Tovi F: Tracheal carcinoma presenting as a thyroid tumor. J Surg Oncol 26:268, 1984.
34. Na DG, Han MH, Kim KH, et al: Primary adenoid cystic carcinoma of the cervical trachea mimicking thyroid tumor: CT evaluation. J Comput Assist Tomogr 19:559, 1995.
35. Hatton MQ, Allen MB, Cooke NJ: Pancoast syndrome: An unusual presentation of adenoid cystic carcinoma. Eur Respir J 6:271, 1993.
36. Radhika S, Dey P, Rajwanshi A, et al: Adenoid cystic carcinoma in a bronchial washing: A case report. Acta Cytol 37:97, 1993.
37. Chen KT: Exfoliative cytology of tracheobronchial adenoid cystic carcinoma. Diag Cytopathol 15:132, 1996.
38. Lin O, Harkin TJ, Jagirdar J: Basaloid-squamous cell carcinoma of the bronchus: Report of a case with review of the literature. Arch Pathol Lab Med 119:1167, 1995.
39. Tamura S, Nakano T, Yamaguchi K, et al: A case of adenoid cystic carcinoma of the bronchus producing cancer-associated antigen CA19-9. Intern Med 31:363, 1992.
40. Grillo HC, Mathisen DJ, Wain JC: Management of tumors of the trachea. Oncology 6:61, 1992.
41. Regnard JF, Fourquier P, Levasseur P: Results and prognostic factors in resections of primary tracheal tumors: A multicenter, retrospective study. The French Society of Cardiovascular Surgery. J Thorac Cardiovasc Surg 111:808, 1996.
42. Nomori H, Kaseda S, Kobayashi K, et al: Adenoid cystic carcinoma of the trachea and main-stem bronchus: A clinical, histopathologic, and immunohistochemical study. J Thorac Cardiovasc Surg 96:271, 1988.
43. Fonseca I, Soares J: Adenoid cystic carcinoma: A study of nucleolar organizer region (AgNOR) counts and their relation to prognosis. J Pathol 169:255, 1993.
44. Weiss L, Ingram M: Adenomatoid bronchial tumors: A consideration of the carcinoid tumors and the salivary tumors of the bronchial tree. Cancer 14:161, 1961.
45. Klacsmann PG, Olson JL, Eggleston JC: Mucoepidermoid carcinoma of the bronchus: An electron microscopic study of the low-grade and the high-grade variants. Cancer 43:1720, 1979.
46. Yousem SA, Hochholzer L: Mucoepidermoid tumors of the lung. Cancer 60:1346, 1987.
47. Heitmiller RF, Mathisen DJ, Ferry JA, et al: Mucoepidermoid lung tumors. Ann Thorac Surg 47:394, 1989.
48. Leonardi HK, Jung-Legg Y, Legg MA, et al: Tracheobronchial mucoepidermoid carcinoma: Clinicopathological features and results of treatment. J Thorac Cardiovasc Surg 76:431, 1978.
49. Tsuchiya H, Nagashima K, Ohashi S, et al: Childhood bronchial mucoepidermoid tumors. J Pediatr Surg 32:106, 1997.
50. Turnbull AD, Huvos AG, Goodner JT, et al: Mucoepidermoid tumors of bronchial glands. Cancer 28:539, 1971.
51. Axelsson C, Burcharth F, Johansen AA: Mucoepidermoid lung tumors. J Thorac Cardiovasc Surg 65:902, 1973.
52. Ozlu C, Christopherson WM, Allen JD Jr: Muco-epidermoid tumors of the bronchus. J Thorac Cardiovasc Surg 42:24, 1961.
53. Larson RE, Woolner LB, Payne WS: Mucoepidermoid tumor of the trachea: Report of a case. J Thorac Cardiovasc Surg 50:131, 1965.
54. Dowling EA, Miller RE, Johnson IM, et al: Mucoepidermoid tumors of the bronchi. Surgery 52:600, 1962.
55. Trentini GP, Palmieri B: Mucoepidermoid tumor of the trachea. Chest 62:336, 1972.
56. Sniffen RC, Soutter L, Robbins LL: Muco-epidermoid tumors of the bronchus arising from surface epithelium. Am J Pathol 34:671, 1958.
57. Stafford JR, Pollock WJ, Wenzel BC: Oncocytic mucoepidermoid tumor of the bronchus. Cancer 54:94, 1984.
58. Guillou L, de Luze P, Zysset F, et al: Papillary variant of low-grade mucoepidermoid carcinoma—an unusual bronchial neoplasm: A light microscopic, ultrastructural, and immunohistochemical study. Am J Clin Pathol 101:269, 1994.
59. Patel RG, Norman JR: Unilateral hyperlucency with left lower lobe mass in a patient with bronchial asthma. Chest 107:569, 1995.
60. Barsky SH, Martin SE, Matthews M, et al: "Low-grade" mucoepidermoid carcinoma of the bronchus with "high-grade" biological behavior. Cancer 51:1505, 1983.
61. Metcalf JS, Maize JC, Shaw EB: Bronchial mucoepidermoid carcinoma metastatic to skin: Report of a case and review of the literature. Cancer 58:2556, 1986.
62. Wolf KM, Mehta D, Claypool WD: Mucoepidermoid carcinoma of the lung with intracranial metastases. Chest 94:435, 1988.
63. Moran CA, Suster S, Koss MN: Acinic cell carcinoma of the lung ("Fechner tumor"): A clinicopathologic, immunohistochemical, and ultrastructural study of five cases. Am J Surg Pathol 16:1039, 1992.
64. Ansari MA, Marchevsky A, Strick L, et al: Upper airway obstruction secondary to acinic cell carcinoma of the trachea: Use of Nd:YAG laser. Chest 110:1120, 1996.
65. Katz DR, Bubis JJ: Acinic cell tumor of the bronchus. Cancer 38:830, 1976.
66. Fechner RE, Bentinck BR, Asker JB Jr: Acinic cell tumor of the lung: A histologic and ultrastructural study. Cancer 29:501, 1972.
67. Kay S, Brooks JW: Benign mixed tumor of the trachea with seven-year follow-up. Cancer 25:1178, 1970.
68. Sweeney EC, McDermott M: Pleomorphic adenoma of the bronchus. J Clin Pathol 49:87, 1996.
69. Bizal JC, Righi PD, Kesler KA: Pleomorphic adenoma of the trachea. Otolaryngol Head Neck Surg 116:139, 1997.
70. Moran CA, Suster S, Askin FB, et al: Benign and malignant salivary gland–type mixed tumors of the lung: Clinicopathologic and immunohistochemical study of eight cases. Cancer 73:2481, 1994.
71. Clarke PJ, Dunnill MS, Gunning AJ: Mixed tumours of the lung: A report of three cases. Br J Dis Chest 80:80, 1986.
72. Sakamoto H, Uda H, Tanaka T, et al: Pleomorphic adenoma in the periphery of the lung: Report of a case and review of the literature. Arch Pathol Lab Med 115:393, 1991.
73. Payne WS, Schier J, Woolner LB: Mixed tumors of the bronchus (salivary gland type). J Thorac Cardiovasc Surg 49:663, 1965.

74. Hemmi A, Hiraoka H, Mori Y, et al: Malignant pleomorphic adenoma (malignant mixed tumor) of the trachea: Report of a case. Acta Pathol Jpn 38:1215, 1988.

75. Fechner RE, Bentinck BR: Ultrastructure of bronchial oncocytoma. Cancer 31:1451, 1973.

76. Tashiro Y, Iwata Y, Nabae T, et al: Pulmonary oncocytoma: Report of a case in conjunction with an immunohistochemical and ultrastructural study. Pathol Int 45:448, 1995.

77. Matsuba K, Takizawa T, Thurlbeck WM: Oncocytes in human bronchial mucus glands. Thorax 27:181, 1972.

78. Santos-Briz A, Terron J, Sastre R, et al: Oncocytoma of the lung. Cancer 40:1330, 1977.

79. Black WC III: Pulmonary oncocytoma. Cancer 23:1347, 1969.

80. Heard BE, Corrin B, Dewar A: Pathology of seven mucous cell adenomas of the bronchial glands, with particular reference to ultrastructure. Histopathology 9:687, 1985.

81. Cwierzyk TA, Glasberg SS, Virshup MA, et al: Pulmonary oncocytoma. Acta Cytol 29:620, 1985.

82. Nielsen AL: Malignant bronchial oncocytoma: Case report and review of literature. Hum Pathol 16:852, 1985.

83. Fechner RE, Bentinck BR: Ultrastructure of bronchial oncocytoma. Cancer 31:1451, 1973.

84. England DM, Hochholzer L: Truly benign "bronchial adenoma": Report of 10 cases of mucous gland adenoma with immunohistochemical and ultrastructural findings. Am J Surg Pathol 19:887, 1995.

85. Heard BE, Corrin B, Dewar A: Pathology of seven mucous cell adenomas of the bronchial glands, with particular reference to ultrastructure. Histopathology 9:687, 1985.

86. Emory WB, Mitchell WT Jr, Hatch HB Jr: Mucous gland adenoma of the bronchus. Am Rev Resp Dis 108:1407, 1973.

87. Weinberger MA, Katz S, Davis EW: Peripheral bronchial adenoma of mucous gland type: Clinical and pathologic aspects. J Thorac Surg 29:626, 1955.

88. Spencer H, Dail DH, Arneaud J: Noninvasive bronchial epithelial papillary tumors. Cancer 45:1486, 1980.

CHAPTER 34

Miscellaneous Epithelial Tumors

TRACHEOBRONCHIAL PAPILLOMAS

A *papilloma* can be defined as a branching or coarsely lobulated tumor composed of epithelium-lined fibrovascular papillae that arise from and project above an epithelial surface. Although such tumors within the lungs can be classified histologically into several types, depending largely on the nature of the surface lining,[1] from clinical and radiologic points of view they are best considered under the headings "multiple" and "solitary." These tumors should be distinguished from conditions in which a papillary proliferation of airway epithelium represents a hyperplastic process, as on the surface of some mucous gland adenomas (*see* page 1259) and some inflammatory tracheobronchial polyps (*see* page 1371).

Multiple Papillomas

Multiple papillomas of the respiratory tract occur most commonly in the larynx of children between 18 months and 3 years of age.[2] In the majority of patients, they remain localized and eventually disappear spontaneously, although excised tumors sometimes recur or new ones appear, especially adjacent to a tracheostomy site. Infrequently (about 2% of the combined cases in four large series),[3] they arise in the respiratory tract distal to the larynx, where they can cause partial or complete airway obstruction (Fig. 34–1). Most such cases are limited to the trachea; however, extension into the bronchi, bronchioles, and even alveolar airspaces can occur.[3–5] In one review, the average time between the appearance of lesions in the larynx and the detection of bronchopulmonary disease was 10 years;[6] cases have been reported as having an interval as long as 34 years after the initial appearance of laryngeal papillomas.[7] Rarely, bronchial papillomas precede the appearance of laryngeal or tracheal lesions or develop in their absence.[5, 8, 9] Although the disease usually develops initially in children, it can also present in adults.[10–12]

There is now convincing evidence from immunohistochemical, ultrastructural, and molecular biologic studies that the majority, if not all, cases of multiple airway papillomas are caused by human papillomavirus.[13–15] Although type 11 has been implicated most commonly, a variety of other types may be seen; there is evidence that specific types (e.g., 16 and 18) are more likely to be associated with malignant transformation (*see* farther on).[16] The pathogenesis of papilloma formation in the lower respiratory tract has been debated. The high incidence of tracheal and lower airway involvement in patients with laryngeal papillomatosis who undergo tracheostomy supports the role of local trauma in the spread of disease.[17, 18] Although some investigators have hypothesized that this association is related to implantation of fragments of inhaled papillomas from the larynx,[19] it is perhaps more likely that trauma-induced epithelial metaplasia is responsible.[20] It is also probable that multifocal viral infection is responsible, a hypothesis supported by the find-

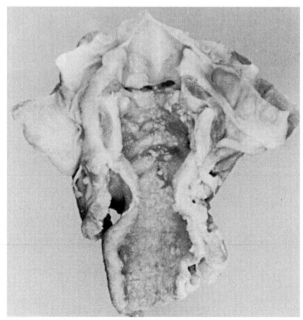

Figure 34–1. Multiple Tracheal Papillomas. The specimen consists of a trachea and larynx from a 26-year-old man who had had recurrent laryngotracheobronchial papillomas since childhood. The entire tracheal mucosa has an irregular, somewhat velvety appearance caused by the presence of innumerable minute papillomas. The narrowing in the midportion of the trachea represents a stricture related to a previous tracheostomy.

ing of papillomavirus DNA in normal mucosa in some cases.[21]

Pathologically, the tumors in the larynx, trachea, and bronchi are identical and consist of sessile or pedunculated papillary growths lined by a flattened squamous epithelium that usually shows normal maturation.[1, 22] Multinucleation and cytoplasmic vacuolation resembling the changes in condylomas of the genital tract can be seen in some cases.[5] Extension into the underlying airway mucosa occurs rarely.[23] Involvement of distal airways or alveolar air spaces may be microscopic or may result in solid or cavitated masses measuring up to several centimeters in diameter.[4, 7, 22, 24] Although true squamous cell carcinoma may be present (*see* farther on), extension into the surrounding parenchyma with filling of alveolar air spaces can be caused by proliferation of the papillomas themselves, simulating malignant invasion.[7] Depending on the extent and location of the tracheobronchial papillomas, the remaining lung can show bronchiectasis, obstructive pneumonitis, patchy fibrosis, or areas of acute inflammation with abscess formation.

Tracheal and bronchial papillomas may be identified on the radiograph and CT scan as small nodules projecting into the lumen of the airway.[25] On CT, the presence of numerous papillomas may be manifested as diffuse nodular thickening of the trachea.[26] The papillomas may lead to bronchial obstruction resulting in atelectasis, obstructive pneumonitis, and bronchiectasis.[27, 28] Involvement of distal airways and parenchyma can result in multiple sharply circumscribed nodules.[28, 29] These tend to be located in the perihilar lung parenchyma and are most numerous in the posterior half of the thorax.[28] The nodules may grow up to several centimeters in diameter, at which point they frequently become cavitated

and have walls measuring 2 to 3 mm in thickness (Fig. 34–2).[25, 28] Fluid levels can sometimes be identified.[28] As indicated previously, many of these cavities are related to papillomatosis; however, they may be caused by a necrotic squamous cell carcinoma[18] or an abscess secondary to obstructive pneumonitis.[30]

Clinically, the diagnosis should be suspected in any patient with a history of laryngeal papillomas who develops cough, hemoptysis, asthma-like symptoms, recurrent pneumonia, or atelectasis.[9, 11]

The prognosis is poor in patients with extensive spread of papillomas in the trachea and lungs;[19] airway obstruction and parenchymal infiltration can result in progressive dyspnea, infection, and, ultimately, death. In addition, there is a significant risk of the papillomas undergoing malignant transformation, not uncommonly in young individuals. As might be expected, the tumor is usually squamous cell carcinoma;[13, 22, 31–33] rarely, patients develop small cell carcinoma.[34] Although this complication occurs most commonly in patients who have a history of exposure to other potentially carcinogenic agents, such as radiation and cigarette smoke,[35] the virus may be the only apparent etiologic factor.[13, 33, 34, 36]

Solitary Papilloma

Solitary papillomas of the tracheobronchial tree are less common than the multiple form. They almost invariably occur in adults, often middle-aged or older, and usually men.[1, 30, 37–40] Using molecular biologic techniques, some

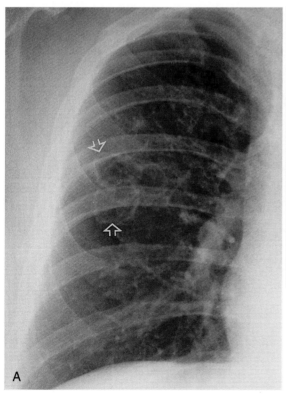

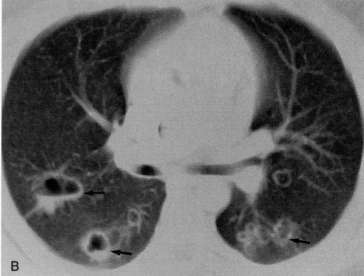

Figure 34–2. Tracheobronchial Papillomatosis. A view of the right lung from a posteroanterior chest radiograph *(A)* reveals several thin-walled cavities *(arrows)*. Similar findings were present in the left lung. A CT scan *(B)* demonstrates bilateral thin-walled cavities, several of which contain air-fluid levels *(arrows)*. The patient was a 31-year-old woman with long-standing papillomatosis. (Case courtesy of Dr. Jim Barrie, University of Alberta Hospital, Edmonton, Alberta.)

investigators have found the presence of human papillomavirus in a large proportion of cases.[16]

The papillomas are usually located in lobar or segmental bronchi, where they appear grossly as filiform or finely corrugated tumors 0.5 to 1.5 cm in diameter (Fig. 34–3); an exceptional tumor has been reported with a diameter of 5 cm.[41] Rare examples have been reported to arise in the trachea.[42] Most are histologically identical to those of the multiple form, consisting of mature squamous epithelium lining thin fibrovascular cores. Cytologic atypia and carcinoma *in situ* may also be seen, either in the papillary tumor itself or in the adjacent airway epithelium;[1, 40, 43] occasionally, clearly invasive squamous cell carcinoma is present.

Several less common but histologically distinctive papillary tumors have also been described, including those lined by transitional cell[1, 44] or columnar[45] epithelium and those lined by apparently normal ciliated respiratory epithelium.[46, 47] (The last-named types are probably best regarded as part of a histologic spectrum of inflammatory polyps [*see* page 1371]). Some bronchial gland tumors also have a surface papillary component.[48] Rarely, metastatic papillary adenocarcinoma occurs in an endobronchial location.[1]

The radiologic manifestations depend on the size and location of the papilloma. Many of those that occur in the trachea or main bronchi measure less than 1 cm in diameter and are not detected on the chest radiograph.[49] When radiologic and CT findings are evident, they usually consist of a polypoid mass projecting into the airway lumen (Fig. 34–4).[25, 50] Partial bronchial obstruction may result in reflex vasoconstriction leading to decreased perfusion and hyperlucency of the affected lung or lobe (Fig. 34–5). Complete obstruction is manifested by atelectasis and obstructive pneumonitis (Fig. 34–6).

A history of repeated or unresolved pneumonia or, occasionally, hemoptysis may be obtained. Sometimes, the tumor appears to undergo autoamputation at the site of its attachment to the airway wall, in which case the papilloma may be coughed up and the distal pneumonia will clear. As indicated, some papillomas are complicated by the development of dysplasia or carcinoma; there is evidence that the

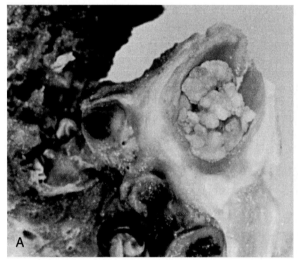

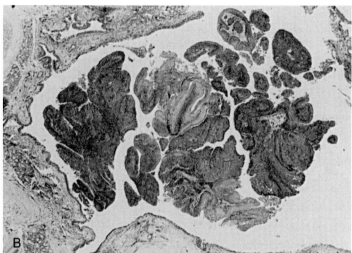

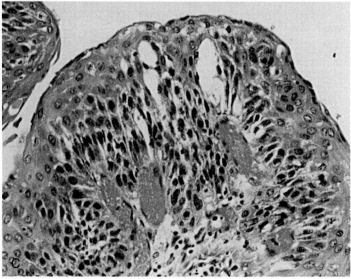

Figure 34–3. Solitary Bronchial Papilloma. A lower lobe bronchus *(A)* is almost completely occluded by a coarsely lobulated tumor confined to the airway lumen (Bar = 4 mm). Histologic sections at two different magnifications *(B* and *C)* show branching papillary projections lined by stratified squamous epithelium; there is mild cytologic atypia in the basal layer. Although this tumor was solitary, an identical histologic appearance is seen in the multiple form. *(B,* ×12; *C,* ×250.)

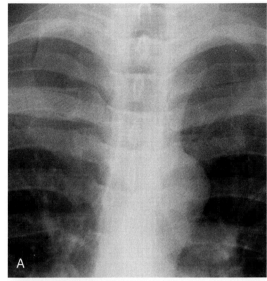

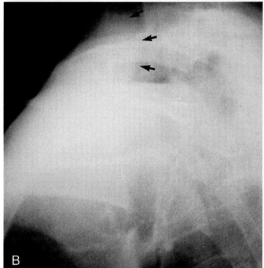

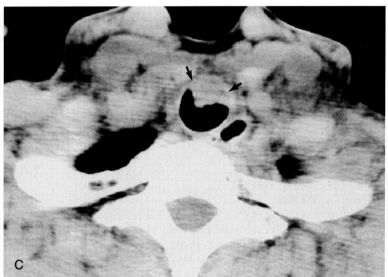

Figure 34–4. Tracheal Papilloma. Views of the trachea from posteroanterior *(A)* and lateral *(B)* chest radiographs demonstrate an endotracheal soft tissue mass. The tumor is best seen on the lateral view *(arrows)*. A CT scan *(C)* demonstrates a soft tissue tumor originating from the anterior aspect of the trachea *(arrows)*. There is no evidence of extension beyond the tracheal wall. The diagnosis of papilloma was confirmed at surgery. The patient was a 35-year-old woman.

presence of human papillomavirus types 16 and 18 is associated with this process, whereas type 11 papillomas remain benign.[16]

PULMONARY ADENOMAS

True adenomas of the lung are rare.* Some occur predominantly in the proximal airways and are believed to arise from the tracheobronchial mucous glands; these include pleomorphic, oxyphilic, and mucous gland adenomas *(see* page 1259). Other tumors are located predominantly in the lung periphery and appear to be derived from bronchiolar or alveolar epithelium; these include mucinous cystadenoma, papillary and alveolar adenomas, and (possibly) pneumocytoma (sclerosing hemangioma, *see* page 1364).

---

*As discussed elsewhere (*see* page 1229), use of the term *adenoma* to refer to carcinoid tumor, adenoid cystic carcinoma, or mucoepidermoid carcinoma is both semantically and conceptually inaccurate and should be avoided.

Mucinous Cystic Tumor

Mucinous cystic tumor (mucinous cystadenoma) is an unusual pulmonary tumor that has been hypothesized to represent a spectrum of neoplasia analagous to mucinous tumors of the appendix and ovary.[51-53] Most patients are between 40 and 70 years of age;[53] many have a history of cigarette smoking.

Reported tumors have ranged in size from 1 to 15 cm.[51, 52] Histologically, they consist of a unilocular (occasionally multilocular) cyst filled with mucus and enclosed by a fibrous capsule of variable thickness. The capsule itself is lined predominantly by a single layer of columnar, mucus-secreting epithelial cells. Focally, the epithelium may be absent or piled up in papillary projections. Mucus, sometimes containing small clusters of detached epithelial cells, may be present in and occasionally outside the capsule. Typically, mitotic figures are sparse, and cytologic atypia is minimal. However, nuclear pleomorphism may be evident focally (*see* farther on).

Radiologic features are nonspecific, most often consisting of a well-circumscribed nodule or mass. Slow

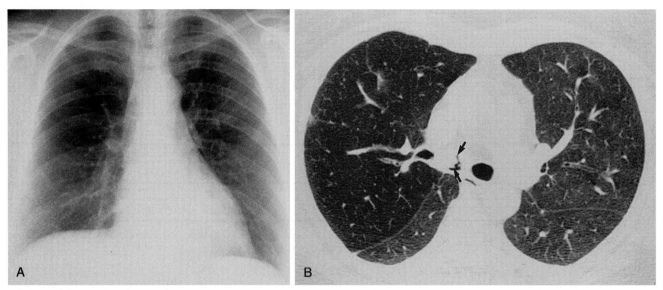

Figure 34–5. Endobronchial Papilloma. A posteroanterior chest radiograph *(A)* in a 51-year-old woman reveals subtle decrease in vascularity and hyperlucency of the right upper lobe, features that are easier to appreciate on the HRCT scan *(B)*. The latter also demonstrates a soft tissue tumor *(arrows)* within the right main bronchus. The patient presented with a history of progressive wheezing and had been diagnosed as having asthma. The diagnosis of endobronchial papilloma was confirmed by bronchoscopic biopsy and resection.

growth—in one case by several centimeters over an 11-year period[53]—may be evident. Patients may be asymptomatic or present with cough or signs and symptoms of pneumonia. One patient who had a 15-cm cyst in the lower lobe presented with chest pain.[51]

The presence of a well-developed fibrous capsule lined by a single layer of cytologically bland epithelial cells is consistent with the designation *cystadenoma.* However, some tumors also show foci of increased epithelial proliferation, cytologic atypia, or, occasionally, frank carcinoma.[54, 55] As a result, it has been proposed that there is a spectrum of neoplasia analogous to benign, borderline, and malignant mucinous tumors of the ovary and appendix. Patients with the clearly benign form of cyst can be expected to be

cured following complete surgical excision. However, the prognosis appears to be excellent even for patients in whom there is local spread of tumor (e.g., in the pleural space).[51]

Papillary Adenoma

Papillary adenoma is a rare pulmonary neoplasm characterized pathologically by a well-circumscribed, sometimes encapsulated[56] nodule that compresses the adjacent lung parenchyma and is composed of numerous branching papillary projections.[1, 57, 58] Cells lining the papillae are cuboidal or columnar, with uniform nuclei; there are few mitotic figures and no necrosis is seen. Ultrastructural[57, 59] and immunohisto-

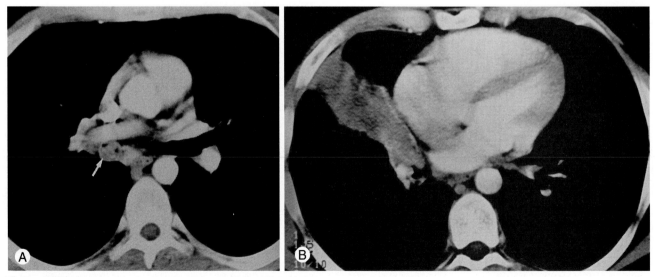

Figure 34–6. Endobronchial Papilloma. A contrast-enhanced CT scan at the level of the bronchus intermedius *(A)* demonstrates almost complete obstruction of the bronchus by a soft tissue mass *(arrow)*. A CT scan at the level of the right middle lobe bronchus *(B)* reveals extension of tumor into this airway associated with right middle lobe atelectasis and obstructive pneumonitis.

chemical[57, 56] studies of some tumors have shown evidence of type II cell and/or Clara cell differentiation; oncocytic features have been documented occasionally.[60] Similar tumors can arise spontaneously or be induced experimentally in animals.[61, 62]

Most reported cases have occurred in adults. The typical presentation is as a peripheral nodule 1 to 4 cm in diameter in an asymptomatic person. The tumor is benign and may show minimal growth radiographically over many years.[59]

Alveolar Adenoma

Another benign neoplasm of bronchioloalveolar cells has been termed *alveolar adenoma.* Histologically, the tumor consists of numerous variably sized cystic spaces lined by cuboidal or flattened epithelium without cytologic atypia.[63–65] The tumor may be confused with lymphangioma[66] and has been speculated to represent a variant of sclerosing hemangioma.[67] Cytogenetic analysis in one case provided evidence of clonal proliferation.[68] In one series of six patients, the mean age at presentation was 59 years;[63] all were asymptomatic and none had evidence of recurrence of the tumor following resection.

TRACHEOBRONCHIAL MELANOMA

Primary tracheobronchial melanoma is exceedingly rare.[69–71] Reviews of the literature have documented fewer than 25 cases,[81] in some of which the possibility of metastasis cannot be definitely excluded.[72, 73] The histogenesis of the lesion is uncertain. Some observers consider that the tumor is derived from melanocytic cells that originate in the primitive foregut and migrate into the tracheobronchial tree during early fetal life;[69, 72, 74] however, such cells have not been demonstrated in the absence of melanoma. The finding of melanin production in some carcinoid tumors suggests that the epithelium of the tracheobronchial tree is able to undergo melanocytic differentiation,[75, 76] and it is conceivable that the tumor is related to the normal airway neuroendocrine cell. Finally, it has been suggested that the tumor might arise in foci of melanocytic metaplasia in the tracheobronchial glands.[81]

Those tumors likely to represent primary melanoma usually arise in proximal bronchi and grow as polypoid, obstructing lesions. Possible origin in the trachea has also been described,[77, 78] in some cases associated with a flat gross appearance.[73] The histologic pattern is the same as melanoma arising in an extrapulmonary location.[81]

Clinical signs and symptoms are related to airway obstruction; hemoptysis may occur. Radiographic features are those of other endobronchial tumors. The prognosis is variable. In one review of 18 patients, approximately half died as a result of the tumor;[73] however, disease-free survival up to 11 years was documented.

Before a pulmonary origin can be concluded, the possibility of an extrapulmonary source must be eliminated by thorough investigation. The diagnosis should be questioned if there is a history of excision of a skin lesion, especially when pigmented and no matter how remote. Primary sites other than the skin, principally the eyes and the mucosa of the anal canal, pharynx, vagina, and esophagus, must also be considered.[79] Although the presence of melanocytic cells in the airway mucosa adjacent to the melanoma suggests an origin at this site, this appearance has also been described in association with melanoma.[80] In one series of 8 cases reported from the Armed Forces Institute of Pathology, the following criteria were considered necessary for inclusion as primary pulmonary melanoma:[81] (1) a solitary, centrally located lesion; (2) melanocytic differentiation confirmed by immunohistochemical and/or ultrastructural examination; (3) absence of a past history of excision or fulgaration of a cutaneous, mucosal, or ocular lesion; and (4) absence of melanoma elsewhere at the time of diagnosis.

REFERENCES

1. Spencer H, Dail DH, Arneaud J: Noninvasive bronchial epithelial papillary tumors. Cancer 45:1486, 1980.
2. Editorial: Multiple papillomas of the larynx in children. Lancet 1:367, 1981.
3. Singer DB, Greenberg SD, Harrison GM: Papillomatosis of the lung. Am Rev Resp Dis 94:777, 1966.
4. Kirchner JA: Papilloma of the larynx with extensive lung involvement. Laryngoscope 61:1022, 1951.
5. Rubel LR, Reynolds RE: Cytologic description of squamous cell papilloma of the respiratory tract. Acta Cytol 23:227, 1979.
6. Smith L, Gooding CA: Pulmonary involvement in laryngeal papillomatosis. Pediatr Radiol 2:161, 1974.
7. Moore RL, Lattes R: Papillomatosis of larynx and bronchi: Case report with 34-year follow-up. Cancer 12:117, 1959.
8. Stein AA, Volk BM: Papillomatosis of trachea and lung: Report of a case. AMA Arch Pathol 68:124, 1959.
9. Kaufman G, Klopstock R: Papillomatosis of the respiratory tract. Am Rev Resp Dis 88:839, 1963.
10. Nikolaidis ET, Trost DC, Buchholz CL, et al: The relationship of histologic and clinical factors in laryngeal papillomatosis. Arch Pathol Lab Med 109:24, 1985.
11. Khan MA, Mathur AP, Allen A, et al: Tracheobronchial papillomatosis. N Y State J Med 77:2073, 1977.
12. Rahman A, Ziment I: Tracheobronchial papillomatosis with malignant transformation. Arch Intern Med 143:577, 1983.
13. Helmuth RA, Strate RW: Squamous carcinoma of the lung in a nonirradiated, nonsmoking patient with juvenile laryngotracheal papillomatosis. Am J Surg Pathol 11:643, 1987.
14. Hartley C, Hamilton J, Birzgalis AR, et al: Recurrent respiratory papillomatosis–the Manchester experience, 1974–1992. J Laryngol Otol 108:226, 1994.
15. Tachezy R, Hamsikova E, Valvoda J, et al: Antibody response to a synthetic peptide derived from the human papillomavirus type 6/11 L2 protein in recurrent respiratory papillomatosis: Correlation between Southern blot hybridization, polymerase chain reaction, and serology. J Med Virol 42:52, 1994.
16. Popper HH, el-Shabrawi Y, Wockel W, et al: Prognostic importance of human papillomavirus typing in squamous cell papilloma of the bronchus: Comparison of in situ hybridization and the polymerase chain reaction. Hum Pathol 25:1191, 1994.
17. Siegel SE, Cohen SR, Isaacs H Jr, et al: Malignant transformation of tracheobronchial juvenile papillomatosis without prior radiotherapy. Ann Otol Rhinol Laryngol 88(Part 1):192, 1979.
18. Brach BB, Klein RC, Mathews AJ, et al: Papillomatosis of the respiratory tract: Upper airway obstruction and carcinoma. Arch Otolaryngol 104:413, 1978.
19. Kramer SS Wehunt WD, Stocker JT, et al: Pulmonary manifestations of juvenile laryngotracheal papillomatosis. Am J Roentgenol 144:687, 1985.
20. Kashima H, Mounts P, Leventhal B, et al: Sites of predilection in recurrent respiratory papillomatosis. Ann Otol Rhinol Laryngol 102:580, 1993.
21. Steinberg BM, Topp WC, Schneider PS, et al: Laryngeal papillomavirus infection during clinical remission. N Engl J Med 308:1261, 1983.
22. Al-Saleem T, Peale AR, Norris CM: Multiple papillomatosis of the lower respiratory tract: Clinical and pathologic study of eleven cases. Cancer 22:1173, 1968.
23. Fechner RE, Fitz-Hugh GS: Invasive tracheal papillomatosis. Am J Surg Pathol 4:79, 1980.
24. Kerley SW, Buchon-Zalles C, Moran J, et al: Chronic cavitary respiratory papillomatosis. Arch Pathol Lab Med 113:1166, 1989.
25. McCarthy MJ, Rosado-de-Christenson ML: Tumors of the trachea. J Thorac Imaging 10:180, 1995.
26. Takasugi JE, Godwin JD: The airway. Semin Roentgenol 26:175, 1991.
27. Kramer SS, Wehunt WD, Stocker JT, et al: Pulmonary manifestations of juvenile laryngotracheal papillomatosis. Am J Roentgenol 144:687, 1985.
28. Rosenbaum HD, Alavi SM, Bryant LR: Pulmonary parenchymal spread of juvenile laryngeal papillomatosis. Radiology 90:654, 1968.
29. Laubscher FA: Solitary squamous cell papilloma of bronchial origin. Am J Clin Pathol 52:599, 1969.
30. Drennan JM, Douglas AC: Solitary papilloma of a bronchus. J Clin Pathol 18:401, 1965.
31. Byrne JC, Tsao M, Fraser RS, et al: Human papillomavirus-11 DNA in a patient with chronic laryngotracheobronchial papillomatosis and metastatic squamous cell carcinoma of the lung. N Engl J Med 317:873, 1987.
32. Guillou L, Sahli R, Chaubert P, et al: Squamous cell carcinoma of the lung in a nonsmoking, nonirradiated patient with juvenile laryngotracheal papillomatosis: Evidence of human papillomavirus-11 DNA in both carcinoma and papillomas. Am J Surg Pathol 15:891, 1991.
33. Wilde E, Duggan MA, Field SK: Bronchogenic sqamous cell carcinoma complicating localized recurrent respiratory papillomatosis. Chest 105:1887, 1994.
34. Blackman F, Chung HR, McDonald RJ, et al: Oat cell carcinoma with multiple tracheobronchial papillomatous tumors. Chest 83:817, 1983.
35. DiMarco AF, Montenegro H, Payne CB Jr, et al: Papillomas of the tracheobronchial tree with malignant degeneration. Chest 74:464, 1978.
36. Simma B, Burger R, Uehlinger J, et al: Squamous cell carcinoma arising in a nonirradiated child with recurrent respiratory papillomatosis. Eur J Pediatr 152:776, 1993.
37. Maxwell RJ, Gibbons JR, O'Hara MD: Solitary squamous papilloma of the bronchus. Thorax 40:68, 1985.
38. Zimmermann A, Lang HR, Muhlberger F, et al: Papilloma of the bronchus. Respiration 39:286, 1980.
39. Smith JR, Dexter D: Papillary neoplasms of the bronchus of low-grade malignancy. Thorax 18:340, 1963.
40. Laubscher FA: Solitary squamous cell papilloma of bronchial origin. Am J Clin Pathol 52:599, 1969.
41. Maxwell RJ, Gibbons JR, O'Hara MD: Solitary squamous papilloma of the bronchus. Thorax 40:68, 1985.
42. Naka Y, Nakao K, Hamaji Y, et al: Solitary squamous cell papilloma of the trachea. Ann Thorac Surg 55:189, 1993.
43. Sochocky S: Papilloma of the bronchus. Am Rev Tuberc 78:916, 1958.
44. Assor D: A papillary transitional cell tumor of the bronchus. Am J Clin Pathol 55:761, 1971.
45. Basheda S, Gephardt GN, Stoller JK: Columnar papilloma of the bronchus: Case report and literature review. Am Rev Respir Dis 144:1400, 1991.
46. Ashmore PG: Papilloma of the bronchus. J Thorac Surg 27:293, 1954.
47. Ashley DJB, Danino EA, Davies HD: Bronchial polyps. Thorax 18:45, 1963.
48. Guillou L, de Luze P, Zysset F, et al: Papillary variant of low-grade mucoepidermoid carcinoma—an unusual bronchial neoplasm: A light microscopic, ultrastructural, and immunohistochemical study. Am J Clin Pathol 101:269, 1994.
49. Kwong JS, Adler BD, Padley SPG, et al: Diagnosis of diseases of the trachea and main bronchi: Chest radiography versus CT. Am J Roentgenol 161:519, 1993.
50. Kwong JS, Müller NL, Miller RR: Diseases of the trachea and main-stem bronchi: Correlation of CT with pathologic findings. RadioGraphics 12:645, 1992.
51. Gowar FJS: An unusual mucous cyst of the lung. Thorax 33:796, 1978.
52. Kragel PJ, Devaney KO, Meth BM, et al: Mucinous cystadenoma of the lung: A report of two cases with immunohistochemical and ultrastructural analysis. Arch Pathol Lab Med 114:1053, 1990.
53. Dixon AY, Moran JF, Wesselius LJ, et al: Pulmonary mucinous cystic tumor: Case report with review of the literature. Am J Surg Pathol 17:722, 1993.
54. Graeme-Cook F, Mark EJ: Pulmonary mucinous cystic tumors of borderline malignancy. Hum Pathol 22:185, 1991.
55. Davison AM, Lowe JW, Da Costa P: Adenocarcinoma arising in a mucinous cystadenoma of the lung. Thorax 47:129, 1992.
56. Yamamoto T, Horiguchi H, Shibagaki T, et al: Encapsulated type II pneumocyte adenoma: A case report and review of the literature. Respiration 60:373, 1993.
57. Noguchi M, Kodama T, Shimosato Y, et al: Papillary adenoma of type 2 pneumocytes. Am J Surg Pathol 10:134, 1986.
58. Hegg CA, Flint A, Singh G: Papillary adenoma of the lung. Am J Clin Pathol 97:393, 1992.
59. Fantone JC, Geisinger KR, Appelman HD: Papillary adenoma of the lung with lamellar and electron-dense granules. Cancer 50:2839, 1982.
60. Fine G, Chang C-H: Adenoma of type 2 pneumocytes with oncocytic features. Arch Pathol Lab Med 115:797, 1991.
61. Kauffman SL, Alexander L, Sass L: Histologic and ultrastructural features of the Clara cell adenoma of the mouse lung. Lab Invest 40:708, 1979.
62. Palmer KC: Clara cell adenomas of the mouse lung: Interaction with alveolar type 2 cells. Am J Pathol 120:455, 1985.
63. Yousem SA, Hochholzer L: Alveolar adenoma. Hum Pathol 17:1066, 1986.
64. Bohm J, Fellbaum C, Bautz W, et al: Pulmonary nodule caused by an alveolar adenoma of the lung. Virchows Arch 430:181, 1997.
65. Oliveira P, Moura Nunes JF, Clode AL, et al: Alveolar adenoma of the lung: Further characterization of this uncommon tumour. Virchows Arch 429:101, 1996.
66. Al-Hilli F: Lymphangioma (or alveolar adenoma?) of the lung. Histopathology 11:979, 1987.
67. Semeraro D, Gibbs AR: Pulmonary adenoma: A variant of sclerosing haemangioma of the lung? J Clin Pathol 42:1222, 1989.
68. Roque L, Oliveira P, Martins C, et al: A nonbalanced translocation (10;16) demonstrated by FISH analysis in a case of alveolar adenoma of the lung. Cancer Genet Cytogenet 89:34, 1996.
69. Salm R: A primary malignant melanoma of the bronchus. J Pathol Bacteriol 85:121, 1963.
70. Cagle P, Mace ML, Judge DM, et al: Pulmonary melanoma: Primary versus metastatic. Chest 85:125, 1984.
71. Carstens PH, Kuhns JG, Ghazi C: Primary malignant melanomas of the lung and adrenal. Hum Pathol 15:910, 1984.
72. Robertson AJ, Sinclair DJM, Sutton PP, et al: Primary melanocarcinoma of the lower respiratory tract. Thorax 35:158, 1980.
73. Jennings TA, Axiotis CA, Kress Y, et al: Primary malignant melanoma of the lower respiratory tract: Report of a case and literature review. Am J Clin Pathol 94:649, 1990.
74. Jensen OA, Egedorf J: Primary malignant melanoma of the lung. Scand J Resp Dis 48:127, 1967.
75. Cebelin MS: Melanocytic bronchial carcinoid tumor. Cancer 46:1843, 1980.
76. Grazer R, Cohen SM, Jacobs JB, et al: Melanin-containing peripheral carcinoid of the lung. Am J Surg Pathol 6:73, 1982.
77. Reid JD, Mehta VT: Melanoma of the lower respiratory tract. Cancer 19:627, 1966.
78. Mori K, Cho H, Som M: Primary "flat" melanoma of the trachea. J Pathol 121:101, 1977.
79. Reed RJ, Kent EM: Solitary pulmonary melanomas: Two case reports. J Thorac Cardiovasc Surg 48:226, 1964.
80. Littman CD: Metastatic melanoma mimicking primary bronchial melanoma. Histopathology 18:561, 1991.
81. Wilson RW, Moran CA: Primary melanoma of the lung: A clinicopathologic and immunohistochemical study of eight cases. Am J Surg Pathol 21:1196, 1997.

CHAPTER 35

Lymphoproliferative Disorders and Leukemia

PULMONARY LYMPHOID HYPERPLASIA

Focal Lymphoid Hyperplasia

Focal lymphoid hyperplasia (nodular lymphoid hyperplasia, pseudolymphoma) is an uncommon and somewhat controversial abnormality characterized pathologically by a localized, polymorphous proliferation of cytologically mature mononuclear cells. The hypothesis that most such lesions represent a benign (possibly reactive) process was proposed by Saltzstein in 1963.[1] Although acknowledging that some histologic subtypes of primary pulmonary lymphoma (such as large cell lymphoma) could be confidently recognized as malignant, this author argued that the presence of prominent germinal centers, the absence of regional lymph node involvement, and the generally good prognosis of localized small lymphocytic proliferations implied that the majority were not true neoplasms; hence the term *pseudolymphoma*.

Although many pathologists and clinicians accepted this viewpoint and the term became widespread in published reports, it was clear that there were important problems with this concept. For example, some patients who had lesions histologically consistent with "pseudolymphoma" as defined by Saltzstein eventually developed disseminated lymphoma.[2, 3] In addition, immunologic and immunohistochemical studies in the 1970s and 1980s showed that many lymphoid aggregates considered histologically to be "pseudolymphoma" were associated with serologic or immunohistochemical evidence of a monoclonal B-cell proliferation, implying neoplasia.[4, 5] Because lesions in which such monoclonality was identified were otherwise identical clinically, radiologically, and pathologically to those in which it had not been assessed, it was suggested that the majority, if not all, of such tumors represent a malignant process.[5–7] This view is currently held by most authorities.

Despite these observations, in the absence of immunohistochemical or molecular confirmation of lymphoma, some investigators prefer to be less dogmatic by referring to these lesions in such noncommittal terms as *small (well-differenti-*

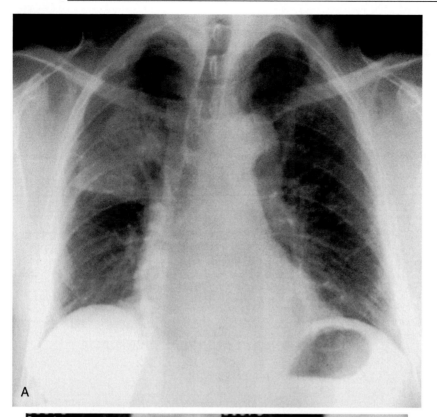

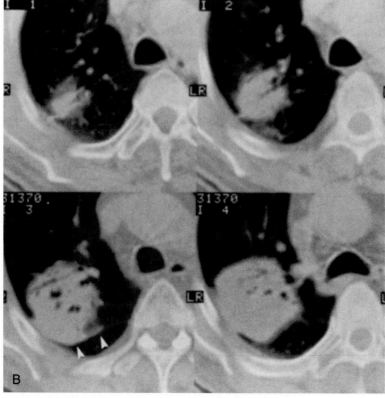

Figure 35–1. Focal Lymphoid Hyperplasia. A posteroanterior chest radiograph *(A)* demonstrates an area of air-space consolidation in the posterior segment of the right upper lobe. The right hilum and mediastinum are normal. Sequential 10-mm collimation CT scans through the posterior segmental lesion *(B)* reveal a nodular area of consolidation that abuts the major fissure *(arrowheads)* and contains an air bronchogram. Pathologic study of the resected lobe disclosed features compatible with lymphoid hyperplasia. The patient was a 57-year-old man.

ated) lymphocytic proliferation.[8, 9] Because occasional cases of true localized lymphoid hyperplasia undoubtedly exist,[10–12] there is some justification for this approach. Some of these lesions are eventually followed by the development of lymphoma in the lung or elsewhere, despite evidence of poly-

clonality on initial examination; it is possible that they represent a form of lymphoid dysplasia analogous to the dysplasia seen in many epithelia prior to the development of invasive carcinoma.

Microscopic examination shows a mixture of lymphocytes, plasma cells, and histiocytes;[13] germinal centers are common but by no means imply a benign process. Granulomas and isolated multinucleated giant cells are seen in many cases.[3] Necrosis is uncommon. By definition, immunohistochemical and molecular studies show a polyclonal population of lymphoid cells.

The most frequent radiologic manifestations consist of a solitary nodule or a focal area of consolidation usually limited to one lobe (Fig. 35–1).[14, 15] The tumors usually measure 2 to 5 cm in diameter,[13] although masses and infiltrates ranging up to 10 cm in diameter have been described.[16] Virtually all lesions contain air bronchograms.[15, 16] Less common manifestations include multiple nodules or multiple infiltrates and cavitation.[15, 16] There is no associated lymphadenopathy; its presence or the finding of pleural effusion should suggest a diagnosis of lymphoma.[14]

Most lesions arise in adults, the majority of whom are asymptomatic;[3] some patients have presented with cough or hemoptysis.[10] A small number (10% to 15%) have evidence of an underlying autoimmune abnormality, such as Sjögren's syndrome or systemic lupus erythematosus. Polyclonal hypergammaglobulinemia is seen in some patients. Because of the polymorphous histologic nature of the lesion, diagnosis usually requires surgical excision with thorough histologic sampling and appropriate immunohistochemical and molecular analyses to exclude low-grade B-cell lymphoma (*see* farther on). The prognosis of excised lesions is generally excellent; however, local recurrence and lymphoma eventually occur in some cases, and close follow-up is advisable.

Diffuse Lymphoid Hyperplasia

Two varieties of diffuse pulmonary lymphoid hyperplasia have been described depending on the anatomic location; the first affects predominantly the parenchymal interstitium (lymphoid or lymphocytic interstitial pneumonia) and the second predominantly the interstitium adjacent to conducting airways (follicular bronchitis and bronchiolitis).[17] Although the two have traditionally been considered as separate entities, it has been argued that they may represent a spectrum of reactive histologic changes to a variety of stimuli.[17]

Lymphoid Interstitial Pneumonia

Lymphoid interstitial pneumonia (LIP) is probably the more common of the two reaction patterns. From both pathologic and clinical points of view, it resembles focal lymphoid hyperplasia. As with the latter condition, however, it is clear from immunologic,[17, 18] immunohistochemical,[7] and molecular[17, 20] studies that some lesions are, in fact, low-grade lymphoma. It is not known whether cases that appear initially to be reactive and that subsequently come to be recognized as lymphoma[21] represent a premalignant condition or a malignancy that is difficult to diagnose at the outset.[20, 22]

The etiology and pathogenesis of the condition are likely varied. The possibility that LIP represents an immunologic disorder is supported by the observation that many cases are associated with other conditions in which there are abnormalities of immune function. The most common of these are Sjögren's syndrome[23, 33] and acquired immunodeficiency syndrome (AIDS) (*see* page 1685);[24–26] however,

cases have also been reported in association with chronic active hepatitis,[27] renal tubular acidosis,[28] primary biliary cirrhosis,[27] myasthenia gravis,[23] systemic lupus erythematosus,[30] autoimmune thyroiditis,[31] and allogeneic bone marrow transplantation.[32] Because of the presence of granulomatous inflammation, it has been speculated that some cases may actually represent lymphocyte-rich examples of extrinsic allergic alveolitis.[17] The possibility that the condition is caused by a virus has also been considered. As indicated previously, some cases are associated with human immunodeficiency virus (HIV) infection, in which case it is conceivable that the pulmonary reaction represents a direct effect of the infection. Experimental studies in sheep infected with ovine lentivirus (an organism related to HIV) support this hypothesis.[34] There is also evidence that Epstein-Barr virus infection may be involved in some cases.[36, 37]

Pathologically, LIP is characterized by a more or less diffuse interstitial infiltrate of mononuclear cells, in the typical case predominantly lymphocytes (Fig. 35–2);[27] plasma cells are occasionally prominent.[38, 39] Although the infiltrate is present in the alveolar interstitium, involvement of interstitial tissue adjacent to small vessels and airways is common. Focal nodular accumulations of lymphoid cells can be seen, some of which may develop germinal centers. Interstitial fibrosis is also present in some cases and can become severe

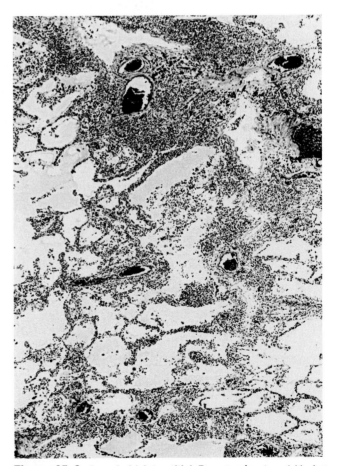

Figure 35–2. Lymphoid Interstitial Pneumonia. A variable but overall moderately severe infiltrate of mononuclear inflammatory cells is present in perivascular and alveolar interstitial tissue. The cells were seen on higher magnification to be mostly mature lymphocytes, with occasional plasma cells. (×40.)

enough to have a honeycomb appearance.[40] Cytologically, the cells show minimal nuclear atypia. Air spaces are uninvolved by the mononuclear infiltrate, although focal bronchiolar obstruction can result in findings of obstructive pneumonitis. Rare cases have been reported of coexistent nodular pulmonary amyloidosis.[23, 41] The diagnosis of a reactive process is supported by the presence of polyclonality on immunohistochemical and molecular analysis,[42] which should be performed in all cases.

The most frequently reported radiographic findings consist of a reticular or reticulonodular pattern involving mainly the lower lung zones.[27, 43] In some cases, branching and linear opacities consistent with interlobular septal thickening have been described in the periphery of the lung;[40] however, such thickening is more suggestive of lymphoma than LIP. Other radiographic patterns include bilateral areas of ground-glass opacity[44] or consolidation (Fig. 35–3).[45] A nodular pattern may also occur,[43] most commonly in patients with AIDS.[14, 46] Although hilar and mediastinal lymph node enlargement has been described in patients who have AIDS and LIP,[46, 47] this finding is seldom present in those without AIDS.[14, 45, 48] Pleural effusion is rare. Fibrosis and honeycombing, although also rare, develop in some patients.[23, 40]

The CT features of LIP have been described in a small number of patients.[44, 46, 47, 49] The most frequent abnormality consists of bilateral areas of ground-glass attenuation (*see* Fig. 35–3); less common findings include air-space consolidation, small nodules, and cysts (Fig. 35–4). The last-mentioned are usually located deep within the lung parenchyma and presumably result from partial bronchiolar obstruction caused by peribronchiolar lymphocyte infiltration.[44, 49]

With the exception of AIDS, in which affected patients are most often children, most patients with LIP are adults, a mean age of 52 years being found in 18 patients reviewed in one series.[27] A female predominance has been noted.[27] Dyspnea and cough are the major complaints. Some patients also have systemic symptoms, such as fever, weight loss, and arthralgias. Cyanosis and clubbing were present in roughly half the patients described in one study.[49] Hypergammaglobulinemia—usually both IgG and IgM—is common;[27] hypogammaglobulinemia is seen occasionally.[23]

The prognosis depends to some extent on the nature of the underlying disease. Patients with AIDS often die of infectious or neoplastic abnormalities associated with their underlying disease rather than LIP itself; however, about a third experience progressive respiratory failure.[50] In some

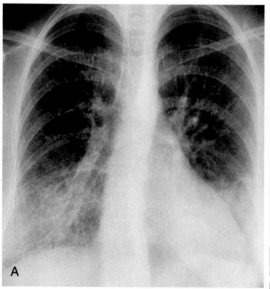
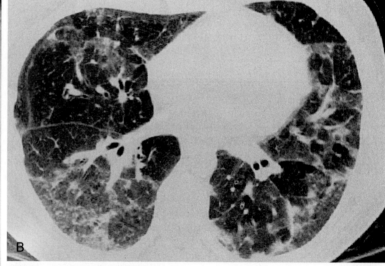
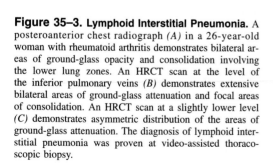
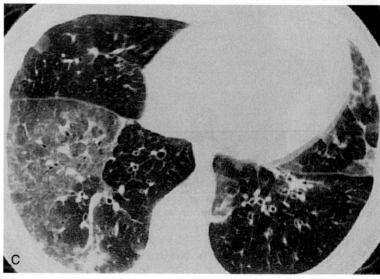

Figure 35–3. Lymphoid Interstitial Pneumonia. A posteroanterior chest radiograph *(A)* in a 26-year-old woman with rheumatoid arthritis demonstrates bilateral areas of ground-glass opacity and consolidation involving the lower lung zones. An HRCT scan at the level of the inferior pulmonary veins *(B)* demonstrates extensive bilateral areas of ground-glass attenuation and focal areas of consolidation. An HRCT scan at a slightly lower level *(C)* demonstrates asymmetric distribution of the areas of ground-glass attenuation. The diagnosis of lymphoid interstitial pneumonia was proven at video-assisted thoracoscopic biopsy.

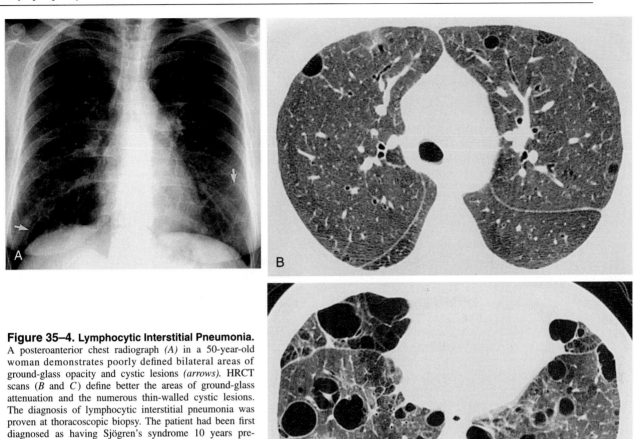

Figure 35–4. Lymphocytic Interstitial Pneumonia.
A posteroanterior chest radiograph *(A)* in a 50-year-old woman demonstrates poorly defined bilateral areas of ground-glass opacity and cystic lesions *(arrows)*. HRCT scans *(B* and *C)* define better the areas of ground-glass attenuation and the numerous thin-walled cystic lesions. The diagnosis of lymphocytic interstitial pneumonia was proven at thoracoscopic biopsy. The patient had been first diagnosed as having Sjögren's syndrome 10 years previously and had been experiencing increasing systemic symptoms and progressive dyspnea over the previous year. (Case courtesy of Dr. Jim Barrie, University of Alberta, Edmonton, Alberta, Canada.)

individuals not affected by AIDS, there is also progression of disease within the lung, sometimes associated with fibrosis and an evolution similar to that of idiopathic pulmonary fibrosis; in others, the disease evolves into clear-cut low-grade or high-grade lymphoma.[51, 52]

Follicular Bronchitis and Bronchiolitis

Follicular bronchitis and bronchiolitis are characterized histologically by a mononuclear cell infiltrate (again predominantly lymphocytes, with lesser numbers of plasma cells and histiocytes) in the interstitial tissue adjacent to bronchi and bronchioles. As the name suggests, germinal center formation is common, resulting in a distinctly nodular appearance to the abnormality (Fig. 35–5).[53] As with LIP, many patients have a history of an underlying immunodeficiency disorder or connective tissue disease, particularly Sjögren's syndrome or rheumatoid arthritis;[53] in the latter disease, bronchiolitis appears to be particularly more common in adolescents (juvenile rheumatoid arthritis) (*see* page 1451).

The chest radiograph characteristically shows a diffuse reticular or reticulonodular pattern.[53, 54] CT may demonstrate small nodular opacities in a peribronchovascular and centri-

lobular distribution.[55-57, 59] In the majority of cases, these measure 1 to 3 mm in diameter (Fig. 35–6),[55] although focal nodular areas of consolidation up to 1 cm in diameter may be seen (Fig. 35–7). Centrilobular nodules, also presumably caused by follicular bronchiolitis, have also been described on HRCT in approximately 20% of patients with rheumatoid arthritis.[56]

A preponderance of males has been found in some studies;[17] however, most patients with underlying connective tissue disease are female.[53, 54] The most common clinical finding is progressive shortness of breath;[53, 57] cough, fever, and recurrent pneumonia are occasionally present. Leukocytosis with prominent eosinophilia is seen in some patients, suggesting to some investigators the possibility of a hypersensitivity reaction.[53] Pulmonary function studies reveal evidence of obstruction, restriction, or combined restriction and obstruction.[53, 58, 59]

NON-HODGKIN'S LYMPHOMA

The most frequent manifestation of thoracic involvement in non-Hodgkin's lymphoma is mediastinal or hilar lymph node enlargement, a feature that was evident radio-

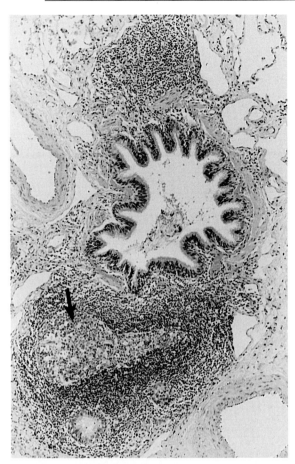

Figure 35–5. Follicular Bronchiolitis. The interstitial tissue adjacent to a membranous bronchiole is expanded by an infiltrate of lymphoid cells, focally with germinal center formation *(arrow)*. Similar disease was present in relation to many other bronchioles. The patient had rheumatoid disease.

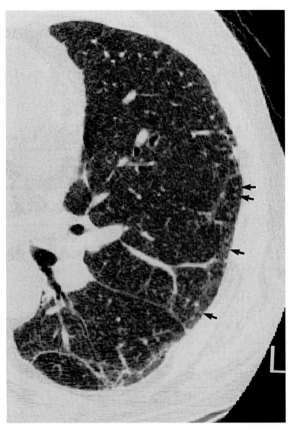

Figure 35–6. Follicular Bronchiolitis. A view of the left lung from an HRCT scan demonstrates centrilobular subpleural nodules measuring 1 to 3 mm in diameter *(arrows)*. Evidence of mild fibrosis with irregular linear opacities and thickening of interlobular septa, particularly in the left lower lobe, is also noted. The patient was a 64-year-old man with progressive systemic sclerosis. Subpleural centrilobular nodules are frequently seen on HRCT scans in patients with progressive systemic sclerosis and are presumed to reflect the presence of follicular bronchiolitis.

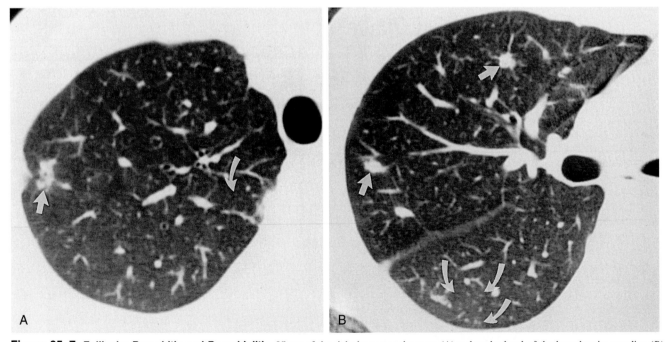

Figure 35–7. Follicular Bronchitis and Bronchiolitis. Views of the right lung near the apex *(A)* and at the level of the bronchus intermedius *(B)* from a HRCT scan demonstrate focal nodular consolidation surrounding bronchi *(straight arrows)* and a few small centrilobular nodular opacities *(curved arrows)* resulting from follicular bronchiolitis. The patient was a 24-year-old woman with rheumatoid arthritis.

graphically in 36% of 1,269 cases in one study.[60] Although pulmonary parenchymal disease is less common, it is also evident in many patients. The following description is limited largely to the latter form of disease and can be conveniently considered in two groups: cases in which lymphoma is apparently limited to the lungs (with or without mediastinal lymph node involvement) at the time of diagnosis (primary pulmonary lymphoma), and cases in which concomitant or previous extrathoracic lymphoma is evident as well (secondary pulmonary lymphoma). Intrathoracic lymphoma developing either primarily or secondarily in the pleura or mediastinum is discussed separately (*see* pages 1291 and 2838).

Primary Pulmonary Lymphoma

The criteria for designating a lymphoma as primary in the lung are variable. Perhaps the most widely accepted are those of Saltzstein,[1] who considered lymphoma to be primary if it affected the lung (with or without involvement of hilar and mediastinal lymph nodes) and showed no evidence of extrathoracic dissemination for at least 3 months after the initial diagnosis. Although many authors abide by these criteria or minor modifications thereof, some are more restrictive, accepting, for example, only hilar and not mediastinal node involvement. Others are more liberal in their definition, for example, accepting the simple criterion of clinical presentation within the lung regardless of the presence or absence of extrathoracic lymphoma.[61] As a result of these different definitions, the true incidence of primary pulmonary lymphoma is difficult to ascertain. Nevertheless, it is clearly an uncommon neoplasm: in the study of 1,269 cases of lymphoma,[60] only 0.34% were deemed to have a pulmonary origin. Overall, the tumors have been estimated to comprise only 3% to 4% of all extranodal lymphomas.[63] Although a variety of morphologic subtypes can be seen,[64] the most common is low-grade (small lymphocytic) B-cell lymphoma; high-grade (large cell) B-cell lymphoma and predominantly T-cell angioimmunoproliferative lesions (lymphomatoid granulomatosis) comprise most of the remaining tumors.

Low-Grade B-Cell Lymphoma

It is now widely believed that many primary extranodal lymphomas, including those that arise in the lung, are derived from mucosa-associated lymphoid tissue (MALT); hence the term *maltoma* that is sometimes used to describe the tumors.[13, 65–68] In addition to a characteristic morphology (*see* farther on), these tumors lack immunohistochemical reactivity for CD5 and CD10 as well as evidence of *bcl*-1 and *bcl*-2 gene rearrangements, features that are typically present in follicular and mantle cell lymphomas of lymph node origin.[65, 66] In the lung, the tumors are believed to arise from marginal zone cells (centrocyte-like cells) that are present in normal or hyperplastic bronchus-associated lymphoid tissue (BALT).[66]

As indicated previously, this form of lymphoma is clearly the most frequent to involve the lungs as a primary tumor: in four series comprising 147,[3] 36,[62] 69,[63] and 62[64] patients, this variant was found in 92%, 58%, 88%, and 69%, respectively. The vast majority of tumors occur in

adults, with a mean age at diagnosis of about 55 to 60 years.[7, 8, 10] Men and women are equally affected.

The etiology and pathogenesis of these tumors are unclear. It has been speculated that some background stimulus, such as cigarette smoke or infection, leads to BALT hyperplasia, which is then followed by neoplastic transformation.[69] Many patients are nonsmokers, however, and histologic evidence of local or diffuse lymphoid hyperplasia is evident only occasionally,[63] in which case there is usually a history of an immunologic abnormality, such as rheumatoid disease, Sjögren's syndrome, or systemic lupus erythematosus; rarely, HIV infection has been implicated.[70] An association between lymphoproliferative disease and asbestos exposure has also been reported;[71, 72] occasionally, lymphocytic neoplasia and mesothelioma have occurred simultaneously in patients who had known asbestos exposure.[73] Contrary to high-grade B-cell lymphoma, there appears to be no association of the low-grade form with Epstein-Barr virus.[74]

Pathologic Characteristics

Grossly, low-grade lymphoma typically appears as a single white or tan lesion that varies from a well-circumscribed nodule to a relatively ill-defined infiltrate in all or part of a lobe (Fig. 35–8).[7, 8, 62–64, 69] Occasionally, there are multiple foci of disease.[75] Rarely, tumor is present predominantly within the tracheobronchial lumen.[76–78]

Malignant cells are found predominantly within intersti-

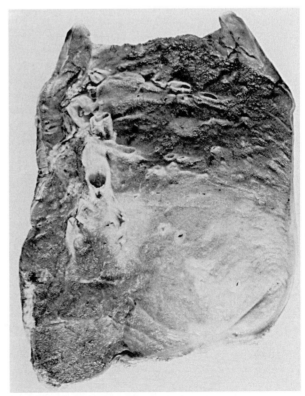

Figure 35–8. Primary Pulmonary Low-Grade B-Cell Lymphoma. A slice of right lower lobe shows an ill-defined tumor in its basal portion. The difference in shade is related to the amount of tumor in the underlying lung, the more white area having a large amount (effectively obliterating the underlying parenchyma) and the paler region showing only partial involvement.

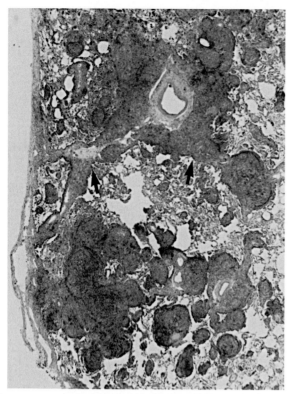

Figure 35–9. Primary Pulmonary Low-Grade B-Cell Lymphoma.
A section from the periphery of an area of poorly defined parenchymal consolidation shows abundant lymphoid cells within the interstitial tissue of an interlobular septum *(arrows)*. The nodular infiltrate in the centrilobular region to the right is centered predominantly about transitional airways, although focal extension into alveolar interstitium is also present. (×14.)

of the larger masses, expansion and confluence of the interstitial infiltrate and invasion into air spaces frequently result in a more or less solid appearance. Extension from interlobular septa into the pleura is frequent where the tumor abuts this structure. Although infiltration of the walls of small vessels and of the bronchiolar epithelium by tumor cells is also common histologically (in the latter site resulting in so-called lymphoepithelial lesions [Fig. 35–10]),[63, 69] macroscopically identifiable stenosis of bronchi and larger pulmonary arteries is usually not evident.[63]

Tumor cells consist of small lymphocyte-like cells with round (less commonly cleaved) uniform nuclei, small nucleoli, and rare mitotic figures (Fig. 35–11). Cytoplasm is usually scanty but can be moderately abundant and have a plasmacytoid appearance.[63] Mature plasma cells, immunoblasts, and macrophages are usually sparse; when their numbers are considerable, the possibility of a reactive (benign) process becomes more likely. Germinal centers may be seen, occasionally in large numbers (Fig. 35–12).[7, 79] Inflammatory changes of obstructive pneumonitis, reflecting small airway obstruction, are fairly common; poorly defined granulomas are sometimes present.[7, 63] Necrosis is unusual. Immunohistochemical analysis shows positive reactions for CD20 and CD3 in the atypical lymphoid cells in virtually all tumors, confirming B-cell differentiation;[69] clusters of nonneoplastic T lymphocytes can also be found admixed with the malignant B cells in many cases.[63, 69, 80] Cytogenetic abnormalities have been documented occasionally.[81, 82]

Because the degree of cytologic atypia of the lymphoid cells is usually slight and because of the admixture of normal inflammatory cells and germinal centers in some cases, the diagnosis may be difficult on the basis of histology alone, particularly in small biopsy specimens. For example, in one retrospective study of 83 previously diagnosed primary pulmonary lymphomas, 14 cases were excluded from analysis by reviewing pathologists, 6 because of insufficient material and 8 because of disagreement with the original diagnosis.[63] In these difficult cases, ancillary immunohistochemical and molecular biologic studies are often helpful, the identification of monoclonality in the lymphoid cells usually being

tial tissue, a feature seen most clearly at the periphery of tumor nodules in relation to bronchovascular bundles and interlobular septa, where cell aggregates frequently result in a micronodular appearance (Fig. 35–9). Extension also occurs into the parenchymal interstitium, albeit usually to a lesser extent than in the former sites. In the central portions

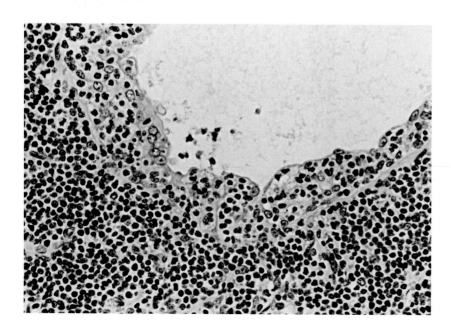

Figure 35–10. Low-Grade B-Cell Lymphoma — Lymphoepithelial Lesion. A portion of a membranous bronchiole whose wall is thickened by a monomorphic population of small lymphoid cells is shown. The cells extensively infiltrate the airway epithelium (the larger, paler cells adjacent to the airway lumen).

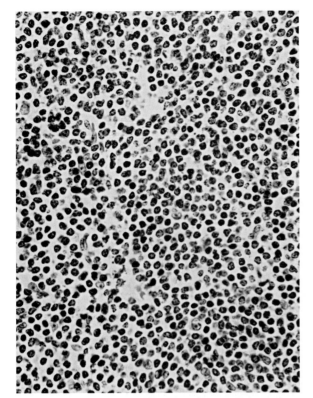

Figure 35–11. Primary Pulmonary Low-Grade B-Cell Lymphoma. The section shows a monomorphous population of small lymphocyte-like cells with mild nuclear atypia, an appearance typical of low-grade B-cell lymphoma. (×400.)

accepted as a reliable indicator of malignancy. Monoclonal light chain production can sometimes be shown on paraffin-embedded tissue, usually in tumors with plasmacytoid differentiation. Immunohistochemical identification of monoclonal surface immunoglobulin on fresh-frozen tissue sections or dispersed cells derived directly from the tumor is a more reliable technique.[6, 61, 83, 84] Monoclonal gene rearrangements can also be detected using molecular biologic techniques, such as polymerase chain reaction and restriction enzyme DNA digestion;[69, 85, 86] such techniques are particularly useful in small biopsy samples, such as those obtained by bronchoscopy.[87]

When interpreting the results of these studies, it is important to remember that some lesions with apparent polyclonal immunohistochemical profiles have subsequently progressed to clear-cut lymphoma associated with a change to a monoclonal pattern.[9] It should also be recognized that it may be impossible to categorize precisely a particular tumor as benign or malignant; in this instance, it may be preferable to refer to the lesion by the relatively noncommittal term *small (well-differentiated) lymphocytic proliferation.*[8, 9]

Radiologic Manifestations

The most common radiologic manifestation of primary low-grade B-cell lymphoma consists of a solitary nodule or a poorly defined focal opacity measuring from 2 to 8 cm in diameter (Fig. 35–13).[88–90] Air bronchograms are visible on the radiograph or CT in approximately 50% of cases (Fig. 35–14).[91] Other patterns of lung involvement include a local-

ized area of consolidation—which may range from a small subsegmental area to an entire lobe—or, less commonly, multiple nodules or infiltrates (Fig. 35–15).[88, 89, 92, 92a] The parenchymal abnormalities typically show an indolent course with slow growth over months or years.[91, 93]

On CT, the bronchi within affected lung parenchyma may appear stretched and slightly narrowed.[92] Rarely, airway involvement is manifested by bronchial wall thickening and marked narrowing of the bronchial lumen.[94] Magnetic resonance (MR) imaging performed in one case demonstrated signal intensity similar to muscle on T1-weighted images and signal intensity slightly higher than muscle on T2-weighted images.[95]

Pleural effusion is present in approximately 10% of cases, usually in association with evidence of parenchymal involvement.[88, 89, 91] Lymphadenopathy is evident radiographically in less than 5% of cases at presentation.[88]

Clinical Manifestations

Approximately 40% to 50% of patients with primary low-grade B-cell lymphoma are asymptomatic when first seen, their disease being discovered on a screening chest radiograph.[64] When present, pulmonary symptoms include cough, dyspnea, and (less commonly) chest pain and hemoptysis. Systemic symptoms, such as fever, night sweats, or weight loss, are present in 20% to 40% of patients;[64] although these may be seen with localized disease, they should suggest the possibility of extrathoracic involvement. Additional systemic symptoms may be seen in patients who have an underlying connective tissue disease, such as Sjögren's syndrome.[18] Other conditions rarely seen in association with the neoplasm are Langerhans' cell granulomatosis and sarcoidosis.[97]

Laboratory Findings

Fiberoptic bronchoscopy is often abnormal and may reveal significant bronchial stenosis. Bronchoscopic biopsy of such areas may yield diagnostic tissue. The diagnosis has also been made by cytologic examination of bronchial washings,[98] transthoracic needle aspiration specimens,[99] and bronchoalveolar lavage fluid.[29, 100] As with tissue samples, the use of flow cytometric analysis, gene rearrangement analysis, and immunohistochemistry to subtype lymphocytes and demonstrate monoclonality can be particularly valuable for diagnostic purposes in all of these relatively small samples.[35, 100, 101]

Pleural effusion is usually an exudate;[102] cytologic examination of aspirated fluid and pleural biopsy specimens is diagnostic in many patients. The use of immunohistochemical techniques again may be helpful in differentiating between benign and malignant causes of the effusion: in the former, lymphocytes are predominantly T cells, whereas in the latter, monoclonal B cells predominate.[103, 104]

In a minority of patients, serum immunoelectrophoresis shows a monoclonal gammopathy, typically IgM;[7, 8, 10, 19, 62, 64] affected patients often have tumors that show prominent plasmacytoid differentiation.[19] The same monoclonal immunoglobulin may be found in samples of bronchoalveolar lavage fluid. Free light chains, including Bence Jones proteins, are found in the urine in some cases.[105] The blood

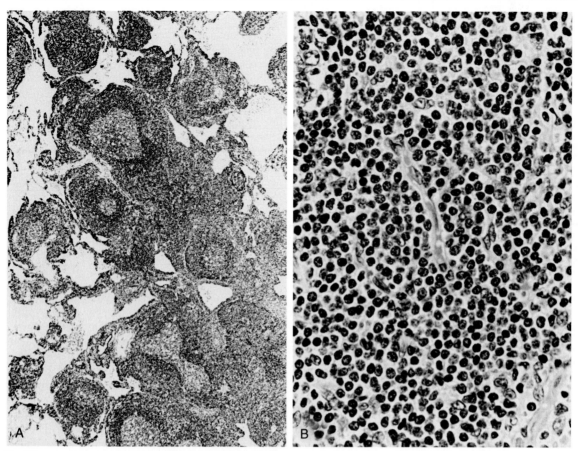

Figure 35–12. Primary Pulmonary Lymphoma B-Cell Lymphoma with Prominent Germinal Center Formation. A section from an ill-defined upper lobe nodule *(A)* shows abundant lymphoid cells in the parenchymal and perivascular interstitium; numerous germinal centers are evident. Examination of the infiltrate between the germinal centers at higher magnification *(B)* shows a uniform population of small lymphoid cells confirmed by immunohistochemical analysis to be a monoclonal B-cell proliferation.

leukocyte count is usually within normal limits, an absolute lymphocytosis being rare.[8, 19, 62] A single case associated with autoantibody-mediated hemolytic anemia has been reported.[106] Pulmonary function tests occasionally show obstructive or restrictive abnormalities; however, they are normal in the majority of patients.

Prognosis and Natural History

As the name suggests, patients with pulmonary low-grade B-cell lymphoma generally have an excellent prognosis.[7, 62, 107] For example, in one study of 43 patients, the overall 5-year survival was 84%, a value equivalent to that of the appropriate unaffected (control) population.[64] (Despite this, patients with systemic symptoms, including fever, night sweats, or weight loss, had a significantly worse prognosis, the 5-year survival being only about 55%.) In another investigation of 61 patients, the overall 5-year survival was 94%.[63] Recurrence in the lung after surgical resection occurs in a minority of patients; however, even in this circumstance or in the absence of definitive treatment, prolonged survival can occur.[96]

Occasional cases appear to progress to a high-grade B-cell lymphoma within the lung.[63, 64] An association between low-grade B-cell lymphoma and lymphoid proliferation in extrapulmonary mucosal sites, particularly the stomach and

upper respiratory tract, has also been noted in a number of patients,[6, 9] the pulmonary abnormality presenting either first or after the other mucosal lesion.[108] Some cases are also complicated by the development of extrapulmonary large cell lymphoma, sometimes many years after the initial diagnosis of the pulmonary tumor.[8]

High-Grade Lymphoma

Most cases of primary high-grade pulmonary lymphoma are of B-cell type; occasional cases of anaplastic (Ki-1) lymphoma[109] or peripheral T-cell[110, 111] lymphoma have also been reported. An underlying abnormality can be identified in a number of patients. Some tumors appear to be derived from the low-grade B-cell lymphoma described previously.[13] Others occur in patients who have organ transplants (post-transplant lymphoproliferative disorder; *see* page 1711) or AIDS.[112]

The histologic diagnosis of primary high-grade lymphoma usually is easily made by means of traditional pathologic features, including a monomorphic cellular infiltrate, cytologic atypia, mitotic activity, and necrosis. In some cases, an admixture of benign inflammatory cells, particularly T cells (T-cell–rich B-cell lymphoma),[113] may make the diagnosis more difficult. In contrast to low-grade lymphoma, high-grade tumors tend to show a less prominent interstitial

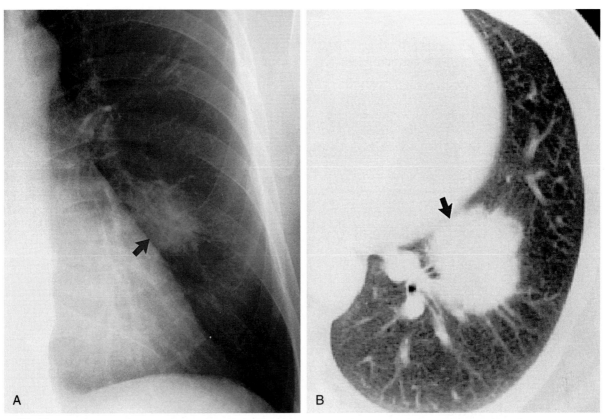

Figure 35–13. Low-Grade B-Cell Lymphoma. Close-up views of the left lung from a posteroanterior chest radiograph *(A)* and a CT scan *(B)* demonstrate a 3-cm nodule *(arrows)* in the left lower lobe. The nodule has poorly defined lobulated margins. At surgery, the nodule was shown to originate in the left lower lobe and extend into the lingula across the major fissure. Histologic assessment revealed low-grade B-cell lymphoma. The patient was a 52-year-old man.

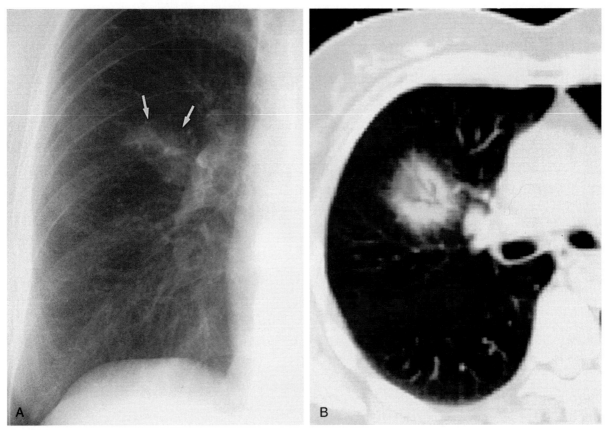

Figure 35–14. Primary Low-Grade B-Cell Lymphoma. Close-up views of the right lung from a posteroanterior chest radiograph *(A)* and a conventional CT scan *(B)* demonstrate a 3-cm area of consolidation in the right upper lobe *(arrows)*. An air bronchogram is clearly visible on the CT scan. The diagnosis of low-grade B-cell lymphoma was proven at surgery. The patient was a 68-year-old woman.

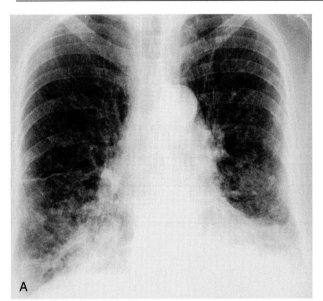

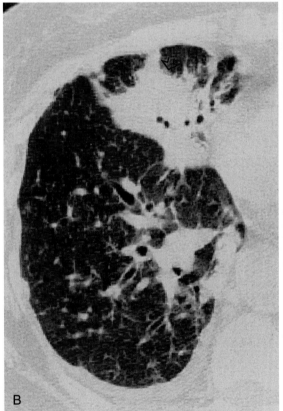

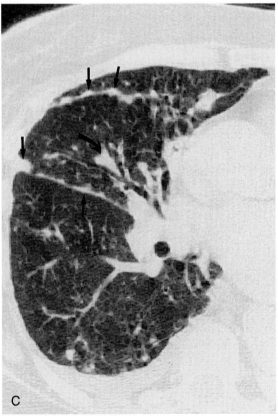

Figure 35–15. Primary Pulmonary Low-Grade B-Cell Lymphoma. A posteroanterior chest radiograph *(A)* reveals poorly defined nodular opacities throughout both lungs and areas of consolidation in the lower lung zones. Also noted are small bilateral pleural effusions. Magnified views of the right lung from HRCT scans *(B* and *C)* demonstrate nodular thickening of the interlobar fissures *(straight arrows)* and bronchovascular bundles *(curved arrows)*. Also present are a focal area of consolidation *(open arrow)* with air bronchograms in the right middle lobe and a small right pleural effusion. Similar findings were present in the left lung. The patient was a 73-year-old woman who presented with a 6-month history of dry cough and progressive shortness of breath.

growth pattern, fewer germinal centers, and more frequent necrosis and vascular infiltration.[8, 10] Rarely, tumor is mistaken for poorly differentiated carcinoma.[113a] Concomitant involvement of regional lymph nodes is common.[10]

Radiologic manifestations of high-grade lymphoma are nonspecific and include localized opacities with or without air bronchograms, bilateral consolidation, or a diffuse reticulodular pattern.[114] Occasionally, the pattern progresses from a localized opacity to extensive bilateral consolidation within a few weeks of initial presentation;[115] associated respiratory failure is common.

In contrast to patients with low-grade lymphoma, al-most all those with high-grade lesions have systemic as well as pulmonary symptoms. In one study of nine patients, bronchoscopy was abnormal in seven, and bronchial biopsy yielded diagnostic tissue in five. As might be expected, the prognosis is worse than for low-grade tumors;[8, 116] the 5-year survival ranges from 45% to 60% in some studies[62, 64] to 0 in others.

Angiocentric Immunoproliferative Lesion

The term *angiocentric immunoproliferative lesion* (AIL, angioimmunoproliferative lesion, lymphomatoid granulomatosis) refers to a group of abnormalities characterized histologically by a lymphoreticular infiltrate that has a variable degree of cytologic atypia and polymorphism and shows prominent vascular infiltration. The condition has been subdivided into three forms or grades. Grade 1 lesions consist predominantly of lymphocytes with minimal cytologic atypia; in the lung, the abnormality corresponds to the condition initially described by the term *benign lymphocytic angiitis and granulomatosis*.[117, 118] Grade 2 lesions consist of a polymorphous infiltrate of lymphocytes, plasma cells, histiocytes, and a variable number of large, cytologically atypical lymphoid cells; in the lung, this form corresponds to the entity termed *lymphomatoid granulomatosis*.[68, 119, 120] Grade 3 lesions consist of a monomorphous infiltrate of large lymphoid cells, all of which have significant atypia; this variant is clearly malignant and has been appropriately termed *lymphoma*.[121, 122]

The concept that AIL represents a histologic spectrum of neoplastic disease is supported by cases in which there is transition over time of one form into another and by cases in which more than one histologic pattern is present in the same lesion. These combinations have been documented most commonly for Grades 2 and 3 lesions. Cytogenetic and molecular studies have also provided evidence of clonal proliferation in many lesions,[123] and it is now widely believed that the vast majority of Grade 2 tumors are neoplastic.[119, 120, 124] An association of Grade 1 lesions with higher grade forms, however, is unusual.[125] In addition, molecular investigations of some low-grade and intermediate-grade lesions have failed to identify evidence of clonal proliferation.[126, 127] As a result, it has been suggested that at least some of these tumors may represent a nonneoplastic lymphoid proliferation to one or more as yet unidentified stimuli.[126]

Immunophenotypic analyses of Grades 2 and 3 AIL lesions have shown that some appear to be clonal proliferations of T cells;[125, 128, 129] however, the neoplastic proliferation appears to be composed of B cells in most cases.[129] An association with Epstein-Barr virus infection has been identified in the latter cases.[129–131, 131a]

Pathologically, Grade 1 lesions consist of poorly defined foci of perivascular and peribronchiolar interstitial lymphocytic infiltrates; other inflammatory cells are usually few in number, and cytologic atypia is minimal. Grade 2 lesions (lymphomatoid granulomatosis) usually consist of multiple nodules with variable degrees of necrosis and cavitation. Histologically, the lung parenchyma is replaced by a diffuse proliferation of lymphocytes with lesser numbers of plasma cells and histiocytes; a variable number of large, cytologically atypical lymphoreticular cells are admixed (Fig. 35–16).[118, 119, 132] Infiltration of the walls of vessels of medium to small size is prominent and can be so marked that the vascular lumens are obliterated; in such a situation, elastic tissue stains may be useful to identify the angiocentric nature of the infiltrate. Grade 3 lesions are grossly and histologically similar to the Grade 2 forms except for the presence of more numerous atypical cells and fewer benign lymphocytes. Because there is a variation in the number of atypical cells in different cases, precise classification of a particular lesion as Grade 2 or 3 may be difficult.

The most common radiologic manifestation of lymphomatoid granulomatosis (seen in 70% to 80% of patients) is one of multiple nodules or masses ranging in size from 0.5 to 8 cm in diameter.[133–135, 135a] In some patients, the initial abnormality consists of poorly defined opacities, which then progress over a number of weeks to form nodules or masses (Fig. 35–17). The nodules frequently have ill-defined margins and show a tendency to coalesce (Fig. 35–18);[134] although they may be diffuse throughout both lungs, they tend to be most numerous in the lower lung zones.[119, 134] Some abut the pleura and mimic the appearance of pulmonary infarcts.[134] Spontaneous pneumothorax may occur,[137] presumably as a result of rupture of one of these necrotic subvisceral pleural nodules.[134] Cavitation is present in 30% to 40% of cases.[119, 133, 134] Neither the nodules nor masses contain air bronchograms.[134]

Other radiologic findings include areas of consolidation (described in as many as 50% of patients)[133] and a reticulonodular pattern (in approximately 20%).[133, 134] Pleural effusions are present in 10% to 25% of patients.[133–135] Hilar lymph node enlargement is uncommon, being seen in only 14 out of a total of 284 (5%) patients reported in four studies.[120, 133, 134, 136] Rapid progression of any of the parenchymal abnormalities may be seen.

Most patients with Grade 2 or 3 lesions are between 40 and 60 years of age.[120, 138] Thoracic symptoms (cough, dyspnea, chest pain) and systemic complaints (fever, weight loss, malaise) are present in the majority at the time of diagnosis.[117, 120] Concomitant or subsequent involvement of the skin and central nervous system is common: neurologic manifestations—consisting of signs of cerebral involvement and cranial and peripheral neuropathies—are present in 30% of patients, and cutaneous disease—manifested by either an erythematous rash or skin nodules—is present in 40%.[119, 120] Other less common manifestations include features of retroperitoneal fibrosis, lytic and blastic bone lesions,[139] diabetes insipidus,[140] and polyarthritis.[141] One exceptional case has been reported in which AIL was associated with asbestos-related interstitial fibrosis and glomerulonephritis.[142] Clinical evidence of involvement of lymph nodes, liver, and spleen is unusual except in the late stage of disease.

The prognosis of AIL is variable. As might be expected, patients with Grade 1 lesions generally do well, whereas those with higher grade lesions generally fare much worse. In one series, approximately two thirds of the latter patients died, with a median survival time of only 14 months;[120] in another, the 5-year survival rate was approximately 20%.[118] In many instances, death is related to progressive pulmonary or central nervous system disease.[118]

Secondary Pulmonary Lymphoma

Pleuropulmonary involvement with lymphoma in patients known to have disease outside of the thorax is much more common than the primary condition; for example, in one series of 1,269 cases, the pleura was affected in 21% and the lungs in 29%.[60] In another review of 651 patients, 54 (8%) had histologically documented pulmonary involvement.[143] As with carcinoma, such disease can develop by direct spread from involved mediastinal or hilar lymph nodes or by intravascular dissemination (metastasis). (One unusual example of the latter mechanism was reported in a patient who underwent autologous bone marrow transplantation for immunoblastic lymphoma;[144] subsequent massive recurrence

Text continued on page 1287

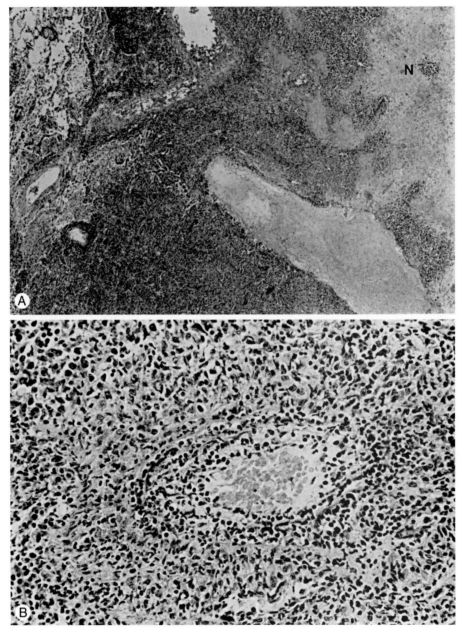

Figure 35–16. Angiocentric Immunoproliferative Lesion (Lymphomatoid Granulomatosis). A section *(A)* of a (grossly) poorly defined lung nodule shows a diffuse lymphoid infiltrate effacing normal lung architecture. There is prominent necrosis on the right (n). The limits of the wall of a small pulmonary artery *(B)* are hardly recognizable as a result of marked cellular infiltration.

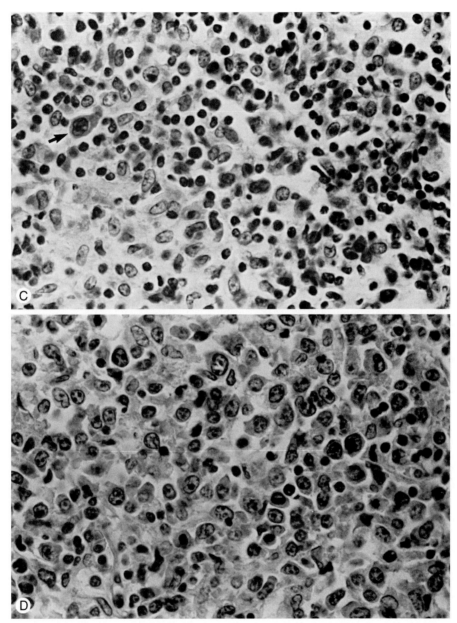

Figure 35–16 *Continued.* The cytologic appearance of the majority of the infiltrate *(C)* consisted of a polymorphic population of lymphocytes, histiocytes, plasma cells, and occasional atypical plasmacytoid cells *(arrow).* Other areas demonstrated a more extensive proliferation of atypical cells *(D),* which proved to be monoclonal on immunohistochemical investigation. (A, ×50; B, ×100; C, D, ×600.)

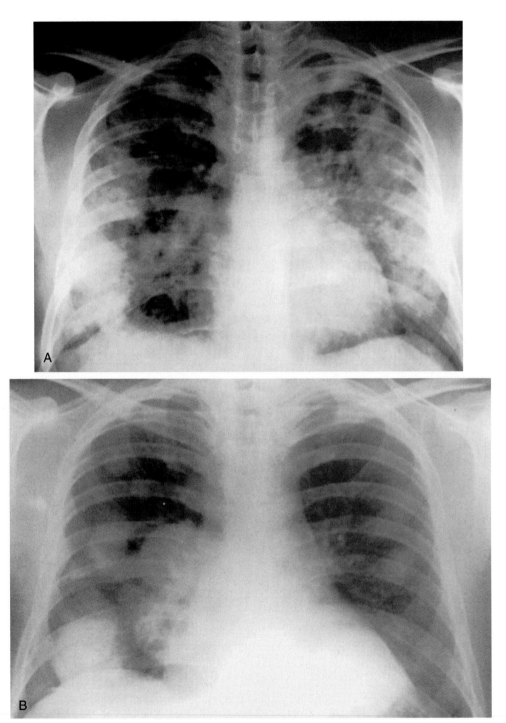

Figure 35–17. Angiocentric Immunoproliferative Lesion (Lymphomatoid Granulomatosis). A posteroanterior chest radiograph *(A)* shows multiple isolated and confluent nodular opacities in both lungs consistent with an air space–filling process. The lesions tend to be situated peripherally rather than centrally. The left hilum is obscured by the parenchymal abnormalities, and the right hilum is slightly prominent, suggesting lymph node enlargement. Two months later, a chest radiograph *(B)* disclosed some improvement in the features seen earlier, but both lungs were now the site of large, well-defined nodules; the lesions are homogeneous except for a single nodule in the right lower lobe that contains a central radiolucency, suggesting cavitation. (Courtesy of Dr. Max Palayew, Jewish General Hospital, Montreal, Canada.)

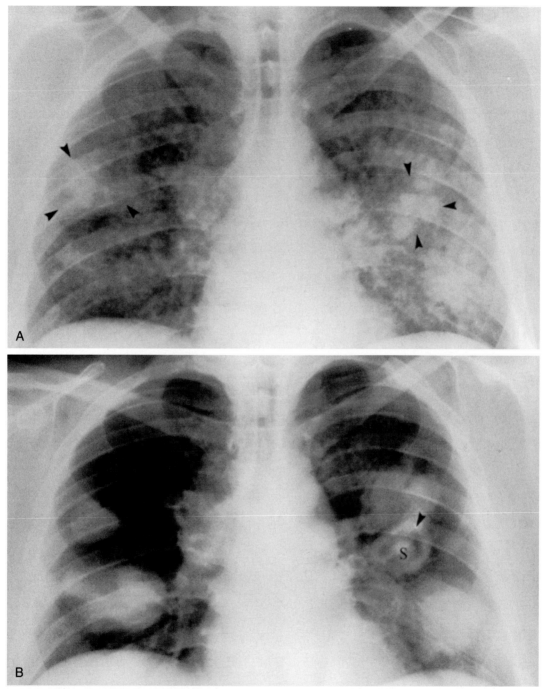

Figure 35–18. Angiocentric Immunoproliferative Lesion (Lymphomatoid Granulomatosis.) A posteroanterior chest radiograph *(A)* demonstrates bilateral confluent and isolated nodular opacities; some of the larger opacities *(arrowheads)* possess features of air-space consolidation. Bilateral hilar lymph node enlargement is present, and the aortopulmonary window is prominent, suggesting mediastinal node involvement. Two months later, a repeat chest radiograph *(B)* shows that the diffuse disease has resolved but has been replaced by large cavitary and noncavitary nodules. One cavitary lesion on the left *(arrowhead)* contains a central loose body (S) that could represent infarcted tissue or a blood clot. Several of the nodules relate to the more confluent areas of consolidation identified in *A*. Open-lung biopsy revealed infarcts caused by involvement of peripheral vessels by lymphomatoid granulomatosis. The patient was a 52-year-old man.

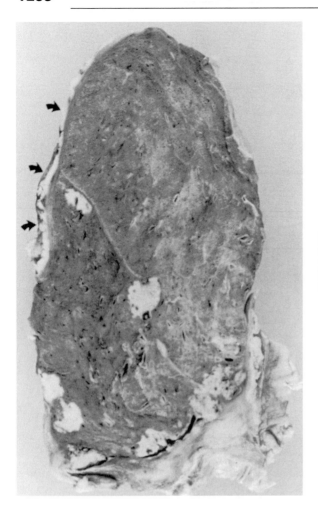

Figure 35–19. Secondary Pulmonary Lymphoma. Multiple, irregularly shaped but well-demarcated nodules are located predominantly adjacent to the pleura. The latter is also diffusely infiltrated *(arrows)*. The patient had disseminated large cell lymphoma and had been treated with systemic chemotherapy; most of the tumor was necrotic.

Figure 35–20. Secondary Pulmonary Lymphoma. A section of right lung removed at autopsy reveals three small parenchymal nodules and diffuse consolidation of most of the middle lobe and the anterior basal segment of the lower lobe. Disseminated large cell lymphoma.

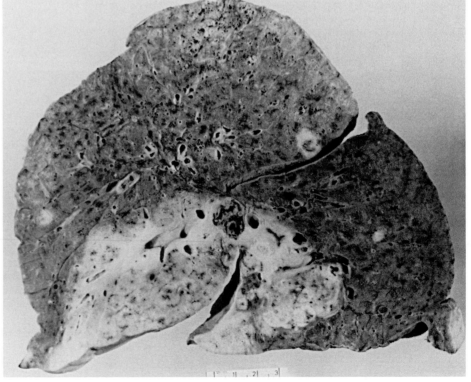

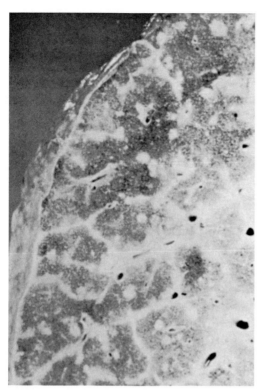

Figure 35–21. Secondary Pulmonary Lymphoma—Lymphangitic Spread. A magnified view of the anterior portion of a slice of upper lobe shows extensive thickening of interlobular septal and perivascular interstitial tissue as a result of lymphomatous infiltration.

in the lungs was attributed to spread of tumor from involved marrow at the time of transplantation.) Pulmonary involvement by non-Hodgkin's lymphoma in AIDS occurs in about 8% of cases;[145] although such involvement can be primary in the lung, more often there is concomitant evidence of extrapulmonary disease.

Any of the histologic subtypes of lymphoma can be responsible for pleuropulmonary disease; because the gross pathologic, radiologic, and clinical manifestations tend to be similar, the following discussion applies to all. Specific features of some of the more distinctive disorders are discussed separately.

Pathologic Characteristics

Grossly, secondary lymphoma can possess a variety of patterns, including solitary or multiple parenchymal nodules (Fig. 35–19), segmental or lobar consolidation (Fig. 35–20), an endobronchial mass,[145a] and focal or extensive interstitial thickening resembling lymphangitic carcinomatosis (Fig. 35–21). The interstitial pattern commonly results from spread of tumor from involved hilar or bronchopulmonary lymph nodes; peribronchial proliferation or endobronchial extension of such tumor can cause airway narrowing (Fig. 35–22), with secondary atelectasis and obstructive pneumonitis. Histologic features are those of the specific lymphoma type.

Radiologic Manifestations

Pulmonary involvement is apparent radiographically at presentation in approximately 5% of all patients with non-Hodgkin's lymphoma.[146, 147] The typical pattern consists of solitary or multiple nodules or masses ranging from 0.5 to 8 cm in diameter.[146, 147] They are usually most frequent in the lower lobes (Fig. 35–23).[148, 149] The nodules are round, ovoid, or polyhedral in shape and usually possess poorly defined margins, sometimes with linear strands extending into adjacent lung parenchyma. In cases of untreated lymphoma, the masses tend to coalesce, producing an opacity identical to and indistinguishable from that of primary pulmonary lymphoma.[148] Cavitation occurs rarely.[146, 150, 151] In one series of large cell lymphoma, cystlike lesions situated within or contiguous to masses were observed in 17 patients;[1] in 8, the cystic changes resembled cavitation radiographically.

In contrast to primary pulmonary lymphoma, the secondary variety tends to affect the larger airways (in most cases probably reflecting extension from bronchopulmonary lymph nodes as described previously) and may result in

Figure 35–22. Secondary Pulmonary Lymphoma: Interstitial Spread with Airway Compression. This large cell lymphoma involved multiple lymph node groups, including those in the hilar and peribronchial regions; the residua of the latter are indicated by *curved arrows*. The tumor extended into peribronchovascular connective tissue and bronchial mucosa, almost completely occluding two segmental airways *(arrowheads)*. Mucous plugging is evident in one subsegmental bronchus *(straight arrow)*.

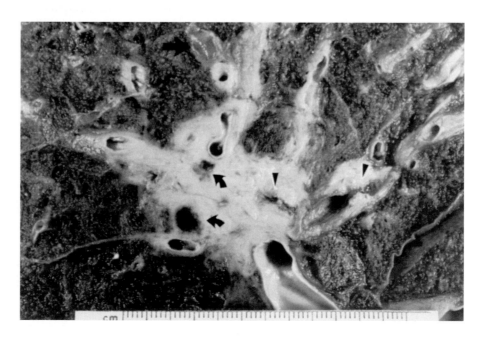

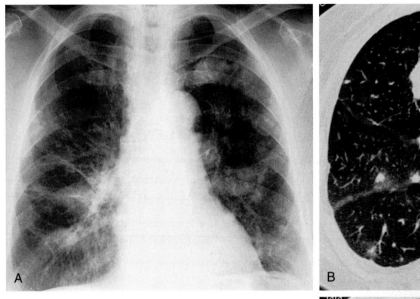

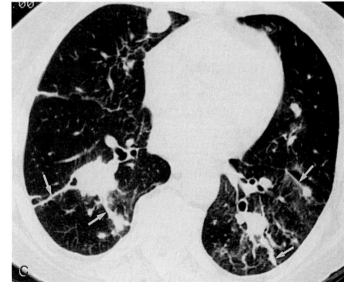

Figure 35–23. Secondary Pulmonary Lymphoma. A posteroanterior chest radiograph *(A)* in a 79-year-old woman demonstrates poorly defined nodular opacities in both lungs. HRCT scans *(B* and *C)* reveal nodules of various sizes in both lungs. The majority of nodules have irregular margins, and several are associated with thickening of the adjacent interlobular septa *(straight arrows)*. An air bronchogram *(curved arrow)* is evident in the nodule in the superior segment of the left lower lobe. The focal areas of ground-glass attenuation, evident particularly in the left lower lobe, are due to interstitial infiltration by lymphoma. The diagnosis of secondary lymphoma was proven by biopsy.

atelectasis and obstructive pneumonitis.[152, 153] A diffuse reticulonodular pattern with thickening of the interlobar septa resembling lymphangitic carcinomatosis sometimes occurs (Fig. 35–24).[90, 148, 154] Less common findings include micronodules, ground-glass opacities, and air-space consolidation (Fig. 35–25), particularly in patients with recurrent disease.[90, 155]

Pleural involvement can be manifested in several ways. Effusion by itself is uncommon;[156] however, it develops in association with parenchymal lymphoma at some point in the course of the disease in many patients (24 of 54 in one review[143]). Pleural lymphoma may be seen radiologically at the time of presentation or during recurrence (occasionally as the only site).[157] The appearance may consist of plaquelike areas of pleural thickening, focal nodules, pleura-based masses, or, less commonly, diffuse pleural thickening (Fig. 35–26) *(see* page 2838).[157, 158]

Clinical Manifestations

As might be expected, extrathoracic manifestations often predominate in patients with secondary pulmonary lym-

phoma. The most frequent presenting complaints are fever, anorexia, weight loss, and weakness, symptoms that may be rapidly progressive and can suggest complicating infection.[159] Involvement of the upper respiratory tract, particularly the nasopharynx and tonsils, or gastrointestinal tract may simulate carcinoma. Liver and spleen involvement may result in hepatosplenomegaly. Invasion of the spinal cord, cranial nerves, and meninges can result in pain, paresthesia, and paralysis.

As in primary pulmonary lymphoma, intrathoracic manifestations of secondary disease frequently cause no symptoms. Cough (sometimes with hemoptysis), chest pain, and dyspnea are occasionally present,[160, 161] particularly in patients with extensive disease. Evidence of pleuritis and alcohol-induced symptoms are less frequent than in Hodgkin's disease.[162]

Laboratory Findings

The total and differential leukocyte counts are usually within normal limits, although some patients with secondary

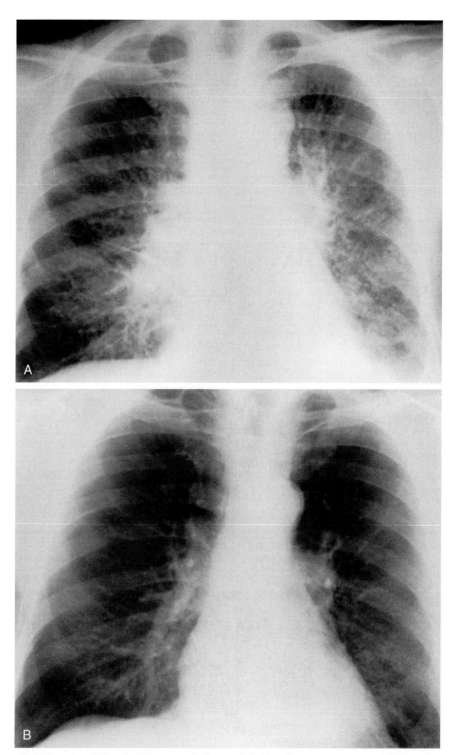

Figure 35–24. Regression of Diffuse Interstitial Disease in Large Cell Lymphoma. A posteroanterior chest radiograph *(A)* reveals bilateral hilar lymph node enlargement, thickening and loss of definition of the bronchovascular bundles, Kerley A lines, and small nodules. Small pleural effusions are present bilaterally. The superior mediastinum is widened as a result of lymph node enlargement. Two years later after chemotherapy, the abnormal features have completely cleared *(B)*. The patient was a 32-year-old man.

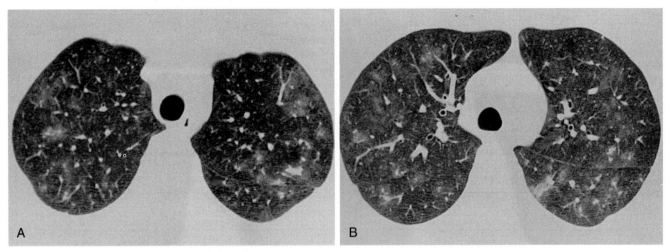

Figure 35–25. Secondary Pulmonary T-Cell Lymphoma. HRCT scans (*A* and *B*) demonstrate bilateral areas of ground-glass attenuation. The diagnosis of pulmonary T-cell lymphoma was confirmed by open-lung biopsy. The patient was a 35-year-old man who had presented 1 year previously with extensive mediastinal lymph node enlargement but no evidence of pulmonary involvement on the radiograph or CT scan. At the time of relapse, he presented with progressive shortness of breath; mediastinal and hilar lymph nodes were normal in size.

hypersplenism have hemolytic anemia, leukopenia, or thrombocytopenia. In the late stage of disease, leukemia may develop. When associated with hypereosinophilia, the clinical picture may simulate simple pulmonary eosinophilia (Loeffler's syndrome).[163, 164] Most pleural effusions are serous or serosanguineous; a few are chylous or pseudochylous.[165] In the setting of known extrathoracic lymphoma, the diagnosis of pleuropulmonary involvement can be made by cytologic examination of sputum,[166, 167] bronchial washings and brushings, and pleural fluid.[168, 169]

Specific Secondary Lymphomas

Waldenström's Macroglobulinemia

Waldenström's macroglobulinemia is a relatively uncommon form of lymphoma that is characterized by anemia, infiltration of the bone marrow by malignant lymphoplasmacytoid cells, and monoclonal IgM gammopathy. Hepatomegaly, splenomegaly, and peripheral lymph node enlargement

are common. The lungs are involved uncommonly.[170] Histologically, there is an interstitial infiltrate of small lymphoid cells, many of which show plasmacytoid differentiation and some of which show characteristic periodic acid–Schiff–positive intranuclear inclusions. The diagnosis can be confirmed by immunohistochemical demonstration of intracytoplasmic IgM on tissue specimens or in cells recovered by bronchial lavage.[171]

The chest radiograph has been reported to show a diffuse reticulonodular pattern or, less commonly, local homogeneous consolidation.[170, 172–175] Pleural effusion is present in about 50% of cases.[175] An unusual case has been reported in which the disease remained localized in mediastinal lymph nodes for a period of 9 years without the development of pulmonary disease.[176] When considering the diagnosis, it should be remembered that rare patients develop systemic amyloidosis, which may affect the lung.[177]

The disease occurs predominantly in the elderly and usually has an insidious onset. Of 15 patients with pulmonary involvement in one review, 6 were asymptomatic, and

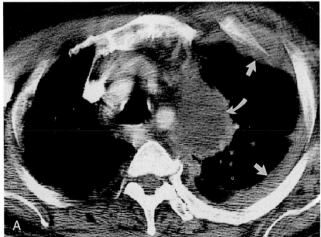
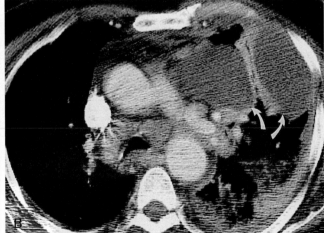

Figure 35–26. T-Cell Lymphoma with Diffuse Pleural Involvement. Contrast-enhanced spiral CT scans (*A* and *B*) demonstrate left pleural thickening *(straight arrows)* and loculated left pleural effusions *(curved arrows)* as well as enlargement of paratracheal lymph nodes. The patient was a 74-year-old man who presented with a 6-month history of low-grade fever and left chest pain. He had undergone repeated thoracentesis and was clinically suspected of having an empyema. After decortication, histologic analysis demonstrated diffuse pleural involvement with T-cell lymphoma.

the other 9 complained of dyspnea and cough at the time an abnormality was recognized radiologically.[170] Hyperviscosity syndrome may develop, and sausage-like segmentation of the retinal veins may occur, reducing visual acuity.[175] IgM monoclonal spikes were found in the sera of all 15 patients in the review cited and in the pleural effusion of 3 of the 6 patients with this complication in whom the pleural fluid was examined using protein electrophoresis.[170] Both exudative effusion[178] and chylothorax[179] have been documented. One unusual case has been reported in a canary breeder in whom the monoclonal IgM antibody was specific for an antigen in canary droppings.[180]

Burkitt's Lymphoma

An autopsy study of 17 individuals with Burkitt's lymphoma showed pleuropulmonary disease in 11;[181] the visceral pleura was generally more densely infiltrated than the lung parenchyma. Pulmonary parenchymal involvement was patchy and predominantly interstitial in location. In another review of the radiographic manifestations in 40 patients, abnormalities within the thorax were observed in 12.[182] Pleural effusion was the most common abnormality, being present in 9 of the 12 patients; however, in 7 of these, it was associated with ascites and thus was not necessarily attributable to direct involvement of the pleura by neoplasm. The remaining three patients manifested mediastinal lymph node enlargement, one with associated hilar node involvement.

Malignant Histiocytosis

Malignant histiocytosis is an uncommon malignancy characterized by the proliferation of atypical histiocytes predominantly in the liver, spleen, lymph nodes, and bone marrow. As a result of immunohistochemical studies, some cases previously considered to be this entity are now believed to be better classified as anaplastic large cell or T-cell lymphoma.

Evidence of intrathoracic involvement is found during life in 30% to 40% of patients reported to have malignant histiocytosis[183, 184] and may be the initial manifestation of the disease.[185, 186] Pathologically, the malignant cells are most prominent in the peribronchovascular, interlobular, and pleural connective tissue; adjacent airways, vessels, and parenchyma.[185] Individual cells resemble histiocytes with varying degrees of nuclear atypia; erythrophagocytosis is common. The pathologic diagnosis can be difficult to make, especially in those tumors with minimal cytologic atypia;[185] in these cases, the condition must be differentiated from virus-associated hemophagocytic syndrome, an abnormality that also affects the lungs and shows similar clinical and radiographic features.[187]

The most frequent radiographic manifestations are hilar and mediastinal lymph node enlargement, a reticular or reticulonodular interstitial pattern, and pleural effusion.[183–185, 188] Respiratory symptoms are usually overshadowed by systemic effects of the disease, particularly fever, weight loss, and generalized lymph node enlargement. Cough and dyspnea may be present, and extensive pulmonary disease occasionally causes respiratory failure.[186] Inappropriate antidi-

uretic hormone secretion has been noted in a number of patients.[183, 185]

Mycosis Fungoides

Mycosis fungoides is a T-cell lymphoma with prominent skin involvement. Dissemination of disease, including leukemia (Sézary's syndrome), occurs in the late stage. Pulmonary involvement is present at autopsy in approximately 50% of patients.[189–191] It may be a manifestation of generalized dissemination of the lymphoma in several tissues or associated with Sézary's syndrome.[192, 193] The usual pathologic findings consist of bilateral nodular aggregates of tumor cells within lung parenchyma;[190, 191] less commonly, there is predominantly peribronchovascular interstitial infiltration or an angiocentric distribution of disease.[194] Hilar and mediastinal lymph nodes are usually involved.[190]

Radiographic manifestations are nonspecific and include parenchymal nodules, patchy areas of consolidation, a diffuse reticulonodular pattern, and pleural effusion.[194–196] As in some cases of large cell lymphoma, air-space consolidation can develop rapidly and can simulate acute pneumonia.[192, 197, 198] Concomitant hilar or mediastinal (or both) lymphadenopathy is often present.

Dyspnea on exertion and a nonproductive cough are the usual symptoms of pulmonary disease.[196] Although the diagnosis may be suggested by examination of bronchial secretions or bronchoalveolar lavage specimens[199] or of tissue obtained by transbronchial biopsy or transthoracic needle aspiration,[196, 200] definitive diagnosis often requires an open-lung biopsy. When pulmonary involvement is present, there is usually disseminated disease and little response to therapy, and the prognosis is poor.[196, 199]

Intravascular Lymphomatosis

Intravascular lymphomatosis (angiotropic lymphoma, angioendotheliomatosis) is a rare disorder characterized pathologically by a malignant proliferation of lymphoid cells within the lumen of capillaries, arterioles, and venules; involvement of the adjacent extravascular tissue is typically absent or minimal. Immunophenotypic analysis has shown most cases to be composed of B cells;[201] however, a T-cell phenotype can also be seen.[201a] Clinically, the disease is manifested most often in the central nervous system (progressive dementia and multiple neurologic defects) and the skin (plaques and nodules). Pulmonary involvement has been reported in several cases in the absence of skin and central nervous system involvement, the clinical features including hypoxemia and fever of unknown origin,[201] progressive dyspnea,[202, 203] and pulmonary hypertension.[204] An interstitial reticular or reticulonodular pattern can be seen on chest radiographs.[201a, 202] HRCT has shown areas of ground-glass attenuation and intralobular linear opacities.[210, 210a] Diffuse gallium uptake and an abnormal perfusion scan have been reported in one case.[203] The diagnosis has been made by transbronchial biopsy.[205]

Mediastinal Lymphoma

As with pulmonary disease, lymphoma involving the mediastinum may be part of a generalized process or may occur exclusively or predominantly at this site; in the latter situation, the tumor is sometimes known as *primary mediastinal lymphoma.* Although virtually any histologic type of tumor may present in the mediastinum,[206] the two most common forms are lymphoblastic lymphoma and diffuse large cell lymphoma. The radiologic manifestations of these two are similar and are thus described together; however, the clinical and pathologic differences between them are sufficient to justify separate consideration.

Lymphoblastic Lymphoma

Lymphoblastic lymphoma comprises about 60% of cases of apparently primary mediastinal non-Hodgkin's lymphoma,[207] and approximately 50% to 80% of patients with this neoplasm have a prominent mass in the mediastinum at the time of presentation.[208] Lymphoblastic leukemia is pathologically and immunologically identical to lymphoblastic lymphoma, differing from the latter tumor only by having prominent bone marrow and blood involvement (often defined as > 25% marrow relacement by malignant cells); approximately 10% to 20% of affected patients present with a mediastinal mass.[209] The majority of patients with either form of tumor are children or adolescents, frequently male; immunologic studies show most tumors to have features of thymic T cells.

Signs and symptoms related to mediastinal involvement are common and include respiratory distress (as a result of airway compression) and superior vena cava syndrome. Pleural and pericardial effusions are also frequent.[209] Both leukemic and lymphomatous forms are aggressive tumors that are usually associated with widespread dissemination, especially to extrathoracic lymph nodes and the central nervous system; a leukemic phase also commonly develops in patients who initially present with lymphoma. Despite these features, current therapy results in remission in the majority of patients and a 3-year disease-free survival of approximately 55%.[209]

Diffuse Large Cell Lymphoma

Diffuse large cell lymphoma is a histologic variant of mediastinal lymphoma that is also associated with characteristic clinicopathologic features.[211–216] Grossly, the tumors are large, averaging almost 12 cm in diameter in one review.[213] Invasion of contiguous mediastinal structures, chest wall, and lung is common at the time of presentation.[213] As the name suggests, the majority of the neoplasms are composed of large cleaved or noncleaved cells; a pattern of immunoblastic sarcoma is present in some cases.[213] Immunohistochemical examination shows most tumors to have features of B-cell differentiation. Sclerosis, manifested by either diffuse increase in reticulin or relatively broad bands of fibrous tissue, is a prominent feature in many cases. Histologic differentiation from other mediastinal neoplasms, particularly thymoma and germ cell tumors, can be difficult, especially with small tissue samples.

The majority of large cell lymphomas occur in young adults. In most series, the sex incidence is about equal, although in some there is a predominance of women.[213, 214] Symptoms referable to the thorax, particularly dyspnea and pain, are present in the majority of patients. Superior vena cava syndrome also occurs in many individuals (e.g., 38

[40%] of 93 patients in three series[213, 216, 217]); compression of the vena cava in the absence of the full-blown clinical syndrome can be identified in some patients.[216] Compression of the main pulmonary artery also is seen in some patients.[217a] Although the diagnosis can be made on specimens obtained by fine-needle aspiration,[218, 219] this may be difficult, and mediastinoscopic or open biopsy is often necessary. With aggressive chemotherapy and radiation therapy, most investigators have found a complete remission rate of about 80% and a 50% to 60% 5-year survival.

Radiologic Manifestations

Radiologically, the most commonly involved lymph nodes in mediastinal lymphoma are the anterior mediastinal and paratracheal nodes;[146, 147] in one investigation of 181 consecutive patients with no previous treatment, involvement of these groups was apparent radiographically in 24% of cases and on CT in 34%.[147] Other nodal stations that may be involved include, in decreasing order of frequency, the subcarinal, hilar, internal mammary, pericardial, and posterior mediastinal (Fig. 35–27).[147] The lymphadenopathy may be noncontiguous and in 40% of cases involves a single nodal group.[146] The enlarged nodes may have homogeneous soft tissue attenuation (Fig. 35–28) or, less commonly, a central area of decreased attenuation and rim enhancement (*see* Fig. 35–27). They may encase major vessels and lead to obstruction of the superior vena cava (Fig. 35–29). Irradiation or chemotherapy (or both) can result in a rapid resolution of intrathoracic disease. After treatment, particularly radiotherapy, dystrophic calcification may occur, most commonly in lymph nodes in the anterior mediastinum.[220] Rarely, nodal calcification is present at the time of initial diagnosis.[114]

The contribution of CT to the initial staging of patients with non-Hodgkin's lymphoma was assessed in one study of 181 consecutive individuals.[147] Intrathoracic abnormalities were seen in 45%. Prevascular and paratracheal lymph node enlargement was the most common abnormality, being present in approximately 75% of patients with intrathoracic disease. (As might be expected, adenopathy was seen more commonly on CT than on radiography; CT was particularly helpful in the detection of subcarinal and pericardial node enlargement.) Pulmonary parenchymal involvement was evident on CT in 24 patients (13%); in approximately one third of these, the parenchymal abnormalities were not evident on radiography. The most common findings included nodules, masses, and focal areas of air-space consolidation; less commonly, direct parenchymal infiltration from adjacent mediastinal lymph nodes was evident (Fig. 35–30).[147] Pleural effusion was evident on CT in 36 (20%) patients, focal soft tissue pleural masses in 9 (5%), and chest wall involvement in 9. Overall, the findings on routine chest CT increased the stage in 16 patients (9%) compared with chest radiography. The additional CT findings, however, did not influence the need for combination chemotherapy. The authors concluded that CT may be of additional value in defining prognostic subsets and in selecting poor-risk patients for investigative therapies.

MR imaging shows the same anatomic features as CT. Lymphoma usually has a homogeneous appearance on MR, the signal intensity being slightly greater than muscle on T1-

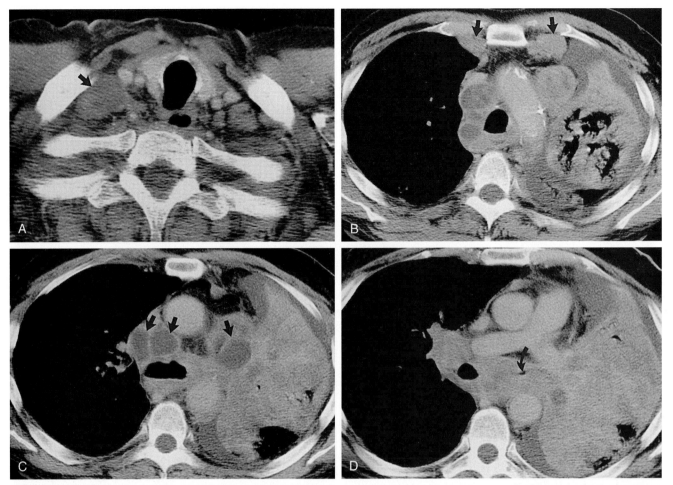

Figure 35–27. Mediastinal and Supraclavicular B-Cell Lymphoma. A contrast-enhanced CT scan demonstrates enlargement of right supraclavicular lymph nodes (*arrow* in *A*); internal mammary nodes (*arrows* in *B*); and anterior mediastinal, aortopulmonary window, paratracheal, subcarinal, and hilar nodes (*C* and *D*). The right supraclavicular and internal mammary nodes have homogeneous soft tissue attenuation, whereas the paratracheal and aortopulmonary window nodes (*arrows* in *C* and *D*) have low attenuation centers with rim enhancement suggestive of central necrosis. The enlarged nodes are associated with marked extrinsic compression of the left main bronchus (*curved arrow* in *D*) leading to obstructive pneumonitis and loss of volume. Also noted is a small left pleural effusion. The patient was a 58-year-old man. The diagnosis of large cell lymphoma was proven by biopsy of the right supraclavicular lymph nodes.

weighted and T2-weighted images.[221] Although the technique enables greater soft tissue contrast than CT, it is seldom used in the initial assessment of patients with lymphoma. It may be helpful, however, in patients who are allergic to intravenous contrast agents or who have a superior vena cava syndrome, or in the assessment of pericardial or chest wall invasion. In one study of 57 patients with biopsy-proven lymphoma or Hodgkin's disease, chest wall involvement was evident on MR imaging in 20 patients and on CT in 7;[222] pleural disease was seen on MR in 14 patients and on CT in 5 patients. Of the 15 patients in the study who had chest wall disease and were treated with radiation therapy, 3 (20%) had the portals changed because of the MR findings.[222]

Gallium 67 scintigraphy is inferior to CT in the initial assessment of patients who have lymphoma. The procedure has an important role, however, in the evaluation of patients who have a residual tumor mass after treatment, uptake being present in residual lymphoma but not in necrotic tumor or fibrotic tissue.[223–225] Preliminary results suggest that fludeoxyglucose F 18 positron-emission tomography imaging may be superior to CT in the demonstration of

nodal involvement in both non-Hodgkin's lymphoma and Hodgkin's disease.[226] Fludeoxyglucose F 18 is a glucose analogue that is metabolized in proportion to the glycolytic metabolic rate, which is elevated in tumors;[227] uptake of the substance in non-Hodgkin's lymphoma has been shown to correlate with both tumor grade and prognosis.[228–230]

PLASMA CELL NEOPLASMS

Multiple Myeloma

Thoracic disease in multiple myeloma is common: in one review of 958 patients, evidence of skeletal or pleuropulmonary abnormality was found at some time during the course of the disease in 443 (46%);[231] radiographic abnormalities were present in 25% at the time of diagnosis. The pathogenesis of these abnormalities is multifactorial and may be related to either a direct effect of the neoplastic plasma cells or indirect effects caused by disease in other organs. Pathologically, the former disease is characterized by a proliferation of plasma cells with varying degrees of atypia.[232, 233]

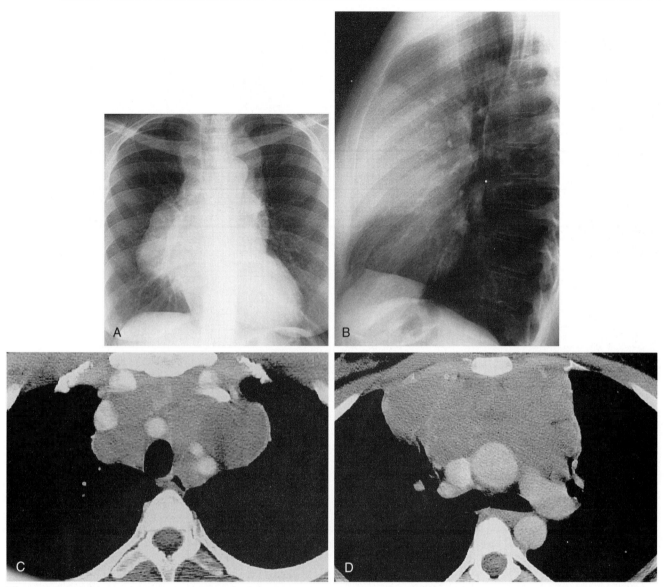

Figure 35–28. Mediastinal B-Cell Lymphoma. Posteroanterior *(A)* and lateral *(B)* chest radiographs reveal a large, lobulated anterior mediastinal mass. The absence of hilar lymphadenopathy is noted, the interlobar arteries being clearly seen through the soft tissue masses ("hilum overlay" sign). Contrast-enhanced spiral CT scans *(C* and *D)* demonstrate diffuse enlargement of the anterior mediastinal and paratracheal lymph nodes with obliteration of the fat planes between the nodes. Despite the extensive lymphadenopathy, there is no evidence of compression of the vascular structures. Mediastinoscopy revealed diffuse large cell lymphoma. The patient was a 31-year-old woman.

Neoplastic infiltration of the skeleton is undoubtedly the most common manifestation of thoracic disease, being identified as an isolated finding (without adjacent chest wall invasion) in 257 (28%) patients in the series cited previously;[231] in 15%, it was the initial abnormality. The ribs are most frequently affected, although involvement of the vertebrae and sternum, either alone or in combination with the ribs, is also fairly common.

The usual radiographic appearance consists of one or more well-defined, osteolytic lesions; diffuse osteoporosis, fracture, or a combination of lesions can also be seen. The involved rib may show focal expansion (Fig. 35–31). Extension and proliferation of tumor in the adjacent chest wall result in a rather typical radiologic appearance of a smooth homogeneous soft tissue mass protruding into the thorax and compressing the lung (Fig. 35–32). Such tumor

masses can grow to a large size, sometimes almost completely opacifying a hemithorax.[234] The association of an osteolytic lesion in a rib with a soft tissue mass protruding into the thorax should strongly suggest the diagnosis;[235] however, this combination can also occur with metastatic carcinoma, with other primary chest wall diseases (such as osteomyelitis), and with lesions originating in the lung (such as pulmonary carcinoma and fungal infections).

Infiltration of the lungs or pleura by neoplastic cells is much less common than that of the skeleton. Pleural effusion caused by malignant infiltration has been reported rarely;[236–239] for reasons that are unclear, this appears to occur more often on the left side. Pleural thickening and nodularity are sometimes evident in addition to the effusion.[241] Pulmonary parenchymal or airway involvement is also uncommon. This can take the form of one or more localized masses that are

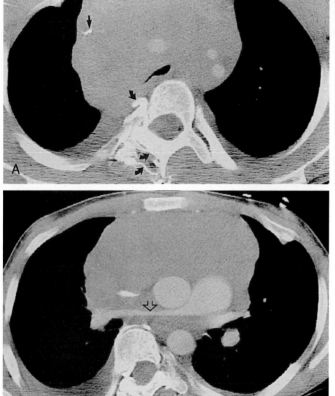

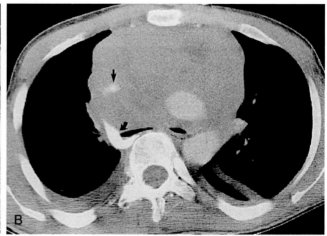

Figure 35–29. Mediastinal Lymphoblastic T-Cell Lymphoma with Superior Vena Cava Obstruction. A contrast-enhanced CT scan through the upper chest *(A)* demonstrates diffuse soft tissue infiltration of the mediastinum resulting in marked compression and deformity of the trachea. Intravenous contrast material can be seen within an encased and markedly narrowed right brachiocephalic vein *(straight arrow)* and within collateral veins *(curved arrows)*. Small bilateral pleural effusions are also evident. A CT scan at the level of the main bronchi *(B)* reveals encasement of the superior vena cava *(straight arrow)* and prominent collateral circulation through the azygos vein *(curved arrow)*. A further scan at the level of the bronchus intermedius *(C)* demonstrates narrowing and elongation of the right pulmonary artery *(open arrow)*. The patient was an 18-year-old man who presented with progressive shortness of breath and clinical findings of superior vena cava obstruction.

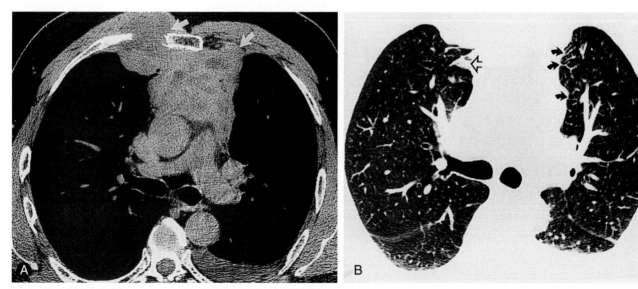

Figure 35–30. B-Cell Lymphoma with Chest Wall and Pulmonary Invasion. A CT scan *(A)* in a 51-year-old man demonstrates inhomogeneous enlargement of the anterior mediastinal nodes with extension into the chest wall *(arrows)*. A small left pleural effusion is also evident. Lung windows *(B)* demonstrate thickening of interlobular septa *(curved arrows)* adjacent to the enlarged mediastinal lymph nodes, consistent with direct extension of lymphoma into the lungs. The focal area of consolidation in the right lung *(open arrow)* is also presumed to represent secondary lymphoma.

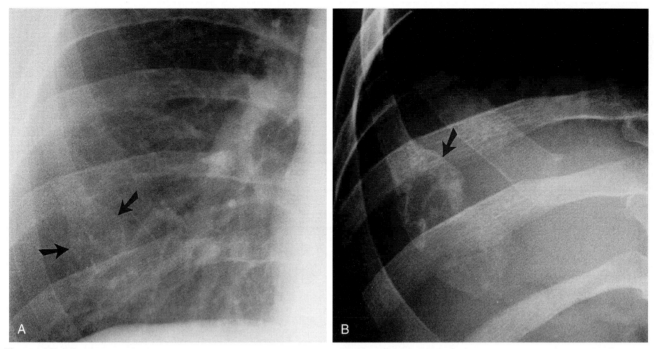

Figure 35–31. Multiple Myeloma. A view of the right chest from a posteroanterior radiograph *(A)* demonstrates a focal expansile lesion *(arrows)* involving the right anterior sixth rib. The abnormality is better seen on the overexposed rib view *(B)*.

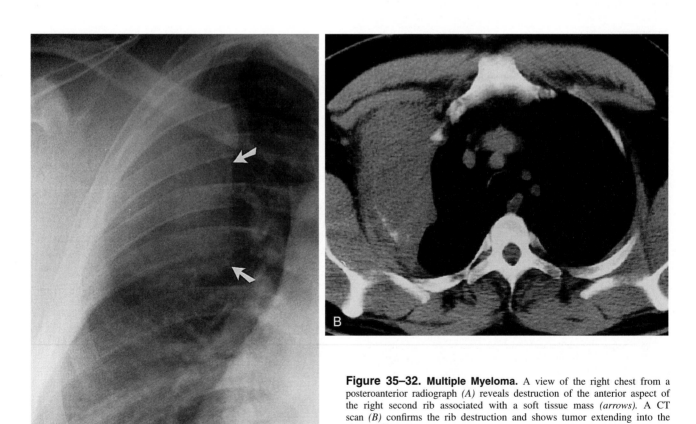

Figure 35–32. Multiple Myeloma. A view of the right chest from a posteroanterior radiograph *(A)* reveals destruction of the anterior aspect of the right second rib associated with a soft tissue mass *(arrows)*. A CT scan *(B)* confirms the rib destruction and shows tumor extending into the chest wall.

typically somewhat lobulated in contour and homogeneous in density,[240] relatively diffuse parenchymal infiltration, or an endobronchial or endotracheal tumor, sometimes associated with atelectasis and obstructive pneumonitis.[232, 233] One or more of these patterns was identified in only 11 (1%) of the 958 patients in the review cited previously.[231] Other intrathoracic abnormalities that have been described include multiple pulmonary nodules mimicking metastases and mediastinal lymph node enlargement.

Although the most common thoracic abnormalities in multiple myeloma are caused by direct neoplastic infiltration, other mechanisms are also involved. For example, pleural effusion was considered to be caused by congestive heart failure more often than by tumor infiltration in the large series cited previously;[231] the cause of the failure was identified as cardiac amyloidosis in 18 (31%) of the 58 patients with effusion. Pulmonary amyloidosis—usually of the diffuse alveolar septal type—can also occur as part of generalized amyloid deposition.[242] Pneumonia is not infrequent, most often from *Streptococcus pneumoniae* and gram-negative organisms.[231] Pulmonary thromboembolism has also been reported to have an increased frequency.[231] Rarely, myeloma is associated with metastatic calcification of the lungs.[243, 244]

The majority of patients with multiple myeloma are symptomatic when first seen, by which time their disease is usually widely disseminated. Occasionally, the diagnosis is made in asymptomatic patients by finding a monoclonal peak on electrophoresis carried out for some other reason. Thoracic signs and symptoms depend on the location of the lesion. Rib involvement can cause local tenderness and pain on respiration. Pulmonary parenchymal, bronchial, and tracheal involvement may be manifested by cough, chest pain, or dyspnea. Signs and symptoms of extrathoracic disease are also common;[245] in one review of 869 cases, these included bone pain (68%), palpable liver (21%), and palpable spleen (5%).[246]

Laboratory abnormalities are frequent; in the previously cited review, they included anemia (62%), renal insufficiency (55%), hypercalcemia (30%), and proteinuria (88%, Bence Jones type in 49%). Virtually all patients have evidence of monoclonal gammopathy.[246] In approximately 60% of symptomatic patients, it is related to IgG and in 20% to IgA; the remainder manifest Bence Jones proteinuria or proteinemia, as determined by immunoelectrophoresis.[246, 247] Definitive diagnosis is most often made by bone marrow biopsy. Pleural involvement may be detected by cytologic examination of the fluid[248] or biopsy.[236] Pulmonary disease has been identified by the finding of monoclonal plasma cell population on bronchoalveolar lavage.[249]

As might be expected, the prognosis of patients who have multiple myeloma is considerably better in those with one or two localized lesions than in those with generalized disease. The former may respond to irradiation,[247] although the disease may recur many years later, sometimes in the lungs.[240] Most patients eventually die from infection (usually bacterial)[246, 250] or renal insufficiency.[246, 251] In some patients who appear clinically stable, an aggressive terminal phase has been described characterized radiographically by parenchymal consolidation resembling pneumonia and clinically by fever, pancytopenia, and enlarging soft tissue masses.[252]

Plasmacytoma

A plasmacytoma can be defined as a more or less well-defined neoplastic proliferation of plasma cells in the absence of a generalized plasma cell disorder. As such, it excludes the far more common situation in which a localized plasma cell tumor is a manifestation of multiple myeloma. These tumors can consist of an isolated expansile osteolytic lesion of bone or a visceral or soft tissue mass, the latter often termed *extramedullary plasmacytoma*. The majority of such tumors are located in the upper respiratory tract, particularly the pharynx; in one large review of 272 cases, only 13 (4.7%) were situated in the lungs or trachea.[253] In a literature review in 1992, only 19 well-documented examples were identified in the lower respiratory tract.[254]

Pathologically, the tumors typically consist of sheets of plasma cells with variable degrees of atypia. Occasionally, amorphous eosinophilic material is present between tumor cells. In most such cases, this material represents amyloid; rarely, it is immunoglobulin (IgG, κ).[255, 255a] (In one unusual example of the latter form of disease, there were few plasma cells, and the κ chains were largely present within macrophages and alveolar epithelial cells.[256]) It is important to ensure that the cellular proliferation is monomorphous and to adhere to strict criteria of plasma cell differentiation to be certain of the diagnosis; in fact, it is likely that some reported cases of plasmacytoma are in reality B-cell lymphoma with plasmacytoid differentiation or plasma cell granuloma. Immunohistochemical demonstration of a monoclonal proliferation of plasma cells can be helpful in distinguishing a neoplastic from a reactive process, especially in small biopsy samples obtained by endoscopy or fine-needle aspiration.[257, 258]

Pulmonary parenchymal plasmacytomas present radiographically as a nodule or somewhat lobulated mass indistinguishable from pulmonary carcinoma. Eleven cases of tracheal plasmacytoma had been reported by 1995;[259] although the tumor may not be detected on the radiograph, it can be seen as a focal polypoid lesion on CT (Fig. 35–33).[259] Large lesions can cause airway obstruction, either inspiratory or expiratory, depending on their location within the neck or thorax. Endobronchial tumors can cause atelectasis or obstructive pneumonitis.[260, 261] Ossification is occasionally identified.[234, 255] Pleural effusion is rare.[262]

Clinical symptoms depend on the location of the lesion. Parenchymal and endobronchial tumors can either cause no symptoms or be accompanied by hemoptysis, cough, dyspnea, or chest pain.[234] Tracheal involvement can cause dyspnea and wheezing. The majority of tumors are not associated with abnormal levels of serum or urine immunoglobulins; occasionally—usually with large tumors—M protein can be detected.[263, 264] The diagnosis has been made in occasional patients by examination of specimens obtained by transthoracic needle aspiration.[265] Additional plasma cell tumors or overt multiple myeloma develop in some patients; however, prolonged survival without these complications may be seen.[253]

Light and Heavy Chain Disease

Heavy chain disease is associated with monoclonal gammopathies related to the Fc fragments of heavy chains from IgG, IgA, or IgM. In IgG heavy chain disease, enlarge-

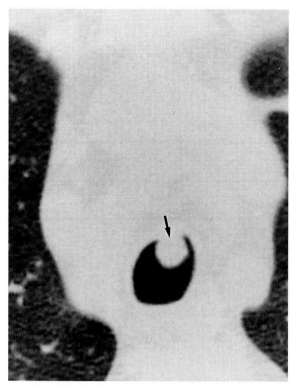

Figure 35–33. Primary Plasmacytoma of the Trachea. An HRCT scan through the upper thoracic trachea demonstrates a polypoid endotracheal mass *(arrow)* measuring 1 cm in diameter. The patient was a 51-year-old man who presented with hemoptysis; there was no clinical or laboratory evidence of multiple myeloma at presentation or on a 1-year follow-up.

ment of lymph nodes (including those in the mediastinum) is common and typically is accompanied by hepatosplenomegaly, anemia, and leukopenia. Most affected patients die from pneumonia within a year of diagnosis.[266] IgA heavy chain disease is usually associated with an abdominal neoplasm and severe malabsorption syndrome;[267] rare cases associated with pulmonary parenchymal involvement and mediastinal lymph node enlargement have been documented.[268] An unusual case of systemic light chain disease has been reported in which there were multiple pulmonary nodules composed of amyloid-like material secondary to deposition of light chain protein.[269]

HODGKIN'S DISEASE

Intrathoracic involvement in Hodgkin's disease is common, most often in the form of mediastinal and hilar lymph node enlargement. In one series of 659 patients, mediastinal lymph node enlargement was present in 405 (61%) and hilar lymph node enlargement in 193 (29%) at the time of diagnosis.[270] Evidence of pleuropulmonary involvement is present at the time of diagnosis in 10% to 15% of patients[270, 271] and at some time during the course of the disease in 15% to 40%.[272] The majority of cases are of the nodular sclerosis subtype: in one review of 89 patients with lung involvement, 77 of these were from the 460 patients who had nodular sclerosis, whereas only 6 occurred in the 146 patients who had the mixed cellularity subtype.[270] Since the advent of multiagent chemotherapy, the incidence of thoracic Hodg-

kin's disease at autopsy has decreased;[273] nevertheless, in one review of 80 patients who died between 1972 and 1977, residual disease was present in the lung in 39% and intrathoracic lymph nodes in 59%.[274]

Intrathoracic involvement is usually associated with evidence of Hodgkin's disease elsewhere in the body; for example, in one series of 1,470 consecutive patients, only 44 (3%) were found to have purely intrathoracic disease after appropriate clinical and pathologic staging.[275] Primary pulmonary Hodgkin's disease (unassociated with clinical or radiologic evidence of disease in lymph nodes or other tissues) is even more uncommon:[272, 275] in a study of 155 cases of Hodgkin's disease from Yale University between 1980 and 1987, only one case was identified; a review of the literature published at the same time documented only 60 additional reports.[272] According to this review, there is a slight female predominance (1.4:1) and a bimodal peak incidence between 21 and 30 years and 60 and 80 years.[272] For unknown reasons, such primary pulmonary disease has a pronounced predilection for the upper lobes.[272]

Pathologic Characteristics

Pulmonary involvement in Hodgkin's disease probably occurs most often by direct extension from affected hilar or bronchopulmonary lymph nodes; thus, the most common pathologic appearance is thickened peribronchovascular interstitial tissue (Fig. 35–34). The infiltrate can extend from this location into adjacent bronchial mucosa, resulting in a

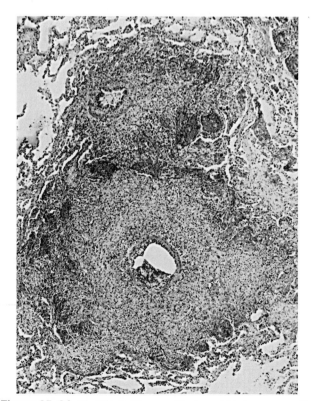

Figure 35–34. Hodgkin's Disease. The interstitial tissue surrounding a small bronchiole and its accompanying pulmonary artery is greatly expanded because of an infiltrate of inflammatory cells and scattered malignant Hodgkin's cells. Early extension into adjacent parenchyma is noted. (×40.)

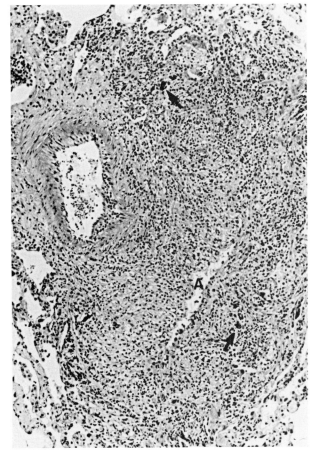

Figure 35–35. Hodgkin's Disease—Bronchiolar Obstruction. The entire wall of this membranous bronchiole is involved with an infiltrate of Hodgkin's disease. (Reed-Sternberg cells are identifiable as relatively large, darkly staining cells [*arrows*]). The bronchiolar lumen (A) has been reduced to a narrow slit.

plaquelike elevation or (less commonly) an endobronchial polypoid tumor, both of which can cause airway narrowing with distal atelectasis and obstructive pneumonitis;[273, 276] rarely, this is the first manifestation of the disease.[272] Similar luminal obstruction can be seen in membranous bronchioles (Fig. 35–35).

The peribronchovascular interstitial infiltrate can also extend into adjacent lung parenchyma; enlargement and coalescence of such foci undoubtedly account for most of the localized nodules or masses seen grossly.[278] Interlobular septa, pleura, and their adjacent lung parenchyma can also be infiltrated. Extensive lobar involvement simulating acute air-space pneumonia and multiple small nodules simulating miliary disease are infrequent manifestations.[273, 276] Fibrous nodules, representing foci of healed disease, can be found in any of the aforementioned locations in patients who have received chemotherapy.[274]

Microscopically, the infiltrate is identical to that seen in affected lymph nodes, the pattern varying with the different histologic subtypes; as noted previously, nodular sclerosis is by far the most frequent of these. The disease can be confused histologically with peripheral T-cell lymphoma, large cell lymphoma of the mediastinum,[279] and (rarely) thymoma or germ cell tumors (the latter particularly in the "syncytial" variant of nodular sclerosis, which tends to have bulky

mediastinal disease[280]). Use of a panel of immunohistochemical markers is of value in making the distinction between these conditions and Hodgkin's disease. Microscopic foci of disease may be apparent in hilar or mediastinal (or both) lymph nodes of normal size,[272, 281] and these should ideally be examined before a case of isolated (primary) pulmonary disease is accepted. Granulomatous inflammation can be seen both in relation to the parenchymal and interstitial infiltrates and in hilar or mediastinal lymph nodes unaffected by Hodgkin's disease itself;[278] in some cases, the appearance is suggestive of concomitant sarcoidosis.[282]

Radiologic Manifestations

The incidence of various intrathoracic abnormalities identifiable on plain chest radiographs was assessed in a study of 300 consecutive patients who had untreated Hodgkin's disease and non-Hodgkin's lymphoma.[146] Hodgkin's disease was found to be associated with a higher incidence of intrathoracic disease at presentation (67% compared with 43%), manifested predominantly by bulky anterior mediastinal lymph node enlargement. In this study, lung involvement was also more common in Hodgkin's disease (approximately 12% versus 4%) and was always accompanied by mediastinal or hilar lymph node enlargement or both.

Mediastinal Lymph Node Enlargement

Mediastinal lymph node enlargement is seen on the initial chest radiograph in 60% to 80% of patients (Fig. 35–36).[146, 270, 283] Involvement of the anterior mediastinal and paratracheal lymph nodes is four times more common in Hodgkin's disease than in non-Hodgkin's lymphoma, being evident at presentation on the chest radiograph in 90% and on CT in 98% of patients with intrathoracic disease.[146, 283] Lymphadenopathy most commonly involves the anterior mediastinal nodes followed in decreasing frequency by paratracheal, hilar, subcarinal, internal mammary, pericardiophrenic, and posterior mediastinal (Figs. 35–37 and 35–38).[146, 283] Involvement of contiguous groups of lymph nodes occurs in approximately 90% of patients.[284, 285] In one investigation of 203 patients with newly diagnosed Hodgkin's disease, intrathoracic lymphadenopathy was evident on the chest radiograph in 78% and on CT in 86%;[283] on CT, the anterior mediastinal and paratracheal nodes were involved in 84% of cases, hilar nodes in 28%, subcarinal nodes in 22%, pericardiophrenic nodes in 8%, internal mammary nodes in 5%, and posterior mediastinal nodes in 5%. Most cases of subcarinal, pericardiophrenic, internal mammary, and posterior mediastinal lymphadenopathy were detected only on CT.[283]

Involvement of the anterior mediastinal and internal mammary nodes may be associated with invasion of the sternum or the parasternal tissues,[286–288] either unilaterally or bilaterally.[289] The results of one study suggest that MR imaging may be superior to CT in the detection of chest wall involvement, either by demonstrating chest wall extension not apparent on CT or by identifying additional sites of chest wall involvement.[222]

On the chest radiograph, involvement of the anterior mediastinal and paratracheal lymph nodes results in widen-

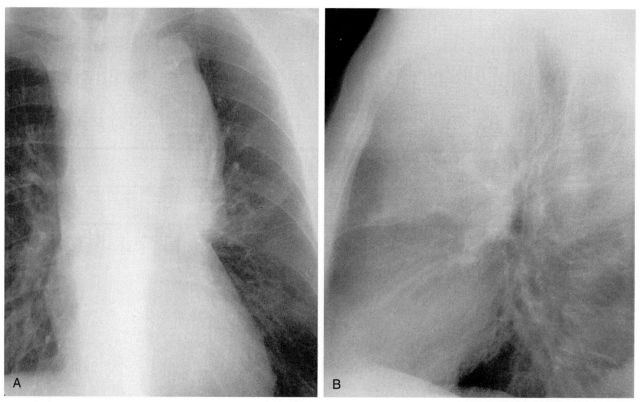

Figure 35–36. Hodgkin's Disease. A close-up view of the mediastinum from a posteroanterior chest radiograph *(A)* reveals asymmetric widening of the mediastinum with a lobulated contour consistent with extensive anterior mediastinal lymph node enlargement. Increased soft tissue opacity in the region of the superior vena cava is consistent with paratracheal lymph node enlargement. A lateral view *(B)* confirms the presence of extensive anterior mediastinal lymphadenopathy. The patient was a 57-year-old man with Hodgkin's disease proven by biopsy of the enlarged paratracheal lymph nodes.

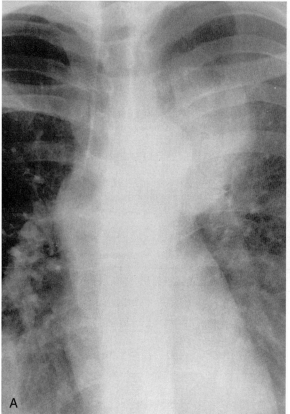

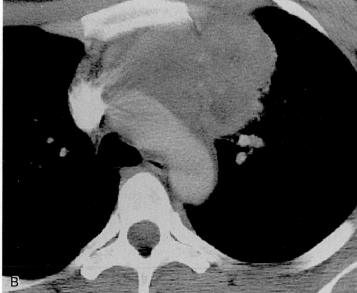

Figure 35–37. Hodgkin's Disease. A close-up view of the mediastinum from a posteroanterior chest radiograph *(A)* demonstrates a focal mass overlying the aortic arch; the appearance mimics a pulmonary mass. A contrast-enhanced spiral CT scan *(B)* demonstrates anterior mediastinal lymph node enlargement; no other site of lymph node involvement was apparent on CT. The patient was a 27-year-old woman.

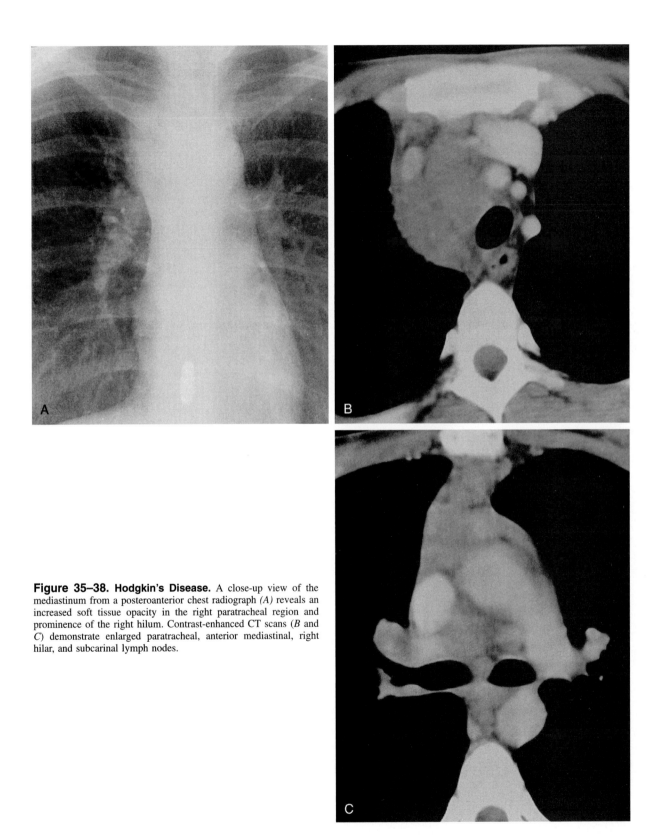

Figure 35–38. Hodgkin's Disease. A close-up view of the mediastinum from a posteroanterior chest radiograph *(A)* reveals an increased soft tissue opacity in the right paratracheal region and prominence of the right hilum. Contrast-enhanced CT scans *(B* and *C)* demonstrate enlarged paratracheal, anterior mediastinal, right hilar, and subcarinal lymph nodes.

ing of the mediastinum and a lobulated contour (*see* Fig. 35–36). The nodal enlargement protrudes into the right and left hemithoraces in an asymmetric fashion (*see* Figs. 35–37 and 35–38). Paravertebral lymph node enlargement results in widening and lobulation of the paraspinal interface (Fig. 35–39), whereas enlargement of the pericardiophrenic lymph nodes is manifested by a lobulated contour or a "double density" of the cardiac silhouette (Figs. 35–40 and 35–41). Ultimately, however, it is necessary to confirm the presence of suspected lymph node involvement by CT. Fat accumulation, particularly in the paraspinal region and pericardiophrenic angles, cannot be distinguished from lymphadenopathy on the chest radiograph; also, CT may demonstrate evidence of lymphadenopathy that is not detectable on the radiograph. For example, in a study of 203 patients with newly diagnosed Hodgkin's disease, CT provided additional evidence of lymph node enlargement in 8%, chest wall

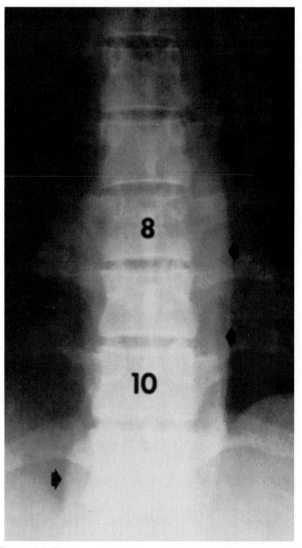

Figure 35–39. Paravertebral Lymph Node Involvement in Hodgkin's Disease. An overexposed radiograph of the mediastinum and spine in a patient with Hodgkin's disease reveals typical feature of paravertebral node enlargement *(arrowheads).* The abnormality is manifested by a lobulated or straightened configuration of the right or left paraspinal lines, or both. Enlarged paravertebral nodes are most often identified in the lower thorax at the T8 to T12 vertebrae.

involvement in 5%, pericardial involvement in 4%, and pleural involvement in 3%.[283] Based on the additional information provided by CT, treatment was altered in 19 of the 203 patients (9%).

An anterior mediastinal mass can be caused by Hodgkin's disease involving the thymus gland rather than by enlarged lymph nodes. Occasionally, it has a cystic appearance, mimicking cystic change in a thymoma or a germ cell tumor. Rarely, a benign cyst of the thymus and Hodgkin's disease occur simultaneously.[290] In patients with Hodgkin's disease, diffuse enlargement of the thymus gland following remission of disease after treatment can also result from "rebound" hyperplasia (*see* page 2877). Another cause of an anterior mediastinal mass in patients with Hodgkin's disease is spontaneous mediastinal hemorrhage associated with radiotherapy and combination chemotherapy.[291]

Dystrophic calcification develops in involved intrathoracic lymph nodes in some cases after mediastinal radiation (Fig. 35–42).[220, 292–295] Although some investigators consider the complication to be unrelated to the degree of radiation,[293] others link it with relatively high doses.[295] The time interval between irradiation and the appearance of calcification may be as short as 1 year or as long as 9 years. Several cases have been described in which lymph node calcification developed after chemotherapy without accompanying radiation.[296]

As with carcinoma, Hodgkin's disease can extend beyond affected lymph nodes into adjacent mediastinal tissue and invade such structures as the esophagus, superior vena cava, and pericardium; corresponding radiologic manifestations, such as pericardial effusion, may be seen.[292, 297] An exception is diaphragmatic paralysis secondary to invasion of the phrenic nerve; in contrast to pulmonary carcinoma, Hodgkin's disease rarely results in this complication.[292, 297, 298]

Pleuropulmonary Disease

Involvement of peribronchovascular tissue by Hodgkin's disease is manifested radiographically by a coarse reticulonodular and linear pattern that extends outward from the hila (Fig. 35–43). Lymphoid tissue at the bifurcation of bronchi and vessels can also be affected,[292, 298] and involvement of the interlobular septa can result in Kerley lines.[298] Consolidation of lung parenchyma remote from the mediastinum is not uncommon (Fig. 35–44).[292] Such disease can develop either in the center of the lung as a nodular opacity or air-space consolidation or beneath the visceral pleura, where it may form a plaquelike mass similar to asbestos-related pleural disease.

Pleural or subpleural nodules or plaques are seen on CT in up to 30% of patients with advanced or recurrent Hodgkin's disease.[157] The size of such nodules ranges widely and may vary with time; individual foci may coalesce to form a large homogeneous nonsegmental mass,[292] sometimes involving a whole lobe.[292, 299, 300] This type of parenchymal consolidation is unassociated with loss of volume (Fig. 35–45); its borders can be shaggy and ill-defined or sharply marginated. Because the airways are unaffected, an air bronchogram may be visible. Such masses can undergo necrosis and form a cavity that may be thin or thick walled (Fig. 35–46); in many cases, they are multiple and are situated in

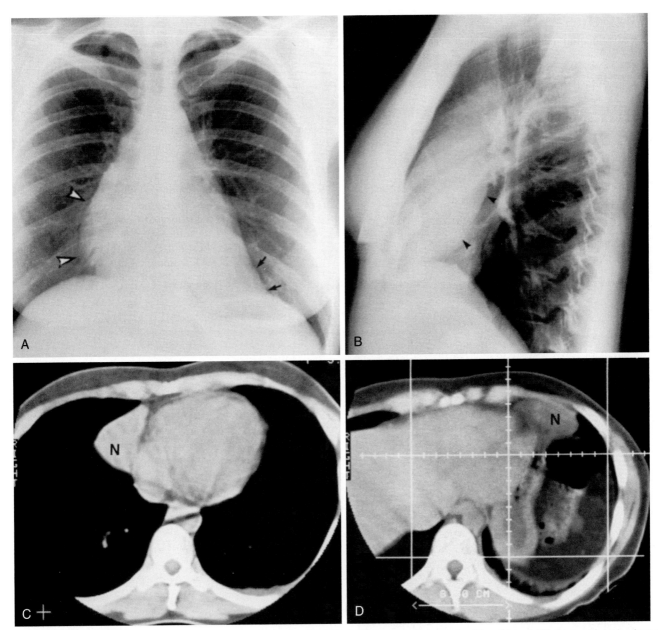

Figure 35–40. Diaphragmatic Lymph Node Involvement in Hodgkin's Disease. Posteroanterior *(A)* and lateral *(B)* chest radiographs show a "double density" of the right cardiac silhouette *(arrowheads)* caused by a paracardiac mass. There is also a small opacity in the vicinity of the cardiac apex that is consistent with a pleuropericardial fat pad *(arrows)*. CT scans *(C and D)* through the lower thorax and upper abdomen reveal enlarged lymph nodes (N) as the cause of the findings in *A* and *B*. Percutaneous biopsy of the right-sided lesion disclosed typical features of Hodgkin's disease. The patient was a young asymptomatic woman.

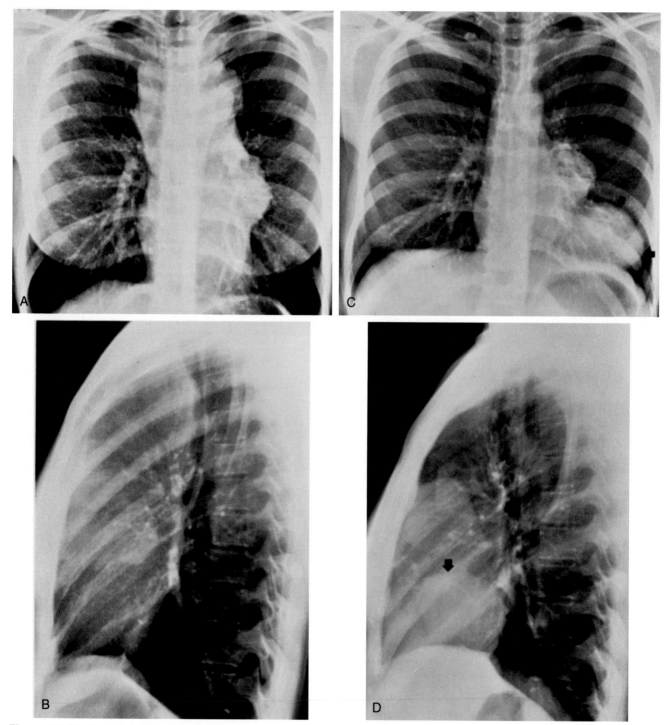

Figure 35–41. Hodgkin's Disease. The initial radiographs on this 28-year-old woman (*A* and *B*) revealed markedly enlarged anterior mediastinal lymph nodes, biopsy of which showed Hodgkin's disease. After treatment, all evidence of anterior mediastinal disease disappeared. Posteroanterior (*C*) and lateral (*D*) chest radiographs 6 months after initial presentation demonstrate recurrence of disease leading to enlargement of the pericardiophrenic lymph nodes (*arrows*).

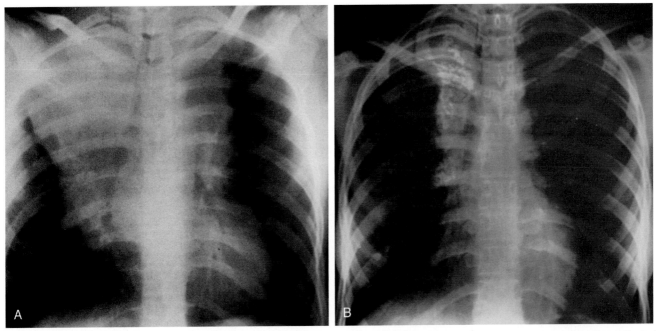

Figure 35–42. Calcification of Mediastinal Lymph Nodes After Irradiation for Hodgkin's Disease. Marked enlargement of anterior mediastinal nodes *(A)* had largely disappeared 3 years later *(B)*, but the nodes had undergone extensive calcification. The patient was a teenage girl.

Figure 35–43. Mixed Interstitial Air-Space Pattern of Pulmonary Involvement in Hodgkin's Disease. A posteroanterior chest radiograph reveals bilateral patchy air-space opacities throughout both lungs, worse on the right. The bronchovascular bundles are thickened, and septal lines are present in both upper and lower lobes. Mediastinal and hilar nodes are enlarged.

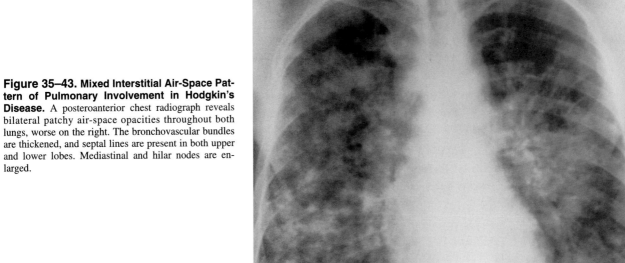

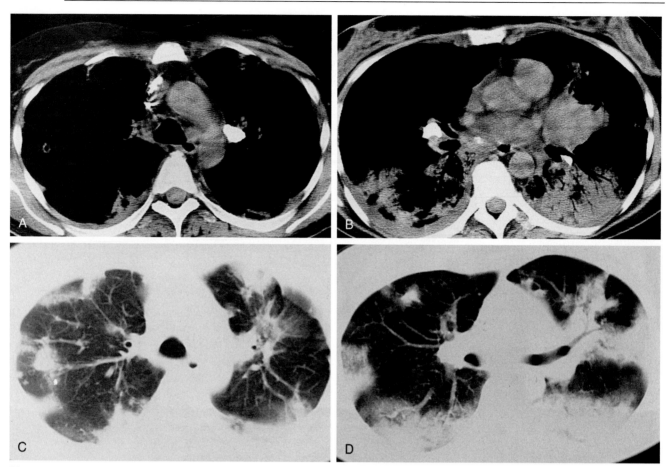

Figure 35–44. Parenchymal Consolidation in Hodgkin's Disease. Conventional CT scans (*A* and *B*) in a 45-year-old woman with previously treated Hodgkin's disease demonstrate calcified mediastinal and hilar lymph nodes and enlarged subcarinal and left hilar lymph nodes. Lung windows (*C* and *D*) reveal peribronchial and peripheral areas of consolidation.

the lower lobes.[301–303] In one patient, cavitated nodules were recurrent.[304]

Rarely, there is a generalized miliary or reticulonodular pattern,[299] in which case differentiation from lymphangitic spread of carcinoma or sarcoidosis may be difficult or impossible without biopsy.[300, 305] Bronchial occlusion is almost always caused by tumor within the airway lumen or wall[306–309] and can result in lobar or segmental atelectasis and obstructive pneumonitis (Figs. 35–47 and 35–48). In one study of six patients, atelectasis was caused by an endobronchial lesion in four, in three of whom endobronchial involvement dominated the initial pulmonary manifestations.[309]

Pleural effusion is seen at presentation in approximately 10% of patients[146, 283] and eventually develops in approximately 30%, most often in association with other intrathoracic manifestations of the disease.[292] The fluid can be serous, chylous, pseudochylous,[310] or (rarely) serosanguineous. The incidence of pneumothorax is increased in patients with Hodgkin's disease; among 1,977 cases of lymphoma, the complication was 10 times higher than expected, the majority of patients being under 30 years of age.[311] Treatment with radiotherapy, lung involvement, radiation fibrosis, and infection appear to be risk factors.

Chest Wall and Other Skeletal Involvement

Approximately 15% of patients with Hodgkin's disease manifest bone involvement radiographically.[312] The thoracic

skeleton is usually[288, 298, 310] but not invariably[289] affected by direct extension of tumor from the mediastinum or lungs. In such cases, destruction of ribs, vertebrae, or the sternum typically results in focal lytic areas (Fig. 35–49). By contrast, vertebral involvement other than by direct extension is often purely osteoblastic (ivory vertebra) (Fig. 35–50). Involvement of the nonthoracic skeleton (most commonly the spine or pelvis) usually results in mixed lytic and blastic lesions.[312]

Occasionally, a large, solitary peripheral tumor originates from a rib and protrudes into the thorax, in which circumstance the destructive lesion in the rib can be masked by the soft tissue element, producing a combination of signs that occurs much more frequently in myeloma or metastatic carcinoma.[310]

Follow-Up

Therapy is usually followed by slow involution of enlarged mediastinal lymph nodes. In one study, 86% of patients with Stage 1 or 2 Hodgkin's disease and mediastinal nodal involvement had a normal-appearing chest radiograph 11 months after treatment.[315] By contrast, in another investigation of 57 patients, residual abnormalities were evident on the chest radiograph in 50 (88%);[316] at a median follow-up of 48 months, 24 of the 57 patients (42%) still had abnormalities. In this study, residual mediastinal abnormalities did not by themselves indicate persistent active disease or an in-

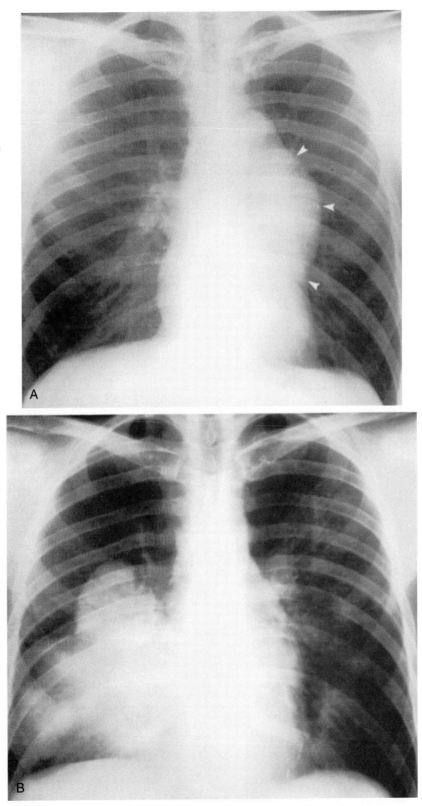

Figure 35–45. Parenchymal Consolidation in Hodgkin's Disease. A posteroanterior chest radiograph *(A)* reveals a smoothly contoured left anterior mediastinal mass *(arrowheads)* caused by Hodgkin's disease involvement of lymph nodes. Five years later, a posteroanterior radiograph *(B)* shows regression of the mediastinal lesion, but in the interim massive consolidation of the right middle and lower lobes caused by direct spread of Hodgkin's disease from hilar and mediastinal nodes had developed. In the left lung, the poorly defined opacities that have developed at a distance from the hilum and mediastinum, characteristic of subpleural parenchymal consolidation, can be noted.

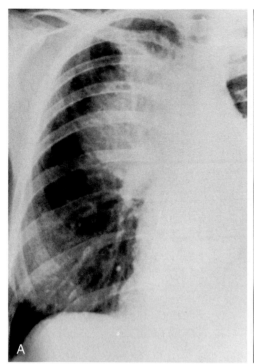
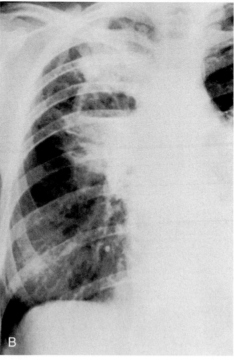

Figure 35–46. Hodgkin's Disease—Cavitation. A close-up view of the right hemithorax from a posteroanterior radiograph *(A)* reveals a poorly defined mass of homogeneous density situated within the right upper lobe contiguous with the mediastinum. Three weeks later, a large cavity had formed within the mass *(B);* the cavity possesses a thick, irregular wall and contains a prominent air-fluid level. The patient was a 26-year-old woman.

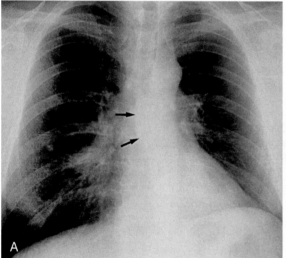
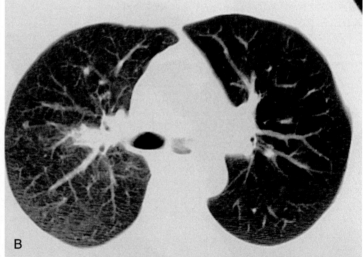
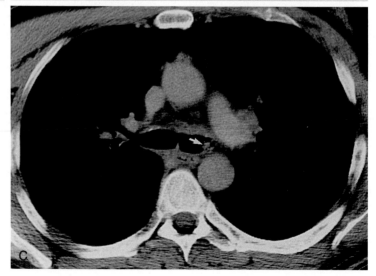

Figure 35–47. Endobronchial Hodgkin's Disease. A posteroanterior chest radiograph *(A)* in a 45-year-old man reveals decreased volume and vascularity of the left lung. Also noted are increased opacity in the subcarinal space and deviation of the azygoesophageal recess interface *(arrows),* consistent with subcarinal lymph node enlargement. A CT scan *(B)* demonstrates decreased attenuation and vascularity of the left lung, increased attenuation within the lumen of the left main bronchus, and two small nodules in the right lung. Soft tissue windows *(C)* demonstrate a soft tissue mass within the lumen of the left main bronchus *(arrow).* The decreased attenuation and vascularity of the left lung were presumably the result of reflex vasoconstriction secondary to decreased ventilation. Endobronchial obstruction by Hodgkin's disease was bronchoscopically proven.

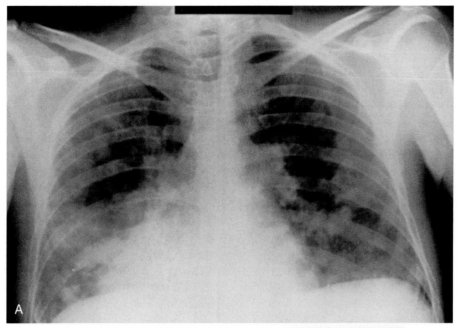

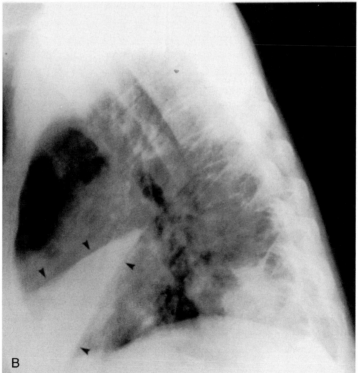

Figure 35–48. Atelectasis Caused by Endobronchial Hodgkin's Disease. Posteroanterior *(A)* and lateral *(B)* chest radiographs show multiple, poorly defined nodular opacities in both lungs. Confluence of several such lesions has created a larger air-space opacity in the right lower lobe. The middle lobe *(arrowheads)* is homogeneously consolidated and partly atelectatic as a result of endobronchial obstruction from Hodgkin's disease. Lymph nodes in the aortopulmonary window and left hilum are moderately enlarged. The patient was a young man with stage IV disease. (Courtesy of Dr. F. R. MacDonald, Foothill's Hospital, Calgary, Alberta, Canada.)

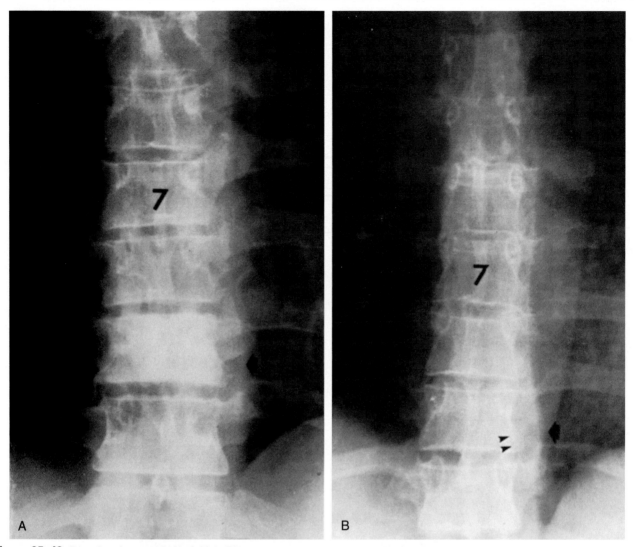

Figure 35–49. Bone Involvement in Hodgkin's Disease. A close-up view of the mediastinum from an overexposed anteroposterior radiograph *(A)* reveals diffuse osteosclerosis of the ninth thoracic vertebral body ("ivory vertebra") accompanied by a focal deformity of the left paraspinal line *(arrowhead)*, indicating enlargement of paravertebral lymph nodes. A similar view *(B)* in another patient also shows deformity of the left paraspinal line *(arrowhead)* as well as erosion of the cortex of the ninth thoracic vertebral body *(small arrowheads)*. Involvement of the thoracic spine in Hodgkin's disease is most common between T7 and T12; osteolytic lesions are more common than osteoblastic ones.

creased risk of relapse.[316] The significance of residual mediastinal masses on chest radiographs was further assessed in a study of 110 patients treated for advanced Hodgkin's disease with chemotherapy, radiation therapy, or both.[317] The relapse rate was not influenced by the rapidity of resolution of the radiographic findings and was similar in patients with normal radiographs and those who had residual radiographic abnormalities 1 year after treatment. These studies indicate that residual abnormalities on the chest radiograph or on CT may represent only nonviable or fibrotic tissue.[317, 318] The distinction of residual tumor from necrotic tumor or fibrotic tissue can usually be made with gallium 67 scintigraphy.[319, 320]

Fibrous tissue can be readily distinguished from tumor on MR imaging because of its low water content leading to a short T2. The procedure initially demonstrates a heterogeneous pattern after treatment, which progresses to low signal intensity on T2-weighted images characteristic of scar tissue.[321] In one study, the decrease in signal intensity on MR images became apparent between 8 and 12 weeks after treatment and was usually associated with tumor shrinkage.[322] Radiation-induced inflammatory changes may also result in increased signal intensity on T2-weighted images.

Features of Recurrent Disease

After radiation therapy, the most frequent sites of relapse are the upper mediastinum and lung parenchyma. Of 254 consecutive, surgically staged patients with Hodgkin's disease in one study, 21 developed intrathoracic recurrence.[323] In 12, the recurrence was primarily in lymph nodes, usually in the upper half of the mediastinum and sometimes in the hilar or diaphragmatic areas; in only 2 of the 12 was there simultaneous involvement of lung parenchyma, one by direct extension from hilar nodes and the other as a discontinuous mass. Pulmonary parenchymal relapses developed in 10 of the 21 patients, in 7 of whom the lung was the only site of recurrence; in only 1 of the 10 was there associated mediastinal lymph node enlargement. Parenchy-

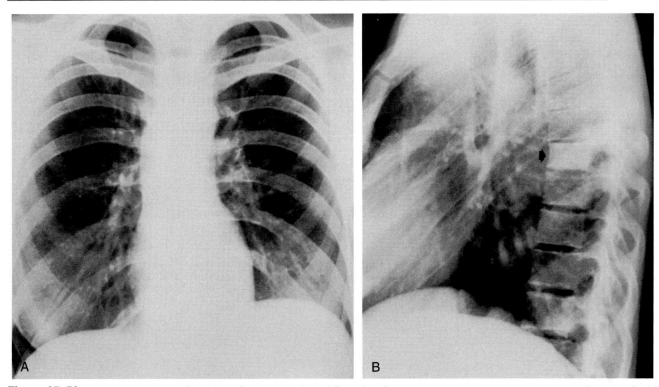

Figure 35–50. Hodgkin's Disease: Combined Splenomegaly and Bone Involvement. Posteroanterior *(A)* and lateral *(B)* radiographs of a 26-year-old woman demonstrate elevation of the left hemidiaphragm as a result of a markedly enlarged spleen. The lungs are clear, and there is no evidence of hilar or mediastinal node enlargement. In lateral projection, the seventh thoracic vertebral body *(arrow)* can be seen to be slightly compressed and to be uniformly dense ("ivory vertebra"); the eleventh thoracic vertebral body is sclerotic in its posterior portion. This combination of changes is highly suggestive of Hodgkin's disease. Some months later, the patient developed massive consolidation of the right lung from Hodgkin's disease.

mal involvement consisted of nodular masses ranging from 1 to 5 cm in diameter and usually not contiguous with the mediastinum. The most common pretreatment radiographic finding in the 21 patients was anterior mediastinal lymph node enlargement, present initially in 18 patients.

The patterns of relapse in the lung were assessed in another CT investigation in 15 patients.[284] At initial presentation, all had mediastinal lymphadenopathy, one had endobronchial disease, and one had pulmonary involvement. At the time of pulmonary relapse, five patients had no evidence of mediastinal lymphadenopathy on CT. Patterns of pulmonary involvement at relapse included nodules in 12 patients, focal areas of consolidation in 4, and direct mediastinal extension into the lung parenchyma in 3. The nodules were multiple in 10 patients and were most commonly located at a bronchial bifurcation; some were connected with thickened interlobular septa. Cavitation was present in a small number of nodules and in one of the areas of consolidation.

Clinical Manifestations

Most patients with Hodgkin's disease seek the advice of a physician when they notice enlarged peripheral lymph nodes. The abnormality is discovered initially in the cervical area in the great majority; primary mediastinal involvement without superficial or retroperitoneal node enlargement occurs in about 3%[275] to 10%[324] of patients. The initial symptom in such patients may be retrosternal pain or a feeling of discomfort. Rare complications of mediastinal disease include a palpable soft tissue mass secondary to direct invasion of the sternum or parasternal area of the chest wall,[288] a bronchoesophageal or tracheoesophageal fistula,[308, 325] and a fistula between internal mammary and pulmonary arteries.[326]

In the review of 60 cases of primary pulmonary Hodgkin's disease cited previously, dry cough and chest discomfort were the most common symptoms;[272] productive cough, dyspnea, hemoptysis, and wheezing were seen less frequently. The chest discomfort was most often described as pleuritic in character. Nine (15%) of the 60 patients were asymptomatic.

Systemic (B) symptoms, such as fever, night sweats, and weight loss, are not uncommon, occurring in about one third of patients at the time of diagnosis.[272] Although fever can be caused by the primary disease, complicating infections should be excluded. The so-called Pel-Ebstein relapsing fever is rare, occurring only once in 124 febrile episodes experienced by 44 patients in one study.[327] Specific symptoms and signs depend on the systems involved. Involvement of bone can produce a pain that, along with other symptoms, may be induced or worsened by the ingestion of alcohol.[162, 328] The spleen and liver are enlarged in about 50% of cases. Neurologic involvement occurs occasionally. Hypertrophic osteoarthropathy associated with clubbing of the fingers and toes is an uncommon manifestation.[313, 314]

In contrast to its occurrence in sarcoidosis, bilateral hilar node enlargement in Hodgkin's disease is usually associated with symptoms, signs, or both. For example, of 100 patients with bilateral hilar node enlargement, all 11 with Hodgkin's disease were symptomatic, and in 9 of these extrathoracic tumor was readily detected on physical examination;[329] by contrast, the 30 patients who were asymptomatic and 50 of the 52 patients who had no physical findings had sarcoidosis.

In its later stages, especially when the patient is receiving corticosteroids or chemotherapeutic agents, Hodgkin's disease may be complicated by infection. The lungs are frequently affected, leading sometimes to difficulty in radiologic interpretation. Tuberculosis, formerly a common complication of Hodgkin's disease, now has a lower incidence than other opportunistic infections.[330, 331] Sepsis caused by encapsulated bacteria after splenectomy develops in some patients, especially children.[332] Herpes zoster involving the skin is a relatively common accompaniment of late-stage disease;[333] involvement of the lungs is rare.

Laboratory Findings

Investigation of the blood usually reveals a slight leukocytosis with neutrophilia, sometimes with eosinophilia and lymphopenia. Normocytic normochromic anemia may develop early, but more often is a late manifestation. A rise in the serum level of alkaline phosphatase may reflect osteoblastic bone lesions or liver disease but can also occur in their absence.[334]

Bronchoscopy is often abnormal in patients with pulmonary disease. In the review of 60 cases of primary disease described earlier, 17 of 35 patients undergoing the procedure had an abnormality;[272] 2 showed an intraluminal mass, 5 showed stenosis or external compression, 11 showed "inflammation," 5 showed distortion of normal architecture, and 2 showed secretions or blood. Despite these findings, the diagnosis is only occasionally established by cytologic examination of sputum,[335–337] bronchial brush,[338, 339] or bronchoalveolar lavage specimens.[340, 341]

Prognosis and Natural History

Major factors influencing prognosis are the stage of disease at the time of diagnosis and the histologic subtype. The outlook is relatively good for patients with nodular sclerosis Hodgkin's disease, particularly in stages I and II, long-term, disease-free remission being possible in the vast majority of patients. In patients with primary lung involvement, the prognosis appears to be related to the extent of pulmonary involvement, those with disease involving more than one lobe tending to fare worse.[272, 297] Other factors that seem to portend a poorer prognosis in these patients are pleural involvement, systemic (B) symptoms, and cavitary disease.[272] A complete response to chemotherapy, radiotherapy, or both is seen in many patients; however, relapse is not uncommon (in 18 of 38 cases in the literature review cited previously).[272] Despite this, pulmonary involvement does not appear to affect survival after autologous bone marrow transplantation.[342] Significant differences in disease-free survival have been found between patients with positive and negative gallium studies after therapy; in one investigation, the mean survival time in patients with negative gallium studies was 20.1 months, whereas in patients with a positive study it was 9.4 months.[343]

A number of investigators have examined the long-term effects of radiotherapy and chemotherapy for Hodgkin's disease on pulmonary function.[344–348] Most have found a significant decrease in several parameters, including forced expiratory volume in 1 second (FEV_1), total lung capacity (TLC), forced vital capacity (FVC), and diffusing capacity. For example, in one retrospective study of 129 patients from Norway, nearly 30% were found to have reductions in these functional measures 5 years or longer after therapy;[344] chemotherapy with bleomycin-anthracyclines was found to be the only significant predictor of functional impairment. By contrast, in another prospective study of 145 patients from the United States, mantle radiotherapy was found to be the only significant predictor of a decrease in FVC and diffusing capacity of the lungs for carbon monoxide (D_{LCO}).[345] Whatever the responsible agents, the clinical consequences of the impaired function appear to be small in most patients and certainly do not outweigh the benefits of the therapy. Other uncommon pulmonary complications that have been reported after radiotherapy for Hodgkin's disease are pneumothorax,[349] hyperlucent lung,[347] and veno-occlusive disease.[347, 350]

Patients with Hodgkin's disease are at increased risk for the development of other malignancies after treatment with radiotherapy and chemotherapy, particularly acute leukemia and non-Hodgkin's lymphoma.[351–354] Among the solid tumors, pulmonary carcinoma is one of the more common.[355, 356] In one study of more than 2,800 patients, the relative risk for developing this cancer 10 years or more after diagnosis was 8.3.[353] The risk in some studies has been found to be associated with both chemotherapy and radiotherapy,[353, 356] whereas in others only radiotherapy has been found to be related.[352, 355] Risk has been shown to increase with increasing radiation dose and to have a strong (multiplicative) association with cigarette smoking.[355, 356] An increased risk for the development of mesothelioma after radiotherapy for Hodgkin's disease has also been found by some investigators.[357] Additional conditions that have been associated with Hodgkin's disease include sarcoidosis,[282] Langerhans' cell histiocytosis,[358] minimal change glomerulonephropathy, and (in one case) Wegener's granulomatosis.[359]

MISCELLANEOUS LYMPHOPROLIFERATIVE DISORDERS

Angioimmunoblastic Lymphadenopathy

Angioimmunoblastic lymphadenopathy (AILD, immunoblastic lymphadenopathy)[360, 361] is a disease of poorly defined cause and pathogenesis that not uncommonly affects mediastinal lymph nodes and occasionally involves the lungs and pleura. As initially defined in 1974, the abnormality has many features suggestive of an autoimmune or hyperimmune disorder, such as polyclonal hypergammaglobulinemia, Coombs'-positive hemolytic anemia, circulating immune complexes, and a variety of serologic abnormalities (including the occasional presence of antinuclear antibodies, rheumatoid factor, cryoglobulins, and cold agglutinins).[362, 363]

Because occasional cases occurred after vaccination[364] and because many patients associated the onset of symptoms with recent drug ingestion,[361, 363] it was initially speculated that the condition might represent an unusual hypersensitivity reaction to a foreign antigen. Subsequent studies, however, revealed that many patients with lymph node changes consistent with AILD also had atypical cellular areas within the affected nodes and a clinical behavior more suggestive of lymphoma.[365] In addition, as with focal pulmonary lymphoid hyperplasia (pseudolymphoma), molecular studies of many cases of AILD (including some without histologic atypia) have shown evidence of clonal T-cell or B-cell expansion;[366] such cases as well as those with histologic evidence of malignancy have come to be termed *AILD-like T-cell lymphoma*. Despite these findings, some cases of AILD do not have molecular or histologic features of malignancy (at least initially); in addition, both B-cell and T-cell clones can apparently appear and disappear during the course of the disease.[367] As a result, some investigators have suggested that the abnormality represents a disorder of immunoregulation with a high propensity to progress to malignancy.[367]

Pathologic changes of AILD are best observed in lymph nodes, the biopsy of which usually provides the diagnosis.[360–362] Typically, there is effacement of the normal lymph node architecture by a proliferation of lymphocytes, plasma cells, eosinophils, and immunoblasts; sometimes, clusters of clear cells also can be identified, in which case the possibility of lymphoma should be considered.[366] This cellular proliferation is accompanied by numerous small blood vessels, usually associated with the deposition of eosinophilic (hyalin) material in the perivascular space. Pulmonary disease is not uncommon; for example, in one review of 34 cases, it was present radiographically in 19 (55%).[368] Although some of these cases probably represent pneumonia, others are caused by infiltration of peribronchovascular and interlobular connective tissue[369] or alveolar septa[370] by a cellular infiltrate identical to that in the lymph nodes.

Thoracic disease in AILD is most commonly manifested radiographically by mediastinal and hilar lymph node enlargement, which is present in 30% to 60% of patients.[59, 371a] The most common lymph node groups to be involved are the paratracheal and bronchopulmonary; however, two of seven patients in one study showed evidence of anterior mediastinal node enlargement on conventional radiographs, and one had increased uptake of gallium in the same location.[372] Involved nodes have been reported to show marked enhancement following intravenous administration of contrast agent.[372a, 372b] Pulmonary involvement most often results in a linear or reticulonodular pattern (Fig. 35–51).[59, 372] Confluence of such interstitial disease may result in an air-space pattern that simulates pneumonia or edema or in multiple confluent nodules.[370] Pleural effusion has been identified in approximately 15% of patients; in some of these, it is directly related to pleural infiltration by a cellular population similar to that in the lymph nodes, detectable by biopsy[373] or by cytologic examination of pleural fluid.[370, 372]

The disease occurs most commonly in patients older than 40 years of age.[362] Constitutional symptoms, including fever, weight loss, sweats, and fatigue, are present in most patients at the outset. Lymph node enlargement is almost invariable; of 29 patients in one series, it was recorded as generalized in 21 and regional in 8.[361] In the latter patients, the most frequent sites were cervical and supraclavicular. A maculopapular rash is also common.[362, 371] Polyclonal gammopathy (including IgG, IgM, and IgA) is present in most patients; in a minority, major increases are noted only in

IgM or IgG. Anemia is present in about 75% of patients[362] and a positive Coombs' test in about 50%. Many patients are lymphocytopenic.[371] Although spontaneous remission and apparent response to corticosteroid therapy have been documented,[362, 370, 374] the course of the disease usually is progressive; most patients die of infection (sepsis or pneumonia) or develop clear-cut lymphoma.[371]

Multicentric Reticulohistiocytosis

Multicentric reticulohistiocytosis is a rare systemic disease of uncertain cause, characterized principally by multiple mucocutaneous papules and deforming polyarthritis.[375, 376] Biopsy specimens of skin and synovium show characteristic infiltrates of closely packed foamy and granular histiocytes interspersed with multinucleated giant cells. Involvement of other tissues and visceral organs has been documented histologically,[376] and several cases have been reported in which pulmonary, pleural, or mediastinal lymph node disease has been suspected.[376, 377] The clinical and radiographic features of these latter cases have not been well described but seem to be related most frequently to pleural effusion. An association with visceral or lymphoreticular malignancy has been reported in about 25% of cases.[376]

LEUKEMIA

Autopsy studies show that thoracic involvement is common in leukemia of all types. Mediastinal and hilar lymph node infiltration is the most frequent finding, particularly in cases of acute lymphoblastic leukemia and chronic lymphocytic leukemia. Pleuropulmonary infiltration has been found at autopsy in up to 64% of cases by some investigators,[378] although most cite an incidence of 20% to 40%.[379–383] Despite these figures, the likelihood that clinical and radiographic abnormalities are related to pleuropulmonary leukemic infiltration itself is low,[384–386] most abnormalities being caused by infectious pneumonia, hemorrhage, drug-induced lung damage, or heart failure.[380, 387–389] Because of their different clinicopathologic manifestations, myeloproliferative and lymphoproliferative disorders are best considered separately.

Myeloproliferative Disorders

Acute and Chronic Myelogenous Leukemia

Pathologic Characteristics

A variety of pathologic abnormalities are associated with pleuropulmonary infiltration by neoplastic myeloid cells. The most frequent is probably infiltration of peribronchovascular, pleural, or (less commonly) alveolar interstitial tissue (Fig. 35–52).[378, 379, 381] Although usually a microscopic finding of no clinical significance, such infiltration is occasionally severe enough to result in significant disease (Fig. 35–53). For example, pleural infiltration can be complicated by effusion and is rarely of a size sufficient to simulate mesothelioma grossly.[379] Similarly, involvement of the alveolar interstitium can cause restrictive functional impairment. Peribronchovascular infiltration is usually limited to the out-

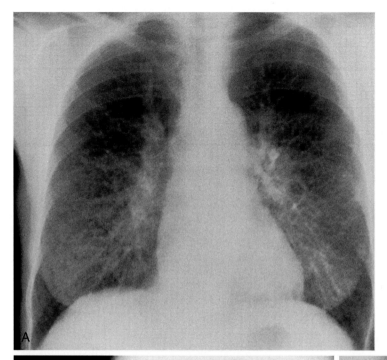

Figure 35–51. Angioimmunoblastic Lymphadenopathy. Posteroanterior *(A)* and lateral *(B)* radiographs show a diffuse interstitial pattern manifested by small nodules, thickened and ill-defined bronchovascular bundles, and Kerley A and B lines. The pattern is seen to better advantage in a magnified view of the left lung *(C)*. Hilar lymph nodes are asymmetrically enlarged. The major fissures are slightly thickened, presumably as a result of involvement of the pleural interstitium. An open-lung biopsy disclosed histologic abnormalities consistent with angioimmunoblastic lymphadenopathy. The patient was a 52-year-old woman who originally presented with generalized lymph node enlargement.

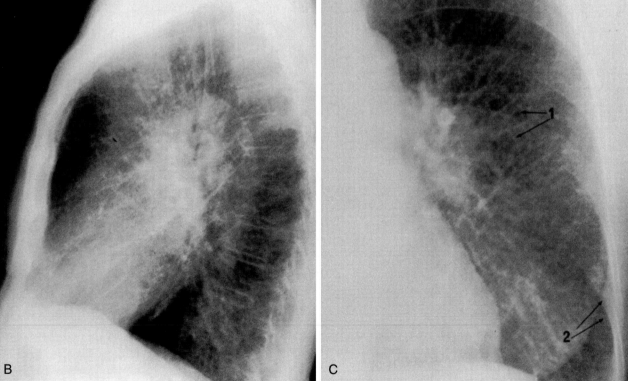

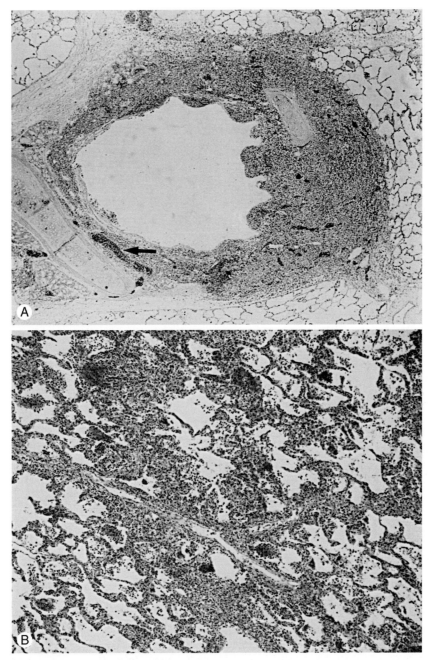

Figure 35–52. Acute Myelogenous Leukemia—Interstitial Infiltration. The mucosal and peribronchial interstitial tissue of this subsegmental bronchus *(A)* is diffusely infiltrated by leukemic blast cells. Bronchial artery branches are plugged by similar cells *(arrow)*. Diffuse parenchymal interstitial infiltration *(B)* by similar cells was evident elsewhere in the lung. *(A,* ×18; *B,* ×40.)

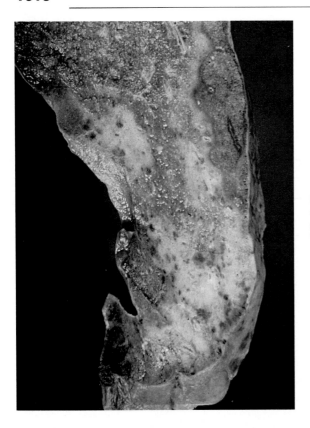

Figure 35–53. Acute Myelogenous Leukemia—Parenchymal Consolidation. A magnified view of the lingula reveals patchy parenchymal consolidation by a white tumor, shown on histologic examination to consist almost entirely of blasts. The patient was a 59-year-old man with acute myelogenous leukemia.

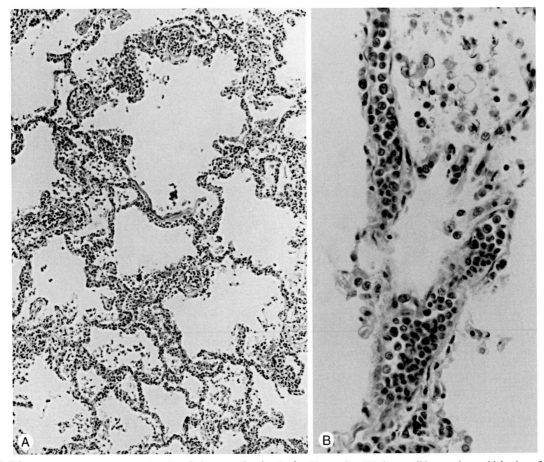

Figure 35–54. Acute Myelogenous Leukemia—Pulmonary Leukostasis. The section *(A)* shows mild to moderate thickening of alveolar septa as a result of the presence of numerous intravascular blasts. A magnified view of two arterioles *(B)* shows the blasts to better advantage.

ermost portions of the airway and vessel walls; occasionally, there is extension into the airway mucosa.[379]

Pulmonary involvement can also take the form of a localized mass of myeloid cells (granulocytic sarcoma). Usually, this presents as a peripheral parenchymal nodule;[390] occasionally a lesion causes endobronchial obstruction[391] or involves the pleura.[392] Such nodules can appear before a diagnosis of myelogenous leukemia has been established (sometimes in the absence of peripheral blood or bone marrow involvement[392]), during the period of clinically evident leukemia, or as a manifestation of relapse.[393]

Pulmonary leukostasis is a distinctive abnormality characterized by the presence of numerous leukemic cells within small pulmonary vessels, often unassociated with tissue invasion.[394–396] It can develop during the course of the leukemia or, less commonly, as a presenting feature; in some cases, it appears to be related to the institution of chemotherapy.[396] The complication usually occurs in patients with acute myelogenous leukemia or with chronic myelogenous leukemia in blast crisis. The total white blood cell count is typically between 100,000 and 500,000/mm³, with a predominance of immature forms;[394, 395] however, in some cases, it is less than 50,000/mm³.[397] (The clinicopathologic features of leukostasis associated with myeloproliferative disorders are also seen rarely in patients whose white cell count is markedly elevated as a result of infection[398] or who have chronic lymphocytic leukemia.[399])

Histologically, pulmonary capillaries, arterioles, and small arteries are distended with blast cells (Fig. 35–54);

occasionally, there is extension into adjacent interstitial tissue. The intravascular leukemic cells are typically tightly clustered together, with or without intermingled strands of fibrin; sometimes, they are associated with well-developed fibrin thrombi.[394, 396] Interstitial and air-space edema can also be present;[394] although this may be unrelated to the leukostasis, it has been suggested that it may be caused by endothelial damage resulting from the release of toxic substances from the static leukemic cells.[396]

The pathogenesis of the leukostasis is incompletely understood. Although blood viscosity can be increased, it is not always so,[394] and it has been speculated that the stasis is caused by mechanical obstruction by the relatively nondeformable blast cells.[394, 395] There is also some evidence that the rapidity with which the white blood cell count increases may be important.[394, 395] The occurrence of leukostasis in some patients shortly after the induction of chemotherapy has led to speculation that the therapy itself may be important in pathogenesis, possibly by damaging the leukemic cells and causing them to agglutinate more easily or to release thromboplastic substances that can, in turn, induce local coagulation.[396] According to the results of one investigation, increased expression of endothelial adhesion molecules does not appear to be a factor.[400]

Because of their large size, megakaryocytes may also be trapped in the pulmonary capillaries in megakaryocytic leukemia or some cases of chronic myelogenous leukemia in blast crisis (Fig. 35–55). In one investigation, alveolar septal fibrosis was observed adjacent to the megakaryocytic

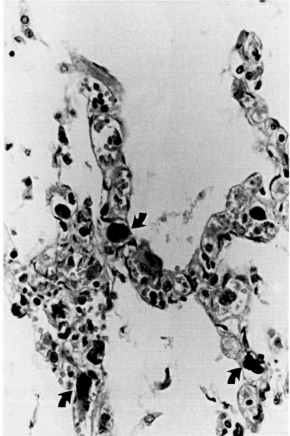

Figure 35–55. Megakaryocytic Leukemia with Platelet and Megakaryocytic Alveolar Capillary Stasis. A high-power view of several alveoli shows moderate septal thickening as a result of capillary dilation. Vascular lumens are filled with numerous platelets; several megakaryocytes are also evident *(arrows)*. The patient had hepatosplenomegaly with numerous sinusoidal megakaryocytes. The chest radiograph showed a fine reticular pattern in the lower lobes.

clusters; it was speculated that leakage of mitogenic factors from abnormal platelet granules may have been responsible.[401]

It has also been suggested that lysis of leukemic myeloid cells may be a cause of localized or diffuse alveolar damage. One group of investigators has described five patients with acute myeloblastic leukemia who developed patchy, often multilobar pneumonia soon after the institution of chemotherapy;[402] lung biopsy specimens showed diffuse alveolar damage associated with leukemic cells in vessels, interstitium, and alveolar exudate (Fig. 35–56). No pathogenic microorganisms were identified by culture or special stains. The authors hypothesized that leukemic cell death secondary to chemotherapy resulted in lysis and release of

enzymes that, in turn, caused the pneumonitis. A similar process might be responsible for more diffuse interstitial damage, in some cases associated with acute respiratory failure (i.e., adult respiratory distress syndrome [ARDS])[397, 403, 403a] or diffuse pulmonary hemorrhage.[404] (The last-named complication may also be related to disseminated intravascular coagulation, particularly when the leukemia is promyelocytic in type.[405])

Radiologic Manifestations

The mediastinum is the most common intrathoracic site affected by myelogenous leukemia.[406] It may be manifested radiographically as a focal mediastinal mass or as general-

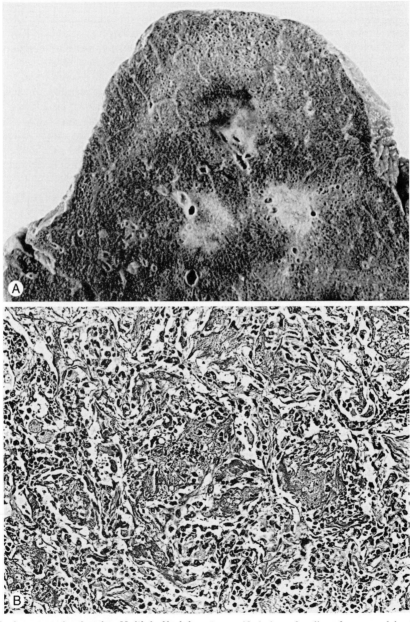

Figure 35–56. Acute Myelogenous Leukemia—Multiple Nodules. A magnified view of a slice of an upper lobe *(A)* shows patchy hemorrhage and three fairly well-demarcated, irregularly shaped foci of white consolidation. A section of one of these foci *(B)* shows filling of alveolar air spaces by a proteinaceous exudate and mild alveolar interstitial thickening; myeloblasts are evident in both locations. The patient had been recently treated for acute myelogenous leukemia and had died unexpectedly of a myocardial infarct. *(B, ×200.)*

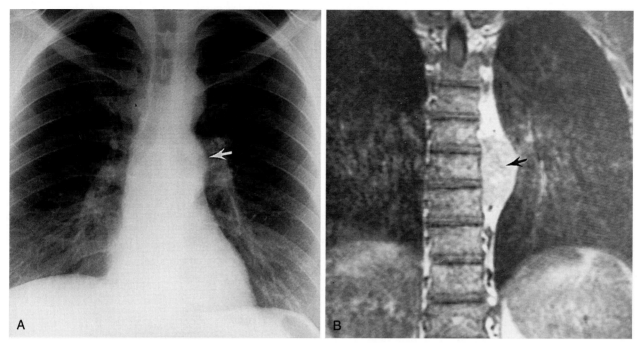

Figure 35–57. Paravertebral Granulocytic Sarcoma. A posteroanterior chest radiograph *(A)* reveals a mediastinal mass *(arrow)*. A T1-weighted MR image *(B)* demonstrates a paravertebral mass *(arrow)* with signal characteristics similar to the involved bone marrow. (Case courtesy of Dr. David Godwin. From Takasugi JE, Godwin JD, Marglin SI, Petersdorf SH: Intrathoracic granulocytic sarcoma. J Thorac Imaging 11:223, 1996.)

ized mediastinal widening. Hilar enlargement is present in approximately 15% of cases, most commonly in association with mediastinal abnormalities.[406] Other findings include cardiac enlargement as a result of a pericardial mass or pericardial effusion, pleural effusions, pleural masses, and lung opacities.[406] On CT, the mediastinal involvement can be shown to be the result of a focal mass, infiltration of mediastinal fat, or lymph node enlargement.[406] MR imaging performed in one patient with mediastinal granulocytic sarcoma demonstrated the same signal intensity within the mediastinal mass as in the involved bone marrow on both T1-weighted and T2-weighted images (Fig. 35–57).[406]

Pleural effusion, usually unilateral, is second only to mediastinal lymph node enlargement in frequency. Although it can be identified in up to 25% of patients,[407] it is probably caused by actual leukemic infiltration in no more than 5%,[379] more likely causes being lymphatic obstruction, cardiac failure, or pulmonary infection.[379, 407]

As indicated previously, pulmonary disease in patients with myelogenous leukemia is most often caused by processes other than leukemic cell infiltration. For example, in one series of 21 patients with abnormal chest radiographs,[379] all of whom were considered during life to have leukemic infiltration of their lungs, only 2 had such a finding at autopsy. The most common pulmonary abnormality is localized or diffuse air-space consolidation, caused almost invariably by pneumonia, edema, or hemorrhage.[379, 403a, 407, 408] In an autopsy review of 60 patients who died from acute or chronic myelogenous or lymphocytic leukemia,[409] radiographically demonstrable disease was related to hemorrhage in 74%, infection in 67%, edema or congestion in 57%, and leukemic infiltration in 26%; only 5% were radiographically normal.

The usual pattern of pulmonary parenchymal involve-

ment caused by pulmonary leukemic cell infiltration or intravascular leukostasis consists of a diffuse bilateral reticulation or linearity that resembles interstitial edema or lymphangitic carcinomatosis.[407] This pattern tends to occur in the terminal stages of the disease and with blast crisis.[379] In a study of 10 patients with pulmonary leukostasis in which terminal chest radiographs were compared with findings at autopsy, no radiographic abnormalities attributable to leukostasis were found in 6;[410] however, in 4 patients there was diffuse air-space consolidation caused by alveolar edema. Rarely, leukemic involvement results in focal areas of air-space consolidation or nodules.[406] One case has been reported of a patient with chronic myelogenous leukemia in whom CT demonstrated several cavitated and noncavitated nodules, one of which had an air crescent; the nodules were shown at autopsy to be the result of leukemic involvement.[411]

Clinical Manifestations

Acute myelogenous leukemia occurs most commonly between the ages of 10 and 40 years. Onset is typically abrupt, with major symptoms and signs related to bleeding or infection. The spleen and liver are often enlarged and bleeding, and oral infection and retinal hemorrhage are frequent manifestations. Fever is almost invariable, as is pallor related to anemia. Neurologic manifestations, such as confusion, somnolence, and personality disturbances, are found in some patients and have been attributed to central nervous system leukostasis, which commonly coexists with pulmonary leukostasis.[395] As indicated previously, pulmonary symptoms—including cough, expectoration, dyspnea, and hemoptysis—usually are the result of infection, especially by opportunistic bacteria and *Aspergillus*, rather than leukemic infiltration.[389] Interstitial infiltration or extensive leukostasis,

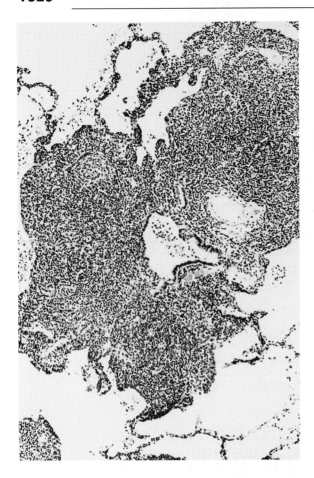

Figure 35–58. Chronic Lymphocytic Leukemia. This section shows the interstitial tissue surrounding a small pulmonary artery and adjacent membranous bronchiole to be infiltrated by a uniform population of small lymphoid cells; focally, these extend into the adjacent alveolar septa.

however, can cause dyspnea and, rarely, respiratory failure.[412] Disseminated intravascular coagulation can occur, particularly in acute promyelocytic leukemia, and can cause respiratory failure secondary to pulmonary hemorrhage.[413, 414] Alveolar proteinosis is also a rare but well-recognized complication.[415]

Chronic myelogenous leukemia occurs most often in individuals between 30 and 60 years of age and typically has a relatively indolent onset, with fatigue, weight loss, and anorexia. Lymph node enlargement and hepatosplenomegaly are present in about 50% of patients. Pulmonary signs and symptoms are even less common than in acute myelogenous leukemia, except when there is transformation to blast crisis.

The diagnosis of leukemia is made by the demonstration of neoplastic cells in peripheral blood or bone marrow. The total leukocyte count is increased in most cases, but may be normal or even reduced, with few immature cells in the peripheral blood. In the latter circumstance, examination of the bone marrow is required to establish the diagnosis. Cytologic or immunocytochemical analysis of pulmonary secretions obtained by bronchoalveolar lavage or bronchial washing[385, 416] or of pleural fluid[417] occasionally demonstrates leukemic cells, thus revealing the cause of the pleuropulmonary manifestations.

Extramedullary Hematopoiesis

Extramedullary hematopoiesis is a relatively common complication of several hematologic conditions that usually affects the spleen and liver but can involve virtually any organ or tissue. Intrathoracic disease is characteristically manifested as a paravertebral mediastinal mass in a patient with hereditary spherocytosis, thalassemia, or myelofibrosis.[418–420] Rare cases of pleural,[421] pulmonary parenchymal,[422] or bronchial wall[423] extramedullary hematopoiesis have also been reported in association with myeloproliferative disorders; some have been associated with evidence of parenchymal interstitial infiltration on radiographs and the development of respiratory insufficiency.[424–426] The condition is discussed further in Chapter 76 (*see* page 2980).

Sweet's Syndrome

Sweet's syndrome is characterized by multiple painful skin plaques that correspond pathologically to a dense neutrophil infiltrate in the dermis.[427, 428] The cause and pathogenesis are unknown; however, an underlying malignancy—most often acute myelogenous leukemia—is present in 10% to 15% of cases; pulmonary carcinoma has been associated rarely.[429, 430] Pulmonary involvement, manifested most often by dyspnea and occasionally by acute respiratory failure, is uncommon.[427] In some patients, ill-defined opacities have been noted on chest radiographs, and infiltrates of polymorphonuclear leukocytes have been found within alveolar air spaces on histologic examination.[427, 428, 431] Analysis of bronchoalveolar lavage fluid in one individual showed a total white cell count of 11.2×10^9 per liter (of which approximately 90% were neutrophils).[427]

Lymphoproliferative Disorders with Leukemia

Pulmonary involvement in leukemic lymphoproliferative disease is probably most common with chronic lymphocytic leukemia;[432] however, a significant number of cases occur in patients who have adult T-cell leukemia[433, 434] or hairy cell leukemia.[435] As with myeloproliferative disorders, the most common pathologic manifestation is an interstitial infiltrate, most often in the peribronchovascular and interlobular septal connective tissue. Occasionally, infiltration in the former site causes airway stenosis, resulting in obstructive pneumonitis[436] or dyspnea.[383] Infiltration of bronchiolar walls with relative sparing of the rest of the lung parenchyma is prominent in some cases (Fig. 35–58).[437] Significant extension from any of these interstitial locations into alveolar air spaces is uncommon; however, localized tumors of neoplastic cells similar to granulocytic sarcoma can occur.[439, 440] Rarely, the lung is the site of transformation of chronic lymphocytic leukemia into high-grade lymphoma (Richter's syndrome).[438]

The most common radiographic sign of lymphoproliferative leukemia within the thorax is mediastinal and hilar lymph node enlargement (Fig. 35–59); this occurs in about 25% of patients,[407, 441] an incidence that is about half that found at autopsy.[441] Less common manifestations include interstitial and air-space infiltrates (Fig. 35–60); although these may be diffuse, they tend to involve mainly the perihilar regions.[442] As discussed previously (*see* page 1292), an anterior mediastinal mass, representing either thymic or lymph node enlargement and sometimes associated with pleural effusion, is often the initial radiographic sign of acute lymphoblastic leukemia;[443] it is also frequently present in young patients with lymphoblastic lymphoma who develop a leukemic phase.[444] Rarely, mediastinal lymph node enlargement occurs in patients with adult T-cell leukemia or lymphoma.[445]

Chronic lymphocytic leukemia usually develops insidiously, manifesting itself by painless lymph node enlargement or hepatosplenomegaly. Clinical manifestations of pulmonary involvement are uncommon; some patients have findings of chronic bronchitis.[446] Rarely, dyspnea and respiratory insufficiency are associated with leukostasis.[399] The course of the disease is often prolonged and associated with few disabling symptoms; however, generalized weakness and loss of weight and appetite develop as the disease progresses. Anemia and hemorrhage resulting from thrombocytopenia occur late. Skin lesions develop in many patients. In one group of 24 patients, decreases in vital capacity, FEV_1, and D_{LCO} were seen in 9, 8, and 7 patients;[446] some of the abnormalities appeared to be related to the number of leuke-

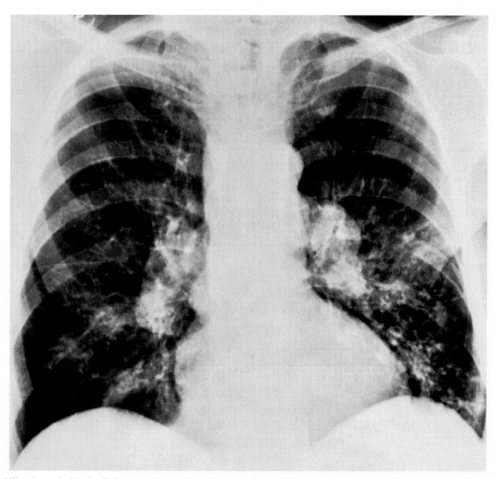

Figure 35–59. Hilar Lymph Node Enlargement in Chronic Lymphocytic Leukemia. A posteroanterior chest radiograph reveals markedly enlarged lymph nodes in both hila and (probably) slight enlargement of the nodes in the paratracheal chain bilaterally. There is no evidence of significant pulmonary or pleural disease (the minor parenchymal changes in the left lower lobe represent resolving bronchopneumonia). The patient was a 65-year-old man with chronic lymphocytic leukemia.

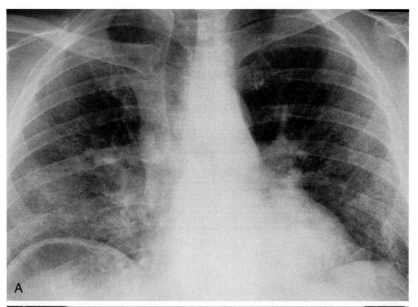

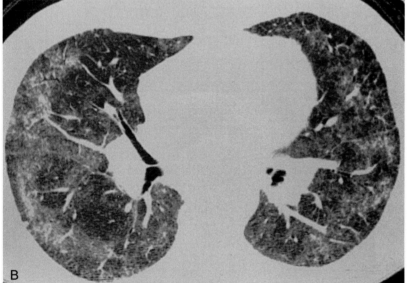

Figure 35–60. Chronic Lymphocytic Leukemia with Pulmonary Involvement. An anteroposterior chest radiograph *(A)* reveals evidence of paratracheal and bilateral hilar lymphadenopathy as well as poorly defined bilateral areas of parenchymal opacification. An HRCT scan *(B)* demonstrates extensive bilateral areas of ground-glass attenuation and a few linear opacities. Soft tissue windows *(C)* demonstrate anterior mediastinal and paratracheal lymph node enlargement. The patient was a 67-year-old man with chronic lymphocytic leukemia and biopsy-proven pulmonary involvement.

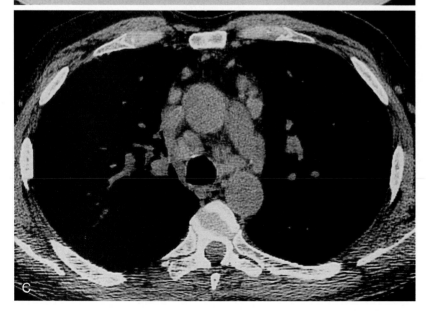

mic cells in the blood. A possible relation between chronic lymphocytic leukemia and the subsequent development of pulmonary carcinoma has been postulated.[447, 448]

Clinical manifestations of other lymphoproliferative disorders are typically more acute and severe than those of chronic lymphocytic leukemia. In one series of 35 patients with adult T-cell leukemia, 14 (40%) were considered to have significant chest radiographic abnormalities at presentation.[434] The incidence of pulmonary infection at some time during the course of the disease is high in all forms of leukemia.[434, 449]

The diagnosis is usually made by examination of peripheral blood. Pleuropulmonary disease in chronic lymphocytic leukemia has been confirmed by detecting abnormal lymphocytes in bronchoalveolar lavage fluid, transbronchial fluid specimens,[432] or pleural fluid. Lack of these cells, however, does not indicate absence of disease; one patient has been described whose pleural biopsy specimen showed a monoclonal B-cell infiltrate consistent with chronic lymphocytic leukemia but whose pleural fluid showed a predominance of T cells and a polyclonal B-cell population, presumably representing a reactive process.[450]

1. Saltzstein SL: Pulmonary malignant lymphomas and pseudolymphomas: Classification, therapy, and prognosis. Cancer 16:928, 1963.

2. Greenberg SD, Heisler JG, Gyorkey F, et al: Pulmonary lymphoma versus pseudolymphoma: A perplexing problem. South Med J 65:775, 1972.

3. Koss MN, Hochholzer L, Nichols PW, et al: Primary non-Hodgkin's lymphoma and pseudolymphoma of lung: A study of 161 patients. Hum Pathol 14:1024, 1983.

4. Chee YC, Yap CH, Poh SC: Pulmonary lymphoma or pseudolymphoma: A diagnostic dilemma. Ann Acad Med Singapore 15:113, 1986.

5. Addis BJ, Hyjek E, Isaacson PG: Primary pulmonary lymphoma: A re-appraisal of its histogenesis and its relationship to pseudolymphoma and lymphoid interstitial pneumonia. Histopathology 13:1, 1988.

6. Herbert A, Wright DH, Isaacson PG, et al: Primary malignant lymphoma of the lung: Histopathologic and immunologic evaluation of nine cases. Hum Pathol 15:415, 1984.

7. Turner RR, Colby TV, Doggett RS: Well-differentiated lymphocytic lymphoma. Cancer 54:2088, 1984.

8. Kennedy JL, Nathwani BN, Burke JS, et al: Pulmonary lymphomas and other pulmonary lymphoid lesions: A clinicopathologic and immunologic study of 64 patients. Cancer 56:539, 1985.

9. Evans HL: Extranodal small lymphocytic proliferation: A clinicopathologic and immunocytochemical study. Cancer 49:84, 1982.

10. Kawahara K, Shiraishi T, Okabayashi K, et al: Nodular lymphoid hyperplasia in the lung. Thorac Cardiovasc Surg 44:210, 1996.

11. Colby TV, Carrington CB: Lymphoreticular tumors and infiltrates of the lung. *In* Sommers SC, Rosen PP (eds): Pathology Annual. Vol. 18, Part I. Norwalk, CT, Appleton-Century-Crofts, 1983.

12. Feoli F, Carbone A, Dina MA, et al: Pseudolymphoma of the lung: Lymphoid subsets in the lung mass and in peripheral blood. Cancer 48:2218, 1981.

13. Koss MN: Pulmonary lymphoid disorders. Semin Diagn Pathol 12:158, 1995.

14. Bragg DG, Chor PJ, Murray KA, et al: Lymphoproliferative disorders of the lung: Histopathology, clinical manifestations, and imaging features. Am J Roentgenol 163:273, 1994.

15. Holland EA, Ghahremani GG, Fry WA, et al: Evolution of pulmonary pseudolymphomas: Clinical and radiologic manifestations. J Thorac Imaging 6:74, 1991.

16. Hutchinson WB, Friedenberg MJ, Saltzstein SL: Primary pulmonary pseudolymphoma. Radiology 82:48, 1964.

17. Nicholson AG, Wotherspoon AC, Diss TC, et al: Reactive pulmonary lymphoid disorders. Histopathology 26:405, 1995.

18. Walters MT, Stevenson FK, Herbert A, et al: Urinary monoclonal free light chains in primary Sjögren's syndrome: An aid to the diagnosis of malignant lymphoma. Ann Rheum Dis 45:210, 1986.

19. Liebow AA, Carrington CB: Diffuse pulmonary lymphoreticular infiltrations associated with dysproteinemia. Med Clin North Am 57:809, 1973.

20. Kurosu K, Yumoto N, Furukawa M, et al: Third complementarity-determining-region sequence analysis of lymphocytic interstitial pneumonia: Most cases demonstrate a minor monoclonal population hidden among normal lymphocyte clones. Am J Respir Crit Care Med 155:1453, 1997.

21. Kradin RL, Young RH, Kradin LA, et al: Immunoblastic lymphoma arising in chronic lymphoid hyperplasia of the pulmonary interstitium. Cancer 50:1339, 1982.

22. Herbert A, Walters MT, Cawley MID, et al: Lymphocytic interstitial pneumonia identified as lymphoma of mucosa associated lymphoid tissue. J Pathol 146:129, 1985.

23. Strimlan CV, Rosenow EC, Weiland LH, et al: Lymphocytic interstitial pneumonitis. Ann Intern Med 88:616, 1978.

24. Grieco MH, Chinoy-Acharya P: Lymphocytic interstitial pneumonia associated with acquired immune deficiency syndrome. Am Rev Respir Dis 131:952, 1985.

25. Morris JC, Rosen MJ, Marchevsky A, et al: Lymphocytic interstitial pneumonia in patients at risk for the acquired immune deficiency syndrome. Chest 91:63, 1987.

26. Travis WD, Fox CH, Devaney KO, et al: Lymphoid pneumonitis in 50 adult patients infected with the human immunodeficiency virus: Lymphocytic interstitial pneumonitis versus nonspecific interstitial pneumonitis. Hum Pathol 23:529, 1992.

27. Koss MN, Hochholzer L, Langloss JM, et al: Lymphoid interstitial pneumonia: Clinicopathological and immunopathological findings in 18 cases. Pathology 19:178, 1987.

28. Helman CA, Keeton GR, Benatar SR: Lymphoid interstitial pneumonia with associated chronic active hepatitis and renal tubular acidosis. Am Rev Respir Dis 115:161, 1977.

29. Poletti V, Romagna M, Gasponi A, et al: Bronchoalveolar lavage in the diagnosis of low-grade, MALT type, B-cell lymphoma in the lung. Monaldi Arch Chest Dis 50:191, 1995.

30. Yood RA, Steigman DM, Gill LR: Lymphocytic interstitial pneumonitis in a patient with systemic lupus erythematosus. Lupus 4:161, 1995.

31. Khardori R, Eagleton LE, Soler NG, et al: Lymphocytic interstitial pneumonitis in autoimmune thyroid disease. Am J Med 90:649, 1991.

32. Perreault C, Cousineau S, D'Angelo G, et al: Lymphoid interstitial pneumonia after allogeneic bone marrow transplantation. Cancer 55:1, 1985.

33. Deheinzelin D, Capelozzi VL, Kairalla RA, et al: Interstitial lung disease in primary Sjögren's syndrome: Clinical-pathological evaluation and response to treatment. Am J Respir Crit Care Med 154:794, 1996.

34. DeMartini JC, Brodie SJ, de la Concha-Bermejillo A, et al: Pathogenesis of lymphoid interstitial pneumonia in natural and experimental ovine lentivirus infection. Clin Infect Dis 17(Suppl 1):S236, 1993.

35. Zaer FS, Braylan RC, Zander DS, et al: Multiparametric flow cytometry in the diagnosis and characterization of low-grade pulmonary mucosa-associated lymphoid tissue lymphomas. Mod Pathol 11:525, 1998.

36. Andiman WA, Martin K, Rubinstein A, et al: Opportunistic lymphoproliferations associated with Epstein-Barr viral DNA in infants and children with AIDS. Lancet 2:1390, 1985.

37. Kaan PM, Hegele RG, Hayashi S, et al: Expression of bcl-2 and Epstein-Barr virus LMP1 in lymphocytic interstitial pneumonia. Thorax 52:12, 1997.

38. Greenberg SD, Haley MD, Jenkins DE, et al: Lymphoplasmacytic pneumonia with accompanying dysproteinemia. Arch Pathol 96:73, 1973.

39. Moran TJ, Totten RS: Lymphoid interstitial pneumonia with dysproteinemia: Report of two cases with plasma cell predominance. Am J Clin Pathol 54:747, 1970.

40. Liebow AA, Carrington CB: The interstitial pneumonias. *In* Simon M, Potchen EJ, Le May M (eds): Frontiers of Pulmonary Radiology. New York, Grune & Stratton, 1969, p 102.

41. Bonner H, Ennis RS, Geelhoed GW, et al: Lymphoid infiltration and amyloidosis of lung in Sjögren's syndrome. Arch Pathol 95:42, 1973.

42. Kawabuchi B, Tsuchiya S, Nakagawa K, et al: Immunophenotypic and molecular analysis of a case of lymphocytic interstitial pneumonia. Acta Pathol Jpn 43:260, 1993.

43. Julsrud PR, Brown LR, Li CY, et al: Pulmonary processes of mature-appearing lymphocytes: Pseudolymphoma, well-differentiated lymphocytic lymphoma, and lymphocytic interstitial pneumonia. Radiology 127:289, 1978.

44. Ichikawa Y, Kinoshita M, Koga T, et al: Lung cyst formation in lymphocytic interstitial pneumonia: CT features. J Comput Assist Tomogr 18:745, 1994.

45. Feigin DS, Siegelman SS, Theros EG, et al: Nonmalignant lymphoid disorders of the chest. Am J Roentgenol 129:221, 1977.

46. McGuinness G, Scholes JV, Jagirdar JS, et al: Unusual lymphoproliferative disorders in nine adults with HIV or AIDS: CT and pathologic findings. Radiology 197:59, 1995.

47. Oldham SAA, Castillo M, Jacobson FL, et al: HIV-associated lymphocytic interstitial pneumonia: Radiologic manifestations and pathologic correlation. Radiology 170:83, 1989.

48. Torii K, Ogawa K, Kawabata Y, et al: Lymphoid interstitial pneumonia as a pulmonary lesion of idiopathic plasmacytic lymphadenopathy with hyperimmunoglobulinemia. Intern Med 33:237, 1994.

49. Carignan S, Staples CA, Müller NL: Intrathoracic lymphoproliferative disorders in the immunocompromised patient: CT findings. Radiology 197:53, 1995.

50. Saldana MJ, Mones JM: Lymphoid interstitial pneumonia in HIV infected individuals. Prog Surg Pathol 12:181, 1992.

51. Banerjee D, Ahmad D: Malignant lymphoma complicating lymphocytic interstitial pneumonia: A monoclonal B-cell neoplasm arising in a polyclonal lymphoproliferative disorder. Hum Pathol 13:780, 1982.

52. Schuurman H-J, Gooszen HC, Tan IWN, et al: Low-grade lymphoma of immature T-cell phenotype in a case of lymphocytic interstitial pneumonia and Sjögren's syndrome. Histopathology 11:1193, 1987.

53. Yousem SA, Colby TV, Carrington CB: Follicular bronchitis/bronchiolitis. Hum Pathol 16:700, 1985.

54. Fortoul TI, Cano-Valle F, Oliva E, et al: Follicular bronchiolitis in association with connective tissue diseases. Lung 163:305, 1985.

55. Remy-Jardin M, Remy J, Wallaert B, et al: Pulmonary involvement in progressive systemic sclerosis: Sequential evaluation with CT, pulmonary function tests, and bronchoalveolar lavage. Radiology 188:499, 1993.

56. Remy-Jardin M, Remy J, Cortet B, et al: Lung changes in rheumatoid arthritis: CT findings. Radiology 193:375, 1994.

57. Kinoshita M, Higashi T, Tanaka C, et al: Follicular bronchiolitis associated with rheumatoid arthritis. Intern Med 31:674, 1992.

58. Yousem SA, Cobly TV, Carrington CB: Lung biopsy in rheumatoid arthritis. Am Rev Respir Dis 131:770, 1985.

59. Gibson M, Hansell DM: Lymphocytic disorders of the chest: Pathology and imaging. Clin Radiol 53:469, 1998.

60. Rosenberg SA, Diamond HD, Jaslowitz B, et al: Lymphosarcoma: A review of 1269 cases. Medicine 40:31, 1961.

61. Weiss LM, Yousem SA, Warnke RA: Non-Hodgkin's lymphomas of the lung. Am J Surg Pathol 9:480, 1985.

62. L'Hoste RJ, Filippa DA, Lieberman PH, et al: Primary pulmonary lymphomas. Cancer 54:1397, 1984.

63. Fiche M, Capron F, Berger F, et al: Primary pulmonary non-Hodgkin's lymphomas. Histopathology 26:529, 1995.

64. Li G, Hansmann M-L, Zwingers T, et al: Primary lymphomas of the lung: Morphological, immunohistochemical and clinical features. Histopathology 16:519, 1990.

65. Burke JS: Extranodal lymphomas and lymphoid hyperplasias. *In* Sarkin Jaffe E (ed): Surgical Pathology of the Lymph Nodes and Related Organs. Vol. 16. Major Problems in Pathology. 2nd ed. Toronto, WB Saunders, 1995.

66. Harris NL: Low-grade B-cell lymphoma of mucosa-associated lymphoid tissue and monocytoid B-cell lymphoma: Related entities that are distinct from other low-grade B-cell lymphomas. Arch Pathol Lab Med 117:771, 1993.
67. Addis BJ, Hyjek E, Isaacson PG: Primary pulmonary lymphoma: A re-appraisal of its histogenesis and its relationship to pseudolymphoma and lymphoid interstitial pneumonia. Histopathology 13:1, 1988.
68. Koss M, Zeren EH: Low-grade B-cell lymphomas of lung and lymphomatoid granulomatosis. Pathology 4:125, 1996.
69. Nicholson AG, Wotherspoon AC, Diss TC, et al: Pulmonary B-cell non-Hodgkin's lymphomas: The value of immunohistochemistry and gene analysis in diagnosis. Histopathology 26:395, 1995.
70. Teruya-Feldstein J, Temeck BK, Sloas MM, et al: Pulmonary malignant lymphoma of mucosa-associated lymphoid tissue (MALT) arising in a pediatric HIV-positive patient. Am J Surg Pathol 19:357, 1995.
71. Kagan E, Jacobson RJ: Lymphoid and plasma cell malignancies: Asbestos-related disorders of long latency. Am J Clin Pathol 80:14, 1983
72. Kagan E, Jacobson RJ, Yeung KY, et al: Asbestos-associated neoplasms of B cell lineage. Am J Med 67:325, 1979.
73. Tondini M, Rocco G, Travaglini M, et al: Pleural mesothelioma associated with non-Hodgkin's lymphoma. Thorax 49:1269, 1994.
74. Hytiroglou P, Strauchen JA, Vrettou E, et al: Epstein-Barr virus and primary lung lymphoma: A study utilizing the polymerase chain reaction. Mod Pathol 6:575, 1993.
75. Elenitoba-Johnson K, Medeiros LJ, Khorsand J, et al: Lymphoma of the mucosa-associated lymphoid tissue of the lung: A multifocal case of common clonal origin. Am J Clin Pathol 103:341, 1995.
76. Kaplan MA, Pettit CL, Zukerberg LR, et al: Primary lymphoma of the trachea with morphologic and immunophenotypic characteristics of low-grade B-cell lymphoma of mucosa-associated lymphoid tissue. Am J Surg Pathol 16:71, 1992.
77. Wiggins J, Sheffield E, Green M: Primary B cell malignant lymphoma of the trachea. Thorax 43:497, 1988.
78. Hardy K, Nicholson DP, Schaefer RF, et al: Bilateral endobronchial non-Hodgkin's lymphoma. South Med J 88:367, 1995.
79. Peterson H, Snider HL, Yam LT, et al: Primary pulmonary lymphoma: A clinical and immunohistochemical study of six cases. Cancer 56:805, 1985.
80. Swanson S, Innes DJ Jr, Frierson HF Jr, et al: T-immunoblastic lymphoma mimicking β-immunoblastic lymphoma. Arch Pathol Lab Med 111:1077, 1987.
81. Kubonishi I, Sugito S, Kobayashi M, et al: A unique chromosome translocation, t(11;12;18) (q13;q13;q12), in primary lung lymphoma. Cancer Genet Cytogenet 82:54, 1995.
82. Wotherspoon AC, Pan LX, Diss TC, et al: Cytogenetic study of B-cell lymphoma of mucosa-associated lymphoid tissue. Cancer Genet Cytogenet 58:35, 1992.
83. Knowles DM II, Halper JP, Jakobiec FA: The immunologic characterization of 40 extranodal lymphoid infiltrates: Usefulness in distinguishing between benign pseudolymphoma and malignant lymphoma. Cancer 49:2321, 1982.
84. Gephardt GN, Tubbs RR, Liu AC, et al: Pulmonary lymphoid neoplasms: Role of immunohistology in the study of cellular immunotypes and in differential diagnosis. Chest 89:545, 1986.
85. Subramanian D, Albrecht S, Gonzalez JM, et al: Primary pulmonary lymphoma: Diagnosis by immunoglobulin gene rearrangement study using a novel polymerase chain reaction technique. Am Rev Respir Dis 148:222, 1993.
86. Shiota T, Chiba W, Ikeda S, et al: Gene analysis of pulmonary pseudolymphoma. Chest 103:335, 1993.
87. Kurosu K, Yumoto N, Mikata A, et al: Monoclonality of B-cell lineage in primary pulmonary lymphoma demonstrated by immunoglobulin heavy chain gene sequence analysis of histologically nondefinitive transbronchial biopsy specimens. J Pathol 178:316, 1996.
88. Koss MN, Hochholzer L, Nichols PW, et al: Primary non-Hodgkin's lymphoma and pseudolymphoma of the lung: A study of 161 patients. Hum Pathol 14:1024, 1983.
89. Turner RR, Colby TV, Doggett RS: Well-differentiated lymphocytic lymphoma: A study of 47 patients with primary manifestation in the lung. Cancer 54:2088, 1984.
90. Lee KS, Kim Y, Primack SL: Imaging of pulmonary lymphomas. Am J Roentgenol 168:339, 1997.
91. Cordier JF, Chailleux E, Lauque D, et al: Primary pulmonary lymphomas: A clinical study of 70 cases in nonimmunocompromised patients. Chest 103:201, 1993.
92. Bozanko CMM, Korobkin M, Fantone JC, et al: Lobar primary pulmonary lymphoma: CT findings. J Comput Assist Tomogr 15:679, 1991.
92a. O'Donnell PG, Jackson SA, Tung KT, et al: Radiological appearances of lymphomas arising from mucosa-associated lymphoid tissue (MALT) in the lung. Clin Radiol 53:258, 1998.
93. Au V, Leung AN: Radiologic manifestations of lymphoma in the thorax. Am J Roentgenol 168:93, 1997.
94. Gollub MJ, Castellino RA: Diffuse endobronchial non-Hodgkin's lymphoma: CT demonstration. Am J Roentgenol 164:1093, 1995.
95. Takashima S, Fujita N, Morimoto S, et al: MR imaging of primary pulmonary lymphoma. Australas Radiol 34:353, 1990.
96. Roggeri A, Agostini L, Vezzani G, et al: Primary malignant non-Hodgkin's lymphoma of the lung arising in mucosa-associated lymphoid tissue (MALT). Eur Respir J 6:138, 1993.
97. Finke R, Lydtin H, Prechtel K: Sarcoidosis and immunocytoma. Am J Med 80:939, 1986.
98. Lorenzetti E, Nardi F: Diagnostic value of bronchial washing in a case of primary pulmonary non-Hodgkin's lymphoma. Appl Pathol 2:277, 1984.
99. Kuruvilla S, Gomathy DV, Shanthi AV, et al: Primary pulmonary lymphoma: Report of a case diagnosed by fine needle aspiration cytology. Acta Cytol 38:601, 1994.
100. Keicho N, Oka T, Takeuchi K, et al: Detection of lymphomatous involvement of the lung by bronchoalveolar lavage: Application of immunophenotypic and gene rearrangement analysis. Chest 105:458, 1994.
101. Betsuyaku T, Munakata M, Yamaguchi E, et al: Establishing diagnosis of pulmonary malignant lymphoma by gene rearrangement analysis of lymphocytes in bronchoalveolar lavage fluid. Am J Respir Crit Care Med 149:526, 1994.
102. Xaubet A, Diumenjo MC, Marin A, et al: Characteristics and prognostic value of pleural effusions in non-Hodgkin's lymphomas. Eur J Respir Dis 66:135, 1985.
103. Yam LT, Lin DG, Janckila AJ, et al: Immunocytochemical diagnosis of lymphoma in serous effusions. Acta Cytol 29:833, 1985.
104. Das DK, Gupta SK, Ayyagari S, et al: Pleural effusions in non-Hodgkin's lymphoma: Cytomorphologic, cytochemical and immunologic study. Acta Cytol 31:119, 1987.
105. Harrison RN: Chronic lymphocytic pulmonary infiltrate and Bence Jones proteinuria. Respiration 46:334, 1984.
106. Liaw YS, Yang PC, Su IJ, et al: Mucosa-associated lymphoid tissue lymphoma of the lung with cold-reacting autoantibody-mediated hemolytic anemia. Chest 105:288, 1994.
107. Tamura A, Komatsu H, Yanai N, et al: Primary pulmonary lymphoma: Relationship between clinical features and pathologic findings in 24 cases. The Japan National Chest Hospital Study Group for Lung Cancer. Jpn J Clin Oncol 25:140, 1995.
108. Kawamata N, Miki T, Fukuda T, et al: Determination of a common clonal origin of gastric and pulmonary mucosa-associated lymphoid tissue lymphomas presenting five years apart. Intern Med 34:220, 1995.
109. Close PM, Macrae MB, Hammond JM, et al: Anaplastic large-cell Ki-1 lymphoma: Pulmonary presentation mimicking miliary tuberculosis. Am J Clin Pathol 99:631, 1993.
110. Cheng AL, Su IJ, Chen YC, et al: Characteristic clinicopathologic features of Epstein-Barr virus-associated peripheral T-cell lymphoma. Cancer 72:909, 1993.
111. Harrison NK, Twelves C, Addis BJ, et al: Peripheral T-cell lymphoma presenting with angioedema and diffuse pulmonary infiltrates. Am Rev Respir Dis 138:976, 1988.
112. Hayashi K, Hoshida Y, Ohnoshi T, et al: Primary pulmonary non-Hodgkin's lymphoma in a Japanese renal transplant recipient. Int J Hematol 57:245, 1993.
113. Brousset P, Chittal SM, Schlaifer D, et al: T-cell rich B-cell lymphoma in the lung. Histopathology 26:371, 1995.
113a. Matsui K, Kitagawa M, Wakaki K, et al: Lung carcinoma mimickiing malignant lymphoma: Report of three cases. Acta Pathol Jpn 43:608, 1993.
114. Lautin EM, Rosenblatt M, Friedman AC, et al: Calcification in non-Hodgkin lymphoma occurring before therapy: Identification on plain films and CT. Am J Roentgenol 155:739, 1990.
115. Eliasson AH, Rajagopal KR, Dow NS: Respiratory failure in rapidly progressing pulmonary lymphoma. Am Rev Respir Dis 141:231, 1990.
116. Kim H, Dorfman RF: Morphological studies of 84 untreated patients subjected to laparotomy for the staging of non-Hodgkin's lymphomas. Cancer 33:657, 1974.
117. Israel HL, Patchefsky AS, Saldana MJ: Wegener's granulomatosis, lymphomatoid granulomatosis, and benign lymphocytic angiitis and granulomatosis of lung: Recognition and treatment. Ann Intern Med 87:691, 1977.
118. Saldana MJ, Patchefsky AS, Israel HI, et al: Pulmonary angiitis and granulomatosis. Hum Pathol 8:391, 1977.
119. Liebow AA, Carrington CRB, Friedman PJ: Lymphomatoid granulomatosis. Hum Pathol 3:457, 1972.
120. Katzenstein A-LA, Carrington CB, Liebow AA: Lymphomatoid granulomatosis. Cancer 43:360, 1979.
121. Nonomura A, Ohta G: Lymphomatoid granulomatosis-like lesions in malignant lymphoma. Acta Pathol Jpn 36:1617, 1986.
122. Colby TV, Carrington CB: Pulmonary lymphomas simulating lymphomatoid granulomatosis. Am J Surg Pathol 6:19, 1982.
123. Donner LR, Dobin S, Harrington D, et al: Angiocentric immunoproliferative lesion (lymphomatoid granulomatosis): A cytogenetic, immunophenotypic, and genotypic study. Cancer 65:249, 1990.
124. Leavitt RY, Fauci AS: Pulmonary vasculitis. Am Rev Respir Dis 134:149, 1986.
125. Tanaka Y, Sasaki Y, Kurozumi H, et al: Angiocentric immunoproliferative lesion associated with chronic active Epstein-Barr virus infection in an 11-year-old boy: Clonotypic proliferation of Epstein-Barr virus-bearing CD4+ T lymphocytes. Am J Surg Pathol 18:623, 1994.
126. Vergier B, Capron F, Trojani M, et al: Benign lymphocytic angiitis and granulomatosis: A T-cell lymphoma? Hum Pathol 23:1191, 1992.
127. Bleiweiss IJ, Strauchen JA: Lymphomatoid granulomatosis of the lung: Report of a case and gene rearrangement studies. Hum Pathol 19:1109, 1988.
128. Minase T, Ogasawara M, Kikuchi T, et al: Lymphomatoid granulomatosis: Light microscopic, electron microscopic and immunohistochemical study. Acta Pathol Jpn 35:711, 1985.
129. Myers JL, Kurtin PJ, Katzenstein AL, et al: Lymphomatoid granulomatosis: Evidence of immunophenotypic diversity and relationship to Epstein-Barr virus infection. Am J Surg Pathol 19:1300, 1995.
130. Katzenstein A-LA, Peiper SC: Detection of Epstein-Barr virus genomes in lymphomatoid granulomatosis: Analysis of 29 cases by the polymerase chain reaction technique. Mod Pathol 3:435, 1990.
131. Nicholson AG, Wotherspoon AC, Diss TC, et al: Lymphomatoid granulomatosis: Evidence that some cases represent Epstein-Barr virus-associated B-cell lymphoma. Histopathology 29:317, 1996.

131a. Haque AK, Myers JL, Hudnall SD, et al: Pulmonary lymphomatoid granulomatosis in acquired immunodeficiency syndrome: Lesions with Epstein-Barr virus infection. Mod Pathol 11:347, 1998.

132. Koss MN, Hochholzer L, Langloss JM, et al: Lymphomatoid granulomatosis: A clinicopathologic study of 42 patients. Pathology 18:283, 1986.

133. Wechsler RJ, Steiner RM, Israel HL, et al: Chest radiograph in lymphomatoid granulomatosis: Comparison with Wegener granulomatosis. Am J Roentgenol 142:79, 1984.

134. Prénovault JMN, Weisbrod GL, Herman SJ: Lymphomatoid granulomatosis: A review of 12 cases. J Can Assoc Radiol 39:263, 1988.

135. Pisani RJ, DeRemee RA: Clinical implications of the histopathologic diagnosis of pulmonary lymphomatoid granulomatosis. Mayo Clin Proc 65:151, 1990.

135a. Donnelly TJ, Tuder RM, Vendegna TR: A 48-year-old woman with peripheral neuropathy, hypercalcemia, and pulmonary infiltrates. Chest 114:1205, 1998.

136. Fauci AS, Haynes BF, Costa J, et al: Lymphomatoid granulomatosis: Prospective clinical and therapeutic experience over 10 years. N Engl J Med 306:68, 1982.

137. Slabbynck H, Mignolet M, Kockx M, et al: Spontaneous pneumothorax in lymphomatoid granulomatosis. Monaldi Arch Chest Dis 51:199, 1996.

138. Koss MN, Hochholzer L, Langloss JM, et al: Lymphomatoid granulomatosis: A clinicopathologic study of 42 patients. Pathology 18:283, 1986.

139. Patton WF, Lynch JP III: Lymphomatoid granulomatosis: Clinicopathologic study of four cases and literature review. Medicine 61:1, 1982.

140. Bushunow PW, Casas V, Duggan DB: Lymphomatoid granulomatosis causing central diabetes insipidus: Case report and review of the literature. Cancer Invest 14:112, 1996.

141. Bergin C, Stein HB, Boyko W, et al: Lymphomatoid granulomatosis presenting as polyarthritis. J Rheumatol 11:537, 1984.

142. Cooke CT, Matz LR, Armstrong JA, et al: Asbestos related interstitial pneumonitis associated with glomerulonephritis and lymphomatoid granulomatosis. Pathology 18:352, 1986.

143. Mentzer SJ, Reilly JJ, Skarin AT, et al: Patterns of lung involvement by malignant lymphoma. Surgery 113:507, 1993.

144. Rossetti F, Deeg HJ, Hackman RC: Early pulmonary recurrence of non-Hodgkin's lymphoma after autologous marrow transplantation: Evidence for reinfusion of lymphoma cells? Bone Marrow Transplant 15:429, 1995.

145. Irwin DH, Kaplan LD: Pulmonary manifestations of acquired immunodeficiency syndrome-associated malignancies. Semin Respir Infect 8:139, 1993.

145a. Hardy K, Nicholson DP, Schaefer RF, et al: Bilateral endobronchial non-Hodgkin's lymphoma. South Med J 88:367, 1995.

146. Filly R, Blank N, Castellino RA: Radiographic distribution of intrathoracic disease in previously untreated patients with Hodgkin's disease and non-Hodgkin's lymphoma. Radiology 120:277, 1976.

147. Castellino RA, Hilton S, O'Brien JP, et al: Non-Hodgkin lymphoma: Contribution of chest CT in the initial staging evaluation. Radiology 199:129, 1996.

148. Robbins LL: The roentgenological appearance of parenchymal involvement of the lungs by malignant lymphoma. Cancer 6:80, 1953.

149. Lewis ER, Caskey CI, Fishman EK: Lymphoma of the lung: CT findings in 31 patients. Am J Roentgenol 156:711, 1991.

150. Van Schoor J, Joos G, Pauwels R: Non-Hodgkin's lymphoma presenting as multiple cavitating pulmonary nodules. Eur Respir J 6:1229, 1993.

151. Jackson SA, Tung KT, Mead GM: Multiple cavitating pulmonary lesions in non-Hodgkin's lymphoma. Clin Radiol 49:883, 1994.

152. Samuels ML, Howe CD, Dodd GD, et al: Endobronchial malignant lymphoma: Report of five cases in adults. Am J Roentgenol 85:87, 1961.

153. Havard CWH, Nichols JB, Stanfeld AG: Primary lymphosarcoma of the lung. Thorax 17:190, 1962.

154. Goldstein J, Burns JC: Lymphoma of lung masquerading as sarcoidosis. Tubercle 42:507, 1961.

155. Brown MJ, Miller RR, Müller NL: Acute lung disease in the immunocompromised host: CT and pathologic examination findings. Radiology 190:247, 1994.

156. Celikoglu F, Teirstein AS, Krellenstein DJ, et al: Pleural effusion in non-Hodgkin's lymphoma. Chest 101:1357, 1992.

157. Shuman LS, Libshitz HI: Solid pleural manifestations of lymphoma. Am J Roentgenol 142:269, 1984.

158. Leung AN, Müller NL, Miller RR: CT in differential diagnosis of diffuse pleural disease. Am J Roentgenol 154:487, 1990.

159. Kennedy P, Buck M, Joshua DE, et al: Rapidly progressive fatal pulmonary infiltration by lymphoma. Aust N Z J Med 15:62, 1985.

160. Rees GM: Primary lymphosarcoma of the lung. Thorax 28:429, 1973.

161. Garrison CO, Dines DE, Harrison EG Jr, et al: The alveolar pattern of pulmonary lymphoma. Mayo Clin Proc 44:260, 1969.

162. Brewin TB: Alcohol intolerance in neoplastic disease. BMJ 2:437, 1966.

163. Bailey CC, Campbell RHA: Lymphosarcoma presenting as Löffler's syndrome. BMJ 1:460, 1973.

164. Reddy SS, Hyland RH, Alison RE, et al: Tumor-associated peripheral eosinophilia: Two unusual cases. J Clin Oncol 2:1165, 1984.

165. Bruneau R, Rubin P: The management of pleural effusions and chylothorax in lymphoma. Radiology 85:1085, 1965.

166. Manoharan A, Ford J, Hill J, et al: Sputum cytology in the diagnosis of pulmonary non-Hodgkin's lymphoma. Thorax 39:392, 1984.

167. Schumann GB, DiFiore K, Johnston JL: Sputum cytodiagnosis of disseminated histiocytic lymphoma. Acta Cytol 27:262, 1983.

168. Yam LT, Lin DG, Janckila AJ, et al: Immunocytochemical diagnosis of lymphoma in serous effusions. Acta Cytol 29:833, 1985.

169. Seidel TA, Garbes AD: Cellules Grumelees: Old terminology revisited. Acta Cytol 29:775, 1985.

170. Winterbauer RH, Riggins RCK, Griesman, FA, et al: Pleuropulmonary manifestations of Waldenström's macroglobulinemia. Chest 66:368, 1974.

171. Kobayashi H, Ii K, Hizawa K, et al: Two cases of pulmonary Waldenström's macroglobulinemia. Chest 88:297, 1985.

172. Aubert L, Detolle P, Sors Ch: Maladie de Waldenström à forme bronchopulmonaire. [Bronchopulmonary form of Waldenström's disease.] J Fr Med Chir Thorac 16:709, 1962.

173. Furgerson WB Jr, Bachman LB, O'Toole WF: Waldenström's macroglobulinemia with diffuse pulmonary infiltration: Lung biopsy and response to chlorambucil therapy. Am Rev Respir Dis 88:689, 1963.

174. Benda R, Mossé A: Sur une "forme pulmonaire" de maladie de Waldenström. [On a "pulmonary form" of Waldenström's disease.] J Fr Med Chir Thorac 16:703, 1962.

175. Major D, Meltzer MH, Nedwich A, et al: Waldenström's macroglobulinemia presenting as a pulmonary mass. Chest 64:760, 1973.

176. Nomura S, Kanoh T: Localized form of Waldenström's macroglobulinemia: Long-term follow-up study. Tonoku J Exp Med 153:37, 1987.

177. Gertz MA, Kyle RA, Noel P: Primary systemic amyloidosis: A rare complication of immunoglobulin M monoclonal gammopathies and Waldenström's macroglobulinemia. J Clin Oncol 11:914, 1993.

178. Beumer HM, Olislagers WP, Djajadiningrat RJ, et al: Pleuropulmonary involvement in Waldenström's macroglobulinemia: Case report. Respiration 45:154, 1984.

179. Rizzo S, Campagnoli M: Chylothorax as a complication of Waldenström's disease. Eur J Respir Dis 65:371, 1984.

180. James JM, Brouet JC, Orvoenfrija E, et al: Waldenström's macroglobulinaemia in a bird breeder: A case history with pulmonary involvement and antibody activity of the monoclonal IgM to canary's droppings. Clin Exp Immunol 68:397, 1987.

181. Banks PM, Arseneau JC, Grainick HR, et al: American Burkitt's lymphoma: A clinicopathologic study of 30 cases: II. Pathologic correlations. Am J Med 58:322, 1975.

182. Dunnick NR, Reaman GH, Head GL, et al: Radiographic manifestations of Burkitt's lymphoma in American patients. Am J Roentgenol 132:1, 1979.

183. Ducatman BS, Wick MR, Morgan TW, et al: Malignant histiocytosis: A clinical, histologic, and immunohistochemical study of 20 cases. Hum Pathol 15:368, 1984.

184. Dunnick NR, Parker BR, Warnke RA, et al: Radiographic manifestations of malignant histiocytosis. Am J Roentgenol 127:611, 1976.

185. Colby TV, Carrington CB, Mark GJ: Pulmonary involvement in malignant histiocytosis. Am J Surg Pathol 5:61, 1981.

186. Wongshaowart B, Kennealy JA, Crissman J, et al: Respiratory failure in malignant histiocytosis. Am Rev Respir Dis 124:640, 1981.

187. Risdall RJ, McKenna RW, Nesbit ME, et al: Virus-associated hemophagocytic syndrome: A benign histiocytic proliferation distinct from malignant histiocytosis. Cancer 44:1002, 1979.

188. Stempel DA, Volberg FM, Parker BR, et al: Malignant histiocytosis presenting as interstitial pulmonary disease. Am Rev Respir Dis 126:726, 1982.

189. Epstein EH Jr, Levin DL, Croft JD Jr, et al: Mycosis fungoides: Survival prognostic features, response to therapy, and autopsy findings. Medicine 51:61, 1972.

190. Rappaport H, Thomas LB: Mycosis fungoides: The pathology of extracutaneous involvement. Cancer 34:1198, 1974.

191. Long JC, Mihm MC: Mycosis fungoides with extracutaneous dissemination: A distinct clinicopathologic entity. Cancer 34:1745, 1974.

192. Foster GH, Eichenhorn MS, Van Slyck EJ: The Sézary syndrome with rapid pulmonary dissemination. Cancer 56:1197, 1985.

193. Nonomura A, Ohta G: Lymphomatoid granulomatosis–like lesions in malignant lymphoma. Acta Pathol Jpn 36:1617, 1986.

194. Marglin SI, Soulen RL, Blank N, et al: Mycosis fungoides: Radiographic manifestations of extracutaneous intrathoracic involvement. Radiology 130:35, 1979.

195. Marglin SI, Soulen RL, Blank N, et al: Mycosis fungoides: Radiographic manifestations of extracutaneous intrathoracic involvement. Radiology 130:35, 1979.

196. Stokar LM, Vonderheid EC, Abell E, et al: Clinical manifestations of intrathoracic cutaneous T-cell lymphoma. Cancer 56:2694, 1985.

197. Rubin DL, Blank N: Rapid pulmonary dissemination in mycosis fungoides simulating pneumonia. Cancer 56:649, 1985.

198. Israel RH: Mycosis fungoides with rapidly progressive pulmonary infiltration. Radiology 125:10, 1977.

199. Milier KS, Sahn SA: Mycosis fungoides presenting as ARDS and diagnosed by bronchoalveolar lavage: Radiographic and pathologic pulmonary manifestations. Chest 89:312, 1986.

200. Rosen SE, Vonderheid EC, Koprowska I: Mycosis fungoides with pulmonary involvement. Acta Cytol 28:51, 1984.

201. Demirer T, Dail DH, Aboulafia DM: Four varied cases of intravascular lymphomatosis and a literature review. Cancer 73:1738, 1994.

201a. Ko YH, Han JH, Go JH, et al: Intravascular lymphomatosis: A clinicopathological study of two cases presenting as an interstitial lung disease. Histopathology 31:555, 1997.

202. Yousem SA, Colby TV: Intravascular lymphomatosis presenting in the lung. Cancer 65:349, 1990.

203. Kamesaki H, Matsui Y, Ohno Y, et al: Angiocentric lymphoma with histologic features of neoplastic angioendotheliomatosis presenting with predominant respiratory and hematologic manifestations. Am J Clin Pathol 94:768, 1990.

204. Snyder LS, Harmon KR, Estensen RD: Intravascular lymphomatosis (malignant

angioendotheliomatosis) presenting as pulmonary hypertension. Chest 96:1199, 1989.

205. Takamura K, Nasuhara Y, Mishina T, et al: Intravascular lymphomatosis diagnosed by transbronchial lung biopsy. Eur Respir J 10:955, 1997.

206. Suster S, Moran CA: Pleomorphic large cell lymphomas of the mediastinum. Am J Surg Pathol 20:224, 1996.

207. Waldron JA Jr, Dohring EJ, Farber LR: Primary large cell lymphomas of the mediastinum: An analysis of 20 cases. Semin Diagn Pathol 2:281, 1985.

208. Trump DL, Mann RB: Diffuse large cell and undifferentiated lymphomas with prominent mediastinal involvement: A poor prognostic subset of patients with non-Hodgkin's lymphoma. Cancer 50:277, 1982.

209. Picozzi VJ, Coleman CN: Lymphoblastic lymphoma. Semin Oncol 17:96, 1990.

210. Nambu A, Kurihara Y, Ichikawa T, et al: Lung involvement in angiotropic lymphoma: CT findings. Am J Roentgenol 170:940, 1998.

210a. Jang H-J, Lee KS, Han J: Intravascular lymphomatosis of the lung: Radiologic findings. J Comput Assist Tomogr 22:427, 1998.

211. Yousem SA, Weiss LM, Warnke RA: Primary mediastinal non-Hodgkin's lymphomas: A morphologic and immunologic study of 19 cases. Am J Clin Pathol 83:676, 1985.

212. Lamarre L, Jacobson JO, Aisenberg AC, et al: Primary large cell lymphoma of the mediastinum: A histologic and immunophenotypic study of 29 cases. Am J Surg Pathol 13:730, 1989.

213. Perrone T, Frizzera G, Rosai J: Mediastinal diffuse large-cell lymphoma with sclerosis: A clinicopathologic study of 60 cases. Am J Surg Pathol 10:176, 1986.

214. Möller P, Lämmler B, Eberlein-Gonska M, et al: Primary mediastinal clear cell lymphoma of B-cell type. Virchows Arch (Pathol Anat) 409:79, 1986.

215. Menestrina F, Chilosi M, Bonetti F, et al: Mediastinal large-cell lymphoma of B-type, with sclerosis: Histopathological and immunohistochemical study of eight cases. Histopathology 10:589, 1986.

216. Lazzarino M, Orlandi E, Paulli M, et al: Primary mediastinal B-cell lymphoma with sclerosis: An aggressive tumor with distinctive clinical and pathologic features. J Clin Oncol 11:2306, 1993.

217. Levitt LJ, Aisenberg AC, Harris NL, et al: Primary non-Hodgkin's lymphoma of the mediastinum. Cancer 50:2486, 1982.

217a. Putterman C, Gilon D, Uretzki G, et al: Right ventricular outflow tract obstruction due to extrinsic compression by non-Hodgkin's lymphoma: Importance of echocardiographic diagnosis and follow up. Leuk Lymphoma 7:211, 1992.

218. Singh HK, Silverman JF, Powers CN, et al: Diagnostic pitfalls in fine-needle aspiration biopsy of the mediastinum. Diagn Cytopathol 17:121, 1997.

219. Silverman JF, Raab SS, Park HK: Fine-needle aspiration cytology of primary large-cell lymphoma of the mediastinum: Cytomorphologic findings with potential pitfalls in diagnosis. Diagn Cytopathol 9:209, 1993.

220. Fishman EK, Kuhlman JE, Jones RJ: CT of lymphoma: Spectrum of disease. Radiographics 11:647, 1991.

221. Negendank WG, Al-Katib AM, Karanes C, et al: Lymphomas: MR imaging contrast characteristics with clinical-pathologic correlations. Radiology 177:209, 1990.

222. Carlsen SE, Bergin CJ, Hoppe RT: MR imaging to detect chest wall and pleural involvement in patients with lymphoma: Effect on radiation therapy planning. Am J Roentgenol 160:1191, 1993.

223. Israel O, Front D, Lam M, et al: Gallium 67 imaging in monitoring lymphoma response to treatment. Cancer 61:2439, 1988.

224. Front D, Israel O, Epelbaum R, et al: Ga-67 SPECT before and after treatment of lymphoma. Radiology 175:515, 1990.

225. Front D, Bar-Shalom R, Epelbaum R, et al: Early detection of lymphoma recurrence with gallium-67 scintigraphy. J Nucl Med 34:2101, 1993.

226. Moog F, Bangerter M, Diederichs CG, et al: Lymphoma: Role of whole-body 2-deoxy-2-[F-18]-fluoro-D-glucose (FDG) PET in nodal staging. Radiology 203:795, 1997.

227. Som P, Atkins HL, Bandophadhyah D: A fluorinated glucose analog, 2-fluoro-2-deoxy-D-glucose (F-18). J Nucl Med 21:670, 1980.

228. Okada J, Yoshikawa K, Imazeki K, et al: Positron emission tomography using fluorine-18-fluorodeoxy-glucose in malignant lymphoma: A comparison with proliferative activity. J Nucl Med 33:325, 1992.

229. Rodriguez M, Rehn S, Ahlström H, et al: Predicting malignancy grade with PEG in non-Hodgkin's lymphoma. J Nucl Med 36:1790, 1995.

230. Lapela M, Leskinen S, Minn H, et al: Increased glucose metabolism in untreated non-Hodgkin's lymphoma: A study with positron emission tomography and fluorine-18 fluorodeoxyglucose. Blood 9:3522, 1995.

231. Kintzer JS, Rosenow EC, Kyle RA: Thoracic and pulmonary abnormalities in multiple myeloma. Arch Intern Med 138:727, 1978.

232. Garewal H, Durie BG: Aggressive phase of multiple myeloma with pulmonary plasma cell infiltrates. JAMA 248:1875, 1982.

233. Gilchrist D, Chan CK, LaRoye GJ, et al: Bronchial mucosal infiltration and unilateral lung collapse: An unusual complication of multiple myeloma. Am J Med 85:74, 1988.

234. Kinare SG, Parulkar GB, Panday SR, et al: Extensive ossification in a pulmonary plasmacytoma. Thorax 20:206, 1965.

235. Wolfe DA, Dennis JM: Multiple myeloma of the chest wall. Am J Roentgenol 89:1241, 1963.

236. Badrinas F, Rodriguez-Roisin R, Rives A, et al: Multiple myeloma with pleural involvement. Am Rev Respir Dis 110:82, 1974.

237. Chee YC, Chea E: IgA myeloma with primary pleural involvement. Eur J Respir Dis 65:136, 1984.

238. Kwan WC, Lam SC, Klimo P: Kappa light-chain myeloma with pleural involvement. Chest 86:494, 1984.

239. Witt DH, Zalusky R, Castella A, et al: Light chain myeloma with meningeal and pleural involvement. Am J Med 80:1213, 1986.

240. Baker WH, Castleman B: Pulmonary mass after 17 years of plasma-cell myeloma. N Engl J Med 286:1256, 1972.

241. Moulopoulos LA, Granfield CAJ, Dimopoulos MA, et al: Extraosseous multiple myeloma: Imaging features. Am J Roentgenol 161:1083, 1993.

242. Iwasaki T, Hamano T, Aizawa K, et al: A case of pulmonary amyloidosis associated with multiple myeloma successfully treated with dimethyl sulfoxide. Acta Haematol 91:91, 1994.

243. Mootz JR, Sagel SS, Roberts TH: Roentgenographic manifestations of pulmonary calcifications: A rare cause of respiratory failure in chronic renal disease. Radiology 107:55, 1973.

244. Weber CK, Friedrich JM, Merkle E, et al: Reversible metastatic pulmonary calcification in a patient with multiple myeloma. Ann Hematol 72:329, 1996.

245. Kapadia SB: Multiple myeloma: A clinicopathologic study of 62 consecutively autopsied cases. Medicine 59:380, 1980.

246. Kyle RA: Multiple myeloma: Review of 869 cases. Mayo Clin Proc 50:29, 1975.

247. Conklin R, Alexanian R: Clinical classification of plasma cell myeloma. Arch Intern Med 135:139, 1975.

248. Favis E, Kerman H, Schildecker W: Multiple myeloma manifested as a problem in the diagnosis of pulmonary disease. Am J Med 28:323, 1960.

249. Menashe P, Stenson W, Reynoso G, et al: Bronchoalveolar lavage plasmacytosis in a patient with a plasma cell dyscrasia. Chest 95:226, 1989.

250. Twomey JJ: Infections complicating multiple myeloma and chronic lymphocytic leukemia. Arch Intern Med 132:562, 1973.

251. A cooperative study by Acute Leukemia Group B. Correlation of abnormal immunoglobulin with clinical features of myeloma. Arch Intern Med 135:46, 1975.

252. Garewal H, Durie BGM: Aggressive phase of multiple myeloma with pulmonary plasma cell infiltrates. JAMA 248:1875, 1982.

253. Wiltshaw E: The natural history of extramedullary plasmacytoma and its relation to solitary myeloma of bone and myelomatosis. Medicine 55:217, 1976.

254. Joseph G, Pandit M, Korfhage L: Primary pulmonary plasmacytoma. Cancer 71:721, 1993.

255. Morinaga S, Watanabe H, Gemma A, et al: Plasmacytoma of the lung associated with nodular deposits of immunoglobulin. Am J Surg Pathol 11:989, 1987.

255a. Piard F, Yaziji N, Jarry O, et al: Solitary plasmacytoma of the lung with light-chain extracellular deposits: A case report and review of the literature. Histopathology 32:356, 1998.

256. Kazzaz B, Dewar A, Corrin B: An unusual pulmonary plasmacytoma. Histopathology 21:285, 1992.

257. Okada S, Ohtsuki H, Midorikawa O, et al: Bronchial plasmacytoma identified by immunoperoxidase technique on paraffin embedded section. Acta Pathol Jpn 32:149, 1981.

258. Husain M, Nguyen GK: Primary pulmonary plasmacytoma diagnosed by transthoracic needle aspiration cytology and immunocytochemistry. Acta Cytol 40:622, 1996.

259. Logan PM, Miller RR, Müller NL: Solitary tracheal plasmacytoma: Computed tomography and pathological findings. Can Assoc Radiol J 46:125, 1995.

260. Mazumdar P, Abraham S, Damodaran VN, et al: Pulmonary plasmacytoma: A case report. Am Rev Respir Dis 100:866, 1969.

261. Tenholder MF, Scialla SJ, Weisbaum G: Endobronchial metastatic plasmacytoma. Cancer 49:1465, 1982.

262. Nagai K, Ando K, Yoshida H, et al: Response of the extramedullary lung plasmacytoma with pleural effusion to chemotherapy. Ann Hematol 74:279, 1997.

263. Baroni CD, Mineo TC, Ricci C, et al: Solitary secretory plasmacytoma of the lung in a 14 year old boy. Cancer 40:2329, 1977.

264. Wile A, Olinger G, Peter JB, et al: Solitary intraparenchymal pulmonary plasmacytoma associated with production of an M-protein. Cancer 37:2338, 1976.

265. Amin R: Extramedullary plasmacytoma of the lung. Cancer 56:152, 1985.

266. Bloch KJ, Lee L, Mills JA, et al: Gamma heavy chain disease—an expanding clinical and laboratory spectrum. Am J Med 55:61, 1973.

267. Pittman FE, Tripathy K, Isobe T, et al: IgA heavy-chain disease: A case detected in the Western hemisphere. Am J Med 58:424, 1975.

268. Stoop JW, Ballieux RE, Hijams W, et al: Alpha-chain disease with involvement of the respiratory tract in a Dutch child. Clin Exp Immunol 9:625, 1971.

269. Kijner CH, Yousem SA: Systemic light chain deposition disease presenting as multiple pulmonary nodules: A case report and review of the literature. Am J Surg Pathol 12:405, 1988.

270. Colby TV, Hoppe RT, Warnke RA: Hodgkin's disease: A clinicopathologic study of 659 cases. Cancer 49:1848, 1981.

271. Filly R, Blank N, Castellino RA: Radiographic distribution of intrathoracic disease in previously untreated patients with Hodgkin's disease and non-Hodgkin's lymphoma. Radiology 120:277, 1976.

272. Radin AI: Primary pulmonary Hodgkin's disease. Cancer 65:550, 1990.

273. Stolberg HO, Patt NL, MacEwen KF, et al: Hodgkin's disease of the lung. Am J Roentgenol 92:96, 1964.

274. Colby TV, Hoppe RT, Warnke RA: Hodgkin's disease at autopsy: 1972–1977. Cancer 47:1852, 1981.

275. Johnson DW, Hoppe RT, Cox RS, et al: Hodgkin's disease limited to intrathoracic sites. Cancer 52:8, 1983.

276. Rottino A, Hoffman G: The pathology of the lung in Hodgkin's disease. Am J Surg 89:550, 1955.

277. Tredaniel J, Peillon I, Ferme C, et al: Endobronchial presentation of Hodgkin's

disease: A report of nine cases and review of the literature. Eur Respir J 7:1852, 1994.

278. Yousem SA, Weiss LM, Colby TV: Primary pulmonary Hodgkin's disease: A clinicopathologic study of 15 cases. Cancer 57:1217, 1986.

279. Suster S, Moran CA: Pleomorphic large cell lymphomas of the mediastinum. Am J Surg Pathol 20:224, 1996.

280. Ben-Yehuda-Salz D, Ben-Yehuda A, Polliak A, et al: Syncytial variant of nodular sclerosis Hodgkin's disease: A new clinicopathologic entity. Cancer 65:1167, 1990.

281. Chetty R, Slavin JL, O'Leary JJ, et al: Primary Hodgkin's disease of the lung. Pathology 27:111, 1995.

282. Merchant TE, Filippa DA, Yahalom J: Sarcoidosis following chemotherapy for Hodgkin's disease. Leuk Lymphoma 13:339, 1994.

283. Castellino RA, Blank N, Hoppe RT, et al: Hodgkin disease: Contributions of chest CT in the initial staging evaluation. Radiology 160:603, 1996.

284. Cobby M, Whipp E, Bullimore J, et al: CT appearances of relapse of lymphoma in the lung. Clin Radiol 41:232, 1990.

285. Rosenberg SA, Kaplan HS: Evidence for an orderly progression in the spread of Hodgkin's disease. Cancer Res 26:1225, 1966.

286. Cropp AJ, DiMarco AF, Lankerani M: False-positive transbronchial needle aspiration in bronchogenic carcinoma. Chest 85:696, 1984.

287. Leading article: Outlook in Hodgkin's disease. BMJ 2:328, 1967.

288. Goldman JM: Parasternal chest wall involvement in Hodgkin's disease. Chest 59:133, 1971.

289. Press GA, Glazer HS, Wasserman TH, et al: Thoracic wall involvement by Hodgkin disease and non-Hodgkin lymphoma: CT evaluation. Radiology 157:195, 1985.

290. Lindfors KK, Meyers JE, Dedrick CG, et al: Thymic cysts in mediastinal Hodgkin disease. Radiology 156:37, 1985.

291. Bethancourt B, Pond GD, Jones SE, et al: Mediastinal hematoma simulating recurrent Hodgkin disease during systemic chemotherapy. Am J Roentgenol 142:1119, 1984.

292. Fisher AMH, Kendall B, Van Leuven BD: Hodgkin's disease: A radiological survey. Clin Radiol 13:115, 1962.

293. Wyman SM, Weber AL: Calcification in intrathoracic nodes in Hodgkin's disease. Radiology 93:1021, 1969.

294. Whitfield AGW, Jones EL: Lymph node calcification in Hodgkin's disease. Clin Radiol 21:259, 1970.

295. Brereton HD, Johnson RE: Calcification in mediastinal lymph nodes after radiation therapy of Hodgkin's disease. Radiology 112:705, 1974.

296. Schnyder PA, Gamsu G: CT of the pretracheal retrocaval space. Am J Roentgenol 136:303, 1981.

297. Whitcomb ME, Schwartz MI, Keller AR, et al: Hodgkin's disease of the lung. Am Rev Respir Dis 106:79, 1972.

298. Martin JJ: The Nisbet Symposium: Hodgkin's disease: Radiological aspects of the disease. Australas Radiol 11:206, 1967.

299. Sheinmel A, Roswit B, Lawrence LR: Hodgkin's disease of the lung: Roentgen appearance and therapeutic management. Radiology 54:165, 1950.

300. Ellman P, Bowdler AJ: Pulmonary manifestations of Hodgkin's disease. Br J Dis Chest 54:59, 1960.

301. Dhingra HK, Flance IJ: Cavitary primary pulmonary Hodgkin's disease presenting as pruritus. Chest 58:71, 1970.

302. Simon G: Intra-thoracic Hodgkin's disease: Part I. Less common intra-thoracic manifestations of Hodgkin's disease. Br J Radiol 40:926, 1967.

303. Madewell JE, Daroca PJ, Reed JC: Pulmonary parenchymal Hodgkin's disease: RPC from the AFIP. Radiology 117:555, 1975.

304. Shahar J, Angelillo VA, Katz D, et al: Recurrent cavitary nodules secondary to Hodgkin's disease. Chest 91:273, 1987.

305. Holeshi S: Unusual x-ray appearances in Hodgkin's disease. Proc R Soc Med 48:1049, 1955.

306. Seward CW, Safdar SH: Endobronchial Hodgkin's disease presenting as a primary pulmonary lesion. Chest 62:649, 1972.

307. Vaughan BF: Endobronchial Hodgkin's disease. Br J Radiol 31:45, 1958.

308. Renzi G, Lesage R: Endobronchial Hodgkin's disease and bronchoesophageal fistula. Chest 61:696, 1972.

309. Samuels ML, Howe CD, Dodd GD, et al: Endobronchial malignant lymphoma: Report of five cases in adults. Am J Roentgenol 85:87, 1961.

310. Strickland B: Intra-thoracic Hodgkin's disease: Part II. Peripheral manifestations of Hodgkin's disease in the chest. Br J Radiol 40:930, 1967

311. Yellin A, Benfield JR: Pneumothorax associated with lymphoma. Am Rev Respir Dis 134:590, 1986.

312. Beachley MC, Lau BP, King ER: Bone involvement in Hodgkin's disease. Am J Roentgenol 114:559, 1972.

313. Adler JJ, Sharma OP: Hypertrophic osteoarthropathy with intrathoracic Hodgkin's disease. Am Rev Respir Dis 102:83, 1970.

314. Hancock BW, Richmond J, Powell T, et al: Intrathoracic Hodgkin's disease presenting as hypertrophic osteoarthropathy. Br J Radiol 49:647, 1976.

315. North LB, Fuller LM, Sullivan-Halley JA, et al: Regression of mediastinal Hodgkin disease after therapy: Evaluation of time interval. Radiology 164:599, 1987.

316. Jochelson M, Mauch P, Balikian J, et al: The significance of the residual mediastinal mass in treated Hodgkin's disease. J Clin Oncol 3:637, 1985.

317. Radford JA, Cowan RA, Flanagan M, et al: The significance of residual mediastinal abnormality on the chest radiograph following the treatment of Hodgkin's disease. J Clin Oncol 6:940, 1988.

318. Canellos GP: Residual mass in lymphoma may not be residual disease (editorial). J Clin Oncol 6:931, 1988.

319. Wylie BR, Southee AE, Joshua DE, et al: Gallium scanning in the management of mediastinal Hodgkin's disease. Eur J Haematol 42:344, 1989.

320. Kramer EL, Divgi CR: Pulmonary applications of nuclear medicine. Clin Chest Med 12:55, 1991.

321. Nyman RS, Rehn SM, Glimelius BLG, et al: Residual mediastinal masses in Hodgkin disease: Prediction of size with MR imaging. Radiology 170:435, 1989.

322. Stebner FC, Bishop CR: Bone marrow scan and radioion uptake of an intrathoracic mass. Clin Nucl Med 7:86, 1982.

323. Costello P, Mauch P: Radiographic features of recurrent intrathoracic Hodgkin's disease following radiation therapy. Am J Roentgenol 133:201, 1979.

324. Ultmann JE, Moran EH: Clinical course and complications in Hodgkin's disease. Arch Intern Med 131:332, 1973.

325. Alba D, Lobato SD, Alvarez-Sala R, et al: Tracheoesophageal fistula as the presenting manifestation of Hodgkin's lymphoma. Postgrad Med J 70:49, 1994.

326. Dunn RP, Wexler L: Systemic-to-pulmonary fistula in intrapulmonary Hodgkin's disease. Chest 66:590, 1974.

327. Lobell M, Boggs DR, Wintrobe MM: The clinical significance of fever in Hodgkin's disease. Arch Intern Med 117:335, 1966.

328. Pinson P, Joos G, Praet M, et al: Primary pulmonary Hodgkin's disease. Respiration 59:314, 1992.

329. Winterbauer RH, Belic N, Moores KD: A clinical interpretation of bilateral hilar adenopathy. Ann Intern Med 78:65, 1973.

330. Arden MJ, Rottino A: Hodgkin's disease complicated by tuberculosis: A twenty-year experience. Am Rev Respir Dis 93:811, 1966.

331. Hatfield PM: Cavitating pulmonary nodules complicating Hodgkin's disease. JAMA 215:1145, 1971.

332. Hays DM, Ternberg JL, Chen TT, et al: Postsplenectomy sepsis and other complications following staging laparotomy for Hodgkin's disease in childhood. J Pediatr Surg 21:628, 1986.

333. Ragozzino MW, Melton LJ III, Kurland LT, et al: Risk of cancer after herpes zoster: A population-based study. N Engl J Med 307:393, 1982.

334. Aisenberg AC: Malignant lymphoma. N Engl J Med 288:883, 1973.

335. Reale FR, Variakojis D, Compton J, et al: Cytodiagnosis of Hodgkin's disease in sputum specimens. Acta Cytol 27:258, 1983.

336. Eisenberg RS, Dunton BL: Hodgkin's disease first suggested by sputum cytology. Chest 65:218, 1974.

337. Suprun H, Koss LG: The cytological study of sputum and bronchial washings in Hodgkin's disease with pulmonary involvement. Cancer 17:674, 1964.

338. Harlan JM, Fennessy JJ, Gross NJ: Bronchial brush biopsy in Hodgkin's disease. Chest 66:136, 1974.

339. Variakojis D, Fennessy JJ, Rappaport H: Diagnosis of Hodgkin's disease by bronchial brush biopsy. Chest 61:326, 1972.

340. Morales FM, Matthews JI: Diagnosis of parenchymal Hodgkin's disease using bronchoalveolar lavage. Chest 91:785, 1987.

341. Fajac I, Cadranel JL, Mariette X, et al: Pulmonary Hodgkin's disease in HIV-infected patient: Diagnosis by bronchoalveolar lavage. Chest 102:1913, 1992.

342. Grimwade DJ, Chopra R, King A, et al: Detection and significance of pulmonary Hodgkin's disease at autologous bone marrow transplantation. Bone Marrow Transplant 13:173, 1994.

343. Front D, Ben-Haim S, Israel O, et al: Lymphoma: Predictive value of Ga-67 scintigraphy after treatment. Radiology 182:359, 1992.

344. Lund MB, Kongerud J, Nome O, et al: Lung function impairment in long-term survivors of Hodgkin's disease. Ann Oncol 6:495, 1995.

345. Horning SJ, Adhikari A, Rizk N, et al: Effect of treatment for Hodgkin's disease on pulmonary function: Results of a prospective study. J Clin Oncol 12:297, 1994.

346. Hassink EA, Souren TS, Boersma LJ, et al: Pulmonary morbidity 10–18 years after irradiation for Hodgkin's disease. Eur J Cancer 29A:343, 1993.

347. Putterman C, Polliack A: Late cardiovascular and pulmonary complications of therapy in Hodgkin's disease: Report of three unusual cases, with a review of relevant literature. Leuk Lymphoma 7:109, 1992.

348. Bossi G, Cerveri I, Volpini E, et al: Long-term pulmonary sequelae after treatment of childhood Hodgkin's disease. Ann Oncol 8(Suppl 1):19, 1997.

349. Penniment MG, O'Brien PC: Pneumothorax following thoracic radiation therapy for Hodgkin's disease. Thorax 49:936, 1994.

350. Swift GL, Gibbs A, Campbell IA, et al: Pulmonary veno-occlusive disease and Hodgkin's lymphoma. Eur Respir J 6:596, 1993.

351. Tawil E, Mercier JP: Second malignancy complicating Hodgkin's disease. J Can Assoc Radiol 34:108, 1983.

352. van Leeuwen FE, Klokman WJ, Hagenbeek A, et al: Second cancer risk following Hodgkin's disease: A 20-year follow-up study. J Cin Oncol 12:312, 1994.

353. Swerdlow AJ, Douglas AJ, Hudson GV, et al: Risk of second primary cancers after Hodgkin's disease by type of treatment: Analysis of 2846 patients in the British National Lymphoma Investigation. BMJ 304:1137, 1992.

354. Swerdlow AJ, Barber JA, Horwich A, et al: Second malignancy in patients with Hodgkin's disease treated at the Royal Marsden Hospital. Br J Cancer 75:116, 1997.

355. van Leeuwen FE, Klokman WJ, Stovall M, et al: Roles of radiotherapy and smoking in lung cancer following Hodgkin's disease. J Natl Cancer Inst 87:1530, 1995

356. Kaldor JM, Day NE, Bell J, et al: Lung cancer following Hodgkin's disease: A case-control study. Int J Cancer 52:677, 1992.

357. Weissmann LB, Corson JM, Neugut AI, et al: Malignant mesothelioma following treatment for Hodgkin's disease. J Clin Oncol 14:2098, 1996.

358. Shin MS, Buchalter SE, Ho KJ: Langerhans' cell histiocytosis associated with Hodgkin's disease: A case report. J Natl Med Assoc 86:65, 1994.
359. Gratadour P, Fouque D, Laville M, et al: Wegener's granulomatosis with antiproteinase-3 antibodies occurring after Hodgkin's disease. Nephron 64:456, 1993.
360. Frizzera G, Moran EM, Rappaport H: Angio-immunoblastic lymphadenopathy with dysproteinaemia. Lancet 1:1070, 1974.
361. Lukes RJ, Tindle BH: Immunoblastic lymphadenopathy: A hyperimmune entity resembling Hodgkin's disease. N Engl J Med 292:1, 1975.
362. Berris B, Fernandes B, Rother I: Immunoblastic lymphadenopathy: Report of four new cases and review of the literature. Can Med Assoc J 127:389, 1982.
363. Coupland RW, Pontifex AH, Salinas FA: Angioimmunoblastic lymphadenopathy with dysproteinemia. Cancer 55:1902, 1985.
364. Gold JA, Sibbald RG, Phillips MJ, et al: Angioimmunoblastic lymphadenopathy following typhoid AB vaccination and terminating in disseminated infection. Arch Pathol Lab Med 109:1085, 1985.
365. Nathwani BN, Rappaport H, Moran EM, et al: Malignant lymphoma arising in angioimmunoblastic lymphadenopathy. Cancer 41:578, 1978.
366. Feller AC, Griesser H, Schilling CV, et al: Clonal gene rearrangement patterns correlate with immunophenotype and clinical parameters in patients with angioimmunoblastic lymphadenopathy. Am J Pathol 133:549, 1988.
367. Lipford EH, Smith HR, Pittaluga S, et al: Clonality of immunoblastic lymphadenopathy and implications for evolution to malignant lymphoma. J Clin Invest 79:637, 1987.
368. Schauer PK, Straus DJ, Bagley CM, et al: Angioimmunoblastic lymphadenopathy: Clinical spectrum of disease. Cancer 48:2493, 1981.
369. Weisenburger D, Armitage J, Dick F: Immunoblastic lymphadenopathy with pulmonary infiltrates, hypocomplementemia and vasculitis. Am J Med 63:849, 1977.
370. Iseman MD, Schwarz MI, Stanford RE: Interstitial pneumonia in angio-immunoblastic lymphadenopathy with dysproteinemia. Ann Intern Med 85:752, 1976.
371. Pangalis GA, Moran EM, Nathwani BN, et al: Angioimmunoblastic lymphadenopathy. Cancer 52:318, 1983.
371a. Libschitz HI, Clouser M, Zornoza J, et al: Radiographic findings in immunoblastic lymphadenopathy and related immunoblastic proliferations. Am J Roentgenol 129:875, 1977.
372. Limpert J, MacMahon H, Variakojis D: Angioimmunoblastic lymphadenopathy: Clinical and radiological features. Radiology 152:27, 1984.
372a. Locksmith JP, Brannon MH: Diffuse CT contrast enhancement of cervical lymph nodes in angioimmunoblastic lymphadenopathy. J Comput Assist Tomogr 15:703, 1991.
372b. Magnusson A, Andersson T, Larsson B, et al: Contrast enhancement of pathologic lymph nodes demonstrated by computed tomography. Acta Radiol 30:307, 1989.
373. Myers TJ, Cole SR, Pastuszak WT: Angioimmunoblastic lymphadenopathy: Pleural-pulmonary disease. Cancer 44:266, 1978.
374. Price D, Dent RG: Pulmonary involvement in angio-immunoblastic lymphadenopathy. Postgrad Med J 59:728, 1983.
375. Barrow MV, Holubar K: Multicentric reticulohistiocytosis. Medicine 48:287, 1969.
376. Goette DK, Odom RB, Fitzwater JE Jr: Diffuse cutaneous reticulohistiocytosis. Arch Dermatol 118:173, 1982.
377. Fast A: Cardiopulmonary complications in multicentric reticulohistiocytosis. Arch Dermatol 112:1139, 1976.
378. Bodey GP, Powell RD, Hersh E, et al: Pulmonary complications of acute leukemia. Cancer 19:781, 1966.
379. Green RA, Nichlos NJ: Pulmonary involvement in leukemia. Am Rev Respir Dis 80:833, 1959.
380. Ross JS, Ellman L: Leukemic infiltration of the lungs in the chemotherapeutic era. Am J Clin Pathol 61:235, 1974.
381. Nathan DJ, Sanders M: Manifestations of acute leukemia in the parenchyma of the lung. N Engl J Med 252:797, 1955.
382. Doran HM, Sheppard MN, Collins PW, et al: Pathology of the lung in leukaemia and lymphoma: A study of 87 autopsies. Histopathology 18:211, 1991.
383. Rollins SD, Colby TV: Lung biopsy in chronic lymphocytic leukemia. Arch Pathol Lab Med 112:607, 1988.
384. Marsh WL Jr, Bylund DJ, Heath VC, et al: Osteoarticular and pulmonary manifestations of acute leukemia: Case report and review of the literature. Cancer 57:385, 1986.
385. Rossi GA, Balbi B, Risso M, et al: Acute myelomonocytic leukemia: Demonstration of pulmonary involvement by bronchoalveolar lavage. Chest 87:259, 1985.
386. Hildebrand FL Jr, Rosenow EC 3rd, Habermann TM, et al: Pulmonary complications of leukemia. Chest 98:1233, 1990.
387. Maile CW, Moore AV, Ulreich S, et al: Chest radiographic-pathologic correlation in adult leukemia patients. Invest Radiol 18:495, 1983.
388. Suzumiya J, Marutsuka K, Nabeshima K, et al: Autopsy findings in 47 cases of adult T-cell leukemia/lymphoma in Miyazaki prefecture, Japan. Leuk Lymphoma 11:281, 1993.
389. Tenholder MF, Hooper RG: Pulmonary infiltrates in leukemia. Chest 78:468, 1980.
390. Callahan M, Wall S, Askin F, et al: Granulocytic sarcoma presenting as pulmonary nodules and lymphadenopathy. Cancer 60:1902, 1987.
391. Dugdale DC, Salnes TA, Knight L, et al: Endobronchial granulocytic sarcoma causing acute respiratory failure in acute myelogenous leukemia. Am Rev Respir Dis 136:1248, 1987.
392. Hicklin GA, Drevyanko TF: Primary granulocytic sarcoma presenting with pleural and pulmonary involvement. Chest 94:655, 1988.
393. Genet P, Pulik M, Lionnet F, et al: Leukemic relapse presenting with bronchial obstruction caused by granulocytic sarcoma. Am J Hematol 47:142, 1994.
394. Vernant JP, Brun B, Mannoni P, et al: Respiratory distress of hyperleukocytic granulocytic leukemias. Cancer 44:264, 1979.
395. McKee LC, Collins RD: Intravascular leukocyte thrombi and aggregates as a cause of morbidity and mortality in leukemia. Medicine 53:463, 1974.
396. Myers TJ, Cole SR, Klatsky AU, et al: Respiratory failure due to pulmonary leukostasis following chemotherapy of acute nonlymphocytic leukemia. Cancer 51:1808, 1983.
397. Dombret H, Hunault M, Faucher C, et al: Acute lysis pneumopathy after chemotherapy for acute myelomonocytic leukemia with abnormal marrow eosinophils. Cancer 69:1356, 1992.
398. McCarthy VP, Carlile JR: Hyperleukocytosis with pertussis. J Assoc Acad Minor Phys 8:52, 1997.
399. de Fijter CW, Schuur J, Potter van Loon BJ, et al: Acute cardiorespiratory failure as presenting symptom of chronic lymphocytic leukemia. Neth J Med 49:33, 1996.
400. van Buchem MA, Hogendoorn PC, Bruijn JA, et al: Endothelial activation antigens in pulmonary leukostasis in leukemia. Acta Haematol 90:29, 1993.
401. Yamauchi K, Shimamura K: Pulmonary fibrosis with megakaryocytoid cell infiltration and chronic myelogenous leukemia. Leuk Lymphoma 15:253, 1994.
402. Tryka AF, Godleski JJ, Fanta CH: Leukemic cell lysis pneumonopathy. Cancer 50:2763, 1982.
403. Carter JM, Dewar JM, Pease C: Interstitial pneumonitis due to leukaemic cell necrosis. N Z Med J 99:754, 1986.
403a. Bell CM, Stewart TE: Acute respiratory distress syndrome associated with tumour lysis syndrome in acute leukemia. Can Respir J 4:48, 1997.
404. Bernini JC, Timmons CF, Sandler ES: Acute basophilic leukemia in a child: Anaphylactoid reaction and coagulopathy secondary to vincristine-mediated degranulation. Cancer 75:110, 1995.
405. Saka H, Ito T, Ito M, et al: Diffuse pulmonary hemorrhage in acute promyelocytic leukemia. Intern Med 31:457, 1992.
406. Takasugi JE, Godwin JD, Marglin SI, et al: Intrathoracic granulocytic sarcomas. J Thorac Imaging 11:223, 1996.
407. Hartweg H: Das Röntgenbild des Thorax be iden chronischen Leukosen. [The roentgenogram of the thorax in chronic leukoses.] Fortschr Roentgenstr 92:477, 1960.
408. Blank N, Castellino RA, Shah V: Radiographic aspects of pulmonary infection in patients with altered immunity. Radiol Clin North Am 11:175, 1973.
409. Maile CW, Moore AV, Ulreich S, et al: Chest radiographic-pathologic correlation in adult leukemia patients. Invest Radiol 18:495, 1983.
410. van Buchem MA, Wondergem JH, Schultze Kool LJ, et al: Pulmonary leukostasis: Radiologic-pathologic study. Radiology 165:39, 1987.
411. Seynaeve P, Mathijs R, Kockx M, et al: Case report: The air crescent sign in pulmonary leukaemic infiltrate. Clin Radiol 45:40, 1992.
412. Yamauchi K, Omata T: Leukemic pneumonitis as a poor prognostic factor in chronic myelomonocytic leukemia. Respiration 59:119, 1992.
413. Cordonnier C, Vernant JP, Brun B, et al: Acute promyelocytic leukemia in 57 previously untreated patients. Cancer 55:18, 1985.
414. Saka H, Ito T, Ito M, et al: Diffuse pulmonary alveolar hemorrhage in acute promyelocytic leukemia. Intern Med 31:457, 1992.
415. Cordonnier C, Fleury-Feith J, Escudier E, et al: Secondary alveolar proteinosis is a reversible cause of respiratory failure in leukemic patients. Am J Respir Crit Care Med 149:788, 1994.
416. Bardales RH, Powers CN, Frierson HF Jr, et al: Exfoliative respiratory cytology in the diagnosis of leukemias and lymphomas in the lung. Diagn Cytopathol 14:108, 1996.
417. Janckila AJ, Yam LT, Li CY: Immunocytochemical diagnosis of acute leukemia with pleural involvement. Acta Cytol 29:67, 1985.
418. Verani R, Olson J, Moake JL: Intrathoracic extramedullary hematopoiesis. Am J Clin Pathol 73:133, 1980.
419. Gumbs RV, Higginbotham-Ford EA, Teal JS, et al: Thoracic extramedullary hematopoiesis in sickle-cell disease. Am J Roentgenol 149:889, 1987.
420. Papavasiliou C, Gouliamos A, Andreou J: The marrow heterotopia in thalassemia. Eur J Radiol 6:92, 1986.
421. Yazdi HM: Cytopathology of extramedullary hematopoiesis in effusions and peritoneal washings. Diagn Cytopathol 2:326, 1986.
422. Glew RH, Haese WH, McIntyre PA: Myeloid metaplasia with myelofibrosis: The clinical spectrum of extramedullary hematopoiesis and tumor formation. Johns Hopkins Med J 132:253, 1973.
423. Gowitt GT, Zaatari GS: Bronchial extramedullary hematopoiesis preceding chronic myelogenous leukemia. Hum Pathol 16:1069, 1985.
424. Yusen RD, Kollef MH: Acute respiratory failure due to extramedullary hematopoiesis. Chest 108:1170, 1995.
425. Coates GG, Eisenberg B, Dail DH: Tc-99m sulfur colloid demonstration of diffuse pulmonary interstitial extramedullary hematopoiesis in a patient with myelofibrosis: A case report and review of the literature. Clin Nucl Med 19:1079, 1994.
426. Asakura S, Colby TV: Agnogenic myeloid metaplasia with extramedullary hematopoiesis and fibrosis in the lung: Report of two cases. Chest 105:1866, 1994.
427. Bourke SJ, Quinn AG, Farr PM, et al: Neutrophilic alveolitis in Sweet's syndrome. Thorax 47:572, 1992.
428. Fett DL, Gibson LE, Su WP: Sweet's syndrome: Systemic signs and symptoms and associated disorders. Mayo Clin Proc 70:234, 1995.
429. Yamamoto T, Furuse Y, Nishioka K: Sweet's syndrome with small cell carcinoma of the lung. J Dermatol 21:125, 1994.

430. Nielsen I, Donati D, Strumia R, et al: Sweet's syndrome and malignancy: Report of the first case associated with adenocarcinoma of the lung. Lung Cancer 10:95, 1993.

431. Lazarus AA, McMillan M, Miramadi A: Pulmonary involvement in Sweet's syndrome (acute febrile neutrophilic dermatosis). Chest 90:922, 1986.

432. Berkman N, Polliack A, Breuer R, et al: Pulmonary involvement as the major manifestation of chronic lymphocytic leukemia. Leuk Lymphoma 8:495, 1992.

433. Yoshioka R, Yamaguchi K, Yoshinaga T, et al: Pulmonary complications in patients with adult T-cell leukemia. Cancer 55:2491, 1985.

434. Tamura K, Yokota T, Mashita R, et al: Pulmonary manifestations in adult T-cell leukemia at the time of diagnosis. Respiration 60:115, 1993.

435. Vardiman JW, Variakojis D, Golomb HM: Hairy cell leukemia. Cancer 43:1339, 1979.

436. Chernoff A, Rymuza J, Lippman ML: Endobronchial lymphocytic infiltration. Am J Med 77:755, 1984.

437. Palosaari DE, Colby TV: Bronchiolocentric chronic lymphocytic leukemia. Cancer 58:1695, 1986.

438. Snyder L, Cherwitz D, Dykoski R, et al: Endobronchial Richter's syndrome: A rare manifestation of chronic lymphocytic leukemia. Am Rev Respir Dis 138:980, 1988.

439. Huhn D, Oertel J, Serke S, et al: Tumorous manifestation of hairy cell leukemia after long-term treatment with interferon alpha. Ann Hematol 70:103, 1995.

440. Okura T, Tanaka R, Shibata H, et al: Adult T-cell leukemia with a solitary lung mass. Chest 101:1471, 1992.

441. Klatte EC, Yardley J, Smith EB, et al: The pulmonary manifestations and complications of leukemia. Am J Roentgenol 89:598, 1963.

442. Jenkins PF, Ward MJ, Davies P, et al: Non-Hodgkin's lymphoma, chronic lymphatic leukaemia and the lung. Br J Dis Chest 75:22, 1981.

443. Mainzer F, Taybi H: Thymic enlargement and pleural effusion: An unusual roentgenographic complex in childhood leukemia. Am J Roentgenol 112:35, 1971.

444. Nathwani BN, Diamond LW, Winberg CD, et al: Lymphoblastic lymphoma: A clinicopathologic study of 95 patients. Cancer 48:2347, 1981.

445. George CD, Wilson AG, Philpott NJ: The radiologic features of adult T-cell leukaemia/lymphoma. Clin Radiol 49:83, 1994.

446. Rolla G, Bucca C, Chiampo F, et al: Respiratory symptoms, lung function tests, airway responsiveness, and bronchoalveolar lymphocyte subsets in B-chronic lymphocytic leukemia. Lung 171:265, 1993.

447. Rahal PS, Cornelius V: Oat cell carcinoma of the lung in patients with CLL. J Korean Med Assoc 92:183, 1994.

448. Travis LB, Curtis RE, Hankey BF, et al: Second cancers in patients with chronic lymphocytic leukemia. J Natl Cancer Inst 84:1422, 1992.

449. Bouza E, Burgaleta C, Golde DW: Infections in hairy-cell leukemia. Blood 51:851, 1978.

450. Swerdlow SH, Zellner DC, Hurtubise PE, et al: Pleural involvement in B-cell chronic lymphocytic leukemia associated with a T-cell-rich "reactive" pleural effusion. Am Rev Respir Dis 134:172, 1986.

CHAPTER 36

Mesenchymal Neoplasms

Neoplasms of the lung composed of mesenchymal tissue are uncommon, accounting for fewer than 1% of all tumors at this site. With the exception of Kaposi's sarcoma in patients who have acquired immunodeficiency syndrome (AIDS), primary sarcomas comprise only 0.01% to 0.2% of all lung tumors;[1] only 43 patients were seen at the Memorial Sloan-Kettering Cancer Center in New York over a 60-year period.[1] Precise histologic classification of a specific neoplasm can be difficult, and as subsequently discussed, the incidence of particular tumors as reported in the literature may not be accurate. The use of electron microscopic, immu-

nohistochemical, genetic, and molecular studies may ameliorate this situation.[2]

When considering a diagnosis of primary pulmonary sarcoma, it must be remembered that pulmonary carcinoma can sometimes have a sarcomatous appearance (sarcomatoid carcinoma, *see* page 1114), and thorough sampling of a tumor is necessary before a diagnosis of a soft tissue neoplasm can be considered definite. As a corollary, definitive diagnosis of a sarcoma on a bronchial biopsy or needle aspirate specimen is usually not possible. Some epithelial tumors (notably renal cell carcinoma and melanoma) can have a sarcomatous appearance; metastases from such tumors as well as from extrapulmonary sarcomas are undoubtedly more common than primary pulmonary sarcoma, and they must be considered before the diagnosis is accepted. In such cases, a history of a primary extrapulmonary tumor is usually clearly evident; however, a pulmonary metastasis is occasionally the initial manifestation of disease or occurs many years after an extrapulmonary tumor was excised. Simultaneous occurrence of sarcoma and pulmonary carcinoma has been reported rarely.[3]

NEOPLASMS OF MUSCLE

Leiomyoma and Leiomyosarcoma

Judging by the number of reported cases in the literature, neoplasms of smooth muscle are among the most common primary soft tissue tumors of the lung.[4–7] Because smooth muscle is normally found in conducting and transitional airways and in pulmonary vessels larger than arterioles or venules, tumors derived from this tissue can occur in virtually any site and can be conveniently discussed under the headings *parenchymal*, *endobronchial*, and *vascular*. A number of reviews of pulmonary smooth muscle tumors have been published, including those affecting the lower respiratory tract in general[8, 9] as well as those dealing specifically with leiomyoma,[7, 10] parenchymal and endobronchial forms of leiomyosarcoma,[11] and vascular leiomyosarcoma.[12, 13]

Parenchymal Leiomyoma and Leiomyosarcoma

The most common location of pulmonary leiomyosarcoma is in the parenchyma itself.[14] In a 1972 review of the Armed Forces Institute of Pathology (AFIP) files from the years 1945 to 1969, 18 examples were identified;[11] an additional 39 cases were found in the literature. Most tumors occurred in men (about 60% of the non-AFIP cases) more than 50 years of age (65%). Pulmonary leiomyomas appear to be equally distributed between parenchymal and endobronchial locations; most occur in middle-aged adults, with a female-to-male ratio of about 1.5:1.[7, 9]

Grossly, parenchymal smooth muscle tumors are lobulated, often well-circumscribed, white to tan nodules or masses, measuring from 1 to as large as 24 cm in greatest diameter. They are usually located in the periphery of the lung.[4, 11] Necrosis and hemorrhage are frequent in malignant tumors.[15] Microscopically the majority of tumors consist of interlacing fascicles of spindle cells with oval, vesicular nuclei that show varying degrees of atypia.[14] Myxoid degeneration, hyalinization, and an epithelioid cell appearance are seen in some cases.[14] As with metastatic leiomyosarcoma, entrapment of alveolar epithelium at the periphery of the neoplasm can result in a pseudoglandular appearance (*see* page 1409). Electron microscopic and immunohistochemical examinations show characteristic features of smooth muscle differentiation, enabling precise classification.[4, 15, 16]

Radiologically, these tumors are usually sharply defined, smooth or lobulated in contour, and homogeneous in density; cavitation or calcification is seen occasionally.[11, 17] CT performed in seven sarcomas demonstrated cavitation not apparent on radiography in one patient, but yielded no additional information in the remaining six cases.[18] More than 90% of pulmonary parenchymal leiomyomas are incidental findings on chest radiographs.[9] Leiomyosarcoma is more likely to be associated with symptoms (e.g., in 9 of 24 cases in one review), including cough, chest pain, and hemoptysis.[19]

As in smooth muscle tumors in other locations, the precise histologic distinction between benignancy and malignancy may be difficult in some cases. In the AFIP study cited previously, the biologic behavior of tumors depended mostly on the number of mitoses:[11] lesions with 12 or more mitotic figures per 10 high-power fields tended to metastasize, whereas those with 8 or fewer either remained stationary or grew slowly. In a more recent investigation from the same institution, it was proposed that a mitotic rate of five per 50 high-power fields indicates malignancy.[15] The necessity for thorough histologic sampling of a tumor so as not to miss focal areas of increased mitotic activity has been emphasized.[15]

In the 1972 AFIP review, size itself did not seem to predict the likelihood of metastasis: six of nine cases ranging in diameter from 3 to 10 cm and three of five cases greater than 10 cm in diameter had metastatic disease at autopsy;[11] as might be expected, the larger tumors frequently extended locally into the chest wall, mediastinum, or diaphragm and were inoperable. Despite the similar incidence of metastases, the 5-year survival was distinctly worse in patients with the larger neoplasms. There is some evidence that tumors occurring in childhood have a somewhat better prognosis.[11]

The possibility that a smooth muscle neoplasm in pulmonary parenchyma represents a metastasis should always be considered,[15, 20] even in the presence of a bland histologic appearance. This is especially important in patients with multiple tumors and in women with uterine leiomyomas or a history of hysterectomy (*see* page 1409).[21]

Endobronchial and Endotracheal Leiomyoma and Leiomyosarcoma

Endobronchial and endotracheal leiomyosarcomas are encountered uncommonly;[11, 22–24] only eight cases were identified in the 1972 AFIP review of smooth muscle tumors,[11] and only seven cases of tracheal leiomyosarcoma had been reported by 1984.[8] Endobronchial leiomyomas are somewhat more common; approximately 30 were reviewed in one series in 1983,[7] and 85 cases had been reported by 1995.[25]

Pathologically, bronchial tumors are typically located in the main or lobar airways. They are fleshy, are often pedunculated, and more or less completely fill the airway lumen; extension into the underlying tracheobronchial wall is unusual, even in the histologically malignant forms.[11, 26]

Radiographic findings consist of atelectasis and obstructive pneumonitis. Nonobstructive tumors present as sessile or pedunculated soft tissue nodules within the trachea or bronchi. In a review of the literature concerning leiomyomas, the mean age at the time of diagnosis was 39 years.[25] As might be expected, the majority of patients have cough, hemoptysis, or dyspnea. Provided that the tumors can be adequately excised, the prognosis is good even in histologically malignant forms; both local recurrence and metastases are exceptional.[11]

Vascular Leiomyoma and Leiomyosarcoma

Although rare cases of apparent leiomyoma have been reported to arise in the pulmonary vessels,[27] the vast majority of smooth muscle tumors at this site are clearly malignant. Virtually all such tumors originate in the pulmonary valve or large pulmonary arteries; only one example has been reported in an apparent arteriovenous fistula,[28] and we are aware of none arising in the normal distal pulmonary vasculature. Rare tumors have been shown to have an origin in a pulmonary vein.[29, 30, 35] The neoplasms are rare, only about 140 cases having been reported by 1997.[31, 32] Men and women are affected in approximately equal numbers. The average age at the time of diagnosis is about 50 years (range in reported cases, 13 to 81 years).[32]

Because of their similar clinical and radiologic appearance and prognosis, discussions of sarcomas arising in the pulmonary artery have usually included tumors that have a variety of pathologic subtypes:[13] in addition to leiomyosarcoma,[13] histologic diagnoses have included chondrosarcoma,[33] osteosarcoma,[34] fibrosarcoma, malignant fibrous histiocytoma,[36] rhabdomyosarcoma,[37] malignant mesenchymoma, angiosarcoma,[38] liposarcoma, malignant schwannoma, and spindle-cell or anaplastic sarcoma.[31, 39] In most of these cases, particularly those reported before 1980, electron microscopic or immunohistochemical studies were not performed to define the cellular differentiation more precisely, so the histologic classification of individual cases is often in some doubt. Because the majority of tumors that can be adequately typed appear to show smooth muscle differentiation[31, 40, 41] and because the radiologic and clinical features of all forms are more or less similar, we include all histologic varieties in the following discussion.

As indicated, the tumors generally arise from the pulmonary valve, pulmonary trunk, or right or left pulmonary artery. In a review of 138 cases reported by 1997, involvement occurred as follows: the pulmonary trunk in 85%, the

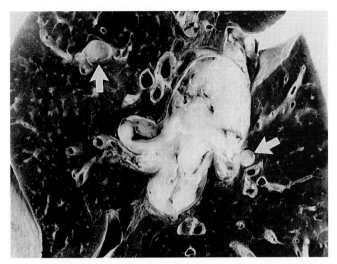

Figure 36–1. Pulmonary Artery Sarcoma. A midsagittal slice of the right lung shows a fleshy mass distending the interlobar artery and extending into several segmental arteries *(arrows)*. The tumor is confined entirely to the arterial lumen. Histologic examination showed undifferentiated (fibrosarcoma-like) sarcoma.

right pulmonary artery in 71%, the left pulmonary artery in 65%, the pulmonary valve in 32%, and the right ventricular outflow tract in 10%.[32] Tumors tend to spread within the vascular lumen and in many cases remain confined to this site (Fig. 36–1).[12, 13] The vessel may be totally occluded by either tumor itself or tumor and overlying thrombus. In other cases, the sarcoma extends across the vessel wall into adjacent bronchial wall, lymph nodes, or lung parenchyma (Fig. 36–2). Microscopic or macroscopic metastases to the lungs are common. Pulmonary infarcts are also frequent,[12] varying from small foci in the lung periphery to involvement of an entire lobe; they are caused by either tumor emboli themselves or thromboemboli induced by the neoplasm. Marked dilation and hypertrophy of the right heart chambers are frequent findings at autopsy, reflecting pulmonary arterial hypertension secondary to vascular occlusion.

The most common radiographic findings are hilar pulmonary artery enlargement (Fig. 36–3), solitary or multiple lung nodules, and enlargement of the cardiopericardial contour.[32] Less common manifestations include focal areas of consolidation and areas of oligemia.[32, 42] In the absence of a mass, both the clinical and the radiographic presentation may be that of acute pulmonary embolism, with or without infarction.[43] Dilation of central pulmonary arteries in this situation may be caused by either neoplastic distention of the vessels or pulmonary arterial hypertension secondary to distal vessel occlusion; in the latter circumstance, the peripheral lung is oligemic.

The most common abnormality on CT consists of an intraluminal soft tissue mass, sometimes associated with expansion of the artery.[34, 44, 44a] Although the mass may be indistinguishable from a thromboembolus, findings that should suggest the diagnosis of sarcoma include extension of the mass into the mediastinum or lung, peripheral pulmonary nodules, or branching soft tissue densities (corresponding to intraluminal tumor growth).[45–47] The magnetic resonance (MR) imaging findings are similar to those of CT (*see* Fig. 36–3). The signal characteristics do not allow distinction

between a sarcoma and a thromboembolus on unenhanced conventional spin-echo images;[47, 48] however, enhancement of sarcoma can be demonstrated after intravenous administration of gadolinium-diethylenetriaminepenta-acetic acid (Gd-DTPA), permitting distinction from thrombus.[49, 49a,b]

Ventilation-perfusion scans usually demonstrate multiple mismatching perfusion defects identical to those seen in pulmonary thromboembolism[42] or absent perfusion of an entire lung.[49b] The most common findings at pulmonary angiography consist of one or more intraluminal filling defects in the proximal pulmonary arteries, again similar to those seen with thromboembolism.[32, 42] Less commonly, angiography shows more specific findings, such as a lobulated intraluminal filling defect, a pedicle, or motion of the tumor during a cine procedure.[42, 50]

Clinical manifestations can be separated into those that occur early and those that occur late in the course of disease.[12] The former include chest pain and dyspnea as prominent features; cough, hemoptysis, fever, and palpitations also occur in about 30% to 50% of patients.[12, 51] Late manifestations are chiefly those of cardiac decompensation and include peripheral edema, hepatomegaly, and cyanosis. A heart murmur can be identified in about 50% of cases,[51] and weight loss, syncope, and unilaterally decreased breath sounds are noted in about a quarter.[52] For obvious reasons, a clinical picture resembling acute or chronic thromboembolism is not uncommon.[53, 54] Unusual presentations or complications include cardiac tamponade secondary to hemopericardium,[51] bleeding diathesis,[55] polycythemia and thrombocytopenia,[56] pericardial effusion,[57] and a pheochromocytoma-like picture.[58]

As might be expected, the prognosis is generally poor, the median survival in patients without surgery having been said to be only 1.5 months.[53] Although there is evidence that surgical removal of involved vasculature can prolong life,[41, 53] long-term survivors are uncommon even with apparent "curative" excision and adjuvant radiotherapy and chemotherapy. Patients who have tumors that are smaller and have a lower histologic grade appear to have a better outcome.[41] It has also been suggested that tumors with cartilaginous or osseous differentiation may have a better prognosis.[40] Death is usually related to pulmonary complications; systemic metastases occur uncommonly.[52, 59]

Diagnosis of Pulmonary Smooth Muscle Neoplasms

Preoperative or premortem diagnosis of a smooth muscle tumor of the lung is made infrequently. In contrast to pulmonary carcinoma, diagnostic procedures such as cytologic examination of sputum or bronchial washings or brushings are usually unrewarding, although the diagnosis has occasionally been made by these techniques.[60] Transthoracic needle aspiration of a parenchymal mass is more likely to provide a diagnosis,[61] although interpretation of cells obtained from benign or low-grade malignant neoplasms may be difficult. The diagnosis of an endotracheal or endobronchial smooth muscle neoplasm should be considered when any predominantly intraluminal tumor possesses a smooth, apparently nonneoplastic epithelial surface; bronchoscopic biopsy often suggests the diagnosis in these cases. It should be remembered, however, that the presence of a sarcoma-like histologic pattern on an endobronchial biopsy specimen

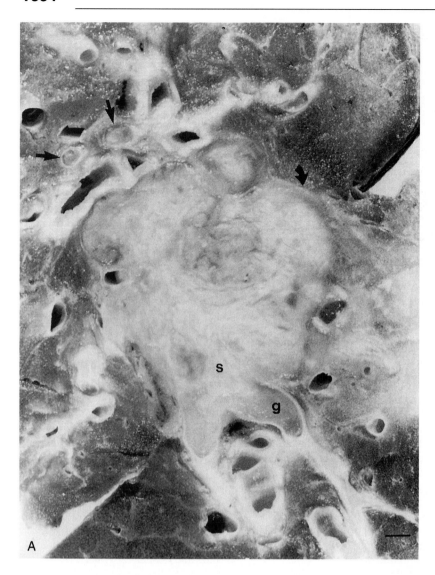

Figure 36–2. Pulmonary Artery Leiomyosarcoma. A magnified view *(A)* of resected right lung reveals occlusion of segmental and subsegmental branches of the pulmonary artery by gelatinous (g) and more solid white tissue (s), consisting of thrombus and sarcoma. Superiorly the tumor has spread outside the vessel wall, forming a solid mass and invading parenchyma *(curved arrow)* and several bronchi (not illustrated on this slice). A few smaller vessels separate from the mass itself also contain tumor *(straight arrows)* (bar = 5 mm).

is more likely to represent sarcomatous change in a bronchial carcinoma (sarcomatoid carcinoma; *see* page 1114) than a primary sarcoma, particularly in cigarette smokers.

The diagnosis of pulmonary arterial sarcoma should be considered if there is a perihilar mass associated with evidence of pulmonary arterial hypertension; in this situation, bronchoscopy is often uninformative, revealing only displacement of segmental bronchi. Contrast-enhanced CT and gadolinium-enhanced MR imaging are the investigative procedures of choice. The diagnosis can be confirmed by biopsy or aspiration of cells during pulmonary angiography.[49b]

Rhabdomyosarcoma

Neoplasms of striated muscle are among the rarest of all pulmonary tumors, only 14 cases having been documented in the literature by 1980.[62] The presence of rhabdomyosarcoma in an organ in which skeletal muscle is not normally found is not well understood. One theory proposes that the neoplasm is derived from primitive mesenchyme that has the capacity for rhabdomyoblastic differentiation.[63] An alternative explanation is that the tumors arise from displaced skeletal muscle derived from the pharynx during embryonic development.[63] Support for the latter hypothesis has been provided by the identification of mature striated muscle cells in some developmental pulmonary anomalies.[64] It is also possible that some tumors are the result of rhabdomyoblastic differentiation in a sarcomatoid carcinoma or a malignant teratoma.[73]

Pathologically, these tumors are usually bulky, relatively well-defined but infiltrating solid or cystic masses in which a precise site of origin cannot be identified.[62, 65–67] Occasional tumors appear to arise in the pulmonary artery and have predominantly intravascular spread[37] or are attached by a pedicle to the airway wall and have an entirely endobronchial or endotracheal growth.[63, 68, 69] Possible origin in the pleura and mediastinum has also been documented.[70] The usual histologic classification is pleomorphic rhabdomyosarcoma; however, occasional examples of alveolar[70] and embryonal[71] subtypes have also been described.

There appear to be two peaks of incidence—one in childhood[70] and the other between 50 and 70 years of age;[68] the majority of patients are male.[68, 70] Clinical and radiologic features are nonspecific; the rare pedunculated endobronchial tumors can cause cough and dyspnea and radiographic evidence of atelectasis or obstructive pneumonitis.[63, 69] Spontaneous pneumothorax has been reported.[66] In one patient, a

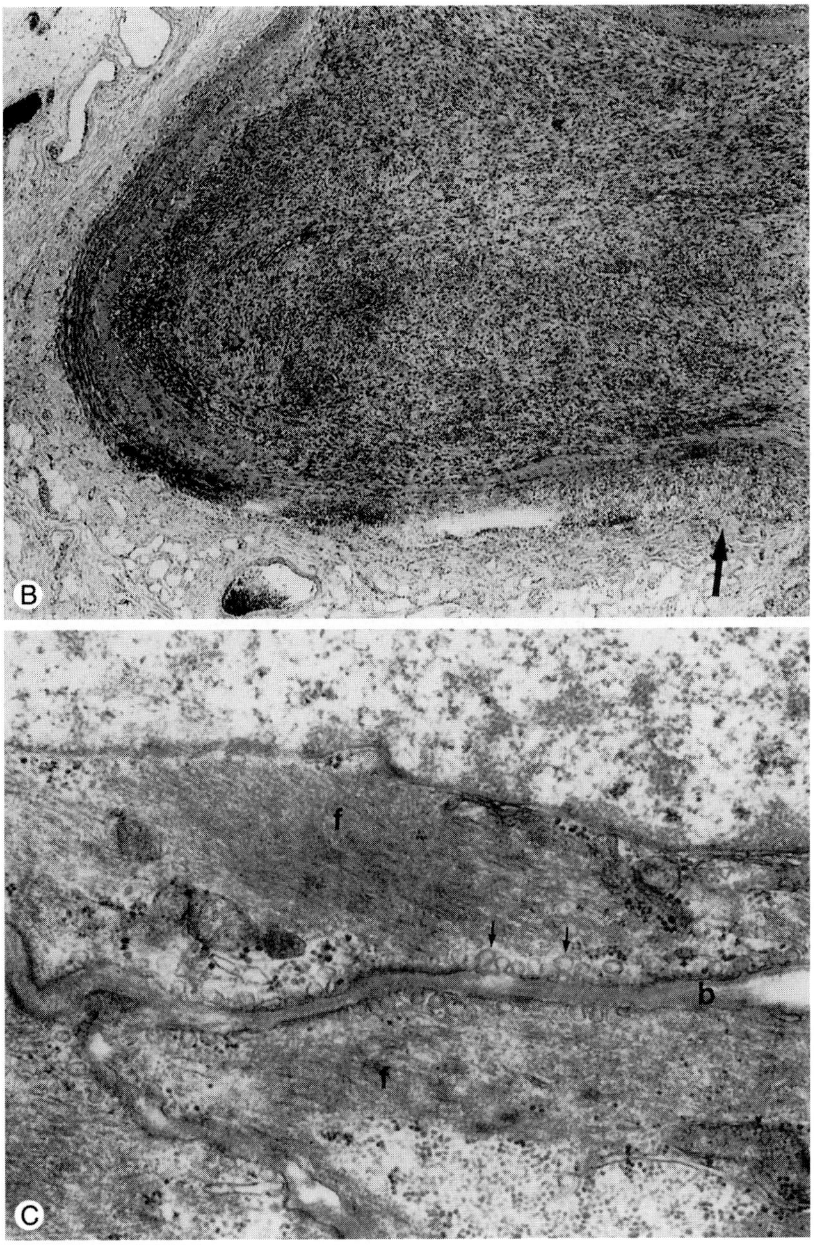

Figure 36–2 *Continued.* A branch of a segmental pulmonary artery *(B)* is completely filled by spindle cell sarcoma. Although most of the tumor is confined to the vessel lumen, extramural extension is present focally *(arrow)*. Ultrastructurally *(C)*, there is evidence of an intercellular basal lamina (b), pinocytotic vesicles *(arrows)*, and numerous cytoplasmic filaments (f), confirming the smooth muscle nature of the tumor. This 46-year-old man presented with hemoptysis. *(B, ×25; C, ×43,000.)*

mobile mass occluded both main bronchi at the carina, resulting in death.[72]

The tumors are often limited to the thorax, either entirely within the pulmonary parenchyma, airway lumen, or vasculature or accompanied by local extension into the mediastinum, diaphragm, or chest wall; however, systemic metastases do occur, not uncommonly in unusual sites, such as the heart and small intestine.[62, 67, 74] Because of the limited number of cases that have been described, it is difficult to make definitive statements regarding prognosis; however, the tumor appears to behave in an aggressive fashion in most patients.[67]

NEOPLASMS OF VASCULAR TISSUE

Glomus Tumor

Glomus tumor (glomangioma) is an uncommon neoplasm usually found in the nail bed of the fingers or toes

and believed to be derived from specialized smooth muscle cells of the glomus body. The latter consists of an arteriovenous anastomosis composed, in part, by a thick-walled channel whose wall contains several layers of large epithelioid cells termed *glomus cells*. The structure and location of the glomus body indicate a role in temperature regulation, a function that is thought to be modulated by the contractile glomus cells. Histologically, neoplasms derived from these cells consist of numerous, somewhat irregular vascular lumens surrounded by clusters or sheets of large polygonal cells with pale eosinophilic or clear cytoplasm; mitotic figures and nuclear atypia are absent. Ultrastructural, immunohistochemical, and tissue culture studies show features of smooth muscle differentiation.[75, 75a]

Although the skin is the most common site of origin, neoplasms with an identical histologic and ultrastructural appearance have been described in a variety of internal organs, including the lungs and trachea.[75–79] The presence of arteriovenous anastomoses in the normal lung (*see* page

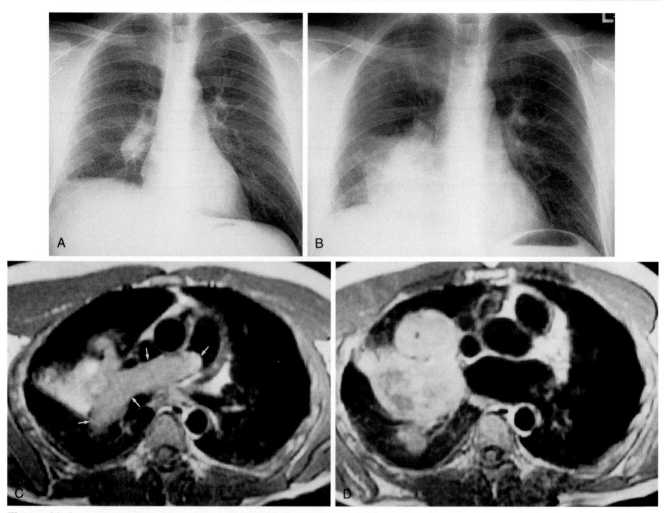

Figure 36–3. Primary Leiomyosarcoma of the Pulmonary Artery. A posteroanterior (PA) chest radiograph *(A)* in a 38-year-old man who presented with shortness of breath demonstrates a prominent right hilum and elevation of the right hemidiaphragm. A ventilation-perfusion scan performed at this time demonstrated no perfusion of the right lung. The findings were interpreted as being due to a large thromboembolus. A PA radiograph 1 year later *(B)* demonstrates increased size of the right hilum and a large mass in the middle lobe. MR imaging *(C)* demonstrates tumor within the right main and interlobar pulmonary arteries *(arrows)* with growth into the adjacent lung parenchyma. MR imaging at the level of the left atrium *(D)* demonstrates extensive tumor growth in the right middle and lower lobes. The MR images were obtained using spin-echo technique, cardiac gating, 5-mm sections, TR 2250, TE 20. The patient underwent right pneumonectomy and complete resection of the tumor within the pulmonary artery.

77) and the documentation in one report of a structure in the tracheal wall similar to a normal glomus body[80] lend some support to the occurrence of neoplasms in these locations.

The majority of tumors occur as polypoid intraluminal masses, particularly in the trachea (most often in the membranous portion[75]) and less commonly in the proximal bronchi. In these locations, they are often associated with hemoptysis or signs and symptoms of partial or complete airway obstruction, including "asthma" and "chronic bronchitis."[75, 80, 81] Rare tumors present as a parenchymal nodule or mass in a patient without respiratory complaints.[75a, 78]

Extrapulmonary glomus tumors are almost always benign, and there is little evidence that the behavior of pulmonary tumors differs. One exceptional case has been reported of a solitary parenchymal nodule in a 19-year-old that was interpreted as a glomus tumor;[82] subcutaneous and lymph node tumors subsequently developed, but it was thought possible that one of the subcutaneous lesions represented the primary tumor site. The neoplasm can be confused histologi-

cally with hemangiopericytoma and carcinoid tumor,[76] and definitive diagnosis should be confirmed by ultrastructural or immunohistochemical examination.

Hemangiopericytoma

Hemangiopericytoma is a mesenchymal tumor that occurs most commonly in the soft tissues of the upper and lower extremities, pelvis, and retroperitoneal space and seldom in visceral organs. One group of investigators documented 247 cases, of which 28 were considered to be primary in the lungs;[83] occasional tumors have been reported to arise in the trachea.[84] Not all reported cases have been convincingly proven pathologically, and electron microscopic and immunohistochemical investigations generally have not been performed. Thus, although acceptable examples of pulmonary tumors consistent with hemangiopericytoma undoubtedly exist[85–88] and approximately 100 examples had been reported by 1993,[88a] the true incidence of these neoplasms is difficult to determine. Most reported cases have occurred in patients between 40 and 60 years of age, about equally in men and women;[87] however, some investigators have found a female predominance (about 2:1) and a higher incidence in younger individuals.[88b]

As the name indicates, hemangiopericytomas are believed to be derived from the vascular pericyte. When primary in the lung, they occur most often within parenchyma and pathologically appear as solitary, usually well-defined nodules or masses unrelated to major airways or vessels.[87] A large size—sometimes as large as an entire hemithorax[89]—is not uncommon.[83] Microscopically the tumors consist of numerous vascular spaces of variable size and shape separated by aggregates of tightly packed oval to spindle-shaped cells with bland nuclei. Mitotic figures and nuclear atypia are variable in number and degree.

The radiographic appearance is that of a nodule or mass that may be round or lobulated (Fig. 36–4).[88a, 90] Calcification is infrequent.[87] Rarely, the tumor occupies most of the hemithorax and is associated with pleural effusion.[88a] In one CT study of four patients, the tumors were found to have an inhomogeneous appearance with central areas of low attenuation and peripheral rim enhancement after intravenous administration of contrast material;[88a] eccentric areas of speckled calcification were present in one case. MR imaging performed in two cases demonstrated heterogeneous signal intensity.

Approximately 50% of patients are asymptomatic when the tumor is discovered. When present, symptoms include cough and hemoptysis;[91] chest pain can result if the tumor extends to a pleural surface. One unusual example, considered to be primary in the lung, presented with hundreds of metastatic nodules in virtually every organ and tissue, including the lungs.[92]

Although some hemangiopericytomas behave in a benign fashion, many are locally invasive at the time of diagnosis or recur after surgical excision; some metastasize and cause death.[89, 93] In one review, one of these outcomes was present in 11 of 18 cases.[87] The malignant forms have been reported to be characterized by a larger size, increased cellularity and mitotic rate, and necrosis.[87, 94]

Kaposi's Sarcoma

Kaposi's sarcoma is a neoplasm with variable clinicopathologic features that is believed to be derived from primitive vasoformative mesenchyme or from endothelial or pericytic cells of small vessels. The tumors occur in two clinical settings: (1) in children and young adults, especially Africans and individuals who have AIDS, in which lymph node and visceral involvement (including the lung) is common, and an aggressive course is the rule (*see* page 1676); and (2) in non-African individuals of advanced age, in which the lesions usually are multiple and are confined to the skin of the lower extremities, and the course is relatively indolent. Rarely, the tumor develops in young individuals who have an underlying immunocompromising condition other than AIDS (particularly renal transplantation)[95] or who are apparently immunocompetent.[96] There is strong evidence for an etiologic association with herpesvirus 8 (*see* page 1677).[97]

Involvement of thoracic structures is not uncommon in disseminated Kaposi's sarcoma, whether or not it is associated with AIDS; for example, this was observed in 6 of 14 autopsy cases in a 1959 review.[98] The incidence of pulmonary involvement in patients with AIDS who have Kaposi's sarcoma has been estimated to be about 25% to 35%.[99] Although most often associated with a concomitant mucosal

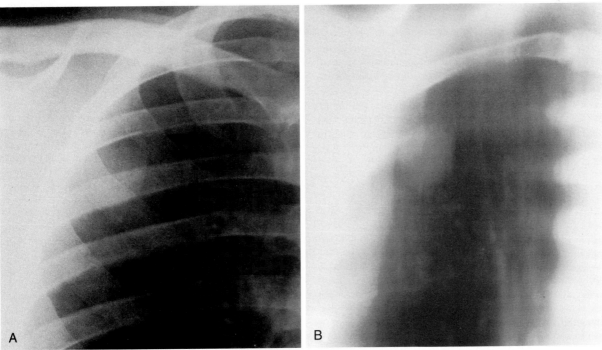

Figure 36–4. Pulmonary Hemangiopericytoma. Detail views of the upper half of the right lung from a posteroanterior chest radiograph *(A)* and an anteroposterior tomogram *(B)* reveal a 3-cm nodular lesion that relates to the visceral pleura. The lesion is well defined and of homogeneous soft tissue density. The patient was a 28-year-old physician.

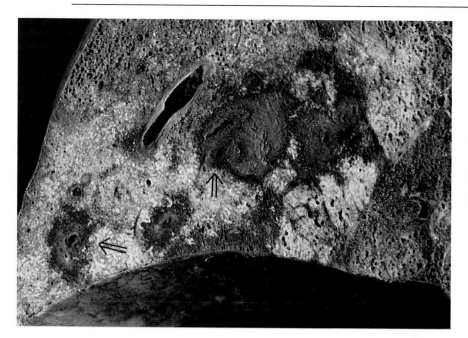

Figure 36–5. Kaposi's Sarcoma—Gross Appearance. A magnified view of the basal aspect of a slice of lower lobe shows a patchy hemorrhagic tumor, in some areas intimately associated with a vessel *(arrows)*. This distribution is similar to that of lymphangitic carcinomatosis.

or skin tumor, the disease occasionally presents in the lung or pleura.[100, 101]

Pulmonary disease in Kaposi's sarcoma is typically most prominent in the pleural or bronchovascular interstitium.[102] This may result in a gross appearance similar to lymphangitic carcinomatosis except that regions involved by Kaposi's sarcoma have a red rather than a white appearance and are usually larger (Fig. 36–5). Involvement of the parenchymal interstitium occurs occasionally.[101] When present in airway mucosa, the lesions commonly appear as purplish, plaquelike elevations;[103, 104] uncommonly, there is significant airway stenosis.[105] Expansion of tumor outside the bronchovascular interstitium may result in nodules or, occasionally, ill-defined areas of parenchymal "consolidation." Histologically, the tumors are composed of clusters of cytologically atypical spindle cells between which are numerous, small, slitlike vascular spaces containing hemosiderin-laden macrophages and red blood cells.

The most common radiographic findings of pulmonary Kaposi's sarcoma consist of thickened bronchoarterial bundles and bilateral, poorly marginated small nodular opacities or a diffuse reticular or reticulonodular pattern.[106–108] Less common manifestations include focal, unilateral or bilateral areas of consolidation.[107] The latter areas may represent pulmonary hemorrhage and may develop suddenly in an area of previous normal lung or around a tumor nodule.[107] Hilar lymph node enlargement is identified radiographically in 10% to 20% of patients and pleural effusion in approximately 35%.[106, 108] The radiographic findings of thoracic Kaposi's sarcoma in patients without AIDS are similar to those in patients with this disease (Fig. 36–6).[109]

The characteristic CT manifestations of Kaposi's sarcoma consist of bronchial wall thickening and multiple bilateral irregular lesions or nodules with poorly defined margins in a predominantly peribronchovascular distribution.[108a, 110, 111] Other parenchymal abnormalities include interlobular septal thickening, mass lesions, and focal areas of consolidation.[110–112]

Pleural effusions and hilar or mediastinal lymph node enlargement have each been reported in 10% to 50% of cases.[110–112] The CT findings are similar in patients who have and who do not have AIDS (Fig. 36–7).

Pulmonary involvement usually is associated with few symptoms or signs; however, hoarseness, cough, dyspnea,

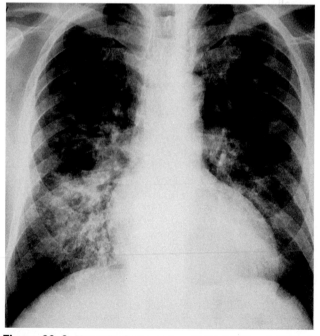

Figure 36–6. Kaposi's Sarcoma in a Patient Without AIDS. An anteroposterior chest radiograph in a 64-year-old man demonstrates poorly defined small nodular opacities in both lungs, focal areas of consolidation, and septal lines (particularly in the right lung base). The patient had emigrated to Canada from Tanzania 10 years previously and presented with a history of progressive shortness of breath and malaise. The diagnosis was proven by open-lung biopsy.

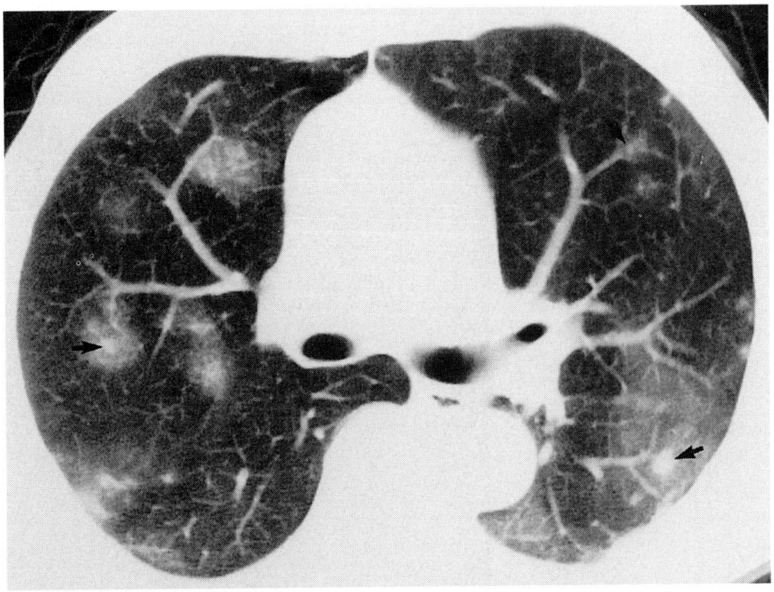

Figure 36–7. Kaposi's Sarcoma Not Related to AIDS. A CT scan in an 83-year-old patient demonstrates bilateral poorly defined nodules *(arrows)* closely related to vessels. Focal areas of ground-glass attenuation surround the nodules. On open-lung biopsy, the abnormalities were shown to be due to Kaposi's sarcoma with surrounding areas of hemorrhage. The patient was human immunodeficiency virus negative.

stridor, hemoptysis, and (rarely) fatal pulmonary hemorrhage may occur.[104, 113] On bronchoscopy, cherry-red or purple, slightly raised areas can be seen; although some investigators find biopsy of such lesions rarely to be of diagnostic value,[113, 114] others have found it to be useful.[99, 103] Preliminary results suggest that analysis of bronchoalveolar lavage (BAL) fluid for the presence of herpesvirus 8 antigen also may be useful in diagnosis.[141]

Epithelioid Hemangioendothelioma

Epithelioid hemangioendothelioma is an uncommon, typically multifocal pulmonary neoplasm first recognized in 1975.[115, 116] Although the tumor was initially believed to be of epithelial origin and to represent an unusual form of bronchioloalveolar neoplasm characterized by extensive intravascular spread (hence the rather cumbersome designation *intravascular bronchioloalveolar tumor [IVBAT]*),[117] subsequent electron microscopic[116–119] and immunohistochemical[117, 120, 121] studies have indicated endothelial differentiation. A variety of names have been proposed to reflect this evidence, including *sclerosing interstitial vascular sarcoma*,[122] *sclerosing endothelial tumor*,[117] *sclerosing epithelioid angiosarcoma*,[123] and *epithelioid hemangioendothelioma*;[124, 125] the last of these is currently believed by most authorities to be the most appropriate.

The explanation for the multifocality of the neoplasm is unclear. The typical absence of both a dominant pulmonary tumor and an extrapulmonary primary, both at presentation and over time, and the similarity in size of the pulmonary nodules suggest that the tumor originates in a multifocal fashion within the lung.[125] Support for this hypothesis was given by one group of investigators who found that the basement membrane material in hepatic and pulmonary nodules of one patient was similar to that found in normal liver and lung, respectively.[126] Some authors, however, have reported evidence for a primary extrapulmonary origin,[127, 128] suggesting that the lung nodules may represent metastases in at least some cases.

The usual pathologic manifestations consist of multiple well-demarcated parenchymal nodules ranging in diameter from 0.3 to 3.0 cm.[117, 123, 125] Cut sections may have a firm, almost cartilaginous, consistency. Light microscopic appearances are characteristic. Under low magnification, a hypocellular sclerotic central portion is surrounded by a somewhat nodular, more cellular periphery (Fig. 36–8). At higher magnification, the latter area can be seen to consist of loose aggregates of plump, oval to spindle-shaped cells. Small intracellular lumens believed to represent vascular differentiation may be seen within the tumor cells (Fig. 36–9). Peribronchial lymphatic and blood vessel invasion is common. Dystrophic calcification and ossification may occur in the acellular region, although it is only occasionally recognizable radiographically.[129] The tumor cells typically show a positive immunohistochemical reaction for factor VIII and vimentin and a negative reaction for cytokeratin.

Radiographic manifestations simulate metastases or infarcts (Fig. 36–10) and consist of multiple well-defined or ill-defined nodules measuring up to 2 cm in diameter.[117] Although these sometimes show little or no growth on serial radiographs,[130] they can also enlarge slowly and eventually cause respiratory insufficiency.[131] There is usually no evidence of hilar or mediastinal lymph node enlargement. Pleural effusion is uncommon.[117, 132] The CT findings in two patients with long-standing tumors consisted of nodules with a perivascular distribution and foci of calcification.[133] In one patient that we have observed, the nodules were situated close to a pleural surface and were surrounded by hemorrhage and edema that were apparent only on CT; although the nodular opacities partially resolved with antineoplastic chemotherapy, many eventually recurred.

Approximately 80% of cases occur in women,[117] many younger than 40 years of age, an association that has been speculated to be related to a hormonal effect.[134, 135] Most patients are initially asymptomatic, the lesions being discovered as an incidental finding on a screening radiograph. Occasionally, there is a history of cough, chest pain, increasing dyspnea, malaise, and weight loss.[116] One patient has been reported who presented with a clinical picture of throm-

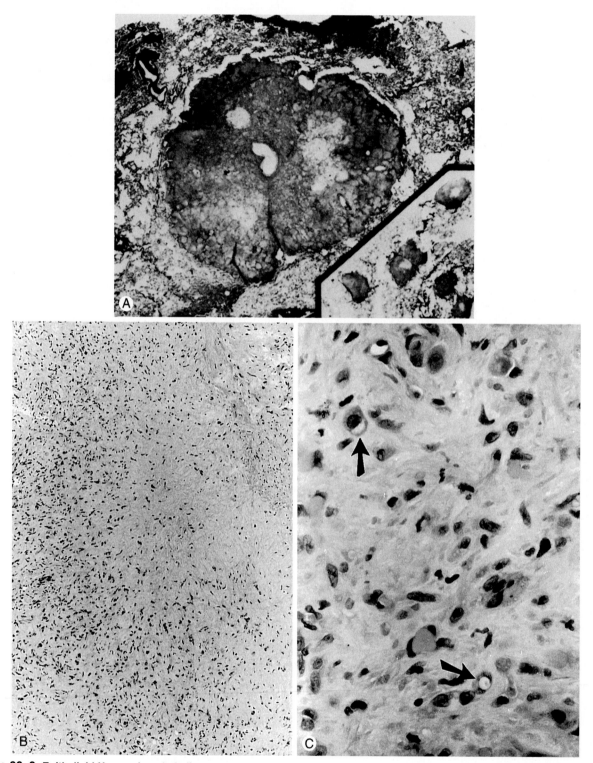

Figure 36–8. Epithelioid Hemangioendothelioma. A low-power view *(A)* of a sharply circumscribed nodule shows several pale foci of sclerosis in its central region; *inset* reveals multiplicity of nodules. A magnified view *(B)* shows an area of sclerosis (S) blending imperceptibly with the more cellular portion of the tumor. Tumor cells themselves (C) are present singly or in small clusters and are quite variable in shape; some *(arrows)* have small intracytoplasmic lumens. (*A* from Bhagaran BJ, et al: Am J Surg Pathol 6:41, 1982.)

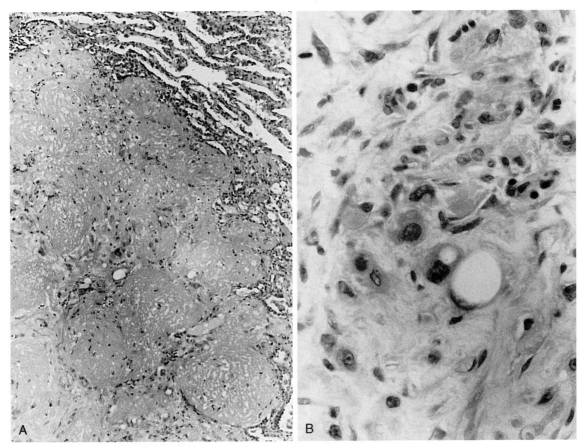

Figure 36–9. Epithelioid Hemangioendothelioma. Sections are from a young woman who had patchy lower lobe opacities on radiographs initially interpreted as pneumonia. The alveolar air spaces *(A)* are obliterated by a somewhat lobulated hypercellular mass that appears to be composed predominantly of fibrous tissue. Higher magnification of another, more cellular focus of disease *(B)* shows scattered inflammatory cells and fibroblasts as well as several neoplastic cells with larger, irregular nuclei. Two of these cells contain intracytoplasmic vacuoles, thought to represent endothelial differentiation. (Courtesy of Dr. Yves Gagnon, Complexe Hospitalier de la Sagamie, Chicoutimi, Québec.)

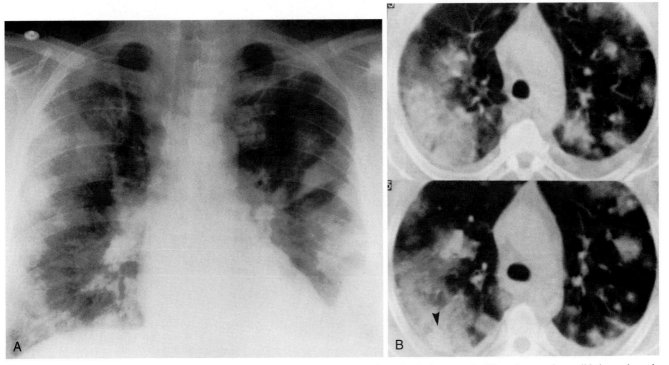

Figure 36–10. Epithelioid Hemangioendothelioma. A posteroanterior chest radiograph *(A)* shows patchy bilateral areas of consolidation and poorly defined nodular opacities. The hila are slightly enlarged, consistent with lymphadenopathy. Small bilateral pleural effusions are present. CT scans *(B)* demonstrate confluent consolidation in the right upper lobe, focal areas of consolidation in the left upper lobe, and isolated nodular opacities *(arrowhead)*. Small pleural effusions are present bilaterally. An open-lung biopsy disclosed epithelioid hemangioendothelioma. The patient died of massive pleural hemorrhage 3 weeks later.

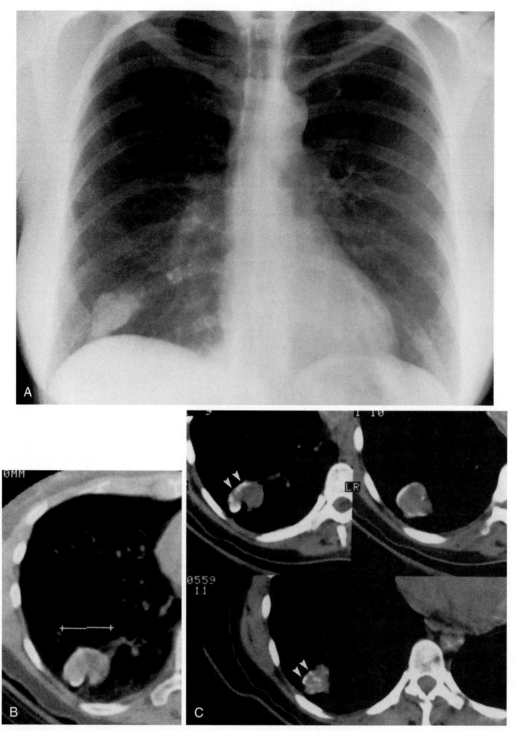

Figure 36–11. Pulmonary Chondroma. A posteroanterior chest radiograph *(A)* demonstrates an elongated, well-defined nodular opacity. CT scans *(B, C)* with lung and mediastinal windows show a bilobed lesion in the posterolateral part of the lower lobe measuring 3.3 cm in diameter. A central soft tissue core (CT attenuation value of +35 HU) is surrounded by a curvilinear rind of calcification *(arrowheads)*. The pathologic diagnosis after surgical resection was chondroma. The patient was a 52-year-old woman.

boembolism and pulmonary hypertension.[136] The initial diagnosis is usually metastatic carcinoma; when investigations fail to yield a source, tissue obtained from the lung or other site shows the characteristic morphology.

The tumors are best considered low-grade sarcomas; in addition to their infiltrative growth pattern histologically, both intrathoracic spread and systemic metastases have been

well documented.[116, 117, 137–139] It has been suggested that the presence of diffuse involvement of the liver may represent synchronous appearance of tumor in this organ rather than metastases.[134] The tumors are often slow growing, and survival may be prolonged even with widespread pulmonary involvement.[117, 140] Despite this, a rapid course can occur,[135] and approximately 40% of patients for whom follow-up information has been recorded have died, usually as a result of respiratory failure.[125]

Angiosarcoma

Angiosarcoma is an extremely rare pulmonary neoplasm whose characteristics have been poorly documented.[142-147] Some reported cases that have been interpreted as primary pulmonary angiosarcoma are probably better regarded as examples of the vascular change in primary pulmonary hypertension,[148] hereditary hemorrhagic telangiectasia,[149] or pulmonary carcinoma with a "pseudovascular" pattern.[150] As might be expected, the usual clinical presentation is hemoptysis. One tumor has been described to arise in the pulmonary artery.[38] Confirmation of the diagnosis requires careful investigation to exclude metastases from the heart, pulmonary artery, or extrathoracic sites.[145, 151, 152] A case has also been described in which a small lung nodule

that was stable in size over a period of 8 years suddenly grew; after resection, the histologic appearance was considered to be consistent with lymphangiosarcoma.[153]

NEOPLASMS OF BONE AND CARTILAGE

Chondroma

As discussed elsewhere (*see* page 1350), it is possible that the majority of benign cartilaginous tumors within the lungs represent one-sided development of neoplasms derived from a bronchial mesenchymal cell (i.e., they are analogous to so-called hamartomas).[154-156] Tumors that might be regarded as true chondromas (i.e., those composed of pure cartilage in continuity with and apparently arising from underlying tracheobronchial cartilage) are rare.[157] Radiographic findings are those of a solitary nodule or mass (Fig. 36–11), with or without airway obstruction (Fig. 36–12). On CT, they may or may not exhibit calcification.

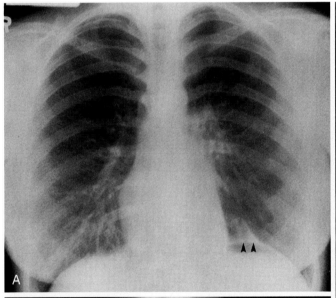

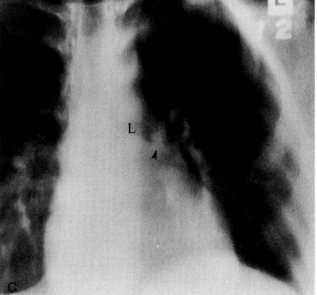

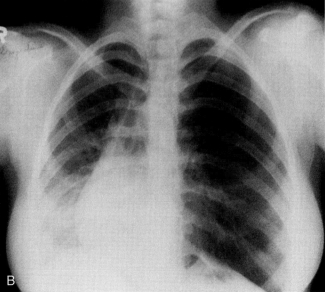

Figure 36–12. Endobronchial Chondroma. Posteroanterior chest radiographs in full inspiration *(A)* and expiration *(B)* show air trapping on the left consistent with a central bronchial obstructing lesion. On the inspiratory film the reduction in volume of the left hemithorax, the slight elevation of the left hemidiaphragm, and an ipsilateral juxtaphrenic peak *(arrowheads)* are noted, all of which signify partial atelectasis of the left lung. The vasculature of the left lung is slightly diminished as a result of hypoxic vasoconstriction. A linear tomogram in anteroposterior projection *(C)* reveals a round intraluminal mass *(arrowhead)* in the left (L) main bronchus. Pathologic examination of this lesion after surgical excision disclosed an intrabronchial chondroma. The patient was a 27-year-old woman with a left-sided wheeze.

An exception to this interpretation may be tumors that occur as part of Carney's "triad," an unusual condition consisting of pulmonary chondromas, gastric epithelioid leiomyosarcoma (leiomyoblastoma), and extra-adrenal paraganglioma.[158, 159] The abnormality is usually seen between the ages of 10 and 30 years; almost all patients have been female. The tumors are frequently multiple and can develop synchronously or metachronously, sometimes being separated by many years (as long as 14 years in one case).[160] Although commonly referred to as Carney's "triad," only two of the three types of tumor have been documented in approximately two thirds of cases.[160–163]

Pulmonary tumors consist of well-demarcated nodules of mature cartilage, often calcified or ossified and sometimes with intraosseous adipose tissue (Fig. 36–13). In contrast to the typical chondromatous hamartoma, epithelial-lined clefts between the cartilaginous lobules are usually absent. This histologic difference and the frequent multiplicity suggest that the pathogenesis of these tumors may be different from the more common chondromatous hamartoma.

Radiographic manifestations consist of single or multiple, unilateral or bilateral, smoothly marginated, round or slightly lobulated nodules (Fig. 36–14).[164, 165] Approximately 30% are calcified.[166] The calcification may be nodular and within the tumor or, more characteristically, at the periphery.[164–166] Rarely, bronchial compression causes distal pneumonitis and abscess formation.[167a] When Carney's triad is suspected, iodine-123 metaiodobenzylguanidine (^{123}I-MIBG) scintigraphy may be helpful in the detection of extra-adrenal paragangliomas.[166]

Pulmonary symptoms are usually absent, the chondromas being discovered on a screening radiograph or as part of a workup or follow-up of a previously diagnosed gastric leiomyosarcoma. In the latter situation, they may be incorrectly interpreted as metastases from the gastric neoplasm. Extra-adrenal paragangliomas can arise in any of the usual sites, but are most common within the thorax; paroxysmal headaches, hypertension, and tachycardia are frequent findings, and vanillylmandelic acid and total catecholamine levels are typically elevated.

Although the follow-up period has not been long in most cases, the condition appears to have a better prognosis than the multiplicity of neoplasms might suggest. Despite the clear-cut malignant nature of the gastric tumors—recurrence and metastases are common—their behavior appears to be less aggressive than the usual solitary gastric leiomyosarcoma.[167] In patients suspected of having the disease, transthoracic needle aspiration of pulmonary nodules is the diagnostic method of choice to exclude pulmonary metastases.[168]

Chondrosarcoma

Although the ribs are not an uncommon site of origin of primary chondrosarcoma, occurrence of the neoplasm within the lung or trachea is rare; in a 1993 review of the English and Japanese literature, only 16 cases were identified.[169] Although several additional examples have been reported, in our opinion and that of others, the majority probably should not be accepted because of inadequate clinical or histologic documentation or inappropriate pathologic classification.[170, 171] Rarely, chondrosarcoma of the extremities presents as a pulmonary metastasis.[172] As indicated previously, occasional cases of pulmonary artery sarcoma with a cartilaginous component have also been reported.[33]

Primary pulmonary chondrosarcomas are believed to be derived from normal tracheobronchial cartilage, although origin from a bronchial chondroma or chondromatous hamartoma has also been considered possible. Grossly, the tumor can present as a polypoid intraluminal growth within the trachea[173] or major bronchi[170, 174, 175] or as a more or less round, lobulated mass within the lung parenchyma.[171] The histologic appearance consists of foci of myxoid or cartilaginous tissue containing chondrocytic cells that have variably pleomorphic nuclei and mitotic activity. Foci of calcification or ossification may be seen.[171]

Radiographic manifestations are those of an intrapulmonary mass (that may or may not be calcified) or atelectasis and obstructive pneumonitis secondary to airway obstruction. Tumors have been described in patients of both sexes

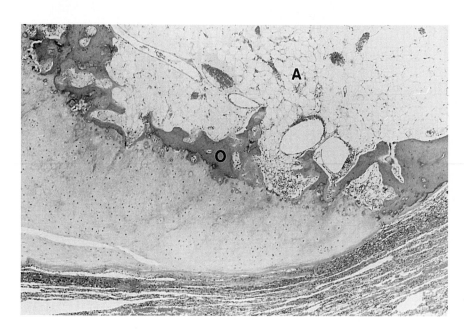

Figure 36–13. Pulmonary Chondroma— Carney's Syndrome. A section of the nodule illustrated in Figure 36–14 shows cartilage with focal ossification (O) and adipose tissue (A). The nodule is well circumscribed and appears to compress the adjacent lung parenchyma.

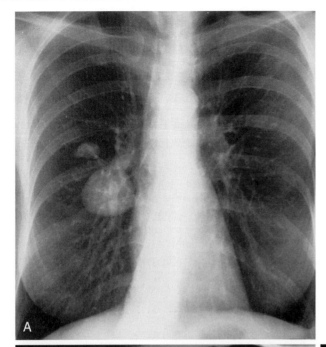

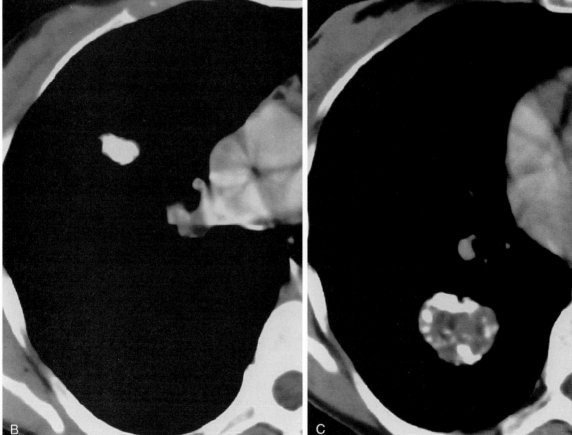

Figure 36–14. Carney's Triad. A posteroanterior chest radiograph *(A)* in a 42-year-old woman demonstrates two smoothly marginated nodules in the right lung. Blunting of the left costophrenic sulcus is present related to previous left gastrectomy for a leiomyosarcoma. Views of the right lung from conventional CT scans *(B, C)* demonstrate diffuse calcification of one of the nodules and focal areas of coarse calcification in the other. At surgery, the nodules were proven to be chondromas with extensive ossification *(see* Fig. 36–13).

from early to late adulthood; the average age in the literature review cited previously was 55 years.[169] The usual presenting symptom is cough, chest pain, or dyspnea.[171] Adequate surgical excision may result in cure, particularly in low-grade tumors. Metastases may develop, but are uncommon; fatality from the neoplasm is usually caused by local intrathoracic spread.[176]

Osteosarcoma

Primary osteosarcoma of the lung is one of the rarest of all pulmonary neoplasms. In a 1971 review, investigators reported two cases and found only three others in the literature;[177] few cases have been described since that date.[178–181] Occasional examples of pulmonary artery osteosarcoma have been documented.[34] Histologically, the tumors are composed of variable amounts of cytologically malignant myxomatous, chondroid, and osteoid tissue. Tumors must be sampled extensively to exclude carcinosarcoma.[178]

It is somewhat surprising that calcification was evident radiographically in only one of the nine cases reported by 1990.[180] In this case, a presumptive preoperative diagnosis of primary pulmonary osteosarcoma was made on the basis of intense radionuclide uptake on a technetium-99m-methylenediphosphonate bone scan.[180] In another case, speckled calcification was evident within the tumor on CT even though it was not apparent on the radiograph.[181] Clinical features are nonspecific.

NEOPLASMS OF NEURAL TISSUE

Neurofibroma, Schwannoma, and Neurogenic Sarcoma

Although not uncommon in the paravertebral region, primary neurogenic neoplasms rarely occur in the lungs. In one review of 1,664 patients who had pulmonary neoplasms, only 4 (0.2%) had the abnormality;[182] by 1983, only 50 cases had been described in the literature.[182] Because of the histologic similarities among many spindle cell neoplasms and the lack of electron microscopic or immunohistochemical studies performed in many of the reported cases, classification as a neurogenic neoplasm may not be correct in all instances, and the true incidence may be even lower than the aforementioned figures suggest. As might be expected, patients with neurofibromatosis are at increased risk for development of these tumors.[183, 184]

The majority of lesions present as solitary, smooth or lobulated nodules within pulmonary parenchyma; less often, they grow as a polypoid mass within the tracheobronchial lumen.[185–188] Multiple tumors are rare. Microscopically, most lesions have been classified as neurofibroma,[185, 190] schwannoma (rarely with atypical architectural or cytologic features ["ancient" schwannoma][184, 189]) being second in frequency;[191, 192] about 20% to 25% have been diagnosed as neurogenic sarcoma.[182] Ganglioneuroma and ganglioneuroblastoma are exceedingly rare.[193] One unusual case has been reported of an amputation neuroma originating in an arm stump and presenting as a mass in the apex of the right lung.[194]

The neoplasms are usually manifested radiographically as a solitary nodule; less commonly, atelectasis or obstructive pneumonitis is seen as a result of bronchial obstruction.[190] Most patients are asymptomatic;[182] cough, pleuritic pain, exertional dyspnea, and hemoptysis have been reported occasionally.[182, 186, 195] Severe hypoxemia resulting from right-to-left shunting was described in one 62-year-old woman with multiple neurofibromas.[196]

Granular Cell Tumor

Granular cell tumors can be found in many sites, but are most common in the tongue, skin, subcutaneous tissue, and breast. Their presence in the lungs has been documented in about 5% of cases;[197] approximately 100 pulmonary examples had been reported by 1995.[198] Multicentric bronchial tumors occur in 5% to 10% of patients.[198–200] Additional tumors are seen in mediastinal lymph nodes (rarely)[200] and outside the thorax (occasionally) in association with pulmonary tumors.[202–204]

The original description of the neoplasm as granular cell "myoblastoma" is now believed to be inappropriate because there is little evidence to link it histogenetically with either striated or smooth muscle. Instead, immunohistochemical, electron microscopic, and histochemical observations are most suggestive of a neural origin from either the neural sheath or, more likely, Schwann's cell.[205, 206] Tumors morphologically similar to granular cell neoplasms have been induced in the uterine cervix of mice that have been treated with estrogen,[207] suggesting a possible role for hormones in the pathogenesis; although support for this thesis was provided by a report of a rapidly growing tracheal lesion in a pregnant woman,[208] the slight male predominance and exceptional association with pregnancy make a hormonal influence of questionable importance.

Most respiratory tract tumors arise in the larynx or main bronchi,[209, 210] in the latter often at or near bifurcations; origin in pulmonary parenchyma or the trachea is unusual.[200, 210, 211] The tumors are usually small (1 to 2 cm), although a diameter of 6 cm has been recorded.[197] Grossly, they are not encapsulated and appear as a white, plaquelike thickening of the bronchial wall or as polypoid projections into the airway lumen associated with a variable degree of obstruction. The cut surface is characteristically somewhat yellowish in appearance.

Microscopically, the tumor consists of nests or large aggregates of polygonal cells of moderate size containing central, round, often hyperchromatic nuclei and granular eosinophilic cytoplasm.[197, 206] Although extension into the submucosa and peribronchial interstitial tissue is frequent, involvement of adjacent lung parenchyma is exceptional.[212] The cytoplasm is periodic acid–Schiff positive and diastase resistant and contains numerous granules with varying ultrastructural characteristics.[206] A positive immunohistochemical reaction for protein S-100 is the rule.[198]

The tumors show no sex predominance. About two thirds of cases occur between the ages of 30 and 49 years.[197, 198, 199] In a review of 20 cases in the files of the AFIP, approximately half the patients were asymptomatic.[198] The major symptoms are cough, chest pain, and findings of pneumonia; hemoptysis occurs occasionally. As with other tumors of the major airways, the clinical picture may simulate asthma.[210] A single case has been described in which a tumor was associated with hypercalcemia.[213] Radiographically, the tumors present as solitary nodules or as atelectasis or obstructive pneumonitis.[214–216] The diagnosis is usually made by bronchoscopic biopsy; neoplastic cells can sometimes be identified in bronchial washings or brushings.[217, 218]

The prognosis is usually excellent; however, neoplasms excised bronchoscopically can recur.[209, 219] Although about 5% of extrapulmonary granular cell tumors are malignant, we are unaware of any pulmonary tumors that have behaved in such a fashion.[198] Metastases to the lungs from an extrapulmonary primary have been documented.[220] The occasional association with pulmonary carcinoma,[221] sarcoidosis,[222] and human immunodeficiency virus infection[223] is probably coincidental.

NEOPLASMS OF ADIPOSE TISSUE

Lipoma

Pulmonary lipomas originate most commonly in the trachea or bronchi and only rarely in the lung parenchyma.[225, 226] They have been estimated to compose about 0.1% of all pulmonary tumors.[224] Because many tumors do not consist solely of adipose cells but instead contain a mixture of myxomatous, fibroblastic, chondroid, or smooth muscle elements,[227] it has been argued that they should be considered a variant of hamartoma rather than a distinct neoplasm (*see* page 1350).[157] However, the identification in one tumor of a supernumerary chromosome consisting of segments of chromosome 12, an abnormality that has also been found in soft tissue adipose tumors, suggests that at least some pulmonary lipomas are not hamartoma variants.[201]

Pathologically, parenchymal lipomas consist of well-circumscribed, yellowish nodules composed of mature adipose cells.[226, 228] Most endobronchial tumors occur in lobar or segmental airways.[226] They may be situated chiefly within the airway lumen or can extend in a dumbbell fashion between cartilage plates into the surrounding peribronchial interstitium and (occasionally) into the lung parenchyma.[229] Atypical giant cells similar to those seen in soft tissue pleomorphic lipomas have been identified occasionally.[230]

Radiographically, the tumor typically presents as a solitary nodule; atelectasis or obstructive pneumonitis may result from airway obstruction by an endobronchial lesion.[231] The diagnosis can be made without difficulty by CT, the low attenuation values of fat providing conclusive evidence of their differentiation.[232–234] The tumors also have a tendency to sequester xenon 133.[232]

Endobronchial lipomas can give rise to symptoms and signs of atelectasis or recurrent pneumonia; as with other mesenchymal neoplasms, tracheal lesions can result in a clinical picture that simulates bronchial asthma.[233] Patients with parenchymal tumors may be asymptomatic or present with cough, chest pain, or dyspnea.[226]

Liposarcoma

Primary pulmonary liposarcoma is rare.[234, 235] In one case, a 76-year-old man presented with a tracheal polyp;[236] in another, a 9-year-old girl with adrenogenital syndrome developed a parenchymal mass.[237] In a case that we have observed over a number of years, multiple tumors were seen to involve the lungs, pleura, and mediastinum (Fig. 36–15).

NEOPLASMS OF FIBROUS TISSUE

Myxoma

Pulmonary myxomas are exceedingly rare tumors composed entirely of stellate or elongated fibroblast-like cells with abundant intercellular myxoid material. Cases have been described in endobronchial,[238] endotracheal,[239] and intraparenchymal[240] locations. As with fibromas, chondromas, and lipomas, it is possible that these tumors represent part of a spectrum of histologic change seen with hamartomas.

Intrapulmonary Fibrous Tumor (Fibroma)

The term *intrapulmonary fibrous tumor* has been applied to neoplasms that resemble solitary fibrous tumor of the pleura (*see* page 2828) but that occur within the lung.[241, 242] Because many of these tumors are intimately associated with the visceral pleura, it is possible that their origin is the same as that hypothesized for the more common pleural form. Similar to lipomas and chondromas, some fibromas that occur in the lung parenchyma distant from the pleura or in the airways[243] may simply represent a one-sided histologic expression of a hamartoma. It is also possible that some of these cases represent a predominantly fibrous form of benign fibrous histiocytoma.

Grossly, the lesions are well circumscribed and range in size from 1 to 8 cm. Histologically, they consist of spindle-shaped, fibroblast-like cells embedded in a variable amount of collagen.[241, 244] Nuclear atypia is minimal, and mitotic figures are sparse or absent. Entrapped alveolar epithelium is common in the expanding periphery of the tumor.

Intrapulmonary fibrous tumors are similar to other benign pulmonary neoplasms in their radiographic and clinical manifestations. Those in an endobronchial location can cause atelectasis or obstructive pneumonitis; intratracheal lesions can simulate asthma.[243] Parenchymal lesions are usually asymptomatic. Tumors that are incompletely excised may recur. As with solitary tumors of the pleura, intrapulmonary fibrous tumors that have a high mitotic count may behave in a more aggressive fashion; it is possible that such neoplasms are better termed fibrosarcoma outright.

Malignant Fibrous Histiocytoma

Although malignant fibrous histiocytoma is one of the most common soft tissue neoplasms of adults, primary involvement of thoracic structures is infrequent; in the latter instance, an origin from the chest wall is most common, being observed in 15 (7.5%) of 200 cases in one series.[245] By 1996, approximately 50 cases apparently arising within the lungs had been reported,[246] including 22 cases in a 1987 report based on a review of files at the AFIP.[247] Because the lesion has been recognized histologically only since the 1970s, it is probable that the total number of reported cases is greater, some tumors previously being designated fibrosarcoma, leiomyosarcoma, myxosarcoma, or unclassified sarcoma. Sometimes, it is difficult to categorize a pulmonary fibrohistiocytic tumor as benign or malignant on the basis of the histologic appearance; such neoplasms have been designated *borderline* and may represent a variant intermediate between benign fibrous histiocytoma (*see* page 1371) and the clearly malignant tumor described in this section.[248]

The histogenesis of malignant fibrous histiocytoma is uncertain,[249] some investigators believing the progenitor cell to be a histiocyte capable of assuming fibroblastic activities and others a primitive mesenchymal cell capable of differentiation into both histiocytic and fibroblastic forms; still others have suggested independent fibroblastic and histiocytic proliferation.[250] The cause is generally unknown. In one patient, a tumor developed in the right lower lobe 7 years after chemotherapy and mediastinal and lower chest radiation for

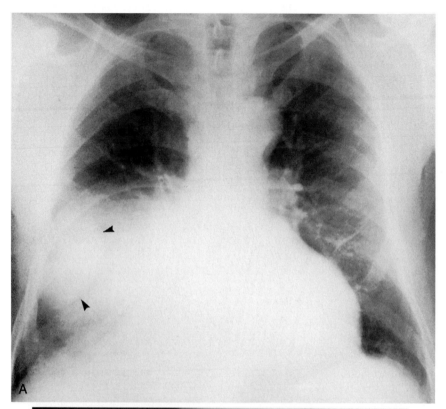

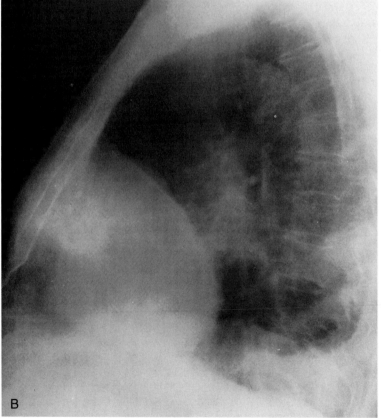

Figure 36–15. Pulmonary and Mediastinal Liposarcoma. Posteroanterior *(A)* and lateral *(B)* chest radiographs in a 55-year-old man reveal a large homogeneous opacity of soft tissue density occupying the right cardiophrenic angle and contiguous anterior chest wall, features consistent with a paracardiac, anterior mediastinal mass. A second, smaller mass *(arrowheads)* is located posterolaterally in the right lower lobe. There is a small right pleural effusion. Thoracotomy and biopsy disclosed a liposarcoma that involved the right side of the mediastinum as well as the lung and intervening pleura.

lymphoma;[251] in another, it arose in the right lower lobe 30 years after exposure to asbestos.[252]

Pathologically, these tumors typically consist of well-circumscribed, smooth or lobulated masses, usually without an obvious site of origin from an airway or vessel wall.[247] Rarely, the pulmonary artery appears to be the primary site.[253] Four histologic subtypes have been described: storiform-pleomorphic, myxoid, giant cell, and inflammatory.[249] The first of these is the pattern usually seen within the lung[247] and consists of fascicles of spindle-shaped cells arranged in a storiform or cartwheel appearance. Interspersed between the fascicles are polygonal ("histiocytic") cells possessing pleomorphic nuclei; mitotic figures are frequent. Atypical multinucleated giant cells are also common. Electron microscopic examination reveals cells that possess fibroblastic or histiocytic differentiation (or both);[249] undifferentiated mesenchymal cells are present in lesser numbers.

Radiologically, most tumors appear as solitary, smooth or lobulated nodules or masses within the lung parenchyma.[247, 252, 254] Less commonly, they present as pulmonary infiltrates or bilateral masses.[247, 254] Calcification has not been reported in adults, although it has been demonstrated on CT in a single pediatric patient.[255] We are not aware of any reports of cavitation within primary tumors, although it has been described in a pulmonary metastasis.[256] Approximately 20% of patients have ipsilateral pleural effusion.[247, 254]

Most of the recognized cases have been in older adults, the mean age of patients in the AFIP series being 52 years;[247] there is no sex predominance. There appears to be a predilection for whites over African Americans.[247] Although many patients are asymptomatic, cough, dyspnea, hemoptysis, and chest pain may be present. A mistaken diagnosis of pulmonary infarction usually reflects either origin from or invasion of the pulmonary vasculature.[257, 258] The diagnosis is usually made after surgical excision; occasionally, it has been suggested preoperatively on specimens obtained by transthoracic needle aspiration.[259]

When the neoplasm is limited to the thorax, the prognosis is difficult to predict; apparent cure after surgical excision has been noted in some patients,[260] whereas survival is measured in months in others. As might be expected, extension into the chest wall or mediastinum and metastases are poor prognostic signs.[247, 248] When metastases develop, the brain is a frequent site; in such cases, death usually ensues rapidly. According to the authors of one study of 13 patients, additional features suggestive of a poor course are local recurrence after surgery and the presence of necrosis in the primary tumor.[248] Another group of investigators found no association between prognosis and histologic subtype.[246]

Fibrosarcoma

Fibrosarcoma is probably the second most common histologic diagnosis that has been given to soft tissue sarcomas of the lung (the most frequent being leiomyosarcoma). In a review of the AFIP files from 1945 to 1969, 13 cases were found, and an additional 44 cases were identified in the literature.[11] As with many other pulmonary sarcomas reported during this period, ultrastructural and immunohistochemical studies were not performed, and it is likely that some tumors would not be classified as fibrosarcoma today.

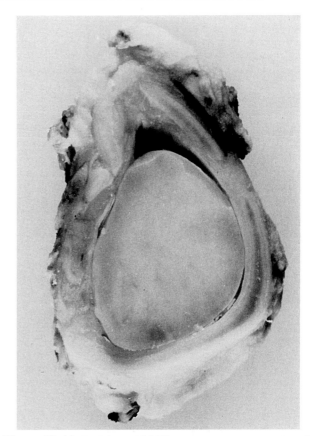

Figure 36–16. Endobronchial Fibrosarcoma. A cross-section of a right main bronchus shows a solid tumor without necrosis or hemorrhage. The tumor was attached by a broad pedicle to the underlying bronchial wall (not shown here); invasive sarcoma extended into the mucosa. Histologic examination showed interlacing fascicles of spindle-shaped cells; immunohistochemical and ultrastructural studies showed no specific differentiation.

In fact, some authors have stated that true pulmonary fibrosarcoma is extremely rare.[14]

Similar to leiomyosarcoma, fibrosarcoma can arise in the trachea, bronchus (Fig. 36–16), pulmonary parenchyma, or pulmonary artery. Most endobronchial tumors occur in lobar or main bronchi of children and young adults.[11] Histologically, they are composed of fascicles of spindle-shaped cells arranged in a characteristic herringbone pattern; mitotic figures are usually evident and may be numerous. There is a variable amount of intercellular collagen. Patients most often present with cough, hemoptysis, or chest pain. Radiographic findings are those of atelectasis or obstructive pneumonitis. Intrapulmonary tumors tend to arise in middle-aged or elderly adults and often do not cause symptoms, especially when smaller;[11] radiographically, they present as a smooth or lobulated mass indistinguishable from other pulmonary nodules.

Endobronchial tumors are often amenable to local surgical excision, after which long-term survival is the rule.[11] By contrast, intrapulmonary lesions often behave in a highly malignant fashion, with death occurring within 2.5 years; in the AFIP series, larger tumors (>8 cm) tended to kill by local extension into adjacent thoracic structures without associated metastatic disease, whereas smaller ones developed extensive metastases.[11] Fibrosarcomas with eight or more mitotic figures per 10 high-power fields were most likely to behave in an aggressive fashion; those with fewer than eight per 10 high-power fields either remained stationary or grew slowly.

MISCELLANEOUS SOFT TISSUE NEOPLASMS

Hamartoma

A hamartoma is a tumor-like malformation composed of tissues that are normally present in the organ in which the tumor occurs, but in which the tissue elements, although mature, are disorganized. In the lung, the term has traditionally been used to refer to a parenchymal tumor that is somewhat lobulated in contour and consists predominantly of cartilage and adipose tissue; similar tumors occur occasionally in endobronchial and exceptionally in endotracheal[261] locations. Despite the widespread use of the term, the belief that these lesions represent true hamartomas has been questioned,[157, 262–264] and it is now generally believed that they are better regarded as benign neoplasms, probably derived from a bronchial wall mesenchymal cell. The results of several clinical and pathologic investigations support this hypothesis.

1. The tumors appear to have an onset in adult life: the peak age incidence is in the fifties,[265, 266] and they are identified uncommonly in individuals less than 30 years of age[265] and virtually never in infants.[263] In addition, tumors can be identified radiographically in adults whose previous chest radiographs have been normal;[267] in one investigation, tumor size correlated with patient age.[268]

2. Serial radiographs sometimes reveal slow[264, 270] and (occasionally) rapid[269] growth; in one study, tumors increased in size by an average of 3.2 mm per year.[268]

3. The results of histologic studies suggest that the peripheral epithelial-lined clefts represent passive entrapment of adjacent airway epithelium within an expanding mesenchymal proliferation rather than a separate element of a hamartomatous process.[262] Additional support for this interpretation

has been provided by electron microscopic studies that have demonstrated a fairly consistent basement membrane underlying the entrapped epithelium[272, 273] and by the occasional small tumor composed entirely of cartilage or other mesenchymal elements (Fig. 36–17).

4. Foci of apparently undifferentiated mesenchymal or fibroblast-like cells are commonly present at the periphery of the cartilaginous lobules; moreover, apparent transition can be demonstrated between the two tissues on both light microscopic (Fig. 36–18)[263] and electron microscopic[273] examination.

5. The results of cytogenetic analyses have shown several chromosomal abnormalities,[274, 275] most commonly in the q13–q15 region of chromosome 12;[276, 277] similar abnormalities have been documented in other benign soft tissue neoplasms, implying that pulmonary hamartoma is also neoplastic.

On the strength of these observations, it appears that the diagnostic label "hamartoma" may be nosologically incorrect and that these tumors are described more appropriately by a term such as *mesenchymoma*.[278] Because of the widespread use of the designation hamartoma, however, this nomenclature is retained in this book, recognizing that the true nature of the tumor may be other than its name implies.

There is also some difference of opinion as to whether the histologic varieties of hamartoma represent separate entities or simply different morphologic expressions of the same process. This issue has been debated especially in relation to the difference between parenchymal and endobronchial tumors; most investigators have argued in favor of the second hypothesis and have provided evidence of histologic overlap between tumors in the two locations.[157, 262, 267, 279] There is also some question regarding the separate existence of other benign pulmonary tumors, such as fibromas, chondromas, and lipomas; the tissue composing each of these occurs in varying proportion in the typical chondromatous hamartoma, and it is conceivable that the former tumors might represent simply a one-sided expression of mesenchymal differentiation in a hamartoma. Although it is not entirely

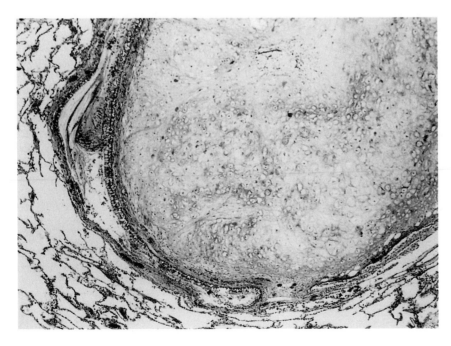

Figure 36–17. Pulmonary Hamartoma (Chondroma). A small nodule of cartilaginous tissue measuring 2 mm in diameter compresses both lung parenchyma and bronchiolar lumen. This lesion was an incidental finding at autopsy, and although descriptively it could be termed a chondroma, it most likely represents an early counterpart of the more typical chondromatous hamartoma before incorporation of epithelial clefts within the mesenchymal tissue. (×40.)

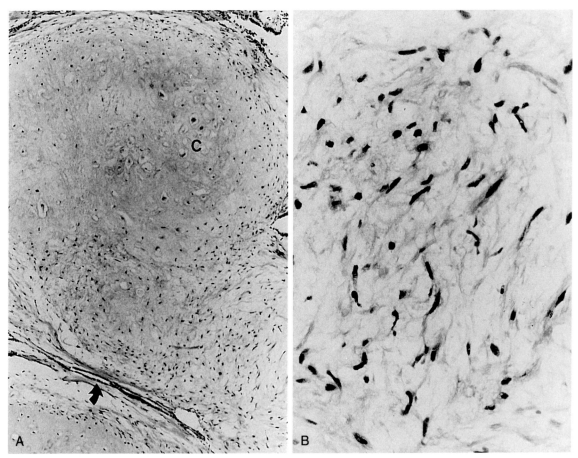

Figure 36–18. Pulmonary Hamartoma. A magnified view *(A)* of a typical chondromatous hamartoma shows cartilage (C), epithelium-lined cleft *(arrow)*, and spindle cells within a loose stroma (seen to better advantage in *B*). The gradual transition between the spindle cells and the cartilage is clearly evident.

clear why some regional differences exist (e.g., the greater proportion of adipose tissue in endobronchial tumors), it seems likely that all these tumors are derived from the same primitive mesenchymal cell that has the ability to differentiate into a variety of distinct adult tissues.

In addition to the typical endobronchial and parenchymal hamartomas discussed in this section, there are several rare tumors that are histologically distinctive and that have also been described as hamartoma.[280–283] One unusual variant is angiofibroma, a lesion consisting of dilated capillaries surrounded by loose fibrous tissue that is most often seen in the skin in patients with tuberous sclerosis; a single example has been described in an endobronchial location in a patient with this disease.[283] Cowden's disease (multiple hamartoma syndrome) is a rare autosomal dominant dermatosis characterized by multiple hamartomas of ectodermal, mesodermal, and endodermal origin and (sometimes) fibrocystic disease or carcinoma of the breast, thyroid tumors, and ovarian cysts;[284] mucocutaneous and gastrointestinal sites are the most frequent, but hamartomas of the lung occur rarely.[285] So-called mesenchymal cystic hamartoma is also a rare pulmonary abnormality that has been hypothesized to represent a developmental condition *(see* page 1373).

Epidemiology

Hamartomas are uncommon pulmonary tumors. In one review of 7,972 autopsies, only 20 examples were found,

for an incidence of 0.25%.[286] In another study of 2,958 solitary lung tumors, 5.7% were found to be hamartomas.[287] As indicated previously, most are discovered in adulthood, with a peak incidence in the fifties;[265] rare cases have been reported in children.[289] The tumors are identified most often in males, the sex predominance being 2 to 3:1.[265, 290] Endobronchial hamartomas are much less common than parenchymal lesions, accounting for about 1.5%[291] and 8%[278] of all pulmonary hamartomas in two large series.

Pathologic Characteristics

The majority of lesions are solitary; in one series of 154 patients, only 4 (2.5%) were multiple.[264] As indicated previously, most are located within the parenchyma, usually in a peripheral location. At this site, they are well-circumscribed, slightly lobulated tumors that can often be "shelled out" of the surrounding, somewhat compressed lung. Although the majority of tumors are less than 4 cm in diameter,[265, 266, 292] occasional examples have been reported to measure as much as 10 cm.[267, 293] Cut sections show lobules of firm, white, cartilaginous-appearing tissue (Fig. 36–19). Histologically, the lobules are often composed of a central area of well-developed cartilage surrounded by a zone of loose (myxomatous) fibroblastic tissue *(see* Fig. 36–18). Adipose tissue, smooth muscle, seromucinous bronchial-type glands, and mononuclear inflammatory cells may also be

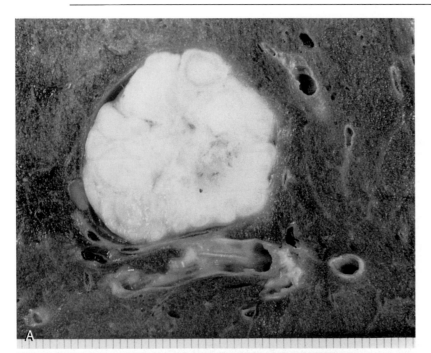

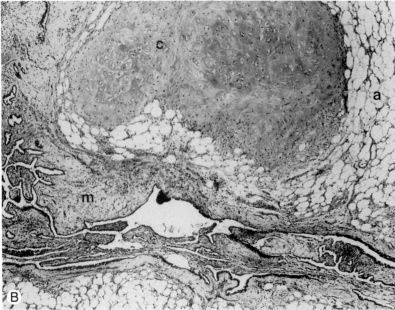

Figure 36–19. Pulmonary Hamartoma. A magnified view of an excised lower lobe *(A)* reveals a well-circumscribed peribronchial tumor that consists of lobules of cartilage separated by thin bands of connective tissue. A section *(B)* demonstrates mature cartilage (c), adipose tissue (a), undifferentiated mesenchymal tissue (m), and multiple epithelium-lined clefts. (*B*, ×40.)

seen in variable proportions. Calcification and ossification can be present and are occasionally extensive. Thin, slitlike spaces or clefts lined by ciliated columnar or cuboidal epithelium are frequently seen between the lobules, most prominently at the periphery of the tumor (*see* Fig. 36–19). One unusual example has been reported in which part of the tumor resembled sclerosing hemangioma.[288]

Although endobronchial hamartomas can be morphologically identical to the parenchymal variety (Fig. 36–20),[262, 279] more often they appear as fleshy, polypoid tumors attached to the bronchial wall by a narrow stalk (Fig. 36–21). Histologically, they often lack epithelial clefts and possess a smooth or slightly undulating surface lined by normal respiratory or metaplastic squamous epithelium. The central portion is usually composed of a core of adipose tissue surrounded by somewhat compressed myxoid tissue. Smooth

muscle and seromucinous glands may be admixed. Cartilage is often absent or present in small amounts;[279] bone is seen occasionally.[271] The tumor is usually attached to the bronchial wall by a narrow base that blends with the normal bronchial mucosa; only rarely is it continuous with bronchial cartilage plates.[157]

Radiologic Manifestations

Pulmonary hamartomas typically are well-circumscribed, smoothly marginated solitary nodules without lobar predilection (Fig. 36–22).[287, 295] The majority are smaller than 4 cm in diameter.[265, 287] Although calcification has been identified pathologically in as many as 15% of tumors in some series,[291] it is visible on the chest radiograph in less than 10% of cases; for example, it was identified on the

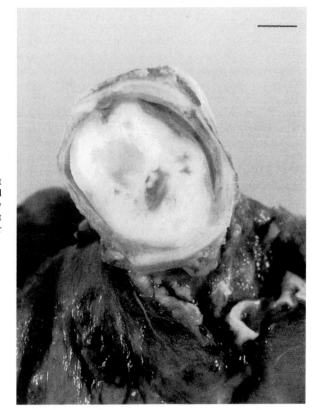

Figure 36–20. Endobronchial Hamartoma. A cross-section of the right upper lobe bronchus shows it to be completely occluded by a well-circumscribed intraluminal tumor. Except for an absence of epithelial clefts, it was histologically similar to the more common parenchymal hamartoma; the white areas represent mature cartilage, and the gray region represents adipose and fibrous tissue. (Bar = 5 mm.)

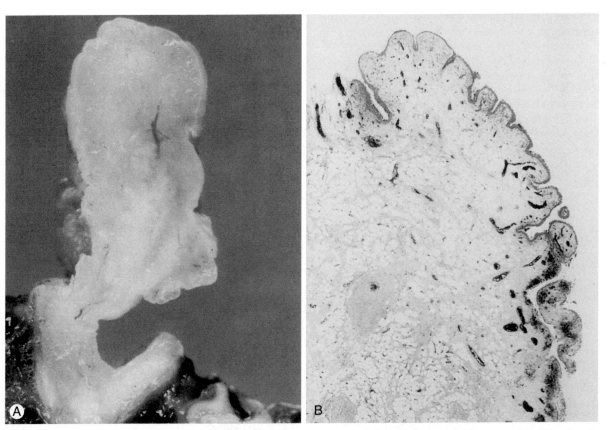

Figure 36–21. Endobronchial Hamartoma (Lipoma). A fleshy polypoid tumor *(A)* is joined by a narrow stalk to a segmental bronchus. A section *(B)* shows the lesion to be composed predominantly of fibroadipose tissue. Note the absence of deep epithelium-lined clefts. This appearance has also led to a designation of lipoma or fibroepithelial polyp. (*B*, ×22.)

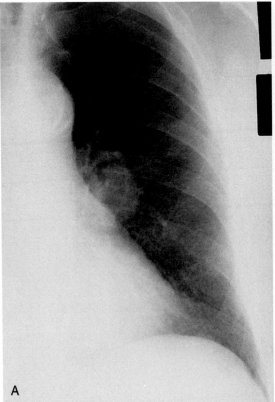

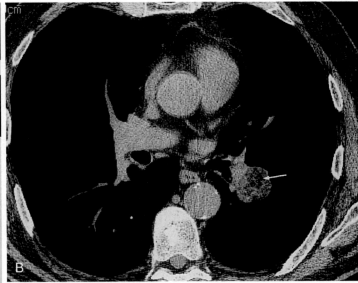

Figure 36–22. Pulmonary Hamartoma. A view of left lung from a postero-anterior chest radiograph *(A)* shows a 3-cm diameter nodule adjacent to the left hilum. An HRCT scan *(B)* performed through the center of the nodule demonstrates focal areas of fat *(arrow)*. This CT appearance is diagnostic of pulmonary hamartoma.

preoperative radiograph in only 2 of 65 tumors,[295] 1 of 17 tumors,[296] and 7 of 80 tumors[297] in three series. The radiographic pattern of calcification may resemble popcorn (Fig. 36–23); although virtually diagnostic, this appearance is relatively uncommon. As indicated previously, serial radiography films may reveal slow or (exceptionally) rapid growth,[269, 270, 298, 299] increasing the difficulty in differentiation from pulmonary carcinoma. Cavitation is extremely rare.[300, 301]

The CT findings were reported in a study of 31 proved and 16 presumed tumors.[302] CT was performed using thin sections (2-mm collimation); the criteria permitting a diagnosis of hamartoma included a smoothly contoured nodule 2.5 cm or less in diameter and focal collections of fat (CT numbers between -40 and -120 HU in at least eight voxels) or fat alternating with areas of calcification (CT numbers >175 HU) *(see* Fig. 36–22). Of the 47 tumors, 17 showed no discernible calcium or fat (the diagnosis being made by other means), 2 revealed diffuse calcification, 18 displayed areas of fat, and 10 showed foci of calcium and fat; thus, 28 (60%) of the 47 hamartomas were correctly

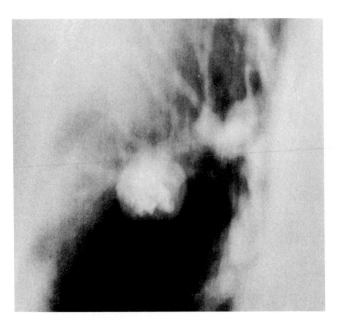

Figure 36–23. Calcification in Pulmonary Hamartoma. A conventional linear tomogram in anteroposterior projection shows a 3-cm, well-defined nodule in the anterior segment of the right upper lobe. The lesion contains a large central area of so-called popcorn ball calcification characteristic of hamartoma (presumptive diagnosis in a 52-year-old man).

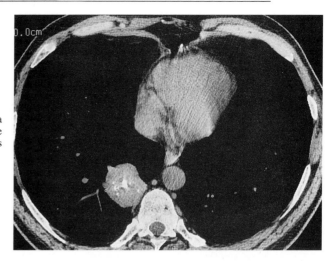

Figure 36–24. Pulmonary Hamartoma. An HRCT scan demonstrates a 4-cm-diameter tumor in the right lower lobe; several foci of calcification are evident. The diagnosis of hamartoma was proven at surgery. The patient was an asymptomatic 52-year-old man.

diagnosed by CT without the necessity of a more invasive procedure. Occasionally, hamartomas demonstrate focal areas of calcification without evidence of fat (Fig. 36–24).

MR imaging has a limited role in assessment. In a review of the findings in six patients, fat was not evident in any, and focal areas of calcification caused signal void or were missed.[303] The hamartomas had intermediate signal intensity (higher than that of skeletal muscle but lower than that of fat) on T1-weighted images and high signal intensity on T2-weighted images. They frequently contained septa that had high signal intensity on T1-weighted images and low signal intensity on T2-weighted images.

Parenchymal hamartomas occasionally grow to a large size (Fig. 36–25). One case has been reported of a tumor 10 cm in diameter that had grown slowly (by an estimated 125 times) over 19 years;[293] selective bronchial arteriography demonstrated a rich blood supply to the tumor. The authors reasoned that most hamartomas, because of their slow growth and origin from the bronchial wall, must receive their blood supply from a systemic vessel. A case has also been reported of a remarkable "tumor" that measured 30 cm in diameter and appeared to be composed of a multitude of small hamartomas.[304]

As might be expected, endobronchial hamartomas are usually manifested radiographically by the effects of airway obstruction. Rarely, they are unassociated with peripheral collapse, as in one patient who was followed for almost 10 years with a diagnosis of emphysema.[154] The CT findings have been described in a small number of cases. The tumors may appear to be composed entirely of fat,[305, 306] a mixture of fat and soft tissue,[305] or areas of fat and calcification (Fig. 36–26)[307] or may have homogeneous soft tissue attenuation.[305] There is usually evidence of associated obstructive atelectasis or pneumonitis.[305, 306]

Clinical Manifestations and Diagnosis

Because of their predominant peripheral location, most hamartomas usually do not cause symptoms.[268, 290] When they do, hemoptysis—rarely massive[308, 309]—is the most common. In the cases in which the lesion obstructs a bronchus, signs and symptoms may be the result of pneumonitis—fever, cough, expectoration, and chest pain.[292, 294] In such circumstances, bronchoscopy and biopsy usually reveal the

diagnosis. In the absence of the characteristic popcorn pattern of calcification radiographically or evidence of focal areas of fat attenuation on CT, the differential diagnosis must include all other solitary pulmonary nodules, particularly carcinoma. Although thoracotomy may be required for definitive diagnosis, transthoracic needle aspiration can provide adequate tissue for diagnosis in many cases.[310–312]

Prognosis and Natural History

Hamartomas are benign, and adequate surgical excision results in cure in the vast majority of patients. For example, in one series of 215 patients, there were no recurrent tumors in the follow-up period of 2 to 192 months;[290] in another review of 154 patients, there were only two recurrences (after 10 and 12 years), each after tumor enucleation.[264] Exceptional cases of the development of additional hamartomas have been reported. Rarely, a sarcoma or carcinoma appears to arise in relation to and possibly from the tumor stroma or entrapped epithelium.[313–315] (An even more unusual event is metastasis to a hamartoma, as reported in one patient with prostatic carcinoma.[316]) Some investigators have suggested that there may be an increased risk for the subsequent development of pulmonary carcinoma in patients who have hamartoma.[317]

Miscellaneous Sarcomas

A study of 25 patients with predominantly spindle cell neoplasms has been reported in which the authors proposed that the tumors were best designated *monophasic synovial sarcoma*.[294] Tumors were mostly intraparenchymal and well circumscribed; necrosis, hemorrhage, and cyst formation were common. Immunohistochemical examination revealed a positive reaction for keratin and epithelial membrane antigen in almost all tumors. The mean age at presentation was 38 years, and there was no sex predominance. Approximately 80% of patients were symptomatic (chest pain, hemoptysis, dyspnea, and cough). Ten patients died as a result of tumor between 1 and 7 years after the initial diagnosis. The detection of a characteristic X;18 translocation has been used in diagnosis.[2]

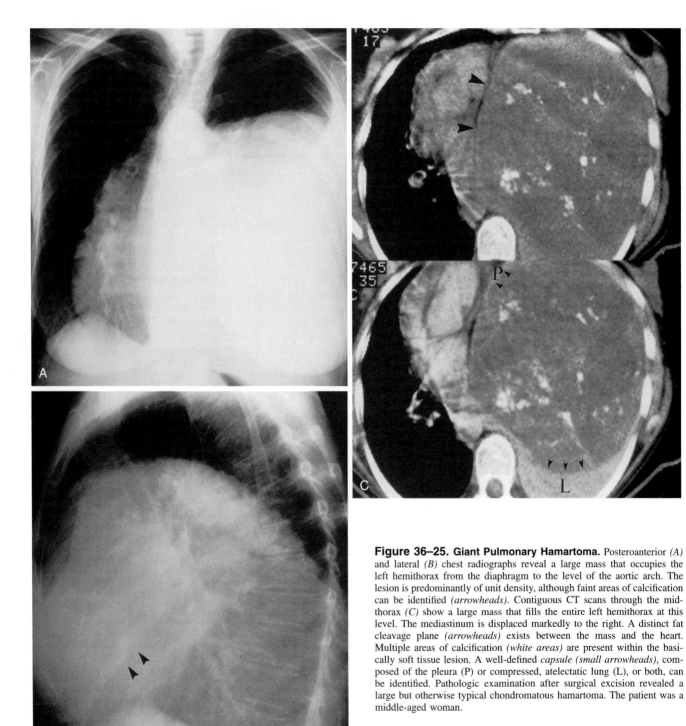

Figure 36–25. Giant Pulmonary Hamartoma. Posteroanterior *(A)* and lateral *(B)* chest radiographs reveal a large mass that occupies the left hemithorax from the diaphragm to the level of the aortic arch. The lesion is predominantly of unit density, although faint areas of calcification can be identified *(arrowheads)*. Contiguous CT scans through the mid-thorax *(C)* show a large mass that fills the entire left hemithorax at this level. The mediastinum is displaced markedly to the right. A distinct fat cleavage plane *(arrowheads)* exists between the mass and the heart. Multiple areas of calcification *(white areas)* are present within the basically soft tissue lesion. A well-defined *capsule (small arrowheads)*, composed of the pleura (P) or compressed, atelectatic lung (L), or both, can be identified. Pathologic examination after surgical excision revealed a large but otherwise typical chondromatous hamartoma. The patient was a middle-aged woman.

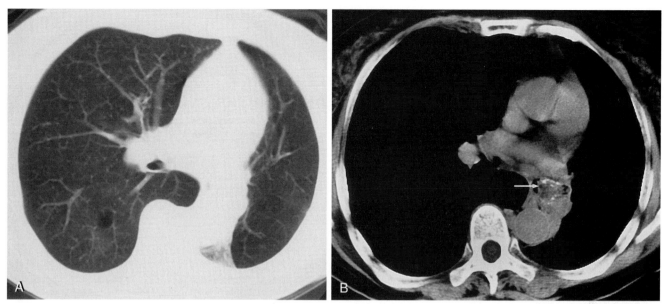

Figure 36–26. Endobronchial Hamartoma. A conventional CT scan *(A)* in a 62-year-old woman demonstrates obstruction of the distal left main and lower lobe bronchi with associated left lower lobe atelectasis. A CT scan photographed at soft tissue windows *(B)* demonstrates an endobronchial tumor with focal areas of fat attenuation *(arrow)* and calcification. (From Kwong JS, Müller NL, Miller RR: Diseases of the trachea and main-stem bronchi: Correlation of CT with pathologic findings. RadioGraphics 12:645, 1992.)

There have been two reports of pulmonary *alveolar soft part sarcoma*, one involving the parenchyma[318] and the other a pulmonary vein.[319] An unusual tumor termed *malignant mesenchymoma* has been reported in the right main bronchus of a 62-year-old man.[320] The tumor was composed of an admixture of osteosarcoma, chondrosarcoma, rhabdomyosarcoma, and undifferentiated mesenchyme, unaccompanied by embryonal or malignant epithelial elements.

REFERENCES

1. Martini N: Invited commentary. Ann Thorac Surg 58:1155, 1994.
2. Roberts CA, Seemayer TA, Neff JR, et al: Translocation (X;18) in primary synovial sarcoma of the lung. Cancer Genet Cytogenet 88:49, 1996.
3. Mann M, Asuncion C: Simultaneous primary lung sarcoma and carcinoma. J Surg Oncol 49:270, 1992.
4. Wick MR, Scheithauer BW, Piehler JM, et al: Primary pulmonary leiomyosarcomas: A light and electron microscopic study. Arch Pathol Lab Med 106:510, 1982.
5. Henrichs KJ, Wenisch HJC, Hofmann W, et al: Leiomyosarcoma of the pulmonary artery: A light and electron microscopical study. Virchows Arch [Pathol Anat Histol] 383:207, 1979.
6. Ramanathan T: Primary leiomyosarcoma of the lung. Thorax 29:482, 1974.
7. Vera-Roman JM, Sobonya RE, Gomez-Garcia JL, et al: Leiomyoma of the lung: Literature review and case report. Cancer 52:936, 1983.
8. Yellin A, Rosenman Y, Lieberman Y: Review of smooth muscle tumours of the lower respiratory tract. Br J Dis Chest 78:337, 1984.
9. White SH, Ibrahim NB, Forrester-Wood CP, et al: Leiomyomas of the lower respiratory tract. Thorax 40:306, 1985.
10. Orlowski TM, Stasiak K, Kolodziej J: Leiomyoma of the lung. J Thorac Cardiovasc Surg 76:257, 1978.
11. Guccion JG, Rosen SH: Bronchopulmonary leiomyosarcoma and fibrosarcoma: A study of 32 cases and review of the literature. Cancer 30:836, 1972.
12. Moffat RE, Chang CHJ, Slaven JE: Roentgen considerations in primary pulmonary artery sarcoma. Radiology 104:283, 1972.
13. Burke AP, Virmani R: Sarcomas of the great vessels: A clinicopathologic study. Cancer 71:1761, 1993.
14. Suster S: Primary sarcomas of the lung. Semin Diagn Pathol 12:140, 1995.
15. Gal AA, Brooks JSJ, Pietra GG: Leiomyomatous neoplasms of the lung: A clinical, histologic, and immunohistochemical study. Mod Pathol 2:209, 1989.
16. Pritchett PS, Fu Y-S, Kay S: Unusual ultrastructural features of a leiomyosarcoma of the lung. Am J Clin Pathol 63:901, 1975.
17. Lillo-Gil R, Albrechtsson U, Jakobsson B: Pulmonary leiomyosarcoma appearing as a cyst: Report of one case and review of the literature. Thorac Cardiovasc Surg 33:250, 1985.
18. Janssen JP, Mulder JJS, Wagenaar SS, et al: Primary sarcoma of the lung: A clinical study with long-term follow-up. Ann Thorac Surg 58:1151, 1994.
19. Moller-Pedersen V, Schulze S, Hoier-Madsen K, et al: Primary pulmonary leiomyosarcoma: Review of the literature and report of a case. Scand J Thorac Cardiovasc Surg 18:251, 1984.
20. Martin E: Leiomyomatous lung lesions: A proposed classification. Am J Roentgenol 141:269, 1983.
21. Ogawa J, Inoue H, Koide S, et al: Leiomyoma of the lung: Report of a case. Tokai J Exp Clin Med 8:129, 1983.
22. Morgan PGM, Ball J: Pulmonary leiomyosarcomas. Br J Dis Chest 74:245, 1980.
23. Gil-Zuricalday P, Lor F, Gil-Turner C: Primary pedunculated leiomyosarcoma of the lung. Thorax 37:153, 1982.
24. Chen KT: Leiomyoma of the trachea. Am J Otolaryngol 4:144, 1983.
25. Ayabe H, Tsuji H, Tagawa Y, et al: Endobronchial leiomyoma: Report of a case treated by bronchoplasty and a review of the literature. Surg Today 25:1057, 1995.
26. Fleetham JA, Lynn RB, Munt PW: Tracheal leiomyosarcoma: A unique cause of stridor. Am Rev Respir Dis 116:1109, 1977.
27. Peters P, Trotter SE, Sheppard MN, et al: Primary leiomyoma of the pulmonary vein. Thorax 47:393, 1992.
28. Wang N-S, Seemayer TA, Ahmed MN, et al: Pulmonary leiomyosarcoma associated with an arteriovenous fistula. Arch Pathol 98:100, 1974.
29. Kaiser LR, Urmacher C: Primary sarcoma of the superior pulmonary vein. Cancer 66:789, 1990.
30. Tsutsumi Y, Deng Y: Alveolar soft part sarcoma of the pulmonary vein. Acta Pathol Jpn 41:771, 1991.
31. Nonomura A, Kurumaya H, Kono N, et al: Primary pulmonary artery sarcoma: Report of two autopsy cases studied by immunohistochemistry and electron microscopy, and review of 110 cases reported in the literature. Acta Pathol Jpn 38:883, 1988.
32. Cox JE, Chiles C, Aquino SL, et al: Pulmonary artery sarcomas: A review of clinical and radiologic features. J Comput Assist Tomogr 21:750, 1997.
33. Lowell LM, Tuhy JE: Primary chondrosarcoma of the lung. J Thorac Surg 18:476, 1949.
34. Murthy MSN, Meckstroth CV, Merkle BH, et al: Primary intimal sarcoma of pulmonary valve and trunk with osteogenic sarcomatous elements. Arch Pathol Lab Med 100:649, 1976.
35. Gyhra AS, Santander CK, Alarcon EC, et al: Leiomyosarcoma of the pulmonary veins with extension to the left atrium. Ann Thorac Surg 61:1840, 1996.
36. Kern WH, Hughes RK, Meyer BW, et al: Malignant fibrous histiocytoma of the lung. Cancer 44:1793, 1979.
37. Emmert-Buck MR, Stay EJ, Tsokos M, et al: Pleomorphic rhabdomyosarcoma arising in association with the right pulmonary artery. Arch Pathol Lab Med 118:1220, 1994.
38. Goldblum JR, Rice TW: Epithelioid angiosarcoma of the pulmonary artery. Hum Pathol 26:1275, 1995.
39. Hopwood D, McNeill G: Spindle cell sarcoma of the pulmonary trunk: A case report with histochemistry and electron microscopy. J Pathol 128:71, 1979.
40. Johansson L, Carlen B: Sarcoma of the pulmonary artery: Report of four cases with electron microscopic and immunohistochemical examinations, and review of the literature. Virchows Arch 424:217, 1994.
41. Janssen JP, Mulder JJ, Wagenaar SS, et al: Primary sarcoma of the lung: A clinical study with long-term follow-up. Ann Thorac Surg 58:1151, 1994.
42. Britton PD: Primary pulmonary artery sarcoma: A report of two cases, with special emphasis on the diagnostic problems. Clin Radiol 41:92, 1990.
43. Olsson HE, Spitzer RM, Erston WF: Primary and secondary pulmonary artery neoplasia mimicking acute pulmonary embolism. Radiology 118:49, 1976.
44. Van Damme H, Vaneerdeweg W, Schoofs E: Malignant fibrous histiocytoma of the pulmonary artery. Ann Surg 205:203, 1986.
44a. Lamers RJS, Hochstenbag MMH, van Belle AF, Wouters EFM: Unilateral hilar mass. Chest 108:1444, 1995.
45. FitzGerald PM: Case report: Primary sarcoma of the pulmonary trunk: CT findings. J Comput Assist Tomogr 7:521, 1983.
46. Crass JR, Letourneau JG, Day DL, Golberg ME: Chest case of the day. Am J Roentgenol 148:638, 1987.
47. Smith WS, Lesar MS, Travis WD, et al: Case report: MR and CT findings in pulmonary artery sarcoma. J Comput Assist Tomogr 13:906, 1989.
48. Scully RE: Case records of the Massachusetts General Hospital. N Engl J Med 312:1242, 1985.
49. Weinreb JC, Davis SD, Berkmen YM, et al: Case report: Pulmonary artery sarcoma: Evaluation using Gd-DTPA. J Comput Assist Tomogr 14:647, 1990.
49a. Kauczor H-U, Schwickert HC, Mayer E, et al: Pulmonary artery sarcoma mimicking chronic thromboembolic disease: Computed tomography and magnetic resonance imaging findings. Cardiovasc Intervent Radiol 17:185, 1994.
49b. Winchester PA, Khilnani NM, Trost DW, et al: Endovascular catheter biopsy of a pulmonary artery sarcoma. Am J Roentgenol 167:657, 1996.
50. Hynes JK, Smith HC, Holmes DR, et al: Preoperative angiographic diagnosis of primary sarcoma of the pulmonary artery. Circulation 66:672, 1982.
51. Al-Robaish A, Lien DC, Slatnik J, et al: Sarcoma of the pulmonary artery trunk: Report of a case complicated with hemopericardium and cardiac tamponade. Can J Cardiol 11:707, 1996.
52. Baker PB, Goodwin RA: Pulmonary artery sarcomas: A review and report of a case. Arch Pathol Lab Med 109:35, 1985.
53. Anderson MB, Kriett JM, Kapelanski DP, et al: Primary pulmonary artery sarcoma: A report of six cases. Ann Thorac Surg 59:1487, 1995.
54. Delany SG, Doyle TC, Bunton RW, et al: Pulmonary artery sarcoma mimicking pulmonary embolism. Chest 103:1631, 1993
55. Wackers FJT, Van Dershoot JV, Hample JF: Sarcoma of the pulmonary trunk associated with hemorrhagic tendency: A case report and review of the literature. Cancer 23:339, 1969.
56. Green J, Crevasse LE, Shanklin DR: Fibrosarcoma of the pulmonary artery associated with syncope, intractable heart failure, polycythemia and thrombocytopenia. Am J Cardiol 12:547, 1964.
57. Thijs LG, Kroon TAJ, Van Leeuwen TM: Leiomyosarcoma of the pulmonary trunk associated with pericardial effusion. Thorax 29:490, 1974.
58. Wolf PC, Dickenman RC, Langston JD: Fibrosarcoma of the pulmonary artery masquerading as pheochromocytoma. Am J Cin Pathol 34:146, 1960.
59. Wackers FJT, Van Der Schoot JB, Hampe JF: Sarcoma of the pulmonary trunk associated with hemorrhagic tendency: A case report and review of the literature. Cancer 23:339, 1969.
60. Sawada K, Fukuma S, Seki Y, et al: Cytologic features of primary leiomyosarcoma of the lung: Report of a case diagnosed by bronchial brushing procedure. Acta Cytol 21:770, 1977.
61. Krumerman MS: Leiomyosarcoma of the lung primary cytodiagnosis in two consecutive cases. Acta Cytol 21:103, 1977.
62. Lee SH, Rengachary SS, Paramesh J: Primary pulmonary rhabdomyosarcoma: A case report and review of the literature. Hum Pathol 12:92, 1981.
63. Ho K-L, Rassekh ZS: Rhabdomyosarcoma of the trachea: First reported case. Hum Pathol 11:572, 1980.
64. Aterman K, Patel S: Striated muscle in the lung. Am J Anat 128:341, 1970.
65. Drennan JM, McCormack RJM: Primary rhabdomyosarcoma of the lung. J Pathol Bacteriol 79:147, 1960.
66. Allan BT, Day DL, Dehner LP: Primary pulmonary rhabdomyosarcoma of the lung in children. Cancer 59:1005, 1987.
67. Przygodzki RM, Moran CA, Suster S, et al: Primary pulmonary rhabdomyosarcomas: A clinicopathologic and immunohistochemical study of three cases. Mod Pathol 8:658, 1995.
68. Fallon G, Schiller M, Kilman JW: Primary rhabdomyosarcoma of the bronchus. Ann Thorac Surg 12:650, 1971.
69. Eriksson A, Thunell M, Lundqvist G: Pendulating endobronchial rhabdomyosarcoma with fatal asphyxia. Thorax 37:390, 1982.
70. Crist WM, Raney RB Jr, Newton W, et al: Intrathoracic soft tissue sarcomas in children. Cancer 50:598, 1982.
71. Ueda K, Gruppo R, Unger F, et al: Rhabdomyosarcoma of lung arising in congenital cystic adenomatoid malformation. Cancer 40:383, 1977.
72. Eriksson A, Thunell M, Lundqvist G: Pendulating endobronchial rhabdomyosarcoma with fatal asphyxia. Thorax 37:390, 1982.
73. Ishizuka T, Yoshitake J, Yamada T, et al: Diagnosis of a case of pulmonary carcinosarcoma by detection of rhabdomyosarcoma cells in sputum. Acta Cytol 32:658, 1988.

74. Avagnina A, Elsner B, De Marco L, et al: Pulmonary rhabdomyosarcoma with isolated small bowel metastasis: A report of a case with immunohistochemical ultrastructural studies. Cancer 53:1948, 1984.

75. Garcia-Prats MD, Sotelo-Rodriguez MT, Ballestin C, et al: Glomus tumour of the trachea: Report of a case with microscopic, ultrastructural and immunohistochemical examination and review of the literature. Histopathology 19:459, 1991.

75a. Koss MN, Hochholzer L, Moran CA: Primary pulmonary glomus tumor: A clinicopathologic and immunohistochemical study of two cases. Mod Pathol 11:253, 1998.

76. Heard BE, Dewar A, Firmin RK, et al: One very rare and one new tracheal tumor found by electron microscopy: Glomus tumour and acinic cell tumour resembling carcinoid tumours by light microscopy. Thorax 37:97, 1982.

77. Alt B, Huffer WE, Belchis DA: A vascular lesion with smooth muscle differentiation presenting as a coin lesion in the lung: Glomus tumor versus hemangiopericytoma. Am J Clin Pathol 80:765, 1983.

78. Tang C-K, Toker C, Foris NP, et al: Glomangioma of the lung. Am J Surg Pathol 2:103, 1978.

79. Fabich DR, Hafez G-R: Glomangioma of the trachea. Cancer 45:2337, 1980.

80. Kim YI, Kim JH, Suh J-S, et al: Glomus tumor of the trachea: Report of a case with ultrastructural observation. Cancer 64:881, 1989.

81. Garcia-Prats MD, Sotelo-Rodriguez MT, Ballestin C, et al: Glomus tumour of the trachea: Report of a case with microscopic, ultrastructural and immunohistochemical examination and review of the literature. Histopathology 19:459, 1991.

82. Mackay B, Legha SS: Coin lesion of the lung in a 19 year old male. Ultrastruct Pathol 2:289, 1981.

83. Meade JB, Whitwell F, Bickford BJ, et al: Primary haemangiopericytoma of lung. Thorax 29:1, 1974.

84. Gavilan J, Rodriquez-Peralto JT, Tomas HO, et al: Hemangiopericytoma of the trachea. J Laryngol Otol 101:738, 1987.

85. McCormack LJ, McIsaac WM, Ragde H, et al: "Functioning" pulmonary neoplasms: I. The carcinoid tumor. II. The hemangiopericytoma. Cleve Clin Q 28:145, 1961.

86. Vidrine A Jr, Welsh RA: Hemangiopericytoma: 5 cases. Surgery 56:912, 1964.

87. Yousem SA, Hochholzer L: Primary pulmonary hemangiopericytoma. Cancer 59:549, 1987.

88. Razzuk MA, Nassur A, Gradner MA, et al: Primary pulmonary hemangiopericytoma. J Thorac Cardiovasc Surg 74:227, 1977.

88a. Halle M, Blum U, Dinkel E, Brugger W: CT and MR features of primary pulmonary hemangiopericytomas. J Comput Assist Tomogr 17:51, 1993.

88b. Kuroya M, Yokomise H, Inui K, et al: Resection of primary pulmonary hemangiopericytoma: A report of two cases. Surg Today 26:208, 1996.

89. Rusch VW, Shuman WP, Schmidt R, et al: Massive pulmonary hemangiopericytoma: An innovative approach to evaluation and treatment. Cancer 64:1928, 1989.

90. Feldman F, Seaman WB: Primary thoracic hemangiopericytoma. Radiology 82:998, 1964.

91. Rothe TB, Karrer W, Gebbers JO: Recurrent haemoptysis in a young woman: A case of a malignant haemangiopericytoma of the lung. Thorax 49:188, 1994.

92. van Assendelft AH, Strengell-Usanov L, Kastarinen S: Pulmonary haemangiopericytoma with multiple metastases. Eur J Respir Dis 65:380, 1984.

93. Hart LL, Weinberg JB: Metastatic hemangiopericytoma with prolonged survival. Cancer 60:916, 1987.

94. Enzinger FM, Smith BH: Hemangiopericytoma: An analysis of 106 cases. Hum Pathol 7:61, 1976.

95. Khan GA, Klapper P: Pulmonary haemorrhage following renal transplantation. Thorax 50:98, 1995.

96. Antman KH, Nadler L, Mark EJ, et al: Primary Kaposi's sarcoma of the lung in an immunocompetent 32-year-old heterosexual white man. Cancer 54:1696, 1984.

97. Cesarman E, Knowles DM: Kaposi's sarcoma–associated herpesvirus: A lymphotropic human herpesvirus associated with Kaposi's sarcoma, primary effusion lymphoma, and multicentric Castelman's disease. Semin Diag Pathol 14:54, 1997.

98. Cox FH, Helwig EB: Kaposi's sarcoma. Cancer 12:289, 1959.

99. Hamm PG, Judson MA, Aranda CP: Diagnosis of pulmonary Kaposi's sarcoma with fiberoptic bronchoscopy and endobronchial biopsy. Cancer 59:807, 1987.

100. Misra DP, Sunderrajan EV, Hurst DJ, et al: Kaposi's sarcoma of the lung: Radiography and pathology. Thorax 37:155, 1982.

101. Nash G, Fligiel S: Kaposi's sarcoma presenting as pulmonary disease in the acquired immunodeficiency syndrome: Diagnosis by lung biopsy. Hum Pathol 15:999, 1984.

102. Stats D: The visceral manifestations of Kaposi's sarcoma. J Mount Sinai Hosp 12:971, 1946.

103. Fouret PJ, Touboul JL, Mayaud CM, et al: Pulmonary Kaposi's sarcoma in patients with acquired immune deficiency syndrome: A clinicopathological study. Thorax 42:262, 1987.

104. Dantzig PI, Rayhanzadeh S, Richardson D, et al: Thoracic involvement of non-African Kaposi's sarcoma. Chest 66:522, 1974.

105. Chin R Jr, Jones DF, Pegram PS, et al: Complete endobronchial occlusion by Kaposi's sarcoma in the absence of cutaneous involvement. Chest 105:1581, 1994.

106. Sivit CJ, Schwartz AM, Rockoff SD: Kaposi's sarcoma of the lung in AIDS: Radiologic/pathologic analysis. Am J Roentgenol 148:25, 1987.

107. Goodman PC: Kaposi's sarcoma. J Thorac Imaging 6:43, 1991.

108. Naidich DP, McGuinness G: Pulmonary manifestations of AIDS: CT and radiographic correlations. Radiol Clin North Am 29:999, 1991.

108a. McGuinness G: Changing trends in the pulmonary manifestations of AIDS. Radiol Clin North Am 35:1029, 1997.

109. Mandel C, Silberstein M, Hennessy O: Case report: Fatal pulmonary Kaposi's sarcoma and Castleman's disease in a renal transplant recipient. Br J Radiol 66:264, 1993.

110. Wolff SD, Kuhlman JE, Fishman EK: Thoracic Kaposi sarcoma in AIDS: CT findings. J Comput Assist Tomogr 17:60, 1993.

111. Hartman TE, Primack SL, Müller NL, Staples CA. Diagnosis of thoracic complications in AIDS: Accuracy of CT. Am J Roentgenol 162:547, 1994.

112. Khalil AM, Carette MF, Cadranel JL, et al: Intrathoracic Kaposi's sarcoma: CT findings. Chest 108:1622, 1995.

113. Medur GU, Stover DE, Lee M, et al: Pulmonary Kaposi's sarcoma in the acquired immune deficiency syndrome. Am J Med 81:11, 1986.

114. Lacquet LK, Mouli AC, Jongerius CM, et al: Intrathoracic chemodectoma with multiple localisations. Thorax 32:203, 1977.

115. Dail D, Liebow A: Intravascular bronchioloalveolar tumor. Am J Pathol 78:6a, 1975.

116. Taguchi T, Tsuji K, Matsuo K, et al: Intravascular bronchioloalveolar tumor: Report of an autopsy case and review of literature. Acta Pathol Jpn 35:631, 1985.

117. Dail DH, Liebow AA, Gmelich JT, et al: Intravascular, bronchiolar, and alveolar tumor of the lung (IVBAT): An analysis of twenty cases of a peculiar sclerosing endothelial tumor. Cancer 51:452, 1983.

118. Corrin B, Manners B, Millard M, et al: Histogenesis of the so-called "intravascular bronchioloalveolar tumour." J Pathol 128:163, 1979.

119. Weldon-Linne CM, Victor TA, Christ ML, et al: Angiogenic nature of the "intravascular bronchioloalveolar tumor" of the lung: An electron microscopic study. Arch Pathol Lab Med 105:174, 1981.

120. Corrin B, Harrison WJ, Wright DH: The so-called intravascular bronchioloalveolar tumour of the lung (low grade sclerosing angiosarcoma): Presentation with extrapulmonary deposits. Diagn Histopathol 6:229, 1983.

121. Sugiyama Y, Yamaguchi K, Oka T, et al: Intravascular bronchiolo-alveolar tumor (IVBAT): Case report with the immunological analysis. Jpn J Med 25:80, 1986.

122. Azumi N, Churg A: Intravascular and sclerosing bronchioloalveolar tumor: A pulmonary sarcoma of probable vascular origin. Am J Surg Pathol 5:587, 1981.

123. Bhagavan BS, Dorfman HD, Murthy MSN, et al: Intravascular bronchioloalveolar tumor (IVBAT): A low-grade sclerosing epithelioid angiosarcoma of lung. Am J Surg Pathol 6:41, 1982.

124. Weiss SW, Enzinger FM: Epithelioid hemangioendothelioma: A vascular tumor often mistaken for a carcinoma. Cancer 50:970, 1982.

125. Eggleston JC: The intravascular bronchioloalveolar tumor and the sclerosing hemangioma of the lung: Misnomers of pulmonary neoplasia. Semin Diagn Pathol 2:270, 1985.

126. Nerlich A, Berndt R, Schleicher E: Differential basement membrane composition in multiple epithelioid haemangioendotheliomas of liver and lung. Histopathology 18:303, 1991.

127. Verbeken E, Beyls J, Moerman P, et al: Lung metastasis of malignant epithelioid hemangioendothelioma mimicking a primary intravascular bronchioalveolar tumor. Cancer 55:1741, 1985.

128. Corrin B, Dewar A, Simpson CG: Epithelioid hemangioendothelioma of the lung. Ultrastruct Pathol 20:345, 1996.

129. Yousem SA, Hochholzer L: Unusual thoracic manifestations of epithelioid hemangioendothelioma. Arch Pathol Lab Med 111:459, 1987.

130. Sherman JL, Rykwalder PJ, Tashkin DP: Intravascular bronchioloalveolar tumor. Am Rev Respir Dis 123:468, 1981.

131. Sicilian L, Warson F, Carrington CB, et al: Intravascular bronchioloalveolar tumor (IV-BAT). Respiration 44:387, 1983.

132. Buggage RR, Soudi N, Olson JL, et al: Epithelioid hemangioendothelioma of the lung: Pleural effusion cytology, ultrastructure, and brief literature review. Diagn Cytopathol 13:54, 1995.

133. Luburich P, Ayuso MC, Picado C, et al: CT of pulmonary epithelioid hemangioendothelioma. J Comput Assist Tomogr 18:562, 1994.

134. Nakatani Y, Aoki I, Misugi K: Immunohistochemical and ultrastructural study of early lesions of intravascular bronchioloalveolar tumor with liver involvement. Acta Pathol Jpn 35:1453, 1985.

135. Bollinger BK, Laskin WB, Knight CB: Epithelioid hemangioendothelioma with multiple site involvement: Literature review and observations. Cancer 73:610, 1994.

136. Yi ES, Auger WR, Friedman PJ, et al: Intravascular bronchioloalveolar tumor of the lung presenting as pulmonary thromboembolic disease and pulmonary hypertension. Arch Pathol Lab Med 119:255, 1995.

137. Wenisch HJC, Lulay M: Lymphogenous spread of an intravascular bronchioloalveolar tumour: Case report and review of literature. Virchows Arch [Pathol Anat Histol] 387:117, 1980.

138. Borlee-Hermans G, Bury T, Grand JL, et al: Intravascular bronchioloalveolar tumour. Eur J Respir Dis 66:341, 1985.

139. Miyauchi J, Mukai M, Yamazaki K, et al: Bilateral ovarian hemangiomas associated with diffuse hemangioendotheliomatosis: A case report. Acta Pathol Jpn 37:1347, 1987.

140. Teo SK, Chiang SC, Tan KK: Intravascular bronchioloalveolar tumour: A 20-year survival. Med J Aust 142:220, 1985.

141. Tamm M, Reichenberger F, McGandy CE, et al: Diagnosis of pulmonary Kaposi's sarcoma by detection of human herpesvirus 8 in bronchoalveolar lavage. Am J Respir Crit Care Med 157:458, 1998.

142. Tralka GA, Katz S: Hemangioendothelioma of the lung. Am Rev Respir Dis 87:107, 1963.

143. Hall EM: A malignant hemangioma of the lung with multiple metastases. Am J Pathol 11:343, 1935.
144. Spragg RG, Wolf PL, Haghighi P, et al: Angiosarcoma of the lung with fatal pulmonary hemorrhage. Am J Med 74:1072, 1983.
145. Yousem SA: Angiosarcoma presenting in the lung. Arch Pathol Lab Med 110:112, 1986.
146. Mullick SS, Mody DR, Schwartz MR: Angiosarcoma at unusual sites: A report of two cases with aspiration cytology and diagnostic pitfalls. Acta Cytol 41:839, 1997.
147. Sheppard MN, Hansell DM, Bois RM, et al: Primary epithelioid angiosarcoma of the lung presenting as pulmonary hemorrhage. Hum Pathol 28:383, 1997.
148. Plaut A: Case reports: Hemangioendothelioma of the lung: Report of two cases. Arch Pathol 29:517, 1940.
149. Wollstein M: Malignant hemangioma of the lung with multiple visceral foci. Report of a case. Arch Pathol 12:562, 1931.
150. Nappi O, Swanson PE, Wick MR: Pseudovascular adenoid squamous cell carcinoma of the lung: Clinicopathologic study of three cases and comparison with true pleuropulmonary angiosarcoma. Hum Pathol 25:373, 1994.
151. Ebi N, Yamamoto H, Sakai J, et al: Angiosarcoma of the heart presenting as fatal pulmonary hemorrhage. Intern Med 36:191, 1997.
152. Nara M, Sasaki T, Shimura S, et al: Diffuse alveolar hemorrhage caused by lung metastasis of ovarian angiosarcoma. Intern Med 35:653, 1996.
153. Kayser K, Bauer M, Lueillig H, et al: Long-term development of a primary lung sarcoma, probably lymphangiosarcoma: A case report. J Thorac Cardiovasc Surg 32:178, 1984.
154. Kaufman J: Endobronchial chondroma: Clinical and physiologic improvement following excision. Am Rev Respir Dis 100:711, 1969.
155. Davidson M: A case of primary chondroma of the bronchus. Br J Surg 28:571, 1941.
156. Walsh TJ, Healy TM: Chondroma of the bronchus. Thorax 24:327, 1969.
157. Tomashefski JF Jr: Benign endobronchial mesenchymal tumors: Their relationship to parenchymal pulmonary hamartomas. Am J Surg Pathol 6:531, 1982.
158. Carney JA, Sheps SG, Go VL, et al: The triad of gastric leiomyosarcoma, functioning extra-adrenal paraganglioma and pulmonary chondroma. N Engl J Med 296:1517, 1977.
159. Carney JA: The triad of gastric epithelioid leiomyosarcoma, functioning extra-adrenal paraganglioma, and pulmonary chondroma. Cancer 43:374, 1979.
160. Dajee A, Dajee H, Hinrichs S, et al: Pulmonary chondroma, extra-adrenal paraganglioma, and gastric leiomyosarcoma. J Thorac Cardiovasc Surg 84:377, 1982.
161. Mishkin FS, Vasinrapee P, Vore L, et al: Carney's triad: Radiographic diagnosis, natural history and importance of pulmonary chondromas. J Can Assoc Radiol 38:264, 1985.
162. Keyhani-Rofagha S, O'Dorisio TM, Lucas JG, et al: Extra-adrenal paraganglioma and pulmonary chondroma: A case report and review of the literature. J Surg Oncol 35:89, 1987.
163. Raafat F, Salman WD, Roberts K, et al: Carney's triad: Gastric leiomyosarcoma, pulmonary chondroma and extra-adrenal paraganglioma in young females. Histopathology 10:1325, 1986.
164. Mishkin FS, Vasinrapee P, Vora L, et al: Carney's triad: Radiographic diagnosis, natural history and importance of pulmonary chondromas. Can Assoc Radiol J 36:264, 1985.
165. Schmutz GR, Fisch-Ponsot C, Sylvestre J: Carney syndrome: Radiologic features. Can Assoc Radiol J 45:148, 1994.
166. Lancha C, Diez L, Mitjavila M, et al: A case of complete Carney's syndrome. Clin Nucl Med 19:1008, 1994.
167. Tisell L-E, Angervall L, Dahl I, et al: Recurrent and metastasizing gastric leiomyoblastoma (epithelioid leiomyosarcoma) associated with multiple pulmonary chondro-hamartomas: Long survival of a patient treated with repeated operations. Cancer 41:259, 1978.
167a. Converry RP, Grainger AJ, Bhatnagar NK, et al: Lung abscess complicating chondromas in Carney's syndrome. Eur Respir J 11:1409, 1998.
168. Case Report: Carney's triad: Role of transthoracic needle biopsy. Am Rev Respir Dis 128:311, 1983.
169. Hayashi T, Tsuda N, Iseki M, et al: Primary chondrosarcoma of the lung: A clinicopathologic study. Cancer 72:69, 1993.
170. Yellin A, Schwartz L, Hersho E, et al: Chondrosarcoma of the bronchus: Report of a case with resection and review of the literature. Chest 84:224, 1983.
171. Morgan AD, Salama FD: Primary chondrosarcoma of the lung: Case report and review of the literature. J Thorac Cardiovasc Surg 64:460, 1972.
172. D'Ambrosio FG, Shiu MH, Brennan MF: Intrapulmonary presentation of extraskeletal myxoid chondrosarcoma of the extremity: Report of two cases. Cancer 58:1144, 1986.
173. Fallahnejad M, Harrell D, Tucker J, et al: Chondrosarcoma of the trachea: Report of a case and five-year follow-up. J Thorac Cardiovasc Surg 65:210, 1973.
174. Daniels AC, Conner GH, Straus FH: Primary chondrosarcoma of the tracheobronchial tree: Report of a unique case and brief review. Arch Pathol 84:615, 1967.
175. Sun C-CJ, Kroll M, Miller JE: Primary chondrosarcoma of the lung. Cancer 50:1864, 1982.
176. Jazy FK, Cormier WJ, Panke TW, et al: Primary chondrosarcoma of the lung: A report of two cases. Clin Oncol 10:273, 1984.
177. Reingold IM, Amromin GD: Extraosseous osteosarcoma of the lung. Cancer 28:491, 1971.
178. Colby TV, Bilbao JE, Battifora H, et al: Primary osteosarcoma of the lung: A

reappraisal following immunohistologic study. Arch Pathol Lab Med 113:1147, 1989.
179. Loose JH, el-Naggar AK, Ro JY, et al: Primary osteosarcoma of the lung: Report of two cases and review of the literature. J Thorac Cardiovasc Surg 100:867, 1990.
180. Petersen M: Radionuclide detection of primary pulmonary osteogenic sarcoma: A case report and review of the literature. J Nucl Med 31:1110, 1990.
181. Stark P, Smith DC, Watkins GE, Chun KE: Primary intrathoracic extraosseous osteogenic sarcoma: Report of three cases. Radiology 174:725, 1990.
182. Roviaro G, Montorsi M, Varoli F, et al: Primary pulmonary tumours of neurogenic origin. Thorax 38:942, 1983.
183. Unger PD, Geller GA, Anderson PJ: Pulmonary lesions in a patient with neurofibromatosis. Arch Pathol Lab Med 108:654, 1984.
184. McCluggage WG, Bharucha H: Primary pulmonary tumours of nerve sheath origin. Histopathology 26:247, 1995
185. Thijs-Van Nies A, Van De Brekel B, Buytendijk HJ, et al: Neurofibroma of the trachea: A case report. Thorax 33:121, 1978.
186. Horovitz AG, Khalil KG, Verani RR, et al: Primary intratracheal neurilemoma. J Thorac Cardiovasc Surg 85:313, 1983.
187. Thijs-van Nies A, Van de Brekel B, Buytendijk HJ, et al: Neurofibroma of the trachea: A case report. Thorax 33:121, 1978.
188. Feldhaus RJ, Anene C, Bogard P: A rare endobronchial neurilemmoma (schwannoma). Chest 95:461, 1989.
189. Nesbitt JC, Vega DM, Mackey B: Cellular schwannoma of the bronchus. Ultrastruct Pathol 20:349, 1996.
190. Bartley TD, Arean VM: Intrapulmonary neurogenic tumors. J Thorac Cardiovasc Surg 50:114, 1965.
191. Silverman JF, Leffers BR, Kay S: Primary pulmonary neurilemoma: Report of a case with ultrastructural examination. Arch Pathol Lab Med 100:644, 1976.
192. Muhrer KH, Fischer HP: Primary pulmonary neurilemoma. J Thorac Cardiovasc Surg 31:313, 1983.
193. Cooney TP: Primary pulmonary ganglioneuroblastoma in an adult: Maturation, involution and the immune response. Histopathology 5:451, 1981.
194. Donnal JF, Coblentz CL, Bergin CJ: Stump neuroma masquerading as recurrent malignancy on chest roentgenogram. Chest 95:684, 1989.
195. Meredith HC, Valicenti JF Jr: Solitary neurofibroma of the trachea: A case report. Br J Radiol 51:218, 1978.
196. O'Donohue WJ Jr, Edland J, Mohiuddin SM, et al: Multiple pulmonary neurofibromas with hypoxemia: Occurrence due to pulmonary arteriovenous shunts within the tumors. Arch Intern Med 146:1618, 1986.
197. Oparah SS, Subramanian VA: Granular cell myoblastoma of the bronchus: Report of 2 cases and review of the literature. Ann Thorac Surg 22:199, 1976.
198. Deavers M, Guinee D, Koss MN, et al: Granular cell tumors of the lung: Clinicopathologic study of 20 cases. Am J Surg Pathol 19:627, 1995.
199. Valenstein SL, Thurer RJ: Granular cell myoblastoma of the bronchus: Case report and literature review. J Thorac Cardiovasc Surg 76:465, 1978.
200. Thomas de Montpreville V, Dulmet EM: Granular cell tumours of the lower respiratory tract. Histopathology 27:257, 1995.
201. Stey CA, Vogt P, Russi EW: Endobronchial lipomatous hamartoma. A rare cause of bronchial occlusion. Chest 113:254, 1998.
202. Ivatury R, Shah D, Ascer E, et al: Granular cell tumor of larynx and bronchus. Ann Thorac Surg 33:69, 1982.
203. Bush RW, Plain GL: Granular cell tumors (myoblastomas) involving the bronchus and skin: Report of a case. Am J Clin Pathol 50:563, 1968.
204. O'Connell DJ, MacMahon H, De Meester TR: Multicentric tracheobronchial and oesophageal granular cell myoblastoma. Thorax 33:596, 1978.
205. Stefansson K, Wollmann RL: S-100 protein in granular cell tumors (granular cell myoblastomas). Cancer 49:1834, 1982.
206. Sobel HJ, Marquet E: Granular cells and granular cell lesions. Pathol Annu 9:43, 1974.
207. Block SR, Christian CL: The pathogenesis of systemic lupus erythematosus. Am J Med 59:453, 1975.
208. Benisch BM, Abt AB, Abramson A: Granular cell myoblastoma of trachea associated with pregnancy. Chest 63:832, 1973.
209. Mikaelian DD, Cohn H, Israel H, et al: Granular cell tumor of the trachea. Ann Otol Rhinol Laryngol 93:457, 1984.
210. Muthuswamy PP, Alrenga DP, Marks P, et al: Granular cell myoblastoma: Rare localization in the trachea: Report of a case and review of the literature. Am J Med 80:714, 1986.
211. Alvarez-Fernandez E, Carretero-Albinana L: Bronchial granular cell tumor: Presentation of three cases with tissue culture and ultrastructural study. Arch Pathol Lab Med 111:1065, 1987.
212. Hebert WM, Seale RH, Samson PC: Primary granular-cell myoblastoma of the bronchus: Report of a case with resection. J Thorac Surg 34:409, 1957.
213. Gabriel JB Jr, Thomas L, Kondlapoodi P, et al: Granular cell tumor of the bronchus: A previously unreported cause of hypercalcemia. J Surg Oncol 24:338, 1983.
214. Campbell DC Jr, Smith EP Jr, Hood RH Jr: Benign granular-cell myoblastoma of the bronchus: Review of the literature and report of a case. Dis Chest 46:729, 1964.
215. Schulster PL, Khan FA, Azueta V: Asymptomatic pulmonary granular cell tumor presenting as a coin lesion. Chest 68:256, 1975.
216. Korompai FL, Awe RJ, Beall AC, et al: Granular cell myoblastoma of the bronchus: A new case, 12-year followup report, and review of the literature. Chest 66:578, 1974.

217. Glant MD, Wall RW, Ransburg R: Endobronchial granular cell tumor: Cytology of a new case and review of the literature. Acta Cytol 23:477, 1979.

218. Thomas L, Risbud M, Gabriel JB, et al: Cytomorphology of granular-cell tumor of the bronchus: A case report. Acta Cytol 28:129, 1984.

219. Majmudar B, Thomas J, Gorelkin L, et al: Respiratory obstruction caused by a multicentric granular cell tumor of the laryngotrache-obronchial tree. Hum Pathol 12:283, 1981.

220. Steffelaar JW, Nap M, von Haelst UJGM: Malignant granular cell tumor: Report of a case with special reference to carcinoembryonic antigen. Am J Surg Pathol 6:665, 1982.

221. Hurwitz SS, Conlan AA, Gritzman MCD, et al: Coexisting granular cell myoblastoma and squamous carcinoma of the bronchus. Thorax 37:392, 1982.

222. Liebman J, Linthicum CM: Granular cell myoblastoma (schwannoma) of the carina in a patient with sarcoidosis. South Med J 69:1613, 1976.

223. Ganti S, Marino W: Granular cell myoblastoma in an HIV positive patient. N Y State J Med 91:265, 1991.

224. Schraufnagel DE, Morin JE, Wang NS: Endobronchial lipoma. Chest 75:97, 1979.

225. Politis J, Funahashi A, Gehlsen JA, et al: Intrathoracic lipomas: Report of three cases and review of the literature with emphasis on endobronchial lipoma. J Thorac Cardiovasc Surg 77:550, 1979.

226. Hirata T, Reshad K, Itoi K, et al: Lipomas of the peripheral lung—a case report and review of the literature. Thorac Cardiovasc Surg 37:385, 1989.

227. Palvio D, Egeblad K, Paulsen SM: Atypical lipomatous hamartoma of the lung. Virchows Arch [Pathol Anat] 405:253, 1985.

228. Plachta A, Hershey H: Lipoma of the lung: Review of the literature and report of a case. Am Rev Respir Dis 86:912, 1962.

229. Touroff ASW, Seley GP: Lipoma of the bronchus and the lung: A report of two unusual cases. Ann Surg 134:244, 1951.

230. Matsuba K, Saito T, Ando K, et al: Atypical lipoma of the lung. Thorax 46:685, 1991.

231. Eastridge CE, Young JM, Steplock AL: Endobronchial lipoma. South Med J 77:759, 1984.

232. Spindel E, Man GCW, Sproule BJ: Intrathoracic liposarcoma: Abnormal regional xenon-133 V/Q study. J Can Assoc Radiol 33:116, 1982.

233. Spinka J, Zwetschke O: Tracheal lipoma simulating the picture of severe bronchial asthma. Cas Lek Cesk 101:395, 1962.

234. Ruiz-Palomo F, Calleja JL, Fogue L: Primary liposarcoma of the lung in a young woman. Thorax 45:908, 1990.

235. Sawamura K, Hashimoto T, Nanjo S, et al: Primary liposarcoma of the lung: Report of a case. J Surg Oncol 19:243, 1982.

236. Van Den Beukel JTI, Wagenaar SJSC, Vanderschueren R: Short reports: Liposarcoma of the trachea. Thorax 34:817, 1979.

237. Wu JP, Gilbert EF, Pellett JR: Pulmonary liposarcoma in a child with adrenogenital syndrome. Am J Clin Pathol 62:791, 1974.

238. Wang NS, Morin J: Recurrent endobronchial soft tissue tumors. Chest 85:787, 1984.

239. Pollak ER, Naunheim KS, Little AG: Fibromyxoma of the trachea. Arch Pathol Lab Med 109:926, 1985.

240. Littlefield JB, Drash EC: Myxoma of the lung. J Thorac Surg 37:745, 1959.

241. Yousem SA, Flynn SD: Intrapulmonary localized fibrous tumor: Intraparenchymal so-called localized fibrous mesothelioma. Am J Clin Pathol 89:365, 1988.

242. Goodlad JR, Fletcher CD: Solitary fibrous tumour arising at unusual sites: Analysis of a series. Histopathology 19:515, 1991.

243. Miller MAL, Toma GA: Fibroma of the trachea. Br J Dis Chest 53:177, 1959.

244. Kovarik JL, Prather Ashe SM: Intrapulmonary fibroma. Am Rev Respir Dis 88:539, 1963.

245. Weiss SW, Enzinger FM: Malignant fibrous histiocytoma: An analysis of 200 cases. Cancer 41:2250, 1978.

246. Halyard MY, Camoriano JK, Culligan JA, et al: Malignant fibrous histiocytoma of the lung: Report of four cases and review of the literature. Cancer 78:2492, 1996.

247. Yousem SA, Hochholzer L: Malignant fibrous histiocytoma of the lung. Cancer 60:2532, 1987.

248. Gal AA, Koss MN, McCarthy WF, et al: Prognostic factors in pulmonary fibrohistiocytic lesions. Cancer 73:1817, 1994.

249. Weiss SW: Malignant fibrous histiocytoma: A reaffirmation. Am J Surg Pathol 6:773, 1982.

250. Yonemoto T, Takenouchi T, Tokita H, et al: Establishment and characterization of a human malignant fibrous histiocytoma cell line. Clin Orthop Rel Res 320:159, 1995.

251. Chowdhury LN, Swerdlow MA, Jao W, et al: Postirradiation malignant fibrous histiocytoma of the lung: Demonstration of alpha₁ antitrypsin-like material in neoplastic cells. Am J Clin Pathol 74:820, 1980.

252. Reifsnyder AC, Smith HJ, Mulhollan TJ, Lee EL: Malignant fibrous histiocytoma of the lung in a patient with a history of asbestos exposure. Am J Roentgenol 154:65, 1990.

253. Kern WH, Hughes RK, Meyer BW, et al: Malignant fibrous histiocytoma of the lung. Cancer 44:1793, 1979.

254. McDonnell T, Kyriakos M, Roper C, Mazoujian G: Malignant fibrous histiocytoma of the lung. Cancer 61:137, 1988.

255. Ismailer I, Khan A, Leonidas J, et al: Computed tomography of primary malignant fibrohistiocytoma of the lung. Comput Radiol 11:37, 1987.

256. Gilman JK, Sievers DB, Thornsvard CT: Malignant fibrous histiocytoma manifesting as a cavitary lung metastasis. South Med J 79:376, 1986.

257. Misra DP, Sunderrajan EV, Rosenholtz MJ, et al: Malignant fibrous histiocytoma in the lung masquerading as recurrent pulmonary thromboembolism. Cancer 51:538, 1983.

258. Tanino M, Odashima S, Sugiura H, et al: Malignant fibrous histiocytoma of the lung. Acta Pathol Jpn 35:945, 1985.

259. Kawahara E, Nakanishi I, Kuroda Y, et al: Fine needle aspiration biopsy of primary malignant fibrous histiocytoma of the lung. Acta Cytol 32:226, 1988.

260. Lee JT, Shelburne JD, Linder J: Primary malignant fibrous histiocytoma of the lung: A clinicopathologic and ultrastructural study of five cases. Cancer 53:1124, 1984.

261. Suzuki N, Ohno S, Ishii Y, et al: Peripheral intrapulmonary hamartoma accompanied by a similar endotracheal lesion. Chest 106:1291, 1994.

262. Bateson EM: Histogenesis of intrapulmonary and endobronchial hamartomas and chondromas (cartilage-containing tumours): A hypothesis. J Pathol 101:77, 1970.

263. Bateson EM: So-called hamartoma of the lung—a true neoplasm of fibrous connective tissue of the bronchi. Cancer 31:1458, 1973.

264. Van Den Bosch JMM, Wagenaar SS, Corrin B, et al: Mesenchymoma of the lung (so called hamartoma): A review of 154 parenchymal and endobronchial cases. Thorax 42:790, 1987.

265. Bateson EM, Abbott EK: Mixed tumors of the lung, or hamarto-chondromas: A review of the radiological appearances of cases published in the literature and a report of fifteen new cases. Clin Radiol 11:232, 1960.

266. Koutras P, Urschel HC, Paulson DL: Hamartoma of the lung. J Thorac Cardiovasc Surg 61:768, 1971.

267. Butler C, Kleinerman J: Pulmonary hamartoma. Arch Pathol 88:584, 1969.

268. Hansen CP, Holtveg H, Francis D, et al: Pulmonary hamartoma. J Thorac Cadiovasc Surg 104:674, 1992.

269. Sagel SS, Ablow RC: Hamartoma: On occasion a rapidly growing tumor of the lung. Radiology 91:971, 1968.

270. Jensen JG, Schiodt T: Growth conditions of hamartoma of the lung: A study based on 22 cases operated on after radiographic observation for from one to 18 years. Thorax 13:233, 1958.

271. Stey CA, Vogt P, Russi EW: Endobronchial lipomatous hamartoma: A rare cause of bronchial occlusion. Chest 113:254, 1998.

272. Perez-Atayde AR, Seiler MW: Pulmonary hamartoma. Cancer 53:485, 1984.

273. Incze JS, Lui PS: Morphology of the epithelial component of human lung hamartomas. Hum Pathol 8:411, 1977.

274. Fletcher JA, Pinkus GS, Donovan K, et al: Clonal rearrangement of chromosome band 6p21 in the mesenchymal component of pulmonary chondroid hamartoma. Cancer Res 52:6224, 1992.

275. Johansson M, Heim S, Mandahl N, et al: t(3;6;14) (p21;p21;q24) as the sole clonal chromosome abnormality in a hamartoma of the lung. Cancer Genet Cytogenet 60:219, 1992.

276. Schoenmakers EF, Geurts JM, Kools PF, et al: A 6-Mb yeast artificial chromosome contig and long-range physical map encompassing the region on chromosome 12q15 frequently rearranged in a variety of benign solid tumors. Genomics 29:665, 1995.

277. Fejzo MS, Yoon SJ, Montgomery KT, et al: Identification of a YAC spanning the translocation breakpoints in uterine leiomyomata, pulmonary chondroid hamartoma, and lipoma: Physical mapping of the 12q14-q15 breakpoint region in uterine leiomyomata. Genomics 26:265, 1995.

278. Van Den Bosch JMM, Wagenaar SS, Corrin B, et al: Mesenchymoma of the lung (so-called hamartoma): A review of 154 parenchymal and endobronchial cases. Thorax 42:790, 1987.

279. Bateson EM: Relationship between intrapulmonary and endobronchial cartilage-containing tumors (so-called hamartomata). Thorax 20:447, 1965.

280. Jones CJ: Unusual hamartoma of the lung in a newborn infant. Arch Pathol 48:150, 1949.

281. Scully RE, Mark EJ, McNeely BU: Case report: Case #32-1985. N Engl J Med 313:374, 1985.

282. Holden WE, Mulkey DD, Kessler S: Multiple peripheral lung cysts and hemoptysis in an otherwise asymptomatic adult. Am Rev Respir Dis 126:930, 1982.

283. Freedman AP, Radocha RF, Shinnick JP: Bronchial angiofibromata in a suspected case of tuberous sclerosis. Chest 76:469, 1979.

284. Thyresson HN, Doyle JA: Cowden's disease (multiple hamartoma syndrome). Mayo Clin Proc 56:179, 1981.

285. Sasaki M, Hakozaki H, Ishihara T: Cowden's disease with pulmonary hamartoma. Intern Med 32:39, 1993.

286. McDonald JR, Harrington SW, Clagett OT: Hamartoma (often called chondroma) of the lung. J Thorac Cardiovasc Surg 14:128, 1945.

287. Bateson EM: An analysis of 155 solitary lung lesions illustrating the differential diagnosis of mixed tumours of the lung. Clin Radiol 16:51, 1965.

288. Grayson W, Leiman G, Cooper K: Exuberant fibroadenomatoid proliferation in a pulmonary mesenchymoma (hamartoma): Report of a lesion mimicking a sclerosing pneumocytoma. Gen Diagn Pathol 142:247, 1997.

289. Gudbjerg CF: Pulmonary hamartoma. Am J Roentgenol 86:842, 1961.

290. Gjevre JA, Myers JL, Prakash UB: Pulmonary hamartomas. Mayo Clin Proc 71:14, 1996.

291. Gjevre JA, Myers JL, Prakash UBS: Pulmonary hamartomas. Mayo Clin Proc 71:14, 1996.

292. Peleg H, Pauzner Y: Benign tumors of the lung. Dis Chest 47:179, 1965.

293. Darke CS, Day P, Grainger RG, et al: The bronchial circulation in a case of giant hamartoma of the lung. Br J Radiol 45:147, 1972.

294. Zeren H, Moran CA, Suster S, et al: Primary pulmonary sarcomas with features of monophasic synovial sarcoma: A clinicopathological, immunohistochemical, and ultrastructural study of 25 cases. Hum Pathol 26:474, 1995.

295. Steele JD: The solitary pulmonary nodule: Report of a cooperative study of resected asymptomatic solitary pulmonary nodules in males. J Thorac Cardiovasc Surg 46:21, 1963.

296. Poirier TJ, Van Ordstrand HS: Pulmonary chondromatous hamartomas: Report of seventeen cases and review of the literature. Chest 59:50, 1971.

297. Shah JP, Choudhry KU, Huvos AG, et al: Hamartomas of the lung. Surg Gynecol Obstet 136:406, 1973.

298. Weisel W, Glicklich M, Landis FB: Pulmonary hamartoma, an enlarging neoplasm. Arch Surg 71:128, 1955.

299. Madani MA, Dafoe CS, Ross CA: Multiple hamartomata of the lung. Thorax 21:468, 1966.

300. Doppman J, Wilson G: Cystic pulmonary hamartoma. Br J Radiol 38:629, 1965.

301. Demos TC, Armin A, Chandrasekhar AJ, et al: Cystic hamartoma of the lung. J Can Assoc Radiol 34:149, 1983.

302. Siegelman SS, Khouri NF, Scott WW, et al: Pulmonary hamartoma: CT findings. Radiology 160:313, 1986.

303. Sakai F, Sone S, Kiyono K, et al: MR of pulmonary hamartoma: Pathologic correlation. J Thorac Imaging 9:51, 1994.

304. Petheram IS, Heard BE: Unique massive pulmonary hamartoma: Case report with review of hamartomata treated at Brompton Hospital in 27 years. Chest 75:95, 1979.

305. Ahn JM, Im JG, Seo JW, et al: Endobronchial hamartoma: CT findings in three patients. Am J Roentgenol 163:49, 1994.

306. Davis WK, Roberts L Jr, Foster WL Jr, et al: Computed tomographic diagnosis of an endobronchial hamartoma. Invest Radiol 23:941, 1988.

307. Kwong JS, Müller NL, Miller RR: Diseases of the trachea and main-stem bronchi: Correlation of CT with pathologic findings. RadioGraphics 12:645, 1992.

308. Kleinman J, Zirkin H, Feuchtwanger MM, et al: Benign hamartoma of the lung presenting as massive hemoptysis. J Surg Oncol 33:38, 1986.

309. Sharkey RA, Mulloy EM, O'Neill S: Endobronchial hamartoma presenting as massive haemoptysis. Eur Respir J 9:2179, 1996.

310. Dahlgren S: Needle biopsy of intrapulmonary hamartoma. Scand J Respir Dis 47:187, 1966.

311. Ludwig ME, Otis RD, Cole SR, et al: Fine needle aspiration cytology of pulmonary hamartomas. Acta Cytol 26:671, 1982.

312. Dunbar F, Leiman G: The aspiration cytology of pulmonary hamartomas. Diagn Cytopathol 5:174, 1989.

313. Poulsen JT, Jacobsen M, Francis D: Probable malignant transformation of a pulmonary hamartoma. Thorax 34:557, 1979.

314. Karpas CM, Blackman N: Adenocarcinoma arising in a hamartoma (adenolipomyoma) of the bronchus associated with multiple benign tumors. Am J Clin Pathol 48:383, 1967.

315. Basile A, Gregoris A, Antoci B, et al: Malignant change in a benign pulmonary hamartoma. Thorax 44:232, 1989.

316. King TC, Myers J: Isolated metastasis to a pulmonary hamartoma. Am J Surg Pathol 19:472, 1995.

317. Ribet M, Jaillard-Thery S, Nuttens MC: Pulmonary hamartoma and malignancy. J Thorac Cadiovasc Surg 107:611, 1994.

318. Sonobe H, Ro JY, Macay B, et al: Pulmonary alveolar soft-part sarcoma. Int J Surg Pathol 2:57, 1994.

319. Tsutsumi Y, Deng Y: Alveolar soft part sarcoma of the pulmonary vein. Acta Pathol Jpn 41:771, 1991.

320. Kalus M, Rahman F, Jenkins DE, et al: Malignant mesenchymoma of the lung. Arch Pathol 95:199, 1973.

CHAPTER 37

Neoplasms of Uncertain Histogenesis and Nonneoplastic Tumors

In addition to the neoplasms described in previous chapters, there are a number of tumors whose cell of origin and/or pathway of cellular differentiation are uncertain, rendering logical classification somewhat difficult. Because of their rarity, pathologic diagnosis of these tumors can also be problematic. A variety of nonneoplastic abnormalities that may present as a nodule or a mass simulating a true neoplasm are also discussed at this point.

NEOPLASMS OF UNCERTAIN HISTOGENESIS

Clear Cell Tumor

Clear cell tumor is a rare pulmonary neoplasm of which only 27 cases had been reported in the English literature by 1990.[1, 2] The histogenesis is uncertain: electron microscopic and immunohistochemical studies have been variably interpreted as providing evidence for a neuroendocrine,[1, 3] bronchiolar (Clara cell),[4] smooth muscle, or pericytic[5] origin.

Evidence of melanocytic differentiation can also be found in some cases.[6, 7] Most patients have been adults; there is a slight female predominance. An association with tuberous sclerosis and pulmonary lymphangioleiomyomatosis has been described in one patient.[7a]

Pathologically, the tumors appear as well-delimited but nonencapsulated nodules, in most cases measuring 1 to 3 cm in diameter (although one example of 6 cm has been reported).[8] Necrosis is seen rarely.[9] Microscopically, they consist of sheets of polygonal cells within a richly vascular stroma (Fig. 37–1). Nuclei are usually central and show little pleomorphism; mitotic figures are rare. The cytoplasm is abundant and appears clear or finely vacuolated. Special stains usually reveal a high-glycogen content; electron microscopic studies have shown the glycogen to be free in the cytoplasm in a monogranular or rosette form and within membrane-bound vesicles in a solely monogranular form.[3, 9, 10] The latter appearance is similar to that seen in Pompe's disease (glycogenosis type II), suggesting that the tumor cells might have an enzyme deficiency.[3] Immunohistochemical studies have shown positive reactions for cathepsin B, protein S-100, neuron-specific enolase, and HMB-45 in many tumors;[1, 7] reactions to keratins and carcinoembryonic antigen are typically negative.

The majority of patients are asymptomatic, the lesion being discovered as a peripheral, well-circumscribed nodule on a screening radiograph. Dyspnea on exertion, cough, and hemoptysis occurred in one patient with a tracheal tumor.[11] Almost all tumors have behaved in a benign fashion, unassociated with recurrence or distant spread; however, one patient developed metastases and died 17 years after the initial diagnosis.[12]

Histologically, the tumors must be differentiated from the more common pulmonary carcinoma with clear cell change, metastatic clear cell carcinoma (especially from the kidney), and the rare clear cell variant of carcinoid tumor. The characteristic immunohistochemical and ultrastructural features of benign clear cell tumor should make the distinction relatively straightforward in most cases.

Paraganglioma

Paragangliomas (chemodectomas) are uncommon neoplasms that arise from the extra-adrenal paraganglia of the

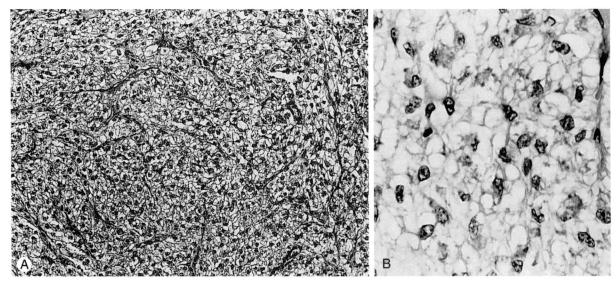

Figure 37–1. Pulmonary Clear Cell Tumor. Sections from a 1.5-cm nodule excised from an asymptomatic 48-year-old woman show tumor cells separated by thin-walled vessels and containing abundant clear cytoplasm. (*A*, ×100; *B*, ×500.)

autonomic nervous system. Histologically, they consist of small, well-defined nests of round-to-oval tumor cells with abundant cytoplasm that is clear or lightly eosinophilic. The clusters are separated by a well-developed vascular network, resulting in an organoid structure that is particularly well demonstrated by reticulin stains. Ultrastructural examination shows membrane-bound, electron-dense neuroendocrine granules.

Within the thorax, paragangliomas are most commonly found near the ascending or transverse portion of the aortic arch where chemoreceptor tissue is normally believed to occur (*see* page 2942). Although these tumors are clearly mediastinal in origin, radiographically they may appear to lie within lung parenchyma, particularly when they arise extrapleurally in the paravertebral sulcus.[13]

Although rare, neoplasms with a histologic appearance identical to mediastinal paragangliomas have also been described in the trachea and lungs. Only five tracheal lesions had been reported by 1993;[14, 15] all patients were older adults, two of whom presented with dyspnea and three with hemoptysis. Fluorescent and biochemical analysis in two cases demonstrated significant quantities of norepinephrine.[14, 16] These tumors have been considered to arise from true tracheal paraganglionic tissue or from aberrant paraganglia normally present in the larynx.[14]

Rare intrapulmonary neoplasms interpreted as paragangliomas have also been reported.[17, 18] However, despite their histologic resemblance to extrapulmonary paragangliomas, it is not certain that all of these represent true neoplasms of paraganglionic tissue. On both the light and electron microscopy, the morphologic appearance of carcinoid tumors can be virtually identical to that of mediastinal paragangliomas; it is thus possible that some, if not all, intrapulmonary tumors that have been designated paraganglioma might more correctly be labeled carcinoid tumor. As a justification for considering these neoplasms to be paragangliomas is the supposition that they arise from "minute pulmonary chemodectomas" or from the chemoreceptor tissue from which such chemodectomas might originate; however, as discussed

farther on, ultrastructural investigations have shown that these "chemodectomas" are probably not related to the paraganglionic system, and this histogenesis is unlikely. Despite these objections, the intimate relationship to the adventitia of a segmental pulmonary artery in one case[19] and the presence of norepinephrine in some tumors suggest that some of these neoplasms may in fact be true paragangliomas.

Most patients reported to have intrapulmonary paragangliomas have been women 40 to 70 years of age.[18] Many have been asymptomatic; when present, symptoms include cough and, occasionally, dyspnea. The majority of tumors have behaved in a benign fashion; however, the follow-up period in many cases has been rather short, and some cases have been reported to be aggressive.[17] Substantial hemorrhage related to the tumor's vascularity has occurred during biopsy and surgery in some tracheal tumors.[14]

Sclerosing Hemangioma

Sclerosing hemangioma (pneumocytoma) is an unusual pulmonary neoplasm whose histogenesis has been controversial since its original description by Liebow and Hubbell in 1956.[20] These authors proposed that the tumor represents a vascular neoplasm, an opinion later supported by several electron microscopic studies.[21, 22] The results of histochemical and immunohistochemical studies suggested to other workers that the tumor might have a mesenchymal,[23] neuroendocrine,[24] or mesothelial[25] derivation. However, the majority of ultrastructural[28] and immunohistochemical[26–30] investigations have provided evidence that the tumor is derived from alveolar or bronchiolar epithelium; the term *sclerosing pneumocytoma* has been proposed to emphasize this hypothesis.[31, 32] Whatever its origin and nature, it is generally agreed that the tumor is neoplastic[37] and distinct from conditions such as fibrous histiocytoma and plasma cell granuloma, with which it has been confused.

Although uncommon, the tumor has comprised a substantial proportion of cases in some series; for example in one review of 45 surgically excised benign neoplasms, 10 (22%) were considered to be this type.[33] There is a female-to-male predominance of approximately 4 to 5:1,[31, 33, 34, 35] a gender difference that may be related to the presence of estrogen receptors in some tumors.[29] Most lesions are discovered in patients between 30 and 50 years of age.

Pathologically, sclerosing hemangioma typically consists of a solitary well-limited, round-to-oval nodule from 1 to 4 cm in diameter. A variegated yellow, red, and gray appearance is often seen on cut sections (Fig. 37–2).[31, 34, 36] Multiple lesions have been described occasionally, suggesting either multicentric origin or bronchogenic spread.[38, 39] Most tumors arise in the peripheral lung parenchyma, commonly in a subpleural location. The microscopic appearance is variable, usually consisting of a combination of solid or papillary cellular areas, relatively acellular sclerotic regions, and dilated blood-filled spaces (Fig. 37–2).[32–34] The proliferating cells are round to oval in shape and contain abundant eosinophilic or clear cytoplasm and bland nuclei. Although nuclear atypia can occur, it is usually mild. Admixed inflammatory cells, especially mast cells and foamy histiocytes, may be abundant focally;[34, 40] a granulomatous inflammatory reaction has also been reported.[41] Papillary structures similar to those in sclerosing hemangioma have also been described in some cases of chondromatous hamartoma.[42]

Radiographically, the tumor characteristically presents as a well-defined, homogeneous nodule or mass without preference for any lobe (Fig. 37–3).[43, 44] Most are juxtapleural in location.[44, 45] Although seldom seen radiographically,[43, 44] calcification was identified on CT in three of eight patients in one series.[44] Cavitation does not occur; however, two cases have been reported in which an air-meniscus sign was identified.[46] Histologically, the meniscus represented dilated, ruptured, and coalesced distal air spaces postulated by the authors to be the result of tumor-related bronchial compression and air trapping. Despite the designation "hemangioma," no connection is visible between the lesion and the pulmonary vasculature. The CT findings consist of a smoothly marginated nodule or mass.[44] In one series of eight tumors, seven showed enhancement following injection of intravenous contrast agent.[44] The enhancement may be homogeneous, ranging from 96 to 157 HU,[44, 45, 59] or there may be localized areas with relatively low attenuation.[43, 44]

The majority of patients are asymptomatic, the abnormality being discovered on a screening chest radiograph.[33] Occasionally, a history of cough or of recent or remote hemoptysis has been obtained.[39] The tumor can be diagnosed on specimens obtained by transthoracic needle aspiration (TTNA);[47, 48] however, confusion with bronchioloalveolar carcinoma can occur.[49] In fact, because of the papillary or clear cell areas, some cases have been mistaken for primary or metastatic carcinoma on histologic evaluation.[34, 50]

Most tumors appear to behave in a benign fashion.[35] In fact, slow growth is not uncommon; in 14 of 51 patients reviewed in one series, the lesions had been apparent radiographically an average of 5 years (in some cases as long as 14 years) before definitive surgery.[34] Despite these observations, occasional cases have been associated with metastases to regional lymph nodes or apparent spread within the lung.[32, 38, 40]

Pulmonary Germ Cell Neoplasms

Intrathoracic germ cell tumors are uncommon and almost invariably develop in the mediastinum; in fact, some tumors reported as being primary in the lung may have been the result of direct extension or metastasis of a mediastinal tumor. In addition, since pulmonary carcinomas can secrete human chorionic gonadotropin (hCG) or α-fetoprotein,[51, 52] it is possible that some primary "germ cell tumors" have been misclassified. Despite these comments, occasional well-documented cases of pure primary pulmonary teratoma and choriocarcinoma have been reported. Rare cases have also been reported of combined germ cell tumor and carcinoma[53] or blastoma.[54]

The origin of intrapulmonary germ cell tumors is not understood. According to one theory, a teratomatous focus situated in the embryonic mediastinum is incorporated in the foregut lung bud and eventually develops into a recognizable tumor within the lung parenchyma.[55] An alternative possibility is that the tumor develops from aberrant tissue derived from the third pharyngeal pouch that migrates along the developing bronchi.[56] The occasional case in which intrapulmonary teratoma is associated with thymic tissue (which itself is derived from the third pharyngeal pouch) has been cited as evidence in support of the latter hypothesis.[56, 57]

Teratoma

By 1992, approximately 30 cases of apparently primary pulmonary teratoma had been described.[58, 61] Pathologically, these neoplasms usually consist of well-circumscribed, cystic masses measuring 3 to 8 cm in diameter and filled with sebaceous material. They are most often intraparenchymal, although endobronchial forms have been described.[60] Histologically, a variety of tissue types may be seen, representing endodermal, ectodermal, and mesodermal derivatives. As in mediastinal teratomas, pancreatic tissue is present more frequently than in extrathoracic teratomas. Foci of carcinoma or sarcoma are seen occasionally.

The radiographic presentation is a peripheral mass, often lobulated and most commonly located in the upper lobe.[60, 61, 62] Of the 30 cases reported by 1992, radiography revealed calcification within the mass in 4 and cavitation or a peripheral crescent-shape lucency in 5.[61] The CT findings have been described in two patients.[61, 63] In one, they consisted of an encapsulated low-attenuation mass in the right lower lobe and a high-attenuation mass at the suprahilar level;[63] at autopsy, this was shown to be a single, pear-shaped solid teratoma that involved all three lobes of the right lung. In a second case, CT scanning demonstrated a poorly defined, heterogeneous mass measuring 4 cm in diameter that was interpreted as representing a conglomeration of fibrotic lung and tumor.[61] We have seen one low-grade tumor in which CT demonstrated a 6-cm-diameter inhomogeneous soft tissue mass containing small areas of calcification (Fig. 37–4).

Most patients come to clinical attention between 20 to 40 years of age, although tumors have been described in individuals as young as 10 months[55] and as old as 68 years.[62] Presenting features include hemoptysis and (rarely) expectoration of hair (trichophytosis). Occasionally, hair has been identified endoscopically projecting from a bronchus.[58] Ap-

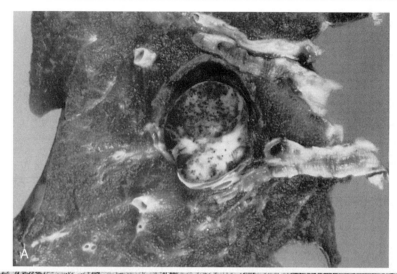

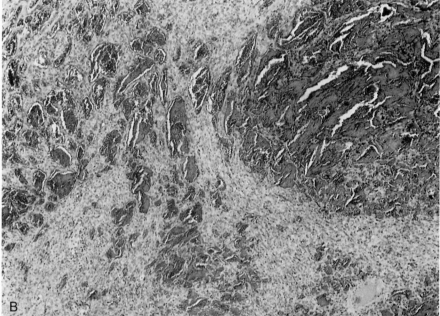

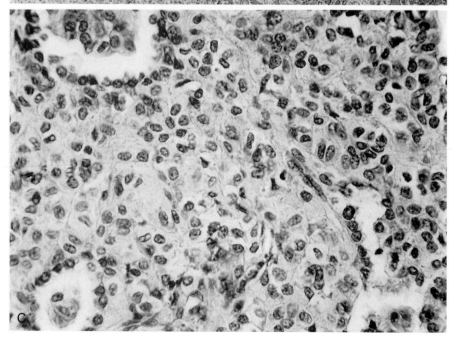

Figure 37–2. Sclerosing Hemangioma.
Grossly *(A)*, a well-circumscribed nodule, partly separated from surrounding lung parenchyma, possesses a variegated appearance. A histologic section *(B)* reveals sheets of tumor cells and multiple hemorrhagic foci. The cells are located in the alveolar interstitium and contain ample cytoplasm and uniform round to oval nuclei *(C)*. *(B,* ×90; *C,* ×600.) (Modified from Katzenstein, A-LA, Weise DL, Fulling K, et al: Am J Surg Pathol 7:3, 1983.)

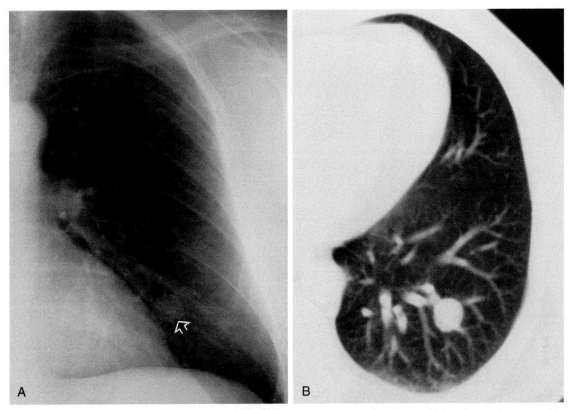

Figure 37–3. Sclerosing Hemangioma. A view from a posteroanterior chest radiograph *(A)* in a 42-year-old man demonstrates a smoothly marginated, 1.5-cm-diameter nodule in the left lower lobe *(arrow).* A CT scan *(B)* essentially confirms the radiographic findings. Homogeneous enhancement was observed following intravenous administration of contrast medium. The nodule was detected incidentally on a chest radiograph. *(B* from Pulmonary sclerosing hemangioma: Unusual cause of a solitary pulmonary nodule. Reprinted from, by permission of the publisher, *CARJ,* 1990; 41(6), pp. 372–4.)

proximately two thirds of tumors have behaved in a benign fashion.[61]

Choriocarcinoma

Primary pulmonary choriocarcinoma has been described rarely;[64–66] as indicated previously, it is possible that some cases represent poorly differentiated pulmonary carcinoma. It has been hypothesized that this tumor may be the result of trophoblastic pulmonary embolism at the time of abortion or delivery; however, this thesis obviously would not apply to the rare occurrence of this neoplasm in men.[65, 68] It is also possible that some tumors represent "overgrowth" of choriocarcinoma in a pulmonary carcinoma, since occasional cases of combined adenocarcinoma and choriocarcinoma have been reported.[53]

Pathologically, the tumors are typically hemorrhagic and necrotic; histologic features are identical to choriocarcinoma arising at other sites. Clinical and radiologic features are nonspecific. One exceptional case has been reported of an apparent primary pulmonary tumor initially interpreted as a metastatic gestational trophoblastic neoplasm.[69] Most patients have been male and have presented with symptoms such as dyspnea, weight loss, and hemoptysis;[70] an elevated level of hCG is common.

Pulmonary Blastoma

Pulmonary blastoma is a malignant tumor of uncertain histogenesis that histologically recapitulates the developing lung in early fetal life. The fundamental nature of the tumor and the terminology that has been applied to it has been controversial and somewhat complicated. Because of the tumor's resemblance to fetal tissue, Spencer hypothesized that it developed from immature pulmonary "blastema," pleuripotential tissue believed to be capable of differentiating into both mesenchymal and epithelial portions of the lung periphery.[71] The development of neoplasia in this tissue was thought to be analogous to that of Wilms' tumor (nephroblastoma) from primitive renal blastema, and the term *pulmonary blastoma* was proposed to emphasize this hypothesis.[71] However, there has been objection to this concept of histogenesis on the basis of a number of observations that instead suggest a derivation from endodermal tissue.[72–75] It has also been suggested that the tumor originates in a pleuripotential stem cell.[76, 77] Pulmonary blastoma should not be confused with pleuropulmonary blastoma of childhood, which is now believed to be a distinct entity and which may be a more appropriate analogue of Wilms' tumor in the lung.[78, 79]

A number of investigators consider pulmonary blastoma to represent a variant of carcinosarcoma (see page 1114).[72, 80–83] The occasional reports of tumors that resemble a combination of both tumors support this hypothesis.[82, 84] Despite this, the characteristic histologic resemblance of pulmonary blastoma to fetal lung during the pseudoglandular period and the relatively large number of cases discovered at a young age[85, 86] suggest that it may be fundamentally different from the neoplasm that is usually called carcinosarcoma; we thus feel that it is justified to continue the use of the term *blastoma* and to consider the tumor as a separate entity. It

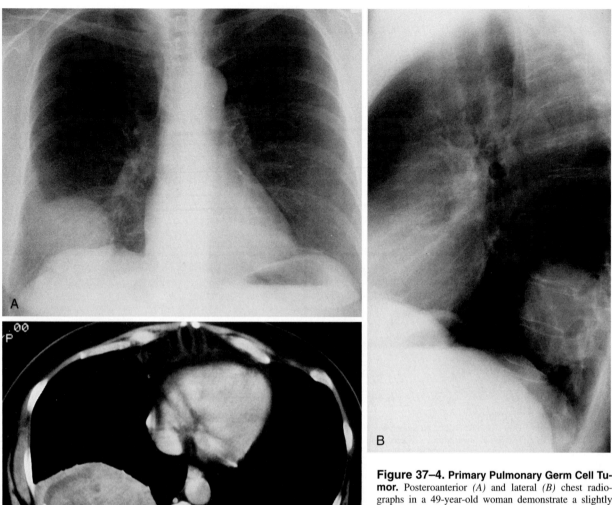

Figure 37–4. Primary Pulmonary Germ Cell Tumor. Posteroanterior *(A)* and lateral *(B)* chest radiographs in a 49-year-old woman demonstrate a slightly lobulated 6-cm-diameter soft tissue tumor in the right lower lobe. A CT scan *(C)* performed following intravenous administration of contrast agent demonstrates inhomogeneous enhancement of the tumor and a small area of calcification. Although the tumor contains areas of low density, these are of greater attenuation than that of subcutaneous fat. Histologic assessment of the resected specimen demonstrated a malignant teratoma.

should be noted, however, that it is grouped with pleomorphic carcinoma and carcinosarcoma in the 1999 World Health Organization (WHO) classification of pulmonary tumors.[87]

To complicate matters even further, an unusual tumor has also been described that resembles pulmonary blastoma without its sarcomatous stroma.[88, 89] Termed *well-differentiated fetal adenocarcinoma* (pulmonary adenocarcinoma of fetal type[90] or pulmonary endodermal tumor resembling fetal lung[89, 91]), this lesion is believed by many observers to represent a variant of blastoma. This hypothesis is supported by the occasional tumor in which both histologic patterns have been identified.[92] Despite this, blastoma and fetal adenocarcinoma are considered by some authors to represent separate entities, and the latter is grouped with other adenocarcinomas in the 1999 WHO classification.[87]

Pulmonary blastoma is rare; only about 120 cases had been documented by 1987,[77] and it is possible that some of these would more correctly have been labeled carcinosar-coma. A review of the files of the Armed Forces Institute of Pathology (AFIP) in 1991 revealed 52 cases: 24 of the classic (biphasic) type and 28 of the fetal type.[92] Tumors occur from childhood to old age, the average age at diagnosis being about 35 to 40 years.[82, 92] A male-to-female predominance of about 2.5 to 1 has been found by some investigators; however, in the AFIP review, the sex incidence was approximately equal.[92] Approximately 80% of patients give a history of cigarette smoking.[92]

Well-Differentiated Fetal Adenocarcinoma

Well-differentiated fetal adenocarcinoma tends to occur in the periphery of the lung and is about half the size of the classic blastoma (mean, about 5 cm);[92] rare examples have been reported to arise in an endobronchial location.[94] Grossly, the tumor is typically well-delimited and has a soft, somewhat gelatinous appearance. Histologically, it consists of numerous complex branching tubules lined by a layer of columnar cells with basal nuclei and clear cytoplasm (Fig. 37–5), the latter caused by the presence of abundant glycogen. Neuroendocrine cells are usually present within the epithelium. Rarely, the neuroendocrine cell aggregates resemble small carcinoid tumors or small cell carcinoma.[95] In addition to the glandular structures, solid clusters of cells somewhat resembling those of endometrial adenosquamous carcinoma (morules) can be seen in many tumors.[89, 90] These cells tend to have prominent clear nuclei that, for unknown reasons, appear to be rich in biotin.[96] Stroma is typically scanty and always benign in appearance. One case has been reported in which there was concomitant yolk sac tumor.[97] One group has described a high-grade form of tumor characterized by disorganized glands, cytologic atypia, absence of morules, presence of necrosis, and overexpression of p53 protein.[197]

Radiologic findings are nonspecific, consisting most often of a peripheral nodule or mass. Pleural effusion is rare.[98] Compared with biphasic blastoma, the fetal variant is more often asymptomatic (approximately 55% to 60% of patients).[92] In the AFIP series, only 3 (14%) of 21 patients with follow-up died of tumor, after 2 to 34 months.[92] In contrast with biphasic tumors, size does not appear to be related to behavior.

Biphasic Blastoma

Biphasic blastomas are typically large, well-delimited masses located in the periphery of the lung;[71, 92, 204] in one review of 39 cases, 17 were larger than 10 cm in diameter.[73] Growth within a bronchial lumen occurs in about 25% of cases.[71, 99, 100] Hemorrhage and necrosis are frequent. Microscopically, the tumor consists of an admixture of primitive-appearing epithelium and stroma that superficially resembles the pseudoglandular period of lung development (Fig. 37–6).[92] The epithelial cells are arranged in small, slitlike spaces or branching tubules and are surrounded by polygonal or spindle-shaped stromal cells with hyperchromatic, pleomorphic nuclei; the latter cells may appear to be more numerous immediately adjacent to the epithelial elements. Occasionally, the stromal cells show chondroid, osteoid, or skeletal differentiation.[100–102]

The most common radiologic manifestation consists of a single well-circumscribed nodule or mass in the periphery of the lung.[103, 104] Rarely, tumors are cavitated, calcified, or multiple.[104] Reported examples have ranged in diameter from 2.5 cm to almost 25 cm.[104, 105] CT scans performed in a small number of cases have demonstrated homogeneous soft tissue attenuation,[104] or a heterogeneous appearance with areas of low attenuation.[106] Pleural effusion occurs in a minority of cases.[92]

Although some patients are asymptomatic, hemoptysis, cough, and chest pain are frequent complaints (in approximately 80% of patients in the AFIP series).[92] Examination of sputum samples and bronchial washings and brushings is often unrewarding; when they do contain malignant cells, these are usually interpreted as carcinoma.[107, 108] Percutaneous aspiration biopsy is more likely to contain diagnostic cells suggestive of a mixed epithelial/mesenchymal neoplasm.[107]

The prognosis of this variant appears to be much worse than that of the fetal type. In the AFIP series, 12 (52%) of 23 patients with adequate follow-up died of their tumor, 9 within 1 year.[92] In another review of 39 patients, 17 (44%) developed metastases, and only 2 of these survived longer than 2 years.[73] Despite this, occasional patients have prolonged survival, even in the presence of metastatic disease.[73, 71, 67, 109] There is evidence that the prognosis is better in women and in patients who have smaller primary tumors.[73, 92]

Pulmonary Thymoma

The presence of tumors histologically resembling thymoma but situated entirely within the lung parenchyma, the pleura or the lung and adjacent hilum has been reported rarely;[110–112] the authors of one review in 1995 documented 29 cases.[70] Although these locations are clearly unusual sites for such a tumor, the presence of myasthenia gravis in some patients,[113] the finding of aberrant thymic tissue in relation

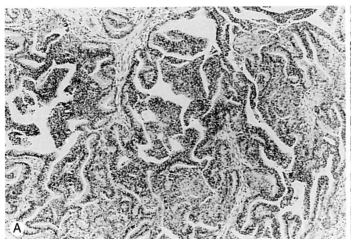
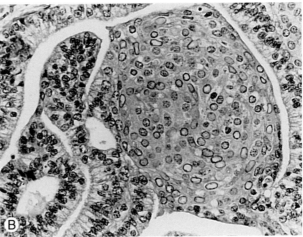

Figure 37–5. Well-Differentiated Fetal Adenocarcinoma. A section of a well circumscribed 2.5-cm tumor *(A)* shows numerous branching tubules lined by columnar cells and separated by a benign fibrous stroma. A magnified view *(B)* shows the columnar cells to have clear apical cytoplasm; a nodule of cells with abundant, relatively dense cytoplasm and nuclei showing prominent central clearing (morule) is also evident.

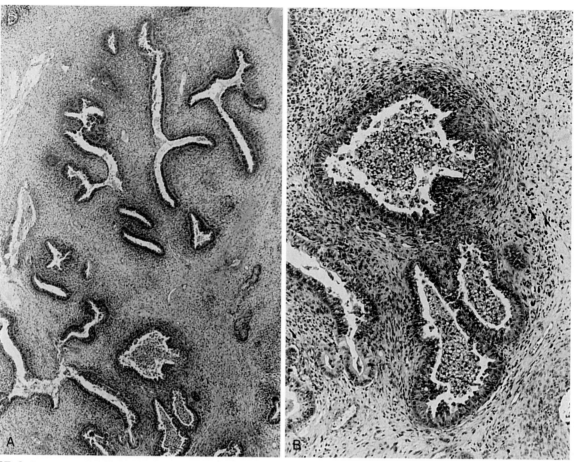

Figure 37–6. Pulmonary Biphasic Blastoma. A low-magnification view of a 6-cm upper lobe mass *(A)* shows several ill-defined lobules containing branching epithelial-lined slits. A higher magnification view *(B)* shows the epithelium to be columnar and the stromal cells spindle shaped; significant nuclear atypia is present in both cell types. Note the increased density of the malignant stromal tissue adjacent to the epithelium, an appearance similar to that of fetal lung in the pseudoglandular stage *(see* Fig. 4–2, page 138).

to the hilum in other patients,[114] and the histologic appearance of the tumors all suggest that the diagnosis is valid.

The right lung appears to be more commonly affected.[70] Histologic features are identical to the more common anterior mediastinal tumor.[112] Radiologic findings are nonspecific. When considering the diagnosis, it is important to remember that a thymoma originating in the mediastinum may mimic a primary lung tumor. In one such case, an 8-cm-diameter pedunculated thymoma was misdiagnosed as a primary lung tumor on the chest radiograph and on gallium 67 scanning;[115] the pedicle and the mediastinal origin were correctly identified on CT.

Most patients are between 30 to 60 years of age and are asymptomatic; rarely, there is a history of myasthenia gravis. Like their mediastinal counterpart, pulmonary thymomas appear to be slow-growing tumors for which cure can be expected in almost all patients following complete excision.[112]

Pulmonary Meningioma

Meningioma can be seen in the lung as a primary lesion or as a metastasis.[116] The former—which is extremely rare—typically presents during adulthood as an asymptomatic nodule in the periphery of the lung.[117–119] One patient had a history of neurofibromatosis.[120] Pathologic features are identical to those of the more common intracranial tumor. The origin of the tumor is uncertain but has been speculated to be from pluripotential subpleural mesenchyme or from embryonic rests of arachnoid cells.[119] As discussed elsewhere *(see* page 1374), it is possible that the tumor is related to pulmonary meningothelial-like nodules.

Pulmonary Ependymoma

A single case has been reported of an apparently primary pulmonary neoplasm that histologically and immunohistochemically resembled an ependymoma.[121] The cell of origin of such a tumor in the lung is unclear.

TUMORS OF NONNEOPLASTIC OR UNCERTAIN NATURE

In this section are described a variety of nonneoplastic abnormalities that can simulate pulmonary neoplasms radiologically and, in some cases, clinically and endoscopically. It should be noted that many other conditions—particularly infections—can also cause localized tumor-like nodules or masses that can be confused with a neoplasm; these are discussed elsewhere in the text in the appropriate section. Rarely, foreign material within the lung is also the inciting cause of a tumor-like growth, as for example in a suture granuloma at the stump of an excised pulmonary lobe,[122] granulation issue around aspirated food,[123] and retained cotton material (*gossypiboma*) following cardiac surgery.[124]

Inflammatory Tracheobronchial Polyps

Inflammatory polyps of the tracheobronchial tree are uncommon, comprising only seven (11%) of 63 benign tracheobronchial tumors in one series.[125] There are likely several pathogenetic mechanisms. In some cases, a history of chronic bronchitis or bronchiectasis has suggested that the polyps represent an exaggerated but localized inflammatory reaction to chronic airway irritation.[127, 128] In others, aspirated foreign material,[126, 129] broncholithiasis,[130] or thermal injury[131, 132] has resulted in the formation of exuberant granulation tissue that constitutes the polypoid mass. Polyps that are associated with asthmatic symptoms are more likely to be the cause of the "asthma" than a tissue manifestation of that disease;[134, 135] however, an edematous stroma and eosinophilic infiltrate similar to nasal allergic polyps have occasionally been demonstrated.[136, 137] Despite the foregoing, in most cases there is no history of concomitant abnormality to explain polyp formation. Some authors have likened these "idiopathic" lesions to fibroepithelial polyps of the skin or uterine cervix.[127, 134]

The polyps are usually solitary, although rare examples of multiple synchronous lesions have been reported.[135] They tend to possess a somewhat lobulated, reddish surface,[125, 128] and may be pedunculated or attached to the airway wall by a broad base. Histologically, the surface epithelium often shows squamous metaplasia and is occasionally ulcerated.[125, 128] Although papillary projections may be evident, they are typically relatively broad and few in number compared with those of squamous papillomas. The bulk of the polyp consists of stroma whose appearance is variable depending on the number of blood vessels, the nature of the connective tissue (which may be either dense collagen or myxoid), and the severity of inflammatory cellular infiltrate.

Radiographic manifestations are those of airway obstruction and include bronchiectasis, atelectasis, and obstructive pneumonitis. Most patients are between 30 and 60 years of age. Clinical findings include hemoptysis, cough (frequently with sputum production), and dyspnea.[131, 132] Wheezing can simulate asthma; occasional patients have been treated for this disease for many years before the culpable polyp is discovered.[135] (However, as indicated previously, some polyps are likely a manifestation of asthma). A history of recurrent pneumonia is not uncommon. In one patient, an unusually large pedunculated polyp caused severe, acute dyspnea by prolapsing from its origin in a right upper lobe segmental bronchus into the left main bronchus.[138]

Plasma Cell Granuloma/Fibrous Histiocytoma (Inflammatory Pseudotumor)

Plasma cell granuloma and *fibrous histiocytoma* are terms that refer to a group of pulmonary tumors character-

ized histologically by a mixture of fibroblasts, histiocytes, lymphocytes, and plasma cells. Since the proportion of these cells varies considerably from tumor to tumor, a variety of terms has been employed to describe them and a dual concept of their pathogenesis has been considered. Those with a predominance of plasma cells have been felt to represent an unusual inflammatory reaction to an unidentified agent[139–141] or a reparative process secondary to a pulmonary infection[142] and have been termed *plasma cell granuloma* or *inflammatory pseudotumor.* By contrast, those with a relative absence of inflammatory cells have been interpreted by some authorities as being neoplastic, tumors with approximately equal numbers of fibroblasts and histiocytes having been designated *fibrous histiocytoma* or *fibroxanthoma,* those containing predominantly histiocytic cells being called *histiocytoma* or *xanthoma,* and those composed chiefly of fibroblasts labeled *fibroma.*

Despite these views, there is in fact considerable histologic overlap between the two "forms" of tumor, those composed predominantly of fibroblasts containing focal areas characteristic of plasma cell granuloma, and vice versa.[139] As a result, it is now widely believed that these tumors represent an unusual inflammatory reaction with a variable histologic appearance and that they should all be termed *inflammatory pseudotumor*[143] or *inflammatory myofibroblastic tumor.*[144] Nevertheless, recurrence,[145–147] local tissue infiltration and destruction,[148, 149] atypical histologic features,[150] and cytogenetic abnormalities[133, 151] have suggested that some lesions may be neoplastic. One group of investigators found molecular evidence of the production of interleukin-1-β and interleukin-6 by the tumor as well as high-serum levels of the same substances;[152] they speculated that abnormal regulation of cytokine production might be involved in tumor development.

Pathologically, the tumors are usually well demarcated and situated in the lung parenchyma;[141, 153, 154] endobronchial[155, 156] or endotracheal[148, 157] locations occur occasionally. Depending on the amount of fibrosis and the degree of histiocytic, lymphocytic, or plasmacytic infiltration, the color can be gray, tan, or yellow. Most nodules range from 2 to 5 cm in diameter; however, occasional examples as large as 12 cm have been recorded.[142] Extension across the pleura into the mediastinum or chest wall can occur.[139, 141]

As indicated, tumors designated plasma cell granuloma are characterized by a predominance of plasma cells with lesser numbers of histiocytes, lymphocytes, and multinucleated giant cells (Fig. 37–7); mast cells and neutrophils also may be present[158] and rarely predominate.[159, 160] Foci of calcification, ossification and organizing pneumonia are frequent.[143] Tumors with a relative paucity of plasma cells and lymphocytes (histiocytoma, fibrous histiocytoma) typically consist of a combination of spindle-shaped, fibroblast-like cells with a variable amount of intervening collagen and polygonal-to-round cells containing granular eosinophilic or foamy cytoplasm. As in plasma cell granuloma, mast cells are occasionally abundant.[161] In general, cytologic features are bland and mitotic figures are rare in both "variants." However, atypia is present occasionally, and some neoplasms have been designated "borderline" to indicate a possible stage intermediate between clearly benign tumors and malignant fibrous histiocytoma.[150] Obviously, it is necessary to distinguish such tumors from inflammatory sarcoma.[162] Cyto-

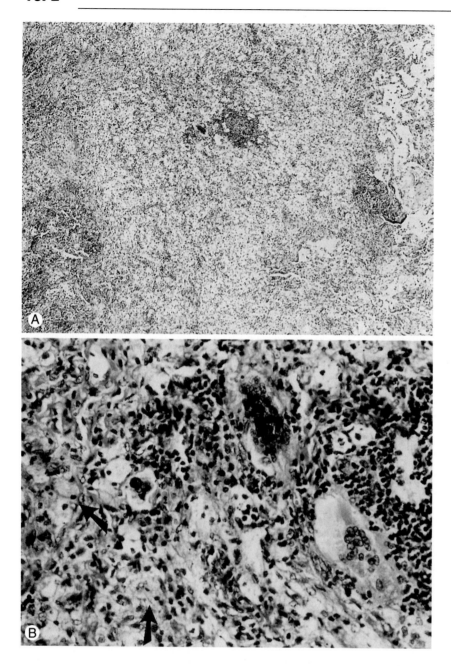

Figure 37–7. Plasma Cell Granuloma ("Inflammatory Pseudotumor"). A diffuse infiltrate of foamy histiocytes, lymphocytes, and scattered fibroblasts *(A)* obliterates the normal lung architecture. At higher power *(B)* foamy histiocytes *(arrows),* lymphocytes, occasional plasma cells, and multinucleated giant cells can be identified. (*A,* ×40; *B,* ×250.)

logic findings in specimens obtained by TTNA have been described.[163]

Radiologic manifestations consist of either a solitary pulmonary nodule or a focal area of consolidation that can mimic a primary or metastatic carcinoma (Fig. 37–8).[164–167] Calcification is present occasionally[166, 168] and cavitation rarely.[141] Endobronchial tumors can cause obstructive pneumonitis. In a review of 60 patients who had inflammatory pseudotumors from the AFIP, 52 (87%) were found to have presented with solitary peripheral nodules or masses, 3 (5%) with multiple nodules, 2 with mediastinal masses, 1 each with an endotracheal or endobronchial tumor, and 1 with a sharply defined circumscribed pleural mass.[187] Tumors were larger than 3 cm in diameter in 31 patients. Secondary airway luminal involvement by a parenchymal lesion was identified in 6 patients and lobar atelectasis in 5. Hilar or mediastinal lymphadenopathy and pleural effusion occurred

in a small number of cases. On CT, the lesions had smooth or lobulated margins, homogeneous or heterogeneous attenuation, and either no enhancement or homogeneous, heterogenous, or peripheral rim enhancement following intravenous administration of contrast medium. Heterogeneous signal intensity was evident on T1-weighted MR images and high-signal intensity on T2-weighted images; the endotracheal tumor showed heterogeneous enhancement following administration of gadolinium.

In one review of 181 cases, there was an age range of 1 to 72 years and no sex predominance;[169] however, a high proportion occur in children and adolescents and they have been considered the most common primary pulmonary "tumor" in this age group.[141] Many patients are asymptomatic,[170] the lesion being discovered on a screening chest radiograph. When present, symptoms include cough, hemoptysis, and chest pain;[141] signs and symptoms of bronchial or

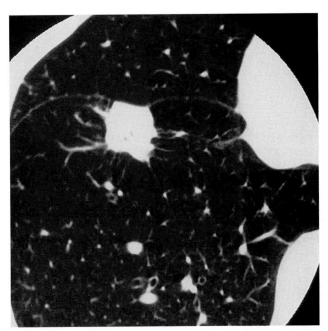

Figure 37–8. Inflammatory Pseudotumor. An HRCT scan demonstrates a lobulated, spiculated soft tissue lesion in the right lower lobe. Small areas of low attenuation consistent with air (bubble lucencies) are evident within the lesion. Histologic assessment of the resected specimen demonstrated an inflammatory pseudotumor. The patient was asymptomatic.

tracheal obstruction are present in some patients.[171] In some instances, a history of recent acute respiratory illness suggests that the process represents a stage in the resolution of acute pneumonia.[139, 141, 158, 172] Rare cases have been associated with hypercalcemia[173] or hypertrophic osteoarthropathy.[174]

Long-term follow-up usually shows no change in size or configuration of these lesions; occasionally, they increase in size over time,[141] sometimes rapidly.[175] In some patients in whom the diagnosis has been established by biopsy only, the lesions have been seen to regress either with or without steroid therapy;[176, 177] however, in others, recurrence has developed following apparent complete surgical excision.[175] In addition, in a minority of patients, there is evidence of locally aggressive behavior, including infiltration of pulmonary vessels, chest wall, and mediastinum.[145, 146, 148]

Pulmonary Hyalinizing Granuloma

The term *pulmonary hyalinizing granuloma* was first employed in 1977 to describe an unusual pulmonary tumor characterized histologically by numerous regularly arranged lamellae of hyalinized collagen.[178] The condition is uncommon; apart from the initial report of 20 patients and more recent series of 4[179] and 24 cases,[180] only scattered case reports have appeared.[181–186]

The etiology and pathogenesis are unclear. Some lesions have been reported to show weak Congo red staining and birefringence consistent with amyloid,[178] and an association with clear-cut pulmonary vascular amyloidosis has been noted in some instances.[189] Despite this, most nodules show no evidence of amyloid deposition,[178, 180] and the overall histologic appearance is unlike that of the typical nodule of

pulmonary amyloid. It has been suggested that the nodules represent an exaggerated host reaction to one of a number of agents,[178] such as *Histoplasma capsulatum*.[180] The presence of Castleman's disease,[190] multiple sclerosis,[191] and serologic abnormalities[180, 181] in some patients suggests the possibility of an underlying derangement of immune function. Concomitant retroperitoneal[178, 182, 186] or mediastinal[178, 180] fibrosis, or both, have also been reported in a number of patients and it is possible that the pulmonary nodules represent a similar disease process in these individuals.

Pathologically, the nodules are well demarcated and often "shell out" easily from surrounding lung parenchyma (Fig. 37–9). Histologically, they consist of numerous interconnecting lamellae of homogeneous, hyalinized collagen.[178, 180] Plasma cells and occasional lymphocytes and multinucleated giant cells are present in small numbers between the lamellae and adjacent to blood vessels. Necrosis is present in some cases and is probably related to ischemia; calcification occurs rarely.[180]

Radiographically, the nodules are usually round, homogeneous, and well defined;[188] cavitation has been noted occasionally.[178, 179] The nodules are frequently multiple and 2 to 4 cm in diameter; calcification is infrequent.[180] Serial radiographs may reveal slow growth;[180] when associated with multiple nodules, the appearance resembles that of metastases (Fig. 37–10).[184, 187]

The tumors occur most often in adults. Many patients are asymptomatic;[178] however, cough, dyspnea, chest pain, and hemoptysis can occur.[178, 180] Circulating immune complexes and a variety of autoantibodies have been identified, typically unaccompanied by evidence of a specific connective tissue disease.[180, 181, 185] The condition is usually benign, although progressive pulmonary disease consisting of increasing dyspnea and enlarging nodules was noted in 6 of 19 patients in one series.[180]

Mesenchymal Cystic Hamartoma

Mesenchymal cystic hamartoma is a rare pulmonary disease first described in 1986 in a report of five patients.[192] It is usually manifested as multiple nodules that slowly increase in size and become cystic. Most patients have been middle aged; however, examples have been documented in boys 1½ and 14 years old.[192, 193] The precise nature of the abnormality is uncertain. Although it was initially hypothesized to be hamartomatous on the basis of pathologic observations,[192] a similar appearance has been seen with metastatic sarcoma,[194] and the possibility that it represents an unusual neoplasm might also be considered.

Pathologically, the initial lesion appears to be composed of an interstitial proliferation of undifferentiated mesenchymal cells separated by anastomosing epithelial-lined slits resembling airways.[192] These lesions correspond to the solid nodules seen grossly and measure up to about 10 mm in diameter. Larger lesions—which may measure up to 10 cm—are composed of cysts lined by a layer of ciliated or metaplastic squamous squamous epithelium; mesenchymal cells identical to those in the smaller nodules can be seen in a dense layer adjacent to the epithelium.

Radiologic findings consist of bilateral nodules or cysts, the latter sometimes resembling those of lymphangioleiomy-

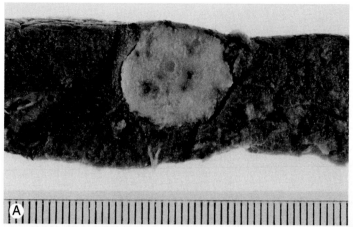

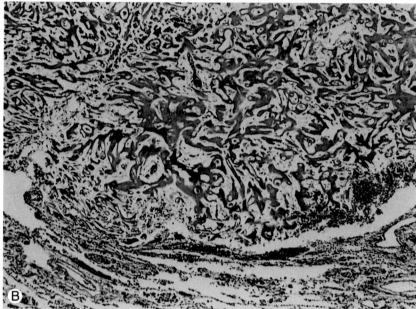

Figure 37–9. Pulmonary Hyalinizing Granuloma. A well-circumscribed, finely granular nodule *(A)* is present in the immediate subpleural region. A section *(B)* shows lamellae of hyalinized collagen separated by a fine fibrovascular stroma and scattered plasma cells. *(B,* ×64.)

omatosis.[195] Pneumothorax and, occasionally, hydropneumothorax, may be seen.[192] Some patients have been asymptomatic, the lesions being discovered on a screening radiograph;[196] however, most have presented with hemoptysis or chest pain related to pneumothorax.[192, 193, 195] Although the condition may be slowly progressive, the prognosis appears to be good in most patients. However, fatality as a result of massive hemoptysis has been reported.[195]

Pulmonary Meningothelial-Like Nodules

So-called pulmonary meningothelial-like nodules (minute pulmonary chemodectomas) consist of intraparenchymal "tumors" usually discovered incidentally on microscopic examination of lungs removed surgically or at autopsy; occasionally, they are recognized grossly as graywhite or yellow-tan nodules measuring 1 to 3 mm in diameter.[198–200] They are usually multiple and, in fact, hundreds have sometimes been identified within several pulmonary lobes.[197] Microscopically, they are often closely associated with small pulmonary veins and consist of nests of rather

uniform, oval or spindle-shaped cells separated by thin strands of fibrous tissue (Fig. 37–11). The nests are situated in perivenous connective tissue and adjacent alveolar interstitium but do not extend into the air spaces themselves. Cell nuclei are oval or spindle shaped and show no atypia or mitotic figures.

The nature of these tumors is uncertain. Although it was originally hypothesized that they were the result of a proliferation of intrapulmonary chemoreceptor tissue,[197] the results of several ultrastructural[198, 199, 201] and immunohistochemical[200] studies indicate a lack of neuroendocrine characteristics and the presence of a number of features that are not normally evident in chemoreceptor tissue. Although some observers have instead suggested an origin in mesothelial[201] or muscle cells,[202] most have interpreted the pathologic features of these tumors as most closely resembling meningiomas,[198, 203] and it has been proposed that the lesions are best designated *pulmonary meningothelial-like nodules*.[200] (It is not clear whether the rare tumor designated pulmonary meningioma that is large enough to be recognized grossly and radiographically [*see* page 1370] represents an exaggerated form of "minute chemodectoma" or a different entity alto-

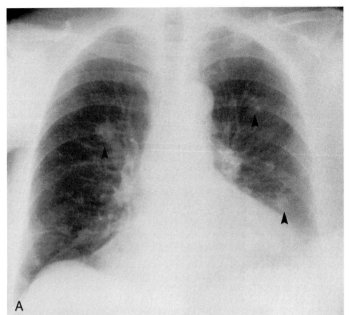

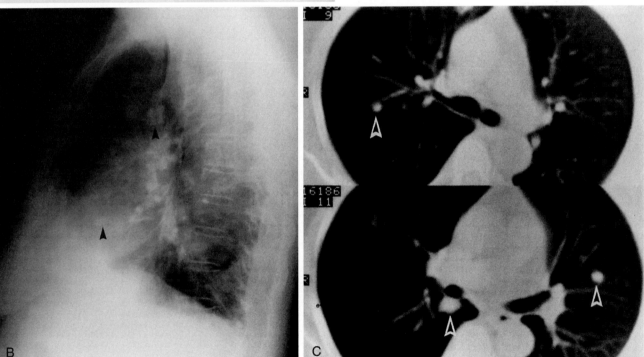

Figure 37–10. Pulmonary Hyalinizing Granuloma. Posteroanterior *(A)* and lateral *(B)* radiographs disclose multiple nodules *(arrowheads)* of variable size in both lungs. The patient was a middle-aged woman with a history of right mastectomy for adenocarcinoma of the breast; the initial radiologic impression was "metastatic carcinoma." CT scans through the hila *(C)* confirm the presence of multiple nodules *(arrowheads)* in both lungs, with no distinguishing features. An open lung biopsy revealed typical findings of hyalinizing granuloma.

gether). Whatever the histogenesis of these tumors, their small size and multiplicity argue for a hyperplastic rather than a neoplastic pathogenesis.

These lesions were identified in only 12 of 3,635 autopsies retrospectively reviewed in one series.[197] However, if looked for prospectively, the true incidence would likely be much higher.[200] The majority are found in patients between 40 to 60 years of age; there is a marked female preponderance, 46 of 55 patients in five series being of this gender.[198] Since all cases have been discovered incidentally, coexistent disease is common, particularly chronic pulmonary and cardiac disease and malignancy;[198, 205] a high incidence of thromboembolism has been noted by some authors.[206] Because of their small size, they cannot be identified radio-

graphically; however, it is conceivable that they could be visualized on HRCT. They are of no known clinical significance.

Endometriosis

Thoracic endometriosis is manifested clinically most often by pneumothorax *(see page 2767).* However, in about 5% of cases the abnormality presents as a pulmonary nodule that may be confused with a neoplasm.[207] Such parenchymal involvement tends to occur at an older age than other manifestations of thoracic endometriosis (mean age of 38 years in one review[207]) and is most often on the right side.

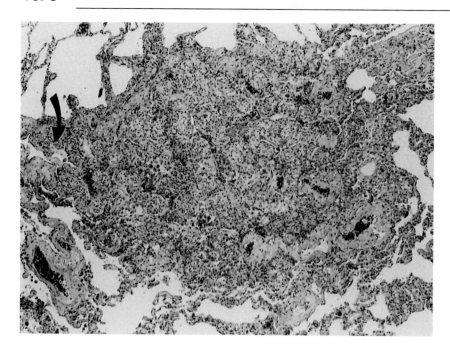

Figure 37–11. Pulmonary Meningothelial-Like Nodule. A small, highly vascular tumor is present in relation to an interlobular septum near the lung periphery (a portion of a pulmonary vein is identifiable at the edge *[arrow]*). The tumor itself is composed of multiple small nodules of oval- to spindle-shaped cells with ample cytoplasm. This was an incidental finding in a 64-year-old woman with congestive heart failure. (×86.)

There is evidence that some cases are the result of embolization of endometrial tissue from the uterus to the lungs via the pulmonary arteries.[208] Experimental studies have shown that endometrial tissue injected intravenously can survive and proliferate within pulmonary vessels and the adjacent parenchyma.[209] Fragments of decidua have occasionally been identified within the lungs of postpartum women,[210, 211] and it is conceivable that glands as well as stromal tissue could also be transported at the same time during labor or surgical trauma. Support for this mechanism was provided in one review of 65 cases of pleural and parenchymal endometriosis in which all patients with evidence of pulmonary parenchymal involvement had a history of at least one spontaneous vaginal delivery or gynecologic operation.[212] In addition, although the right hemithorax was affected in 93% of the 54 patients with pleural endometriosis, this laterality was seen in only 64% of those considered to have parenchymal disease, suggesting that the pathogenesis is different at the two sites and that the parenchymal form may be related to pulmonary blood flow. In fact, it is likely that other mechanisms, such as transdiaphragmatic migration of endometrial tissue or metaplasia of pleural connective tissue, are involved in the development of pleural endometriosis in at least some cases (*see* page 2767); it is possible that extension of disease from this site into the adjacent lung may be responsible for some cases that present as parenchymal disease.

Most foci of disease appear to be entirely within pulmonary parenchyma; occasionally, one is intimately related to the pleura or a bronchus.[213] Pathologic examination reveals a variable amount of fibrous tissue associated with irregularly shaped endometrial glands and stroma. Diagnostic tissue has occasionally been identified in specimens obtained by TTNA.[214]

The radiographic appearance is that of a solitary nodule measuring up to 4 cm in diameter.[215, 216] Cystic change may be seen.[217] In clinically suspected cases, CT may be of value in identifying lesions that are not apparent on conventional radiographs.[218] In one 26-year-old woman, CT performed before menses demonstrated multiple 0.5- to 1.5-cm smoothly marginated nodules with thin-walled cavities;[219] in several nodules, the cavities were eccentric. CT during menses demonstrated focal areas of consolidation, presumably representing blood, surrounding the nodules. Occasionally, nodules also can be seen to increase and decrease in size with the menstrual cycle.[220] Decidualization of stromal cells also may occur during pregnancy and can result in an increase in the size of nodules.[208] One case has been reported in which airway obstruction was associated with recurrent episodes of atelectasis.[213]

Patients usually present with a history of recurrent episodes of hemoptysis (catamenial hemoptysis); occasionally, a lesion is discovered in an asymptomatic patient on a screening chest radiograph. Onset of symptoms is usually within 24 to 48 hours of the beginning of menstruation. An exceptional case has been reported of a woman with catamenial hemoptysis, the origin of which proved to be a pulmonary vascular malformation rather than endometriosis.[221]

Hemangioma

Most, if not all, pulmonary tumors designated *hemangioma* probably represent either a developmental or acquired vascular malformation rather than a true neoplasm. In the former instance, the tumor has been more appropriately termed *arteriovenous malformation* when large and *telangiectasia* when small, although there may be no important pathogenetic differences between the two. The tumors may be solitary or multiple and are not infrequently associated with vascular malformations in other viscera, skin, or mucous membranes (hereditary hemorrhagic telangiectasia [*see* page 655]). Acquired fistulas, more appropriately termed *shunts,* may be seen in a variety of circumstances and are discussed in relation to specific disease entities. A single example has been reported of a pulmonary angiomyolipoma similar to the more common renal tumor.[222]

Lymphangioma

Lymphangiomas that originate within the lung are very rare, only nine cases having been documented by 1995.[223, 224]

Most patients are asymptomatic, the lesion being identified on a screening radiograph;[223–225] one example that involved the hilum and perihilar pulmonary parenchyma in a 54-year-old man was associated with hemoptysis.[226] Like hemangiomas, these lesions probably represent developmental malformations rather than true neoplasms. This hypothesis is supported by the occasional lesions discovered in infancy.[227]

REFERENCES

1. Gaffey MJ, Mills SE, Askin FB, et al: Clear cell tumor of the lung: A clinicopathologic, immunohistochemical, and ultrastructural study of eight cases. Am J Surg Pathol 14:248, 1990.
2. Liebow AA, Castleman B: Benign clear cell ("sugar") tumors of the lung. Yale J Biol Med 43:213, 1971.
3. Becker NH, Soifer I: Benign clear cell tumor ("sugar tumor") of the lung. Cancer 27:712, 1971.
4. Andrion A, Mazzucco G, Gugliotta P, et al: Benign clear cell (sugar) tumor of the lung: A light microscopic, histochemical, and ultrastructural study with a review of the literature. Cancer 56:2657, 1985.
5. Lantuejoul S, Isaac S, Pinel N, et al: Clear cell tumor of the lung: An immunohistochemical and ultrastructural study supporting a pericystic differentiation. Mod Pathol 10:1001, 1997.
6. Gaffey MJ, Mills SE, Zarbo RJ, et al: Clear cell tumor of the lung: Immunohistochemical and ultrastructural evidence of melanogenesis. Am J Surg Pathol 15:644, 1991.
7. Gal AA, Koss MN, Hochholzer L, et al: An immunohistochemical study of benign clear cell ("sugar") tumor of the lung. Arch Pathol Lab Med 115:1034, 1991.
7a. Flieder DB, Travis WD: Clear cell "sugar" tumor of the lung: Association with lymphangioleiomyomatosis and multifocal micronodular pneumocyte hyperplasia in a patient with tuberous sclerosis. Am J Surg Pathol 21:1242, 1997.
8. Harbin WP, Mark GJ, Greene RE: Benign clear cell tumor ("sugar" tumor) of the lung: A case report and review of the literature. Radiology 129:595, 1978.
9. Sale GE, Kulander BG: Benign clear cell tumor of lung with necrosis. Cancer 37:2355, 1976.
10. Hoch WS, Patchefsky AS, Takeda M, et al: Benign clear cell tumor of the lung: An ultrastructural study. Cancer 33:1328, 1974.
11. Kung M, Landa JP, Lubin J: Benign clear cell tumor ("sugar tumor") of the trachea. Cancer 54:517, 1984.
12. Sale GE, Kulander BG: "Benign" clear cell tumor (sugar tumor) of the lung with hepatic metastases ten years after resection of pulmonary primary tumor. Arch Pathol Lab Med 112:1177, 1988.
13. Ashley DJB, Evans CJ: Intrathoracic carotid body tumour (chemodectoma). Thorax 21:184, 1966.
14. Liew S-H, Leong AS-Y, Tang HM: Tracheal paraganglioma: A case report with review of the literature. Cancer 47:1387, 1981.
15. Gallimore AP, Goldstraw P: Tracheal paraganglioma. Thorax 48:866, 1993.
16. Blessing MH, Borchard F, Lenz W: Glomustumor (sog. Chemodektom) der lunge Pathologisch-anatomische und biochemische befunde. Virchows Arch [Pathol Anat] 359:315, 1973.
17. Hangartner JR, Loosemore TM, Burke M, et al: Malignant primary pulmonary paraganglioma. Thorax 44:154, 1989.
18. Skodt V, Jacobsen GK, Helsted M: Primary paraganglioma of the lung: Report of two cases and review of the literature. APMIS 103:597, 1995.
19. Singh G, Lee RE, Brooks DH: Primary pulmonary paraganglioma: Report of a case and review of the literature. Cancer 40:2286, 1977.
20. Liebow AA, Hubbell DF: Sclerosing hemangioma (histiocytoma, xanthoma) of the lung. Cancer 9:53, 1956.
21. Haas JE, Yunis EJ, Totten RS: Ultrastructure of a sclerosing hemangioma of the lung. Cancer 30:512, 1972.
22. Kay S, Still WJS, Borochovitz D: Sclerosing hemangioma of the lung: An endothelial or epithelial neoplasm? Hum Pathol 8:468, 1977.
23. Huszar M, Suster S, Herczeg E, et al: Sclerosing hemangioma of the lung: Immunohistochemical demonstration of mesenchymal origin using antibodies to tissue-specific intermediate filaments. Cancer 58:2422, 1986.
24. Xu HM, Li WH, Hou N, et al: Neuroendocrine differentiation in 32 cases of so-called sclerosing hemangioma of the lung: Identified by immunohistochemical and ultrastructural study. Am J Surg Pathol 21:1013, 1997.
25. Katzenstein A-LA, Weise DL, Fulling K, et al: So-called sclerosing hemangioma of the lung: Evidence for mesothelial origin. Am J Surg Pathol 7:3, 1983.
26. Haimoto H, Tsutsumi Y, Nagura H, et al: Immunohistochemical study of so-called sclerosing haemangioma of the lung. Virchows Arch 407:419, 1985.
27. Nagata N, Dairaku M, Ishida T, et al: Sclerosing hemangioma of the lung: Immunohistochemical characterization of its origin as related to surfactant apoprotein. Cancer 55:116, 1985.
28. Heikkila P, Salminen US: Papillary pneumocytoma of the lung: An immunohistochemical and electron microscopic study. Pathol Res Pract 190:194, 1994.
29. Aihara T, Nakajima T: Sclerosing hemangioma of the lung: Pathological study and enzyme immunoassay for estrogen and progesterone receptors. Acta Pathol Jpn 43:507, 1993.
30. Alvarez-Fernandez E, Carretero-Albinana L, Menarguez-Palanca J: Sclerosing hemangioma of the lung: An immunohistochemical study of intermediate filaments and endothelial markers. Arch Pathol Lab Med 113:121, 1989.
31. Chan K-W, Gibbs AR, Lo WS, et al: Benign sclerosing pneumocytoma of lung (sclerosing haemangioma). Thorax 37:404, 1982.
32. Shimosato Y: Lung tumors of uncertain histogenesis. Semin Diagn Pathol 12:185, 1995.
33. Sugio K, Yokoyama H, Kaneko S, et al: Sclerosing hemangioma of the lung: Radiographic and pathological study. Ann Thorac Surg 53:295, 1992.
34. Katzenstein AL, Gmelich JT, Carrington CB: Sclerosing hemangioma of the lung. Am J Surg Pathol 4:343, 1980.
35. Thomas A, Lee CN: Sclerosing haemangioma in Singapore. Ann Acad Med Singapore 15:71, 1986.
36. Eggleston JC: The intravascular bronchioloalveolar tumor and the sclerosing hemangioma of the lung: Misnomers of pulmonary neoplasia. Semin Diagn Pathol 2:270, 1985.
37. Niho S, Suzuki K, Yokose T, et al: Monoclonality of both pale cells and cuboidal cells of sclerosing hemangioma of the lung. Am J Pathol 152:1065, 1998.
38. Spencer H, Nambu S: Sclerosing haemangiomas of the lung. Histopathology 10:477, 1986.
39. Noguchi M, Kodama T, Morinaga S, et al: Multiple sclerosing hemangiomas of the lung. Am J Surg Pathol 101:429, 1986.
40. Tanaka I, Inoue M, Matsui Y, et al: A case of pneumocytoma (so-called sclerosing hemangioma) with lymph node metastasis. Jpn J Clin Oncol 16:77, 1986.
41. Moran CA, Zeren H, Koss MN: Sclerosing hemangioma of the lung: Granulomatous variant. Arch Pathol Lab Med 118:1028, 1994.
42. Grayson W, Leiman G, Cooper K: Exuberant fibroadenomatoid proliferation in a pulmonary mesenchymoma (hamartoma): Report of a lesion mimicking a sclerosing pneumocytoma. Gen Diagn Pathol 142:247, 1997.
43. Sugio K, Yokoyama H, Kaneko S, et al. Sclerosing hemangioma of the lung: Radiographic and pathologic study. Ann Thorac Surg 53:295, 1992.
44. Im JG, Kim WH, Han MC, et al: Sclerosing hemangiomas of the lung and interlobar fissures: CT findings. J Comput Assist Tomogr 18:34, 1994.
45. Dawson WB, Müller NL, Miller RR: Pulmonary sclerosing hemangioma: Unusual cause of a solitary pulmonary nodule. Can Assoc Radiol J 41:372, 1990.
46. Bahk YW, Shinn KS, Choi BS: The air meniscus sign in sclerosing hemangioma of the lung. Radiology 128:27, 1978.
47. Kaw YT, Nayak RN: Fine-needle aspiration biopsy cytology of sclerosing hemangioma of the lung: A case report. Acta Cytol 37:933, 1993.
48. Wojcik EM, Sneige N, Lawrence DD, et al: Fine-needle aspiration cytology of sclerosing hemangioma of the lung: Case report with immunohistochemical study. Diagn Cytopathol 9:304, 1993.
49. Wang SE, Nieberg RK: Fine-needle aspiration cytology of sclerosing hemangioma of the lung, a mimicker of bronchioloalveolar carcinoma. Acta Cytol 30:51, 1986.
50. Mikuz G, Szinicz G, Fischer H: Sclerosing angioma of the lung: Case report and electron microscope investigation. Virchows Arch [Pathol Anat Histol] 385:93, 1979.
51. Metz SA, Weintraub B, Rosen SW, et al: Ectopic secretion of chorionic gonadotropin by a lung carcinoma: Pituitary gonadotropin and subunit secretion and prolonged chemotherapeutic remission. Am J Med 65:325, 1978.
52. Arnould L, Drouot F, Fargeot P, et al: Hepatoid carcinoma of the lung: Report of a case of an unusual α-fetoprotein–producing lung tumor. Am J Surg Pathol 21:1113, 1997.
53. Adachi H, Aki T, Yoshida H, et al: Combined choriocarcinoma and adenocarcinoma of the lung. Acta Pathol Jpn 39:147, 1989.
54. Siegel RJ, Bueso-Ramos C, Cohen C, et al: Pulmonary blastoma with germ cell (yolk sac) differentiation: Report of two cases. Mod Pathol 4:566, 1991.
55. Pound AW, Willis RA: A malignant teratoma of the lung in an infant. J Pathol 98:111, 1969.
56. Day DW, Taylor SA: An intrapulmonary teratoma associated with thymic tissue. Thorax 30:582, 1975.
57. Holt S, Deverall PB, Boddy JE: A teratoma of the lung containing thymic tissue. J Pathol 126:85, 1978.
58. Prauer HW, Mack D, Babic R: Intrapulmonary teratoma 10 years after removal of a mediastinal teratoma in a young man. Thorax 38:632, 1983.
59. Nakanishi K, Kohzaki S, Fujimoto S, et al: Pulmonary sclerosing hemangioma: Report of a case with emphasis on dynamic MR imaging findings. Radiat Med 15:117, 1997.
60. Jamieson MPG, McGowan AR: Endobronchial teratoma. Thorax 37:157, 1982.
61. Morgan DE, Sanders C, McElvein RB, et al: Intrapulmonary teratoma: A case report and review of the literature. J Thorac Imaging 7:70, 1992.
62. Gautam HP: Intrapulmonary malignant teratoma. Am Rev Resp Dis 100:863, 1969.
63. Berghout A, Mallens WMC, Velde J, et al: Teratoma of the lung in a hemophilic patient. Acta Haematol 70:330, 1983.
64. Tanimura A, Natsuyama H, Kawano M, et al: Primary choriocarcinoma of the lung. Hum Pathol 16:1281, 1985.
65. Whitcomb RW, Schimke RN, Kyner JL, et al: Endocrine studies in a male patient with choriocarcinoma and gynecomastia. Am J Med 81:917, 1986.
66. Pushchak MJ, Farhi DC: Primary choriocarcinoma of the lung. Arch Pathol Lab Med 111:477, 1987.
67. Cutler CS, Michel RP, Yassa M, et al: Pulmonary blastoma: Case report of a patient with a 7-year remission and review of chemotherapy experience in the world literature. Cancer 82:462, 1998.
68. Sullivan LG: Primary choriocarcinoma of the lung in a man. Arch Pathol Lab Med 113:82, 1989.
69. Van Nostrand KM, Lucci JA III, Liao SY, et al: Primary lung choriocarcinoma masquerading as a metastatic gestational neoplasm. Gynecol Oncol 53:361, 1994.
70. Marchevsky AM: Lung tumors derived from ectopic tissues. Semin Diagn Pathol 12:172, 1995.
71. Spencer H: Pulmonary blastomas. J Pathol 82:161, 1961.

72. McCann MP, Fu Y-S, Kay S: Pulmonary blastoma: A light and electron microscopic study. Cancer 38:789, 1976.

73. Fung CH, Lo JW, Yonan TN, et al: Pulmonary blastoma: An ultrastructural study with a brief review of literature and a discussion of pathogenesis. Cancer 39:153, 1977.

74. Tamai S, Kameya T, Shimosato Y, et al: Pulmonary blastoma: An ultrastructural study of a case and its transplanted tumor in athymic nude mice. Cancer 46:1389, 1980.

75. Muller-Hermelink HK, Kaiserling E: Pulmonary adenocarcinoma of fetal type: Alternating differentiation argues in favour of a common endodermal stem cell. Virchows Arch A 409:195, 1986.

76. Berean K, Truong LD, Dudley AW Jr, et al: Immunohistochemical characterization of pulmonary blastoma. Am J Clin Pathol 89:773, 1988.

77. Korbi S, M'Boyo A, Dusmet M, et al: Pulmonary blastoma: Immunohistochemical and ultrastructural studies of a case. Histopathology 11:753, 1987.

78. Dehner LP: Pleuropulmonary blastoma is the pulmonary blastoma of childhood. Semin Diagn Pathol 11:144, 1994.

79. Manivel JC, Priest JR, Watterson J, et al: Pleuropulmonary blastoma: The so-called pulmonary blastoma of childhood. Cancer 62:1516, 1988.

80. Barson AJ, Jones AW, Lodge KV: Pulmonary blastoma. J Clin Pathol 21:480, 1968.

81. Stackhouse EM, Harrison EG Jr, Ellis FH Jr: Primary mixed malignancies of lung: Carcinosarcoma and blastoma. J Thorac Cardiovasc Surg 57:385, 1969.

82. Roth JA, Elguezabal A: Pulmonary blastoma evolving into carcinosarcoma: A case study. Am J Surg Pathol 2:407, 1978.

83. Wick MR, Ritter JH, Humphrey PA: Sarcomatoid carcinomas of the lung: A clinicopathologic review. Am J Clin Pathol 108:40, 1997.

84. Olenick SJ, Fan CC, Ryoo JW: Mixed pulmonary blastoma and carcinosarcoma: Histopathology 25:171, 1994.

85. Addis BJ, Corrin B: Pulmonary blastoma, carcinosarcoma, and spindle-cell carcinoma: An immunohistochemical study of keratin intermediate filaments. J Pathol 147:291, 1985.

86. Ashworth TG: Pulmonary blastoma, a true congenital neoplasm. Histopathology 7:585, 1983.

87. Travis WD, Colby TV, Corrin B, et al, and Collaborators from 14 Countries: World Health Organization Pathology Panel: World Health Organization. Histological Typing of Lung and Pleural Tumors: International Histological Classification of Tumors, 3rd ed, Berlin, Springer-Verlag. In press.

88. Kodama T, Shimosato Y, Watanabe S, et al: Six cases of well-differentiated adenocarcinoma simulating fetal lung tubules in pseudoglandular stage. Am J Surg Pathol 8:735, 1984.

89. Nakatani Y, Dickersin GR, Mark EJ: Pulmonary endodermal tumor resembling fetal lung: A clinicopathologic study of five cases with immunohistochemical and ultrastructural characterization. Hum Pathol 21:1097, 1990.

90. Muller-Hermelink HK, Kaiserling E: Pulmonary adenocarcinoma of fetal type: Alternating differentiation argues in favor of a common endodermal stem cell. Virchows Arch [Pathol Anat] 409:195, 1986.

91. Kradin RL, Young RH, Dickersin GR, et al: Pulmonary blastoma with argyrophil cells and lacking sarcomatous features (pulmonary endodermal tumor resembling fetal lung). Am J Surg Pathol 6:165, 1982.

92. Koss MN, Hochholzer L, O'Leary T: Pulmonary blastomas. Cancer 67:2368, 1991.

93. Korbi S, Boyo AM, Dusmet M, et al: Pulmonary blastoma: Immunohistochemical and ultrastructural studies of a case. Histopathology 11:753, 1987.

94. Babycos PB, Daroca PJ Jr: Polypoid pulmonary endodermal tumor resembling fetal lung: Report of a case. Modern Pathol 8:303, 1995.

95. Mardini G, Pai U, Chavez AM, et al: Endobronchial adenocarcinoma with endometrioid features and prominent neuroendocrine differentiation: A variant of fetal adenocarcinoma. Cancer 73:1383, 1994.

96. Nakatani Y, Kitamura H, Inayama Y, et al: Pulmonary endodermal tumor resembling fetal lung: The optically clear nucleus is rich in biotin. Am J Surg Pathol 18:637, 1994.

97. Siegel RJ, Bueso-Ramos C, Cohen C, et al: Pulmonary blastoma with germ cell (yolk sac) differentiation: Report of two cases. Mod Pathol 4:566, 1991.

98. Chin NK, Lee CN, Lee YS, et al: Pulmonary blastoma in an adult presenting as a chronic loculated effusion: A diagnostic problem. Thorax 49:838, 1994.

99. Berho M, Moran CA, Suster S: Malignant mixed epithelial/mesenchymal neoplasms of the lung. Semin Diagn Pathol 12:123, 1995.

100. Jacobsen M, Francis D: Pulmonary blastoma: A clinicopathological study of eleven cases. Acta Pathol Microbiol Scand [A] 88:151, 1980.

101. Henry K, Keal EE: Pulmonary blastoma with a striated muscle component. Br J Dis Chest 60:87, 1966.

102. Heckman CJ, Truong LD, Cagle PT, et al: Pulmonary blastoma with rhabdomyosarcomatous differentiation: An immunohistochemical study. Am J Surg Pathol 12:35, 1988.

103. Thompson TT: Roentgen manifestations of pulmonary blastoma. Chest 62:104, 1972.

104. Weisbrod GL, Chamberlain DW, Tao LC: Pulmonary blastoma: Report of three cases and a review of the literature. J Can Assoc Radiol 39:130, 1988.

105. Peacock MJ, Whitwell F: Pulmonary blastoma. Thorax 31:197, 1976.

106. Senac MO, Wood BP, Isaacs H, et al: Pulmonary blastoma: A rare childhood malignancy. Radiology 179:743, 1991.

107. Francis D, Jacobsen M: Pulmonary blastoma: Preoperative cytologic and histologic findings. Acta Cytol 23:437, 1979.

108. Spahr J, Draffin RM, Johnston WW: Cytopathologic findings in pulmonary blastoma. Acta Cytol 23:454, 1979.

109. Weinblatt ME, Siegel SE, Isaacs H: Pulmonary blastoma associated with cystic lung disease. Cancer 49:669, 1982.

110. Green WR, Pressoir R, Gumbs RV: Intrapulmonary thymoma. Arch Pathol Lab Med 111:1074, 1987.

111. Fukayama M, Maeda Y, Funata N, et al: Pulmonary and pleural thymoma: Diagnostic application of lymphocyte markers to the thymoma of unusual site. Am J Clin Pathol 89:617, 1988.

112. Moran CA, Suster S, Fishback NF, et al: Primary intrapulmonary thymoma: A clinicopathologic and immunohistochemical study of eight cases. Am J Surg Pathol 19:304, 1995.

113. Kung ITM, Loke SL, So SY, et al: Intrapulmonary thymoma: Report of two cases. Thorax 40:471, 1985.

114. Patterson RL, Heller EL: Aberrant thymic tissue in the lung—with bronchial compression and sudden death during anesthesia. Anesthesiology 4:233, 1943.

115. Kaplan IL, Swayne LC, Widmann WD, Wolff M: CT demonstration of "ectopic" thymoma. J Comput Assist Tomogr 12:1037, 1988.

116. Kodama K, Doi O, Higashiyama M, et al: Primary and metastatic pulmonary meningioma. Cancer 67:1412, 1991.

117. Chumas JC, Lorelle CA: Pulmonary meningioma: A light- and electron-microscopic study. Am J Surg Pathol 6:795, 1982.

118. Robinson PG: Pulmonary meningioma: Report of a case with electron microscopic and immunohistochemical findings. Am J Clin Pathol 97:814, 1992.

119. Flynn SD, Yousem SA: Pulmonary meningiomas: A report of two cases. Hum Pathol 22:469, 1991.

120. Unger PD, Geller GA, Anderson PJ: Pulmonary lesions in a patient with neurofibromatosis. Arch Pathol Lab Med 108:654, 1984.

121. Crotty TB, Hooker RP, Swensen SJ, et al: Primary malignant ependymoma of the lung. Mayo Clin Proc 67:373, 1992.

122. Fink G, Herskovitz P, Nili M, et al: Suture granuloma simulating lung neoplasm occurring after segmentectomy. Thorax 48:405, 1993.

123. Chopra S, Simmons DH, Cassan SM et al: Case reports: Bronchial obstruction by incorporation of aspirated vegetable material in the bronchial wall. Am Rev Respir Dis 112:717, 1975.

124. Patel AM, Trastek VF, Coles DT: Gossypibomas mimicking echinococcal cyst disease of the lung. Chest 105:284, 1994.

125. Caldarola VT, Harrison EG Jr, Clagett OT, et al: Benign tumors and tumorlike conditions of the trachea and bronchi. Ann Otol 73:1042, 1964.

126. Greene JG, Tassin L, Saberi A: Endobronchial epithelial papilloma associated with a foreign body. Chest 97:229, 1990.

127. Ashley DJB, Danino EA, Davies HD: Bronchial polyps. Thorax 18:45, 1963.

128. Peroni A: Inflammatory tumors of the bronchi. Arch Otolaryngol 19:1, 1934.

129. Berman DE, Wright ES, Edstrom HW: Endobronchial inflammatory polyp associated with a foreign body. Chest 86:483, 1984.

130. Barzo P, Molnar L, Minik K: Bronchial papillomas of various origins. Chest 92:132, 1987.

131. Adams C, Moisan T, Chandrasekhar AJ, et al: Endobronchial polyposis secondary to thermal inhalational injury. Chest 75:643, 1979.

132. Williams DD, Vanecko RM, Glassroth J: Endobronchial polyposis following smoke inhalation. Chest 84:774, 1983.

133. Su LD, Atayde-Perez A, Sheldon S, et al: Inflammatory myofibroblastic tumor: Cytogenetic evidence supporting clonal origin. Mod Pathol 11:364, 1998.

134. Drennan JM, Douglas AC: Solitary papilloma of a bronchus. J Clin Pathol 18:401, 1965.

135. Kahn B, Amer NS: Multiple bronchial polyps. Chest 57:279, 1970.

136. Shale DJ, Lane DJ, Fisher CWS, et al: Endobronchial polyp in an asthmatic subject. Thorax 38:75, 1983.

137. Niimi A, Amitani R, Ikeda T, et al: Inflammatory bronchial polyps associated with asthma: Resolution with inhaled corticosteroid. Eur Resp J 8:1237, 1995.

138. Vontz FK, Vitsky BH: Giant bronchial polyp treated by emergency thoracotomy. Chest 66:102, 1974.

139. Spencer H: The pulmonary plasma cell/histiocytoma complex. Histopathology 8:903, 1984.

140. Alvarez-Fernandez E, Escalona-Zapata J: Pulmonary plasma cell granuloma: An electron microscopic and tissue culture study. Histopathology 7:279, 1983.

141. Bahadori M, Liebow AA: Plasma cell granulomas of the lung. Cancer 31:191, 1973.

142. Chen HP, Lee SS, Berardi RS: Inflammatory pseudotumor of the lung: Ultrastructural and light-microscopic study of a myxomatous variant. Cancer 54:861, 1984.

143. Matsubara O, Tan-Liu NS, Kenney RM, et al: Inflammatory pseudotumors of the lung: Progression from organizing pneumonia to fibrous histiocytoma or to plasma cell granuloma in 32 cases. Hum Pathol 19:807, 1988.

144. Pettinato G, Manivel JC, De Rosa N, et al: Inflammatory myofibroblastic tumor (plasma cell granuloma): Clinicopathologic study of 20 cases with immunohistochemical and ultrastructural observations. Am J Clin Pathol 94:538, 1990.

145. Wang NS, Morin J: Recurrent endobronchial soft tissue tumors. Chest 85:787, 1984.

146. Lund C, Sorensen IM, Axelsen F, et al: Pulmonary histiocytomas. Eur J Resp Dis 64:141, 1983.

147. Weinberg PB, Bromberg PA, Askin FB: "Recurrence" of a plasma cell granuloma 11 years after initial resection. South Med J 80:519, 1987.

148. Sandstrom RE, Proppe KH, Trelstad RL: Fibrous histiocytoma of the trachea. Am J Clin Pathol 70:429, 1978.

149. Warter A, Satge D, Roeslin N: Angioinvasive plasma cell granulomas of the lung. Cancer 57:435, 1987.

150. Gal AA, Koss MN, McCarthy WF, et al: Prognostic factors in pulmonary fibrohistiocytic lesions. Cancer 73:1817, 1994.

151. Snyder CS, Dell'Aquila M, Haghighi P, et al: Clonal changes in inflammatory pseudotumor of the lung: A case report. Cancer 76:1545, 1995.

152. Rohrlich P, Peuchmaur M, Cocci SN, et al: Interleukin-6 and interleukin-1-beta production in a pediatric plasma cell granuloma of the lung. Am J Surg Pathol 19:590, 1995.

153. Sajjad SM, Begin LR, Dail DH, et al: Fibrous histiocytoma of lung: A clinicopathological study of two cases. Histopathology 5:325, 1981.

154. Katzenstein A-L, Maurer JJ: Benign histiocytic tumor of lung: A light- and electron-microscopic study. Am J Surg Pathol 3:61, 1979.

155. Armstrong P, Elston C, Sanderson M: Endobronchial histiocytoma: Case reports. Br J Radiol 48:221, 1975.

156. Aisner SC, Albin RJ, Templeton PA, et al: Endobronchial fibrous histiocytoma. Ann Thorac Surg 60:710, 1995.

157. Hakimi M, Pai RP, Fine G, et al: Fibrous histiocytoma of the trachea. Chest 68:367, 1975.

158. Harjula A, Mattila S, Kyosola K, et al: Plasma cell granuloma of lung and pleura. Scand J Thorac Cardiovasc Surg 20:119, 1986.

159. Herczeg E, Weissberg D, Almog C, et al: Inflammatory fibrous histiocytoma of the bronchus. Chest 73:669, 1978.

160. Sherwin RP, Kern WH, Jones JC: Solitary mast cell granuloma (histiocytoma) of the lung. Cancer 18:634, 1965.

161. Charrette EE, Mariano AV, Laforet EG: Solitary mast cell "tumor" of lung: Its place in the spectrum of mast cell disease. Arch Intern Med 118:358, 1966.

162. Ledet SC, Brown RW, Cagle PT: p53 immunostaining in the differentiation of inflammatory pseudotumor from sarcoma involving the lung. Mod Pathol 8:282, 1995.

163. Thunnissen FB, Arends JW, Buchholtz RT, et al: Fine-needle aspiration cytology of inflammatory pseudotumor of the lung (plasma cell granuloma): Report of four cases. Acta Cytol 33:917, 1989.

164. Strutynsky N, Balthazar EJ, Klein RM: Inflammatory pseudotumours of the lung. Br J Radiol 47:94, 1974.

165. Schwartz EE, Katz SM, Mandell GA: Postinflammatory pseudotumors of the lung: Fibrous histiocytoma and related lesions. Radiology 136:609, 1980.

166. McCall IH, Woo-Ming M: The radiological appearances of plasma cell granuloma of the lung. Clin Radiol 29:145, 1978.

167. Unger JM, Peters ME, Hinke ML: Chest case of the day: Case 1. Plasma cell granuloma of the lung. Am J Roentgenol 146:1080, 1986.

168. Doyle AJ: Plasma cell granuloma of the lung. Australas Radiol 32:144, 1988.

169. Berardi RS, Lee SS, Chen HP, et al: Inflammatory pseudotumors of the lung. Surg Gynecol Obstet 156:89, 1983.

170. Shirakusa T, Kusano T, Montonaga R, et al: Plasma cell granuloma of the lung: Resection and steroid therapy. J Thorac Cardiovasc Surg 35:185, 1987.

171. Jayne D, Bridgewater B, Lawson RA: Endobronchial inflammatory pseudotumor exacerbating asthma. Postgrad Med J 73:98, 1997.

172. Vanderheyden M, Van Meerbeeck J, Van Bouwel E, et al: A rare case of inflammatory pseudotumour of the bronchus, occurring in an achondroplastic woman. Eur Respir J 7:826, 1994.

173. Helikson MA, Havey AD, Zerwekh JE, et al: Plasma-cell granuloma producing calcitriol and hypercalcemia. Ann Intern Med 105:379, 1986.

174. Mas Estelles F, Andres V, Vallcanera A, et al: Plasma cell granuloma of the lung in childhood: Atypical radiologic findings and association with hypertrophic osteoarthropathy. Pediatr Radiol 25:369, 1995.

175. Pearl M: Postinflammatory pseudotumor of the lung in children. Radiology 105:391, 1972.

176. Mandelbaum I, Brashear RE, Hull MT: Surgical treatment and course of pulmonary pseudotumor (plasma cell granuloma). J Thorac Cardiovasc Surg 82:77, 1981.

177. Bando T, Fujimura M, Noda Y, et al: Pulmonary plasma cell granuloma improves with corticosteroid therapy. Chest 105:1574, 1994.

178. Engleman P, Liebow AA, Gmelich J, et al: Pulmonary hyalinizing granuloma. Am Rev Resp Dis 115:997, 1977.

179. Chalaoui J, Grégoire P, Sylvestre J, et al: Pulmonary hyalinizing granuloma: A cause of pulmonary nodules. Radiology 152:23, 1984.

180. Yousem SA, Hochholzer L: Pulmonary hyalinizing granuloma. Am J Clin Pathol 87:1, 1987.

181. Schlosnagle DC, Check IJ, Sewell CW, et al: Immunologic abnormalities in two patients with pulmonary hyalinizing granuloma. Am J Clin Pathol 78:231, 1982.

182. Dent RG, Godden DJ, Stovin PG, et al: Pulmonary hyalinizing granuloma in association with retroperitoneal fibrosis. Thorax 38:955, 1983.

183. Maijub AG, Giltman LI, Verner JL, et al: Pulmonary hyalinizing granuloma. Ann Allergy 54:227, 1985.

184. Macedo EV, Adolph J: Pulmonary hyalinizing granulomas. J Can Assoc Radiol 36:66, 1985.

185. Guccion JG, Rohatgi PK, Saini N: Pulmonary hyalinizing granuloma: Electron microscopic and immunologic studies. Chest 85:571, 1984.

186. Dent RG, Godden DJ, Stovin PG, et al: Pulmonary hyalinizing granuloma in association with retroperitoneal fibrosis. Thorax 38:955, 1983.

187. Agrons GA, Rosado-de-Christenson ML, Kirejczyk WM, et al: Pulmonary inflammatory pseudotumor: Radiologic features. Radiology 206:511, 1998.

188. Eschelman DJ, Blickman JG, Lazar HL, et al: Pulmonary hyalinizing granuloma: A rare cause of a solitary pulmonary nodule. J Thorac Imaging 6:54, 1991.

189. Drasin H, Blume MR, Rosenbaum EH, et al: Pulmonary hyalinizing granulomas in a patient with malignant lymphoma, with development nine years later of multiple myeloma and systemic amyloidosis. Cancer 44:215, 1979.

190. Atagi S, Sakatani M, Akira M, et al: Pulmonary hyalinizing granuloma with Castleman's disease. Intern Med 33:689, 1994.

191. John PG, Rahman J, Payne CB: Pulmonary hyalinizing granuloma: An unusual association with multiple sclerosis. South Med J 88:1076, 1995.

192. Mark EJ: Mesenchymal cystic hamartoma of the lung. N Engl J Med 315:1255, 1986.

193. van Klaveren RJ, Hassing HH, Wiersma-van Tilburg JM, et al: Mesenchymal cystic hamartoma of the lung: A rare cause of relapsing pneumothorax. Thorax 49:1175, 1994.

194. Abrams J, Talcott J, Corson JM: Pulmonary metastases in patients with low-grade endometrial stromal sarcoma: Clinicopathologic findings with immunohistochemical characterization. Am J Surg Pathol 13:133, 1989.

195. Chadwick SL, Corrin B, Hansell DM, et al: Fatal haemorrhage from mesenchymal cystic hamartoma of the lung. Eur Respir J 8:2182, 1995.

196. Leroyer C, Quiot JJ, Dewitte JD, et al: Mesenchymal cystic hamartoma of the lung. Respiration 60:305, 1993.

197. Nakatani Y, Kitamura H, Inayama Y, et al: Pulmonary adenocarcinomas of the fetal lung type: A clinicopathologic study indicating differences in histology, epidemiology, and natural history of low-grade and high-grade forms. Am J Surg Pathol 22:399, 1998.

198. Churg AM, Warnock ML: So-called minute pulmonary chemodectoma—a tumor not related to paragangliomas. Cancer 37:1759, 1976.

199. Korn D, Bensch K, Liebow AA, et al: Multiple minute pulmonary tumors resembling chemodectomas. Am J Pathol 7:641, 1960.

200. Gaffey MJ, Mills SE, Askin FB: Minute pulmonary meningothelial-like nodules: A clinicopathologic study of so-called minute pulmonary chemodectoma. Am J Surg Pathol 12:167, 1988.

201. Costero I, Barroso-Moguel R, Martinez-Palomo A: Pleural origin of some of the supposed chemodectoid structures of the lung. Beitr Pathol Bd 146:351, 1972.

202. Torikata C, Mukai M: So-called minute chemodectoma of the lung: An electron microscopic and immunohistochemical study. Virchows Arch A 417:113, 1990.

203. Kuhn C, Askin FB: The fine structure of so-called minute pulmonary chemodectomas. Hum Pathol 6:681, 1975.

204. Majid OA, Rajendran U, Baker LT: Pulmonary blastoma. Ann Thorac Cardiovasc Surg 4:47, 1998.

205. Ichinose H, Hewitt RL, Drapanas T: Minute pulmonary chemodectoma. Cancer 28:692, 1971.

206. Spain DM: Intrapulmonary chemodectomas in subjects with organizing pulmonary thromboemboli. Am Rev Resp Dis 96:1158, 1967.

207. Joseph J, Sahn SA: Thoracic endometriosis syndrome: New observations from an analysis of 110 cases. Am J Med 100:164, 1996.

208. Lattes R, Shepard F, Tovell H, et al: A clinical and pathologic study of endometriosis of the lung. Surg Gynecol Obstet 103:552, 1956.

209. Hobbs JE, Bortnick AR: Endometriosis of the lungs. Am J Obstet Gynecol 40:832, 1940.

210. Park WW: The occurrence of decidual tissue within the lung: Report of a case. J Pathol Bacteriol 67:563, 1954.

211. Hartz PH: Occurrence of decidua-like tissue in the lung (report of a case). Am J Clin Pathol 26:48, 1956.

212. Foster DC, Stern JL, Buscema J, et al: Pleural and parenchymal pulmonary endometriosis. Obstet Gynecol 58:552, 1981.

213. Rodman MH, Jones CW: Catamenial hemoptysis due to bronchial endometriosis. N Engl J Med 266:805, 1962.

214. Granberg I, Willems JS: Endometriosis of lung and pleura diagnosed by aspiration biopsy. Acta Cytol 21:295, 1977.

215. Sturzenegger H: Lungenendometriose unter dem Bild des Rundschattens. [Pulmonary endometriose.] Schweiz Z Tuberk 17:259, 1960.

216. Jelihovsky T, Grant AF: Endometriosis of the lung: A case report and brief review of the literature. Thorax 23:434, 1968.

217. Assor D: Endometriosis of the lung. Am J Clin Pathol 57:311, 1972.

218. Hertzanu Y, Heimer D, Hirsch M: Computed tomography of pulmonary endometriosis. Comput Radiol 11:81, 1987.

219. Volkart JR: Clinical images: CT findings in pulmonary endometriosis. J Comput Assist Tomogr 19:156, 1995.

220. Weittzner S, Oser JF: Granular cell myoblastoma of bronchus. Am Rev Resp Dis 97:923, 1968.

221. Wood DJ, Krishnan K, Stocks P, et al: Catamenial haemoptysis: A rare cause. Thorax 48:1048, 1993.

222. Guinee DG Jr, Thornberry DS, Azumi N, et al: Unique presentation of an angiomyolipoma: Analysis of clinical, radiographic, and histologic features. Am J Surg Pathol 19:476, 1995.

223. Takemura T, Watanabe M, Takagi K, et al: Thoracoscopic resection of a solitary pulmonary lymphangioma: Report of a case. Surg Today 25:651, 1995.

224. Hamada K, Ishii Y, Nakaya M, et al: Solitary lymphangioma of the lung. Histopathol 27:482, 1995.

225. Wada A, Tateishi R, Terazawa T, et al: Lymphangioma of the lung. Arch Pathol 98:211, 1974.

226. Holden WE, Morris JF, Antonovic R, et al: Adult intrapulmonary and mediastinal lymphangioma causing haemoptysis. Thorax 42:635, 1987.

227. Redo SF, Williams JR, Bass R, et al: Respiratory obstruction secondary to lymphangioma of the trachea. J Thorac Cardiovasc Surg 49:1026, 1965.

CHAPTER 38

Secondary Neoplasms

The entire output of the right side of the heart as well as virtually all lymphatic fluid produced by body tissues flows through the pulmonary vascular system. It is not surprising, therefore, that secondary neoplastic involvement of the lungs is extremely common, the incidence of pulmonary metastases ranging from 30% to almost 55% in various series.[1–5] If direct invasion of the lung and trachea and the presence of pulmonary intravascular tumor emboli were included in these figures, the incidence would be even higher. In addition to its frequency, the condition is obviously important because of its serious prognostic implications. Although any malignant neoplasm can metastasize to the lung—including relatively innocuous ones, such as cutaneous basal cell carcinoma[6]—a particularly high incidence is seen in tumors that possess a rich vascular supply and that drain directly into the systemic venous system, such as renal cell carcinoma, sarcomas of bone, and trophoblastic tumors.[4]

PATHOGENESIS

Secondary neoplastic disease of the lungs, pleura, and trachea can occur by two mechanisms: (1) direct extension of tumor, usually from a contiguous neoplasm and occasionally as a continuous intravascular growth between the primary tumor and the lungs; and (2) true metastases, usually via the pulmonary arteries, less commonly via the bronchial arteries or pulmonary lymphatics or across the pleural cavity, and rarely via the airways. Although there is overlap, each of these routes of spread is associated with characteristic pathologic, radiologic, and clinical features.

Direct Extension

Secondary involvement of the lung or trachea by direct neoplastic extension is much less common than by metastasis. It occurs most often by invasion from a primary neoplasm in a contiguous organ or tissue, the most common of which are thyroid,[7] esophagus,[8] and thymus. In addition, any neoplasm metastatic to ribs or mediastinal lymph nodes can extend into the adjacent trachea or lung (Fig. 38–1). Occasionally, such pulmonary invasion simulates primary carcinoma arising in paramediastinal lung. Rarely, direct extension of tumor from its primary site to the lung occurs via the vasculature, either along lymphatic channels or via the vena cava and right side of the heart directly into the pulmonary arteries; the latter mode of spread is seen particularly with renal cell carcinoma and testicular germ cell neoplasms.[4] Another rare form of "direct" tumor spread to the lungs or pleura is by iatrogenic implantation of tumor cells during a diagnostic or therapeutic procedure.[9] Although

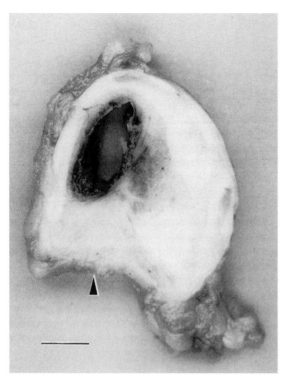

Figure 38–1. Tracheal Stenosis Caused by Invasion of Neoplasm from Contiguous Lymph Nodes. A cross-section of the trachea at autopsy of a 58-year-old man with metastatic colon carcinoma shows severe narrowing of the lumen by tumor (*arrowhead* indicates the membranous portion). This was the result of direct extension into the tracheal wall from deposits of metastatic carcinoma in paratracheal lymph nodes. (Bar = 5 mm.)

the extrapulmonary source of neoplasm is usually evident in all these examples, occasionally it is inapparent.

Metastasis

Metastasis refers to the transport of viable tumor cells from one site in the body to another. Although some consider the term to include evidence of autonomous extravascular growth as well,[4] for purposes of this discussion, we include strictly intravascular tumor emboli as constituting true metastases. The process can occur by four routes.

Spread Via the Pulmonary or Bronchial Arteries

The pulmonary arteries are by far the most common route by which tumor spreads to the lungs. The pathogenesis of metastasis via this conduit is incompletely understood and quite complex;[10] only a brief and rather simplistic overview is attempted here. The initial event clearly must be vascular invasion at the site of the primary neoplasm. In the case of venous invasion, individual cells or fragments of tumor (with or without admixed thrombus) are then dislodged and carried as tumor emboli to the lungs.[11] Although these may be large enough to cause pulmonary infarction or even sudden death (*see* farther on), the vast majority are too small for this and lodge chiefly within small pulmonary arteries or arterioles; it has been estimated that most tumor emboli reaching the lungs via the systemic venous circulation range from 100 to

200 μm in diameter.[4] Such tumor emboli are quite common: in one histologic study of 366 patients who died of choriocarcinoma or of carcinoma of the breast, kidney, liver, or stomach, 95 (26%) showed such involvement.[12] Because it is impossible to view all pulmonary vessels at autopsy, the true incidence is undoubtedly higher.

As might be expected, there is evidence that metastases are more likely to be established when larger numbers of cells reach the pulmonary vessels. Experiments in animals in which malignant cells have been inoculated directly into the cisterna chyli have shown a dose-response relationship—the more numerous the cells, the greater the incidence of viable metastases.[13] Tumor cell surface molecules and the local formation of thrombus may be important for initial adherence within pulmonary vessels.[11] Intrinsic pulmonary disease, such as pneumonitis,[11] and endothelial damage resulting from hyperoxic injury have also been shown experimentally to be associated with an increased number of metastases.

The fate of arrested tumor emboli is variable and likely depends on several factors, including inflammatory and immunologic reactions, the extent and rapidity of organization of any associated thrombus, the viability of tumor cells in their new environment, and the effects on the tumor cells of physical trauma resulting from embolization.[11, 14, 15] In the majority of instances, it is probable that conditions are unsuitable for survival of malignant cells.[14, 15] Occasionally, however, there is proliferation within the vascular lumen and invasion of the adjacent wall. The location of this proliferation, perhaps in addition to properties of the tumor cells themselves,[16] determines the subsequent morphologic appearance of the metastasis. In most cases, there is extension of the newly formed tumor into the surrounding lung parenchyma, forming a relatively well-defined nodule. Less often, tumor cells remain largely confined to the perivascular interstitium, spreading along it and within its lymphatic channels. These are the two principal morphologic manifestations of metastatic cancer in the lung and are discussed in greater detail farther on.

Pulmonary metastasis can also occur via the bronchial arteries, in a fashion analogous to the development of metastases in systemic visceral organs. Although this event is difficult to prove in an individual patient, it is undoubtedly much less common than tumor dissemination via the pulmonary artery. It is likely, however, that some endobronchial metastases arise by this mechanism.

Spread Via the Pulmonary and Pleural Lymphatics

Spread of tumor within the lungs and pleura via lymphatic channels (lymphangitic carcinomatosis) may occur in two ways. As discussed in the previous section, the first is by hematogenous dissemination to small pulmonary arteries and arterioles followed by invasion of the adjacent interstitial space and lymphatics and spread along these pathways toward the hilum or periphery of the lung. That this dissemination is the pathogenetic mechanism in most cases of pulmonary lymphangitic carcinomatosis is suggested by the high frequency of concurrent intravascular cancer or thrombosis[17–21] and by the frequent absence of neoplasm in bronchopulmonary and hilar lymph nodes.[17]

The second mechanism is by retrograde spread of tumor

emboli or continuous cords of tumor within lymphatic channels.[22] In the usual sequence of events, mediastinal lymph nodes are affected first, followed by extension to hilar and bronchopulmonary nodes, and finally by spread into pleural and pulmonary lymphatics. It has been postulated that the pressure within lymphatic channels increases as a result of neoplastic obstruction of hilar lymph nodes, rendering the lymphatic valves incompetent and permitting centrifugal flow of lymph-containing tumor cells.[23] Evidence in favor of this sequence of events has been provided by postmortem lymphangiography.[24] Communicating lymphatic channels between the diaphragmatic and basal lung pleura and the upper abdominal lymph nodes[25] or peritoneal cavity[26] may also provide a route for direct spread of intra-abdominal malignancy.[27]

Spread Via the Pleural Space

Neoplastic spread across the pleural space occurs when individual tumor cells or small tumor fragments are liberated into the pleural space and are carried within pleural fluid to another site. The precise mechanisms of tumor adherence and invasion at the secondary foci are not clear. In one histologic study of peritoneal metastases of ovarian carcinoma, tumor cells were associated with focal mesothelial damage and an underlying inflammatory reaction;[28] the tumor appeared to proliferate in the resulting exudate as it organized, eventually forming a well-developed metastatic nodule. Similar mechanisms presumably prevail in transpleural metastases.

The primary pleural focus may originate by direct tumor extension (e.g., in breast or lung carcinoma) or by spread via lymphatics or blood vessels. The metastases tend to be most numerous in the caudal and posterior parts of the pleural cavities,[4] presumably reflecting the influence of gravity. Metastatic pleural disease is discussed in greater detail in Chapter 69 (*see* page 2756).

Spread Via the Airways

Intrapulmonary growth and invasion of neoplastic cells after inoculation into the airways have been documented in experimental animals.[29] It has also been proposed that this method of tumor dissemination occurs in both extrapulmonary and primary human pulmonary neoplasms.[4] Except for some bronchioloalveolar carcinomas, however, tumor dissemination through the airways is probably rare and difficult to prove in an individual patient.[30, 31]

PATTERNS OF SECONDARY NEOPLASTIC DISEASE

Although metastasis by each of the routes just described is associated with characteristic pathologic and radiologic manifestations, overlap is frequent. For example, tumor that metastasizes via the pulmonary artery can result in either nodular parenchymal or interstitial patterns of growth, or both. Similarly, spread of malignant cells across the pleural space can occur simultaneously with growth within pleural and adjacent pulmonary lymphatics. Thus, although differing in pathogenesis, these routes of metastasis may lead to

similar consequences. Because of this, it is useful to discuss the clinical, pathologic, and radiologic features of pulmonary metastases in terms of patterns of disease, of which five major ones can be recognized: (1) parenchymal nodules; (2) interstitial thickening (lymphangitic carcinomatosis); (3) pulmonary hypertension and infarction (tumor emboli); (4) airway obstruction (endobronchial tumor); and (5) pleural effusion.

Parenchymal Nodules

The most common manifestation of metastatic disease to the lungs consists of one or more nodules within the lung parenchyma. As indicated previously, these are usually derived from small tumor emboli that lodge in peripheral pulmonary arteries or arterioles and subsequently extend into the adjacent lung tissue. Nodules are multiple in the majority of cases (Fig. 38–2) and tend to be most numerous in the basal portions of the lungs, reflecting the effect of gravity on blood flow.[4, 32] They range in size from barely visible to huge growths occupying virtually the entire volume of a lung. Although most often discrete, individual deposits may enlarge and become confluent, resulting in multinodular masses. When multiple, the nodules are usually of varying

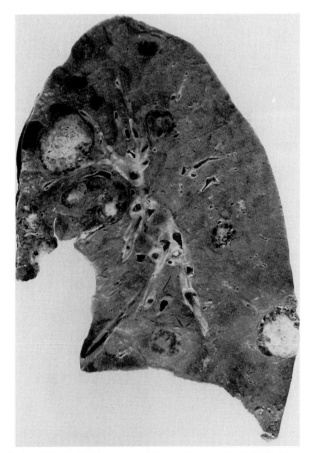

Figure 38–2. Metastatic Choriocarcinoma—Multiple Parenchymal Nodules. A slice of right lung obtained at autopsy of a young man with testicular choriocarcinoma reveals multiple, variably sized, well-circumscribed nodules in the lung parenchyma. Prominent hemorrhage is evident in both tumor and adjacent lung, a characteristic feature of this neoplasm.

size; less often, they are approximately equal, suggesting a single shower of tumor emboli. Rarely, nodular deposits are so numerous and of such minute size as to suggest miliary tuberculosis, both radiographically (Fig. 38–3) and pathologically.[33]

Microscopically, the smallest parenchymal nodules are usually located adjacent to peripheral pulmonary arteries or arterioles, which frequently contain small tumor emboli with or without associated thrombus (Fig. 38–4). Parenchymal growth is usually destructive, grossly visible nodules being composed solely of viable and necrotic neoplastic cells and their attendant stroma (Fig. 38–4). Occasionally the growth pattern is lepidic, the underlying lung architecture being retained in a fashion similar to bronchioloalveolar carcinoma.[34, 35] As in the latter tumor, this type of spread is rarely sufficiently extensive to simulate confluent bronchopneumonia grossly.

Studies of the vascular supply of pulmonary metastases have led to conflicting conclusions. Some authors believe that they are supplied solely from the pulmonary arterial system.[36] However, in one postmortem microarteriographic study, two patterns were found, the blood supply of most peripheral metastases being via the pulmonary vessels and that of most central lesions being via the bronchial circulation.[37] In a study of the blood supply of spontaneous pulmonary metastases in dogs, irregularly dilated pulmonary vessels were found within many small metastases and around the margins of larger ones;[38] tumor tissue infiltrating intact alveoli appeared to be receiving its circulation from the pulmonary capillaries. All new blood vessels were systemic in origin, derived from either bronchial arteries or transpleural collaterals.

Several groups of investigators have demonstrated that CT has a considerably greater sensitivity than either chest radiography or conventional linear tomography in the identification of pulmonary metastases.[39–41] The procedure allows detection of more nodules as well as smaller nodules and has effectively replaced the other two techniques in this setting.[42] The sensitivity of CT is influenced by the technique employed. Using conventional CT with contiguous 10-mm collimation scans, it is approximately 70%;[43] however, detection of nodules is significantly improved with the use of spiral CT,[44] particularly by spacing the scan reconstructions at 4- to 5-mm intervals rather than 8- to 10-mm intervals.[45] Detection can be further improved by cine viewing of spiral CT scans on a workstation as compared to static film–based images.[46] Despite this increased sensitivity, it is obvious that CT does not allow detection of all metastatic nodules; those smaller than 3 mm in diameter are frequently missed.[47, 48]

Although CT is highly sensitive in the detection of pulmonary metastases, it is not specific, many of the nodules identified representing either granulomas or pulmonary lymphoid nodules.[39, 40, 43, 43a] For example, in one study of 91 patients with known extrathoracic malignancy, of whom 31 underwent resection, 27 (87%) were found to have primary or metastatic disease and 4 benign lesions.[39] The likelihood of the nodules representing benign nodules rather than metastases increases if the nodules are seen only on CT and not on chest radiography; in one investigation in which CT was compared with chest radiography, 51 of 64 patients (80%) who had nodules seen both on CT and on chest radiography had metastases, compared to 31 of 69 patients (45%) who had nodules seen only on CT.[41] The specificity

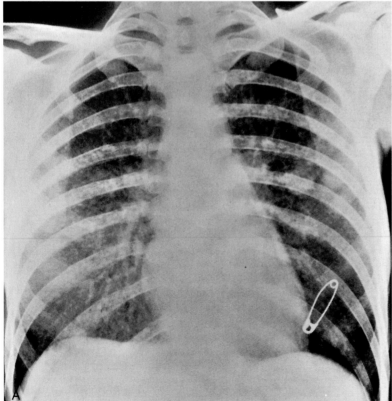

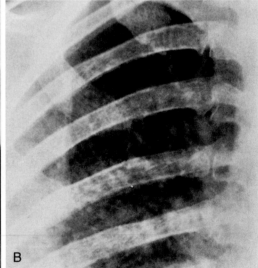

Figure 38–3. Diffuse Micronodular Metastases—Choriocarcinoma. An anteroposterior radiograph *(A)* of a 38-year-old woman reveals widespread nodules distributed evenly throughout both lungs. In some areas, the nodules are sharply circumscribed, but in others they are indistinct and partly coalescent, as revealed to better advantage in the magnified view of the right upper zone *(B)*. At autopsy, the lungs were studded with tiny deposits of metastatic choriocarcinoma and were strikingly hemorrhagic, even in areas not occupied by tumor tissue.

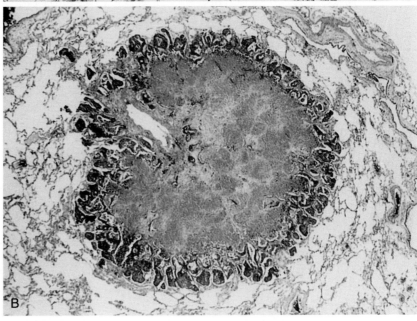

Figure 38–4. Metastatic Carcinoma—Parenchymal Nodules. A small muscular pulmonary artery *(A, arrow)* is completely occluded by organized thrombus and admixed metastatic adenocarcinoma of the colon. The cancer has also grown out of the vessel into adjacent interstitium and alveolar air spaces. In another metastasis *(B)*, there is more extensive parenchymal infiltration and prominent central necrosis. *(A, ×25; B, ×15.)*

of CT in this situation is also higher for newly developed nodules. In one radiologic-surgical correlative study of 84 patients with such nodules, all those detected by both CT and radiography were metastases, compared to 84% of those seen only on CT.[43] In this study, CT detected 173 (73%) of 237 nodules identified at thoracotomy. Because many false-positive diagnoses at CT are related to granulomas, the specificity of CT is also greater in areas in which tuberculosis and fungal disease are not common. For example, in two studies from the United Kingdom, where fungal granulomas are virtually nonexistent, 94% of 200 nodules[49] and 98% of 100 nodules[50] were metastases.

The presence of pulmonary metastases can also be assessed using magnetic resonance (MR) imaging.[51–53] In an early study using spin-echo MR imaging at 0.35 T, small nodules adjacent to vessels were often missed on CT but could be clearly identified with MR imaging.[52] Nodules near the diaphragm were frequently missed because of respiratory motion. In a more recent investigation, the results of MR imaging performed at 0.5 T were compared with those of CT and chest radiography in 11 patients.[53] MR imaging and CT allowed detection of at least one metastatic nodule in all cases, compared to 64% of cases on chest radiography. MR imaging was as sensitive as CT in the detection of individual nodules. Of the various MR sequences used, the short inversion time inversion-recovery (STIR) sequences had the highest sensitivity for the detection of individual nodules. Although no false-positive interpretations were seen on CT, a total of 13 were made on MR imaging; these were most common in the lower lobes, presumably as a result of diaphragmatic motion. Although these studies suggest a potential role for MR imaging in the assessment of pulmonary metastases, we consider that its current shortcomings outweigh its benefits and recommend CT as the imaging modality of choice.

When pulmonary parenchymal nodules are multiple, the probability that they represent metastases is obviously increased; conversely, although a solitary nodule can be a metastasis, the possibility that it represents a primary carcinoma is increased. From a diagnostic viewpoint, therefore, neoplastic parenchymal nodules can be conveniently discussed under the headings *solitary* and *multiple*.

Solitary Nodules

Metastatic neoplasms that present as solitary parenchymal nodules comprise a distinct group that must be differentiated from any other cause of a solitary nodule in the lung (Fig. 38–5). They are relatively uncommon, accounting for approximately 2% to 10% of cases of solitary pulmonary nodules.[54–56] In one study of 634 patients with solitary nodules on CT, 72 (11%) were proven to represent metastases from an extrathoracic neoplasm. Sev-

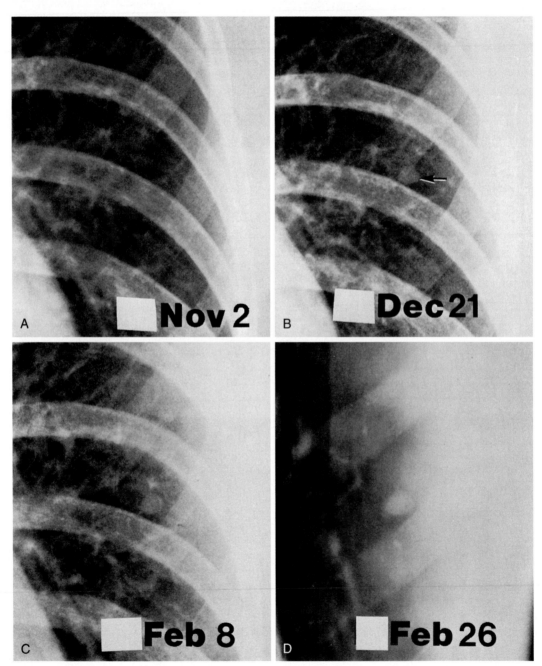

Figure 38–5. Solitary Metastasis from Wilms' Tumor. Detail views of the left midlung zone from four sequential radiographs, covering a span of almost 4 months, are shown. In *A*, an abnormality cannot be identified. Slightly less than 2 months later *(B)*, a tiny nodule measuring 6 mm in diameter had appeared *(arrow)*. Two months later *(C and D)*, the nodule had increased to 8 mm in diameter, representing a doubling in volume. This 19-year-old man had had a left nephrectomy many years previously for Wilms' tumor; subsequently the upper lobe of his right lung and the right lobe of his liver had been resected for metastatic disease. The nodule shown on these radiographs appeared 1 year after the lobectomy and partial hepatectomy. On resection, it proved to be metastatic Wilms' tumor.

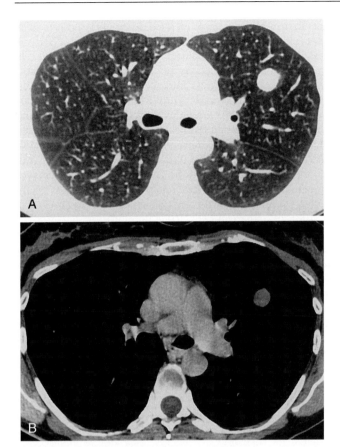

Figure 38–6. Single Metastasis—CT Findings. CT scans *(A, B)* demonstrate a smoothly marginated noncalcified nodule in the left upper lobe; the appearance is indistinguishable from that of a noncalcified granuloma. At thoracotomy, this was proven to be metastatic leiomyosarcoma. The primary site was subsequently determined to be the lower extremity.

enty-one of the 72 metastatic nodules measured between 0.5 and 3 cm in diameter.[55] In another investigation of 275 patients who had CT findings interpreted as consistent with pulmonary carcinoma, 6 (2.2%) proved to have metastatic disease.[56] The vast majority of these solitary metastatic lesions occur in patients aged 45 years and older.[54, 55]

Certain primary neoplasms are more likely than others to produce solitary metastases. These include carcinoma of the colon (particularly of the rectosigmoid area, which accounts for 30% to 40% of all cases);[54, 57] sarcomas (particularly those originating in bone);[3, 54, 57] carcinoma of the kidney, testicle, and breast; and malignant melanoma.[54, 57, 58]

With few exceptions, there are no reliable criteria to distinguish a solitary metastatic nodule from a primary pulmonary carcinoma on the chest radiograph or CT (Fig. 38–6).[55, 56] On HRCT, approximately 50% of metastatic nodules have smooth margins, and 50% have irregular margins.[59, 60] They may be round or oval or have a lobulated contour (Fig. 38–7). Irregular margins with spiculation may result from a desmoplastic reaction or tumor infiltration within the adjacent bronchovascular connective tissue or lymphatics (lymphangitic spread).[59, 60]

Identification of a concomitant primary neoplasm elsewhere or a history of prior neoplasia does not necessarily indicate that a solitary nodule in the lung is metastatic.[61] In one investigation of 50 patients previously treated for a

malignancy and without evidence of metastases elsewhere, 18 had single intrathoracic lesions that proved to be unrelated pulmonary or mediastinal tumors;[62] 9 others had benign pulmonary lesions. In another series of 54 patients with known colonic carcinoma and a solitary pulmonary nodule, only 25 lesions were found to be metastases.[63] In patients with extrathoracic malignancy and only one nodule seen on the radiograph or CT, additional nodules are frequently identified at surgery.[42, 43] For example, in one study of 84 patients with known extrathoracic malignancy, a solitary nodule was seen in 65 lungs on chest radiography;[43] in 21 (32%) of these, more than one nodule was found at CT. In 9 of the remaining 44 lungs (20%) in which only one nodule was demonstrated on CT, additional nodules were found at surgery. In the other 35 (80%), only one nodule was found at surgery.

The distinction between a new primary and metastasis has important prognostic and therapeutic implications, particularly with the increasing use of pulmonary metastasectomy.[64, 65] Although there is debate about the efficacy of this procedure, review of the literature suggests that it is likely to be beneficial in selected patients with certain neoplasms.[66]

Although a definite diagnosis of metastasis versus primary usually cannot be made on clinical and radiologic grounds alone, certain features are associated with an increased probability of one or the other.[67] The nature of the primary extrapulmonary tumor is clearly important: a solitary nodule in a patient with a high-grade sarcoma or deeply invasive melanoma is much more likely to be a metastasis than a new primary. By contrast, such a nodule in a patient with a squamous cell carcinoma of the oropharyngeal region is quite possibly a primary pulmonary carcinoma. The time interval between the initial tumor and the appearance of the pulmonary lesion is also important, although not independent of tumor type. For example, an interval greater than 5 years in a patient with osteosarcoma is almost certain to be associated with a new pulmonary primary; however, in carcinomas originating in the breast or kidney, in which

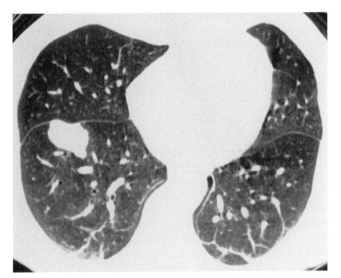

Figure 38–7. Lobulated Metastasis. A CT scan demonstrates a 3-cm-diameter nodule with a lobulated contour within the right lower lobe. At thoracotomy, this was proven to be metastatic adenocarcinoma, the primary site being the colon.

metastases can occur many years after the original tumor is identified, this conclusion is less likely to be correct. Older age and a history of cigarette smoking increase the likelihood that the tumor is primary in the lung.

In those patients who have known extrathoracic malignancy, transthoracic needle aspiration may be helpful in determining the primary or metastatic nature of the pulmonary nodule. Cytologic features alone may enable the pathologist to suspect one or the other strongly;[68] in addition, comparison of the histologic appearance of small tissue fragments in cell blocks with that of the known tumor may prove conclusive. Immunohistochemical examination of cells or tissue fragments, using antibodies directed against protein S-100 (for melanoma), prostate-specific antigen,[69] or a panel of antigens,[70] may also enable precise diagnosis. Identical studies can also be used in tissue obtained at thoracotomy. By demonstrating other pulmonary nodules not visible on plain radiographs, CT can also aid in distinguishing primary from metastatic tumor.

When a solitary pulmonary nodule is identified in a patient without a history of cancer, some physicians put the patient through a battery of radiologic and other diagnostic procedures in an attempt to identify or exclude a primary nonpulmonary malignancy. However, because the great majority of such searches are fruitless,[71, 72] we feel that search for an extrapulmonary primary in the presence of a solitary pulmonary nodule should be limited to cases in which there is specific organ dysfunction.

Multiple Nodules

The radiographic pattern of multiple pulmonary nodules varies from diffuse micronodular shadows resembling miliary disease to large, well-defined cannonball masses (Fig. 38–8). In the former situation, the lesions may be of uniform size, indicating a simultaneous origin in one shower of emboli, or may differ, suggesting embolic events of different ages; the latter pattern is rare in cases of benign nodular disease.[73] Although most individual shadows are fairly sharply defined, some are rather indistinct; when these reach 5 to 6 mm in diameter, they can simulate air-space disease.[74] Mediastinal and hilar lymph nodes are usually not enlarged. An unusual cause of a miliary pattern of metastases was reported in a young boy with neuroblastoma who received an autologous bone marrow transplant;[75] the authors of the report speculated that the pulmonary disease was related to infusion of malignant cells at the time of transplantation.

On CT, pulmonary metastases are most commonly seen in the outer third of the lungs, particularly the subpleural regions of the lower zones.[42, 76, 77] Although nodules less than 2 cm in diameter are frequently round and have smooth margins (Fig. 38–9), they may have various shapes; larger nodules frequently are lobulated and have irregular margins.[78, 79] Irregular margins appear to be particularly common in cases of metastatic adenocarcinoma.[60] Occasionally, a halo of ground-glass attenuation can be seen to surround the nodules. This finding is most common in highly vascular or hemorrhagic tumors, such as angiosarcoma.[80]

Although intravascular tumor emboli can be seen histologically in many patients who have lung metastases, they tend to occur in arterioles or small arteries and therefore are usually not seen on CT.[60] Rarely, they can be identified as nodular or beaded thickening of the peripheral pulmonary arteries (*see* Fig. 38–9).[81] Although this appearance may suggest the diagnosis of metastasis, a similar appearance has

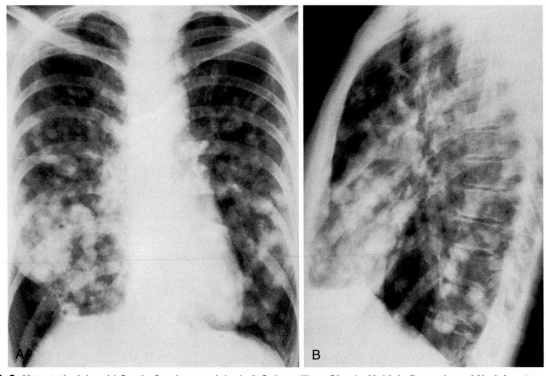

Figure 38–8. Metastatic Adenoid Cystic Carcinoma of the Left Submaxillary Gland—Multiple Parenchymal Nodules. Posteroanterior *(A)* and lateral *(B)* radiographs reveal multiple nodules of homogeneous density ranging in size from 5 mm to 2 cm, distributed widely through both lungs. The apices and bases are relatively less affected than the midzones. There is no evidence of cavitation.

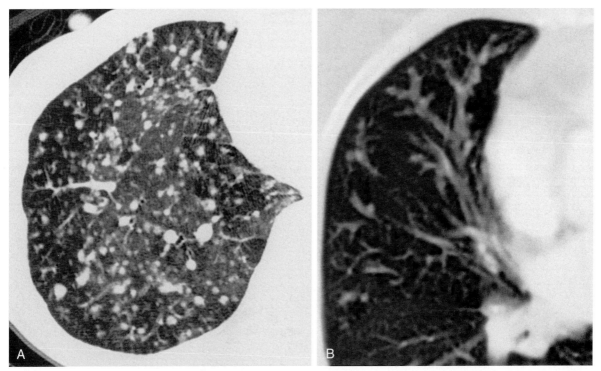

Figure 38–9. Metastatic Carcinoma—CT Appearance. A CT scan *(A)* demonstrates numerous smoothly marginated nodules 2 to 10 mm in diameter in the right lower lobe. The patient was a 70-year-old woman with metastatic adenocarcinoma of unknown primary. A detail view of the right lung from a CT scan in another patient *(B)* shows dilated and beaded pulmonary arteries in the right middle lobe. The appearance is characteristic of intravascular tumor emboli. The patient had metastatic carcinoma of the breast. *(B* courtesy of Drs. Lynn Broderick and Robert Tarver, Indiana University Medical Center, Indianapolis, IN.)

been reported in a patient who had perivascular granulomatous inflammation caused by *Histoplasma capsulatum.*[82] It has also been suggested that pulmonary vessels can often be seen leading directly to a pulmonary metastasis (the *feeding vessel* sign).[83, 84] However, although this finding is certainly seen with metastatic tumors, it is not sensitive. In one analysis of the HRCT and pathologic findings of 190 nodules, including radiographs and stereomicroscopy of autopsy specimens, only 21 (11%) were found to be closely related to a vessel (more specifically, the centrilobular bronchovascular bundle).[85] A total of 130 (68%) nodules were located between the centrilobular bronchovascular bundle and the perilobular structures, and 39 (21%) were in the periphery of the secondary pulmonary lobule. The vessels supplying the metastatic nodule could not be visualized on HRCT.[85]

Cavitation of a nodular metastasis is not as common as with primary lung carcinoma;[86–88] for example, in one report, it was identified in 4% of metastatic deposits and 9% of primary neoplasms.[88] As with primary pulmonary tumors, the complication occurs most often in squamous cell carcinoma and is more common in the upper than the lower lobes. The site of the primary neoplasm is most frequently in the head and neck in men (Fig. 38–10) and the cervix in women.[88, 89] Although uncommon, cavitation can also occur in metastatic adenocarcinoma, particularly in lesions originating in the large bowel,[88, 90] and in metastatic sarcoma, particularly osteogenic; excavation of the latter may account for the relatively high incidence of concomitant pneumothorax in this tumor (*see* farther on).

Calcification of metastatic lesions is rare and almost invariably indicates that the primary neoplasm is osteogenic sarcoma, chondrosarcoma, or synovial sarcoma (Fig. 38–11).[91] If small, such metastases can mimic benign lesions; for example, in one patient with metastatic synovial sarcoma, one nodule simulated a hamartoma and two others granulomas.[91] Calcification can develop at the site of pulmonary metastases that have "vanished" after successful chemotherapy.[92] This chemotherapeutic effect can also be manifested as persistent nodules that, on histologic examination, show only necrosis and fibrosis without residual viable neoplastic tissue.[93, 94] Metastatic testicular neoplasms are particularly prone to this outcome (*see* page 1407).

At least 80% to 90% of patients with multiple pulmonary metastases have a previously diagnosed extrathoracic neoplasm or clinical findings directly referable to a synchronous primary. Signs and symptoms related to parenchymal nodules themselves are uncommon; occasionally, extension of tumor into an adjacent bronchial wall results in cough, hemoptysis, or wheezing. Similarly, extension into the pleura may lead to painful respiration, and invasion of the apical chest wall can result in Pancoast's syndrome.[95] When tumor volume is substantial, dyspnea may result. Hypertrophic pulmonary osteoarthropathy develops in a small number of patients;[96] approximately half have sarcomas, and the remainder a variety of carcinomas.[97] Symptoms may be dramatically relieved by intrathoracic or cervical vagotomy.[96]

The occurrence of spontaneous pneumothorax in association with metastatic disease to the lungs should suggest sarcoma as the primary neoplasm. Although a variety of tumors have been reported,[98, 99] the incidence is especially high in osteogenic sarcoma;[98–100] in one study of 552 patients who had this tumor, pneumothorax developed in 5% who

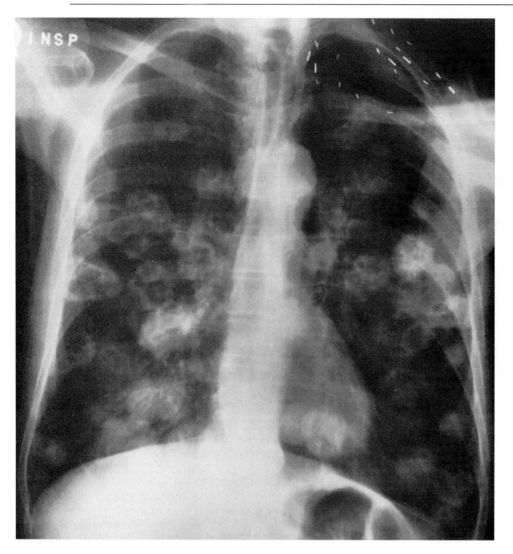

Figure 38–10. Cavitation in Metastatic Carcinoma. A posteroanterior radiograph reveals multiple nodules throughout both lungs ranging from 5 mm to 3 cm in diameter. The majority of the nodules are cavitated. For an unknown reason, such thin-walled cavities tend to occur in metastases from primary neoplasms arising in the head and neck, at least in men (in women, the primary neoplasm tends to be in the genital tract). In this patient, the primary carcinoma was in the pharynx. (The surgical clips over the left supraclavicular region are from a previous radical neck dissection.)

had pulmonary metastases.[101] It has been suggested that the complication is more frequent in patients undergoing chemotherapy.[102] It may occur before radiographic visibility of metastases.[99, 103]

Interstitial Thickening (Lymphangitic Carcinomatosis)

This pattern of tumor spread is frequent: in one study of 174 cases of metastatic pulmonary disease, it was seen in 97 (55%); in more than half the cases, it was the predominant mode of spread.[20] In another investigation of 222 consecutive autopsies of patients with solid tumors, the abnormality was found in 78 (35%) cases.[104] Although virtually any metastatic neoplasm can show lymphangitic spread, the most common originate in the breast, stomach, pancreas, and prostate;[17, 18] in addition, it is not uncommon for primary pulmonary carcinoma, particularly small cell carcinoma and adenocarcinoma, to spread by this route.

Grossly, lymphangitic spread varies from a slight accentuation of the interlobular septa and peribronchovascular connective tissue to obvious thickening (5 to 10 mm) of these structures (Fig. 38–12). Associated pleural involvement is common. Microscopically, neoplastic cells are usu-

ally readily identifiable as small clusters or cords of cells within the lymphatic spaces and in a less well-defined architecture in the peribronchovascular and interlobular interstitium (Fig. 38–13).[17–19] Edema or a desmoplastic reaction to the tumor can contribute significantly to the interstitial thickening. Tumor emboli are frequently present in adjacent small arteries and arterioles, sometimes associated with thrombus. Although often confined solely to the interstitium and lymphatic spaces, the neoplasm can spread outside these structures into the adjacent parenchyma, resulting in parenchymal nodules that can alter the typical pattern. Extension can also occur into the airway mucosa, resulting in stenosis or occlusion with consequent atelectasis and obstructive pneumonitis (*see* Fig. 38–12). In such cases, bronchoalveolar lavage fluid may contain a substantial increase in the number of lymphocytes.[105]

The characteristic radiographic pattern consists of coarsened bronchovascular markings of irregular contour, sometimes indistinctly defined, simulating interstitial pulmonary edema. Although the pattern is uniform throughout both lungs in most patients, it tends to be more obvious in the lower zones (Fig. 38–14). Septal lines (Kerley B lines) are present in most cases (Fig. 38–15).[106] The linear accentuation is sometimes associated with a nodular component, resulting

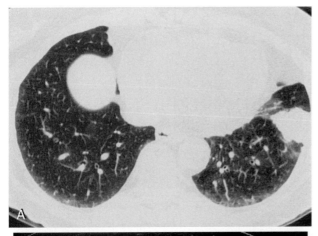

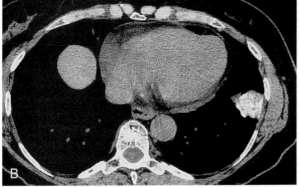

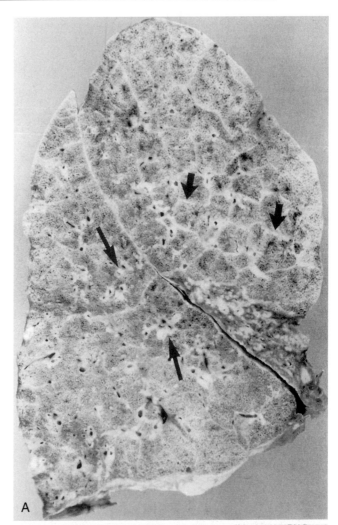

Figure 38–11. Calcified Metastatic Osteosarcoma. A 71-year-old woman with previously resected primary osteosarcoma of the femur developed two new pulmonary nodules. A CT scan through the lower lung zones *(A, B)* demonstrates a 2.5-cm-diameter lobulated nodule in the left lower lobe. It is extensively calcified. A CT scan 6 months previously had been normal.

from intraparenchymal extension of tumor, thus creating a coarse reticulonodular pattern. Although often bilateral, the abnormality may be confined to one lung or even one lobe, as was the case in 28 of 100 patients in one series;[107] 21 of the 28 patients had primary pulmonary carcinoma. Hilar and mediastinal lymphadenopathy is seen radiographically in 20% to 40% of patients and pleural effusion in 30% to 50%.[17, 108] Although characteristic, these findings lack both specificity and sensitivity. In one study, an accurate diagnosis of lymphangitic carcinomatosis was suggested on the chest radiograph in only 20 of 87 (23%) patients.[109] Furthermore, the chest radiograph is normal in 30% to 50% of patients who have pathologically proven lymphangitic carcinomatosis.[17, 109, 110]

Lymphangitic carcinomatosis also has a characteristic HRCT appearance, consisting of smooth or nodular thickening of the interlobular septa and peribronchovascular interstitium with preservation of normal lung architecture (Fig. 38–16).[108, 111] The thickened interlobular septa may be seen as peripheral lines extending to the pleural surface or centrally as polygonal arcades, frequently with a nodular or beaded appearance.[108, 112, 113] This nodular thickening is highly suggestive of the diagnosis and is not seen in pulmonary edema or interstitial fibrosis.[113] Lymphangitic carcinomatosis may also be associated with interstitial pulmonary

Text continued on page 1396

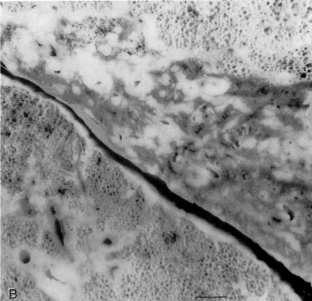

Figure 38–12. Lymphangitic Spread—Carcinoma of the Breast. A section of left lung *(A)* shows extensive infiltration of interlobular septa *(short arrows)* and peribronchovascular tissue *(long arrows)* by breast carcinoma. A magnified view *(B)* reveals a focus of atelectasis in the lingula caused by invasion and compression of small airways by the expanding interstitial neoplasm.

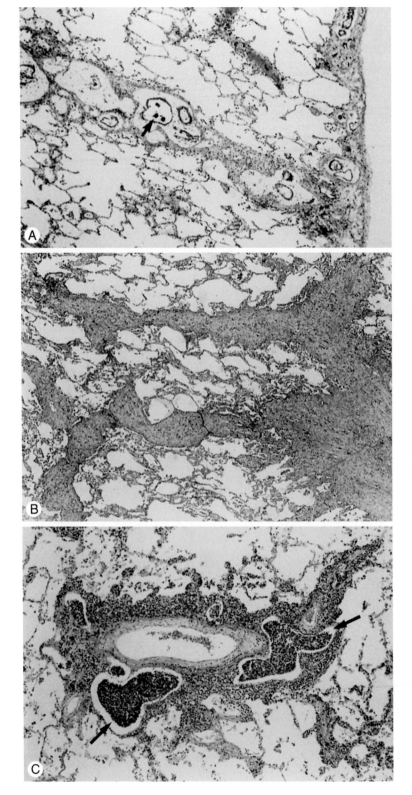

Figure 38–13. Metastatic Carcinoma—Lymphatic and Interstitial Infiltration. Three patterns of lymphangitic carcinomatosis are illustrated. An interlobular septum *(A)* is thickened as a result of lymphatic dilation caused by mucus secretion by a bronchioloalveolar cell carcinoma. Nests of tumor cells, some with psammoma bodies *(arrow)*, can be seen floating within the mucus. There is no tumor outside the lymphatic spaces. Interlobular septa *(B)* are similarly thickened, in this case, primarily as a result of increased collagen induced by metastatic breast carcinoma (desmoplastic reaction). Lymphatic permeation is absent. In the most common pattern *(C)*, the tissue surrounding a pulmonary vein is thickened by a combination of intralymphatic tumor plugs *(arrows)* and interstitial tumor infiltration. The tumor also extends into the parenchymal interstitium at the lower right. (*A*, ×40; *B*, ×25; *C*, ×52.)

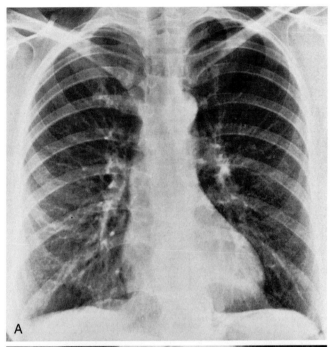

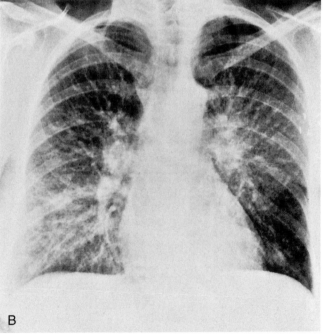

Figure 38–14. Lymphangitic Spread—Carcinoma of the Breast. At the time of the normal radiograph *(A)*, this 50-year-old woman was discovered to have a carcinoma of the left breast, and a modified radical mastectomy was carried out. Seven months later, at which time she was complaining of progressively increasing dyspnea, a radiograph *(B)* revealed extensive involvement of both lungs by a coarse linear and reticular pattern associated with bilateral hilar lymph node enlargement. Loss of lung volume has occurred in this interval as a result of reduced compliance.

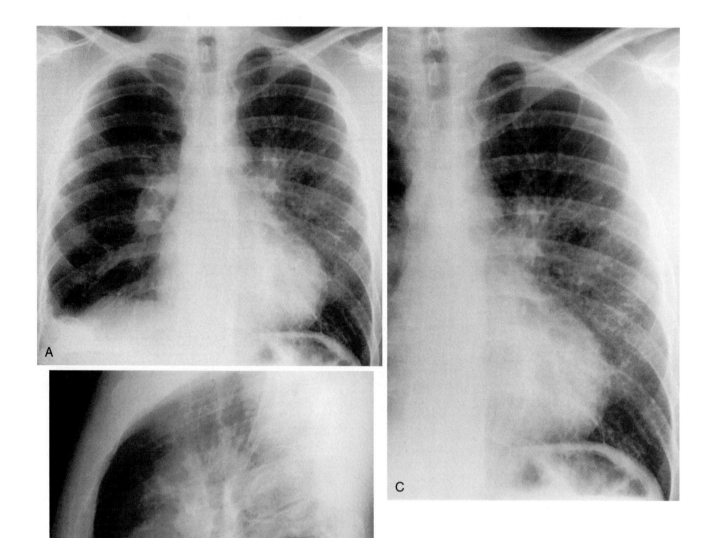

Figure 38–15. Lymphangitic Carcinomatosis. Posteroanterior *(A)* and lateral *(B)* radiographs disclose an interstitial pattern with left-sided predominance consisting of well-formed Kerley A and B lines and thickened, ill-defined bronchoarterial bundles. The right hilum is moderately enlarged as a result of lymph node involvement, although the left hilum is only questionably enlarged. There are small bilateral pleural effusions. A detail view *(C)* of the left lung in *A* shows the same pattern as in *A* and *B*.

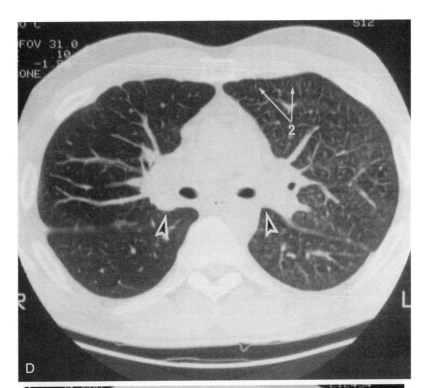

Figure 38–15 *Continued.* CT scans *through the hilum (D) and the left upper lobe (E) reveal predominantly left-sided features of lymphangitic carcinomatosis. Note the Kerley A (1) and B (2) lines and thickened bronchoarterial bundles (closed arrows) that typify this condition. Minimal lesions of a similar nature are visible in the right lung. Lymph nodes are enlarged in both hila (arrowheads), and multiple mediastinal lymph nodes were enlarged on other CT scans (not shown). The patient was a 37-year-old man. An open-lung biopsy of a right lung nodule several months previously had revealed adenocarcinoma, and it is possible that this was the primary lesion.*

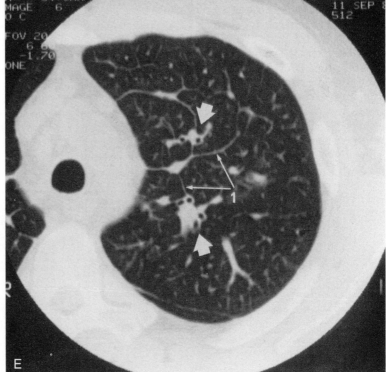

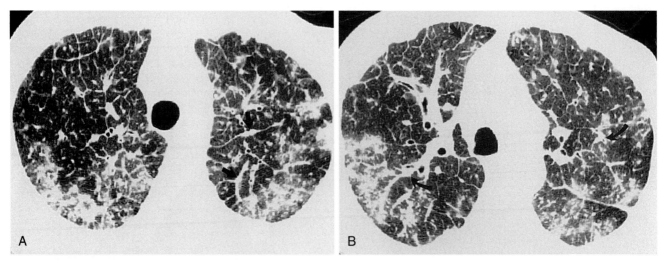

Figure 38–16. Lymphangitic Carcinomatosis. HRCT scans *(A, B)* demonstrate smooth and nodular *(straight arrow)* thickening of the interlobular septa and nodular thickening along the bronchovascular bundles *(curved arrows)*. The patient was a 72-year-old man with dyspnea and poorly differentiated adenocarcinoma of the rectum.

edema, in which case the thickened interlobular septa may have a smooth appearance (Fig. 38–17). Thickening of interlobular septa of adjacent lobules leads to an appearance of polygonal arcades.[108, 112] Characteristically, the arcades are associated with a prominent central dot, representing thickening of the interstitium along the centrilobular bronchovascular bundles.[108, 111] Tumor and edema in the pleural interstitial tissue lead to smooth or nodular thickening of the interlobar fissures. Discrete nodules separate from the interlobular septa may also be seen but are relatively uncommon.[108] Pleural effusion is seen on CT at presentation in approximately 30% of cases and hilar or mediastinal lymph node enlargement in approximately 40%.[108]

At the time of diagnosis, the HRCT findings of lymphangitic carcinomatosis are unilateral or markedly asymmetric in up to 50% of cases (Fig. 38–18).[108, 114] As indicated previously, such unilateral disease is particularly common in patients with pulmonary carcinoma. In some, the abnormalities involve predominantly the peripheral portion of the lung, leading to prominent thickening of the interlobular septa; in others, they involve predominantly the central bronchovascular bundles.[114] As might be expected, patients with diffuse abnormalities on HRCT have considerably more functional impairment and a worse prognosis than those with predominantly central peribronchovascular involvement.[114] In some patients, both radiographic and HRCT findings transiently stabilize or regress with chemotherapy.[115]

HRCT findings may be seen in patients with normal or nonspecific radiographic findings.[111, 116] For example, in one study of 12 patients with pathologically proven lymphangitic carcinomatosis, 3 (25%) had normal chest radiographs and characteristic CT abnormalities.[111] The diagnostic accuracy of CT was compared to that of chest radiography in a study of 118 consecutive patients with various chronic diffuse interstitial lung disease.[116] The CT and radiographic findings were independently assessed by three observers without knowledge of clinical or pathologic data. Of 18 patients with lymphangitic carcinomatosis, a confident diagnosis was made on the chest radiograph in 20% of cases; this interpretation was correct in 64% of readings. By contrast, a confi-

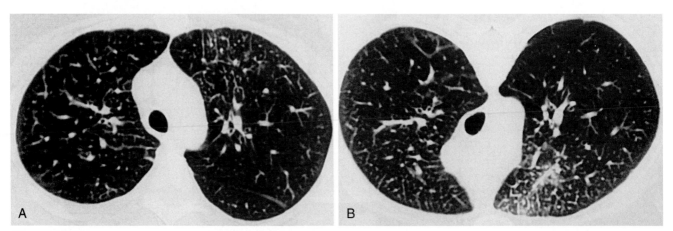

Figure 38–17. Lymphangitic Carcinomatosis—Change with Body Position. HRCT scan performed with the patient supine *(A)* demonstrates bilateral interlobular septal thickening and a small right pleural effusion. With the patient prone *(B)*, there is considerably more interlobular septal thickening anteriorly and less septal thickening evident posteriorly. This change in appearance with body position suggests that at least some of the findings may be the result of interstitial edema secondary to lymphatic obstruction. (Courtesy of Dr. Michael Lefcoe, Victoria Hospital, London, Ontario, Canada.)

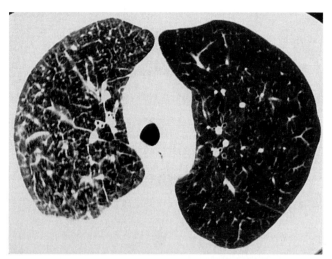

Figure 38–18. Asymmetric Lymphangitic Carcinomatosis. HRCT scan demonstrates interlobular septal thickening throughout the right upper lobe. Also present is a small right pleural effusion. The left lung demonstrates only a few thickened interlobular septa and evidence of emphysema. The patient was a 67-year-old woman with lymphangitic carcinomatosis proven by transbronchial biopsy. (From Leung AN, Staples CA, Müller NL: Chronic diffuse infiltrative lung disease: Comparison of diagnostic accuracy of high-resolution and conventional CT. Am J Roentgenol 157:693, 1991.)

dent diagnosis of lymphangitic carcinomatosis was suggested on CT in 54% of readings, the interpretation being correct in 93% of cases. The relative value of clinical, chest radiographic, and CT findings in making a specific diagnosis of chronic diffuse interstitial lung diseases was assessed in another investigation of 208 consecutive patients, of whom 13 had pathologically proven lymphangitic carcinomatosis.[117] A confident diagnosis was made based on a combination of clinical and radiographic findings in 54% of patients (the assessment being correct in 92%) and on a combination of clinical, radiographic, and CT findings in 92% (correct in all instances).[117] A confident diagnosis was not made on clinical grounds alone in any case.

The most common clinical manifestation of lymphangitic carcinomatosis is dyspnea; although typically insidious in onset, it progresses rapidly and within a few weeks can cause severe disability. In our experience, patients who present with dyspnea that progresses over a period of weeks to months and radiographic evidence of a coarse linear or reticulonodular pattern frequently have pulmonary lymphangitic carcinomatosis, even in the absence of a clinically recognized primary tumor. Cough is seen in some patients.[104] Sometimes, the clinical picture resembles asthma.[118, 119]

The diagnosis is usually evident in patients with a history of carcinoma. Open-lung or transbronchial biopsy is often needed to establish the diagnosis in the absence of a known primary. Transthoracic needle aspiration[120] and intravascular cytology[121] have also been used successfully. As might be expected, the prognosis is usually poor; of 62 patients reported in one study, half died within 3 months, and only 15% survived beyond 6 months.[27]

Pulmonary Hypertension and Infarction (Intravascular Emboli)

Intravascular metastatic neoplasm is not uncommon in the lungs at autopsy; in one study of 366 patients who died

of choriocarcinoma or carcinoma of the breast, kidney, liver, or stomach, 95 (26%) showed tumor within the pulmonary arterial tree.[12] In the investigation of 222 autopsies cited previously, it was identified in 53 cases (24%).[104] The complication is seen most often with adenocarcinoma,[21, 101] especially of the breast or stomach; an unusually high frequency is seen in hepatocellular carcinoma, out of proportion to the incidence of the neoplasm.[12, 101] As many as 10% of cases of primary lung carcinoma also harbor metastatic intravascular tumor at autopsy; as might be expected, the frequency and extent of vascular involvement are higher in patients who have concomitant liver metastases.[12, 122]

Most often, tumor is identified only histologically. Medium-sized to small-sized muscular arteries and arterioles are usually affected; rarely, alveolar septal capillaries are involved.[123, 124] Microscopically, small clusters of malignant cells can be identified within vascular spaces, either free or associated with recent or organizing thrombus (Fig. 38–19).[12, 21, 125] Intimal fibrosis is often present and may be extensive. As indicated previously, concomitant lymphangitic carcinomatosis is common, either focally or widespread.[21, 104, 126] Occasionally, grossly visible emboli can be identified in segmental or larger arteries (Fig. 38–20).[12, 21, 127] Such tumor emboli can result in infarction[12] or sudden death,[128, 129] manifestations that occur most often in association with hepatocellular or renal cell carcinoma. Rarely, a right-sided atrial myxoma[130, 131] or primary vena cava sarcoma[142] has the same effects.

Although intravascular tumor emboli are usually accompanied by radiographic evidence of another pattern of pulmonary involvement (most often lymphangitic carcinomatosis), they may be the sole manifestation of metastatic pulmonary disease. In such cases, the chest radiograph may be entirely normal[132] or may show dilation of central pulmonary arteries and the right ventricle, reflecting pulmonary hypertension. As indicated previously, emboli are rarely identified on CT as nodular or beaded thickening of the pulmonary arteries (*see* Fig. 38–9, page 1389).[81] The propensity for tumor emboli to obstruct arterioles can result in an abnormal radionuclide perfusion lung scan characterized by mismatching ventilation-perfusion defects that are virtually indistinguishable from thromboembolic disease.[133]

Clinical symptoms caused by tumor emboli alone are usually absent, and the condition is not regarded as a common cause of death.[12] The most common symptom is dyspnea;[12] signs of relatively recent-onset cor pulmonale are often present. Occasionally, pleuritic chest pain and hemoptysis indicate the presence of infarction. When symptoms are present, there is usually a past history of carcinoma or evidence of a coexisting extrathoracic primary; occasionally, the diagnosis of metastatic cancer is not evident initially, especially in cases of hepatoma.[12, 134] Differentiation between pulmonary hypertension secondary to thromboemboli and hypertension from tumor emboli may be difficult,[135] particularly because patients with cancer have an increased risk of thromboembolism.[136]

Airway Obstruction (Bronchial and Tracheal Metastasis)

As with the patterns just discussed, neoplastic infiltration of a bronchial wall is common in patients with meta-

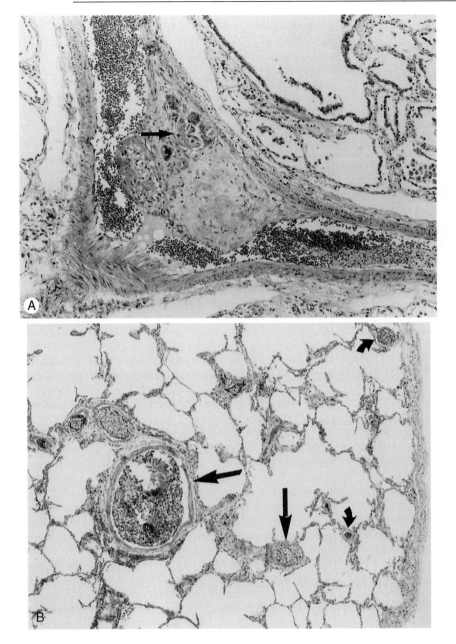

Figure 38–19. Metastatic Carcinoma—Tumor Emboli. A medium-sized pulmonary artery *(A)* contains a small aggregate of metastatic carcinoma *(arrow)* surrounded by partly organized thrombus. Sections of peripheral lung *(B)* show complete occlusion of pulmonary arteries *(straight arrows)* and arterioles *(curved arrows)* by plugs of poorly differentiated carcinoma. Interstitial or parenchymal invasion is absent in both *A* and *B*. (*A,* ×100; *B,* ×40.)

static carcinoma to the lung studied at autopsy: in two reports in which the frequency of such involvement was investigated, the incidence was 51% (97 of 189 cases[5]) and 19% (20 of 109 cases[137]). It is usually caused by direct extension from a parenchymal tumor or an involved lymph node in the hilum or by more or less diffuse mucosal infiltration as part of lymphangitic carcinomatosis (*see* Fig. 38–12).

The majority of cases are incidental findings seen by the pathologist at autopsy or the bronchoscopist during endoscopy; even those grossly visible are usually of such small size and limited extent that they are not manifested either radiographically or clinically. Although most endobronchial tumors large enough to be identified grossly are associated with other metastases, occasionally they appear as isolated tumors, leading to an erroneous diagnosis of primary pulmonary carcinoma (Fig. 38–21).[5] Although virtually any tumor

can present in this way,[138–141] the most common are breast, colorectum, kidney, and melanoma.[143–146]

When present, the usual radiologic findings are those of bronchial obstruction, either partial (causing oligemia and expiratory air trapping) or complete (with atelectasis and obstructive pneumonitis) (Figs. 38–22 and 38–23). In most cases, the primary site is clinically apparent before symptoms related to endobronchial metastases develop.[147] When they occur, symptoms consist of wheeze, hemoptysis, and persistent cough.[146] The last-named can result in expectoration of tumor fragments;[146a] rarely, this is the first indication of disease, especially in renal cell carcinoma.[143]

Hematogenous metastases to the trachea are rare. As with endobronchial metastases, the most common primary sites are kidney, breast, colon, and melanoma.[148, 149] Occasionally, a metastasis is detected as a polypoid soft tissue mass on the chest radiograph or CT (Fig. 38–24).[150] Symp-

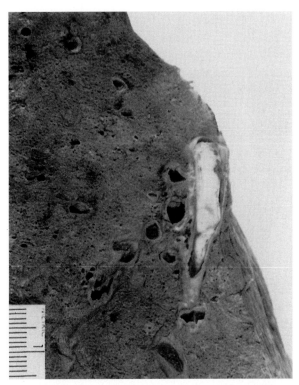

Figure 38–20. Metastatic Carcinoma—Tumor Embolus. A medium-sized pulmonary artery is occluded by an elongated fragment of carcinoma and admixed thrombus; the adjacent lung parenchyma is unremarkable. This was an incidental finding at autopsy of a man with renal cell carcinoma; no parenchymal metastases were evident.

toms include cough, hemoptysis, and, in larger tumors, dyspnea. In one unusual case, a freely mobile, pedunculated endotracheal metastasis from a renal cell carcinoma caused acute upper airway obstruction.[151]

Pleural Effusion

Metastatic spread to the pleura is discussed in detail on page 2756. Briefly, many pleural metastases from sites other than the lung or breast represent tertiary spread from hepatic metastases, particularly when pleural involvement is bilateral.[152] As discussed previously, carcinoma can also reach the basal pleura directly from upper abdominal lymph nodes or the abdominal cavity via transdiaphragmatic lymphatic channels.[25, 26] Of considerable importance is the fact that serous pleural effusions can result from lymphatic obstruction secondary to neoplastic infiltration of mediastinal lymph nodes; in such circumstances, the effusion is not related to direct pleural invasion by neoplastic cells. Effusions usually are hemorrhagic when caused by direct neoplastic involvement of pleural surfaces and serous when secondary to lymphatic obstruction.[152]

SPECIFIC PRIMARY SITES AND TUMORS

Lung

Studies of patients with pulmonary carcinoma have shown lung metastases at autopsy in 7% to 50%.[21, 153–155] In one investigation of 51 cases, 31 were confined to the lungs without evidence of systemic involvement;[154] the ipsilateral lung alone was involved in roughly half, the contralateral lung in about a quarter, and both lungs in the remainder. In this study, pulmonary metastases ranked next in frequency to pleural and osseous sites. The high incidence in these series reflects a thorough pathologic search for tumor deposits, many of which would doubtless be undetectable on chest radiography.

As might be expected, poorly differentiated carcinomas are the most common to be complicated by pulmonary metastasis, possibly because of the frequency of concomitant systemic metastases. The exception is bronchioloalveolar carcinoma, in which bilateral and often extensive lung involvement is not uncommon as a result of spread via the airways.[156] Metastases to the opposite lung in small cell carcinoma have been found at the time of diagnosis in as many as 8% of patients in some studies.[157] Apart from this tumor, radiographically detectable lung metastases at presentation are uncommon. In most instances, the presence of lung metastases can be identified with certainty only in the presence of multiple nodules; when only two tumor masses are seen, and there is no evidence of systemic metastases, they most likely represent separate primaries rather than a primary and solitary metastasis. Lung metastases from pulmonary carcinoma can occur by several routes, of which the most common are probably (1) via the systemic veins and pulmonary arteries from established visceral metastases, particularly in the liver; and (2) via the pulmonary lymphatics to mediastinal lymph nodes and thence to the subclavian vein and pulmonary arteries.

Kidney

The lung is a common site for metastases from renal cell carcinoma: in two autopsy reviews of 523 and 1,828 patients, they were present in 55%[158] and 77%,[159] respectively, for an incidence higher than that associated with any other site. Because approximately 30% of all cases of renal cell carcinoma have distant metastases when first seen,[160] and because as many as 30% to 40% of patients with pulmonary metastases have no symptoms referable to the kidney,[161] differentiation of a solitary metastasis from a primary pulmonary carcinoma can be a problem, especially if the metastasis is predominantly endobronchial. Compounding the diagnostic difficulty is the histologic variability of renal cell carcinoma; although most tumors show a classic clear cell pattern,[162] some have a sarcomatous or other histologic appearance that may not readily suggest a renal primary.

The most common radiographic presentation of metastatic renal cell carcinoma in the thorax is solitary or multiple pulmonary nodules. Not uncommonly, tumors are endobronchial, in which circumstance they may be associated with radiographic evidence of partial or complete airway obstruction. Mediastinal and hilar node enlargement has been reported at autopsy and radiologically in approximately 20% of patients.[159, 163] Although usually associated with pulmonary metastases, paratracheal and bilateral hilar node enlargement is occasionally the sole radiographic manifesta-

Text continued on page 1404

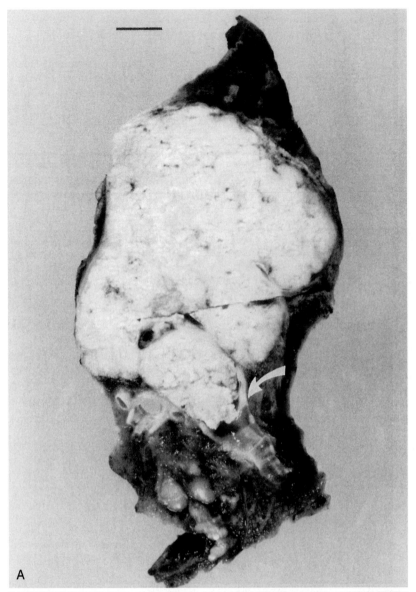

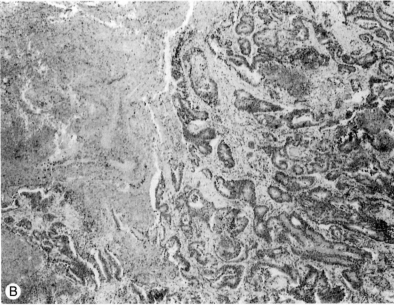

Figure 38–21. Metastatic Carcinoma—Endo-bronchial Extension. A slice from a surgically re-sected lower lobe *(A)* shows a well-delimited parenchy-mal mass with prominent intrabronchial extension *(arrow)*. The appearance is suggestive of a primary squamous cell carcinoma. (Bar = 1 cm.) Microscopi-cally *(B)*, the tumor shows extensive necrosis and easily identifiable glands lined by columnar cells, an appear-ance suggestive of colonic adenocarcinoma. The patient had had a colectomy for a Duke B carcinoma 2 years previously. (×40.)

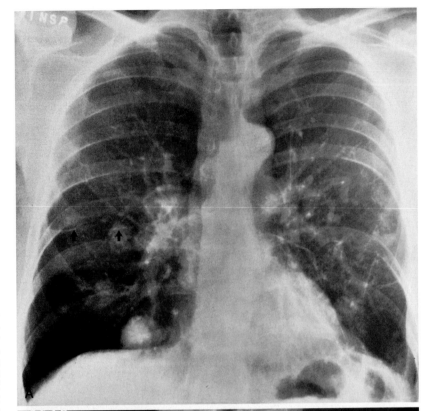

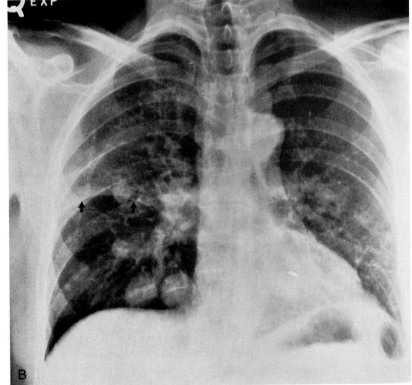

Figure 38–22. Air Trapping in Metastatic Malignant Melanoma. A posteroanterior radiograph exposed at full inspiration *(A)* reveals multiple, sharply circumscribed nodules in the lower portion of both lungs and in the right hilum. Pleural fibrosis is present over the lower half of the left lung, owing to recent thoracotomy. At full expiration *(B)*, the lower half of the right lung has undergone little change in either density or volume because of trapping of air in the right middle and lower lobes. Note that the distance from the horizontal fissure *(arrows* in both views) to the right hemidiaphragm has changed little from inspiration to expiration. This is an uncommon manifestation of metastatic cancer and most commonly results from metastasis to the bronchial wall itself rather than from lymph node compression (except in bronchogenic carcinoma).

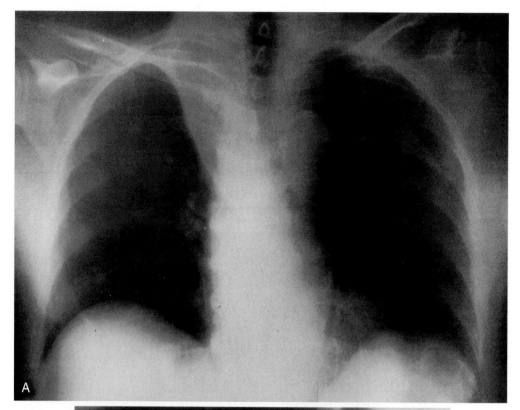

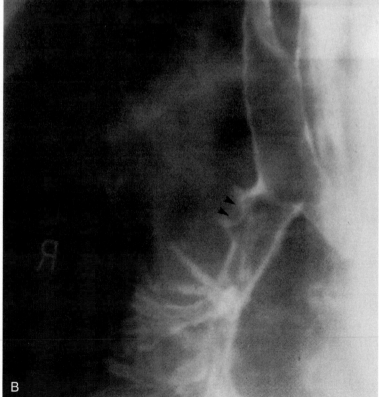

Figure 38–23. Atelectasis Caused by Endobronchial Metastasis from Renal Cell Carcinoma. A posteroanterior chest radiograph *(A)* shows typical features of right upper lobe atelectasis. A bronchogram in slight right posterior oblique projection *(B)* demonstrates amputation of the upper lobe bronchus by an endobronchial mass *(arrowheads)* that protrudes into the right main bronchus. A bronchoscopic biopsy specimen revealed characteristic histopathologic features of renal adenocarcinoma. The patient was a 65-year-old woman.

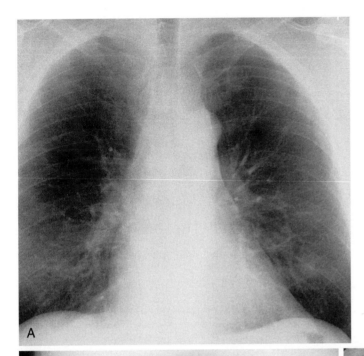

Figure 38–24. Endotracheal Metastasis. Posteroanterior *(A)* and lateral *(B)* chest radiographs demonstrate a 1.5-cm diameter focal soft tissue opacity abutting the posterior wall of the trachea. This is poorly seen on the posteroanterior radiograph but is clearly identified on the lateral view *(arrow)*. A CT scan *(C)* confirms the presence of the endotracheal tumor. The diagnosis of metastatic melanoma was confirmed by bronchoscopy. The patient was a 56-year-old man with a known history of melanoma. (From Kwong JS, Adler BD, Padley SPG, Müller NL: Diagnosis of diseases of the trachea and main bronchi: Chest radiography versus CT. Am J Roentgenol 161:519, 1993.)

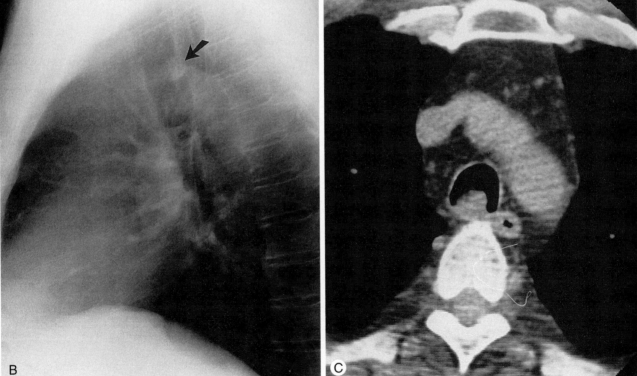

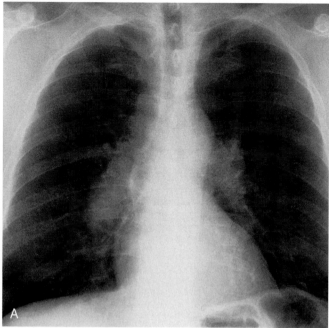

Figure 38–25. Metastatic Renal Cell Carcinoma Mimicking Sarcoidosis. Posteroanterior *(A)* and lateral *(B)* chest radiographs in a 56-year-old man demonstrate extensive paratracheal and bilateral hilar lymphadenopathy. Lymph node biopsy confirmed the diagnosis of metastatic renal cell carcinoma.

tion,[164, 165] resulting in a misdiagnosis of sarcoidosis (Fig. 38–25).[166]

Although patients are usually asymptomatic, those with an endobronchial metastasis may have cough and hemoptysis; in this situation, the diagnosis has been made in several cases on expectorated fragments of neoplasm.[143, 162] Hypertrophic pulmonary osteoarthropathy has been reported rarely.[167] A history of previous renal cell carcinoma or evidence of a synchronous tumor is usually apparent; however, as noted previously, many patients have no symptoms referable to the kidney when the carcinoma is discovered.

Metastatic renal cell carcinoma should be suspected in any patient with radiographic evidence of thoracic metastases and a history of renal cell carcinoma, however remote. Presentation up to 50 years after excision of the primary tumor has been documented.[162] The diagnosis should also be considered whenever a biopsied or excised tumor reveals a prominent clear cell component. Minimal investigations in these cases include urinalysis and excretory urography; the latter may yield false-negative results, and ultrasonography or contrast-enhanced CT may be indicated in patients in whom there is a strong clinical suspicion.

Renal cell carcinoma is one of the more common neoplasms to undergo spontaneous regression;[168, 172, 173] in addition, metastatic nodules occasionally grow slowly over a long period of time. Improved survival appears to be associated with a long disease-free interval between nephrectomy and discovery of metastases, particularly when the metastases are confined to the lungs.[171] Resection of solitary pulmonary metastases has been reported to be associated with a 30% to 35% 5-year survival rate.[169, 170] Renal cell carcinoma is the most common recipient of a tumor-to-tumor metastasis, and pulmonary carcinoma is most often the metastatic "donor."[174]

Colorectum

Metastases to the lung in colorectal carcinoma are second in frequency only to the liver, ranging from approximately 5% to 45% of cases in various series;[175] the overall frequency is probably between 15% and 20%. Carcinoma of the colorectum accounts for 30% to 40% of all solitary metastatic neoplasms to the lung,[54, 57] and is much more likely than other primaries to be the cause of such a nodule. Despite this, in a patient with a solitary nodule and known colonic carcinoma, the metastatic nature of the nodule is not at all certain; for example, in one series of 54 such patients, the nodule was a metastasis in only 25.[63] Metastasis to the bronchus and trachea occurs occasionally.[176]

Histologic differentiation of metastatic colonic carcinoma from primary pulmonary carcinoma is usually straightforward in well-differentiated or moderately differentiated tumors, which comprise the vast majority of cases; electron microscopy, immunohistochemistry,[177] phospholipid analysis,[178] and mucin histochemistry[179] may aid the distinction in selected cases. In one investigation of 22 patients with pulmonary metastases from colorectal carcinoma, satisfactory sputum samples were obtained in 17;[180] of these, 11

(65%) were shown to contain malignant cells on cytologic examination.

Symptoms and radiologic appearance are generally identical to those of other metastatic tumors. One exceptional case has been reported of a patient who had bronchorrhea associated with lymphangitic spread of the carcinoma.[181] In most patients, a primary colorectal tumor has already been recognized;[182] the majority also have evidence of concomitant liver metastases. Survival after resection of pulmonary tumors has been reported to be 40% at 5 years and 30% at 10 years.[183] As might be expected, patients with a single metastasis survive appreciably longer than those with several metastases.[184, 185]

Liver

Pulmonary metastases in hepatocellular carcinoma have been reported in almost two thirds of patients in some series.[186] Their presence is closely related to intrahepatic vascular invasion. Tumor emboli, especially those grossly visible, are particularly common;[187] as indicated previously, they may result in infarction, sudden death, or pulmonary hypertension.[134]

Head and Neck

The incidence of distant metastases in head and neck cancer varies with the site of the primary lesion; in one series of 169 patients with relatively advanced disease, figures ranged from 10% to 20% for carcinomas of the floor of the mouth, tongue, and oropharynx to 30% for the hypopharynx and almost 60% for the larynx.[188] In patients with lower-stage disease, the incidence is undoubtedly much smaller. As might be expected, the lung is the most common site of such metastases; however, hilar and mediastinal lymph node involvement is also common.[188a] Because carcinomas of the head and neck region and the lung often coexist,[189] and because the majority show squamous differentiation histologically, distinguishing a primary from a metastatic carcinoma can, at times, be difficult. The presence of a peripheral tumor unassociated with an airway and concomitant metastases in cervical lymph nodes favors the diagnosis of metastasis; however, even in these situations, the possibility of a primary lung tumor cannot always be excluded.

The 5-year survival after resection of pulmonary metastases of squamous cell carcinoma of the head and neck has been reported to be in the range of 40% to 50%.[66, 190] It is slightly better with metastatic adenoid cystic carcinoma (63%).[190]

Breast

Although breast carcinoma can affect the pleura and lungs by direct extension across the chest wall, such an event is uncommon with current diagnostic and therapeutic techniques, and metastatic disease is much more frequent. Metastasis can occur both hematogenously and by lymphatic spread, the latter probably being the more common. In one autopsy study of 26 patients who died of disseminated breast carcinoma, macroscopically visible infiltration of visceral pleural and parenchymal lymphatics and interstitial tissue was present in 39 of the 52 lungs (75%).[191] By contrast, neoplasm was found in a solely intravascular or pulmonary parenchymal location in only 6 of the 52 lungs. In this series, detailed examination of mediastinal lymph nodes suggested that the mechanism of spread in many of the cases was direct lymphatic extension from the breast to mediastinal nodes and thence to the pleura and lung.

Clinically significant endobronchial metastases occur with considerable frequency compared with other tumors (a finding more likely related to the high prevalence of breast carcinoma than to its intrinsic biologic properties). Although a rare presenting feature, they occasionally complicate the course of a known carcinoma, sometimes as the first indication of recurrence[142, 192] and sometimes many years after the original diagnosis.[192a] In one review of 42 patients with endobronchial metastases of carcinoma of the breast, the average time interval between diagnosis of the breast primary and discovery of the endobronchial metastasis was 77 months.[193] Cough was present in 30 patients (71%) and wheezing and hemoptysis in 10 (25%); atelectasis or obstructive pneumonitis was identified radiographically in 24 (57%).

Pleural effusion is also a common manifestation of intrathoracic spread; in one series of approximately 220 patients with metastatic breast carcinoma seen over a 5-year period, this complication was evident in almost 15%. Most effusions were unilateral and were located on the same side as the affected breast; the median interval from diagnosis of breast cancer to detection of pleural effusion was 32 months.

Isolated (nodular) pulmonary metastases have been said to occur in as many as 15% to 25% of cases.[194] As with other tumors, the presence of a solitary nodule in a patient with known breast carcinoma does not necessarily indicate metastasis; in one investigation of 44 patients, a benign cause was found in 3 (7%).[195] Resection of isolated pulmonary metastases has been associated with a 5-year survival rate of 30% to 50%.[194, 195]

Thyroid

Direct extension of tumor into the trachea is a common occurrence in patients with anaplastic thyroid carcinoma[7] and is often an important factor in causing death; pulmonary metastases are also frequent.[196] Although tracheal invasion also occurs occasionally in papillary and follicular carcinomas,[7, 197] pulmonary metastases are relatively uncommon, presumably reflecting the good prognosis associated with these variants; in three series of 716,[196] 831,[198] and 731[199] patients, they were present in only 87 (12%), 58 (7%), and 73 (10%) cases within the follow-up period recorded. Of 1,127 cases of well-differentiated thyroid carcinoma seen over a 30-year period at the University of Texas M. D. Anderson Hospital and Tumor Institute, 10% had documented pulmonary metastases; the primary tumors in these patients were classified as papillary (67%), follicular (22%), or Hurthle cell (11%). In another report of 831 patients with differentiated thyroid carcinoma, 58 (7%) had pulmonary metastases;[200] the complication occurred in 10% of follicular and 5% of papillary tumors.

Radiographically, the usual pattern consists of paren-

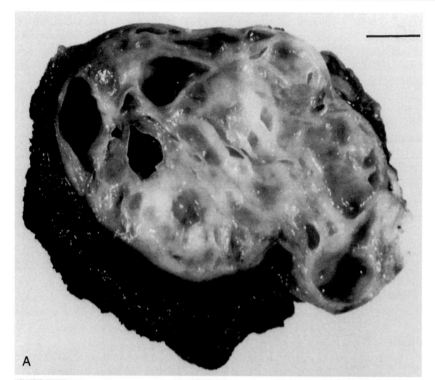

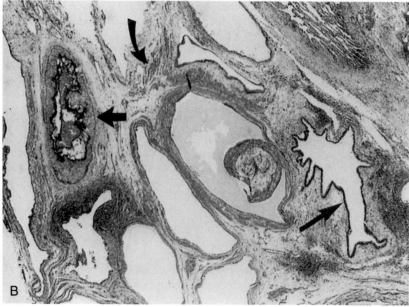

Figure 38–26. Metastatic Testicular Germ Cell Tumor. A wedge excision of lung *(A)* shows a multicystic nodule that is well delimited from adjacent parenchyma, an appearance that might be mistaken for an unusual developmental abnormality. (Bar = 5 mm.) A microscopic section *(B)* shows multiple fluid-filled spaces, some lined by respiratory epithelium *(long arrow)*. Foci of smooth muscle *(curved arrow)* and squamous epithelium *(short arrow)* are also present. This 35-year-old man had had a testicular embryonal choriocarcinoma excised 1 year previously. Standard chemotherapy had been administered. The tumor represents a metastasis from the testicular tumor in which the primitive elements underwent differentiation into mature (teratomatous) tissue. No embryonal carcinoma or choriocarcinoma was identified in the lung specimen. *(B, ×22.)*

chymal nodules of unequal size ranging from 0.5 to 3 cm in diameter.[196, 199] Less commonly, a micronodular pattern (resembling miliary tuberculosis) or a reticulonodular pattern (simulating interstitial fibrosis) is present.[198, 199] Micronodular opacities identified in the lungs on CT scans can persist after treatment with radioactive iodine, reflecting the replacement of tumor by fibrous tissue.[201] Occasionally, the conventional radiograph is normal, the presence of metastasis being established by radioactive iodine imaging[202, 203] or CT.[201] Hilar and mediastinal lymph nodes were enlarged in 17 of 58 cases (29%) in one study.[198] Because of its relatively low grade of malignancy, papillary carcinoma may appear radio-

graphically as a veritable snowstorm of metastatic deposits and yet remain unchanged for a long time.[204]

Among well-differentiated neoplasms, metastases are about equally distributed between papillary and follicular forms.[196, 198] The former tends to be associated with the micronodular pattern; although cervical lymph node metastases are often present, additional systemic spread is typically absent. By contrast, metastases from follicular carcinoma tend to present as larger parenchymal nodules and are not infrequently associated with concomitant skeletal metastases.[196, 198] The diagnosis of thyroid carcinoma as the site of origin of pulmonary metastases is usually evident from the presence of a thyroid mass; however, this is occasionally not appreciable.[205]

Testis

Mediastinal lymph node enlargement is a common intrathoracic manifestation of metastatic testicular seminoma: in a review of the CT scans of 200 patients with pure testicular seminoma, evidence of intrathoracic metastatic disease was found in 30 (15%)—mediastinal node enlargement in 21, pulmonary metastases in 12, pleural effusions in 6, and pleural masses in 2.[206] CT showed metastatic disease in five patients who had normal chest radiographs, as well as additional sites of disease in four other patients whose chest radiographs were abnormal. Mediastinal and hilar lymphadenopathy is also common with other testicular tumors, being seen in 5 of 17 patients in one study.[163]

Pulmonary metastases also occur with considerable frequency with all the histologic variants of malignant testicular neoplasms and usually take the form of solitary or multiple parenchymal nodules.[206a] Histologic examination of nodules excised after chemotherapy has shown three patterns:[128, 207, 208] (1) poorly differentiated or anaplastic tumor; (2) fibrosis or necrosis without evidence of histologically viable tumor; or (3) mature, usually teratomatous tissue (Fig. 38–26). In some instances, the last-named has been confused with primary lung tumors, such as chondromatous hamartoma or developmental cysts;[207] it has been hypothesized that the histologic appearance of this variety results from selective chemotherapeutic destruction of the more malignant elements of the tumor, leaving the more mature components intact.[207, 209] Metastases are multiple in the majority of patients. CT scans reveal enlarged, low-attenuation abdominal and pelvic lymph nodes in almost 50% of patients with testicular cancers. Low-attenuation hilar and mediastinal nodes and pulmonary parenchymal nodules are less common (Fig. 38–27).[210]

Most patients are asymptomatic. Some patients with metastatic choriocarcinoma have suffered massive hemoptysis.[211] A history of a testicular primary is present in the vast majority of patients.[212] Resection of metastases has been reported to be associated with a 60% 5-year survival.[213]

Melanoma

Although intrathoracic metastases are common at autopsy of patients with melanoma,[214] they are seen in a relatively small proportion of all patients with the disease; for example, in one review of more than 7,500 cases, they were identified in only 954 (12%).[215] In this study, the probability of developing a pulmonary metastasis was estimated to be 0.1, 0.13, and 0.17 at 5, 10, and 15 years. This apparent discrepancy between autopsy and in vivo findings is explained by the large number of cases of low-stage disease, in which cure is common.

In one series of 65 patients, 63 had an abnormal radiograph, consisting of pulmonary metastases in 57, enlarged lymph nodes in 28, and pleural effusion in 10.[215] Of the patients with pulmonary involvement, 14 had a solitary nodule; 41, multiple nodules; 8, a miliary pattern; and 5, lymph-

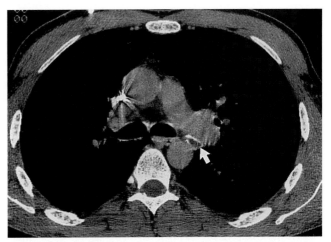

Figure 38–27. Metastatic Testicular Germ Cell Tumor. A 40-year-old man developed increased levels of α-fetoprotein 15 years after surgical resection of a malignant testicular germ cell tumor. The only abnormality seen on extensive investigation was a slightly enlarged lymph node adjacent to the left pulmonary artery (*arrow*). On HRCT, this lymph node can be seen to have a peripheral rim of calcification with a lower attenuation center. At thoracotomy, the node was shown to contain both histologically mature and malignant germ cell components. After surgery, the serum levels of α-fetoprotein returned to normal.

angitic carcinomatosis. Ill-defined air-space disease resembling pneumonia or edema has also been described.[216] Involvement of hilar or mediastinal lymph nodes is also relatively common; in one investigation of 65 patients, it was present in 35 (54%), in 28 of whom it was radiographically visible;[217] in only 3 of the 28 patients was there no radiographic evidence of metastases within the lungs. Lymph node enlargement was frequently asymmetric and sometimes unilateral. Melanoma is also a rare cause of endotracheal metastasis.[148, 149]

When the diagnosis is in doubt, transthoracic needle aspiration may be indicated;[218] tumor cells characteristically show strong immunohistochemical reactions for protein S-100 and HMB-45, and a definitive diagnosis of the metastatic nature of a nodule can usually be made. Five-year survival rates after resection of metastases range from 5% to 25%.[219–221]

Endometrium

Endometrial adenocarcinoma metastasizes to the lungs infrequently; for example, in one series of 470 patients, only 11 (2.3%) developed pulmonary metastases within the follow-up period of 2 to 12 years.[222] Most have concomitant disease in other viscera or lymph nodes. Low-grade endometrial stromal sarcoma is well known to be capable of recurrence many years after initial resection, occasionally in the lungs; some such cases have been confused with mesenchymal cystic hamartoma.[223]

Uterine Cervix

The incidence of pulmonary metastases in patients with invasive cervical carcinoma is probably between 5% and

10%,[224–226] although a figure as high as 33% has been reported.[227] The incidence is higher for adenocarcinoma (15% to 20%) than for squamous carcinoma (approximately 5%).[226, 228] The frequency of pulmonary involvement correlates with the stage of the disease with squamous cell carcinoma;[224, 226] however, there is evidence that metastases develop in patients with adenocarcinoma regardless of the stage at diagnosis.[228] Although pulmonary metastases are usually accompanied by evidence of extrathoracic disease, the lung may be the sole site, as was the case in 40 (12%) of 341 patients in one study.[224] In one review, approximately 95% of metastases were detected within 2 years of identification of the primary tumor.[226]

Although multiple nodules are the usual manifestation, solitary nodules and a lymphangitic pattern have also been described.[229] Rarely, mediastinal or hilar lymph node enlargement is the sole manifestation.[230] Pleural effusion is sometimes apparent.[231]

Ovary

Analysis of 357 patients with ovarian cancer in one investigation revealed thoracic metastases in 169 (45%).[232] Pleural effusion was the most common manifestation (126 of the 169 patients [75%]). In another study of 255 patients, 63 (25%) were found to have malignant pleural effusion.[233] It is likely that the high incidence of pleural disease is the result of direct spread from the peritoneal cavity through diaphragmatic lymphatics.[26] Pulmonary parenchymal metastases have been identified in 7%[233] to 39%[234] of patients; in most cases, they are contiguous with pleural metastases and probably represent direct extension from these sites rather than independent hematogenous deposits.[234] Lymphangitic spread within the lung is uncommon. Some cases of pulmonary tumor emboli have been documented after peritoneovenous shunting for malignant ascites.[235]

Prostate

The incidence of spread of prostatic carcinoma to the lungs is fairly high at autopsy; for example, in one series of 104 patients, it was identified in 40 (38%).[236] Despite this, radiographically detectable lesions are uncommon; in the latter series, of the 27 patients with pulmonary metastases and available chest radiographs, only 4 had radiologic evidence of disease. The frequency of pulmonary metastases is particularly low in patients without other organ involvement: in one series of 1,885 autopsy cases,[237] it was identified in only 5%; however, the incidence increased linearly in accordance with the number of organs involved, being recorded in almost 50% of patients in whom metastases were present in three or more organs. Pulmonary nodules may represent metastatic prostatic carcinoma even in the absence of positive findings on bone scintigraphy performed to detect skeletal metastases.[238] Confusion with a primary pulmonary carcinoma is uncommon.[239, 240] Endobronchial metastases are rare.[241]

In one review of the chest radiographs of 198 patients with Stage D carcinoma, 48 (24%) had intrathoracic abnormalities attributable to the metastases.[242] Of these, 22% had pleural effusion; 16%, reticular opacities; 3.5%, reticulonodular opacities; 8%, isolated or discrete pulmonary nodules; and 4.5%, lymph node enlargement. (The authors considered that about a third of the effusions and half of the reticular opacities were best attributed to concomitant disease rather than to metastases.) Focal or diffuse osteoblastic metastases to the thoracic skeleton may be present either with or without lung or mediastinal involvement.

Radioactive antibodies against prostatic acid phosphatase have been used to differentiate primary pulmonary carcinoma from metastases in patients with pulmonary nodules on radiography.[243] More commonly, the tumor is definitively identified in biopsy or cytology specimens by a positive immunohistochemical reaction for prostate-specific antigen;[240] rarely the presence of characteristic crystalloid material in the neoplastic glands suggests the diagnosis.[244]

Gestational Trophoblastic Neoplasms

The term *gestational trophoblastic neoplasia* refers to three related abnormalities of placental tissue—hydatidiform mole, invasive mole, and choriocarcinoma. The first of these by definition is limited to the uterus, and the second only rarely metastasizes; thus, the remainder of this discussion is concerned principally with the last variant. Although less common, nongestational choriocarcinoma can result in identical clinicopathologic and radiologic patterns of disease.

Pulmonary metastases in gestationally related choriocarcinoma are common,[245] being identified in as many as 85% of patients in some studies.[127] They are invariably hematogenous and are usually manifested by multiple parenchymal nodules (*see* Fig. 38–2, page 1383); occasionally, there is a miliary pattern.[33, 127] Intravascular tumor emboli, sometimes quite large, can also occur.[127, 245] In one investigation, parenchymal nodules were relatively frequent in the apical portion of the lungs, suggesting to the author that tumor dissemination may have occurred during uterine curettage when the patient was recumbent.[246] Therapy usually results in complete regression of parenchymal nodules, although fibrosis (with or without dystrophic calcification) occasionally marks the site of previous disease.[92, 247, 248]

Because of the highly vascular nature of choriocarcinoma, arteriovenous shunting through the lesions is probably common.[249] Persistent arterial oxygen unsaturation can provide convincing physiologic evidence of this process. The marked vascularity is also apparent pathologically by extensive hemorrhage in tumor nodules and adjacent lung parenchyma. Radiographically and on conventional CT, the nodules may have smooth margins or a characteristic fluffy appearance, the latter also the result of hemorrhage.[250, 251] On HRCT, the hemorrhage is characterized by a halo of ground-glass attenuation.[80, 252]

Symptoms are usually absent, although dyspnea may develop in the presence of extensive intravascular tumor embolization, and hemoptysis can occur as a result of intrapulmonary hemorrhage.[127] The determination of chorionic gonadotropin levels is invaluable in diagnosis and in indicating response to treatment. Immunoperoxidase staining of material obtained by needle biopsy may be diagnostic.[253] Gamma scintigraphy using technetium-99m–labeled antibody to human chorionic gonadotropin has also been recom-

1409

mended as a method of identifying both the primary neoplasm and the metastatic pulmonary lesions.[254]

Pulmonary metastases have a remarkable tendency to disappear in response to drug or radiation therapy and, occasionally, after removal of the primary tumor.

Leiomyosarcoma

Metastatic leiomyosarcoma to the lungs may be clearly malignant histologically and clinically, in which circumstance there is usually a well-defined history of an extrathoracic primary (most often of the uterus[255]); in this situation, the diagnosis is usually straightforward. Sometimes, however, diagnostic difficulties can arise when an excised pulmonary nodule of apparent smooth muscle origin possesses a bland histologic appearance and there is no clear-cut evidence of a concomitant or prior extrathoracic neoplasm. The remainder of the discussion is concerned with this variant.

Several interpretations have been given for these tumors. Some have been presumed to represent primary pulmonary smooth muscle neoplasms. Others have been referred to as *pulmonary fibroleiomyomas* and have been hypothesized to represent an unusual form of hamartoma. A further group of tumors with an identical histologic appearance but associated with uterine "leiomyomas" has been considered to represent metastases from this site and has been known as *benign metastasizing leiomyoma*. In fact, it is likely that the majority of these tumors represent metastatic well-differentiated leiomyosarcoma.[256-258] There are three reasons for this conclusion

1. The tumors are frequently associated with extrathoracic smooth muscle neoplasms, usually of the uterus. For example, in one review of 50 patients, a history of previous uterine surgery was found in 39.[257] In most of these patients, the initial diagnosis of the uterine tumor was solitary or multiple leiomyomas; however, subsequent local recurrence and lymph node metastases in some clearly indicated the malignant nature of the neoplasms. Because histologic sampling of the uterine tumors may have been incomplete in some cases, their true nature at the time of the primary surgery might have been misinterpreted.

2. The well-documented increase in size of pulmonary nodules radiographically, the occasional cases of death secondary to pulmonary insufficiency,[257] and the presence of concomitant metastases in sites such as omentum and lymph nodes[256] all indicate the essential malignant behavior of the tumor.

3. Admixed epithelial elements within the smooth muscle component, once believed to be evidence for a hamartomatous nature of the tumors, have been shown on ultrastructural examination to represent normal pulmonary epithelium entrapped by the expanding smooth muscle neoplasm.[257-260]

By far the most common primary site of these neoplasms is the uterus. As indicated, the usual diagnosis in this site is leiomyoma, the tumor not being deemed malignant by criteria of invasion or increased mitotic count. Uncommonly, other primary sites, such as the diaphragm, skin, soft tissues of the extremities,[257] and systemic veins,[257, 261] also have been reported. Rare instances of intravenous leiomyomatosis of

the uterus have also been associated with pulmonary metastases.[262]

The pulmonary nodules are usually fairly well demarcated grossly (Fig. 38–28) and may even "shell out" of the surrounding lung parenchyma.[256, 257] Cyst formation may occur in larger tumors.[263] Histologically, they consist of interlacing fascicles of spindle-shaped cells with a variable admixture of collagen. Nuclei are typically uniform in size and shape with little hyperchromasia; mitotic figures are often few in number. The periphery of the tumor characteristically contains somewhat irregular round or slitlike spaces lined by cuboidal or columnar cells (*see* Fig. 38–28), representing entrapped pulmonary epithelium.

Radiographically, the tumors are usually multiple and bilateral and range from 0.5 to 5.0 cm in diameter (Fig. 38–29).[257] Rarely, the pattern is micronodular[264, 265] or miliary.[266] The nodules can increase both in size and in number[267, 267a] or can remain fairly stable over long periods of time.[267] New nodules may appear, while others shrink and actually disappear;[268, 269] occasionally, such regression has been seen to follow termination of pregnancy[258, 264] or progestin withdrawal,[270] implying a hormonal effect on tumor growth. Although the nodules may show calcification histologically, this is usually not evident radiographically.

Because of the frequency of a uterine primary, these tumors occur almost exclusively in women: only 3 of 59 patients in one series were men.[257] Although the pulmonary nodules can be present at the same time the uterine neoplasm is recognized, more often they appear after hysterectomy, sometimes after an interval as long as 20 to 30 years. Metastases usually do not produce symptoms and are discovered incidentally on a screening chest radiograph; occasionally, there is dyspnea, cough, or chest pain.[257] Rarely, tumors are sufficient in size and number to cause severe pulmonary function impairment[265] or respiratory failure.[257, 268] The diagnosis has been confirmed by cytologic examination of sputum.[270a]

The prognosis is variable and difficult to predict. The authors of one review found an excellent prognosis in patients with only a few nodules.[256] Even with extensive pulmonary involvement, however, both long-term and short-term survivors were identified.

Other Soft Tissue Sarcomas

The lung is the most common site of metastasis from a variety of other soft tissue sarcomas.[271, 272] In most instances, a primary source is clearly evident, and the diagnosis of metastasis can be established by plain radiography; if doubt exists, transthoracic needle aspiration should provide an answer in most cases.[273] Rarely, one or more lung nodules is evident before the clinical appearance of the primary sarcoma,[274] notably with alveolar soft part sarcoma.[275, 276] As with other tumors, metastases occasionally develop many years after the primary is recognized.[277]

Metastatic angiosarcoma to the lungs is uncommon. In one review of 15 cases, the most common primary sites were breast and heart;[278] the median age at the time of diagnosis was 45 years, and the most common presenting symptom was hemoptysis. One case has been reported that

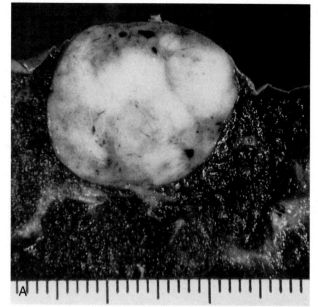

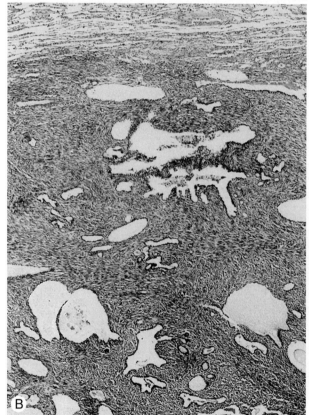

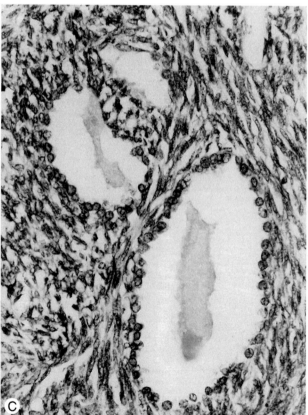

Figure 38–28. Metastatic Leiomyosarcoma—Solitary Nodule. A gross specimen of lung *(A)* reveals a well-circumscribed nodule in a subpleural location, apparently compressing rather than invading lung parenchyma. A histologic section *(B)* shows a spindle cell neoplasm containing numerous, irregularly shaped glandular spaces. At higher magnification *(C)*, these spaces are seen to be lined by cuboidal epithelial cells (hyperplastic type II cells), representing inclusions of lung tissue within the expanding neoplasm. This was an autopsy specimen from a 50-year-old woman with leiomyosarcoma of the uterus. *(B, ×40; C, ×340.)*

was complicated by the development of cavities and hemo-pneumothorax.[279]

As with some carcinomas, excision of isolated metastases of soft tissue sarcomas has been attempted to prolong life. In one retrospective study of 255 patients, the overall 3- and 5-year survival rates after metastasectomy were 54% and 38%;[280] the disease-free survival rates were 42% and 35%. Favorable prognostic factors included disease-free intervals of 2.5 years or more, microscopically free margins, age less than 40 years, and Grade I and II tumors.

Sarcomas of Bone

Metastases to the lungs from sarcomas of bone are frequent, especially from osteosarcoma; in one series of 552 patients with this tumor, 10% had the complication at the time of initial diagnosis.[281] In another study of 255 patients with high-grade osteosarcoma, 107 developed metastases.[282] Seventy-seven had tumor apparently confined to the lungs, and 17 had tumor in both lungs and elsewhere; only 13 did not show pulmonary involvement. Giant cell tumor of bone,

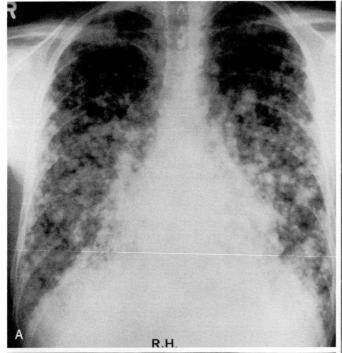

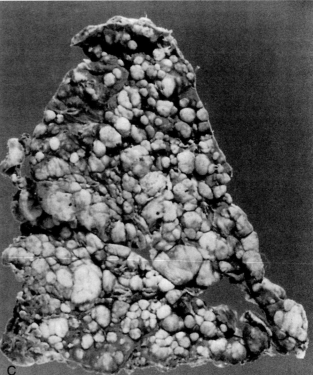

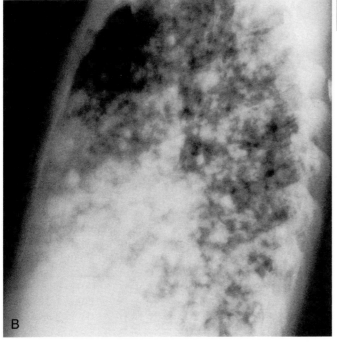

Figure 38–29. Metastases from Leiomyosarcoma—Radiographic Manifestations. Posteroanterior *(A)* and lateral *(B)* chest radiographs disclose multiple discrete and confluent nodular opacities throughout both lungs. The lesions are roughly symmetrically distributed in the two lungs but are more numerous in the mid and lower lung zones, reflecting gravity-induced blood flow distribution. Several weeks later, the patient died; at autopsy, a sagittal section *(C)* through the right lung reveals extensive replacement of parenchyma by sarcoma. The patient was a 24-year-old man with a leiomyosarcoma of the retroperitoneum.

a neoplasm that is usually benign, is occasionally associated with metastases to the lungs.[282a]

Most metastases appear radiographically as parenchymal nodules; in one study, approximately 70% were bilateral.[283] Calcification can be seen occasionally and cavitation rarely.[284] A history of synchronous or previous primary bone neoplasm is almost invariable.[283] Although usually asymptomatic, tumor deposits can be so numerous as to cause respiratory insufficiency.[283] Spontaneous pneumothorax is also a well-recognized complication of metastatic osteogenic sarcoma.[285] The 5-year survival after metastasectomy of the last-named tumor ranges from 20% to 57%.[66]

Central Nervous System and Associated Neoplasms

Metastasis of central nervous system tumors outside of the neuraxis is extremely rare; in one review of 8,000 primary central nervous system neuroectodermal neoplasms, only 35 well-documented cases were identified, of which 16 were to the lungs.[286] All patients had had prior neurosurgery, a finding supporting the hypothesis that it is this procedure rather than the inherent invasive properties of the tumors themselves that is responsible for metastasis.

Although apparently primary neoplasms resembling meningioma have been reported in lung parenchyma *(see* page 1370), most often such tumors represent a metastasis from a spinal or cranial source.[287] In the majority of such cases, there is a history of previous surgery,[288, 289] the presence of pulmonary tumor again most likely representing the effect of therapy rather than the biologic behavior of the meningioma. Exceptionally, no prior surgery has been performed, and the tumors in both pulmonary and cranial sources have a histologically benign appearance.[288]

LABORATORY FINDINGS

Cytology

Malignant cells can be detected in sputum or bronchial washings in 35% to 50% of patients who have metastatic cancer to the lungs.[290–292] Cytologic examination of pleural fluid of malignant origin gives a somewhat higher yield, most authors reporting an accuracy of about 50%.[293, 294] In most instances, the distinction between primary and metastatic neoplasm cannot be made; however, cytologic features occasionally suggest a specific extrapulmonary source.[295] The diagnosis of lymphangitic carcinomatosis has also been made on cytologic examination of blood obtained from a wedged pulmonary artery catheter.[296]

Of greater importance in the cytologic diagnosis of metastatic disease is transthoracic needle aspiration, which, in the hands of experienced practitioners, yields a positive diagnosis in 85% to 95% of cases.[297–299] In fact, when the site of the extrathoracic primary is known, a definitive cytologic diagnosis is frequently possible. In some neoplasms, such as renal cell or colorectal carcinoma, cytologic features alone may be sufficiently characteristic to suggest the site of origin; in other cases, comparison of tissue fragments within a cell block with samples of the known primary tumor is confirmatory. In selected tumors, the use of immunohistochemical techniques is also valuable in determining the primary or metastatic nature of the disease.

Bronchoscopy

Although bronchoscopic examination is not as productive in the diagnosis of pulmonary metastases as in primary pulmonary carcinoma, diagnostic rates between 50% and 60% have been reported by several groups of investigators.[300–302] As might be expected, a positive yield is highest in tumors with endobronchial extension, an event that appears to be much more often than might be predicted by clinical and radiographic findings.[301] In one study of all patients with lung metastases who underwent bronchoscopy over a 66-month period in five community teaching hospitals, the likelihood of a positive diagnosis was highest in colorectal (79%) and breast carcinoma (57%) and lowest in genitourinary cancer (33%).[300] Biopsy, washing, and brushing are complementary procedures in diagnosis.[301]

Pulmonary Function Tests

During the early stages of the disease, the great majority of patients with pulmonary metastases have normal pulmonary function. In fact, parenchymal metastases may be widespread before patients note the onset of dyspnea, at which time stage function testing shows appropriate abnormalities. One group of investigators compared the results of function tests in patients with predominantly nodular and lymphangitic patterns of metastatic disease.[303] Lung volumes were reduced in both groups, and all the patients had hypoxemia at rest; the inhalation of 100% oxygen for 15 minutes corrected the hypoxemia in all but the few patients in whom venous-to-arterial shunting was indicated. Both diffusing capacity and lung compliance were uniformly reduced in all patients with lymphangitic spread, but were reduced in those with nodules only if these were exceptionally numerous. Pulmonary resistance was slightly increased in two of the four patients with lymphangitic spread; in one of these, carbon dioxide retention developed as the disease progressed.

SPONTANEOUS REGRESSION OF METASTASES

The spontaneous disappearance of lung metastases is rare but well documented.[304] Tumors can disappear after removal of the primary tumor, during or after irradiation or drug therapy at levels ordinarily considered no more than palliative, or for no apparent reason.[305] In most cases, the primary lesions are renal cell carcinoma[168] or choriocarcinoma.[306, 307]

REFERENCES

1. Woodard PK, Dehdashti F, Putman CE: Radiologic diagnosis of extrathoracic metastases to the lung. Oncology 12:431, 1998.
2. Putnam JB Jr, Roth JA: Surgical treatment for pulmonary metastases from sarcoma. Hematol Oncol Clin North Am 9:869, 1995.
3. Johnson RM, Lindskog GE: 100 cases of tumor metastatic to the lung and mediastinum. JAMA 202:94, 1967.
4. Willis RA: In Willis RA (ed): The Spread of Tumours in the Human Body. 3rd ed. London, Butterworth, 1973.
5. Rosenblatt MB, Lisa JR, Trinidad S: Pitfalls in the clinical and histologic diagnosis of bronchogenic carcinoma. Dis Chest 49:396, 1966.
6. Akiyama S, Imaizumi M, Sakamoto J, et al: Basal cell carcinoma with lung metastasis. Jpn J Surg 15:215, 1985.
7. Tsumori T, Nakao K, Miyata M, et al: Clinicopathologic study of thyroid carcinoma infiltrating the trachea. Cancer 56:2843, 1985.
8. Sons HU, Borchard F: Esophageal cancer. Arch Pathol Lab Med 108:983, 1984.
9. Zerbey AL, Mueller PR, Dawson SL, et al: Pleural seeding from hepatocellular carcinoma: A complication of percutaneous alcohol ablation. Radiology 193:81, 1994.
10. Carter RL: Some aspects of the metastatic process. J Clin Pathol 35:1041, 1982.
11. Wallace AC, Chew E-C, Jones DS: Arrest and extravasation of cancer cells in the lung. In Weiss L, Gilbert HA (eds): Pulmonary Metastasis. Boston, GK Hall, 1978, p 26.
12. Winterbauer RH, Elfenbein IB, Ball WC Jr: Incidence and clinical significance of tumor embolization to the lungs. Am J Med 45:271, 1968.
13. Burn JI, Watne AL, Moore GE: The role of the thoracic duct lymph in cancer dissemination. Br J Cancer 16:608, 1962.
13a. Adamson IYR, Young L, Orr FW: Tumor metastasis after hyperoxic injury and repair of the pulmonary endothelium. Lab Invest 57:71, 1987.
14. Weiss L: Factors leading to the arrest of cancer cells in the lungs. In Weiss L, Gilbert HA (eds): Pulmonary Metastasis. Boston, GK Hall, 1978, p 5.
15. Orr FW, Adamson IYR, Young L: Pulmonary inflammation generates chemotactic activity for tumor cells and promotes lung metastasis. Am Rev Respir Dis 131:607, 1985.
16. Kim U: Pathogenesis of lung metastases. In Weiss L, Gilbert HA (eds): Pulmonary Metastasis. Boston, GK Hall, 1978, p 76.
17. Janower ML, Blennerhassett JB: Lymphangitic spread of metastatic cancer to the lung: A radiologic-pathologic classification. Radiology 101:267, 1971.
18. Harold JT: Lymphangitis carcinomatosa of the lungs. QJM 83:353, 1952.
19. Morgan AD: The pathology of subacute cor pulmonale in diffuse carcinomatosis of the lungs. J Pathol Bacteriol 61:75, 1949.
20. Hagerstrand I, Fichera G: The small lymph vessels of the lungs in lymphangiosis carcinomatosa. Acta Pathol Microbiol Scand 65:505, 1965.
21. Gonzalez-Vitale JC, Garcia-Bunuel R: Pulmonary tumor emboli and cor pulmonale in primary carcinoma of the lung. Cancer 38:2105, 1976.
22. Zeidman I: Experimental studies on the spread of cancer in the lymphatic system: IV. Retrograde spread. Cancer Res 19:1114, 1959.
23. Heitzman ER, Markarian B, Raasch BN, et al: Pathways of tumor spread through the lung: Radiologic correlations with anatomy and pathology. Radiology 144:3, 1982.
24. Hendin AS, Deveney CW: Postmortem demonstration of abnormal deep pulmonary lymphatic pathways in lymphangitic carcinomatosis. Cancer 33:1558, 1974.
25. Meyer KK: Direct lymphatic connections from the lower lobes of the lung to the abdomen. J Thorac Surg 35:726, 1958.
26. Feldman GB, Knapp RC: Lymphatic drainage of the peritoneal cavity and its significance in ovarian cancer. Am J Obstet Gynecol 119:991, 1974.
27. Yang S-P, Lin C-C: Lymphangitic carcinomatosis of the lungs: The clinical significance of its roentgenologic classification. Chest 62:179, 1972.
28. Sampson JA: Implantation peritoneal carcinomatosis of ovarian origin. Am J Pathol 7:423, 1931.
29. Epstein SS: Lung as a transplant site for malignant tumors in rodents. Cancer 19:454, 1966.
30. Vorzimer J, Perla D: An instance of adamantinoma of the jaw with metastases to the right lung. Am J Pathol 8:445, 1932.
31. Pickren JW, Katz AD: Aspiration metastases from basal cell carcinoma. Cancer 11:783, 1958.
32. Crow J, Slavin G, Kreel L: Pulmonary metastasis: A pathologic and radiologic study. Cancer 47:2595, 1981.
33. Burton RM: A case of chorion-epithelioma with pulmonary complications. Tubercle 44:487, 1963.
34. Rossmann P, Vortel V: Pulmonary metastases imitating alveolar-cell carcinoma. J Pathol Bacteriol 81:313, 1961.
35. Rosenblatt MB, Lisa JR, Collier F: Primary and metastatic bronchiolo-alveolar carcinoma. Dis Chest 52:147, 1967.
36. Cudkowicz L: Bronchial arterial circulation in man: Normal anatomy and responses to disease. In Moser KM (ed): Pulmonary Vascular Diseases. New York, Marcel Dekker, 1979, p 111.
37. Milne ENC: Circulation of primary and metastatic pulmonary neoplasms: A postmortem microarteriographic study. Am J Roentgenol 100:603, 1967.
38. Friedman PJ, Jonas AM, Carrington CB: Observations on the vascularization of secondary pulmonary neoplasms. Invest Radiol 9:227, 1974.
39. Muhm JR, Brown LR, Crowe JR, et al: Comparison of whole lung tomography for detecting pulmonary nodules. Am J Roentgenol 131:981, 1978.
40. Lund G, Heilo A: Computed tomography of pulmonary metastases. Acta Radiol Diagn 23:617, 1982.
41. Gross BH, Glazer GM, Bookstein FL: Multiple pulmonary nodules detected by computed tomography: Diagnostic implications. J Comput Assist Tomogr 9:880, 1985.
42. Davis SD: CT evaluation for pulmonary metastases in patients with extrathoracic malignancy. Radiology 180:1, 1991.
43. Peuchot M, Libshitz HI: Pulmonary metastatic disease: Radiologic-surgical correlation. Radiology 164:719, 1987.
43a. Yokomise H, Mizuno H, Ike O, et al: Importance of intrapulmonary lymph nodes in the differential diagnosis of small pulmonary shadows. Chest 113:703, 1998.
44. Remy-Jardin M, Remy J, Giraud F, Marquette CH: Pulmonary nodules: Detection with thick-section spiral CT versus conventional CT. Radiology 187:513, 1993.
45. Buckley JA, Scott WW, Siegelman SS, et al: Pulmonary nodules: Effect of increased data sampling on detection with spiral CT and confidence in diagnosis. Radiology 196:395, 1995.
46. Tillich M, Kammerhuber F, Reittner P, et al: Detection of pulmonary nodules with helical CT: Comparison of cine and film-based viewing. Am J Roentgenol 169:1611, 1997.
47. Schaner EG, Chang AE, Doppman JL, et al: Comparison of computed and conventional whole lung tomography in detecting pulmonary nodules: A prospective radiologic-pathologic study. Am J Roentgenol 131:51, 1978.
48. Chang AE, Schaner EG, Conkle DM, et al: Evaluation of computed tomography in the detection of pulmonary metastases: A prospective study. Cancer 43:913, 1979.
49. Williams MP, Husband JE, Heron CW: Intrathoracic manifestations of metastatic testicular seminioma: A comparison of chest radiographic and CT findings. Am J Roentgenol 149:473, 1987.
50. Edwards SE, Kelsey-Fry I: Prevalence of nodules on computed tomography of patients without known malignant disease. Br J Radiol 55:715, 1982.
51. Berquist TH, Brown LR, May GR, et al: Magnetic resonance imaging of the chest: A diagnostic comparison with computed tomography and hilar tomography. Magn Reson Imaging 2:315, 1984.
52. Müller NL, Gamsu G, Webb WR: Pulmonary nodules: Detection using magnetic resonance and computed tomography. Radiology 155:687, 1985.
53. Feuerstein IM, Jicha DL, Pass HI, et al: Pulmonary metastases: MR imaging with surgical correlation—a prospective study. Radiology 182:123, 1992.
54. Steele JD: The solitary pulmonary nodule: Report of a cooperative study of resected asymptomatic solitary pulmonary nodules in males. J Thorac Cardiovasc Surg 46:21, 1963.
55. Siegelman SS, Khouri NF, Leo FP, et al: Solitary pulmonary nodules: CT assessment. Radiology 160:307, 1986.
56. Primack SL, Lee KS, Logan PM, et al: Bronchogenic carcinoma: Utility of CT in the evaluation of patients with suspected lesions. Radiology 193:795, 1994.
57. Clagett OT, Woolner LB: Surgical treatment of solitary metastatic pulmonary lesion. Med Clin North Am 48:939, 1964.
58. Paglicci A: Metastatic tumours of the lung: A study of 152 cases. Radiol Med (Tor) 422:184, 1956.
59. Zwirewich CV, Vedal S, Miller RR, Müller NL: Solitary pulmonary nodule: High-resolution CT and radiologic-pathologic correlation. Radiology 179:469, 1991.
60. Hirakata K, Nakata H, Haratake J: Appearance of pulmonary metastases on high-resolution CT scans: Comparison with histopathologic findings from autopsy specimens. Am J Roentgenol 161:37, 1993.
61. Peuchot M, Libshitz HI: Pulmonary metastatic disease: Radiologic-surgical correlation. Radiology 164:719, 1987.
62. Adkins PC, Wesselhoeft CW Jr, Newman W, et al: Thoracotomy on the patient with previous malignancy: Metastasis or new primary? J Thorac Cardiovasc Surg 56:351, 1968.
63. Cahan WG, Castro B El, Hajdu SI: The significance of a solitary lung shadow in patients with colon carcinoma. Cancer 33:414, 1974.
64. Girard P, Baldeyrou P, Le Chevalier T, et al: Surgical resection of pulmonary metastases: Up to what number? Am J Respir Crit Care Med 149:469, 1994.
65. Heij HA, Vos A, de Kraker J, et al: Prognostic factors in surgery for pulmonary metastases in children. Surgery 115:687, 1994.
66. Matthay RA, Arroliga AC: Resection of pulmonary metastases. Am Rev Respir Dis 148:1691, 1993.
67. Askin FB: Something old? Something new? Second primary or pulmonary metastasis in the patient with known extrathoracic carcinoma. Am J Clin Pathol 100:4, 1993.
68. Sinner WN: Fine needle biopsy of solitary pulmonary metastasis. Eur J Radiol 4:9, 1984.
69. Bartziota EV: Fine needle aspiration cytology of prostatic adenocarcinoma metastatic to the lung confirmed by the immunoperoxidase technique. Acta Cytol 30:497, 1986.
70. Raab SS, Berg LC, Swanson PE, et al: Adenocarcinoma in the lung in patients with breast cancer: A prospective analysis of the discriminatory value of immunohistology. Am J Clin Pathol 100:27, 1993.
71. Nystrom JS, Weiner JM, Wolf RM, et al: Identifying the primary site in metastatic cancer of unknown origin. JAMA 241:381, 1979.

72. Steckel RJ, Kagan AR: Diagnostic persistence in working up metastatic cancer with an unknown primary site. Radiology 134:367, 1980.

73. Willis RA: The spread of tumours in the human body. *In* Willis RA (ed): Secondary Tumours of the Lungs. London, Butterworth, 1952, pp 169–177.

74. Ziskind MM, Weill H, Payzant AR: The recognition and significance of acinus-filling processes of the lungs. Am Rev Respir Dis 87:551, 1963.

75. Graeve JLA, De Alarcon PA, Sato Y, et al: Miliary pulmonary neuroblastoma: A risk of autologous bone marrow transplantation? Cancer 62:2125, 1988.

76. Scholten ET, Kreel L: Distribution of lung metastases in the axial plane. Radiol Clin 46:248, 1977.

77. Crow J, Slavin G, Kreel L: Pulmonary metastasis: A pathologic and radiologic study. Cancer 47:2595, 1981.

78. Friedmann G, Bohndorf K, Kruger J: Radiology of pulmonary metastases: Comparison of imaging techniques with operative findings. Thorac Cardiovasc Surg 34:120, 1986.

79. Shirakusa T, Tsutsui M, Motonaga R, et al: Resection of metastatic lung tumor: The evaluation of histologic appearance in the lung. Am Surg 54:655, 1988.

80. Primack SL, Hartman TE, Lee KS, et al: Pulmonary nodules and the CT halo sign. Radiology 190:513, 1994.

81. Shepard JO, Moore EH, Templeton PA, McLoud TC: Pulmonary intravascular tumor emboli: Dilated and beaded peripheral pulmonary arteries at CT. Radiology 187:797, 1993.

82. Kaste SC, Winer-Muram HT, Jenkins III JJ: Pulmonary nodules with a linear and beaded appearance: A nonspecific finding. Radiology 195:874, 1995.

83. Meziane MA, Hruban RH, Zerhouni EA, et al: High-resolution CT of the lung parenchyma with pathologic correlation. RadioGraphics 8:27, 1988.

84. Milne ENC, Zerhouni EA: Blood supply of pulmonary metastases. J Thorac Imaging 2:15, 1987.

85. Murata K, Takahashi M, Mori M, et al: Pulmonary metastatic nodules: CT-pathologic correlation. Radiology 182:331, 1992.

86. LeMay M, Piro AJ: Cavitary pulmonary metastases. Ann Intern Med 62:59, 1965.

87. Deck FW, Sherman RS: Excavation of metastatic nodules in the lung: Roentgenographic considerations. Radiology 72:30, 1959.

88. Dodd GD, Boyle JJ: Excavating pulmonary metastases. Am J Roentgenol 85:277, 1961.

89. Don C, Gray DG: Cavitating secondary carcinoma of the lung. J Can Assoc Radiol 18:310, 1967.

90. Chaudhuri MR: Cavitary pulmonary metastases. Thorax 25:375, 1970.

91. Zollikofer C, Castaneda-Zuniga W, Stenlund R, et al: Lung metastases from synovial sarcoma simulating granulomas. Am J Roentgenol 135:161, 1980.

92. Cockshott WP, deV Hendrickse JP: Pulmonary calcification at the site of trophoblastic metastases. Br J Radiol 42:17, 1969.

93. Vogelzang NJ, Stenlund R: Residual pulmonary nodules after combination chemotherapy of testicular cancer. Radiology 146:195, 1983.

94. Libshitz HI, Jing B-S, Wallace S, et al: Sterilized metastases: A diagnostic and therapeutic dilemma. Am J Roentgenol 140:15, 1983.

95. Omenn GS: Pancoast syndrome due to metastatic carcinoma from the uterine cervix. Chest 60:268, 1971.

96. Firooznia H, Seliger G, Genieser NB, et al: Hypertrophic pulmonary osteoarthropathy in pulmonary metastases. Radiology 115:269, 1975.

97. Amin R: Hypertrophic osteoarthropathy in association with pulmonary metastases from carcinoma of the bladder. Urology 26:581, 1985.

98. D'Angio GJ, Iannaccone G: Spontaneous pneumothorax as a complication of pulmonary metastases in malignant tumors of childhood. Am J Roentgenol 86:1092, 1961.

99. Dines DE, Cortese DA, Brennan MD, et al: Malignant pulmonary neoplasms predisposing to spontaneous pneumothorax. Mayo Clin Proc 48:541, 1973.

100. Sherman RS, Brant EE: An x-ray study of spontaneous pneumothorax due to cancer metastases to the lungs. Dis Chest 26:328, 1954.

101. Kane RD, Hawkins HK, Miller JA, et al: Microscopic pulmonary tumor emboli associated with dyspnea. Cancer 36:1473, 1975.

102. Smevik B, Olbjorn K: The risk of spontaneous pneumothorax in patients with osteogenic sarcoma and testicular cancer. Cancer 49:1734, 1982.

103. Spittle MF, Heal J, Harmer C, et al: The association of spontaneous pneumothorax with pulmonary metastases in bone tumours of children. Clin Radiol 19:400, 1968.

104. Soares FA, Pinto PFE, Magnani GA, et al: Pulmonary tumor embolism to arterial vessels and carcinomatous lymphangitis: A comparative clinicopathological study. Arch Pathol Lab Med 117:827, 1993.

105. Fedullo AJ, Ettensohn DB: Bronchoalveolar lavage in lymphangitic spread of adenocarcinoma to the lung. Chest 87:129, 1985.

106. Levin B: Subpleural interlobular lymphectasia reflecting metastatic carcinoma. Radiology 72:682, 1959.

107. Youngberg AS: Unilateral diffuse lung opacity. Radiology 123:277, 1977.

108. Munk PL, Müller NL, Miller RR, et al: Pulmonary lymphangitic carcinomatosis: CT and pathologic findings. Radiology 166:705, 1988.

109. Goldsmith SH, Bailey HD, Callahan EL, Beattie EJ Jr: Pulmonary metastases from breast carcinoma. Arch Surg 94:483, 1967.

110. Sadoff L, Grossman J, Weiner N: Lymphangitic pulmonary metastasis secondary to breast cancer with normal chest x-rays and abnormal perfusion lung scans. Oncology 31:164, 1975.

111. Stein MG, Mayo J, Müller N, et al: Pulmonary lymphangitic spread of carcinoma: Appearance on CT scans. Radiology 162:371, 1987.

112. Zerhouni EA, Naidich DP, Stitik FP, et al: Computed tomography of the pulmonary parenchyma: II. Interstitial disease. J Thorac Imaging 1:54, 1985.

113. Ren H, Hruban RH, Kuhlman JE, et al: Computed tomography of inflation-fixed lungs: The beaded septum sign of pulmonary metastases. J Comput Assist Tomogr 13:411, 1989.

114. Johkoh T, Ikezoe J, Tomiyama N, et al: CT findings in lymphangitic carcinomatosis of the lung: Correlation with histologic findings and pulmonary function tests. Am J Roentgenol 158:1217, 1992.

115. Ikezoe J, Godwin JD, Hunt KJ, et al: Pulmonary lymphangitic carcinomatosis: Chronicity of radiographic findings in long-term survivors. Am J Roentgenol 165:49, 1995.

116. Mathieson JR, Mayo JR, Staples CA, Müller NL: Chronic diffuse infiltrative lung disease: Comparison of diagnostic accuracy of CT and chest radiography. Radiology 171:111, 1989.

117. Grenier P, Chevret S, Beigelman C, et al: Chronic diffuse infiltrative lung disease: Determination of the diagnostic value of clinical data, chest radiography, and CT with bayesian analysis. Radiology 191:383, 1994.

118. Harold JT: Lymphangitis carcinomatosa of the lungs. QJM 21:353, 1952.

119. Mendeloff AI: Severe asthmatic dyspnea as the sole presenting symptom of generalized endolymphatic carcinomatosis: Report of two cases with autopsy findings and review of the pertinent literature. Ann Intern Med 22:386, 1945.

120. Weisbrod GL, Stoneman MR, Tao LO: Diagnosis of diffuse malignant infiltration of lung (lymphangitic carcinomatosis) by percutaneous fine-needle aspiration biopsy. J Can Assoc Radiol 36:38, 1985.

121. Masson RG, Ruggieri J: Pulmonary microvascular cytology: A new diagnostic application of the pulmonary artery catheter. Chest 88:908, 1985.

122. Burnett RA: Cor pulmonale due to tumour embolism derived from intrasinusoidal metastatic liver carcinoma. J Clin Pathol 28:457, 1975.

123. Soares FA, Magnani LGA, Mello de Oliveira JA: Pulmonary tumor embolism to alveolar septal capillaries: A prospective study of 12 cases. Arch Pathol Lab Med 115:127, 1991.

124. Soares FA, Magnani LGA, Mello de Oliveira JA: Pulmonary tumor embolism to alveolar septal capillaries: An unusual cause of sudden cor pulmonale. Arch Pathol Lab Med 116:187, 1992.

125. Saphir O: The fate of carcinoma emboli of the lung. Am J Pathol 23:245, 1947.

126. Chakeres DW, Spiegel PK: Fatal pulmonary hypertension secondary to intravascular metastatic tumor emboli. Am J Roentgenol 139:997, 1982.

127. Bagshawe KD, Noble MIM: Cardiorespiratory aspects of trophoblastic tumours. QJM 35:39, 1966.

128. Parker KM, Embry JH: Sudden death due to tricuspid valve myxoma with massive pulmonary embolism in a 15-month old male. J Forensic Sci 42:524, 1997.

129. Dada MA, Van Velden DJ: Sudden death caused by testicular germ cell tumour. Med Sci Law 35:357, 1995.

130. Heath D, Mackinnon J: Pulmonary hypertension due to myxoma of the right atrium with special reference to the behavior of emboli of myxoma in the lung. Am Heart J 68:277, 1964.

131. De Carli S, Sechi LA, Ciani R, et al: Right atrial myxoma with pulmonary embolism. Cardiology 84:368, 1994.

132. Altemus LR, Lee RE: Carcinomatosis of the lung with pulmonary hypertension: Pathoradiologic spectrum. Arch Intern Med 119:32, 1967.

133. Bates SC, Tranum BL: Perfusion lung scan: An aid in detection of lymphangitic carcinomatosis. Cancer 50:232, 1982.

134. Brisbane JU, Howell DA, Bonkowsky HL: Pulmonary hypertension as a presentation of hepatocarcinoma. Am J Med 68:466, 1980.

135. Yutani C, Imakita M, Ishibashi-Ueda H, et al: Pulmonary hypertension due to tumor emboli: A report of three autopsy cases with morphological correlations to radiological findings. Acta Pathol Jpn 43:135, 1993.

136. Goldhaber SZ, Dricker E, Buring JE, et al: Clinical suspicion of autopsy-proven thrombotic and tumor pulmonary embolism in cancer patients. Am Heart J 114:1432, 1987.

137. King DS, Castleman B: Bronchial involvement in metastatic pulmonary malignancy. J Thorac Surg 12:305, 1943.

138. Lisa JR, Trinidad S, Rosenblatt MB: Pulmonary manifestations of carcinoma of the pancreas. Cancer 17:395, 1964.

139. Varkey B, Heckman MG: Diagnosis of a case of embryonal carcinoma by bronchial biopsy. Chest 62:758, 1972.

140. Coaker LA, Sobonva RE, Davis JR: Endobronchial metastases from uterine cervical squamous carcinoma. Arch Pathol Lab Med 108:300, 1984.

141. Flynn KJ, Kim HS: Endobronchial metastasis of uterine leiomyosarcoma. JAMA 240:2080, 1978.

142. Shaw GR, Lais CJ: Fatal intravascular synovial sarcoma in a 31-year-old woman. Hum Pathol 24:809, 1993.

143. Jariwalla AG, Seaton A, McCormack RJM, et al: Intrabronchial metastases from renal carcinoma with recurrent tumour expectoration. Thorax 36:179, 1981.

144. Albertini RE, Ekberg NL: Endobronchial metastasis in breast cancer. Thorax 35:435, 1980.

145. Amer E, Guy J, Vaze B: Endobronchial metastases from renal adenocarcinoma simulating a foreign body. Thorax 36:183, 1981.

146. Sutton FD Jr, Vestal RE, Creagh CE: Varied presentations of metastatic pulmonary melanoma. Chest 65:415, 1974.

146a. Zias EA, Owen RP, Borczuk A, et al: An unusual presentation of metastatic colon cancer to the lung. Chest 113:244, 1998.

147. Braman SS, Whitcomb ME: Endobronchial metastasis. Arch Intern Med 135:543, 1975.

148. Morency G, Chalaoui J, Samson SJ: Malignant neoplasms of the trachea. J Can Assoc Radiol 40:198, 1989.

149. Kwong JS, Müller NL, Miller RR: Diseases of the trachea and main-stem bronchi: Correlation of CT with pathologic findings. RadioGraphics 12:647, 1992.

150. Kwong JS, Adler BD, Padley SPG, Müller NL: Diagnosis of diseases of the trachea and main bronchi: Chest radiography vs CT. Am J Roentgenol 161:519, 1993.

151. MacMahon H, O'Connell DJ, Cimochowski GE: Pedunculated endotracheal metastasis. Am J Roentgenol 131:713, 1978.

152. Meyer PC: Metastatic carcinoma of the pleura. Thorax 21:437, 1966.

153. Warren S, Gates O: Lung cancer and metastasis. Arch Pathol 78:467, 1964.

154. Dragoni G, Viganotti G: Metastasi polmonari da neoplasie primitive del polmone. [Pulmonary metastasis of primary lung neoplasia.] Radiol Med 57:119, 1971.

155. Onuigbo WIB: Contralateral pulmonary metastases in lung cancer. Thorax 29:132, 1974.

156. Bell JW, Knudtson KP: Observations on the natural history of bronchioloalveolar carcinoma: Experience with twenty-one cases. Am Rev Respir Dis 83:660, 1961.

157. Hirsch FR: Histopathologic Classification and Metastatic Pattern of Small Cell Carcinoma of the Lung. Copenhagen, Munksgaard, 1983.

158. Bennington JL, Beckwith JB: Tumors of the kidney, renal pelvis, and ureter. *In* Atlas of Tumor Pathology. Second Series, Vol. 12. Washington, DC, Armed Forces Institute of Pathology, 1975, p 168.

159. Saitoh H: Distant metastasis of renal adenocarcinoma in patients with a tumor thrombus in the renal vein and/or vena cava. J Urol 127:652, 1982.

160. Holland JM: Cancer of the kidney—natural history and staging. Cancer 32:1030, 1973.

161. Latour A, Shulman HS: Thoracic manifestations of renal cell carcinoma. Radiology 121:43, 1976.

162. Katzenstein A-L, Purvis R Jr, Gmelich J, et al: Pulmonary resection for metastatic renal adenocarcinoma. Cancer 41:712, 1978.

163. McLoud TC, Kalisher L, Stark P, Greene R: Intrathoracic lymph node metastases from extrathoracic neoplasms. Am J Roentgenol 131:403, 1978.

164. Reinke RT, Higgins CB, Niwayama G, et al: Bilateral pulmonary hilar lymphadenopathy: An unusual manifestation of metastatic renal cell carcinoma. Radiology 121:49, 1976.

165. King TE, Fisher J, Schwarz MI, et al: Bilateral hilar adenopathy: An unusual presentation of renal cell carcinoma. Thorax 37:317, 1982.

166. Kutty K, Varkey B: Metastatic renal cell carcinoma simulating sarcoidosis: Analysis of 12 patients with bilateral hilar lymphadenopathy. Chest 85:533, 1984.

167. Goldstraw P, Walbaum PR: Hypertrophic pulmonary osteoarthropathy and its occurrence with pulmonary metastases from renal carcinoma. Thorax 31:205, 1976.

168. Markewitz M, Taylor DA, Veenema RJ: Spontaneous regression of pulmonary metastases following palliative nephrectomy: Case report. Cancer 20:1147, 1967.

169. Cerfolio RJ, Alen MS, Deschamps C, et al: Pulmonary resection of metastatic renal cell carcinoma. Ann Thorac Surg 57:339, 1994.

170. Kierney PC, van Heerden JA, Segura JW, et al: Surgeon's role in the management of solitary renal cell carcinoma metastases occurring subsequent to initial curative nephrectomy: An institutional review. Ann Surg Oncol 1:345, 1994.

171. Maldazys JD, deKernion JB: Prognostic factors in metastatic renal carcinoma. J Urol 136:376, 1986.

172. Abubakr YA, Chou TH, Redman BG: Spontaneous remission of renal cell carcinoma: A case report and immunological correlates. J Urol 152:156, 1994.

173. MacManus MP, Harte RJ, Stranex S: Spontaneous regression of metastatic renal cell carcinoma following palliative irradiation of the primary tumour. Ir J Med Sci 163:461, 1994.

174. Sella A, Ro JY: Renal cell cancer: Best recipient of tumor-to-tumor metastasis. Urology 30:35, 1987.

175. August DA, Ottow RT, Sugarbaker PH: Clinical perspective of human colorectal cancer metastasis. Cancer Metastasis Rev 3:303, 1984.

176. Conti JA, Kemeny N, Klimstra D, et al: Colon carcinoma metastatic to the trachea: Report of a case and a review of the literature. Am J Clin Oncol 17:227, 1994.

177. Tan J, Sidhu G, Greco MA, et al: Villin, cytokeratin 7, and cytokeratin 20 expression in pulmonary adenocarcinoma with ultrastructural evidence of microvilli with rootlets. Hum Pathol 29:390, 1998.

178. Itoh K, Natori H, Suzuki A, et al: Differentiation of primary or metastatic lung carcinoma by phospholipid analysis. Cancer 57:1350, 1986.

179. Culling CFA, Reid PE, Burton JD, et al: A histochemical method of differentiating lower gastrointestinal tract mucin from other mucins in primary or metastatic tumors. J Clin Pathol 28:656, 1975.

180. Radford D, Petrelli N, Herrera L, et al: Sputum cytology for the detection of pulmonary metastases from colorectal carcinoma. Dis Colon Rectum 30:678, 1987.

181. Shimura S, Takishima T: Bronchorrhea from diffuse lymphangitic metastasis of colon carcinoma to the lung. Chest 105:308, 1994.

182. Berg HK, Petrelli NJ, Herrera L, et al: Endobronchial metastasis from colorectal carcinoma. Dis Colon Rectum 27:745, 1984.

183. McCormack PM, Burt ME, Bains MS, et al: Lung resection for colorectal metastases: 10-year results. Arch Surg 127:1403, 1992.

184. Mansel JK, Zinsmeister AR, Pairolero PC, et al: Pulmonary resection of metastatic colorectal adenocarcinoma: A ten year experience. Chest 89:109, 1986.

185. McAfee MK, Allen MS, Trasteck VP, et al: Colorectal lung metastases: Results of surgical excision. Ann Thorac Surg 53:780, 1992.

186. Sawabe M, Nakamura T, Kanno J, et al: Analysis of morphological factors of hepatocellular carcinoma in 98 autopsy cases with respect to pulmonary metastasis. Acta Pathol Jpn 37:1389, 1987.

187. Kane RD, Hawkins HD, Miller JA, et al: Microscopic pulmonary tumor emboli associated with dyspnea. Cancer 36:1473, 1975.

188. Papac RJ: Distant metastases from head and neck cancer. Cancer 53:342, 1984.

188a. Daly BD, Leung SF, Cheung H, et al: Thoracic metastases from carcinoma of the nasopharynx: High frequency of hilar and mediastinal lymphadenopathy. Am J Roentgenol 160:241, 1993.

189. Shibuya H, Hisamitsu S, Shiori S, et al: Multiple primary cancer risk in patients with squamous cell carcinoma in the oral cavity. Cancer 60:3038, 1987.

190. Mazer TM, Robbins KT, McMurtney MJ, et al: Resection of pulmonary metastases from squamous carcinoma of the head and neck. Am J Surg 156:238, 1988.

191. Thomas JM, Redding WH, Sloane JP: The spread of breast cancer: Importance of the intrathoracic lymphatic route and its relevance to treatment. Br J Cancer 40:540, 1979.

192. Fitzgerald RH Jr: Endobronchial metastases. South Med J 70:440, 1977.

192a. Pikoulis E, Varelas PN, Lechago J, et al: Metastatic breast disease 40 years after initial diagnosis. Chest 114:639, 1998.

193. Ettensohn DB, Bennett JM, Hyde RW: Endobronchial metastases from carcinoma of the breast. Med Pediatr Oncol 13:9, 1985.

194. Friedel G, Linder A, Toomes H: The significance of prognostic factors for the resection of pulmonary metastases of breast cancer. Thorac Cardiovasc Surg 42:71, 1994.

195. Lanza LA, Natarajan G, Roth JA, et al: Long-term survival after resection of pulmonary metastases from carcinoma of the breast. Ann Thorac Surg 54:244, 1992.

196. Nemec J, Pohunkova D, Zamrazil V, et al: Pulmonary metastases of thyroid carcinoma. Czech Med 2:78, 1979.

197. Shin D-H, Mark EJ, Suen HC, et al: Pathologic staging of papillary carcinoma of the thyroid with airway invasion based on the anatomic manner of extension to the trachea: A clinicopathologic study based on 22 patients who underwent thyroidectomy and airway resection. Hum Pathol 24:866, 1993.

198. Massin J-P, Savoie J-C, Garnier H, et al: Pulmonary metastases in differentiated thyroid carcinoma. Cancer 53:982, 1984.

199. Høie J, Stenwig AE, Kullmann G, et al: Distant metastases in papillary thyroid cancer. Cancer 61:1, 1988.

200. Massin JP, Savoie J-C, Garnier H, et al: Pulmonary metastases in differentiated thyroid carcinoma: Study of 58 cases with implications for the primary tumor treatment. Cancer 53:982, 1984.

201. Piekarski JD, Schlumberger M, Leclere J, et al: Chest computed tomography (CT) in patients with micronodular lung metastases of differentiated thyroid carcinoma. Int J Radiat Oncol Biol Phys 11:1023, 1985.

202. Bonte FJ, McConnell RW: Pulmonary metastases from differentiated thyroid carcinoma demonstrable only by nuclear imaging. Radiology 107:585, 1973.

203. Samaan NA, Schultz PN, Haynie TP, et al: Pulmonary metastasis of differentiated thyroid carcinoma: Treatment results in 101 patients. J Clin Endocrinol Metab 60:376, 1985.

204. McGee AR, Warren R: Carcinoma metastatic from the thyroid to the lungs: A twenty-four year radiographic follow-up. Radiology 87:516, 1966.

205. Strate SM, Lee EL, Childers JH: Occult papillary carcinoma of the thyroid with distant metastases. Cancer 54:1093, 1984.

206. Williams MP, Husband JE, Heron CW: Intrathoracic manifestations of metastatic testicular seminioma: A comparison of chest radiographic and CT findings. Am J Roentgenol 149:473, 1987.

206a. Xiao H, Liu D, Bajorin DF, et al: Medical and surgical management of pulmonary metastases from germ cell tumors. Chest Surg Clin North Am 8:131, 1998.

207. Madden M, Goldstraw P, Corrin B: Effect of chemotherapy on the histological appearances of testicular teratoma metastatic to the lung: Correlation with patient survival. J Clin Pathol 37:1212, 1984.

208. Moran CA, Travis WD, Carter D, et al: Metastatic mature teratoma in lung following testicular embryonal carcinoma and teratocarcinoma. Arch Pathol Lab Med 117:641, 1993.

209. Logothetis CJ, Samuels ML, Trindade A, et al: The growing teratoma syndrome. Cancer 50:1629, 1982.

210. Yousem DM, Scatarige JC, Fishman EK, et al: Low-attenuation thoracic metastases in testicular malignancy. Am J Roentgenol 146:291, 1986.

211. Motzer RJ, Bosl GJ: Hemorrhage: A complication of metastatic testicular choriocarcinoma. Urology 30:119, 1987.

212. Cespedes RD, Caballero RL, Peretsman SJ, et al: Cryptic presentations of germ cell tumors. J Am Coll Surg 178:261, 1994.

213. Anyanwu E, Krysa S, Buezebruck H, et al: Pulmonary metastasectomy as secondary treatment for testicular tumors. Ann Thorac Surg 57:1222, 1994.

214. Das Gupta T, Brasfield H: Metastatic melanoma: A clinicopathological study. Cancer 17:1323, 1964.

215. Webb WR, Gamsu G: Thoracic metastasis in malignant melanoma. Chest 71:176, 1977.

216. Dwyer AJ, Reichert CM, Woltering EA, et al: Diffuse pulmonary metastasis in

melanoma: Radiographic-pathologic correlation. Am J Roentgenol 143:983, 1984.

217. Webb WR: Hilar and mediastinal lymph node metastases in malignant melanoma. Am J Roentgenol 133:805, 1979.

218. Perry MD, Gore M, Seigler HF, et al: Fine needle aspiration biopsy of metastatic melanoma. Acta Cytol 30:385, 1986.

219. Karp NS, Boyd A, DePan HJ, et al: Thoracotomy for metastatic malignant melanoma of the lung. Surgery 107:256, 1990.

220. Karakousis CP, Velez A, Driscoll DL, et al: Metastasectomy in malignant melanoma. Surgery 115:295, 1994.

221. Wong JH, Euhus DM, Morton DL: Surgical resection for metastatic melanoma to the lung. Arch Surg 123:1091, 1988.

222. Ballon SC, Donaldson RC, Growdon WA, et al: Pulmonary metastases in endometrial carcinoma. *In* Weiss L, Gilbert HA (eds): Pulmonary Metastasis. Boston, GK Hall, 1978, p 182.

223. Abrams J, Talcott J, Corson JM: Pulmonary metastases in patients with low-grade endometrial stromal sarcoma: Clinicopathologic findings with immunohistochemical characterization. Am J Surg Pathol 13:133, 1989.

224. Carlson V, Delclos L, Fletcher GH: Distant metastases in squamous-cell carcinoma of the uterine cervix. Radiology 88:961, 1967.

225. Tellis CJ, Beechler CR: Pulmonary metastasis of carcinoma of the cervix: A retrospective study. Cancer 49:1705, 1982.

226. Imachi M, Tsukamoto N, Matsuyama T, et al: Pulmonary metastasis from carcinoma of the uterine cervix. Gynecol Oncol 33:189, 1989.

227. Badib AO, Kurohara SS, Webster JH, et al: Metastasis to organs in carcinoma of the uterine cervix. Cancer 21:434, 1968.

228. Sostman HD, Matthay RA: Thoracic metastases from cervical carcinoma: Current status. Invest Radiol 15:113, 1980.

229. Braude S, Thompson PJ: Solitary pulmonary metastases in carcinoma of the cervix. Thorax 38:953, 1983.

230. Scott I, Bergin CJ, Müller NL: Mediastinal and hilar lymphadenopathy as the only manifestation of metastatic carcinoma of the cervix. J Can Assoc Radiol 37:52, 1986.

231. D'Orsi CJ, Bruckman J, Mauch P, et al: Lung metastases in cervical and endometrial carcinoma. Am J Roentgenol 133:719, 1979.

232. Kerr VE, Cadman E: Pulmonary metastases in ovarian cancer: Analysis of 357 patients. Cancer 56:1209, 1985.

233. Dauplat J, Hacker NF, Nieberg RK, et al: Distant metastases in epithelial ovarian carcinoma. Cancer 60:1561, 1987.

234. Dvoretsky PM, Richards KA, Angel C, et al: Distribution of disease at autopsy in 100 women with ovarian cancer. Hum Pathol 19:57, 1988.

235. Fildes J, Narvaez GP, Baig KA, et al: Pulmonary tumor embolization after peritoneovenous shunting for malignant ascites. Cancer 61:1973, 1988.

236. Elkin M, Mueller HP: Metastases from cancer of the prostate. Cancer 7:1246, 1954.

237. Saitoh H, Hida M, Shimbo T, et al: Metastatic patterns of prostatic cancer: Correlation between sites and number of organs involved. Cancer 54:3078, 1984.

238. Petras AF, Wollett FC: Metastatic prostatic pulmonary nodules with normal bone image. J Nucl Med 24:1026, 1983.

239. Cohen O, Leibovici L, Wysenbeek AL: Carcinoma of the prostate presenting as interstitial lung disease. Respiration 51:158, 1987.

240. Gentile PS, Carloss HW, Huang T-Y, et al: Disseminated prostatic carcinoma simulating primary lung cancer: Indications for immunodiagnostic studies. Cancer 62:711, 1988.

241. Lee DW, Ro JY, Sahin AA, et al: Mucinous adenocarcinoma of the prostate with endobronchial metastasis. Am J Clin Pathol 94:641, 1990.

242. Apple JS, Paulson DF, Baber CB, et al: Advanced prostatic carcinoma: Pulmonary manifestations. Radiology 154:601, 1985.

243. Goldenberg DM, DeLand FH, Bennett SJ, et al: Radioimmunodetection of prostatic cancer: In vivo use of radioactive antibodies against prostatic acid phosphatase for diagnosis and detection of prostatic cancer by nuclear imaging. JAMA 250:630, 1983.

244. Molberg KH, Mikhail A, Vuitch F: Crystalloids in metastatic prostatic adenocarcinoma. Am J Clin Pathol 101:266, 1994.

245. Bagshawe KD, Garnett ES: Radiological changes in the lungs of patients with trophoblastic tumours. Br J Radiol 36:673, 1963.

246. Hendin AS: Gestational trophoblastic tumors metastatic to the lung. Cancer 53:58, 1984.

247. Swett HA, Westcott JL: Residual nonmalignant pulmonary nodules in choriocarcinoma. Chest 65:560, 1974.

248. Xu LT, Sun CF, Wang YE, et al: Resection of pulmonary metastatic choriocarcinoma in 43 drug-resistant patients. Ann Thorac Surg 39:257, 1985.

249. Green JD, Carden TS Jr, Hammond CB, et al: Angiographic demonstration of arteriovenous shunts in pulmonary metastatic choriocarcinoma. Radiology 108:67, 1973.

250. Libshitz HI, Baber CE, Hammond CB: The pulmonary metastases of choriosarcoma. Obstet Gynecol 49:412, 1977.

251. Wagner BJ, Woodward PJ, Dickey GE: From the Archives of the AFIP: Gestational trophoblastic disease: Radiologic-pathologic correlation. RadioGraphics 16:131, 1996.

252. Hirakata K, Nakata H, Nakagawa T: CT of pulmonary metastases with pathologic correlation. Semin Ultrasound CT MR 16:379, 1995.

253. Craig ID, Shum DT, Desrosiers P, et al: Choriocarcinoma metastatic to the lung: A cytologic study with identification of human choriogonadotropin with an immunoperoxidase technique. Acta Cytol 27:647, 1983.

254. Morrison RT, Lyster DM, Alcorn LN, et al: Gamma scintigraphy using Tc-99m labeled antibody to human chorionic gonadotropin. Clin Nucl Med 9:20, 1984.

255. Levenback C, Rubin SC, McCormack PM, et al: Resection of pulmonary metastases from uterine sarcomas. Gynecol Oncol 45:202, 1992.

256. Bachman D, Wolff M: Pulmonary metastases from benign-appearing smooth muscle tumors of the uterus. Am J Roentgenol 127:441, 1976.

257. Wolff M, Gordon K, Silva F: Pulmonary metastases (with admixed epithelial elements) from smooth muscle neoplasms. Am J Surg Pathol 3:325, 1979.

258. Horstmann JP, Pietra GG, Harman JA, et al: Spontaneous regression of pulmonary leiomyomas during pregnancy. Cancer 39:314, 1977.

259. Burkhardt A, Otto HF, Kaukel E: Multiple pulmonary (hamartomatous?) leiomyomas. Virchows Arch [Pathol Anat] 394:133, 1981.

260. Herrera GA, Miles PA, Greenberg H, et al: The origin of the pseudoglandular spaces in metastatic smooth muscle neoplasm of uterine origin. Chest 83:270, 1983.

261. Wray RC Jr, Dawkins H: Primary smooth muscle tumors of the inferior vena cava. Ann Surg 174:1009, 1971.

262. Norris HJ, Parmley T: Mesenchymal tumors of the uterus: V. Intravenous leiomyomatosis. Cancer 36:2164, 1975.

263. Gotti G, Haid MM, Paladini P, et al: Pedunculated pulmonary leiomyoma with large cyst formation. Ann Thorac Surg 56:1178, 1993

264. Boyce CR, Buddhdev HN: Pregnancy complicated by metastasizing leiomyoma of the uterus. J Obstet Gynecol 42:252, 1973.

265. Barnes HM, Richardson PJ: Benign metastasizing fibroleiomyoma. J Obstet Gynaecol Br Commonw 80:569, 1973.

266. Lipton JH, Fong TC, Burgess KR: Miliary pattern as presentation of leiomyomatosis of the lung. Chest 91:781, 1987.

267. Sargent EN, Barnes RA, Schwinn CP: Multiple pulmonary fibroleiomyomatous hamartomas: Report of a case and review of the literature. Am J Roentgenol 110:694, 1970.

267a. Maredia R, Snyder BJ, Harvey LAC, Schwartz AM: Benign metastasizing leiomyoma in the lung. RadioGraphics 18:779, 1998.

268. Kaplan C, Katoh A, Shamoto M, et al: Multiple leiomyomas of the lung: Benign or malignant? Am Rev Respir Dis 108:656, 1973.

269. Del Pozo E, Mattei IR: Multiple pulmonary leiomyomatous hamartomas: A case report. Am Rev Respir Dis 100:388, 1969.

270. Cohen JD, Robins HI: Response of "benign" metastasizing leiomyoma to progestin withdrawal: Case report. Eur J Gynaecol Oncol 14:44, 1993.

270a. Ali SZ, Kronz JD, Plowden KM, et al: Metastatic pulmonary leiomyosarcoma: Cytopathologic diagnosis on sputum examination. Diagn Cytopathol 18:280, 1998.

271. Vezeridis MP, Moore R, Karakousis CP: Metastatic patterns in soft-tissue sarcomas. Arch Surg 118:915, 1983.

272. Robinson MH, Sheppard M, Moskovic E, et al: Lung metastasectomy in patients with soft tissue sarcoma. Br J Radiol 67:129, 1994.

273. Kim K, Naylor B, Han IH: Fine needle aspiration cytology of sarcomas metastatic to the lung. Acta Cytol 30:688, 1986.

274. D'Ambrosio FG, Shiu MH, Brennan MF: Intrapulmonary presentation of extraskeletal myxoid chondrosarcoma of the extremity. Cancer 58:1144, 1986.

275. Hurt R, Bates M, Harrison W: Alveolar soft part sarcoma. Thorax 37:877, 1982.

276. Cordier JF, Bailly C, Tabone E, et al: Alveolar soft part sarcoma presenting as asymptomatic pulmonary nodules: Report of a case with ultrastructural diagnosis. Thorax 40:203, 1985.

277. Going JJ, Brewin TB, Crompton GK, et al: Soft tissue sarcoma: Two cases of solitary lung metastasis more than 15 years after diagnosis. Clin Radiol 37:579, 1986.

278. Patel AM, Ryu JH: Angiosarcoma in the lung. Chest 103:1531, 1993.

279. Nomura M, Nakaya Y, Saito K, et al: Hemopneumothorax secondary to multiple cavitary metastasis in angiosarcoma of the scalp. Respiration 61:109, 1994.

280. van Geel AN, Pastorino U, Jauch KW, et al: Surgical treatment of lung metastases: The European Organization for Research and Treatment of Cancer—Soft Tissue and Bone Sarcoma Group study of 255 patients. Cancer 77:675, 1996.

281. McKenna RJ, Schwinn CP, Soong KY, et al: Sarcomata of the osteogenic series (osteosarcoma, fibrosarcoma, chondrosarcoma, parosteal osteogenic sarcoma, and sarcomata arising in abnormal bone). J Bone Joint Surg 48A:1, 1966.

282. Huth JF, Eilber FR: Patterns of recurrence after resection of osteosarcoma of the extremity: Strategies for treatment of metastases. Arch Surg 124:122, 1989.

282a. Kay RM, Eckardt JJ, Seeger LL, et al: Pulmonary metastasis of benign giant cell tumor of bone: Six histologically confirmed cases, including one of spontaneous regression. Clin Orthop 302:219, 1994.

283. McKenna RJ, McKenna RJ Jr: Patterns of pulmonary metastases—an orthopedic hospital experience. *In* Weiss L, Gilbert HA (eds): Pulmonary Metastasis. Boston, GK Hall, 1978, p 168.

284. Nomori H, Kobayashi R, Morinaga S: Solitary, thin-walled cavitary lung metastasis of osteogenic sarcoma. Scand J Thorac Cardiovasc Surg 29:95, 1995.

285. Dines DE, Cortese DA, Brennan MD, et al: Malignant pulmonary neoplasms predisposing to spontaneous pneumothorax. Mayo Clin Proc 48:541, 1973.

286. Smith DR, Hardman JM, Earle KM: Metastasizing neuroectodermal tumors of the central nervous system. J Neurosurg 31:50, 1969.

287. Stoller JK, Kavuru M, Mehta AC, et al: Intracranial meningioma metastatic to the lung. Cleve Clin J Med 54:521, 1987.

288. Miller DC, Ojemann RG, Proppe KH, et al: Benign metastasizing meningioma: Case report. J Neurosurg 62:763, 1985.

289. Tognetti F, Donati R, Bollini C: Metastatic spread of benign intracranial meningioma. J Neurosurg Sci 31:23, 1987.

290. Fontana RS, Carr T, Woolner LB, et al: An evaluation of methods of inducing sputum production in patients with suspected cancer of the lung. Proc Mayo Clin 37:113, 1962.
291. Rosenberg F, Spjut HJ, Gedney MM: Exfoliative cytology in metastatic cancer of the lung. N Engl J Med 261:226, 1959.
292. Johnston WW, Frable WJ: Other neoplasms of the lung, primary and metastatic. *In* Diagnostic Respiratory Cytopathology. Paris, Masson Publishing, 1979.
293. Light RW, Erozan YS, Ball WC Jr: Cells in pleural fluid: Their value in differential diagnosis. Arch Intern Med 132:854, 1973.
294. Naylor B, Schmidt RW: The case for exfoliative cytology of serous effusions. Lancet 1:711, 1964.
295. Kern WH, Schweizer CW: Sputum cytology of metastatic carcinoma of the lung. Acta Cytol 20:514, 1976.
296. Masson RG, Ruggieri J: Pulmonary microvascular cytology: A new diagnostic application of the pulmonary artery catheter. Chest 88:908, 1985.
297. Tao LC, Pearson FG, Delarue NC, et al: Percutaneous fine-needle aspiration biopsy: 1. Its value to clinical practice. Cancer 45:1480, 1980.
298. Poe RH, Tobin RE: Sensitivity and specificity of needle biopsy in lung malignancy. Am Rev Respir Dis 122:725, 1980.
299. Allison DJ, Hemingway AP: Percutaneous needle biopsy of the lung. BMJ 282:875, 1981.
300. Poe RH, Ortiz C, Israel RH: Sensitivity, specificity, and predictive values of bronchoscopy in neoplasm metastatic to lung. Chest 88:84, 1985.
301. Mohsenifar Z, Chopra SK, Simmons DH: Diagnostic value of fiberoptic bronchoscopy in metastatic pulmonary tumors. Chest 74:369, 1978.
302. Chuang MT, Padilla ML, Teirstein AS: Flexible fiberoptic bronchoscopy in metastatic cancer to the lungs. Cancer 52:1949, 1983.
303. Emirgil C, Zsoldos S, Heinemann H: Effect of metastatic carcinoma to the lung on pulmonary function in man. Am J Med 36:382, 1964.
304. Ogihara Y, Takeda K, Yanagawa T, et al: Spontaneous regression of lung metastases from osteosarcoma. Cancer 74:2798, 1994.
305. Francis KC, Hutter RVP, Phillips RK, et al: Osteogenic sarcoma: Sustained disappearance of pulmonary metastases after only palliative irradiation. N Engl J Med 266:694, 1962.
306. Evans KT, Cockshott WP, Hendrickse P deV: Pulmonary changes in malignant trophoblastic disease. Br J Radiol 38:161, 1965.
307. Mark LK, Moel M: Pulmonary metastasis from trophoblastic tumors. Radiology 76:601, 1961.

Index

Note: Page numbers in *italics* refer to illustrations; numbers followed by t indicate tables; numbers followed by n indicate notes.

Vol. 2 ISBN 0-7216-6196-3

90071